DISEASES OF THE LIVER

Contributing Authors

David H. Alpers

Theodore L. Althausen

Archie H. Baggenstoss

Barbara H. Billing

David G. Bragg

A. Joseph Brough

Albert R. Burchell

James B. Carey, Jr.

Burton Combes

David C. Dahlin

Charles S. Davidson

Michael E. De Bakey

John A. Evans

Jay C. Fish

William T. Foulk

George J. Gabuzda

John T. Galambos

Edward A. Gall

Urs Peter Haemmerli

Kurt J. Isselbacher

George L. Jordan, Jr.

Gerald Klatskin

Steven P. Mistilis

Leon Morgenstern

James W. Mosley

Arthur J. Patek, Jr.

Hans Popper

Aron M. Rappaport

Oscar D. Ratnoff

Telfer B. Reynolds

Louis M. Rousselot

Victor M. Sborov

Fenton Schaffner

Steven Schenker

Leon Schiff

Sheila Sherlock

Maurice H. Stauffer

W. H. J. Summerskill

John M. Walshe

Henry O. Wheeler

Roger D. Williams

Wolf W. Zuelzer

DISEASES of the LIVER

Edited by **LEON SCHIFF**, *M.D., Ph.D.*

Professor of Medicine, University of Cincinnati, College of Medicine;
Director, Gastric Laboratory, Cincinnati General Hospital

Third Edition

J. B. LIPPINCOTT COMPANY
Philadelphia • Toronto

Distributed in Great Britain by
Blackwell Scientific Publications, Oxford and Edinburgh

Library of Congress Catalog Card Number 68-8704

Printed in the United States of America

6   5   4   3   2

Dedicated to

Cecil J. Watson

for his contributions, both clinical and
investigative, to the field of liver disease

Contributing Authors

David H. Alpers, M.D.
Assistant Professor of Medicine, Washington University School of Medicine; Director, Gastrointestinal Division, Barnes Hospital, St. Louis, Mo.; formerly, Massachusetts General Hospital, Boston, Mass.

Theodore L. Althausen, M.D.
Professor and Chairman, Emeritus, Department of Medicine, University of California School of Medicine; formerly, Physician-in-Chief, University of California Hospitals, San Francisco, Calif.

Archie H. Baggenstoss, M.D.
Consultant, Section of Experimental and Anatomic Pathology, Mayo Clinic; Professor of Pathology, Mayo Foundation Graduate School of Medicine (University of Minnesota), Rochester, Minn.

Barbara H. Billing, Ph.D.
Reader in Biochemistry Applied to Medicine, University of London Department of Medicine, at the Royal Free Hospital School of Medicine, London

David G. Bragg, M.D.
Chairman, Department of Diagnostic Radiology, Memorial Sloan-Kettering Cancer Center; Assistant Professor of Radiology, Cornell University Medical College, New York, N. Y.

A. Joseph Brough, M.D.
Associate Pathologist and Executive Director of Laboratories, Children's Hospital of Michigan; Assistant Professor, Wayne State University School of Medicine, Detroit, Mich.

Albert R. Burchell, M.D.
Assistant Attending Surgeon, St. Vincent's Hospital and Medical Center of New York; Assistant Professor of Clinical Surgery, New York University School of Medicine, New York, N.Y.

James B. Carey, Jr., M.D., Ph.D.
Professor of Medicine, Section of Gastroenterology, University of Minnesota Health Sciences Center, Minneapolis, Minn.

Burton Combes, M.D.
Professor of Internal Medicine, Department of Internal Medicine, University of Texas Southwestern Medical School at Dallas, Dallas, Texas

David C. Dahlin, M.D.
Consultant, Section of Surgical Pathology, Mayo Clinic; Professor of Pathology, Mayo Foundation Graduate School of Medicine (University of Minnesota), Rochester, Minn.

Charles S. Davidson, M.D.
Professor of Medicine, Harvard University; Associate Director, Thorndike Memorial Laboratory, and Second and Fourth (Harvard) Medical Services, Boston City Hospital, Boston, Mass.

Michael E. De Bakey, M.D.
President, Baylor University College of Medicine, Houston, Texas; Professor and Chairman, Cora and Webb Mading Department of Surgery, Baylor University College of Medicine; Director, Cardiovascular Research and Training Center, Methodist Hospital, Houston, Texas

John A. Evans, M.D.
Professor and Chairman, Department of Radiology, Cornell University Medical College and Radiologist-in-Chief, The New York Hospital, New York, N.Y.

Jay C. Fish, M.D.
Assistant Professor of Surgery, University of Texas Medical Branch, Galveston, Texas

William T. Foulk, M.D.
Consultant, Section of Medicine, Mayo Clinic; Associate Professor of Medicine, Mayo Foundation Graduate School of Medicine (University of Minnesota), Rochester, Minn.

George J. Gabuzda, M.D.
Professor of Medicine, Case Western Reserve University School of Medicine; Associate Director, Department of Medicine, Cleveland Metropolitan General Hospital, Cleveland, Ohio

John T. Galambos, M.D.
Professor of Medicine, and Coordinator, Division of Digestive Diseases, Emory University School of Medicine, Atlanta, Ga.

Edward A. Gall, M.D.
Professor of Pathology and Director, Department of Pathology, College of Medicine, University of Cincinnati and the Cincinnati General Hospital, Cincinnati, Ohio

Urs Peter Haemmerli, M.D.
Oberarzt, Medizinische Universitätsklinik, Kantonsspital Zürich, Privat-Dozent in Gastroenterology, University of Zürich, Zürich, Switzerland

Kurt J. Isselbacher, M.D.
Professor of Medicine, Harvard Medical School; Chief, Gastrointestinal Unit, Massachusetts General Hospital, Boston, Mass.

George L. Jordan, Jr., M.D.
Professor, Cora and Webb Mading Department of Surgery, Baylor University College of Medicine, Houston, Texas

Gerald Klatskin, M.D.
David Paige Smith Professor of Medicine, Department of Internal Medicine, Yale University School of Medicine, New Haven, Conn.

Steven P. Mistilis, M.D., M.B.B.S., M.R.A.C.P.
Research Director, The A. W. Morrow Department of Gastroenterology, Royal Prince Alfred Hospital, Camperdown, Australia

Leon Morgenstern, M.D.
Director of Surgery, Cedars of Lebanon Hospital Division, Cedars-Sinai Medical Center, Los Angeles, Calif.

James W. Mosley, M.D.
Chief, Epidemiology and Research Analysis Branch, Foreign Quarantine Program, National Communicable Disease Center, Public Health Service, U.S. Department of Health, Education and Welfare, Atlanta, Ga.

Arthur J. Patek, Jr., M.D.
Chief of Hepatology, Veterans Administration Hospital, Boston, Mass.; Professor of Medicine, Tufts University School of Medicine, Boston, Mass.; formerly, Clinical Professor of Medicine, College of Physicians and Surgeons, Columbia University, New York, N.Y.

Hans Popper, M.D.
Given Foundation Professor and Chairman, Department of Pathology, Mount Sinai School of Medicine of The City University of New York, New York, N.Y.

Aron M. Rappaport, M.D., Ph.D.
Professor, Department of Physiology, University of Toronto, Faculty of Medicine, Toronto, Ontario

Oscar D. Ratnoff, M.D.
Professor of Medicine, Case Western Reserve University School of Medicine; Career Investigator of the American Heart Association; Physician, University Hospitals of Cleveland, Cleveland, Ohio

Telfer B. Reynolds, M.D.
Professor of Medicine, University of Southern California School of Medicine; Chief of the Liver Service, Los Angeles County–University of Southern California Medical Center, Los Angeles

Louis M. Rousselot, M.D.
Deputy Assistant Secretary of Defense for Health Resources and Medical Manpower, The Pentagon, Washington, D.C.; Emeritus Director of Surgery, St. Vincent's Hospital and Medical Center of New York; Emeritus Professor of Clinical Surgery, New York University School of Medicine, New York, N.Y.

Victor M. Sborov, M.D.
Associate Clinical Professor of Medicine, University of California School of Medicine; Assistant Visiting Physician, University of California Hospitals, San Francisco, Calif.

Fenton Schaffner, M.S., M.D.

Professor of Pathology and Medicine, Mount Sinai School of Medicine of The City University of New York; Attending Physician, The Mount Sinai Hospital, New York, N.Y.

Steven Schenker, M.D.

Associate Professor of Internal Medicine, Department of Internal Medicine, University of Texas Southwestern Medical School at Dallas, Texas

Leon Schiff, M.D., Ph.D.

Professor of Medicine, University of Cincinnati College of Medicine; Director, Gastric Laboratory, Cincinnati General Hospital, Cincinnati, Ohio

Sheila Sherlock, M.D., F.R.C.P., F.A.C.P. (Hon.)

Professor of Medicine, University of London Department of Medicine, at The Royal Free Hospital School of Medicine, London

Maurice H. Stauffer, M.D.

Consultant, Section of Medicine, Mayo Clinic; Assistant Professor of Medicine, Mayo Foundation Graduate School of Medicine (University of Minnesota), Rochester, Minn.

W. H. J. Summerskill, D.M., F.R.C.P., F.A.C.P.

Consultant, Section of Medicine; Director, Gastroenterology Unit, Mayo Clinic; Professor of Medicine, Mayo Foundation Graduate School of Medicine (University of Minnesota), Rochester, Minn.

J. M. Walshe, Sc.D., F.R.C.P.

Reader in Metabolic Disease, Department of Investigative Medicine, University of Cambridge, Cambridge, England

Henry O. Wheeler, M.D.

Professor of Medicine, University of California, San Diego; La Jolla, Calif.

Roger D. Williams, M.M.Sc., M.D.

Clinical Professor of Surgery, University of Miami, Miami, Fla.

Wolf W. Zuelzer, M.D.

Professor of Pediatric Research, Wayne State University School of Medicine; Director of Laboratories, Children's Hospital of Michigan; Director, Child Research Center of Michigan, Detroit, Mich.

Preface to the Third Edition

Knowledge of liver disease is rapidly expanding and the time appears opportune for a second revision of *Diseases of the Liver*. Hepatic disorders are assuming increasing importance both from the standpoints of morbidity and mortality, and hepatic research is being carried out on an ever-increasing scale. Many new chapters have been added to this volume, while a few have been discontinued in an effort to limit its expansion.

The editor wishes to welcome the following new contributors (some, of entirely new chapters, some as co-authors) whose co-operation has been deeply appreciated: Fenton Schaffner and Hans Popper, for their chapter on "Electron Microscopy of the Liver"; Henry O. Wheeler, for "Secretion of Bile"; James B. Carey, Jr., for "Bile Salts and Hepatobiliary Disease"; Oscar D. Ratnoff, for "Disordered Hemostasis in Hepatic Disease"; Burton Combes and Steven Schenker, for "Laboratory Tests"; Telfer B. Reynolds, for "Portal Hypertension"; George J. Gabuzda, co-author, for "Hepatic Coma"; James W. Mosley and John T. Galambos, for "Viral Hepatitis"; Steven P. Mistilis, for "Active Chronic Hepatitis" and "Diseases of the Liver Associated with Ulcerative Colitis"; Kurt J. Isselbacher and David H. Alpers, for "Fatty Liver: Biochemistry and Clinical Aspects"; William T. Foulk and Archie H. Baggenstoss for "Biliary Cirrhosis"; John M. Walshe, for "The Liver in Hepatolenticular Degeneration"; George L. Jordan, Jr., co-author, for "Surgery of the Liver"; A. Joseph Brough, co-author, for "Liver Disease in Infancy and Childhood"; David G. Bragg and John A. Evans, for "Roentgen Aspects of Liver and Biliary Tract Diseases"; Urs Peter Haemmerli, for "Jaundice During Pregnancy"; Leon Morgenstern, for "Postoperative Jaundice"; and Jay C. Fish, co-author, for "Diseases of the Gallbladder and Extrahepatic Bile Ducts."

The editor will always be mindful of the valuable and willing co-operation of a number of authors who participated in the 1st and 2nd Editions but who do not appear in the 3rd. He would still refer the reader to the chapters they wrote. He regrets the untimely death of Oscar Creech, Jr.

As an appropriate gesture of our regard for Dr. Cecil J. Watson and his work, the 3rd edition has been dedicated to him. The esteem with which he is regarded by his colleagues was reflected in a two-day symposium on liver disease held in his honor at Minneapolis, Minnesota in May, 1966. Many who participated in this conference, including the editor, owe much to his inspiring help over the years.

The editor wishes to again express his gratitude to his friend and colleague, Edward A. Gall, for his advice; to Miss Olive Mills for her tireless and most valuable editorial assistance; and to Miss Elaine Besterman and Mrs. Margaret Doerflein for their secretarial help.

LEON SCHIFF, M.D.

Preface to the First Edition

In the recent words of Himsworth, the present time seems to be particularly opportune for reviewing our knowledge of liver disease. A partial list of reasons would include the advances made in the fundamental sciences as they pertain to liver structure and function; the advances in the experimental approach to liver disease; the increased knowledge in the field of viral hepatitis; the newer clinical criteria and concept of hepatic coma, with attention focused on disturbance in the metabolism of ammonia; a better understanding of the pathogenesis and the treatment of cirrhosis; a clearer concept of the metabolic defect in hemochromatosis and the apparent effectiveness of depleting iron stores in the treatment of this disorder; the implication of disturbed copper metabolism in hepato-lenticular degeneration; the increasing experience with needle biopsy of the liver; and the surgical attack on portal hypertension.

This book is not intended to be encyclopedic in nature but rather the expression of present-day information pertaining to various aspects of liver disease by a group of authors particularly qualified by their experience, interest and scientific contributions. The reader may discover certain omissions; but he usually will find these to be matters of lesser importance. They will be more than compensated by the quality of the information contained, which deals with those aspects of hepatic disease that are much more apt to concern him, including the description of the principles of treatment, both medical and surgical, by experts in the field. Furthermore, he will frequently find it unnecessary to consult other books, particularly on points dealing with basic concepts.

To the various contributors the editor expresses his deep gratitude for their excellent and willing co-operation. He has considered it good fortune indeed to have been associated with them in this undertaking. He wishes to express his thanks to Cecil J. Watson, Arthur J. Patek, Jr., and to his colleague, Edward A. Gall, for their helpful suggestions. He is particularly indebted to Miss Olive Mills, without whose tireless and able secretarial and editorial assistance he would not have been able to accomplish his task.

In some instances individual authors have appended acknowledgments of assistance to their respective chapters. To those concerned the editor wishes to express his apologies for not having included these expressions of gratitude for the sake of uniformity of composition and conservation of space.

LEON SCHIFF

Contents

xx   Contents

DISEASES OF THE LIVER

1

Anatomic Considerations

ARON M. RAPPAPORT, M.D., PH.D.

The time when anatomy consisted of tabulated data from the dissecting rooms has passed. These data from the "House of the Dead" came to life when each dissected compartment of the body was used to illustrate its activities that contribute to the maintenance of the organism as a whole. Today, the work of anatomists and physiologists interlaces continuously. Indeed, the concepts of the morphology of the liver have changed with the advances in hepatic electron microscopy, physiology and pathology. Experimentalists and clinicians too have added to the knowledge of normal and abnormal morphology. Functional anatomy is thus on the march, and we shall strive to follow it in our presentation.

In the following pages the development of the liver, its lobes, surface, peritoneal connections (ligaments), its micro-anatomy, vessels and nerves are considered. Also, the bile ducts and gallbladder and general topography are discussed.

The liver is covered by the fibrous capsule of Glisson, which, in turn, is invested with serosa. At the porta hepatis this capsule turns deep into the liver substance along the vessels and the biliary ducts, following them to their finest ramifications.

The liver of an adult weighs from 1,400 to 1,600 Gm., comprising one fiftieth of the body weight. In the newborn the greater comparative size of the liver, (one twentieth of the body weight), is due to its blood-forming activity during fetal life.

Although the largest gland of the body, the liver is believed to yield a relatively small amount of secretion (600 to 800 ml. of bile daily).

The hardened adult specimen *in situ* has the appearance of a wedge with the base to the right. The normal liver extends from the right 5th intercostal space in the mid-clavicular line down to the right costal margin. The lower margin of a normal liver usually transgresses the costal border. The greatest longitudinal diameter of the liver is near its right lateral surface, where it measures from 15 to 17 cm.; its greatest thickness (12 to 15 cm.) is at the level of the upper pole of the right kidney; and its greatest transverse diameter is 15 to 20 cm. A convenient site of transthoracic puncture for liver biopsy is in the anterior axillary line at the 7th, 8th, or 9th interspace, always one interspace below the upper limit of liver dullness. The morphologic and topographic variations of the normal liver were studied by Villemin and associates.[238]

EMBRYOLOGY

The liver arises from the entodermal lining of the foregut during the 4th week. The hepatic diverticulum is situated at the ventral side of the foregut, cranial to its opening into the yolk sac. In embryos of 5 to 6 mm. length, the original hepatic diverticulum can be distinguished as differentiating cranially into proliferating hepatic cords and bile ducts, caudally into the gallbladder. The hepatic tubular cords sprout tridimensionally (cranially, ventrally and laterally), penetrating the septum transversum and passing between the 2 layers of splanchnic mesoderm. The latter envelop the sprouting lobules, provide their interstitial connective tissue, and form the liver capsule.

Strands of entodermal epithelium growing into the septum transversum enclose islets of proliferating mesenchymal cells which later sacculate and are transformed into sinusoids. These groups of cells remain always in contact with the rest of the mesenchyma surrounding the liver anlage. In the human liver the latter is never a compact mass.[139] In a human embryo of 26 somites, irregular masses can be observed developing in a frontal plane. Their strandlike form might be due to the early vascularization of the human septum transversum, between the vessels of which the hepatic cords penetrate. These enlarge at their bases later, fuse and arrange themselves into lamellae and plates. Thus the human liver, initially a simple gland, changes into a "composite labyrinthine gland."[29] Although the differentiation of the liver anlage is conditioned by the interrelation of both entodermal and mesenchymal elements, the primary factor remains the proliferation of the epithelium in tubular cords that communicate with the bile ductules.[21] Similar observations have been made by Wilson et al. in the liver of the mouse embryo.[245]

Recent studies of the liver in human fetuses[9] demonstrate that the earliest organized structures formed by the association of hepatocytes and cholangiolar cells are situated around the small portal branches, i.e., zone 1; they represent the anlage of the *liver acinus*.[194]

The prevailing growth, to right or to left, determines the shape of the liver and the relative size of the lobes. Budding parenchyma, by losing continuity with the liver anlage, may give rise to accessory liver masses.

The primordium of the gallbladder is a diverticular dilation of the original outgrowth from the gut, situated caudal to the confluence of the hepatic ducts. Since it elongates quickly and becomes saccular, developmental disturbance in this region can produce malformations of the gallbladder in the presence of a normal liver. Aberrant biliary ducts, *vasa aberrantia*, are considered by most authors to be proliferating branches of primitive tubular liver cords that were arrested in their development.

Anomalies in the blood supply of the liver are due to anomalies of the vascular anlage rather than of the liver anlage.

Summary. The liver is an entodermal outgrowth of the foregut into mesodermal surroundings increasing the metabolic and digestive activities of the gut. The liver grows by tridimensional budding of the primary bile ductules around the smallest portal branches. Thus small parenchymal masses (liver acini) are formed around a central biliovascular axis. The final shape of the liver and its attached excretory apparatus is an expression of the developmental case history of the organ.

LOBES

As distinguished from the multilobulated liver of many mammals, the human liver is one compact and continuous mass. However, it is divided conventionally by the line of insertion of the falciform ligament into 2 lobes. The right lobe is larger and shows on its posterior-inferior surface 2 smaller lobes —the caudate and the quadrate lobes. The former with its caudate process is wedged between the groove of the inferior vena cava and the porta hepatis. The quadrate lobe lies between the round ligament and the gallbladder. Cantlie[38] and Sérégé[221, 222] considered the gallbladder-caval line as the true dividing line of the liver.

Hjortsjö injected the hepatic ducts *in situ* with red lead in celloidin and took stereoscopic cholangiograms.[102, 103] Then he filled the portal vessels with colored celloidin, corroded them and described their course in relation to the stereogram. In his corrosion specimen he saw a fissure running toward the caval area from the right septal fissure, which is situated to the right of the gallbladder fundus. Occasionally, there were other fissures subdividing the left lobe. In fact, these fissures harbor major branches of the hepatic vein and are bridged *in vivo* by sinusoids.[65]

With a view to operations on the parenchyma, Couinaud[47] and Junès[113] have extended the study of the distribution of the vascular and biliary tree within the liver and found it to be strictly segmental. While Couinaud likens the differing segments in the liver to the lobes of the lung, insisting on segmental resections of the liver, Junès objects to this view because the portal and the hepatic venous systems of the liver segments do not coincide in their distribution and orientation (Fig. 1–18). Besides, the segments of the liver are not separated by a serous membrane similar to the visceral pleura enveloping the pulmonary lobes. Thus the liver is *one* parenchymal mass and the lobes are not delimited by any fibrous septum traversing the liver substance. Each conventional hepatic lobe has its own vascular and biliary systems, but there are intercommunications between the respective systems. Surgical anastomosis of a major intrahepatic bile duct of one lobe with an intestinal loop drains the entire liver.[140, 142]

Although preferential blood flow to the right or the left liver lobe has been proved by injection of radioactive phosphorus into the mesenteric vein,[88] there is sufficient mixture in the streamlined flow and intercommunication between the vascular channels to guarantee unity of function of the organ.[151, 218] Also, splenic portography[1] shadows the entire liver at once.[58] Furthermore, of all the liver functions none ever has been attributed to any lobe. However, from a developmental and microstructural viewpoint, the liver is to be considered as lobulated not only on its surface but also into its innermost parts. The accessory lobes scattered in various organs (mesentery, suspensory ligaments, spleen, adrenals) are the remainders of parenchymal clusters around the sprouting bile ductules that have split off from the entire liver mass. Some abnormal lobulation may have been due to pathologic processes during intrauterine life. Riedel's lobe is a downward prolongation of the right liver lobe often caused by an adhesion to the mesocolon.

Summary. The liver consists of a uniform mass of parenchyma which conventionally appears to be divided into lobes by deep vascular or avascular grooves. In spite of the demonstrated bilateral portal blood flow when the intestines are exposed, there is not enough evidence to prove that under normal circumstances the named lobes of the adult liver receive their blood each from a different intestinal area, and that they have distinct functions. On the microscopic level, however, the liver is lobulated throughout.

SURFACE OF THE LIVER

Of the 5 surfaces of the liver (superior, anterior, right lateral, posterior and inferior), the posterior and inferior show more structural features.

The *superior, anterior* and *lateral* surfaces are smooth and convex to fit into the dome of the diaphragm. They are completely covered by peritoneum except for a small triangular area where the 2 layers of the upper part of the falciform ligament diverge.

In the marks of the *posterior* and the *inferior* surfaces of the liver (Fig. 1–1) we can read the glorious past, when the liver represented one fifth of the entire body weight. The groove of the venous ligament separating conventionally the left liver lobe from the rest of the organ is the site where the gastrohepatic omentum is inserted. Once in this furrow lay a main afferent channel that brought oxygenated blood from the umbilical vein into the hepatic sinusoids. Some of the blood in this channel also passed through the venus duct (duct of Arantius) directly into the inferior vena cava and so to the right atrium. The umbilical vein, an arterial channel now obliterated and transformed into the round hepatic ligament, runs in the lower half of its groove. It delimits the quadrate lobe from the left liver lobe. Thus from the beginning the liver, and especially its left lobe, has had arterial blood of first quality.

A third vascular channel, the inferior vena cava, runs through the posterior surface of the liver at the base of its bare area. In some livers the vein passes under a bridge of liver substance. Here the hepatic veins, arranged in a superior group of 3 (left, right, and median hepatic) with a variable inferior group, empty into the inferior vena cava. Thus the coronary ligament attaching the triangular bare area of the right liver lobe to the diaphragm by areolar tissue encloses the above large veins.

The fossa of the gallbladder delimits the quadrate from the right liver lobe. The horizontal portal fissure, which joins the upper ends of the gallbladder fossa and the groove of the round ligament, contains the branches

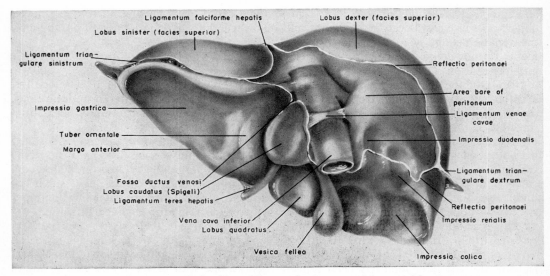

Fig. 1–1. Posterior view of the liver. The marks impressed by neighboring organs upon the liver surface mirror its intricate topographic relation with the surroundings. (Anson, B. J., Maddock, W. G.: Callander's Surgical Anatomy, ed. 3, Philadelphia, Saunders.)

of the hepatic artery and of the portal vein, the hepatic nerve plexus, the hepatic ducts and the lymph vessels.

In the portal fissure the arterial branches lie between the bile ducts in front and the portal branches behind. Had it not been for the caudate process of the same lobe, the noble organ, Hepar, would have had its initial "H" perfectly grooved on its posterior and inferior surface. Grooves are not always the remains of developmental events. They result also from the folding of the liver mass in a limited space.[29]

The diaphragmatic, renal, suprarenal, colic, duodenal, pyloric, gastric, and esophageal areas that we see on a posterior view of the liver are the impressions made by neighboring organs. These imprints should remind us also of a variety of pathologic processes that can involve the liver, together with any of these organs.

Generally speaking, the surface mirrors what is close to it and is exposed to injury from its surroundings.

PERITONEAL CONNECTIONS: LIGAMENTS

The liver is connected to the diaphragm, abdominal wall, stomach and duodenum by bands of connective tissue in peritoneal folds. These have the function of conveying afferent, efferent and collateral blood vessels, lymphatics and nerve plexuses to the liver and helping to maintain the organ in position.

Falciform Ligament. This peritoneal fold connects the liver to the diaphragm and the anterior abdominal wall. It ascends from the umbilicus, from which during fetal life it conducted the umbilical vein to the liver. The obliterated vessel forms the free edge of the sickle-shaped peritoneal fold. It carries between its peritoneal layers the paraumbilical veins, the clinically important collaterals of the portal vein. These veins are often surgically exposed and used as a route for catheterization and radiography of the portal vein, permitting collection of blood samples for metabolic studies.[11, 12, 130] When dilated in cirrhosis and in Cruveilhier-Baumgarten syndrome, blood sampling and visualization of the portal system becomes possible without recourse to catheterization.[226]

Coronary Ligament. The "bare area" of the posterior surface of the liver, connected by areolar tissue with the diaphragm, is enclosed by an upper and a lower layer of peritoneum. The inferior vena cava and the hepatic veins are contained within the coronary ligament.

Hepatorenal Ligament. The lower layer of the coronary ligament, passing along the lower limit of the right posterior hepatic surface, may be reflected on the upper part of the anterior surface of the right kidney, thus forming the hepatorenal ligament. It often contains collateral vessels of the liver.

Right Triangular Ligament. This is the free margin of the coronary ligament.

Left Triangular Ligament. This consists of 2 closely applied layers of peritoneum that continue with the falciform ligament in front and the lesser omentum behind. Both triangular ligaments, besides attaching the liver lobes to the diaphragm, convey collateral branches from the phrenic and the musculophrenic vessels to the liver.

Ligaments are ties that connect the organ with the rest of the organism. Through them nutrients, hormones, raw materials for function, and stimuli are carried in and out by blood and lymph vessels, by ducts and by nerves.

MICRO-ANATOMY

Hepatic Cytology

In describing the minute structure of the liver, a brief discussion of hepatic cytology is essential. It provides the basis for the study of the enzymes and the biochemical changes within the hepatic parenchymal cells and for histochemistry, which has become a routine procedure in the investigation of the physiology and the pathology of the liver. Recalling Soskin's statement that the quantity of tabulated enzymes contained in a muscle cell leaves little or no room for any purely structural protein,[229] one may expect at least a similar balance in the cytoplasm of the metabolizing liver cells. Indeed, because of their rich content in enzymes, hepatic cells are used for the major part of all cytoplasmic and cytochemical studies.

The literature on the microscopic and the electron microscopic studies of hepatic protoplasm is growing; the nomenclature is in flux. Histologists, biologists and biochemists join in their efforts to investigate the function of the protoplasmic organelles, the aspect of which reminds one of the infinite marvels of the deep-sea flora. However, the enthusiast for the great achievements of the electron microscope should bear in mind that the world is infinite not only upward but also downward.[33] If one considers the hepatic cell as a part of this infinity and looks at it through the optical instruments available, the following can be described.

The hepatic parenchymal cell isolated from a fresh piece of liver is more or less rounded. After fixation, it becomes polyhedral, presenting 6 to 8 surfaces. These surfaces are enmeshed by a ring of bile capillaries, excepting the one contiguous with the sinusoids. The diameter of the cell varies between 18 and 26 μ. It contains 1 or 2, rarely several, nuclei that are well developed. Because of intensive metabolic activity the hepatic cell is rich in mitochondria, ergastoplasm and inclusions. It possesses also a Golgi apparatus. (For more details in cellular structure, see Chapter 2, Electron Microscopy of the Liver.)

Cytoplasmic Inclusions. *Glycogen.* The inclusions of the hepatic cell vary with its metabolic state. The glycogen-filled cells of a rabbit that has indulged in carrots before sacrifice, and the biopsy from a dog's liver afford good examples of glycogen inclusions. The tissue has a honeycomb appearance. Glycogen is stored first but released last around the central vein.

Fat inclusions have followed the opposite distribution within the hepatic parenchyma. The "depot-fat" brought into the liver during starvation[10] shows up first in the cells of the area close to the afferent vessels. Accumulation of lipids due to dietary choline deficiency becomes manifest first around the terminal hepatic venules. The first fat droplets are seen at the sinusoidal aspect of the hepatocytes and in the Kupffer cells. Larger fat globules can produce a signet-ring appearance in the cell. Accumulation of fat globules may finally disrupt the cell membrane and form fatty cysts extracellularly.[93, 96] "Fat-storing cells" in zone 1 of the "liver acini" (pp. 6, 9-11) have been described by Ito and Nemoto[107] and Meyer and Hartroft.[165, 166]

Protein inclusions can be demonstrated easily by histochemical methods. During starvation the "pericentral" cells maintain their protein inclusions much longer than the periportal cells. Bile pigments, iron and ceroid material are observed occasionally within the hepatic cytoplasm as a result of earlier or present pathologic changes.

HEPATIC HISTOLOGY

Even in its early stage of development the liver shows the close association of entodermal and mesodermal elements that characterizes this organ. The rows of epithelial cells radiating from the terminal portal vessels to the terminal hepatic ("central") veins are sustained by fine reticulin fibers and sinusoidal capillaries of mesodermal origin. However, the amount of fibrous tissue around the afferent and the efferent channels is in proportion to their size. They are the continuation of Glisson's capsule, a remainder of the septum transversum.

We may well think of the liver as a tree that has grown out from the virgin land of the foregut to increase its metabolic and digestive function. It has spread its crown of parenchyma into the space of the septum transversum but continues to draw its nutrients through the portal capillary roots from the rich soil of the intestine. As the liver anlage develops by tridimensional budding of the bile ducts to the final shape of the organ, small parenchymal clusters remain centered around the spread-out terminal branches of the duct. Here the zonal arrangement of the cells with respect to circulation, function and pathology proves to us, in spite of the doubts of some authors,[64] that lobulation is an essential structural feature of the hepatic parenchyma.

Hepatic lobules were described by Malpighi[158] in 1666, and Mascagni[162] represented them as grapelike bunches attached to the extremities of the portal vein. A more definite concept of hepatic lobulation was introduced by Francis Kiernan in 1833.[121] He described the hexagonal lobule centered around the radicles of the hepatic veins. This lobule is still presented by textbooks of histology as the ultimate unit of the liver. However, the idea of a parenchymal mass filling a hexagonal space around the central vein would not integrate functional unity, either normal or abnormal. Therefore, the existence

of a hexagonal lobule has been questioned by many authors.[5, 63, 64, 157, 179, 193, 199, 212] In spite of its arrangement within a vascular framework, the hexagonal lobule is not conspicuous under microscopic observation of the hepatic circulation *in vivo*. The blood flowing through the pairs of terminal afferent vessels streams into sinusoids of an area extending into *sectors only* of adjacent hexagonal fields.[123] Thus these terminal afferent vessels accompanied by a terminal bile ductule are the orientating landmarks around which the parenchymal tissue is arranged in clumps or small clusters which, under suitable conditions, can be well delimited.

Two differently colored gelatin masses of the same viscosity, injected simultaneously and under the same pressure into the 2 main branches of the portal vein of a dog or a rabbit, sharply delimit parts of the liver. Microscopically, differently colored areas are found to be situated around terminal portal branches, to occupy adjacent parts of neighboring hexagonal fields and to extend from the central vein of one hexagon to the central vein of another (Fig. 1–2). The same arrangement is observed when the colored masses are injected into the 2 branches of the hepatic artery or bile duct. Thus the hexagonal fields are broken down into distinct areas that are the cross sections of berrylike **irregular** parenchymal masses surrounding a trio of axial channels. Of these, the hepatic arteriole and the portal venule bring in the materials for metabolism, while the accompanying terminal bile ductule carries away the product of secretion. Each outlined parenchymal mass represents the hepatic structural and functional unit, which we named the *liver acinus*.

Simple Liver Acinus

The simple liver acinus is a small parenchymal mass, *irregular* in size and shape, and arranged around an axis consisting of a terminal portal venule, hepatic arteriole, bile ductule, lymph vessels and nerves which grow out together from a small triangular portal field. The simple liver acinus lies between 2 (or more) terminal hepatic venules ("central veins") with which its vascular and biliary axis interdigitates. In a two-

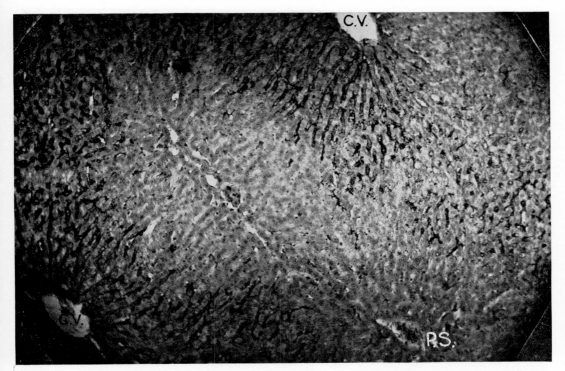

FIG. 1–2. Acinar unit in a rabbit liver. The area clear of India ink is centered around the axial channels that grow out from a small portal space, *P.S.* It extends into 2 adjacent hexagonal fields, the "central veins" of which (*C.V.*) are seen in the left lower and right upper corners. × 100, approx. (Rappaport, A. M., et al.: Anat. Rec. *119*:11.)

dimensional view it occupies sectors of only 2 adjacent hexagonal fields.

If one injects simultaneously the main (lobar) branches of the portal vein and the entire hepatic venous system of the human liver, each with differently colored vinylite acetate, and, after the injection mass has hardened, removes the parenchyma by acid digestion, a three-colored cast is obtained.[20] The cast clearly shows that the area around each terminal hepatic venule ("central vein") is supplied with blood derived from different sources, remote from each other.[196] Hence one cannot consider as a unit the tissue around a terminal hepatic venule (i.e., "central vein" of Kiernan).

Similar casts of the liver of the dog, rabbit, pig and monkey are obtainable also by an injection with vinylite acetate of either the 2 main branches of the portal vein or the hepatic artery or of the bile duct, combined with the simultaneous filling of the hepatic venous system. The terminal branches of the visualized afferent vessels and bile ducts represent the axes around which the hepatic parenchyma is organized. Because of the infinite variety in length, course, and capillary ramification of these terminal branches, the parenchymal masses supplied and drained by them vary likewise.

The width of an acinus is twice the length of a radial sinusoid and measures about ¼ mm. in the *in vivo* transilluminated liver of weanling rats. The plates and cords of the simple acini, although definitely oriented upon their axial channels, are in cellular and capillary continuity with adjacent or overlapping acini. There is no capsular investment around these irregularly shaped microscopic clumps, which would separate them from each other. Nevertheless the terminal afferent and draining channels pervade the entire liver mass in a definite way, subdividing it functionally into small clumps. These

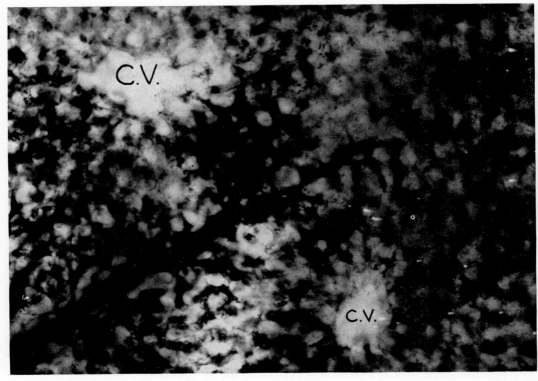

Fɪɢ. 1–3. Liver acinus in a human. The acinus occupies sectors only of 2 adjacent hexagonal fields and reaches their central veins, *C.V.* The axial terminal portal branch of the structural unit is injected with India ink and runs perpendicular to the 2 terminal hepatic (central) venules with which it interdigitates. It is visualized by a fortunate cut parallel with almost its entire length. The central veins lie close to each other in this section. (Thick cleared section × 300.)

clumps, although matted together, hang berrylike on their axial stalks, the dividing line between them being the watershed of biliary drainage. Each acinus empties its biliary secretion into the bile ductule from which it originated, and to which it stays linked. Since the terminal vascular branches, which bring the materials for nutrition and metabolism into the acinus, run along the terminal bile ductule draining the secretory product of the same acinus, structural and functional unity is established in this small clump of parenchyma. In spite of extensive intersinusoidal communication, blood and nutrients are preferentially carried into the sinusoids of each acinus by its parent vessels. This dependence of the parenchyma on the preferential supply lines is evidenced under circulatory (e.g., ischemia) or nutritional (e.g., choline deficiency) stress.*

Figure 1–10 illustrates in the left upper corner the intercommunication of sinusoids at the tip of 2 adjacent acini, the axial vessels of which stem from different portal fields. (The upper portal field is not shown

* For a better illustration of this strict relationship between nutrient vessels, bile duct, and parenchymal clump, I would give the following analogy: Imagine a mat glass wall evenly illuminated from behind by a multitude of small bulbs. Because of the fusion of light one could hardly indicate which small area of the wall is lighted primarily by which bulb. However, if one or several bulbs suddenly emit only a dim light, the specific area they illuminate becomes manifest. Similarly, in the liver, the individual simple, complex, or agglomerated acini become sharply outlined when physiopathologic changes occur.

in the photograph.) This is the area where mutually supplied collateral flow prevails. A lesion (ischemic or fatty) would disunite the tips of the abutting acini and, in an almost vertical sweep, reach both terminal hepatic veins. Since the portal branches we are studying here are of microscopic size, they lie in the realm of an absolutely regular association with similar hepatic arterial and bile duct branches.[66] Thus the injection of the portal system with a colored mass (Fig. 1–3) indicates also the course of the other channel systems and nerves; they are included in our description, though not always mentioned specifically.

Acinar Circulatory Zones. There is a zonal relationship between the cells constituting the acini and their blood supply. The hepatocytes situated close to the axial terminal vascular branches, in zone 1 (Fig. 1–4) are the first to be supplied with fresh blood, rich in oxygen and nutrients. They form the most active and resistant core of the acinus: they are the last to die and the first to regenerate.[84, 85, 214] The more distant the cells are, in any plane, from the site where the terminal portal and arterial branches empty into the sinusoids, the poorer is the quality of blood that bathes them, and the less is their resistance to damage. The greater distance from the supply lines is indicated by the higher order of zones (zones 2 and 3).

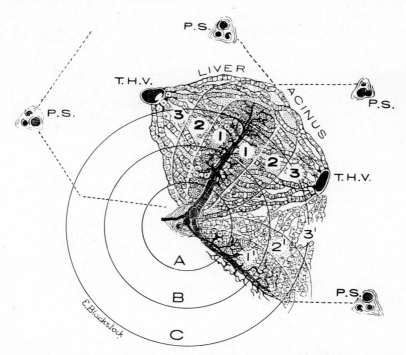

F<small>IG</small>. 1–4. Blood supply of the simple liver acinus and the zonal arrangement of cells. The acinus occupies adjacent sectors of neighboring hexagonal fields. Zones 1, 2 and 3, respectively, represent areas supplied with blood of first, second, and third quality with regard to oxygen and nutrients. These zones center about the terminal afferent vascular branches, terminal bile ductules, lymph vessels, and nerves, and extend into the triangular portal field from which these branches crop out.

Zones 1′, 2′ and 3′ designate corresponding areas in a portion of an adjacent acinar unit. In Zones 1 and 1′ the afferent vascular twigs empty into the sinusoids. Circles B and C indicate peripheral circulatory areas as commonly described around the "periportal" area, A. P.S., portal space; T.H.V., terminal hepatic venules.

The circulatory zones run concentrically around the *terminal* afferent vessels, i.e., around the *smallest* portal *spaces.*

Periportal location is generally assumed to be close to the source of supply, but it is evident that not all cells around portal spaces share equally the supply of fresh blood. Some cells in area B or C (Fig. 1–4), farther away from the portal space, have an excellent blood supply from the terminal afferent vessels branching out from the same portal space. On the other hand, some cells in area A, although close to the triangular portal space, are remote from the terminal arborizations of the afferent vessels, and therefore at a disadvantage with regard to oxygen and nutrients.

Studies of bile formation in the perfused isolated rat liver by Brauer[26] have revealed a zonal blood flow pattern in little clumps of tissue similar to our acini. Also, *in vivo* transillumination of a rat liver, and microscopic observation of the blood flow pattern during circulatory stress, reveals a darkening of the portion of the sinusoid that is remote from the terminal portal venules.

Enzymatic and Metabolic Areas in the Acini. All cells within the liver lobule have always been considered as being of the same kind and showing no functional specificity. Although no particular function can as yet be ascribed to one group of hepatocytes exclusively, their lack of uniformity is evident in histochemical and electron microscopic studies.

Information on the morphologic difference of the cells in zone 1 from those in zone 3 was provided by electron microscopic studies

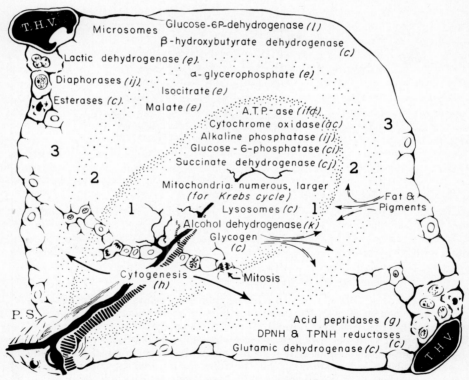

FIG. 1–5. Metabolic areas and their enzymatic pattern. For description, see text. The letters in parentheses indicate corresponding references: *a*, Burstone[35]; *b*, Meyer and Weinmann[167]; *c*, Novikoff and Essner[174]; *d*, Novikoff et al.[175]; *e*, Novikoff et al.[176]; *f*, Padykula and Herman[180]; *g*, Rutenburg and Seligman[211]; *h*, Schepers[214]; *i*, Wachstein[239]; *j*, Schumacher[216]; *k*, Greenberger et al.[82]; *l*, Isselbacher and Jones[106]. *P.S.*, portal space; *T.H.V.*, terminal hepatic venules.

in Porter's biological laboratories. He noticed even intermingling of mitochondria and ergastoplasmic reticulum (ER) in the hepatocytes of zone 1 and ER clusters in the parenchymal cells of zone 3.[187] It is clear that the environment of the cells in the 3 zones shows some difference with regard to pressure, dynamics of flow, and supply of oxygen and of nutrients. Conditions are selective for the presence of some enzymes. As Novikoff and Essner express it: "Just as the distribution of the organelles within each parenchymatous cell is probably related to the direction of cytoplasmic and molecular movement within the cell, so the quantitative differences [in materials and enzymes] among adjacent cells probably reflect the direction of blood flow within the hepatic lobule."[174] Similarly, Schumacher discusses the "topography" of hepatic enzymes as a part of an integrated metabolic system.[216]

Figure 1–5 illustrates and summarizes the distribution of common hepatic enzymes in the circulatory zones. The integration of the enzyme pattern into metabolic systems may enable us in the future to identify the circulatory zones as metabolic areas. A certain metabolic activity is promoted in these areas under normal conditions; as these conditions change, so does the distribution of the enzymes.[60] Immediately after birth there is an increase in activity of many liver enzymes (e.g., glucose-6-phosphatase)[50]; the great change in the intrahepatic circulation due to the occlusion of the arterial ductus Arantii creates suddenly a new environment different for the cells in zone 1 from that in zone 3. It is as if a branch of the Gulf Stream suddenly changed its course; areas of luxurious growth would become barren while in other regions new vegetation would develop.[195]

Activity of respiratory enzymes, such as succinic dehydrogenase and cytochrome oxidase in horse and pig livers and glucose-6-phosphatase in rat livers, has been shown to be particularly concentrated in zone 1.[40, 216] In these cells, containing numerous long mitochondria and exposed first to fresh blood entering the acinus, oxidative processes via the Krebs cycle operate at a high level. Also, the higher level of glucose-6-phosphatase activity makes these cells the first to deposit glycogen. In addition, the abundance of large lysosomes rich in acid phosphatase may facilitate a higher rate of pinocytosis and entrance of proteins and other materials from the nutrient-laden portal blood into the hepatocytes. Zone 3 is the site of the NAD and NADP diaphorases and of glycogen storage, of glycolytic activity and of the formation of fat and pigments, some of them fat-containing. With increasing fat formation the lipid-laden cells will be seen in zone 3, at the periphery of the acinus, and in the adjacent zone 2.

The concept of metabolic heterogeneity in the various zones is in the process of formation and will probably undergo various modifications; nevertheless it has permitted selective microchemical studies on cells from different circulatory zones isolated by microdissection.[171, 223] Similarly, enzymatic specificity and metabolic heterogeneity of the cells in different circulatory zones must be implicated in some way in the selective toxic injury of cells in different parts of the liver acinus.[232, 244] This susceptibility to different degrees of damage by anoxia or malnutrition, characteristic for each zone, enabled us to delimit these zones before their enzymatic pattern was known. Thus the work done independently by histochemists[52] and enzymologists[171, 233] confirms the subdivision of the simple acinus into zones, as evidenced by histopathologic changes in the injured liver of the dog, rat, rabbit, monkey and man.

Cytogenesis after hepatectomy or toxic injury is closely connected with DNA metabolism and is said to occur mainly in zone 1. Schepers, studying cellular gigantism after toxic injury, calls the area close to the terminal afferent vessels the "cytogenic zones," because here the newborn cells are smallest.[214] While the cells are moving toward the "cytoclastic locus" around the terminal hepatic venule, they fulfill their physiologic tasks; they become polyploidic, age, die, and are often eliminated into the hepatic veins. The movement of cells from the cytogenic zone into zone 3 in hepatectomized rats has also been noticed by Grisham.[84] The statement by Leblond and Walker,[131] that mitosis does not take place in the rat liver, is in contradiction to a recent and

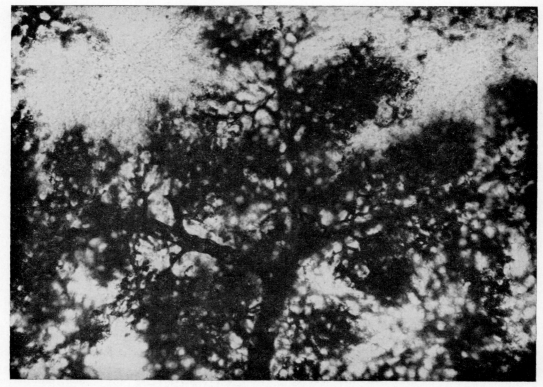

Fɪɢ. 1–6. Human complex acinus. The sinusoids injected with India ink are supplied by 3 terminal portal branches and their parent preterminal vessel. These portal branches form the axial channels of a complex acinus cut longitudinally. (150 μ thick cleared section × 88.)

thorough study by MacDonald[145] of the life span of the liver cell in the rat. His findings agree with what one would expect of an organ whose rapid regeneration has been known since ancient times and was exemplified in the legend of Prometheus. If further proof of the continual rebirth of the liver is added in the future, the notion of the lobule as a static anatomic unit will lose much of its meaning.

Complex Acinus

A complex acinus is a microscopic clump of tissue composed of at least 3 simple acini and a sleeve of parenchyma around the preterminal portal, arterial, and biliary branches, lymph vessels, and nerves that give origin to the terminal axial channels of the simple acini constituting this larger unit.

Figure 1–6 represents a longitudinal cut through a complex liver acinus. A pretermi-

nal portal branch ramifies in 3 directions. Each of its terminal branches forms the axis of a simple acinus. Each acinus has a well-delimited periphery which extends toward the portal space out of which it grew. It drains into 2 areas about terminal hepatic venules (these areas in the upper half of the picture are poorly injected). Also a distinct clump of tissue surrounds the preterminal channels as a sleeve. This sleeve of parenchyma consists of tiny clumps—acinuli —that are nourished by small axial venules and hepatic arterioles branching off from the preterminal vessels. Such vascular twigs have been demonstrated radiologically by Daniel and Prichard[48]: they arborize into a thicket of sinusoids.

A cross section through this complex acinus at the level where the preterminal vessel divides into its terminal branches would produce a picture comparable to

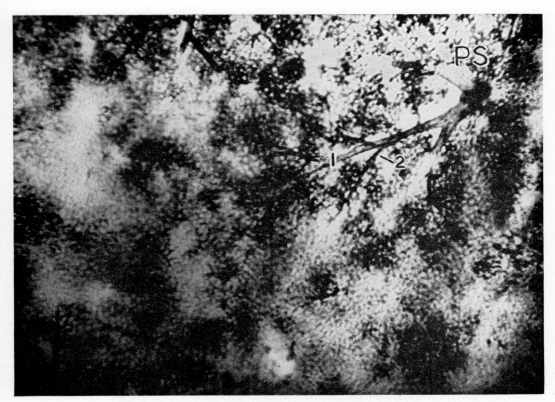

FIG. 1–7. Group of acinar agglomerates. Human liver injected with India ink. Three large portal branches grow out in different directions from a portal space (*P.S.* in right upper corner). One of these runs diagonally through the field and represents the axis of an *acinar agglomerate*. From this portal branch preterminal (*1*) and terminal (*2*) branches grow out and form the axes of the outcropping complex and simple acini, respectively. (100 μ thick cleared section × 18)

Figure 1–10. Note also that the cut would have to be inclined toward the left in order to lay bare the origin of all 3 branches by the same plane of section. The preterminal parent channels supply and drain this complex parenchymal unit (Fig. 1–6). The subdivision of the complex acinus into circulatory zones is difficult to illustrate. Zone 3 continues from one simple acinus into the neighboring one as the circulatory peripheral zone of the complex acinus. As usual zone 3 is prone to ischemia, toxic or nutritional damage, and the localization of these injuries serves indeed to outline the irregular size and shape of the complex acini in the rat, dog, monkey and human. Data on the function of the normal complex acinus as a whole are not available.

Structural and functional unity in these clumps is also demonstrated by the three-colored injection technic[20] mentioned on p. 7. The specimens show that the axial vessels of the simple acini are always of the same color as the parent stems of the complex acini. Indeed, owing to this arrangement, the microscopic segmentation of the liver into differently colored afferent vascular areas is made possible. The complex acini are, of course, parts of greater microscopic clumps of tissue, the acinar agglomerates.

Acinar Agglomerate. The acinar agglomerate is a microscopic parenchymal clump, composed of 3 or 4 complex acini and the acini forming the sleeve of parenchyma around the large portal space containing the supplying and draining channels and nerves of the agglomerate.

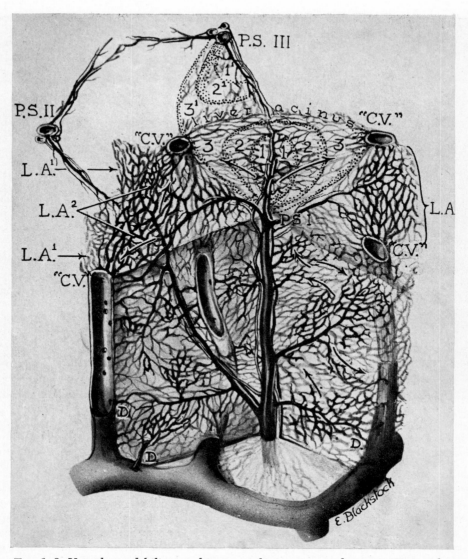

FIG. 1–8. Vascular and biliary architecture of an acinar agglomerate. For explanation, see text. *P.S.I, P.S.II, P.S.III,* portal fields; *L.A., L.A.,*[1] simple liver acinus; *L.A.*[2] simple acinus penetrating a hexagonal field situated well above the level of origin of the acinus, "*C.V.*" (central vein), terminal hepatic venule; *D,* collecting venules of Deysach; 1,2,3, circulatory zones of the simple liver acinus. Note the arcuate courses of the terminal portal branches, the irregularly arranged simple acini, and the short portal vessels that form the axes of tiny acini (acinuli) constituting the mantle of parenchyma around the longitudinally cut portal space.

Figure 1–7 illustrates acinar agglomerates in the human liver. A large portal branch runs diagonally through the field and divides into its preterminal (1) and terminal branches (2). The terminal ramification occurs at the margin of the field. The parenchyma around the preterminal branches forms complex acini composed of simple acini. The tissue organized around such vascular structure and its terminal ramifications is an acinar agglomerate. It has unity because the main route of vascular supply and

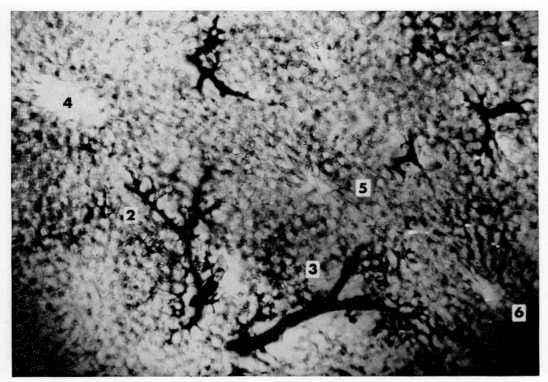

FIG. 1–9. Human liver injected with India ink. Interdigitation of portal and hepatic vein branches. Two horizontal terminal portal branches (*2, 3*), forming the axes of acini, interdigitate with 3 vertical radicles of ("central") hepatic veins (*4, 5, 6*) around which they arch. (Cleared thick section × 110.)

the biliary drainage is common to the whole clump as well as to its subdivisions. Furthermore, the handle of the catapult-like vascular structure originates from a large vascular branch from which other vessels also ramify; they are of appropriate size to form the axis of other acinar agglomerates. Thus the field in Figure 1–7 comprises a group of acinar agglomerates. Vessels and bile ducts that form the axis of a *group of acinar agglomerates* have passed the microscopic threshold and become visible to the naked eye. They should not be included in the microscopic study of liver structure, but it is easy to imagine that several groups of acinar agglomerates may form a small liver lobe in an animal with a multilobulated liver.

Architectural Framework in the Liver

This framework is represented by the afferent vascular trees, closely followed in

their branchings by the bile ducts and ductules as illustrated in Figure 1–8. The blood coming up through the portal space with the respiratory tides in the portal branch and with pulsating jets in the arterial channel disperses like a fountain through their terminal afferent twigs and sinusoids; it waters and nourishes the parenchyma of the liver acini, each of them extending into several adjacent hexagonal fields. The bile secreted by this structural unit and collected in the bile capillaries is drained by the terminal bile ductule and duct accompanying the afferent vascular channels. The latter, and consequently the liver acini, have by no means a rigid geometric arrangement around the central veins; they run in curved rather than straight lines but mainly perpendicular to the terminal hepatic ("central") veins with which they interdigitate. This relationship between the microscopic afferent and

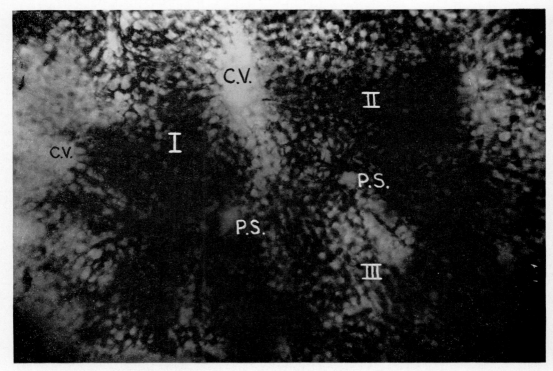

Fig. 1–10. Acinar units and the hexagonal field. Human liver injected with India ink. The tissue around a terminal hepatic venule (*C.V.*, near center of upper half of the field) is composed of parts of acini e.g., I, II and III) which form the lower half of a hexagonal field. Their ink-filled axial vessels grow out from 2 small portal spaces (*P.S.*). The tissue of the upper part of this field stems from other acinar units. Acinus I is seen to be drained by 2 "central" veins (C.V.). (Cleared thick section × 110.)

efferent hepatic vessels (Fig. 1–9) is the same as that observed in the gross specimens where the interdigitating course of the intrahepatic vessels is brought out clearly by injection and corrosion procedures.[19, 62, 65]

The various ways of branching and sinusoidal anastomosing of the terminal afferent vessels with vascular areas situated above and below a hexagonal field indicate that the hepatic structural units (acini) are closely connected with each other (Fig. 1–8). However, each is centered definitely around its main axial bile and vascular channels. This centering can be seen readily in Figure 1–10, a cleared thick section of a human liver, injected with India ink. The cluster of parenchyma is outlined distinctly by the well-filled thicket of sinusoids that extends between the "central veins" of 2 neighboring hexagonal fields (Fig. 1–10, I).

The *portal spaces* can be classified according to their function. The smallest *triangular* portal spaces in a microscopic field contain the *preterminal* branches of portal vein, hepatic artery and bile duct, lymph vessels and nerves. The triangular shape of the portal space is due to the tridimensional outcropping of terminal branches from the channels of the triad and their sheath of connective tissue.[194] In proximity to these triangular spaces and deriving from them, is a number of small, round or oval portal spaces representing the multiple cross sections of the *terminal* channels that supply and drain the simple acini. *These smallest portal spaces are the most important functional landmarks in the hepatic parenchyma* (see pp. 18 and 21). Larger portal spaces, either triangular with rounded edges or roughly oval, are the cross sections of the trio of channels servicing acinar agglomerates or groups of acinar agglomerates. In contradiction to the geometric lobulation taught by the classicists, we must state that the liver acini are *irregular in size and shape* and depend very much on the configuration of their axial channels and ramifying twigs.

The *hexagonal pattern* in the hepatic parenchyma that has fascinated the histologists for over 130 years is seen to be the result of tridimensional budding of the terminal bile ducts and accumulation of connective tissue around them.[193, 199] While some authors deny the existence of the hexagonal lobule,[63, 64, 157, 212] others consider it as a structural unit which, because of its arrangement around a central vein, is most adequate for metabolic activity.[137, 164] But metabolic as well as endocrine exchange takes place in the sinusoid and not in the peripheral veins that drain the capillary network. In the acinar concept the sinusoids cease to be a random network of capillaries. They form the well-delimited (Fig. 1–10, I, II) and distensible framework of a small parenchymal unit which they sustain and supply. Sinusoids are arranged as radial and peripheral channels[63] and are fed by inlet-portal venules and arterioles, offsprings of the acinar axial vessels.

Structural Elements of the Acinar Units. *Hepatic Cords and Plates.* The oversimplified description of a test-tube–like hepatic epithelium arranged in cords, 2 cells thick and comprising a bile canaliculus between them,[153, 154] has been revised by Elias' tridimensional studies of the mammalian liver.[61–63] The parenchyma of the human liver is fashioned in cribriform sheets or plates 1 cell thick. Each cell is surrounded by a polygonal network of bile capillaries which unite in the bile canaliculi. This concept leans on earlier observations of Koelliker (1853),[125] Hering (1872),[98] Braus[29] and Pfuhl.[182] Perhaps it can be challenged by the observations made with intravital fluorescence microscopy.[92] Also, in random sections hepatic cells in sheet arrangement are observed rarely. However, the acinar arrangment of sheets and plates, resulting from the fusion of branched cords that surround axial channels and are situated perpendicular to the central veins, explains why

we find unicellular chains of cells rather than sheets or cords.[199]

Bile Capillaries, Canaliculi, Intermediate Canals of Hering[98] and (Axial) Terminal Bile Duct Branches. The study of the bile capillaries has reached safer ground since Ellinger and Hirt[67] first visualized by fluorescence microscopy the bile capillaries *in vivo*. However, it is to the credit of Grafflin and associate[78] that they recognized certain phenomena in this capillary pattern as abnormal. These phenomena were brought about by abnormal conditions inherent in the method and the prolonged observation. Hanzon[92] too has proved that a capillary plexus surrounds each liver cell in a lamina except for the side exposed to the sinusoids. Bile capillaries empty into bile canaliculi, which in their zigzag course reach the intermediate canal of Hering (Fig. 1–11). As confirmed by electron microscopy[28] the walls of the capillaries and the canaliculi are formed by the modified membranes of the surrounding hepatic cells.

The intermediate canal, *Zwischenstück* of Hering, was reinvestigated by Clara[42] and was studied with the electron microscope.[86, 210, 231, 247] Its wall, endowed with microvilli, is formed by the cell membranes of hepatocytes and of cuboidal epithelial cells lining the smallest bile ductules. These cells are poor in mitochondria and contain a dark-staining argentophilic nucleus. The intermediate canal of Hering is only 2 to 4 cells long; the ampulla-like dilation of its lumen[68] could not be demonstrated by Steiner and Carruthers[231] in their electron micrograms. Its wall is composed of cuboidal, flat epithelial cells containing a dark-staining argentophilic nucleus.

Several intermediate canals join the axial terminal branch of the bile duct. The region of the canal of Hering is richly vascularized, and is the site of parenchymal repair and perhaps of fluid absorption.

Terminal (Axial) Branches of Afferent Vessels. Sinusoids. Radicles of Hepatic Veins.

Portal Vein. Elias[63] introduced a distinctive nomenclature for the finer intrahepatic ramifications of the portal vein. His differentiation into "conducting" and "axial distributing veins," although possible only

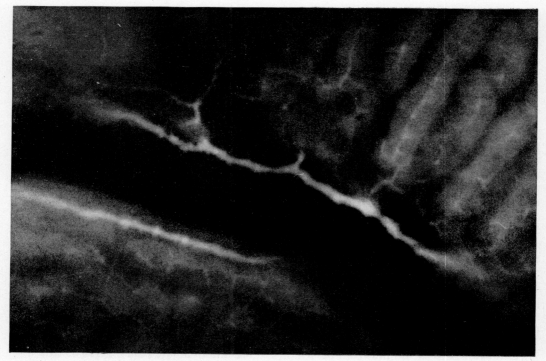

FIG. 1–11. Uranin secretion of the liver cells in a rat. The uranin content of the bile makes visible the bile canaliculi, the intermediate canal of Hering (left upper corner), and the terminal (axial) bile ductules. The latter accompany a terminal (axial) portal branch which courses close to the liver surface. × 500 approx. (Hanzon, V., and Blomqvist, B.: Anatomiska Institutionen, Uppsala, Sweden.)

when these vessels are seen cut longitudinally, is very suitable for practical purposes. However, serial sections of conducting veins reveal the regular branching out of venules to supply a periportal cuff of tissue. Thus the "conducting veins" distribute blood quite regularly to neighboring tissue too. Similar observations were made by Daniel and Prichard.[48] In distinction, however, the "axial distributing vein"[63] is a terminal branch of the portal vein and usually is situated in the axis of an acinar unit, the sinusoidal glomus of which it supplies with its arborizing inlet venules. These venules show sphincter activity that regulates the amount of portal blood in the sinusoids.[124, 197]

Terminal portal venules are easily recognized in the microscopic slide; their cross section is found in the *smallest round* or *oval* portal spaces. *Preterminal* portal branches, the axial vessels of complex acini, lie in small *triangular* portal spaces.

HEPATIC ARTERY. The branches of this vessel supply all the structures in the portal tracts and also the sinusoids. Its terminal ramifications have been the object of many studies and still are debated vividly. There are great differences of opinion as to the actual arterial terminations and the way they join the portal vein. Indeed, two blood streams flow into a firmly encapsulated organ: the arterial under pressure of 120 mm. Hg, the portal under 9 mm. Hg. The question as to how the portal blood streams uphill is not answered fully. We believe that sluice mechanisms raise one stream to the level of the other by means of sphincters at the junction of arterioles and arterial capillaries with portal venules and sinusoids. There are also sphincters at the outlets of the sinusoids into the peripheral veins. Sphincter activity has been observed by several workers,[124, 197, 220, 240] but the information about the histologic features of these sphincters is recent.[45, 63, 241] McCuskey describes the sphincters as consisting of reticuloendothelial cells.[149] These cells when contracted bulge with their nuclear region into the vascular lumen and occlude it.

According to Hale's clear review,[89] the distribution of the terminal (axial) branches of the hepatic artery may be divided into (a) a general plexus within the portal tract, (b) a special capillary plexus surrounding the bile ducts (peribiliary plexus), and (c) the arterial capillaries emptying directly into the sinusoids (Fig. 1–12).

General plexus supplies the structures within the portal tract, except for the terminal branches of the bile duct. These capillaries have a more open network woven around the contents of the portal space, and send branches into the radial or peripheral sinusoids.[37, 141, 177, 224]

Peribiliary plexus consists of a close network around the bile ducts up to their terminal branches. These capillaries play an important role in secretion,[4] absorption and concentration of bile, in regeneration of hepatic parenchyma, and in collateral arterial circulation of the hepatic parenchyma[204] (p. 31). Branches of this plexus pass into radial[8, 177] and peripheral[3, 63] sinusoids, and through capillary connections join the por-

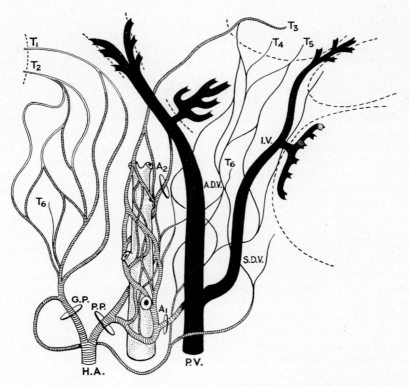

Fig. 1–12. A_1, arteriolar-venular anastomosis between hepatic artery and portal vein; A_2, capillary anastomosis between hepatic artery and portal vein; *A.D.V.*, axial distributing vein; *H.A.*, hepatic artery; *G.P.*, general plexus of hepatic artery; *I.V.*, inlet venule; *P.P.*, peribiliary plexus of hepatic artery; *P.V.*, portal vein; *S.D.V.*, small distributing vein. Branches from general plexus: T_1, emptying into a radial sinusoid; T_2, emptying into the peripheral sinusoid; T_3, intralobular capillary. Branches from peribiliary plexus: T_4, emptying into a radial sinusoid; T_5, emptying into a peripheral sinusoid. Stippled area represents bile ducts. Interrupted lines represent the limits of hexagonal fields. (Hale, A. J.: Glasgow, M. J. 32:283.)

tal vein. These capillaries form so-called "internal radicles of the portal vein."[3, 8, 37, 43, 121, 141] Another connection between arterioles of this plexus and portal venules provided with sphincters important for raising the pressure and speeding the flow has been observed by earlier workers.[105] It has been confirmed through microscopic observation of the intrahepatic circulation *in vivo*.[124, 197, 240]

Arterioles Emptying Directly into Sinusoids. The intralobular arterioles running freely through the hepatic parenchyma were described by earlier workers[29, 41] and by recent investigators.[63, 64, 220] However, the zone in which it lies and its mode of termination never have been described exactly. We have repeatedly observed *in vivo* the activity of hepatic arterioles in zone 1 only.[197]

Summary. The structural complexity of the arterioportal junctions adds to the difficulty of exact understanding of the mechanism of the dual blood supply. However, precise knowledge of the intrahepatic circulation is essential for the solution of many problems of hepatic physiology, pathology and therapy.

SINUSOIDS. Those who consider the aspect of narrow islets of cells between wide capillary canals as being brought about by the penetration of solid parenchymal masses into the omphalomesenteric lakes, may regard the rows of epithelial cells in a microscopic field as the sectioned tips of coral formations whose narrow walls crisscross down deep to the bottom of the lakes, forming a labyrinthine scenery.

Those who are inclined to see in the architecture of the liver lobule the stamp of endocrine rather than exocrine activity[137, 164] are supported in their opinion by the close relationship between parenchyma and capillary network, and by the structure of the sinusoids, but not by their radial course toward the radicles of the hepatic veins. Indeed, as in other endocrine organs, rows of parenchymal cells are bordered by large capillaries into which metabolic products and waste are poured. But endocrine organs, e.g., adrenal and pituitary, show neither radial capillary course nor central veins to drain them. Furthermore, the hepatic capil-

laries are unique in their thin endothelial syncytial lining as their large Kupffer cells.[124, 127, 237] These phagocytic endocytes[249] are attached to the endothelial plasmodium and spread their stellate processes through the capillary lumen toward different points of the wall where they anchor.[246] Besides their role in the production of bilirubin, they are the scavengers of this complex canal system, clearing it of particulate matter, old erythrocytes, bacteria[160] and debris which they engulf.

Kupffer cells (the littoral cells) are seen in the electron microscope as a discontinuous layer[70, 90, 91, 174] of endothelium composed of cells of various types.[215] Some are very thin and extend over 3 or 4 parenchymal cells; some are thicker, up to 800 mμ. Their overlapping cytoplasmic lamellae are separated from each other by narrow passages that provide access to Disse's space for the plasma. Other Kupffer cells are even larger, with an oval nucleus and cytoplasmic projections on their undersurface for interlacing contact and attachment to the microvilli of the parenchymatous cells. These larger Kupffer cells have a few round mitochondria; their endoplasmic reticulum and Golgi apparatus are not prominent; their large lysosomes are rich in acid phosphatase. The endothelium lining the hepatic sinusoids of the rat lacks a basement membrane in zone 2 and in adjacent portions of zones 1 and 3. The fenestrations of the endothelium in this area permit easy passage for macromolecules into Disse's spaces which communicate with the tissue spaces at both ends of the sinusoids.[34]

Active littoral cells have also high ATP-ase activity.[174] Littoral cells show pseudopodlike processes on their sinusoidal as well as on their undersurface for phagocytosis in the sinusoidal and in Disse's spaces. Kupffer cells produce reticular fibers which, together with the concentrated plasma proteins, form a continuous basement membrane beneath the endothelium[90]; reticulum fibers are also seen within human Kupffer cells.[46] Kupffer cells metabolize phagocytized material (pigments, fat, cholesterol, colloids); their nuclei also synthesize protein.[72]

The width of the sinusoids varies from 6 to 30 μ and can increase to 180 μ when necessary. This change in caliber is due to contractility, an exquisite feature of these capillaries, the structural elements of which are not investigated fully. There is also tonic contractility[124] which, together with the inlet and the outlet sphincters, helps to regulate the amount of flow through a vascular area. The activity in the sinusoids is intermittent. Groups of sinusoids shift their work asynchronously. The circulatory activity spreads simultaneously to those sectors of neighboring hexagonal fields that are adjacent to the active axial vessel.[123] This phenomenon explains itself as circulatory activity of single acini (Fig. 1–10, I, II). About 25 per cent of sinusoids are active while the remainder are resting or storing blood.[240] Thus is disclosed the microscopic feature of the function of the liver as a "venesector and blood giver of the circulatory system."[114]

RADICLES OF THE HEPATIC VEINS. The histologic feature of the junction of the sinusoids with the hepatic veins where sphincter activity is observed *in vivo* needs further investigation.[193] Also, the abrupt transition from capillaries to such large vessels as the central veins is unusual in vascular anatomy. Whether the majority of the sinusoids empty individually or through collecting venules into the radicles of the hepatic veins also has not been determined. However, Hanzon's microphotos of the different phases of uranin secretion *in vivo* (his Figs. 16 and 39),[92] demonstrate that different acini around a central vein empty into collecting venules which they border. The central veins are the drainage centers of several collecting venules as well as of individual sinusoids. The sluice channels of Deysach[53] are collecting venules surrounded by sphincters at their site of junction with the preterminal hepatic venules into which they short-circuit a certain amount of sinusoidal blood when needed. The terminal hepatic venules represent the drainage centers into which peripheral and radial sinusoids of different acini empty their blood (Fig. 1–3). The absence of a limiting plate around these veins also indicates that the surrounding tissue is not bound together and lacks unity. Therefore, an area of early necrosis around the central veins produced by hepatic ischemia has a stellate shape.

The walls of the hepatic venous branches have also contractile sphincters. In dogs the smooth muscles in the wall of the hepatic veins contract during shock.[163] The presence of these muscle fibers in dogs and humans was described by early workers[30, 184] and demonstrated later by Popper,[186] who found that an inversely proportional rate of flow is possible in the hepatic veins and in their mural lymphatics.

The interdigitating relationship between the branches of the hepatic vein and the portal vein, observed in the gross specimen, is maintained in the microscopic field between terminal branches of these veins. The terminal (axial) branches of the portal vein and the hepatic artery run mainly perpendicular to the radicles of the hepatic veins which they surround.

Summary. The essential feature of the hepatic parenchyma is its lobulation. It is not a matter of conjecture but a biologic principle that secreting cells have a definite arrangement around the very small afferent vessels on which their function and nutrition depend. They also have an intimate connection with the very small excretory channels through which their products are discharged. This principle is depicted in the *liver acinus*, the above-described hepatic structural and functional unit. It can be demonstrated by special injection technic and is also revealed in the pattern of certain pathologic processes.

ANATOMIC PATTERN OF PATHOLOGIC PROCESSES[200, 201]

The concept of a hexagonal lobule that is situated around a terminal hepatic ("central") vein offers to the pathologist only 2 or 3 landmarks for the orientation of lesions he observes: the "central" vein, the periphery and rarely the midzone.[101] On the other hand, in the acinar concept attention is focused on the dynamic lines along which adequate or deficient nutrients and oxygen are moved into the parenchyma, and the produced bile is carried away (Fig. 1–13A). Noxious agents, ascending infections of bile ducts, and lymph vessels all enter the liver along the same lines. In severe injury, large areas of parenchyma are wiped out, and orientation becomes impossible, but in cases

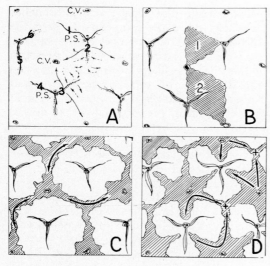

Fig. 1–13. Orienting lines and patterns in the hepatic parenchyma. **A**, the 6 dynamic lines (1 to 6) in an (assumed) regular hexagonal field are the routes of blood supply ($\longrightarrow$) and of bile drainage ($- - \rightarrow$); they are also the principal pathways of invasion of the hepatic parenchyma. *C.V.*, central vein; *P.S.*, portal space. **B, C, D**, patterns of hepatic lesions. (For explanation, see text.) (Rappaport, A. M., and Hiraki, G. Y.: Acta Anat., Basel, 32:126.)

of less damage the pathologic change is patterned on the anatomy of the acini and their circulatory zones:

1. A "paracentral" lesion—necrotic, fatty or fibrous—is a focal lesion occupying about one triangular sector of the hexagon, with the base toward one of its sides.[228] It represents the tangential cut of the damaged periphery of an acinus that lies above or below the plane of section (Fig. 1–13B, 1).[59] Similar lesions were produced experimentally by Kettler and called *Gruppennekrosen*.[118] "Midzonal" lesions have been explained by us[199] as tangential cuts of the damaged periphery of acini. Cheng[39] demonstrated by serial histologic sections that the so-called "midzonal" necrosis produced by experimental intoxication with beryllium sulfate represents the tangential cut of a necrotic area near a terminal afferent vascular branch. If one ceases to consider as a unit the tissue comprised within the imaginary hexagonal field and sees it composed of parts of simple acini surrounding a terminal hepatic vein, "focal" and "midzonal" lesions are easily recognized as sectioned lesions of single acini.

2. A periportal lesion unfolding toward 2 adjacent "central veins" (Fig. 1–13B, 2) represents the transverse section of an acinus entirely diseased, e.g., the necrosis in phosphorus poisoning.

3. The "pericentral" lesions seen in ischemic necrosis (Fig. 1–14), in fatty change[17, 18, 219] and in early dietary cirrhosis demonstrate[94, 95] by their stellate processes extending into adjacent hexagonal fields (Fig. 1–13C, *arrows*), that in reality the progressing damage skirts around the supplying vessels. The lesions are located at the periphery of parenchymal clumps representing complex acini. In advanced lesions the line of damage starts at a small triangular portal space harboring the preterminal channels and runs—as shown, in a horizontal plane (Fig. 1–13D)—toward the terminal hepatic ("central") veins of 2 neighboring hexagonal fields. It extends toward the site where the tips of the terminal channels forming the axes of 2 simple acini abut and dwindle to capillary size (at X in Fig. 1–13D). From here the line of injury curves and reaches the terminal hepatic ("central") vein of the adjacent hexagon, finally to return to its initial preterminal portal space. Necrotic, fatty or cirrhotic lesions, as they progress, broaden (arrows in Fig. 1–13D) and form bands tridimensionally interwoven like baskets containing only Zone 1, the core of the simple acini.[95]

Scanning a wider microscopic area, one can find in the same slide small periportal rims, islets and clumps of surviving parenchyma in the midst of necrotic, fatty, or fibrotic tissue (Fig. 1–15A). It is easily recognized that the surviving cells are oriented around terminal (Fig. 1–15A, 1) and preterminal (Fig. 1–15A, 2) afferent axial vessels and bile ductules. Conversely, the "central" veins have become separated from the normal tissue. A band of damaged tissue connecting several terminal hepatic ("central") veins to each other and to portal fields may arch as the broken line in Fig. 1–15A over many hexagonal fields to surround an

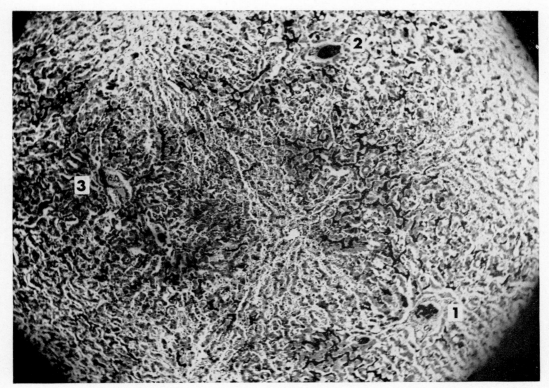

FIG. 1–14. Breakdown of the uniform parenchymal mass into its acinar constituents. Ischemic necrosis developing and progressing along the periphery of the acinar units delineates their boundaries. Note the 3 portal spaces (1, 2, 3) situated in the 3 corners of the field and arranged almost equidistantly on a circle surrounding the "central" vein. Note also the irregular acini (injected with India ink) that grow out from the portal spaces, and a small ink-filled venule leaving space 3. The "central" necrosis has stellate shape, and its projections extend toward and beyond the weakest points of circulation, the site where the capillarized tips of the acini meet each other. A similar distribution of lesions is observed in fatty change and in dietary cirrhosis.

area of healthy tissue that represents the cross section of an "acinar agglomerate" (Fig. 1–15A, 3). Within this area the contiguity of the parenchyma is maintained because the pathologic change is not severe enough to injure the peripheries of complex or simple acini. The lesser degree of damage may be due to the fact that the parenchyma has been spared massive invasion, or that it lies closer to major supply channels. Such orientation can be established by serial sectioning of the area under study. The cleavage of the uniform hepatic parenchyma into regenerating nodules and nodes (Fig. 1–15B) by fatty change or diffuse fibrosis[17] occurs along the peripheries of simple acini,

complex acini and of acinar agglomerates, where the radicles of the hepatic veins are normally situated.

This peculiar position of the central veins at the periphery of the regenerating nodules has been re-emphasized recently.[116] However, no adequate explanation has been given for this "move" of the radicles of hepatic veins from a central to a peripheral position in the tissue. The anatomic explanation is now possible on the basis of the acinar concept, which presents the "central" veins as drainage centers at the outskirts of several acini. In regeneration these veins do not "move"; they just retain their original position. The peripheries of the simple acini

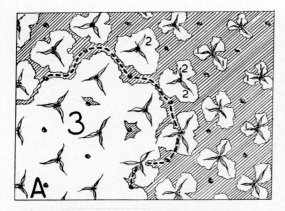

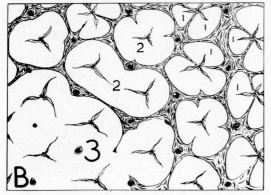

FIG. 1–15. **A,** hepatic damage affecting the peripheries of simple acini (1), of complex acini (2), and of acinar agglomerates (3). The damage is greatest in the right half of the diagram, where only small bands of parenchyma around the terminal axial branches have survived. **B,** regeneration and hyperplasia of acinar remnants have formed nodules of various size and shape: (1) mono-acinar nodules; (2) nodules deriving from the remnant of a complex acinus; (3) node representing the regenerated remnant of an acinar agglomerate. For explanation, see text. (Rappaport, A. M., and Hiraki, G. Y.: Acta Anat., Basel, 32:126.)

surrounding a terminal hepatic ("central") vein are *not* bound together by a limiting plate[63]; this facilitates the cleavage of the individual acini by any damage that spreads in a stellate fashion along the acinar peripheries.

IRREGULARITY OF NODES AND NODULES

The irregularity of regenerating nodes and nodules is usually attributed to the varying degree of regenerating power that the organ has preserved. However, the established irregularity in size and shape of normal simple and complex acini and acinar agglomerates makes clear how nodules deriving from their remnants will likewise show a great variety in magnitude and form. Also, when certain parts of the liver suffer either from a mild injury or from occasional noxious agents and deficiencies, the lesions will affect only the circulatory periphery of an acinar agglomerate or of a group of acinar agglomerates. The lesions will delimit in a wide sweep an area that is serviced by one *major* trio of axial channels. Within this area the circulation is still coherent, and the intrahepatic flow of nutrients is not arrested at the mono-acinar peripheries (Fig. 1–15A & B, 1); they continue to intercommunicate largely, assure the resistance of the hepatic parenchyma and preserve an apparent polygonal pattern. Regeneration in such a region, favored by good supply, is active and produces large nodes (Fig. 1–15B, 3) that have hypertrophied in an "orderly" fashion. However, tissue that by the pathologic processes has undergone subdivision into a complex or mono-acinar pattern will regenerate and form nodes and nodules that are divorced from their "central" veins and give the impression of *pseudo*lobulation (Fig. 1–15B). On the basis of our structural and functional concept we can understand "pseudolobulation" and that it reveals, although in a distorted way, the true acinar lobulation of the liver.

VESSELS OF THE LIVER

EXTRAHEPATIC DISTRIBUTION OF THE HEPATIC VESSELS

The liver receives blood through the portal vein and through the hepatic artery, a branch of the celiac axis. Since the portal vein drains the blood of an area supplied by the other branches of the celiac axis and by the superior and the inferior mesenteric arteries, the amount of blood flowing into the liver depends in fact on the flow in these arteries.

Common Hepatic Artery. This artery, the second major branch of the celiac axis, courses to the right along the upper border of the pancreas in the right gastropancreatic fold, which conducts the artery to the medial border of the hepatoduodenal part of the lesser omentum. It ascends in front of the portal vein and to the left of the bile duct. It divides into the left and the right hepatic arteries to supply the corresponding lobes of the liver. Michels[168] sees the hepatic artery dividing into 3 terminal branches: right, middle (for quadrate lobe), and left. There is an extensive and continuously growing literature[119] on the anomalies of the hepatic artery and its branches. This subject has also been dealt with by Michels[168] and by Johnston and Anson.[112] We shall mention the common anomalies and their relationships to the ducts.

Anomalies of the Hepatic Artery. In about 50 per cent of cases there are aberrant hepatic arteries. The right hepatic artery springs from the superior mesenteric artery, while the left aberrant hepatic artery derives frequently from the left gastric artery. Each of these arteries is often the single hepatic artery, and its injury can damage the liver severely. Knowledge of the anomalies of the hepatic artery is important for any surgery in the hepatic and duodenal area and for an effective chemotherapeutic infusion of a cancerous liver.[119]

Since the cystic artery arises in about 35 per cent of cases from the right hepatic branch only, or from a right hepatic artery, the variations and the topographic relationship of these arteries with the bile duct and the portal vein are important (Fig. 1–16).

Cystic Artery. The cystic artery arises in about a third of cases from the right hepatic artery in the upper part of Calot's triangle formed by the cystic and the hepatic ducts, and therefore has the above relationship to the bile duct and the portal vein as indicated in Fig. 1–16. (For other variations see Daseler and assoc., 1947[49].) The cystic artery divides into a superficial branch that is distributed to the peritoneal surface of the gallbladder and a deep branch that supplies the attached wall of the gallbladder and its bed. The artery is single in 75 per cent of cases and double in 25 per cent. In the latter, the deep and the superficial branches have each a separate origin.

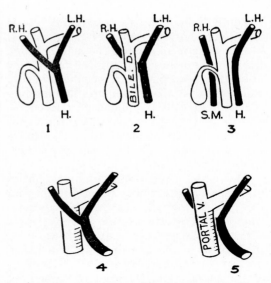

Fig. 1–16. Anomalies of hepatic artery. Their relation to portal vein and bile duct.
1. Anterior to the bile duct, 24%
2. Posterior to the bile duct, 64%   } 100%
3. Arising from superior mesenteric artery, 12%
4. Anterior to the portal vein, 91% } 100%
5. Posterior to the portal vein, 9%

L.H., left hepatic artery; *R.H.*, right hepatic artery; *S.M.*, superior mesenteric artery. (Grant, J. C. B.: Method of Anatomy, ed. 5, Baltimore, Williams & Wilkins.)

Terminal Branches of the Hepatic Artery. These vessels enter the portal fissure and lie here in a plane between the bile ducts and the branches of the portal vein which they flank to the left. Left and right arterial lobar branches anastomose rarely outside the portal fissure but intercommunicate by small twigs present in the deeper folds of the capsule of Glisson within the groove of the round ligament.[77] This explains why, after ligation of one branch of the hepatic artery in the autopsy specimen, the entire liver still can be injected with a barium mass through the other arterial branch.[218] Inside the liver substance the terminal branches of the hepatic artery communicate with each other and the portal vein only through capillaries. The ramifying gastroduodenal and right hepatic arteries, branches of the proper hepatic artery, are of importance as potential collaterals to the liver.

Portal Vein. The valveless portal vein is an afferent nutrient vessel of the liver and in this sense is an arterial channel. Analogy between the portal vein and the pulmonary artery has been based on recent studies by Reeves et al.[207] They compare the lung lobule with its central pulmonary arterial inflow to the liver acinus with its portal venular axis. It carries blood from the entire capillary system of the digestive tract, spleen, pancreas and gallbladder.

The portal vein derives from the omphalomesenteric veins which bring blood from the yolk sac and the intestines to the liver. The omphalic portion of the veins regresses with the disappearance of the yolk sac. With the growth of the intestines the mesenteric portions persist and become the tributaries of the portal vein. Its stem is formed by the omphalomesenteric trunks arranged in a figure-of-8 around the first and third portions of the duodenum. Its spiral course is formed by dropping out the posterior (right) limb of the "8" below and the anterior (left) limb of the "8" above.

Anomalies of the Portal Vein. These are relatively rare. The cavernomatous transformation of the portal vein is considered by some authors as an acquired anatomic anomaly due to early thrombosis and recanalization of the portal system.[227] Others consider it as an atypical development of the plexus of veins between the omphalomesenteric and the hepatic veins during the second month of fetal life.[14, 73] Leger and associates have thoroughly discussed the anatomy and pathogenesis of the portal cavernoma.[133] They stress the viewpoint that the postnatal obliterative process in the umbilical vein and the duct of Arantius may spread to the portal stem and its tributaries. A number of small cavernomatous veins form in the process of bypassing the obliterated vascular area.

Of recent years more frequent operations on the portal vein have led to new investigations of its anatomy.[56, 76, 189] It has been found constant in its length but extremely variable in its tributaries.

Splenic Vein. This vein (0.94 cm. diam.) commences with 5 to 6 branches that return the blood from the spleen and unite to form a single nontortuous vessel. In its course across the posterior abdominal wall it grooves the upper part of the pancreas, from which it collects numerous short tributaries. It can be visualized preoperatively by splenoportography[1, 7, 134] (see Chapter 10). It runs close to the hilum of the left kidney and terminates behind the neck of the pancreas, where it joins at a right angle the superior mesenteric vein. Because of its nearness to the vessels of the left kidney the splenic vein can be anastomosed to the renal vein. Its tributaries are the short gastric veins, the pancreatic veins, the left gastro-epiploic vein and the inferior mesenteric vein.

Inferior Mesenteric Vein. This vein (0.24 cm. diam.) returns blood from the area irrigated by the superior and the inferior left colic and the superior rectal veins.

Superior Mesenteric Vein. This vein (0.78 cm. diam.) is second in diameter to the portal vein itself and well suited for anastomosis with the caval system. It carries blood from the veins of the small intestine, the cecum, the ascending and the transverse colon. The portal trunk (about 2 cm. diameter) is formed behind the neck of the pancreas by the confluence of its roots, i.e., the splenic and the superior mesenteric veins. The length of the portal trunk is approximately 5.5 to 8 cm. (Fig. 1–17). The portal trunk receives also the rootlets of the superior pancreaticoduodenal vein, some accessory pancreatic veins,[56] the pyloric vein, the left gastric (coronary) vein and the cystic vein. Usually there is an upper segment of the portal trunk, averaging 5 cm. in length, which is devoid of major branches.[76] Here surgical dissection can be started without danger of hemorrhage.

The most troublesome tributary of the portal trunk is the left gastric (coronary) vein. It runs upward along the lesser curvature of the stomach, where it receives some esophageal veins. With progressing cirrhosis of the liver these enlarge to form varices that are apt to produce fatal hemorrhage. The portal trunk runs in the hepatoduodenal ligament in a plane dorsal to the bile duct and the hepatic artery and divides into 2 lobar branches before entering the portal fissure. The right lobar branch, short and thick, receives the cystic vein. The left lobar branch, longer and smaller, is joined by the umbilical vein (ligamentum teres) and the

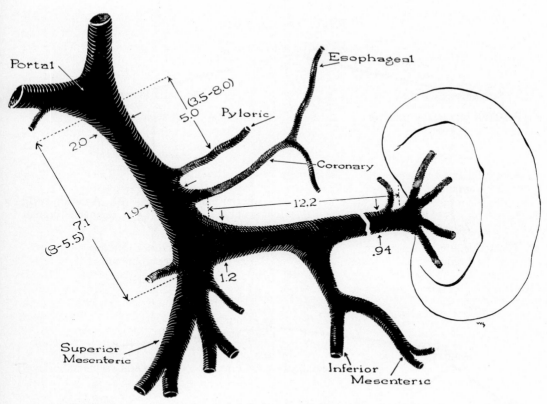

Fig. 1–17. Mensuration of the portal vein and its main branches. Figures are in centimeters. (Gilfillan, R. S.: Arch. Surg. *61*:449.)

associated para-umbilical veins. It connects by the venous ligament (ductus venosus Arantii) with the inferior vena cava. The left lobar branch gives branches to the quadrate lobe and also to the caudate lobe before entering the liver at the left end of the porta hepatis.

INTRAHEPATIC DISTRIBUTION OF THE HEPATIC VESSELS

The topography of the vascular and biliary structures within the liver have been studied by Segall,[218] Hjortsjö[102, 103] and Fainsinger.[69] Elias and Petty,[65] Couinaud,[47] Junès[113] and Bilbey[19] have reinvestigated the gross intrahepatic distribution of portal vein, the hepatic artery and the hepatic vein. We shall follow their description (Fig. 1–18).

Portal Vein. The portal trunk divides in the portal fissure into the left and right hepatic lobar branches, which form an angle of 90° with each other. The left branch is longer than the right and consists of transverse and umbilical parts. The latter is the remainder of the umbilical vein. It has a longitudinal course and continues into the round hepatic ligament. Thus a bend is formed between transverse and umbilical parts of the left lobar branch. The para-umbilical veins, important hepatofugal collaterals within the falciform ligament (p. 4), spring from the umbilical part of the left portal branch.

The injection of multicolored vinylite acetate into the vascular branches and the biliary ducts accessible in the porta hepatis has demonstrated that the liver can be divided into segments according to the distribution of the major or efferent vascular and biliary branches (Fig. 1–18). These branches have been named by Bilbey[19] after the segments of the liver they supply. The outline on page 28 summarizes his nomenclature for the

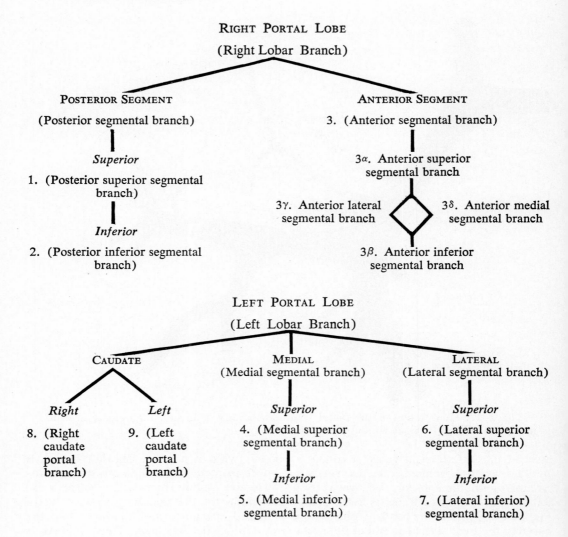

RIGHT PORTAL LOBE

(Right Lobar Branch)

POSTERIOR SEGMENT

(Posterior segmental branch)

Superior

1. (Posterior superior segmental branch)

Inferior

2. (Posterior inferior segmental branch)

ANTERIOR SEGMENT

3. (Anterior segmental branch)

3α. Anterior superior segmental branch

3γ. Anterior lateral segmental branch

3δ. Anterior medial segmental branch

3β. Anterior inferior segmental branch

LEFT PORTAL LOBE

(Left Lobar Branch)

CAUDATE

Right

8. (Right caudate portal branch)

Left

9. (Left caudate portal branch)

MEDIAL
(Medial segmental branch)

Superior

4. (Medial superior segmental branch)

Inferior

5. (Medial inferior) segmental branch)

LATERAL
(Lateral segmental branch)

Superior

6. (Lateral superior segmental branch)

Inferior

7. (Lateral inferior) segmental branch)

intrahepatic branches of the portal vein, the hepatic artery and the bile duct. Superior, inferior, medial and lateral branches of the (right) anterior segment radiate from a common, deeply situated central vessel and are difficult to isolate surgically. The surgical topography of the liver segments has been well presented by Reifferscheid.[208]

Each segment depends on its major vessel for blood supply. There is no anastomosis between the macroscopic branches, but large intercommunication at the level of the sinusoids.

Hepatic Artery. Segall likened the straight intrahepatic arterial branches in the younger individual to those of a maple tree,

and the tortuous branches of the older ones (over 40 years) to those of a bare apple tree.[218] He also described numerous intercommunications between right and left hepatic trunks situated in the capsular folds of the portal fissure. Ligation of one hepatic arterial trunk still permitted him to inject the entire liver through the other truncus.

The intrahepatic arterial branches follow the smaller portal branches closely, "climbing along them like a vine on a tree." This feature can be observed also at the microscopic level.[124] There is an absolute irregularity in the branching of the arterial trunks and the major rami. They do not parallel the corresponding portal channels or the major intrahepatic bile ducts. Co-ordination of the courses of the branches of portal vein, hepatic artery and bile duct is accomplished in the peripheral parts of the liver, at the level where tridimensional branching is the major law for the housing of a maximum of parenchyma in a limited space. Also, the dome-shaped diaphragm may determine the hemispheric shape of the hepatic surfaces underneath which tridimensional growth is favored by ideal conditions.

Hepatic Veins. The hepatic veins empty into the inferior vena cava where it lies in the groove of the posterior surface of the liver. They are enveloped by the coronary ligament. Since catheterization of the hepatic veins for the determination of hepatic blood flow has become a current procedure,[25, 225]

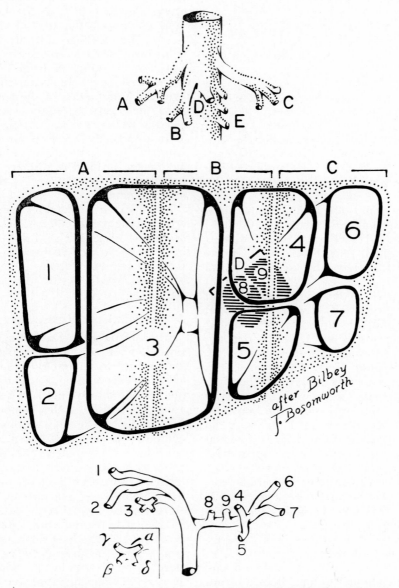

FIG. 1–18. Portal and hepatic venous segments of the liver overlap. For explanation, see text.

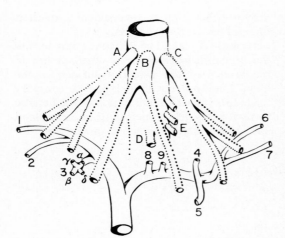

FIG. 1–19. Scheme of interdigitation of hepatic and portal venous trees.

and guided catheterization of the hepatic veins has permitted their roentgenography,[15, 173, 190, 202, 236] a brief outline of the intrahepatic branches of these veins may be useful.

An upper group of 3 major hepatic veins (right, middle and left) empty into the inferior vena cava. They drain 3 hepatic venous segments (Fig. 1–18A, B, C) which interdigitate and overlap the outlined portal segments.

Left Hepatic Vein. This vessel (Fig. 1–18C) drains the left lobe. It is composed of 2 major radicles: an upper one coming from the upper half and a lower from the lower half of the territory they drain.

Middle Hepatic Vein. This vein carries blood from the central parts of the liver (Fig. 1–18B), i.e., from areas irrigated by the right and the left lobar portal branches. The middle vein sometimes unites with the left hepatic vein to form a short common trunk before emptying into the vena cava.

Right Hepatic Vein. This vessel (Fig. 1–18A) is the remainder of the cardiac portion of the right omphalomesenteric vein. It drains the territory to the right of the Sérégé gallbladder-caval line (p. 2).

Several smaller veins (Fig. 1–18D and E) empty below the group of the major 3 or 2 veins into the vena cava. They drain blood from around the gallbladder, from the caudate process and from the posterior portal segment and the lateral portion of the an-

terior portal segment in the right liver lobe.

The intrahepatic course of the valveless hepatic veins is straight and simple. Their smaller branches are in direct contact with the hepatic parenchyma. There are frequent anastomoses among the various branches of the hepatic veins.

There is a definite spatial relationship between the branches of the hepatic veins and those of the portal vein and the hepatic artery. The branches of the hepatic vein interdigitate with the afferent vessels (Fig. 1–19). This architectural arrangement is maintained up to their finest ramifications. A uniform and quick drainage from all parts of the liver is accomplished thereby. The regular interdigitation of the terminal radicles of the hepatic veins (the "central" veins) with the tridimensionally arranged terminal afferent channels, brings about a hexagonal pattern in the hepatic parenchyma at the microscopic level. The distance between 2 such "central" veins is equal to the width of one liver acinus.

This distance is halved by the perpendicularly running pair of afferent axial vessels of the acinus (Fig. 1–3). Now the veins are found to be situated at the periphery of the structure that they drain, an arrangement that corresponds to the rule in vascular anatomy.

HEPATIC COLLATERAL CIRCULATION

Arterial Channels. The frequent fatal outcome after severance of the hepatic artery in humans and in laboratory animals has led for a long time to the belief that the hepatic artery is a terminal vessel. A review of this problem[160] has shown that Haberer[87] in 1905 was the first to prove experimentally that ligation of the hepatic artery proximal to its gastroduodenal branch is not fatal. However, the study of the collateral hepatic circulation did not advance until it was demonstrated that in the dog all branches of the hepatic artery can be ligated with impunity when the animal is treated with antibiotics postoperatively.[161] The liver deprived of the hepatic arterial channels develops a rich collateral arterial supply on which it survives.[75, 81, 83] The literature on this subject has grown at a rapid pace since the hepatic artery was ligated in human patients for the treatment of the sequelae of portal hypertension.[16, 129, 209]

The hepatic artery is provided with collateral flow through its anastomoses with adjacent arteries arising from the celiac axis and the superior mesenteric artery. Good collateral circulation becomes manifest in cases of gradual occlusion of the artery. *The liver as an outgrowth of the gut shares one of its architectural features, the vascular arcade.* The supramesocolic organs are provided with blood by their own vessels and by collaterals that run in modified arcades. In fact, collateral circulation is due to the persistence of modified pathways of fetal circulation.

At the fetal period of our life the organs lie closer together, and their vascular interrelationship is more intimate. Growth increasing the distance between the organs weakens their vascular interconnections. Thus the gastro-epiploic, the pancreaticoduodenal and the primary branches of the colic arteries represent the *dorsal* anastomosis of the embryonic ventral splanchnic arteries, while the left and the right gastric and hepatic arteries are the equivalent of the *ventral* anastomosis of the fetal ventral splanchnic arteries.

The many aberrant hepatic arteries described in about 50 per cent of human cases and their anastomosis with the regular vessels are similarly modified vascular arcades. The frequent and extensive communication between the ultimate and the penultimate terminals of the right, the middle and the left hepatic arteries[168] that takes place in the capsular folds within the fossa for the umbilical vein, and in the region around the caudate lobe,[77] denotes the same arching principle that the splanchnic vessels follow before sending their terminals into the organ. Of course, there are weak points in these anastomosing arcades, and the liver is placed in a "bad corner." Sudden interruption of the hepatic arterial supply through the celiac axis always means putting all hope in collaterals, if any.[16]

Interruption of arterial flow to the cirrhotic liver is absolutely unphysiological[198] and often induces hepatic failure. This operation has now become obsolete. However, the effects of ligation of the hepatic artery or one of its branches in humans are not necessarily fatal in cases with relatively normal hepatic function; adequate perfusion can be provided by portal and remaining arterial flow until arterial collaterals have fully developed.[31]

Michels[169] has listed 26 potential collateral pathways which may develop to supply the human liver deprived of its arterial blood flow: 10 of these are anatomic variations of the hepatic artery. However, only 7 provide sufficient communication between hepatic and nonhepatic vessels to guarantee an immediate collateral supply after occlusion of the hepatic artery.

The main collaterals of the common hepatic artery are: right and left gastrics, right and left gastro-epiploics, gastroduodenal, supraduodenal, retroduodenal, superior and inferior pancreaticoduodenals, aberrant hepatic arteries and inferior phrenic arteries.

In the liver of the rat and the dog, after interruption of the arterial supply, revascularization is provided also by the increasing pericholedochal arterial network.[51, 204] We wonder how much the rich ramifications of the supraduodenal and the inferior pancreaticoduodenal arteries, around the supraduodenal and the retroduodenal parts of the common bile duct, are capable of a similar task in humans. The role of the hepatic arterial collaterals in the relief of experimentally induced hepatic coma was stressed by Rappaport and associates[205]; they further investigated the metabolic role of the hepatic artery[203] and the part it plays in prolonging the survival of depancreatized dogs at no time treated with insulin.[206]

Portal Channels. Pick[183] has divided the portal collaterals into *hepatopetal* and *hepatofugal*. The hepatopetal pathways develop in cases with unimpeded intrahepatic circulation but with extrahepatic blockage of the portal vein. The blood bypasses this obstruction by using normal and anomalous channels which enlarge and accommodate the increasing flow through them.

The number and size of hepatopetal collaterals depend on the site of portal obstruction. They usually consist of: (1) deep cystic veins; (2) epiploic veins of the lesser omentum and the hepatocolic and the hepatorenal ligaments; (3) veins in the wall of the common bile duct; (4) diaphragmatic veins; (5) veins of the suspensory ligament of the liver; (6) the para-umbilical veins.

We found in dogs in which an Eck fistula had been formed by the classic technic, not comprising the complete ligation of the smallest tributaries of the portal stem, that hepatopetal collaterals developed in spite of the portacaval anastomosis. Thus intestinal blood bypassed the portacaval shunt and continued to flow through the narrow intrahepatic pathways.

The hepatofugal collaterals shunt the blood from the abdominal viscera around the intrahepatic obstacle. McIndoe[150] classified these collaterals on an embryologic basis in 3 groups:

1. *Veins located in the gastrointestinal tract at the junction of absorbing epithelium with protective epithelium.* In portal hypertension, varices are formed in the "stomachoesophageal and hemorrhoidal plexuses."[242] The former shunts blood from the left gastric (coronary) veins via the inferior hemiazygos and through the diaphragmatic and the azygos veins into the superior vena cava. The hemorrhoidal plexus transfers blood from the superior rectal (inf. mesent.) vein via the middle and the inferior rectal veins into the inferior vena cava. Both plexuses are vulnerable, but the esophageal plexus mainly gives rise to prolonged bleeding in patients suffering from portal hypertension.

2. *Veins occurring at the site of the obliterated fetal circulation, the so-called accessory portal system of Sappey.* These are the para-umbilical veins in the falciform and the round ligaments. They unite with the epigastric and internal mammary veins as well as with the azygos vein through the diaphragmatic veins. Veins may pass along the round ligament to the umbilicus and there develop prominent varicosities known as the "caput medusae." A large vein over which a loud murmur can be heard is present in cases with Cruveilhier-Baumgarten syndrome. Its superficial tortuous course was displayed by phlebography.[226] Other varieties of collaterals can be observed in the many ramifications of the venous channels in the thoracicoabdominal wall.

3. *Veins in the abdomen found at all sites where the gastrointestinal tract and the glands derived from it become retroperitoneal in their development or adhere to the abdominal wall because of pathologic processes.* These veins of Retzius can arise from the duodenum, omentum, spleen, pancreas, small intestine and colon. They establish connections between the portal bed and the ascending lumbar azygos and renal veins. Of clinical importance is the "portorenal plexus," consisting of anastomoses between the left renal vein and the portal beds in the pancreas, spleen and descending colon.[242] Had its function been understood earlier, the possibility of alleviating portal hypertension by splenorenal anastomosis[138] might have been recognized sooner. Simonds[227] gives a classic description of such a naturally occurring anastomosis which was disturbed during splenectomy with fatal consequences. Other rare portacaval shunts pass via the adrenal vein.[73]

Within the hepatic parenchyma collateral channels are formed by anastomoses between smaller branches of the portal and the hepatic veins, the tributaries of the caval system. Moschcowitz[172] made an extensive study of their genesis and considered them as "intrahepatic Eck fistulae." Their presence was demonstrated by multicolored injection of cirrhotic liver specimens.[186]

Pathways of Hepatic Circulation

The circulation of the liver is characterized by its dual blood supply. As in the similarly supplied lungs, vital metabolic changes of the blood are effected in the liver. From these organs the blood is sent almost directly to the heart for distribution. However, the dynamics in the pulmonary and in the portal circuits differ. Whereas the venous pulmonary stream is driven through its capillary bed by the muscle of the right ventricle, and the pulsatile flow is conditioned by the respiratory phases, the flow in the portal vein could be likened to that of a swampy river. Having its sources in the capillary network of the large splanchnic marsh, the movement of the blood is nonpulsatile and subjected to many fluctuations. The velocity and pressure of the portal stream are very much determined by the flow through the hepatic delta which, in turn, changes with the phases of respiration. If one observes the exposed portal vein of a dog, one is amazed by the sudden gains in speed of the portal blood stream; the latter becomes turbulent during inspiration. Indeed, the hepatic veins within the parenchyma do not collapse during inspiration, and the aspirating force of the thorax has its full effect on the entire sinusoidal network.

The vascular branches of the portal and hepatic veins interdigitate and run close to each other. They are separated by only small parenchymal masses, the length of a sinusoid or half the width of an acinus, that is, the distance between its axial vessels and "central vein." After a person ingests food, the muddy bed of the intestinal capillaries is flooded, and the tide in the portal stream rises. However, during exercise the circulation in the musculocutaneous areas is increased at the expense of that in the splanchnic area, and the hepatic minute volume drops. Thus, inflow into the splanchnic area and outflow from the hepatic sinusoidal network determine the volume of flow and the pressure level in the portal vein. Other factors influencing inflow and outflow are the number and width of collateral venous channels, and the amount of arterial blood flowing through the liver.

There is a vicarious relationship between arterial and portal blood passing through the liver. Competition of inflow is controlled where the hepatic artery meets the portal vein. This junction is arteriolar, capillary or sinusoidal.[149, 188, 197] Thus, as in other vascular areas, the regulation takes place at the terminal vascular branches which, in the liver, we defined as the afferent axial channels of the acinar structural and functional units. The blood coming up in an intermittent flow through the portal branch, and in pulsating jets through the companion arterial twig, disperses like a fountain. It runs through the sinusoids down into the radicles of the hepatic veins and waters and nourishes the parenchyma of liver acini. The various ways of branching and anastomosing of the terminal afferent vessels with vascular areas situated above and below a hexagonal field (Fig. 1–8) indicate that the structural units are intimately connected with each other by their blood vessels and form *one* parenchymal mass.

Inflow and outflow from the sinusoidal delta are regulated by an intricate sluice mechanism, the morphology and the nervous control of which have not been investigated fully. Thanks to this marvelous play of sphincters at the inlet and outlet venules,[124, 197] the arterioles and the capillaries, the arterial and the portal streams, coming into the same compartment under a remarkable pressure difference, further each other's flow instead of inhibiting it. The arterial jets break up the stagnant portal blood in the sinusoids and send it on. The rushing blood column may exert a siphoning effect on communicating lateral sinusoids and empty them. Empty sinusoids opening up offer no resistance to the inflow of low-pressured portal blood. The opening and closing of adjacent blood channels by sphincters has a valvular effect similar to that in the heart cavities, where low-pressured blood is passed to a chamber that is under high pressure later, in its active phase.

Figure 1–20 illustrates how the pressure in the portal vessel (generously assumed to be 8 to 10 mm. Hg) is raised to arteriolar pressure (35 mm. Hg) through intermittent sphincter activity. The sinusoidal area (black in left half of acinus) has been filled with portal blood when the arterioles were closed. The sphincters guarding the arteriolar-portal anastomoses and the inlets of the arterioles into the sinusoids open, the arterial jets (white dotted) increase the *vis a tergo* and sweep the portal blood ahead through open outlet sphincters into the terminal hepatic venules (T.H.V.). During this event flow is speeded up and exerts through intersinusoidal connections a siphoning effect on neighboring sinusoids. When, however, the outlet sphincters are closed, the rich mixture of arterial and portal blood, appropriate for specific metabolic activities, undergoes a thorough chemical exchange with the liver cell. At a later phase when the sphincters of the arterioles and of the arteriolar-portal anastomoses have closed again, portal inlet sphincters open and venous blood may flow into the same area following the pressure gradient between the terminal portal and terminal hepatic venules (approximately 100 mm. H_2O). A comparison with a sluice mechanism is suggestive,

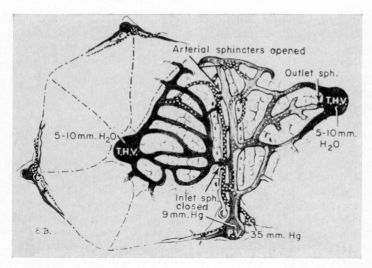

Fig. 1–20. Microcirculation in a liver acinus. The pressure in the terminal portal, arterial and hepatic venous branches is indicated. Note in the left half of the figure an opened arteriolar inlet sphincter that admits arterial (*white dotted*) blood into the sinusoidal area primarily filled with portal (*black*) blood; the outlet sphincters around the terminal hepatic venule (*T.H.V.*) are open. In the right half of the figure all arteriolar-portal and arteriolar-sinusoidal sphincters have opened, admitting blood and thus raising the pressure in all the sinusoids to arteriolar level. One outlet sphincter at the junction of a sinusoid with the terminal hepatic venule (*T.H.V.*) is closed. *P.V.*, portal vein.

since with the reopening of the arteriolar sphincters the low pressure level of the portal stream will be raised to a higher arteriolar level. Flow in single sinusoids, as recorded on film in the *in vivo* transilluminated mammalian liver, is definitely pulsatile.[197] The overall impression of continuous sinusoidal flow is due to random intermittent activity of millions of sphincters in a given time.

Under unknown conditions, the portal stream, which keeps the sinusoidal system filled (sometimes one third of the entire blood volume is stored in it) may detour its blood from the sinusoidal delta and short-circuit it by direct channels into the large hepatic veins. Also, extrahepatic collateral venous channels are used to transfer the blood rapidly into the inferior vena cava.[48] Thus portal circulation time is reduced, and the blood returns more quickly to the heart.

Collateral arterial circulation also plays a definite role in the liver. This becomes manifest under pathologic and experimental conditions. After all branches of the hepatic artery *and* the portal vein in a dog have been ligated in a stepwise procedure, the liver, this huge vascular organ, can survive on collateral circulation alone.[204]

From the related data, much of which has been gathered since the observation of the intrahepatic circulation *in vivo*, [124, 149, 197, 220, 240] one might be inclined to believe that we know a great deal about the hepatic circuit interposed between the splanchnic capillaries and the heart. However, most of the data concern only the changing circulatory phenomena. We lack knowledge of the underlying causes. Further investigation of the morphology and physiology of the sphincter mechanisms that distribute and regulate the blood supply of the hepatic parenchyma, and integration of their function into the regulatory mechanisms of the splanchnic area, will advance the physiology, pathology and therapy of the liver.

LYMPH VESSELS OF THE LIVER

In the human liver a well-developed subserous hepatic network communicates with the lymph vessels of the gallbladder. The deep lymphatic channels run in the portal tracts where they are visible as the spaces of Mall,[157] especially when serous exudation is present.[100] The lymphatics surround the branches of the hepatic artery and the portal vein up to their finest ramifications in the simple liver acini. Also the biliary tree and hepatic lymph vessels are connected intimately. The injection of Chicago blue into the clamped choledochus against the direction of bile flow under 310 mm. H_2O pressure makes the dye appear immediately in the hepatic lymph vessels.[148]

The lymph from these vessels is drained toward the lymph nodes of the hilum of the liver. Frequently, the lymphatics surrounding the tributaries of the hepatic veins are overlooked. They run along the walls of the tributaries of the hepatic veins and drain into the nodes around the inferior vena cava.

Histamine in low doses increases hepatic lymph flow, its protein content and specific gravity by changing the permeability of the endothelial cells lining the sinusoids.[248]

Experimental production of ascites by constriction of the inferior vena cava above the hepatic veins[152] blocks the efferent lymph vessels in the wall of the great vein.

The lymphatic drainage within the hepatic parenchyma and its reticulum is under discussion. Some believe that from a third to one half of the body lymph originates in the liver. Lymph capillaries have not been detected between the parenchymal cells. Disse[54] in 1890 put forward the theory that lymph spaces exist between the longitudinal fibers that surround the hepatic sinusoids. The walls of these clefts consist of a structureless fine ground substance and fine fibrils forming a membrane. These findings are supported by some,[63, 68, 127] while others deny the existence of a perisinusoidal lymph space.[132, 137, 157, 237] Popper[185] considered the perisinusoidal spaces as agonal changes of the tissue.

The question of the site of origin of the lymphatics in the hepatic parenchyma is not answered. Electron microscopy has revealed a continuous tissue space along the sinusoidal linings that terminate at the limiting plates. The connection between the Disse spaces and the lymph vessels in the terminal portal fields has not yet been demonstrated.[90] Lymph capillaries exist in the walls of the portal and the hepatic veins and extend to their endothelial lining. Therefore, one may assume that some lymph percolates from these veins into the lymph vessels of the surrounding connective tissue.

NERVE SUPPLY OF THE LIVER

Sympathetic fibers deriving from bilateral ganglia T 7 to T 10, and synapsing in the semilunar ganglion of the celiac plexus, intermingle with fibers from the right and the left vagus and the right phrenic nerve to form the hepatic arterial nerve plexus.[80] It is known also as the anterior nerve plexus and surrounds the hepatic artery as a thick coat. Other nerve bundles ramify around the portal vein and bile ducts and form a posterior hepatic plexus;[110] both plexuses intercommunicate. Other nerve bundles travel freely in the peritoneal folds associated with the porta hepatis. Some nerve fibers from the plexus around the gallbladder enter the hepatic parenchyma. The arteries are innervated exclusively by the sympathetic fibers, whereas the bile ducts are innervated by both sympathetic and parasympathetic fibers. Some fibers follow the vessels and bile ducts into their finest ramifications and send off branches supplying the structural elements of the portal tracts;[2, 135] they also join the nerve plexus around the hepatic venous branches.[234] Others pass into the parenchyma and form the parenchymal plexus around the cell cords and some end in small knobs around single cells.

Resection of the anterior nervous plexus[147] changes the quality of bile secretion: the concentration of bile salts and pigments increases. Interruption of the anterior nerve plexus prevents the accumulation of fat in the liver. Degeneration of the nerve fibers around the hepatic veins has been observed in the human cirrhotic liver.[104]

STROMA OF THE LIVER

The connective tissue of the liver is called *stroma*. It shows a varying degree of cellularity: fixed histiocytes, monocytes, plasma cells and lymphocytes. It forms the capsule of Glisson, which is attached to the parenchyma by radial processes. The capsule is thick around the inferior vena cava and at the porta hepatis. The branching tree of connective tissue follows the vascular and biliary branches through the porta into the segments of the liver, ramifying in them, and almost joining up at their surface with the capsule. The sparse connective tissue around the hepatic veins merges with the fibrous tissue around the inferior vena cava. The connective tissue carries also the lymphatics and the nerve fibers. There is also the mesh of reticulum fibers suspended among the bundles of connective tissue fibers around the portal and hepatic venous tree. The argentaffin reticulum framework, probably a product of the reticular cells lining the sinusoids, sustains the liver cords and plates. When this framework survives hepatic injury, the hepatocytes can regenerate more rapidly and fill the empty spaces in an orderly fashion. Under the electron microscope the reticulum fibers show a characteristic segmentation that distinguishes them from the collagenous and elastic fibers.

BILIARY SYSTEM

Ducts

Bile excretion starts in the intercellular bile capillaries and canaliculi which empty into the smallest bile ductules. The uniting bile ductules form the terminal "interlobular" ducts. The latter are lined by tall cuboidal epithelium and follow the course of the terminal axial branches of the portal vein surrounding them in a plexiform way. From the confluence of the terminal bile ducts larger ducts arise. Their epithelium is taller and contains mitochondria; their walls are thicker; also, they are surrounded by the larger amount of connective tissue present in the portal tracts. The peribiliary arterial plexus is woven around these ducts and is in intimate connection with the outpocketings of their walls described by Beale (1889).[13]

Plexus and parietal sacculi help concentrate the bile by the absorption of water.[99] Considering the weight of the liver and the volume of hepatic blood flow (1,500 cc./min.), a larger bile secretion than the daily outflow from the bile duct might be expected. An absorptive mechanism in the smaller bile ducts similar to that in the renal tubules was suggested.[192] Brauer,[27] in his studies of bile secretion of the removed and perfused liver, later demonstrated that the bile secreted by the hepatic cells in passing down the biliary tree is afforded an opportunity to reach electrolyte equilibrium with the blood plasma. He further concurred that the prebiliary plexus is an excellent anatomic device for effecting the exchange between blood and bile constituents. Finally, observations with the electron microscope of fine microvilli protruding into the lumen of the bile capillaries,[181] and of the striated border of the isoprismatic epithelium lining the bile ductules,[28] corroborate this suggestion.

Intrahepatic Ducts. The wall of the microscopic intrahepatic bile ducts is formed by dense fibrous tissue which contains many elastic fibers. The mucosa formed by tall to columnar epithelium tends to be folded. The localized occurrence of smooth muscle fibers in the wall of the ducts near the hilum of the liver forms the morphologic basis for the narrowing of the bile ducts seen in the cholangiograms.[230] Topographic studies of the intrahepatic distribution of the bile ducts have been carried out to enable a correct interpretation of the cholangiograms.[65, 102, 103, 230] Exact knowledge of the intrahepatic topography of the major bile channels is required when anastomosis between them and the intestinal lumen must be established in order to bypass a heavily scarred bile duct.

In the hilar region there is no fixed coordination between the major ducts and the major branches of the portal vein. In the peripheral parts of the liver branches of the portal vein, the hepatic artery and bile ducts run together. Of all the major intrahepatic bile ducts the most constant in its course is the lateral superior segmental duct. It runs straight toward the suspensory ligament and is found when the liver is approached from its upper left corner.[65] On the right side the inferior branch is easily accessible.[65]

Extrahepatic Ducts

Common Hepatic Duct. This duct arises from the confluence of the right and left lobar ducts, which leave the liver in the right end of the portal fissure to become the right and left hepatic ducts. The common hepatic duct is 3 cm. long and is situated to the right of the hepatic artery and in front of the portal vein. It is joined by the cystic duct at its right side and in an acute angle to form the bile duct (ductus choledochus). This manner of junction is considered as normal. Anatomic variations in the types of anastomosis between the cystic and hepatic ducts are of surgical importance (Fig. 1–21).

Bile Duct (Ductus Choledochus). The length of the bile duct depends on the site of junction of the cystic duct with the common hepatic duct.[79] If this junction is very low, the choledochus is short (Fig. 1–21). Its average length is quoted as 7 cm.; its diameter, as of the size of a goose quill. The free or supraduodenal part of the choledochus runs downward and slightly to the left and lies in the right border of the lesser omentum, anterior to the aditus to the lesser sac. Usually, surgical revision of the common bile duct is carried out at this free part; also, it is the most common site of strictures.

The *pancreatic part* of the bile duct passes retroperitoneally behind the first portion of the duodenum. It then runs in a groove on the posterior surface of the head of the pancreas, where it is situated in front of the inferior vena cava. At the left side of the duodenum it is joined in 89 per cent of cases by the pancreatic duct (Wirsung) and forms the ampulla of Vater (3 to 5 mm. long).

The *duodenal* or *intramural part* of the choledochus has been the object of many studies aiming to clarify the intricate sphincter mechanism present here.[23, 24, 36, 111, 159, 178, 217] It is destined to regulate a one-way flow of biliary and pancreatic secretion into the intestine. In their passage through the duodenal wall the united bile and pancreatic ducts form a wartlike elevation of the mucosa called the papilla of Vater. A shallow dilation inside the papilla, in average 3 mm. deep and as some believe (Job[111]) inconstant, is called the ampulla of Vater. Cholangiography reveals in about one fourth of the cases a reflux from the bile duct into the pancreatic duct. In these cases the openings of both ducts lead into a common cavity. Then biliary disease can easily reflect upon the pancreas.

SPHINCTER OF ODDI. The circular smooth muscle fibers surrounding these structures are defined as the sphincter of Oddi. It is composed of:

1. *Choledochus Sphincter.* It consists of circular muscle fibers that surround the intramural portion of the common bile duct in its course through the intestinal submucosa. This sphincter, which is always present, constricts the lumen of the bile duct.

2. *Pancreatic Sphincter.* It is present only in 33 per cent of individuals and is not a real muscle ring.[126] Thus the reflux of bile

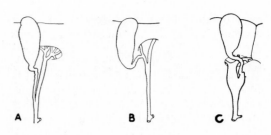

VARIATIONS IN THE CYSTIC DUCT

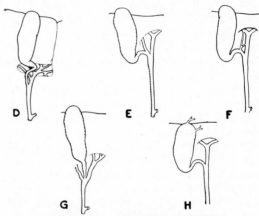

ACCESSORY HEPATIC DUCTS

FIG. 1–21. Anomalies of cystic and bile ducts. Variations in the length and course of the cystic duct: *A,* low junction of cystic duct with bile duct; *B,* high junction of cystic duct with bile duct; *C,* swerving course of cystic duct before joining the common bile duct. *D–H,* accessory right hepatic ducts. (Of 95 gallbladders and bile passages injected *in situ* with melted wax and then dissected, 6 had accessory hepatic ducts in positions of surgical danger. Of these, 3 joined the common hepatic duct near the cystic duct [D], 2 joined the cystic duct [E], and 1 joined the bile duct [G] and the gallbladder [H]. All except H were sketched from specimens.) (Grant, J. C. B.: Method of Anatomy, ed. 5, Baltimore, Williams & Wilkins.)

from the bile duct into the lumen of the pancreatic duct is possible.

3. *Sphincter Ampullae.* This consists of longitudinal fibers surrounding a weak layer of sparse circular fibers.[122] The longitudinal fibers in contracting shorten the ampulla and

raise mucosal folds to prevent reflux of intestinal content into the lumina of the ducts.

GALLBLADDER

The gallbladder is a receptacle for bile (30 to 50 ml.). In the form of a pear-shaped sac 3 cm. wide and 7 cm. long, it lies on the undersurface of the right liver lobe. Its parts are designated as fundus, body and neck. The fundus projects beyond the inferior border of the liver at the site where the lateral margin of the rectus crosses the costal margin. The body is directed upward and to the left. Posteriorly, fundus and body are in close relation with transverse colon and duodenum, respectively. Gallstones can perforate into these viscera.

Where the neck of the gallbladder is attached to the liver by areolar tissue, it is reached by the cystic artery. The neck is curved anteriorly in an S-shape, and when enlarged forms the so-called Hartmann's pouch. The mucous membrane of the neck forms a spiral valve of Heister which continues into the cystic duct. The latter arises from the left upper corner of the pouch and has a proximal valvular and a distal smooth portion. The spiral valve has the function of regulating bile flow both ways—into and out of the gallbladder. During the fasting state the gallbladder receives bile from the hepatic duct through the cystic duct. When stimulated by food or cholecystokinin the gallbladder delivers the concentrated bile through the cystic duct into the common bile duct and the intestine.[108, 109] Some consider the mucosal folds of Heister's valve as an architectural device to prevent distension and collapse of the cystic duct when sudden change of pressure occurs in the gallbladder or the common duct.[136]

Histology of Extrahepatic Ducts and Gallbladder. *The cystic, the hepatic and the common bile ducts* all possess a mucosa, a submucosa and a muscularis. The mucosa consists of a single layer of columnar epithelium and a tunica propria which contains mucous glands. These are of the type of utricular glands, and their openings are visible to the naked eye. They are lined by simple cylindrical epithelium and are surrounded by a wall of connective tissue rich in capillary network. Some believe that they

represent small receptacles in which the bile is concentrated as in the gallbladder. In the dog these *sacculi* dilate and increase in number after cholecystectomy.[235]

The wall of the extrahepatic ducts is formed by a strong layer of connective tissue fibers into which sparse muscle elements are interspersed,[146] except for the region of the neck of the gallbladder and at the lower end of the common duct where muscle rings are conspicuous.[97] Taking into consideration the absorptive and the sphincter mechanisms, it is to be emphasized that the extrahepatic bile ducts are not passive conducting tubes of bile. They take part in the concentration and intermittent discharge of bile.

The *gallbladder* is lined by a mucosa thrown into multiple folds beautifully described by William Boyd.[22] They serve to increase the absorptive capacity of the organ. The epithelial lining of the mucosa is columnar, the cells being provided with a striated border (for absorption). Glands of the tubulo-alveolar type are found in the region of the neck. They are the only glands to produce mucus in the gallbladder. The Rokitansky-Aschoff sinuses are only outpouchings of the mucosa into defects of the muscularis favoring bacterial retention and inflammation. However, the ducts of Luschka are lined with mucosa of the bile duct type.[143] They are situated in the areolar tissues of the hepatic surface of the gallbladder and communicate with intrahepatic bile ducts rather than with the gallbladder cavity. Their presence is an indication for drainage of the gallbladder bed following cholecystectomy. A small amount of areolar tissue separates the mucosa from a skimpy layer of decussated smooth muscle bands well developed only in the fundus and the neck of the organ. Their arrangement is similar to that of the urinary bladder.[6] There are many elastic fibers in the body of the gallbladder. The serosa is attached to the muscularis by a subserous layer of connective tissue that contains the vessels, nerves and lymphatics.

Blood Supply of Bile Ducts and Gallbladder. The arterial supply of the bile ducts comes mainly from the right hepatic artery. The gallbladder may be supplied by 1, 2 or 3 arteries. Its venous network does not accompany the arteries but empties directly into hepatic areas connecting with right and left portal venous branches.[115] Branches of the posterior, superior and postero-inferior pancreaticoduodenal arteries forming abundant anastomotic loops contribute also to the formation of Zuckerkandel's plexus around the common bile duct.[57]

A continuation of this plexus within the liver along the intrahepatic bile ducts forms the peribiliary plexus. In the dog whose hepatic artery has been ligated, these vascular networks become pathways by which the hepatic parenchyma connects with collateral arterial vessels, mainly from the phrenico-abdominal and inferior pancreaticoduodenal arteries. The periductal plexus in such animals has been demonstrated by catheterization and roentgenography of the celiac axis *in vivo*.[191, 204]

The cystic artery usually arises from the right hepatic arterial branch, joins the gallbladder at its neck, divides into 2 branches that run under the serosa of the gallbladder, supplying this organ as a terminal artery. Injury to this vessel or its parent artery is followed by gangrene of the gallbladder. In some cases, where the gallbladder is buried more deeply into the liver substance, collateral blood supply from the hepatic parenchyma may prevent this cataclysm. The anomalies of its arterial supply have been described by Flint,[74] Browne[32] and Michels.[168] The veins of the gallbladder empty into the portal vein or form a vein at the neck of the gallbladder which passes directly into hepatic parenchyma joining the sinusoids.

Lymph Vessels of Bile Ducts and Gallbladder. The lymph vessels of the hepatic, cystic and upper parts of the common bile duct empty into glands of the hilum. Those of the lower part of the common bile duct drain into glands around the head of the pancreas.

The lymph vessels of the gallbladder investigated by Sudler (1901) are connected intimately with the lymph vessels of Glisson's capsule.[233] The importance of this connection for the "liver-gallbladder" syndrome has been stressed by Fazio.[71] The gallbladder, although an outgrowth of the intestine, has no lymph follicles. However, there is a superficial subserous network of lymphatics and a submucous one which does not penetrate the mucosal folds. They empty into the "lymph gland of the neck" of the gallbladder.

Nerves. Nerve fibers supplying the extrahepatic ducts derive mainly from the sympathetic hepatic plexus laced around the hepatic artery. These also receive filaments from the right and left vagus nerves. Some nerve fibers deriving from the plexus can be seen running along the common bile duct. Sparse ganglion cells are present in the muscularis and the mucosa of the gallbladder. Most nerve cells are found in the fibromuscular layer of the cystic duct.[144] Nervous connection with the spinal system is brought about by fibers from the right phrenic and the musculophrenic nerves. Since these nerves derive from the 3rd or 4th cervical nerve, the anatomic basis for shoulder pain in gallbladder disease is seen readily.

Anatomic Variations of Bile Ducts and Gallbladder. These anomalies are much less frequent than those in the vascular supply of the liver and its bile receptacle. The *absence* or the *obliteration* of the bile duct is noticed early in the newborn. It is fatal when not corrected in time. Absence of the gallbladder is normal for the rat, horse and deer. It is rare in humans (1 in 4,000 cases) and in two thirds of cases it shows some symptoms.[55] Usually it is associated with absence of the cystic duct.

Accessory hepatic ducts, low junction of the branches of the hepatic duct, anomalies in the anastomoses between cystic duct and hepatic duct, and congenital cystic dilatation of the common bile duct are the most common malformations of the duct system[155, 213] (Fig. 1–21).

The common hepatic duct can receive accessory hepatic ducts, or it may be completely absent. In the latter case 2 hepatic ducts run separately and join close to the duodenum. Then the right duct anastomoses with the cystic duct[44] (Fig. 1–21).

Double gallbladder usually produces symptoms of biliary disease and sometimes can be discovered by cholecystogram or during operation.[170] This anomaly is due to nonconfluent cavitation of the solid gallbladder anlage. Bilobed, hourglass-constricted gallbladders, those with folded fundus (phrygian cap) or persistent septum, favor retention and inflammation. The gallbladder can be completely buried in liver substance or attached loosely to it by a mesenterium (floating gallbladder). The latter variety is preferred by the surgeon.

TOPOGRAPHY

LIVER

The liver occupies the right hypochondrium and the epigastric space. It extends into the left hypochondrium and into the right lumbar region. Protected in its greater part by the ribs, only a small part of its anterior surface touches the anterior abdominal wall. The organ fits perfectly into the dome of the diaphragm and is held there like a ball in a socket by intra-abdominal pressure. Interposed between diaphragm above and transverse mesocolon and colon below, the liver divides the subdiaphragmatic compartment into a suprahepatic and a subhepatic space.

Suprahepatic Space. The *left* suprahepatic space is separated from the *right* by the falciform ligament. The latter has an anterior division extending between anterior surface of liver, diaphragm and anterior abdominal wall. The posterior *right suprahepatic division* is delimited by the convex hepatic surface, the diaphragm and the coronary ligament. Eighty percent of all infections are found in this latter division.[243]

Subhepatic Space. This space extends between the concave surface of the liver and the transverse mesocolon, the colon, duodenum, stomach and anterior abdominal wall.

The *right subhepatic area* has an anterior and a posterior division. The latter extends between the inferior surface of the liver, the posterior peritoneal reflection of the coronary ligament and the upper pole of the right kidney. Frequently, the anterior subhepatic division is entered by the surgeon to labor in the operating fields of gallbladder and common bile duct.

The *left subhepatic area* is divided by the frontally orientated stomach and the lesser omentum into an anterior and a posterior compartment (lesser sac). All these spaces and their divisions, when infected, can be entered by surgical procedures that follow the extrapleural and extraperitoneal routes in order to avoid the spread of infection in the thoracic and the abdominal cavities.

GALLBLADDER AND BILE DUCTS

The topography of gallbladder and bile ducts is discussed under "Biliary System," and the variations of the hepatic vessels under "Vessels of the Liver." The abnormal topography of the hepatic pedicle results from the frequent anomalies encountered in these structures. Normally, vessels and bile duct are disposed in 2 layers within the hepatoduodenal ligament. The ventral layer contains the bile duct and the hepatic artery, while the portal vein lies in a more dorsal plane. A thoraco-abdominal incision, approaching this vessel from behind, is therefore suitable for carrying out an anastomosis between portal stem and superior vena cava.

The hepatic artery, a vessel much attacked by the surgeons lately, lies in the left border of the hepatoduodenal ligament, at the margin where its thin and transparent gastrohepatic neighbor abuts. As a landmark to identify the site where the knot will be slung around the hepatic artery, Madden[156] advises the exposure of the gastroduodenal artery branching off from the hepatic artery and arching over the portal vein. This large vein, having the hepatic artery on its medial side, and running underneath the gastroduodenal artery, allows the operator to know for certain whether the hepatic artery is ligated proximally or distally to the gastroduodenal artery, an important hepatic collateral.[87]

Summary. Although the liver occupies a shielded corner of the abdominal cavity, because of its size, topography and vascular connections, it shows intricate relationship with almost all abdominal organs. Therefore, pathologic changes in these organs may be reflected first in the liver.

REFERENCES

1. Abeatici, S., and Campi, L.: Sur les possibilités de l'angiographie hépatique, la visualisation du système portal (recherches expérimentales), Acta Radiol. 36:383, 1951.
2. Alexander, W. F.: Innervation of biliary system, J. Comp. Neurol. 72:357, 1940.

3. Andrews, W. H. H., Maegraith, A. G., and Wenyon, C. E. M.: Studies on the liver circulation. II. The micro-anatomy of the hepatic circulation, Ann. Trop. Med. *43*:229, 1949.

4. ———: Excretory function of the liver. A reassessment, Lancet *2*:166, 1955.

5. Arey, L. B.: On the presence of the so-called portal lobules in the seal's liver, Anat. Rec. *51*:315, 1932.

6. Aschoff, L.: Lectures on Pathology, p. 182, New York, Hoeber, 1924.

7. Bahnson, H. T., Sloan, R. D., and Blalock, A.: Splenic-portal venography. A technique utilizing percutaneous injection of radiopaque material into the spleen, Bull. Johns Hopkins Hosp. *92*: 331, 1953.

8. Bailey, F. R.: Bailey's Text-Book of Histology, ed. 12, p. 481, Baltimore, Williams & Wilkins, 1948.

9. Balis, J. U., Chan, A., and Conen, P. E.: Electron microscopy study of the developing human liver, Advances in Hepatology, Trans. Symp. I.A.S.L., Brussels and Leuven, 1964, p. 133, Baltimore, Williams & Wilkins, 1965.

10. Barrett, H. M., Best, C. H., and Ridout, J. H.: A study of the source of liver fat using deuterium as an indicator, J. Physiol. *93*:367, 1938.

11. Bayly, J. H.: The use of the umbilical vein in the diagnosis of upper gastrointestinal bleeding, Am. J. Gastroenterol. *41*:235, 1964.

12. ———: The portal vein and liver portography utilizing the umbilical vein, J. Nat. Med. Ass. *57*:267, 1965.

13. Beale, L. S.: The Liver, p. 30, London, Churchill, 1889.

14. Beitzke, H.: Über einen Fall von kavernöser Umwandlung der Pfortader, Charité-Ann. *34*:466, 1910.

15. Belli, L., Galmarini, D., and Di Francesco, U.: Cateterismo e flebografia epatica selectiva nella esplorazione preoperatoria della ipertensione portale cirrogena, Minerva med. *52*:2399, 1961.

16. Berman, J. K., and Hull, J. E.: Hepatic, splenic, and left gastric arterial ligations in advanced portal cirrhosis, A.M.A. Arch. Surg. *65*:37, 1952.

17. Best, C. H., Hartroft, W. S., Lucas, C. C., and Ridout, J. H.: Liver damage produced by feeding alcohol or sugar and its prevention by choline, Brit. Med. J. *2*:1001, 1949.

18. ———: Effects of dietary protein, lipotropic factors, and realimentation on total hepatic lipids and their distribution, Brit. Med. J. *1*:1439, 1955.

19. Bilbey, D. L. J., and Rappaport, A. M.: Segmental anatomy of human liver, Anat. Rec. *136*:330, 1960.

20. ———: The segmental anatomy of the human liver, Anat. Rec. *136*:165, 1960.

21. Bloom, W.: The embryogenesis of human bile capillaries and ducts, Am. J. Anat. *36*:451, 1925/26.

22. Boyd, W.: Studies in gallbladder pathology, Brit. J. Surg. *10*:337, 1923.

23. Boyden, E. A.: The sphincter of Oddi, Surgery *1*:25, 1937.

24. ———: Hypertrophy of the sphincter choledochus, Surgery *10*:567, 1941.

25. Bradley, S. E., Inglefinger, F. J., Bradley, G. P., and Curry, J. J.: Estimation of hepatic blood flow in man, J. Clin. Invest. *24*:890, 1945.

26. Brauer, R. W.: Observations concerning fluid compartments, blood-flow patterns and bile-formation in the isolated rat liver, J. Nat. Cancer Inst. *15*:1469, 1955.

27. ———: Mechanisms of bile secretion, J.A.M.A. *169*:1462, 1959.

28. Braunsteiner, H., Fellinger, K., and Pakesch, F.: Elektronenmikroskopische Beobachtungen an normalen Leberschnitten sowie nach Gallenstauung, Histamin und Allylformiatvergiftung, Z. ges. exp. Med. *121*:254, 1953.

29. Braus, H.: Anatomie des Menschen, ed. 2, pp. 14 & 324, Berlin, Springer, 1924.

30. Brissaud, E., and Sabourin, C.: Sur la constitution lobulaire du foie et les voies de la circulation sanguine intrahépatique, C. R. Soc. Biol. *40*:757, 1888.

31. Brittain, R. S., Marchioro, T. L., Herman, G., Waddell, W. R., and Starzl, T. E.: Accidental hepatic artery ligation in humans, Am. J. Surg. *107*:822, 1964.

32. Browne, E. Z.: Variations in origin and course of the hepatic artery and its branches, Surgery *8*:424, 1940.

33. Brunner, C.: Die Lehre von den Geistigen und vom Volke, pp. 244-555, Stuttgart, Cotta, 1962.

34. Burkel, W. E., and Low, F. N.: The fine structure of rat liver sinusoids, space of Disse, and associated tissue space, Am. J. Anat. *118*:769, 1966.

35. Burstone, M. S.: New histochemical techniques for the demonstration of tis-

sue oxidase (cytochrome oxidase), J. Histochem. Cytochem. 7:112, 1959.

36. Cameron, A. L., and Noble, J. F.: Reflux of bile up the duct of Wirsung caused by an impacted biliary calculus, J.A.M.A. 82:1410, 1924.

37. Cameron, G. R., and Mayes, B. T.: Ligation of the hepatic artery, J. Path. Bact. 33:799, 1930.

38. Cantlie, J.: On a new arrangement of the right and left lobe of the liver, J. Anat. Physiol. 32:4, 1897.

39. Cheng, K.-K.: Experimental studies on the mechanism of the zonal distribution of beryllium liver necrosis, J. Path. Bact. 71:265, 1956.

40. Chiquoine, A. D.: Distribution of glucose-6-phosphatase in the liver and kidney of the mouse, J. Histochem. Cytochem. 1:429, 1953.

41. Chrzonszczewsky, N.: Zur Anatomie und Physiologie der Leber, Virchows Arch. path. Anat. 35:153, 1866.

42. Clara, M.: Untersuchungen an der menschlichen Leber. Über den Übergang der Gallen-kapillaren in die Gallengänge, Z. mikr.-anat. Forsch. 20:584, 1930.

43. Cohnheim, J., and Litten, M.: Über Circulationsstörungen in der Leber, Virchows Arch. path. Anat. 67:153, 1876.

44. Collett, H. S., Caylor, H. D., and Tirman, W. S.: Choledocholithiasis, Am. J. Surg. 80:514, 1950.

45. Coronini, C.: Über die gefässregulatorischen Einrichtungen im Periportalfeld der Leber, Zbl. allg. Path. 82:241, 1944.

46. Cossel, L.: Beitrag zur Ultrastruktur der Blutgewebsgrenze in der Leber. Elektronenmikroskopische Untersuchungen an Lebern von Mäusen und Leberpunktaten vom Menschen, Beitr. Path. Anat. 120:133, 1958.

47. Couinaud, C.: Les enveloppes vasculobiliaires du foie ou capsule de Glisson. Leur intérêt dans la chirurgie vésiculaire, les résections hépatiques et l'abord du hile du foie, Lyon chir. 49:589, 1954.

48. Daniel, P. M., and Prichard, M. M. L.: Variations in the circulation of the portal venous blood within the liver, J. Physiol. 114:521, 1951.

49. Daseler, E. H., Anson, B. J., Hambley, W. C., and Reimann, A. F.: The cystic artery and constituents of the hepatic pedicle: study of 500 specimens, Surg. Gynec. Obstet. 85:47, 1947.

50. Dawkins, M. J. R.: Glycogen synthesis and breakdown in fetal and newborn rat liver, Ann. N. Y. Acad. Sci. 111:203, 1963.

51. Delong, R. P.: Revascularization of the rat liver following interruption of its arterial supply, Surg. Forum 4:388, 1953.

52. Desmet, V.: Expérimentelle levercarcinogenese, histochemisetic studie, pp. 80, 317, Brussels, Presses Académiques Européenes S.C., 1963.

53. Deysach, L. J.: The nature and location of the "sphincter mechanism" in the liver as determined by drug actions and vascular injections, Am. J. Physiol. 132:713, 1941.

54. Disse, J.: Über die Lymphbahnen der Säugetierleber, Arch. mikr. Anat. 36:203, 1890.

55. Dixon, C. F., and Lichtman, A. L.: Congenital absence of gallbladder, Surgery 17:11, 1945.

56. Douglass, B. E., Baggenstoss, A. H., and Hollinshead, W. H.: The anatomy of the portal vein and its tributaries, Surg. Gynec. Obstet. 91:562, 1950.

57. Douglass, T. C., and Cutter, W. W.: Arterial blood supply of the common bile duct, Arch. Surg. 57:599, 1948.

58. Dreyer, B., and Budtz-Olsen, O. E.: Splenic venography; demonstration of the portal circulation with Diodone, Lancet 262:530, 1952.

59. Dubin, I. N.: Anoxic necrosis of liver in man, Am. J. Path. 33:589, 1957.

60. Eger, W.: Zur Struktur und Funktion des Lebergewebes, Ärztl. Sammelblätter 50:1, 1961.

61. Elias, H.: The liver cord concept after one hundred years, Science 110:470, 1949.

62. ———: A re-examination of the structure of the mammalian liver. I. Parenchymal architecture, Am. J. Anat. 84:311, 1949.

63. ———: A re-examination of the structure of the mammalian liver. II. The hepatic lobule and its relation to the vascular and biliary systems, Am. J. Anat. 85: 379, 1949.

64. ———: Morphology of the liver, p. 134, Tr. 11th Liver Injury Conf., New York, Macy, 1953.

65. Elias, H., and Petty, D.: Gross anatomy of blood vessels and ducts within the human liver, Am. J. Anat. 90:59, 1952.

66. Elias, H., and Sokol, A.: Dependence of

the lobular architecture of the liver on the porto-hepatic blood pressure gradient, Anat. Rec. *115*:71, 1953.

67. Ellinger, P., and Hirt, A.: Mikroskopische Untersuchung an lebenden Organen; Methodik: Intravitalmikroskopie, Z. ges. Anat. (Abt. 1) *90*:791, 1929.

68. Eppinger, H.: Beiträge zur normalen und pathologischen Histologie der menschlichen Gallenkapillaren mit bes. Berücksichtigung der Pathogenese des Ikterus, Beitr. Path. Anat. *31*:230, 1902.

69. Fainsinger, M. H.: The radiology of the intrahepatic biliary tract, S. Afr. J. Med. Sci. *15*:51, 1950.

70. Fawcett, D. W.: Observations on the cytology and electron microscopy of hepatic cells, J. Nat. Cancer Inst. *15*:1475, 1955.

71. Fazio, A.: Connessioni linfatiche tra fegato e cistifellea e loro importanza nella patogenesi della sindrome epatocolecistica, Ann. ital. Chir. *29*:345, 1952.

72. Ficq, A.: Radioautographic studies on nuclear activity in the liver, J. Histochem. Cytochem. *7*:215, 1959.

73. Fleischhauer, H.: Über den chronischen Pfortaderverschluss, Virchows Arch. path. Anat. *286*:747, 1932.

74. Flint, E. R.: Abnormalities of the right hepatic, cystic, and gastro-duodenal arteries, and of the bile ducts, Brit. J. Surg. *10*:509, 1923.

75. Fraser, D., Jr., Rappaport, A. M., Vuylsteke, C. A., and Colwell, A. R., Jr.: Effects of the ligation of the hepatic artery in dogs, Surgery *30*:624, 1951.

76. Gilfillan, R. S.: Anatomic study of the portal vein and its main branches, Arch. Surg. *61*:449, 1950.

77. Glauser, F.: Studies of intrahepatic arterial circulation, Surgery *33*:333, 1953.

78. Grafflin, A. L., and Corddry, E. G.: Further studies of hepatic structure and function by fluorescence microscopy, Bull. Johns Hopkins Hosp. *93*:205, 1953.

79. Grant, J. C. B.: A Method of Anatomy, ed. 4, p. 251, Baltimore, Williams & Wilkins, 1948.

80. Gray, H.: Anatomy of the Human Body, ed. 26, pp. 1328 & 1111, Philadelphia, Lea & Febiger, 1954.

81. Gray, H. K.: Clinical and experimental investigation of circulation of liver, Ann. Roy. Coll. Surg. Engl. *8*:354, 1951.

82. Greenberger, N. J., Cohen, R. B., and Isselbacher, K. J.: The effect of chronic ethanol administration on liver alcohol dehydrogenase activity in the rat, Lab. Invest. *14*:264, 1965.

83. Grindlay, J. H., Mann, F. C., and Bollman, J. L.: Effect of occlusion of blood supply to normal liver; experimental study, A.M.A. Arch. Surg. *62*:806, 1951.

84. Grisham, J. W.: Lobular distribution of hepatic nuclei labeled with tritiated-thymidine in partially hepatectomized rats, Fed. Proc. *18*:478, 1959.

85. ————: Deoxyribose nucleic acid synthesis and cell renewal in regenerating rat liver, J. Histochem. Cytochem. *8*:330, 1960.

86. Grisham, J. W., and Hartroft, W. S.: Morphologic identification by electron microscopy of "oval" cells in experimental hepatic degeneration, Lab. Invest. *10*:317, 1961.

87. Haberer, H.: Experimentelle Unterbindung der Leberarterie, Arch. klin. Chir. *78*:557, 1905.

88. Hahn, P. F., Donald, W. D., and Grier, R. C., Jr.: Physiological bilaterality of portal circulation; streamline flow of blood into liver as shown by radioactive phosphorus, Am. J. Physiol. *143*:105, 1945.

89. Hale, A. J.: The minute structure of the liver: a review, Glasgow Med. J. *32*:283, 1951.

90. Hampton, J. C.: An electron microscope study of hepatic uptake and excretion of submicroscopic particles injected into the blood stream and into the bile duct, Acta Anat. *32*:262, 1958.

91. ————: A re-evaluation of the submicroscopic structure of the liver, Texas Rep. Biol. Med. *18*:602, 1960.

92. Hanzon, V.: Liver cell secretion under normal and pathologic conditions studied by fluorescence microscopy on living rats, Acta physiol. scand. (supp. 101, Fig. 14) *28*:93, 1952.

93. Hartroft, W. S.: Accumulation of fat in liver cells and in lipodiastemata preceding experimental dietary cirrhosis, Anat. Rec. *106*:61, 1950.

94. ————: Discussion of Elias, H.: Morphology of the liver, pp. 169-180, Tr. 11th Liver Injury Conf., New York, Macy, 1953.

95. ————: The trabecular anatomy of late stages of experimental dietary cirrhosis, Anat. Rec. *119*:71, 1954.

96. Hartroft, W. S., and Ridout, J. H.:

Pathogenesis of the cirrhosis produced by choline deficiency. Escape of lipid from fatty hepatic cysts into the biliary and vascular systems, Am. J. Path. *27*: 951, 1951.

97. Hendrickson, W. F.: A study of the musculature of the entire extrahepatic biliary system, Bull. Johns Hopkins Hosp. *9*: 221, 1898.

98. Hering, E.: Manual of Human and Comparative Histology, vol. 2, Tr. by N. Power, Berlin, Stricker, 1872.

99. Higgins, G. M.: The biliary tract of certain rodents with and those without a gallbladder, Anat. Rec. *32*:89, 1926.

100. Hill, K. R.: Liver disease in Jamaican children, p. 263, Tr. 10th Liver Injury Conf., New York, Macy, 1951.

101. Himsworth, H. P.: Lectures on the Liver and its Diseases, pp. 40-42 (Fig. 23A), Cambridge, Mass., Harvard, 1948.

102. Hjortsjö, C. H.: The internal topography of the liver: studies by roentgen and injection technic, Nord. Med. *38*:745, 1948.

103. ———: The topography of the intrahepatic duct system, Acta anat. *11*:599, 1951.

104. Honjo, I., and Hasebe, S.: Studies on the intrahepatic nerves in the cirrhotic liver, Rev. int. Hépat. *15*:595, 1965.

105. Hyrtl, M.: Über das Verhalten der Leberarterie zur Pfortader bei Amphibien und Fischen, Sitzber. Akad. Wiss. Wien. *49*:167, 1864.

106. Isselbacher, K. J., and Jones, W. A.: Alterations of glucose metabolism in viral and toxic liver injury, Gastroenterology *46*:424, 1964.

107. Ito, T., and Nemoto, M.: Über die Kupfferschen Sternzellen und die Fettspeicherungszellen in der Blutkapillarenwand der menschlichen Leber, Okajimas Folia Anat. Jap. *24*:243, 1952.

108. Ivy, A. C.: Factors concerned in the evacuation of the gallbladder, Medicine *11*:345, 1932.

109. Ivy, A. C., Drewyer, G. E., and Orndoff, B. H.: The effect of cholecystokinin on human gallbladder, Am. J. Physiol. *93*: 661, 1930.

110. Jayle, G. E.: Les nerfs du foie, étude anatomique et histologique, Nutrition *7*: 57, 1937.

111. Job, T. T.: The anatomy of the duodenal portion of the bile and pancreatic ducts, Anat. Rec. *32*:212, 1926.

112. Johnston, E. V., and Anson, B. J.: Variations in the formation and vascular relationships of the bile ducts, Surg. Gynec. Obstet. *94*:669, 1952.

113. Junès, M. P.: Les arborisations biliovasculaires intrahépatiques: (étude anatomo-chirurgicale en vue des hépatectomies) d'après 50 moulages hépatiques en matières plastiques, Bordeaux chir. *1*:5, 1954.

114. Katz, L. N., and Rodbard, S.: The integration of the vasomotor responses in the liver with those in other systemic vessels, J. Pharmacol. Exp. Ther. *67*:407, 1939.

115. Kedzior, E., and Kus, J.: The blood vessels of the gallbladder, Folia Morph. (Warszawa) *24*:357, 1965.

116. Kelty, R. H.: Baggenstoss, A. H., and Butt, H. R.: Relation of the regenerated liver nodule to the vascular bed in cirrhosis, Gastroenterology *15*:285, 1950.

117. Kennedy, E. P., and Lehninger, A. L.: Oxidation of fatty acids and tricarboxylic acid cycle intermediates by isolated rat liver mitochondria, J. Biol. Chem. *179*: 957, 1949.

118. Kettler, L. H.: Untersuchungen über die Genese von Lebernekrosen auf Grund experimenteller Kreislaufstörungen, Virchows Arch. path. Anat. *316*: 525, 1949.

119. Khazei, A. M., and Watkins, E., Jr.: Hepatic artery anomalies or deformities managed during infusion chemotherapy of liver cancer, Surg. Clin. N. Amer. *45*: 639, 1965.

120. Kielley, R. K., and Schneider, W. C.: Synthesis of p-amino-hippuric acid by mitochondria of mouse liver homogenates, J. Biol. Chem. *185*:869, 1950.

121. Kiernan, F.: The anatomy and physiology of the liver, Phil. Trans. Roy. Soc. London *123*:711, 1833.

122. Kirk, J.: The sphincter papillae, J. Anat. *78*:118, 1944.

123. Knisely, M. H.: Personal communication, May, 1952.

124. Knisely, M. H., Bloch, E. H., and Warner, L.: Selective phagocytosis. I. Microscopic observations concerning the regulation of blood flow through the liver and other organs and the mechanism and rate of phagocytic removal of particles from the blood, Det. Kong. Dans. Videnskab. Selskab. Biol. Skri. IV.: No. 7, 1948.

125. Koelliker, A.: Manual of Human Histology, Tr. by G. Busk and T. Huxley, London, Sydenham Soc., 1853-54.
126. Kreilkamp, B. L., and Boyden, E. A.: Variability in the composition of the sphincter of Oddi. A possible factor in the pathologic physiology of the biliary tract, Anat. Rec. 76:485, 1940.
127. Krogh, A.: The Anatomy and Physiology of the Capillaries, pp. 94 and 95, New Haven, Yale, 1928.
128. Kühnau, J.: Neuere Erkenntnisse über die Wirkstoffe der Leber, Deutsche Gesell. Verdauungs Krkh. Sonderband, p. 104, 1952.
129. Laufman, H., Ross, A., Bernhard, V. M., Bourdeau, R. V., Furr, W. E., Jr., and Douglass, T. C.: Graded hepatic arterial ligations in experimental ascites, Surg. Gynec. Obstet. 96:409, 1953.
130. Lavoie, P., Jacob, M., Leduc, J., Legaré, A., and Viallet, A.: The umbilicoportal approach for the study of splanchnic circulation: technical, radiological and hemodynamic considerations, Canad. J. Surg. 9:338, 1966.
131. Leblond, C. P., and Walker, B. E.: Renewal of cell populations, Physiol. Rev. 36:255, 1956.
132. Lee, F. C.: On the lymph vessels of the liver, Contr. Embryol. Carneg. Instn. 15: 65, 1923.
133. Leger, L., Colin, A., Sors, C., and Lemaigre, G.: Les cavernomes de la veine porte; étude anatomique, physio-pathogénique, J. Chir. 84:145, 1962.
134. Leger, L., Gally, L., Arway, N., Oudot, J., and Auvert, J.: La portographie. Technique. Étude expérimentale, anatomique et clinique, Presse méd. 59:410, 1951.
135. Lewis, H. P.: Pain in acute and chronic diseases of the liver, Ann. Int. Med. 35:878, 1951.
136. Lichtenstein, M. E., and Ivy, A. C.: The function of the "valves" of Heister, Surgery 1:38, 1937.
137. Lichtman, S. S.: Diseases of the Liver, Gallbladder and Bile Ducts, ed. 3, vol. 1, p. 21, Philadelphia, Lea & Febiger, 1953.
138. Linton, R. R.: The selection of patients for portacaval shunts with a summary of results in 61 cases, Ann. Surg. 134:433, 1951.
139. Lipp, W.: Die Entwicklung der Paren-

chymstruktur der Leber, Anat. Anz. 99: 241, 1952.
140. Lippman, H. N., and Longmire, W. P., Jr.: Intrahepatic cholangiojejunostomy for biliary obstruction, Surg. Gynec. Obstet. 98:363, 1954.
141. Loeffler, L.: Weitere Untersuchungen über die Folgen der Unterbindung der Leberarterie, Arch. klin. Chir. 149:370, 1928.
142. Longmire, W. P., Jr., and Sanford, M. C.: Intrahepatic cholangiojejunostomy with partial hepatectomy for biliary obstruction, Surgery 24:264, 1948.
143. Luschka, H.: Die Anatomie des Menschlichen Bauches, p. 255, Tübingen, Laupp, 1863.
144. Lütkens, U.: Aufbau und Funktion der extrahepatischen Gallenwege, Leipzig, Vogel, 1926.
145. MacDonald, R. A.: "Lifespan" of liver cells. Autoradiographic study using tritiated thymidine in normal, cirrhotic, and partially hepatectomized rats, Arch. Int. Med. 107:335, 1960.
146. Mahour, G. H., Wakim, K. G., Soule, E. H., and Ferris, D. O.: Structure of the common bile duct in man: presence or absence of smooth muscle, Ann. Surg. 166:91, 1967.
147. Mallet-Guy, P., Feroldi, J., Eicholz, L., and Michoulier, J.: Étude expérimentale de la neurectomie périartère hepatique. I. Effets de la résection du "pédicule nerveux antérieure" sur le foie normal, Lyon Chir. 51:45, 1956.
148. Mallet-Guy, P., Michoulier, J., Baev, S., Oleskiewicz, L., and Woszczyk, M.: Recherches expérimentales sur la circulation lymphatique du foie I. Donnés immédiates sur la perméabilité biliolymphatique, Lyon Chir. 58:847, 1962.
149. McCuskey, R. S.: A dynamic and static study of hepatic arterioles and hepatic sphincters, Am. J. Anat. 119:455, 1966.
150. McIndoe, A. H.: Vascular lesions of portal cirrhosis, Arch. Path. Lab. Med. 5:23, 1928.
151. McIndoe, A. H., and Counseller, V. S.: Bilaterality of the liver, Arch. Surg. 15: 589, 1927.
152. McKee, F. W., Schlereb, P. R. Schilling, J. A., Tishkoff, G. H., and Whipple, G. H.: Protein metabolism and exchange as influenced by constriction of the vena cava. Experimental ascites and internal

plasmapheresis, J. Exp. Med. 87:457, 1948.

153. McNee, J. W.: Jaundice; a review of recent work, Quart. J. Med. 16:390, 1923.

154. ———: Discussion on jaundice, Brit. Med. J. 2:495, 1924.

155. McWhorter, G. L.: Congenital cystic dilation of common bile duct, Arch. Surg. 8:604, 1924.

156. Madden, J. L., and Lore, J. M., Jr.: Surgical anatomy of portal system, Surg. Forum 3:133, 1952.

157. Mall, F. P.: A study of the structural unit of the liver, Am. J. Anat. 5:227, 1906.

158. Malpighi, M.: De viscerum structura exercitatio anatomica, London, 1666.

159. Mann, F. C., and Giordano, A. S.: The bile factor in pancreatitis, Arch. Surg. 6:1, 1923.

160. Markowitz, J., and Rappaport, A. M.: The hepatic artery, Physiol. Rev. 31:188, 1951.

161. Markowitz, J., Rappaport, A. M., and Scott, A. C.: Prevention of liver necrosis following ligation of hepatic artery, Proc. Soc. Exp. Biol. Med. 70:305, 1949.

162. Mascagni, P.: Prodromo della grande Anatomia, Firenze, 1819.

163. Mautner, H., and Pick, E. P.: Über die durch Schockgifte erzeugten Zirkulationsstörungen. II. Das Verhalten der überlebenden Leber, Biochem. Z. 127:72, 1922.

164. Maximow, A. A., and Bloom, W.: Textbook of Histology, ed. 6, p. 389, Philadelphia, Saunders, 1952.

165. Meyer, J. S., and Hartroft, W. S.: Hepatic lipid produced by polyphagia in albino rats; Relationship to dietary choline and casein, Am. J. Path. 36:365, 1960.

166. ———: Choline, hepatic fat, and insulin polyphagia, J. Nutr. 70:91, 1960.

167. Meyer, J., and Weinmann, J. P.: Distribution of phosphamidase activity in the male albino rat, J. Histochem. Cytochem. 5:354, 1957.

168. Michels, N. A.: The hepatic, cystic and retroduodenal arteries and their relation to the biliary ducts, Ann. Surg. 133:503, 1951.

169. Michels, N. A.: Collateral arterial pathways to liver after ligation of hepatic artery and removal of celiac axis, Cancer 6:708, 1953.

170. Moore, T. C., and Hurley, A. G.: Congenital duplication of the gallbladder, review of the literature and report of an unusual symptomatic case, Surgery 35:283, 1954.

171. Morrison, G. R.: Personal communication, 1962.

172. Moschcowitz, E.: Laennec's cirrhosis: its histogenesis with special reference to the role of angiogenesis, Arch. Path. 45:187, 1948.

173. Ney, H. R.: Die Kontrastdarstellung der Lebervenen im Röntgenbild, Fortschr. Röntgenstr. 86:302, 1957.

174. Novikoff, A. B., and Essner, E.: The liver cell: some new approaches to its study, Am. J. Med. 29:102, 1960.

175. Novikoff, A. B., Hausman, D. H., and Podber, E.: The localization of adenosine triphosphate in liver: in situ staining and cell fractionation studies, J. Histochem. Cytochem. 6:61, 1958.

176. Novikoff, A. B., Shin, W. Y., and Drucker, J.: Cold acetone fixation for enzyme localization in frozen sections, J. Histochem. Cytochem. 8:37, 1960.

177. Olds, J. M., and Stafford, E. S.: On the manner of anastomosis of the hepatic and portal circulation, Bull. Johns Hopkins Hosp. 47:176, 1930.

178. Opie, E. L.: The relation of cholelithiasis to disease of pancreas, J.A.M.A. 43:1102, 1904.

179. ———: The pathogenesis of tumours of the liver produced by butter yellow, J. Exp. Med. 80:231, 1944.

180. Padykula, H. A., and Herman, E.: The specificity of the histochemical method for adenosine triphosphatase, J. Histochem. Cytochem. 3:170, 1955.

181. Palade, G. E.: The fine structure of mitochondria, Anat. Rec. 114:427, 1952.

182. Pfuhl, W.: Handbuch der Mikroskopischen Anatomie des Menschen, vol. 5, part 2,266, Berlin, Springer, 1932.

183. Pick, L.: Über totale hämangiomatöse Obliteration des Pfortaderstammes, Arch. path. Anat. 197:490, 1909.

184. Pollister, A. W., and Pollister, P. F.: Über Drosselvorrichtungen an Lebervenen, Klin. Wschr. 10:2129, 1931.

185. Popper, H.: Significance of agonal changes in the human liver, Arch. Path. 46:132, 1948.

186. Popper, H., Elias, H., and Petty, D. E.: Vascular pattern of the cirrhotic liver, Am. J. Clin. Path. 22:717, 1952.

187. Porter, K. R.: Personal communication, 1962.

188. Prinzmetal, M., Ornitz, E. M., Jr., Sim-

kin, B., and Bergman, H. C.: Arterio-venous anastomoses in liver, spleen, and lungs, Am. J. Physiol. *152*:48, 1948.

189. Purcell, H. K., Connor, J. J., Alexander, W. F., and Scully, N. M.: Observations on the major radicles of the extrahepatic portal systems, A.M.A. Arch. Surg. *62*:670, 1951.

190. Rappaport, A. M.: Hepatic venography, Acta radiol. *36*:165, 1951.

191. ————: The guided catheterization and radiography of the abdominal vessels, Canad. Med. Ass. J. *67*:93, 1952.

192. ————: Circulatory aspects of liver physiology, Thesis, University of Toronto, 1952.

193. ————: In discussion of Elias, H.: Morphology of the liver, p. 196, Tr. 11th Liver Injury Conf., New York, Macy, 1953.

194. ————: The structural and functional unit in the human liver (liver acinus), Anat. Rec. *130*:673, 1958.

195. Rappaport, A. M.: Liver morphology, Discussion Workshop, Ann. N. Y. Acad. Sci. *111*:527, 1963.

196. Rappaport, A. M., and Bilbey, D. L. J.: Segmentation of the liver at microscopic level, Anat. Rec. *136*:262, 1960.

197. Rappaport, A. M., Black, R. G., Lucas, C. C., Ridout, J. H., and Best, C. H.: Normal and pathologic microcirculation of the living mammalian liver, Rev. int. Hépat. *16*:813, 1966.

198. Rappaport, A. M., Borowy, Z. J., and Lotto, W. N.: Experimental hepatic coma, Surg. Forum *4*:504, 1952.

199. Rappaport, A. M., Borowy, Z. J., Lougheed, W. M., and Lotto, W. N.: Subdivision of hexagonal liver lobules into a structural and functional unit; role in hepatic physiology and pathology, Anat. Rec. *119*:11, 1954.

200. Rappaport, A. M., and Hiraki, G. Y.: Histopathological changes in the structural and functional unit of the human liver, Acta Anat. *32*:240, 1958.

201. ————: The anatomical pattern of lesions in the liver, Acta Anat. *32*:126, 1958.

202. Rappaport, A. M., Holmes, R. B., Stolberg, H. O., McIntyre, J. L., and Baird, R. J.: Hepatic venography, Gastroenterology *46*:115, 1964.

203. Rappaport, A. M., and Knoblauch, M.: The hepatic artery, its structural, circulatory and metabolic functions, 3rd Intern. Symp. Intern. Assoc. Study of Liver, Kyoto, 1966; Tijdschrift voor Gastroenterologie, p. 116, Antwerpen, Belgium, 1967.

204. Rappaport, A. M., Lotto, W. N., and Lougheed, W. M.: Experimental hepatic ischemia, collateral circulation of the liver, Ann. Surg. *140*:695, 1954.

205. Rappaport, A. M., Macdonald, M. H., and Borowy, Z. J.: Hepatic coma following ischemia of the liver, Surg. Gynec. Obstet. 97:748, 1953.

206. Rappaport, A. M., Vranic, M., Campbell, J., Green, G. R., Cowan, J. S., and Wrenshall, G. A.: Effects of hepatic artery ligation on survival and metabolism of depancreatized dogs, Am. J. Physiol. *215*:898, 1968.

207. Reeves, J. T., Leathers, J. E., and Boatright, C.: Microradiography of the rabbit's hepatic microcirculation. The similarity of the hepatic portal and pulmonary arterial circulations, Anat. Rec. *154*:103, 1966.

208. Reifferscheid, M.: Chirurgie der Leber, Stuttgart, Thieme, 1957.

209. Rienhoff, W. F., Jr.: Ligation of the hepatic and splenic arteries in the treatment of portal hypertension with a report of 6 cases, Bull. Johns Hopkins Hosp. *88*:368, 1951.

210. Rouiller, C.: Les canalicules biliaires: étude au microscope électronique, Acta Anat. *26*:94, 1956.

211. Rutenburg, A. M., and Seligman, A. M.: The histochemical demonstration of acid phosphatase by a post-incubation coupling technique, J. Histochem. Cytochem. *3*:455, 1955.

212. Sabourin, C.: Recherches sur l'anatomie normale et pathologique de la glande biliaire de l'homme, Paris, Alcan, 1888.

213. Sachs, A. E.: Absence of common bile duct, J.A.M.A. *149*:1462, 1952.

214. Schepers, G. W. H.: Hepatic cellular gigantism as a manifestation of chemical toxicity, p. 785, Proc. 13th Int. Congr. on Occupational Health, (1961.)

215. Schmidt, F. C.: Electronmikroskopische Untersuchungen an den Sinusoid Wandzellen (Kupfferschen Sternzellen) der weissen Maus, Anat. Anz. *108*:376, 1960.

216. Schumacher, H. H.: Histochemical distribution pattern of respiratory enzymes in the liver lobule, Science *125*:501, 1957.

217. Schwegler, R. A., Jr., and Boyden, E. A.: The development of the pars intestinalis of the common bile duct in the human fetus, with special reference to the origin of the ampulla of Vater and the sphincter of Oddi, Anat. Rec. 68:17, 1937.

218. Segall, H. N.: An experimental anatomical investigation of the blood and bile channels of the liver, Surg. Gynec. Obstet. 37:152, 1923.

219. Sellers, E. A., and You, R. W.: Propylthiouracyl, thyroid and dietary liver injury, J. Nutr. 44:513, 1951.

220. Seneviratne, R. D.: Physiological and pathological responses in blood vessels of liver, Quart, J. Exp. Physiol. 35:77, 1949.

221. Sérégé, H.: Sur la teneur en urée de chaque lobe du foie en rapport avec les phases de la digestion, C. R. Soc. Biol. 54:200, 1902.

222. ———: Variations horaires d'excrétion de l'urée chez l'homme en rapport avec les phases de la digestion, et dissociation fonctionelle de chaque lobe du foie, C. R. Soc. Biol. 54:300, 1902.

223. Shank, R. E., Morrison, G., Cheng, C. H., Karl, I., and Schwartz, R.: Cell heterogeneity within the hepatic lobule (quantitative histochemistry), J. Histochem. Cytochem. 7:237, 1959.

224. Sharpey-Schafer, E. A.: Schafer's Essentials of Histology, ed. 15, pp. 400-401, London, Longmans, 1949.

225. Sherlock, S.: Hepatic vein catheterization in clinical research, Proc. Inst. Med. Chicago 18:335, 1951.

226. Sherlock, S., and Walshe, V.: The use of portal anastomotic vein for absorption studies in man, Clin. Sci. 6:113, 1946.

227. Simonds, J. P.: Chronic occlusion of the portal vein, Arch. Surg., 33:397, 1936.

228. Smetana, H. F., Keller, T. C., and Dubin, I. N.: Symposium on diseases of the liver; histologic criteria for differential diagnosis of liver diseases in needle biopsies, Rev. Gastroenterology 20:227, 1953.

229. Soskin, S.: Carbohydrate Metabolism, p. 27, Chicago, Univ. Chicago Press, 1946.

230. Stahle, J.: Studies on the bile ducts, and the blood vessels in Glisson's capsule; a histological investigation of the incidence of smooth muscle in the intrahepatic bile ducts, Acta Soc. Med. Upsalien. 57:455, 1952.

231. Steiner, J. W., and Carruthers, J. S.: Studies on the fine structure of the terminal branches of the biliary tree, Am. J. Path. 38:639, 1961.

232. Stoner, H. B.: The mechanism of toxic hepatic necrosis, Brit. J. Exp. Path. 37: 176, 1956.

233. Sudler, M. T.: The architecture of the gallbladder, Bull. Johns Hopkins Hosp. 12:126, 1901.

234. Sutherland, S. D.: The intrinsic innervation of the liver, Rev. int. Hepat. 15: 569, 1965.

235. Sweet, J. E.: The gallbladder, its past, present and future, Int. Clin. 1:187, 1924.

236. Tori, G., and Scott, W. G.: Experimental method for visualization of the hepatic vein—venous hepatography, Am. J. Roentgenol. 70:242, 1953.

237. Trowell, O. A.: The experimental production of watery vacuolation of the liver, J. Physiol. 105:268, 1946.

238. Villemin, F., Dufour, R., and Rigaud, A.: Variations morphologiques et topographiques du foie, Arch. Mal. appar. dig. 40:63, 1951.

239. Wachstein, M.: Enzymatic histochemistry of the liver, Gastroenterology 37: 525, 1959.

240. Wakim, K. G., and Mann, F. C.: The intrahepatic circulation of the blood, Anat. Rec. 82:233, 1942.

241. Warner, L.: Morphological changes in liver and spleen following intraperitoneal injection of cevitaminic acid, Anat. Rec. 76 (Supp. 2) 57, 1940.

242. Weiss, S.: Portal hypertension, a critical study of the circulatory system of the liver and the evolution of the syndrome of portal hypertension, Int. Clin. 1:148, 1936.

243. Wellman, J. M., and Maddock, W. G.: Subphrenic abscess, Univ. Hosp. Bull., Ann Arbor 5:10, 1939.

244. Wilson, J. W.: Hepatic structure in Brauer, R. W. (ed.) Liver Function, Am. Inst. Biol. Sci. Pub. No. 4:175, Washington, D.C., 1958.

245. Wilson, J. W., Groat, C. S., and Leduc, E. H.: Histogenesis of the liver, Ann. N.Y. Acad. Sci. 111:8, 1963.

246. Wolf-Heidegger, G., and Beydl, W.: Zur Morphologie und Topographie d. Kup-

fferschen Sternzellen, Acta anat. *19*:15, 1953.

247. Wood, R. L.: The fine structure of the junction between bile canaliculi and bile ducts in mammalian liver, Anat. Rec. *139*:287, 1961.

248. Zeppa, R., and Womack, N. A.: Humoral control of hepatic lymph flow, Surgery *54*:37, 1963.

249. Zimmermann, K. W.: Über das Verhältnis der "Kupfferschen Sternzellen" zum Endothel der Leberkapillaren beim Menschen, Z. mikr. anat. Forsch. *14*: 528, 1928.

2

Electron Microscopy of Liver

FENTON SCHAFFNER, M.D., AND HANS POPPER, M.D.

By increasing resolution, electron microscopy of liver tissue has permitted recognition of structural details not seen before. This, so far, has provided few, if any, diagnostic criteria useful in management of patients, in contrast to organs such as the kidney and small bowel. It has, however, fostered better understanding of abnormal structure and function of the liver by better defining hepatocyte abnormalities such as diffuse injury without necrosis. This is barely appreciable under the conventional microscope but readily identified using electron microscopy. In this respect, light microscopic technics using fixatives, embedding media, and microtomes of electron microscopy (light microscopic "thin-section" technic) have been a valuable link, particularly since these aspects of electron microscopy are usually studied under relatively low magnification. By contrast, investigations explaining the functional significance of structural alterations are carried out more frequently with higher magnification and require correlation with chemical analysis of cellular fractions. Appreciation of the functional significance of morphologic alterations provides a structural explanation of the results of some of the hepatic tests not available from conventional microscopy, and thus may provide a better correlation between liver biopsy findings and the results of hepatic tests than conventional microscopy.

Electron microscopy supplemented by functional studies, mainly chemical analyses of cell fractions, still leaves many problems unanswered for which working hypotheses rather than facts are offered. Some of these result from lack of understanding of morphologic features such as the changes of mitochondria in alcoholic liver injury or the absence of morphologic changes if a biochemical defect is obvious, such as faulty uptake or conjugation of bilirubin in constitutional hyperbilirubinemia. However, absence of a single enzyme from a structure containing many enzymes need not be recognized morphologically.

THE NORMAL LIVER

The liver is composed of interlacing plates of dodecahedral hepatocytes measuring about 25 microns in diameter, the plates being covered by a thin layer of endothelial lining cells demarcating blood sinusoids.[25, 36,45, 135, 149] The collecting system for bile secreted by the hepatocyte starts with the bile canaliculi, which are merely small spaces between 2 or, less often, 3 hepatocytes. (Canaliculi surrounded by more than 3 cells are rare in the normal liver.) The system continues as specialized epithelial structures, the bile ductules, which drain into ducts in the portal tracts. Ductules differ from ducts by having 6 or less cells on cross section, and by the absence of nearby arteries and veins. Only minor differences exist between the ultrastructural appearance of the human liver and that of other mammals.

HEPATOCYTES

These cells, which appear hexagonal in cross section, have 3 distinct types of surfaces.[27, 57] One faces the sinusoid, and its surface area is greatly increased by the extension of numerous irregular microvilli

50

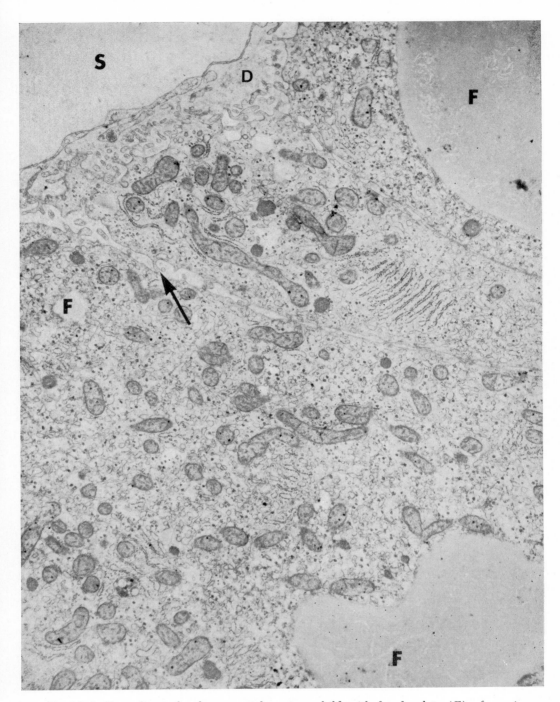

Fɪɢ. 2–1. Fatty liver of unknown etiology in a child with fat droplets (F) of varying size. The sinusoid (S) is separated from the normal space of Disse (D), by a thin endothelial lining cell. Note that the surface of the hepatocyte has numerous finger-like microvilli extending into the space of Disse and into the extension of this space between neighboring cells (arrow). The hepatocellular mitochondria, the ovoid gray bodies, are more variable in size and shape than normal, and the endoplasmic reticulum is more in the form of small vesicles than normal. The black dots represent glycogen which is depleted. × 10,000.

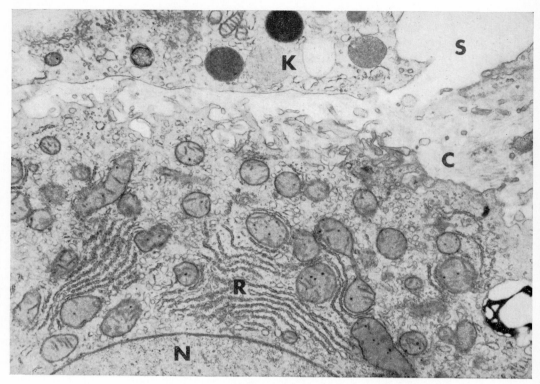

FIG. 2–2. Normal hepatocyte and Kupffer cell in the sinusoidal wall in a patient with long-standing incomplete biliary obstruction. The Kupffer cell (*K*) contains numerous bodies of phagocytic material and projects into the sinusoidal lumen (*S*). The hepatocytic nucleus (*N*) is surrounded by clusters of long profiles of rough endoplasmic reticulum (*R*). A bundle of collagen fibers (*C*) can be seen in the space of Disse with no microvilli on the cell surface below the bundle. × 14,000.

measuring from 0.5 to 1.0 micron in length and 0.1 micron in diameter. The microvilli lie in the narrow tissue space of Disse beneath the sinusoidal endothelial layer (Figs. 2–1 and 2–2). This surface represents the membrane across which blood-liver exchange occurs.

The second surface, which comprises about half the perimeter, faces the adjacent hepatocyte. A part of this surface may be separated from the neighboring cell by a distance of 0.2 to 1.0 micron for one to two thirds of the width of the cell beginning at the sinusoidal surface. The intercellular space is an extension of the perisinusoidal tissue space, and the hepatocytes extend a few microvilli into the space (Fig. 2–1). Most of the remainder of this cell surface lies in close apposition to that of its neigh-

bor, being no more than 0.02 micron away. This approximated portion of the surface is usually straight, although peg and groove configurations are noted occasionally (Fig. 2–3). Whether information can be transmitted directly from one cell to the next across these surfaces is not known.

A small portion of the surfaces between adjacent hepatocytes near the center of the liver cell plates represents the third type of surface, which is adapted for bile secretion. The normal bile canaliculus, which accounts for 6 per cent of the perimeter of the cell, is a space about 1.0 micron in diameter formed by separation of adjacent surfaces when they extend microvilli of about the same length and width as on the sinusoidal surface, but more regularly into the channel thus formed (Fig. 2–3). The bile canalicu-

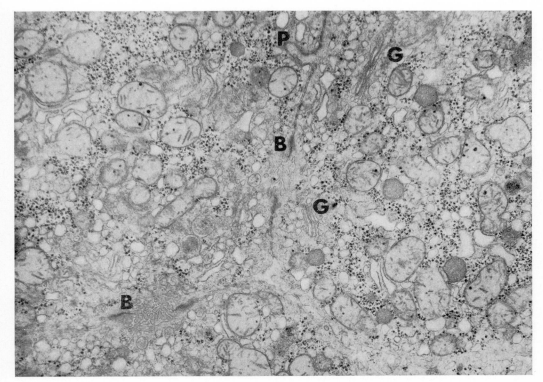

FIG. 2–3. Portion of 3 normal hepatocytes in an alcoholic. Bile canaliculi (*B*) between the 2 upper cells and between the one on the left and the one below are filled with microvilli. The thin lamellae of the Golgi apparatus (*G*) are best seen in the cell on the right. Note a peg (*P*) from the cell on the right extending into its neighbor. The uniformly round, dark gray bodies are microbodies or peroxisomes. × 15,000.

lus is sealed by a specialized area of the adjacent cell surfaces called the junctional complex, which consists of a dense desmosome and a short zone which appears to result from fusion of cells with almost absence of surface membranes. The junctional complex not only seals the canaliculus but anchors one cell to the next. The desmosome also serves as the point of attachment for numerous fine fibrils, or tonofilaments, which radiate into the cytoplasm and may be related to cell tone.

In the center of the cell is a round nucleus about 10 microns in diameter. It is separated from the cytoplasm by a double membrane, the leaves of which are 70 to 80 Å thick and 120 to 140 Å apart.[45] These membranes are fused where they outline numerous small pores, each 0.1 to 0.2 micron apart, measuring 700 ± 300 Å in diameter (Figs. 2–4 and 2–6). These pores are believed to provide the exit into the cytoplasm for the thread-like messenger RNA, particles of ribosomal RNA, and the small transfer RNA, all of which are formed in the nucleus, and to provide the entrance for the necessary nuclear and nucleolar building blocks. With osmium tetroxide fixation, the nucleoplasm is uniform, but with glutaraldehyde fixation the DNA containing nuclear chromatin appears as clumps of densely packed filaments mainly around the nuclear periphery (Fig. 2–7). These filaments are tightly wound coils of 2 fibrils 30 to 500 Å in diameter. Small granules of varying size are found in the remainder of the nucleoplasm; sometimes even in the chromatin clumps. Larger ones, numbering up to 200 per nucleus, are

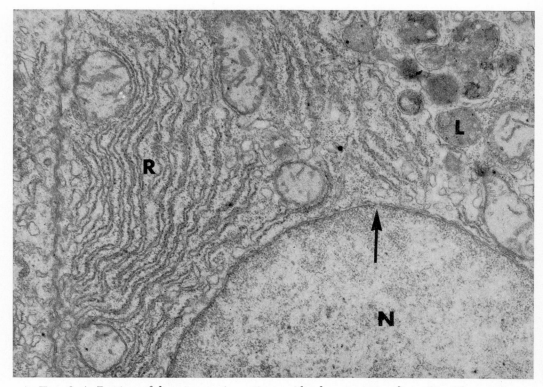

Fig. 2–4. Portion of hepatocyte in patient with chronic active hepatitis. The nucleus (N) is surrounded by a double membrane which has small pores in the membranes (*arrow*), through which nuclear building blocks enter and RNA leaves. In the cytoplasm numerous long profiles of rough endoplasmic reticulum (R) are seen, some of which appears to be forming from alignment of ribosomes. The irregular bodies in the upper right are lysosomes (L). × 18,000.

perichromatin granules 300 to 350 Å in diameter with a clear halo. These contain RNA and DNA. The nature of the smaller interchromatin granules is not known.

In the interior of the nucleus is the nucleolus which is the site of synthesis of the 3 forms of RNA which regulate cytoplasmic protein synthesis. The nucleolus is 2 to 4 microns in diameter and is composed of a nucleolonema with dense granules 50 to 200 Å in diameter and of filaments 80 to 100 Å long by 30 to 50 Å wide. The nucleolonema is RNA protein whereas the pars amorpha is protein only. No membranes are found in or around this organelle.

In the cytoplasm numerous organelles can be recognized. They differ, depending on the location within the lobule. The most

discrete organelle is the mitochondrion, about 800 of which have been calculated to be scattered throughout a single cell. These are rounded or elongated ovoid bodies 0.4 to 0.8 micron wide and up to 5.0 microns long, the longest being near the portal tracts (Fig. 2–4). Mitochondria are surrounded by a double membrane, the inner one having several deep invaginations or cristae. The matrix is slightly more dense than the interorganelle hyaloplasm, and contains 3 to 10 small, dense intramitochondrial granules per section, some containing calcium and some DNA (Fig. 2–5). In the matrix the enzymes and cofactors of the Krebs tricarboxylic acid cycle are located. Crystalloid inclusions are in the matrices of rare mitochondria. These are rods or filaments composed of tightly

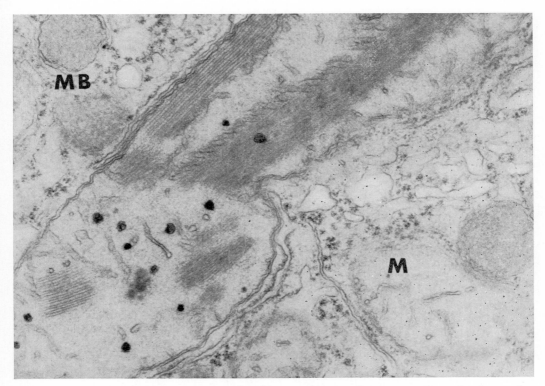

FIG. 2–5. Portion of a giant mitochondrion with crystalline material in the form of parallel fibrils in its matrix along with numerous dense granules. Compare the size with that of a normal mitochondrion (M) below and a microbody (MB) above. The mitochondria are surrounded by a double membrane with invaginations of the inner one, whereas microbodies have only one membrane. × 33,000.

coiled spirals 60 to 80 Å in diameter (Fig. 2–5). The nature and significance of these bodies found in normal persons,[177] apparently normal dogs,[148] and more frequently in various forms of liver injury[127] are not known. On the inner surface of the inner membranes, especially along the cristae, small nobs on short stalks are seen with specialized technics for separating and fragmenting mitochondria. These structures, called elementary particles, contain the flavoproteins and cytochromes of the electron transfer system and the enzymes needed for formation of ATP. This is the site of oxidative phosphorylation and of water formation. This means that here the stored energy of the sun is transformed into biological energy. Mitochondria, which are remarkably similar in all cells of plants and animals, thus constitute the energy sources for cellular functions.

Two related types of membranous structures are found interspersed between mitochondria. The single membrane is about 70 Å thick. Together the 2 membrane systems constitute the endoplasmic reticulum, or ergastoplasm, which is a major portion of the microsomal fraction studied by cytochemists. One system is a series of thin parallel channels usually arranged in several clusters fairly uniformly distributed throughout the cytoplasm (Fig. 2–2). The outer aspect of the membrane is lined by small ribosomal particles 150 to 300 Å in diameter (Figs. 2–4 and 2–10). This is the rough, or granular, form of the endoplasmic reticulum which serves as the template for synthesis of protein primarily for secretion.

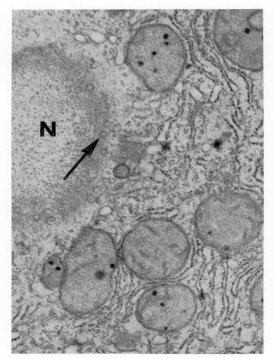

FIG. 2–6. Pores (*arrow*) in the membrane of a tangentially cut nucleus (*N*). Note the profiles of rough endoplasmic reticulum around the ovoid mitochondria. × 22,000.

Each peptide chain is synthesized along a unit called the polyribosome, composed of 12 or more ribosomes aligned on the thin thread of messenger RNA usually in the form of a spiral.[12, 39] The other system is composed of irregular tubules and vesicles without surrounding ribosomes and is the smooth, or agranular, form (Fig. 2–10). This is the site of sterol synthesis, and of conjugation and other chemical alterations including inactivation and detoxification of many endogenous hormones and exogenous drugs. This membrane contains hemoproteins (P450 and b5) which act as the microsomal electron transfer system, and are called the cytoplasmic or microsomal cytochromes. Both rough and smooth endoplasmic reticulum also contain glucose-6-phosphatase,[43, 119] the enzyme responsible for forming glucose for the blood by removing the phosphate which is needed for intracellular metabolism of glu-

cose. Glycogen is scattered throughout the cytoplasm in the form of particles called rosettes, which are clusters of smaller particles 100 to 200 Å in diameter. The smaller particles called the monoparticulate form are found in many cells of the body as well as in hepatocellular nuclei that have undergone glycogen "degeneration."[146]

An organelle that varies in number from 5 to 25 per cell cross section is the microbody. This structure, about 0.5 micron in diameter, is surrounded by a single membrane and is composed of an amorphous matrix more dense than that of mitochondria (Figs. 2–3 and 2–10). In most species, but not in man, a nucleoid is present. In the rat and dog it is a small, lattice-like crystal, in the hamster a central bar, and in other species it is an eccentric plate.[64] The nucleoid has been related to uricase activity, although the crystalline nucleoid is not the enzyme itself. Other enzymes in microbodies are peroxidases like catalase and d-amino acid oxidase. The structures first discovered with the electron microscope have been also called peroxisomes.[42] They are formed from smooth ends of profiles of rough surfaced endo-

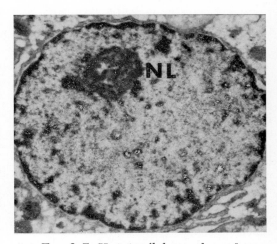

FIG. 2–7. Hepatocellular nucleus after glutaraldehyde fixation. The small dark clusters around the perimeter and scattered in the nucleoplasm are chromatin clumps. The large round body is the nucleolus (NL) surrounded by clumps of nucleolus associated chromatin. Note also the fine granules in the nucleoplasm. × 10,000.

plasmic reticulum,[50] and react to some forms of cell injury by becoming larger and more numerous, the significance of which is unknown.[160]

All cells have organelles called lysosomes specialized for digestion and storage.[94] Primary lysosomes, like the granules in neutrophilic leukocytes, are available without preceding stimuli. Secondary lysosomes, the ones found in hepatocytes, form around material to be acted upon, and are therefore indications of preceding exogenous or endogenous stimuli. The common stimuli for formation of hepatocytic lysosomes are intake by the cell of extraneous, not very soluble material, and focal breakdown of a portion of its own cytoplasm (autophagic vacuole).[48] These organelles are surrounded by a single membrane and contain numerous hydrolytic enzymes with acid pH optima. Acid phosphatase is the most widely used lysosomal marker. These organelles are most numerous between the nucleus and the bile canaliculus. They vary in size, shape, and density according to their contents[17] (Fig. 2–4).

One of the residues of digestion is polymerized, partially oxidized fatty acid which is a component of lipofuscin, the wear and tear pigment. Long-term use of various drugs like phenacetin may cause extensive lipofuscin deposition in otherwise normal livers.[1] This may remain stored in the lysosome for the life of the cell. Other material such as excess iron, copper, or injected colloid such as dextran or Thorotrast[66] may be stored in lysosomes. This function of segregating some material from the rest of the cell has given rise to the name "segresome" for this organelle. When first discovered they were thought to be responsible for cell death if they ruptured and their enzymatic contents were released. Subsequent studies have shown this process to be an unlikely event in the hepatocyte. Indeed, lysosomes may prevent cell death by isolating a focally damaged portion and digesting it, or by segregating noxious agents including viruses.

The cytoplasm around the bile canaliculus differs from that in the rest of the cell. The canaliculus and its surrounding cytoplasm is called the bile secretory apparatus. Little

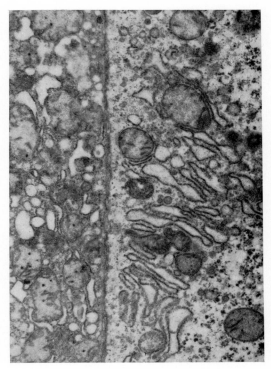

Fig. 2–8. Portions of light and dark cells in a patient with cholangitis. The hyaloplasm in the dark one on the left is dense, and the organelles are tightly packed. In the cell on the right the hyaloplasm is light and the organelles are separated. × 18,000.

glycogen and rough endoplasmic reticulum and few, if any, mitochondria, microbodies, or lysosomes are in this pericanalicular zone. It is demarcated by the Golgi apparatus on one side and the canaliculus 2 to 3 microns away on the other. The Golgi apparatus consists of grouped thin parallel profiles, or lamellae, which are closer together and have narrower internal channels than the endoplasmic reticulum, and of small vesicles, about 0.1 micron in diameter, budding off the ends of the long profiles and scattered about the Golgi lamellae in a random fashion[48, 94] (Fig. 2–3). Granules, possibly protein or lipoprotein, may be present in the lamellae and vesicles, especially in the fed state (Fig. 2–10).

The main functions of the Golgi apparatus

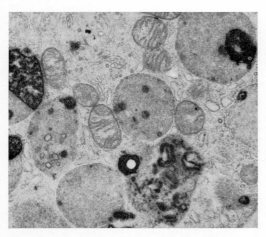

Fig. 2–9. Cytoplasm of a Kupffer cell in a patient recovering from viral hepatitis, with numerous phagocytic vacuoles each differing from the other in size and contents. Some barely recognizable membranous structures are in some of the vacuoles, and probably represent cell breakdown products of hepatocytes. × 13,000.

The exact mode of bile secretion is unknown. Vesicles containing some of the components may move from the endoplasmic reticulum or Golgi apparatus to the canaliculus. The cytoplasm beneath the canalicular membrane is more dense than that in the rest of the cell. This pericanalicular ectoplasm is devoid of organelles and it has been postulated as a zone in which the membranes of the vesicles dissolve, allowing their contents to be moved across the canalicular membrane. This movement was originally thought to occur in a molecular fashion, but more likely substances are moved as micelles with bile salts as the key molecules in these aggregates. The pericanalicular ectoplasm becomes thickened in cholestasis, which suggests that some interference with secretion occurs at this site.

Intralobular Mesenchymal Cells

In the normal liver thin extensions of endothelial cells lining blood sinusoids rest on the microvilli of the hepatocytes (Fig. 2–1). A thin basement membrane is present only close to the portal or central veins, but is missing in 90 per cent of the lobule.[27] Cytoplasm around the nucleus is more bulky and contains most of the organelles. The extensions of these endothelial cells may interweave with one another in a loose network surrounding many gaps through which plasma may flow and bathe the narrow space of Disse between the endothelial cells and hepatocytes.[149] Where the cell membrane of the hepatocyte is in contact with these bundles, it is devoid of microvilli (Fig. 2–2). Although collagen bundles are infrequent in the very thin electron microscope sections, they are numerous in the thin sections viewed under the light microscope, and they merge to form the "basement membrane" demonstrated by silver impregnation of conventional paraffin sections.

Scattered throughout the lobule in the space of Disse, or between hepatocytes, are cells with much rough endoplasmic reticulum and several uniformly small fat droplets in their cytoplasm.[24, 27, 140] The function of these lipocytes is unknown, but they have been said to represent fibroblasts possibly in a resting stage.[140] Their fat content does not parallel that in the hepatocytes.

seem to be to package proteins for export from the cell and to form lysosomes.[13, 94] In the hepatocyte the close proximity to the bile canaliculus suggests that the packaging is for bile secretion. This is supported by the enlargement of the Golgi apparatus in cholestasis. However, what is assembled and how much is also delivered to the sinusoidal surfaces of the cell are unknown. The small vesicles may represent material being delivered to the Golgi zone from the cell surface or from the endoplasmic reticulum, or it may be material leaving the apparatus to canalicular or sinusoidal surfaces. Some of these tiny vesicles are collected in single large vesicles about 1 micron in diameter called multivesicular bodies or vacuoles (Fig. 2–12).

A typical centriole, rarely with a cilium projecting into the canalicular lumen, can sometimes be found near the Golgi apparatus (Fig. 2–12). In cells that have recently divided, microtubules, remnants of the spindle apparatus, are seen.[158] Fat droplets (Fig. 2–1), and large glycogen-smooth membrane complexes or glycogen bodies (Fig. 2–11), are found free in the cytoplasm.

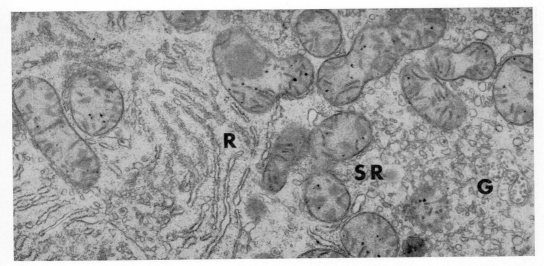

Fig. 2–10. Portion of a hepatocyte of a rat given the pesticide dieldrin for several weeks. The cytoplasm contains many tubules and vesicles of smooth endoplasmic reticulum (SR), some of which appears to be forming from rough endoplasmic reticulum (R). The Golgi apparatus (G) on the left contains several small granules which may be lipoprotein. × 20,000.

In the sinusoidal lumen, in addition to hematic cells, macrophages are found which may comprise a small part of the sinusoidal wall (Fig. 2–2). Kupffer cells in a strict sense are irregular in outline and contain numerous vacuoles of engulfed material, some recognizable as hepatocellular fragments (Fig. 2–9). Occasionally similar cells are seen normally in the tissue spaces.

Portal Tracts

Blood vessels, nerves, and bile ducts and ductules interspersed between thick collagen bundles can be seen in the portal tracts. Macrophages and fibroblasts are seen among the fiber bundles. The arterial vessels are easily recognized by the presence of smooth muscle cells around the endothelium. Occasional small, thick-walled arterial capillaries are readily differentiated from venous channels which are thin and have no muscle cells. All vessels are surrounded by a single basement membrane.

Biliary Epithelium

The bile ductules on cross section are comprised of 2 to 6 cuboidal cells arranged around a lumen which varies in diameter from 1 to 10 microns[129, 157] (Fig. 2–13). The luminal surface has irregularly spaced and usually short microvilli. Pinocytotic vacuoles are common beneath the luminal membrane. Occasionally single cilia are noted arising from the centriole of the cell and projecting into the lumen. The lateral surfaces of neighboring ductular cells are straight for a third to one-half the distance from the lumen when they begin interdigitating with one another, or are slightly separated from each other. Junctional complexes are present only near the luminal surface. Between some ductular cells is a small lumen resembling a bile canaliculus. The basal surfaces are straight and rest on a single, thin basement membrane. The cytoplasm of the ductular cells contains few organelles when contrasted with that of hepatocytes. A prominent Golgi apparatus with lamellae, vesicles and multivesicular vacuoles lies between the centrally situated nucleus and the luminal surface. Mitochondria are sparse and small, and endoplasmic reticulum is scanty. Rarely fat droplets or pigment-containing lysosomes are seen. Tonofilaments are more numerous and obvious than in hepatocytes. Bile duct cells are similar to ductular cells except that they are more columnar and their nuclei are more basal.

Bile ducts and ductules are in close proximity to veins, and at times their basement membranes fuse. Outside the basement membranes fiber bundles are clustered (Fig. 2–13) although in places empty spaces (tissue spaces or artefacts?) are seen.

Ductules are normally found in the parenchyma also, especially near portal tracts. These are more frequent in older persons and are usually accompanied by a few mononuclear inflammatory cells. Bile ductules always are surrounded by a basement membrane, except when they are next to hepatocytes. Here 1 or 2 ductular cells may share a canalicular lumen with the hepatocyte. This represents the origin of the biliary tree and has been called the "ampulla" or "canal of Hering."

Embryonal and Neonatal Liver

In the early embryonal liver no endoplasmic reticulum is found but ribosomes and polyribosomes are numerous.[109] The endoplasmic reticulum appears in midgestation when ribosomes become less numerous. With continued development the distance between the membranes of the endoplasmic reticulum decreases. At birth the liver is rich in glycogen which rapidly disappears except from lysosomes.[70, 108] As the glycogen decreases, smooth endoplasmic reticulum increases. Extramedullary hematopoiesis can be found in islands in the space of Disse and around the hepatic vein tributaries.

ELECTRON MICROSCOPY IN LIVER DISEASE

The ultrastructural pathology of the human liver has not been studied systematically because, with minor exceptions, it is of little diagnostic value clinically. Observations have been made in several diseases with a few attempts at correlation with clinical or functional data.

Cholestasis and Biliary Cirrhosis

When bile secretion ceases because of an obstruction in the extrahepatic ducts or because cholate excretion is interfered with

many bile canaliculi lose their microvilli and dilate, more so in the centrilobular zone[15, 130, 149, 181] (Fig. 2–11). These canaliculi also lose their adenosine triphosphatase activity.[178] In many of the dilated canaliculi dense fibrillar and amorphous deposits develop, often interspersed with small lipid droplets and irregular lamellar membranes[16] (Fig. 2–14). Extensive accumulations are the bile plugs or thrombi of light microscopy. In canaliculi without bile plugs, a fine, faint, amorphous material is seen. About one-third of bile canaliculi remain normal, retaining their normal adenosine triphosphatase activity, even next to dilated ones that contain bile plugs.

Changes in the hepatocellular cytoplasm related to cholestasis are enlargement of the Golgi apparatus with an increase in multivesicular bodies, the presence of lobulated vacuoles containing stringy, dense, lamellated membranes (probably phospholipids), elongation and curling of some mitochondrial cristae, and deposition in the cytoplasm of the same dense fibrillar or amorphous material seen in the bile plugs (Fig. 2–11). The latter material is not enveloped by a membrane and is the intracellular bile pigment noted by light microscopy. The degree of cholestatic alterations varies from hepatocyte to hepatocyte. If the cell is crowded with pigment and phospholipid, it appears vacuolated on light microscopy (feathery degeneration). These variations in appearance indicate different degrees of inhibition of bile secretion in neighboring cells. In cholestasis following administration of various drugs, the smooth endoplasmic reticulum is hypertrophied, probably as an adaptive response of the cell to metabolize the drug (see Adaptation later in this chapter).

Bile canaliculi do not rupture early in the course of cholestasis but only when the cell dies. Since these cells no longer secrete bile, this rupture does not contribute to jaundice. Bile plugs from ruptured canaliculi are engulfed by macrophages. Bile pigment in macrophages is either in the form of engulfed plugs or more commonly in the same form as in hepatocytes, possibly as a result of uptake of excess unconjugated bilirubin or of hepatocellular breakdown products.

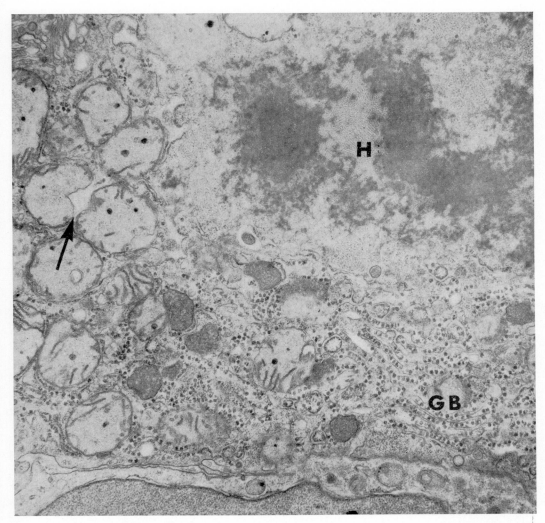

FIG. 2–11. Mallory's alcoholic hyalin (*H*) in acute alcoholic hepatitis. Most of the material appears fibrillar but a more dense central core is also present. The hepatocyte also shows abnormalities of mitochondrial membranes (*arrow*), and a portion of a glycogen body (*GB*), with glycogen particles aligned in single file between long parallel membranes of smooth endoplasmic reticulum. × 13,000.

Bile ductules also are altered in cholestasis.[129] Pinocytotic vacuoles are increased on cell surfaces and multivesicular bodies around the Golgi apparatus are more prominent. In the ductular cell cytoplasm, the same bile pigmented material and phospholipid-containing vacuoles are abundant. The basal halves of neighboring cells are separated, and the basement membrane is duplicated in many places. The collagen envelope is greatly thickened and many fibroblasts, macrophages, and leukocytes are in the vicinity. In places leukocytes can be found inside or entering the basement membrane.

The appearance of many normal bile canaliculi suggests continued bile secretion which makes reabsorption of biliary constituents by the ductules possible. The centrolobular accentuation of cholestasis with formation of bile plugs in this zone can be explained by inspissation of pigments and lipids in the complex polysaccharide nor-

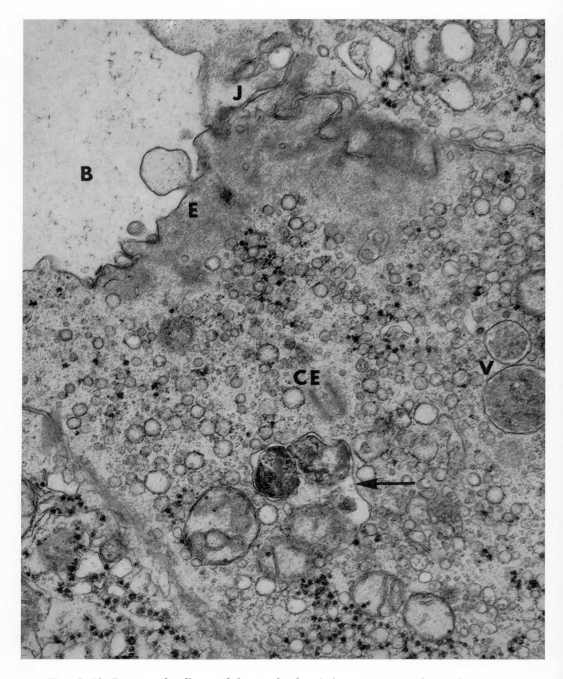

FIG. 2–12. Portion of cell near bile canaliculus (*B*) in patient with intrahepatic cholestasis. The canaliculus is filled with a loose amorphous material and also contains a
single edematous microvillus. The canaliculus is sealed by a junctional complex (*J*) which
in places appears to fuse the 2 cells together. The cytoplasm immediately below the surface membrane, the pericanalicular ectoplasm, is condensed and nearly devoid of any
structures. In the vicinity are a portion of the centriole (*CE*), multivesicular bodies (*V*),
and a lysosome containing remnants of membranous structures (*arrow*). × 18,000.

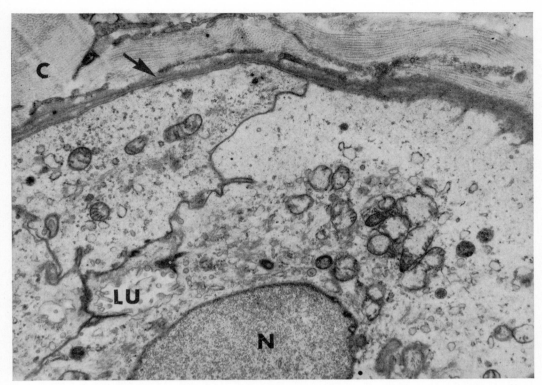

FIG. 2–13. Portion of normal bile ductule in a patient with glycogen storage disease. The lumen (*LU*) is small and contains many microvilli. The lateral cell borders are interdigitated, especially near the lumen. The basal cell border rests on a thin basement membrane (*arrow*), on the other side of which are numerous bundles of collagen (*C*). Note the paucity of cytoplasmic organelles compared to hepatocytes. × 18,000.

mally secreted on the cell surface. The flushing of the system by the few secreting cells is inadequate in the central zone, but the increasing volume of flow cleanses the canalicular system as the bile converges toward the collecting ductules as a result of the combined contribution of all the canaliculi. The periductular inflammation and fibrosis is further evidence of the continued but depressed secretion, permitting reabsorption of an irritating material. Persisting cholestasis can thus lead to sufficient periductular scarring to produce amputation and destruction of ductules. Thus a secondary mechanical component eventually can follow the metabolically induced intrahepatic cholestasis.

This mechanical intrahepatic obstruction causes peripheral cholestasis immediately proximal to the obstruction. The electron microscopic picture of central and peripheral cholestasis is identical. This may occur early in drug induced liver injury and later in any type of icteric hepatitis, and is particularly severe in primary and secondary biliary cirrhosis. Bile duct damage and destruction followed by periductal fibrosis without initial centrilobular cholestasis occurs in primary biliary cirrhosis and, in effect, in congenital biliary atresia.[60] In these diseases hepatocytes are essentially normal on electron microscopy early in the disease, except for hypertrophy of the Golgi zone and occasional phospholipid and bilirubin deposits which are interpreted as an attempt to compensate for the regurgitation of bile through the damaged bile ducts.[74] Ductular cells show also imbibition of bile in their cytoplasm. Cholestasis, if present, is peripheral near the destroyed bile ducts unless the patient has been given drugs, such as anabolic steroids, that might produce centrilobular cholestasis in normal persons.

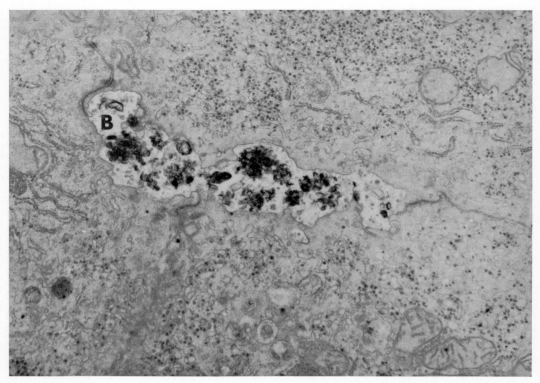

Fig. 2–14. Dilated bile canaliculus (B) containing bile plug in jaundiced patient with stones in the common bile duct. Canalicular microvilli are virtually absent, and the pericanalicular ectoplasm devoid of structure is a fairly broad zone around the canaliculus. × 13,000.

Late in the disease both central and peripheral cholestasis may be found with all the hepatocellular changes seen in all forms of cholestasis. The intralobular mesenchymal reaction in primary biliary cirrhosis is great enough to cause confusion with chronic hepatitis on a light microscopic level, but on the electron microscope level the majority of these cells in primary biliary cirrhosis are intrasinusoidal or immediately perisinusoidal rather than adjacent to damaged hepatocytes. Lymphocytes, macrophages, monocytes—some in transition to macrophages, and plasma cells account for most of the mesenchymal cells.[74]

Electron microscopy has demonstrated that the site of primary injury in centrilobular cholestasis is not the biliary passages but rather the bile secretory apparatus of the hepatocyte. It has not proved to be a useful differential diagnostic tool, however, for separation of the surgically correctable extrahepatic forms from intrahepatic cholestasis. Similarly, differentiation of drug induced cholestasis[84] from that occurring during pregnancy,[2, 47] or idiopathically,[20] or from that which results presumably from viral hepatitis has not been possible by this technic and is still better accomplished, if at all, by light microscopy.

Viral Hepatitis

Fine structurally, the liver cells vary greatly in appearance from one another in acute viral hepatitis, just as under the light microscope.[132] Much of this variation is the result of differences in the degree of hydration and glycogen depletion of the cells. Overhydrated or ballooned cells are recognized by their large size, and by dispersed organelles and glycogen particles. The most uniform change is disruption of the rough endoplasmic reticulum profiles into vesicles (Fig. 2–15). This is associated with a de-

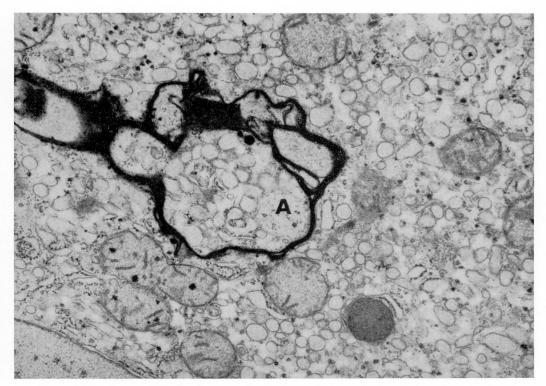

Fig. 2–15. Large autophagic vacuole (A), and extensively disrupted endoplasmic reticulum mainly in the form of vesicles in a patient with acute hepatitis. × 18,000.

tachment of the ribosomes from the profiles. The total number of ribosomes may or may not be diminished, and the degree of reduction determines the eosinophilia of scattered hepatocytes. The light and electron microscopic characteristic variation of neighboring hepatocytes is explained, however, not only by different content of the basophilia, but also by the variation in hydration of cells (light and dark cells) (Fig. 2–8). Eventually the rough endoplasmic reticulum is reduced in mass. The alteration of the rough endoplasmic reticulum seems to correlate best with decreased hepatocellular protein secretion and thus with reduced production of such serum proteins as albumin, alpha globulin, and coagulation proteins. Restoration to normal can be recognized by the presence of many polyribosomes near the nucleus aligning to form new profiles of rough endoplasmic reticulum. The smooth endoplasmic reticulum is variably increased in amount and may be either tubular or vesicular.

Autophagic vacuoles are numerous, several or single large ones being found in almost every cell (Fig. 2–15). As the disease improves, the autophagic vacuoles appear more like bodies of residual pigment clustered around bile canaliculi. Varying degrees of cholestasis are noted with no relationship to the severity of the hepatocellular changes. Mitochondria generally are normal except in severely damaged cells in which they are swollen and clumped. The sinusoidal surface of the hepatocyte has numerous edematous microvilli and pieces of the cytoplasm appear to be shed. Macrophages near these pieces contain bits of hepatocellular cytoplasm in various stages of breakdown surrounded by single membranes (Fig. 2–9). Plasma cells and fibroblasts are often adjacent to the macrophages, more so when the disease is protracted. The Disse spaces are widened and as the duration of disease lengthens, they become filled with thicker fiber bundles.

Necrosis of hepatocytes in hepatitis so

conspicuous on light microscopy is noted in 2 forms under the electron microscope. The first is indicated by almost complete loss of glycogen and endoplasmic reticulum with pyknosis, clumping of swollen mitochondria and giant blebs on the surface membrane of the cell. The seeming liquefaction of the cell interior has given rise to the term colliquation necrosis.[38] The second is formation of acidophilic bodies (structures resembling Councilman bodies).[18, 73] These are mummified whole cells which appear to have become suddenly dehydrated or coagulated.[37] Their hyaloplasm is more dense than normal but endoplasmic reticulum and even glycogen seem preserved. Mitochondria, on the other hand, have irregular limiting membranes and vacuoles in the matrix. The surface of these bodies is smooth and they are attached to neighboring hepatocytes. Nuclei are in various stages of disintegration. The bodies are surrounded by macrophages which contain engulfed pieces that are easily recognizable. Such bodies are not pathognomonic. Ones with identical electron microscopic characteristics have been seen in primary hepatic carcinoma, in drug reactions, in extrahepatic biliary obstruction, and in transplanted canine livers undergoing rejection.[32, 73]

Thus, electron microscopic studies have shown that cytoplasm loses some function in viral hepatitis because of necrosis, shedding and focal degradation in cells. The main clinical and functional features of the disease, however, are explained to a much greater degree by diminished function of the surviving cytoplasm in viable cells. Alterations of the rough endoplasmic reticulum seem to be the most significant structural abnormalities. Viral particles have not been found despite extensive search and several false alarms.

ALCOHOLIC HEPATITIS

Electron microscopic studies of livers of normal persons given large quantities of alcohol reveal that hepatocellular mitochondria become more varied in size and shape (Fig. 2–1), and several giant forms with crystalline inclusions (Fig. 2–5) may be found per cell although not in all cells.[82, 122]

Glycogen is depleted, fat droplets accumulate and coalesce, and smooth endoplasmic reticulum increases. The ribosomes of the rough surfaced endoplasmic reticulum become detached and are free in the hyaloplasm. They may even be decreased in number.

In patients with acute alcoholic hepatitis, the changes described in normal persons given alcohol are also found, only they are more severe.[46, 76, 112] In addition, mitochondrial membranes, especially the outer one, are disrupted and the inner one may be indented, giving the impression of vacuole formation in mitochondria (Fig. 2–11). Giant forms are more numerous, and clumping with interlocking of mitochondria appears. A correlation exists between mitochondrial size and the degree of ethanol abuse.[72] The most distinctive change is the appearance in a few cells of a fibrillar material delimited from the rest of the cytoplasm only in places by a single membrane.[14, 76, 112] In some patients this fibrillar material is loose and not dense, in others it is condensed and the centers appear as solid cores (Fig. 2–11). This is the "alcoholic hyalin" of Mallory. Its source is unknown and origin from degenerated mitochondria[112] or endoplasmic reticulum[14] seems unlikely. The Mallory body may be removed by incorporation of the material into lysosomes.[76] As in viral hepatitis, shedding of hepatocellular cytoplasm from the cell surface is seen. Disse spaces are widened and pericellular collagen deposition is more striking than in viral hepatitis. Furthermore, in alcoholic liver disease, polymorphonuclear leukocytes are numerous among the mesenchymal cells, often near cells containing alcoholic hyalin, some of which may be recognized in neighboring macrophages.

While structural abnormalities of the endoplasmic reticulum best explain the functional derangements in viral hepatitis, in alcoholic disease mitochondrial abnormalities indicative of impaired energy production are morphologically more in the foreground. The functional significance of the mitochondrial alteration is problematic. Furthermore, the interference with hepatocellular perfusion by pericellular fibrosis is an important factor, depriving hepatocytes of nutrients and ready access to the blood stream.

Chronic Hepatitis and Cirrhosis

In chronic active hepatitis not associated with alcoholism all the features of viral hepatitis are noted.[35, 131] In addition, large lymphoid cells are found near and even deeply indenting hepatocytes.[110] These cells have few lysosomes and scant endoplasmic reticulum but numerous ribosomes, single and in polysomes. The role of these cells is unknown. They resemble the cells found in delayed hypersensitivity reactions in other organs. Plasma cells usually near macrophages are numerous in the lobular parenchyma as well as in portal tracts and septa around proliferated ductules.

The bile ductules are more numerous than in acute and subacute hepatitis but otherwise they are similar in that they are surrounded by a single basement membrane and envelopes of collagen bundles interspersed with lymphoid cells and macrophages not adjacent to blood vessels. The cytoplasm of the epithelial cells has larger and more numerous organelles than normal, including lysosomes with phagocytic material of various types.[111] Electron microscopy has clarified the nature of the "pseudo-ductules" frequently found in chronic hepatitis and cirrhosis of any type. They are clusters of hepatocytes that resemble ductules which surround a single large canalicular lumen.[107] These tubular hepatocytes appear similar to embryonal cells with a more polar organization of their organelles, a basal position of the nucleus and a basement membrane enveloping the entire complex. They probably represent a type of cell regeneration.

In advanced but still active alcoholic liver disease, the features of acute alcoholic hepatitis such as alcoholic hyalin and mitochondrial abnormalities remain discernible. Nothing in the electron microscopic study of the liver indicates the irreversible transition into cirrhosis in alcoholic liver disease or in chronic active hepatitis. Nevertheless, when livers with cirrhosis are studied, additional features may be seen. Hepatocytes in

cirrhotic nodules can separate from their neighbors.[105, 106] These hepatocytes differ from acidophilic bodies in that they are of normal or only slightly increased overall density, and the cell membrane has numerous microvilli on its entire circumference. This may represent attempts to increase the cell surface active in transport in the nodule in which circulation is impaired, to compensate for all function lost elsewhere (regenerated nodule).

Another change prominently but not exclusively found in cirrhosis is development of a basement membrane beneath the sinusoidal lining cells converting sinusoids to capillaries.[111, 131] Normally basement membranes, usually incomplete, extend beneath sinusoidal lining cells for a short distance no more than 1 or 2 cells from the central veins and portal veins.[27] In chronic hepatitis and cirrhosis, the membranes are more often complete and extend for distances of many cells. This capillarization of sinusoids and the collagen deposition in the space of Disse provide a barrier to perfusion (Fig. 2–16). When the already inferior circulation of the cirrhotic nodule is added to this microcirculatory change, the effect on the liver and on the body can be great enough to produce a circulatory hepatic insufficiency even in the presence of morphologically normal hepatocytes. In addition to contending with these factors, the hepatocytes must compete for nutrients with the various mesenchymal cells which have a much shorter life span and hence a more rapid turnover. The mesenchymal cells also contribute to the impedance of microcirculation which, indeed, may be significant enough to perpetuate liver disease in the absence of any other factor.

Drug Induced Injury

Isolated examples of cholestasis in man have been studied electron microscopically following administration of chlorpromazine, anabolic and contraceptive steroids and various other unrelated drugs.[16, 84, 166] Aside from the features of cholestasis already described, no other significantly abnormal features were noted except for increased smooth endoplasmic reticulum and occasional focal necrosis. No systematic study is available of

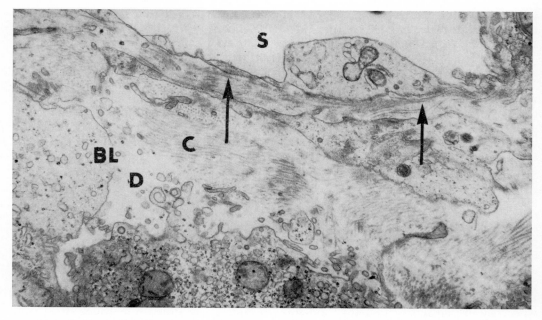

FIG. 2–16. Widened space of Disse (D) containing much collagen (C) in cirrhosis. Beneath the endothelial cell bordering the sinusoid (S), basement membrane material is seen (arrows). The surface of one hepatocyte has a large bleb (BL), and bits of cytoplasm possibly shed from the hepatocyte are nearly in the space of Disse. × 13,000.

the drug induced hepatic injuries resembling viral hepatitis. Following administration of chlofibrate, increases in size and number of microbodies was described.[160]

FATTY LIVER IN PREGNANCY, AFTER TETRACYCLINE, AND IN CHILDREN

In these similar and at times associated conditions, small fat droplets are found scattered through the hepatocellular cytoplasm (Fig. 2–1). Mitochondrial abnormalities have been described,[180] but have been inadequately documented to characterize the conditions morphologically or functionally. No published studies are available of children with fatty liver and fatty degeneration of the brain and kidney (Reyes' syndrome). A case studied by us revealed no abnormalities except for the fat droplets in the hepatocellular cytoplasm. Mitochondrial swelling, depletion of endoplasmic reticulum, cytoplasmic fat droplets with closely approximated mitochondria and insufficient complexes were noted in protein deficient

children affected with kwashiorkor. Protein repletion reversed some of these changes.

PASSIVE CONGESTION

Three factors operate in passive congestion: 1) increased hydrostatic pressure, 2) impaired perfusion, and 3) hypoxia as a result of slow flow. The first 2 seem more important for the liver cell alterations than the third as judged from electron microscopic studies.[128] These showed extensive deposition of collagen in tissue spaces which replaces hepatocytes. The cells disappear partly as a result of pressure atrophy and partly as a result of starvation because of impaired perfusion. This is inferred from loss of glycogen and endoplasmic reticulum without formation of autophagic vacuoles. Necrosis is uncommon in chronic congestion, and mesenchymal cells other than fibroblasts are sparse. Disruption of liver cell plates is seen in the centrilobular zone with rupture of bile canaliculi, although such cells must have ceased forming bile because the patients may not be jaundiced. Cholestasis in passive congestion has not been studied.

ISOLATED HYPERBILIRUBINEMIAS

Direct reacting hyperbilirubinemia as an isolated phenomenon occurs with pigment in the hepatocyte in the Dubin-Johnson syndrome, or without it in the Rotor syndrome.[90, 169] Both result from impaired secretion of all organic anions other than bile salts. The pigment may be a polymer of partially oxidized metanephrine glucuronide as it is in Corriedale sheep with a similar defect.[34] Howler monkeys accumulate a similar appearing pigment derived from their food.[86] Under the electron microscope the pigment-containing lysosomes are larger and more numerous in the centrilobular zone although they can be found in all cells. The pigment is not homogeneous but consists of a varying mixture of dense particles, lipid droplets, moderately dense matrix, and light areas quite distinct from lipofuscin. Bile canaliculi and hepatocellular cytoplasmic organelles are otherwise normal. Kupffer cells may contain pigment granules; bile ductular cells are free of it. In Rotor's syndrome the cells appear normal with excess lipofuscin pigment.

In unconjugated nonhemolytic hyperbilirubinemias, the hepatocytes are normal except for numerous lipofuscin pigment-containing lysosomes around bile canaliculi, particularly in the centrolobular zone.[40] Membrane changes variously described appear to be artefacts. Differences between patients with defects in uptake or in conjugation of bilirubin have not been found.

IRON EXCESS

Ferritin has a characteristic electron microscopic appearance in the form of particles 100 Å in diameter. They are composed of 6 subunits, or micelles. The particles may be free or arranged in crystalline arrays, or aggregated into hemosiderin granules, the latter probably representing an iron-containing lysosome.[18] The crystalline ferritin may also be in lysosomes sometimes mixed with lipofuscin. All iron-containing bodies have been called siderosomes. Some of the iron in the larger aggregates may be inorganic hydrated iron oxide not bound to the protein

apoferritin. When excess iron is present in human livers as a result of iron overload from transfusions, from defective iron utilization in some anemias or from excess iron absorption by the gut, numerous dense irregular granules are noted, mainly in the pericanalicular zone and most in hepatocytes of the lobular periphery. These granules may measure up to several microns in diameter and a limiting membrane can sometimes be recognized. Single ferritin molecules or small clusters are found in the surrounding cytoplasm. Numerous lipofuscin granules are also seen. Usually these are more dense than normal and contain iron particles. Iron-containing granules are also in ductular cells. They are found particularly in Kupffer cells in hemolysis or after blood transfusions. Distinction between the various iron storage diseases by the ultrastructural study of the liver is impossible.

The features of cirrhosis or alcoholic liver disease are the same whether iron is present or not. Around iron-laden macrophages, collagen fiber deposition is extensive, perhaps more so than around macrophages containing other pigment. This has led to the proposal that such macrophages stimulate fiber formation and at the same time serve as a scaffold for its deposition. This may be a factor in the production of cirrhosis in hemochromatosis. Hepatocytes heavily laden with iron, however, may be otherwise normal in appearance and not surrounded by fibers. When patients with excess iron in their livers develop viral hepatitis, acidophilic bodies contain numerous iron granules.

WILSON'S DISEASE

Dense lysosomes containing lipofuscin pigment are numerous in Wilson's disease and may be related to the excessive copper deposition in the liver. Electron probe analysis has revealed copper in these lysosomes.[55] The acid phosphatase content of these structures may appear decreased as a result of interference with certain histochemical reactions by the copper.[85] In addition, some hepatocytes of some patients contain enlarged mitochondria with dense matrices and widened cristae.

GLYCOGEN STORAGE DISEASE

Type II glycogen storage, or Pompe's disease, characterized by absence of lysosomal glucosidase has a unique electron microscopic appearance. Numerous membrane-bound pericanalicular monoparticulate glycogen bodies [59, 67, 87] resemble the neonatal lysosomes.[109] The missing enzyme normally removes glycogen from lysosomes where it is present in late fetal life. In the other forms of glycogen storage disease affecting the liver, the normal cytoplasmic glycogen is increased in amount. This may obscure the endoplasmic reticulum and make the number of mitochondria seem reduced. No specific features distinguish developing cirrhosis in glycogen storage disease from other conditions producing fibrosis save for the excess glycogen and occasional fat droplets. Children fed a high carbohydrate diet or diabetic children overtreated with insulin and sugar present similar pictures of glycogen-laden cells with dispersed organelles.

LIPOIDOSES AND OTHER STORAGE DISEASES

In Niemann-Pick disease, large pericanalicular vacuoles contain a characteristic laminated structure, presumably phospholipid.[172] These bodies are probably lysosomes. The same structures are found in the Niemann-Pick (mesenchymal) cells. In Tay-Sacks disease a few membrane-filled lysosomes may be found in the liver as in the neurons. These findings distinguish these lipoidoses from Gaucher's disease in which numerous large ovoid or elongated bodies up to several microns in length are found in unique large, mesenchymal cells exhibiting much endoplasmic reticulum which is mainly smooth. The bodies contain loosely packed tubules running roughly parallel to the long axis of the body, with a superficial resemblance to mitochondrial cristae. These Gaucher cells lie in the tissue spaces or in the sinusoids. They are not macrophages nor do they contain fat droplets. The stored material is not found in hepatocytes which themselves are normal.

In the group of diseases known as the Hunter-Hurler syndrome associated with storage of mucopolysaccharides, the stored material is a faint fibrillar or amorphous network localized in numerous rounded vacuoles or in coalescing groups of vacuoles. They give an acid phosphatase reaction and often fill much of the cytoplasm of hepatocytes as well as of macrophages.[28, 172] Ultrastructural differences between the various types of this syndrome have not been detected.

AMYLOIDOSIS

Amyloid is deposited in the space of Disse and when abundant compresses the hepatocytes.[21, 142] Its deposition, however, is not associated with altered structure aside from compression. The amyloid is composed of a fibrillar material embedded in an amorphous faint matrix. None is seen within cells. The fibrils are less than 100 Å thick and may have either periodicity or be associated with fine granules that give the appearance of periodicity. No difference has been found between primary and secondary amyloid, or between spontaneously occurring human amyloid and that produced experimentally in animals by hyperimmunization.

PRIMARY HEPATIC CANCER

The electron microscopic appearance of hepatic carcinomas depends on the degree of dedifferentiation or deviation from the norm.[91, 123, 170] Indeed, minimal deviation tumors may be composed of nearly normal appearing hepatocytes with glycogen, rough endoplasmic reticulum and a functioning bile secretory apparatus. Dilated canaliculi may contain bile plugs. Occasional dense acidophilic bodies are seen as in viral hepatitis.

More anaplastic cells also appear more primitive with the electron microscope. Glycogen is often scanty or even absent. Rough endoplasmic reticulum is sparse, although free polysomes and ribosomes may be plentiful. Smooth endoplasmic reticulum is also scanty, but in places it may be in irregular whorls which may be almost as large as nuclei. Mitochondria are less numerous than normal. They have bizzare shapes and irregular arrangements of cristae. Nuclei are often not centrally located. The cell membranes have fewer than normal microvilli, and bile canaliculi may be absent, rudimentary, or have wide lumens so that several cells form acini. The sinusoidal endothelium is either missing in large areas or is continuous and rests on a basement membrane. Fiber bundles in the space of Disse are small and few in number. Diagnostic ultrastructural features, however, have not been described in human tumors.

MISCELLANEOUS DISEASES

Ultrastructural studies have been carried out on isolated examples of various infectious diseases such as malaria,[120] leptospirosis,[41] and kala-azar.[165] In these the organism or some residue of it could be identified. Only leptospirosis revealed hepatocellular changes indicative of cholestasis.[41] Toxicosis of infancy produces cholestasis and fat droplets in hepatocytes.[175] Biopsy specimens obtained during operations may exhibit numerous nonspecific hepatocellular changes mainly on the vascular pole.[89] They have been related to anesthesia rather than to the surgery.

IN VITRO STUDIES OF LIVER

The phenomena related to necrosis and autolysis have been sequentially studied on pieces of liver which have been allowed to stand without any attempt at supporting life.[171] Many of the alterations associated with injury are produced, including autophagic vacuoles, rarefaction of microbody matrix, formation of multivesicular bodies, and nuclear and plasma membrane alterations. Lysosomal alterations were observed although they occurred late, excluding a primary digestive function of these organelles under these circumstances. This militates against such a function in the living liver cell. Lipid transport has been studied in the isolated perfused liver in which the Golgi apparatus was found to participate in the metabolism of very low density lipoproteins in the hepatocyte.[56]

The electron microscopic study of cells grown *in vitro* has shown that mesenchymal cells grow out first and create a carpet upon which the hepatocytes can extend.[19, 173] Ultimately such explant cultures may provide a simplified model for many purposes. The

electron microscopy of cell fractions, important in determining purity of preparations and status of isolated organelles, has as yet no usefulness in the study of liver diseases and therefore is not reviewed here.

EXPERIMENTAL MODELS

Numerous attempts have been made to duplicate human lesions in experimental animals to study time sequences and reduce the role of extraneous factors. In addition, individual biochemical lesions were produced which permitted study of associated structural changes. These correlated ultrastructural and biochemical studies serve as the basis for understanding the more complex changes found in human disease, and assist in the development of a systematic electron microscopic pathology of liver diseases. As yet this can rarely be done on a molecular basis, but rather as the pathology of organelles. The experimental models can be only briefly reviewed and then primarily from the standpoint of their contribution to organelle pathology.

Regeneration. Since repair begins right after injury, those features that belong to the restoration phase must be recognized first. Following partial hepatectomy in the rat, fat and free ribosomes increase in hepatocytes, while the endoplasmic reticulum decreases and autophagic vacuoles form.[9] Their surface membranes are altered and light and dark cells appear.[51] During mitosis, the chromosomes appear as irregularly shaped chromatin clumps.[81] Fine tubular structures, the spindle apparatus, can often be seen, especially near the centriole. The newly formed cells after 30 hours contain fat and free ribosomes but little smooth or rough endoplasmic reticulum and little glycogen.[153] Nuclei and nucleoli are larger than in control specimens. After 36 hours the fat begins to disappear and the rough endoplasmic reticulum begins to reorganize near the Golgi zone. Between 96 and 120 hours the cytoplasm returns to normal while the nuclear enlargement associated with large chromatin clumps and large nucleoli with a prominent small granule fraction persists for several more days. Regeneration after damage of embryonal liver may lead to failure of normal development of the biliary system with resultant canalicular cysts.[11]

During regeneration the cell organization does not apppear to be geared for its mature functions of protein export, detoxification and excretion but rather for its own development.

Adaptation. In addition to regeneration of entire cells or addition of new cells (hyperplasia), cells may become adapted to a change in their milieu, task or substrate. When animals are exposed to various drugs and chemicals such as barbiturates or pesticides , hepatic as well as nonhepatic carcinogens, the liver enlarges.[8] The number of hepatocytes remains constant or slowly increases.[79] The cytoplasmic/nuclear ratio and the parenchyma/tissue space ratio goes up in the liver as the liver weight/body weight ratio also increases. Compared to normal growth, these changes represent disproportionate hypertrophy of hepatocytes following phenobarbital administration or disproportionate hypertrophy with hyperplasia as produced by administration of many substances like halothane[79] or carcinogens.[8]

Parallel with the rise in relative liver weight the microsomal "processing" enzymes usually increase which act on many exogenous and endogenous substances.[54] They interact with the microsomal cytochromes or heme proteins such as P450 and b5. Cholesterol synthesis also increases.[71] Under the electron microscope, much of the cytoplasm of the hypertrophied hepatocyte is occupied by extensive lattice-works of tubular smooth endoplasmic reticulum.[71, 98, 115] The membranes are continuous with the rough endoplasmic reticulum and appear to be derived from the latter (Fig. 2–10). These cells show a concomitant loss of glycogen,[115] and detachment of ribosomes from the rough membranes,[71] along with the absolute gain in smooth membranes. Similar hypertrophy of the smooth endoplasmic reticulum is seen, especially if adverse reactions occur in patients receiving drugs.[137] The changes are reflected by hepatocellular enlargement and diffuse eosinophilic homogenization of the cytoplasm as seen by light microscopy.[99] The cytoplasmic basophilia is mainly perinuclear

and peripheral, since this is where the remaining ribosomes and the rough endoplasmic reticulum are crowded. Distinct eosinophilic cytoplasmic inclusions are also noted after administration of many substances that can induce hypertrophy of the smooth endoplasmic reticulum, including phenobarbital,[26, 31] thio-hydantoin,[58] DDT,[99] and even carbon tetrachloride.[152] On electron microscopy they are whorls of smooth membranes usually with a lipid core in glycogen-depleted areas (myelin figures). These membranes communicate with the tubular smooth reticulum and the entire structure is felt to be another form of hypertrophy. In terms of electron histochemistry, these myelin figures have nonspecific di- and triphosphatase activity.[58] They can be isolated by centrifugation of tissue at least partially fixed. Without fixation the whorls disappear into the microsomal fraction.

Stimuli inducing enzymes and cholesterol synthesis as well as hypertrophy of the smooth endoplasmic reticulum are least effective in the immature liver, are more effective soon after birth than in adults, and are most effective after partial hepatectomy.[31] The process is hormonally regulated, since sex hormones influence the rate of synthesis in castrates.[93] The morphologic response can be exaggerated if other drugs are given along with the initial inducer, even if the second drug is an enzyme inhibitor.[26] In some instances the inducing drug itself or its metabolites inhibit activity of certain enzymes.[88] This does not prevent hypertrophy of the endoplasmic reticulum but results in different enzymes being induced by different drugs despite the similar morphologic picture. Disparity between enzyme activity and amount of membrane also occurs if a large dose of a slowly metabolized inducer binds the enzymes temporarily. Subsequently the enzyme activity rises to match the amount of membranes.[71] Further differences may be caused by regulation of enzyme activity and membrane formation by different although closely correlated genes.[98] For instance, on regression of induction excess membranes persist longer than increased enzyme activity, and membrane disappearance is further delayed by actinomycin D.

Excess membranes disappear gradually without cytoplasmic autophagy. Reinduction may be slower than the original induction because of newly formed repressors.

When the degree of induction needed for adaptation exceeds the capacity of the cell, membranes are more increased than enzyme activity. This is associated with abnormalities of mitochondrial structure and function, and the formation of autophagic vacuoles. The border between beneficial adaptation and injury is where cells can no longer maintain the increase in processing enzymes stimulated by changes in their tasks, substrates or milieu.[8]

Mitochondria also adapt to changes in milieu, for instance to increases in oxygen tension such as encountered in space cabin atmospheres.[133, 136] The number and size of mitochondria increase as well as the amount of mitochondrial membranes. Along with this, mitochondrial enzyme activity and oxidative phosphorylation become hypernormal. Microbodies participate also in this adaptive process, in ways less clearly defined and less well studied. Their size and numbers increase in many conditions and, after salicylate administration, nucleoid and matrix may be altered.[146, 160]

Hepatocellular Injury and Necrosis. Many models of hepatocellular injury have been studied with the hope of learning how poisons interfere with cell function and lead to cell death. The main morphologic features of injury are detachment of ribosomes from membranes, disaggregation of polysomes, swelling of mitochondria, formation of autophagic vacuoles, loss of microvilli, edematous blebs on the cell surface, coagulation necrosis, and disruption of cells.

Ethionine. The most completely understood model is ethionine intoxication. This amino acid which forms nonutilizable s-adenosyl ethionine thus binds ATP irreversibly and prevents its utilization for other metabolic processes.[7] One consequence of this is the inability of the cell to secrete lipoprotein. Triglyceride protein complexes accumulate in small vacuoles of the endoplasmic reticulum called liposomes.[139] These fat droplets coalesce to produce the fatty liver characteristic of the acute ethionine lesion.

These changes can all be prevented by adenine.[7] Nucleoli and nuclei are also altered, which suggests that the biochemical deficit in ATP produced by ethionine also affects DNA and especially RNA synthesis, and ribosomal integrity.[92] Some adaptation to prolonged ethionine administration occurs as evidenced by increases in smooth endoplasmic reticulum, microbodies and nucleolar size, although continuing injury is shown by detachment of ribosomes from membranes of the endoplasmic reticulum, decrease in glycogen content and numerous autophagic vacuoles.[179]

Carbon Tetrachloride. Another widely studied model is carbon tetrachloride intoxication. Ribosomal detachment and disruption of rough endoplasmic reticulum followed by mitochondrial swelling seem to be key features associated with decreased ability to incorporate amino acids into proteins such as albumin.[145] This, too, is accompanied by fat droplets in the cytoplasm, but here the primary action appears to be a direct one of the solvent on the various phospholipid membranes of the cell.[65] Mitochondrial membranes may become more permeable to calcium which may accumulate in these organelles in the form of large granules.[116] Endothelial cells in the sinusoids are said to be affected even before hepatocytes.[121] Starvation increases the severity of the carbon tetrachloride effect.[77] Some adaptation to this agent also occurs in that myelin whorls develop on chronic administration, and in guinea pigs, but not in rats, smooth endoplasmic reticulum increases.

In cirrhosis induced by carbon tetrachloride, the hepatocytes in the nodules have much rough endoplasmic reticulum with many ribosomes, many microbodies, and much glycogen with few autophagic vacuoles.[33] The spaces of Disse are widened and filled with newly formed collagen often around proliferated ductules.[150] Sinusoids become like capillaries by development of a basement membrane beneath the endothelial lining cells, and new blood vessels grow into the areas of fibrosis.[151]

Effects of Ethyl Alcohol in Rats. When labeled glycerol or fatty acid was used, the precursors of triglycerides were seen quickly in the endoplasmic reticulum, and within 10 minutes in the lipid drops in the cell as well as in small droplets in the Golgi zone and smooth endoplasmic reticulum.[147] Rough endoplasmic reticulum and protein synthesis is normal in acute experiments even with steatosis.[5] Following long term feeding, first rough endoplasmic reticulum decreases and smooth increases,[68, 113, 168] and then mitochondria are enlarged and bizarre. These mitochondrial changes, appearing after 2 weeks and persisting,[68] have been considered as equivalent to Mallory bodies in man. When alcohol constitutes more than 30 per cent of the caloric intake, even otherwise adequate diets do not inhibit these changes.[114]

Hypoxia. Exposure of animals to low oxygen tension, simulating hypoxia or ischemia encountered clinically, causes anoxic vacuoles which contain exogenously administered colloid but initially no acid phosphatase.[23] This contrasts with the vacuoles formed after giving sucrose which do not contain acid phosphatase, and probably reflect incorporation of sugar into lysosomes whereas the anoxic vacuoles become lysosomes subsequently. Breakdown of cytoplasm leads to formation of other lysosomes in the form of autophagic vacuoles.[53] Mitochondria become swollen and interlocked, and Golgi vesicles swell but are reduced in number.[159] These changes quickly regress on return to ambient air.

Nutritional Abnormalities. Various dietary imbalances produce ultrastructural changes of questionable specificity in the livers of various species. Protein deficiency in rats,[162] dogs[49] or monkeys[96] decreases the numbers of mitochondria and the amount of endoplasmic reticulum while glycogen and fat increase in the cell. High carbohydrate or saturated fat diets decrease the osmiophilia of fat droplets, indicating the presence of saturated fat, while the reverse is true following diets high in unsaturated fats.[103] Feeding of orotic acid causes breakdown of endoplasmic reticulum with accumulation of fat, all prevented by adenine.[69, 95] Choline deficiency, especially with low protein intake, results in dilatation of the endoplasmic reticulum and loss of ribosomes, mitochondrial swelling and prominence of the Golgi zone.[4, 164] Choline quickly improves this, even on low protein diets.[164]

Nucleoprotein Abnormalities and Carcinoma. Inhibitors of protein synthesis such as actinomycin D[44, 144, 155] and puromycin[156] alter the ribosomes associated with decrease in amino acid incorporation into protein, and the nucleoli usually with separation of their granular and fibrillar components. Other agents such as mithramycin[78] and acridine orange[117] have similar effects. Aflatoxin[161] and related fungal toxins[167] may also produce nucleolar changes along with hypertrophy of the smooth endoplasmic reticulum, and formation of compact masses of smooth membranes. Azo dyes[80, 100] and other carcinogens[6] have a somewhat similar effect. The appearance of the resulting tumors[62] or even of spontaneous tumors[61] in rats depends on the rate of growth. The faster growing ones have a simpler organization and small mitochondria containing few cristae; the slower growing ones resemble normal hepatocytes. Animals with nonhepatic tumors have more hepatocellular lysosomes and mitochondrial interlocking as death approaches.[104]

Miscellaneous Drugs and Chemicals. Animals have been exposed to various other substances or circumstances encountered by man, either in his daily life or as a patient. These include dimethylsulfoxide,[141] the antioxidant butylated hydroxytoluene,[83] triparanol,[63] pyrrolizidine alkaloids,[163] ionizing radiation,[52] and endotoxin.[22, 29] The changes produced were nonspecific, involving the endothelial cell as well as the hepatocyte. Mitochondrial swelling and increases in the smooth endoplasmic reticulum were most often encountered.

Viral Hepatitis. Studies of animal viral hepatitides concerned mostly mouse viral hepatitis,[124] but viral disease has even been induced in resistant rats by prior partial hepatectomy.[126] Viral particles are found in vacuoles in the hepatocyte, in the space of Disse, and in Kupffer cells.[174] Glycogen decreases and focal cytoplasmic degradation is found. Mitochondria swell and smooth endoplasmic reticulum increases. Corticosteroids enhance necrosis.[125] Despite some similarities to human viral hepatitis, the differences are too great to provide useful models for the human disease. A chronic murine reovirus hepatitis showed pericellular fibrosis with capillarization of sinusoids and nonspecific hepatocellular changes, although viral particles were no longer seen.[102]

Mesenchymal Reaction. For the examination of various aspects of the mesenchymal reaction, runt disease in rats,[3, 138] canine homotransplant rejection,[75] phagocytosis of foreign particles,[30] steroid induced reticuloendothelial blockade[176] and granuloma formation around schistosome eggs[154] have been used. In general the response evoked mainly concerns macrophages and fibroblasts. The participation of leukocytes or lymphoid cells depends on the nature of the stimulus. The macrophages have many phagosomes with acid phosphatase activity and may also be responsible for extracellular digestion. Their proliferation may obstruct the flow of blood in sinusoids, and thus cause hepatocellular damage.

Cholestasis. One of the early experimental models was bile duct ligation designed to show that rupture of bile canaliculi was not responsible for jaundice in extrahepatic biliary obstruction. Loss of canalicular microvilli, dilatation of canaliculi, curling of mitochondrial cristae, enlargement of the Golgi apparatus, and phospholipid-containing vacuoles were noted. In addition, proliferated bile ductules and connections between canaliculi and ductules were studied in detail. All the changes were similar to those that occur in man with extrahepatic biliary obstruction. Regurgitation through intact cells is observed if colloidal heavy metal particles are injected into bile ducts in a retrograde fashion with ligation of the ducts.

Many drugs known to produce cholestasis in man, when given to animals, alter canaliculi as in cholestasis. This is associated with diminished ability to secrete Bromsulfalein. No special chemical configuration could be found responsible, although 17 alpha alkyl substitution in androgenic steroids increased their icterogenic potential. These steroids also produce internal rearrangements of organelles within the hepatocytic cytoplasm.[97] Since none of the drugs produced jaundice

in the animals, tests were carried out with substances that did. If the bile acid taurolithocholate, derived from the primary bile acid taurochenodeoxycholate by action of enteric bacteria, is given intravenously just in excess of the body cholate pool, it interferes with bile secretion within minutes, and it elevates serum bilirubin for a day in rats and hamsters. Within 1 hour after taurolithocholate injection, the hepatocytes lose their bile canalicular microvilli, their pericanalicular ectoplasm widens, and their Golgi lamellae and vesicles are dilated.[134] Subsequently the canaliculi dilate and endoplasmic reticulum and mitochondrial membranes are altered. By 24 hours, canaliculi begin to return to normal but ductules are now abnormal with loss of luminal microvilli and straightening of lateral cell borders. All is normal by 48 hours.

Chronic feeding of lithocholate leads to bile duct hyperplasia and gallstone formation.[101] These findings are of interest because lithocholate is present in all species as a secondary or even primary bile acid. Many species can easily reconvert it to chenodeoxycholate or to other dihydroxy bile acids. Lithocholate is a poor micelle former and probably acts by interfering with salt and water secretion mainly mediated by bile salts. The other organic anions such as the glucuronides of steroids and bilirubin as well as neutral lipids, including phospholipid, continue to be secreted to some extent. These substances may complex or precipitate with the polysaccharides of the cell surface to form bile plugs in which phospholipid and bile pigment components are recognized.[16] This model has thus served in elucidation of the pathogenesis of centrilobular cholestasis.

ORGANELLE PATHOLOGY AND THE ROLE OF ELECTRON MICROSCOPY IN LIVER DISEASES

Electron microscopy has permitted the development of Organelle Pathology. This means the recognition of structural abnormalities in viable cells which are more frequently responsible for functional changes rather than necrosis of hepatocytes. Unfortunately, almost all studies have to be carried out on biopsy material since cytoplasmic integrity is quickly lost after death. The correlation of electron microscopic and biochemical observations permits the delineation of a series of processes. One of the processes defined by electron microscopy as a disturbance of the bile secretory apparatus was cholestasis. Moreover, abnormal results of liver function tests can also be better explained by alterations of organelles detected by electron microscopy. A chain of events may take place in the liver cells as a result of injury initiated originally in one group of organelles. An initially local injury may have extensive consequences in organs and organ systems, and the same may occur in organelles of cells having several main functions. This is less frequently the case in cells like mesenchymal cells, each of which has one major function. A change in the task of the hepatocyte, or changes in its milieu or regulators, or the presence of exogenous agents such as drugs may initiate an anabolic reaction as well as a catabolic one as far as hepatocytes are concerned. Hepatocellular alterations, either necrosis or damage of viable cells, provoke a secondary mesenchymal response. An agent may interfere with transcription of DNA to RNA or translation of RNA to protein.[143] Actinomycin D, dimethylnitrosamine, ethionine, puromycin, thioacetamide or carbon tetrachloride may all initially interfere with the integrity of the rough endoplasmic reticulum by processes that interfere with the formation or function of messenger RNA or with the integrity of ribosomes, or that alter the phospholipid membrane. The initial lesion as seen with the electron microscope may thus be almost identical as the result of a catabolic effect of all these various agents. Mitochondrial swelling is usually a secondary response. The initial lesion in a group of organelles can be removed by segregation and digestion of the injured structures in autophagic vacuoles. Removal of a group of organelles, or "cellular house cleaning," also occurs in preparation for cell division when cell structure is simplified, and some, but not all,[10] somatic functions are temporarily suspended.

Anabolic intracellular regeneration may take place with replacement of damaged organelles, as for instance, when polysomes line up to form new rough endoplasmic reticulum. An anabolic adaptive response also results in that hypertrophy of smooth endoplasmic reticulum provides extra processing enzymes for the extracellular or intracellular material requiring metabolic handling. If this adaptation is overstressed, however, secondary damage may result. Hypertrophy, the enlargement of the cells, may also be followed by new formation of cells, or hyperplasia. If this becomes uncontrolled, the structure of the cell becomes oversimplified with permanent deletion of many functions. This occurs in carcinoma.

In human diseases we rarely have the opportunity to study a chain of events because the specimen under study usually is obtained long after the initial injury has occurred. What we observe is the primary effect plus the initial response, the secondary intracellular changes, and the extracellular inflammatory reaction. The ultrastructural study of liver disease provides sets of changes, no one of which is diagnostic but, just as with light microscopy, the pattern may serve to suggest the pathogenesis. Although the electron microscope has not offered diagnostic possibilities in liver disease, it has an important function in the recognition of organelle changes. With this information, future therapy may be properly directed to the altered biochemical pathways associated with each disease.

REFERENCES

1. Abrahams, C., Wheatley, A., Rubenstein, A. H., and Stables, D.: Hepatocellular lipofuscin after excessive ingestion of analgesics, Lancet 2:621, 1964.
2. Adlercreutz, H., Svanborg, A., and Anberg, A.: Recurrent jaundice in pregnancy. I. A clinical and ultrastructural study, Am. J. Med. 42:335, 1967.
3. Arakawa, K., Jézéquel, A.-M., Macvie, S. I., Johnston, R., Perz, Z. M., and Steiner, J. W.: The liver in murine transplantation (runt) disease, Am. J. Path. 49:257, 1966.
4. Asai, J.: Histological and electron microscopic investigation of the liver in the choline deficient guinea pig, Nagoya J. Med. Sci. 28:81, 1965.

5. Ashworth, C. T., Johnson, C. F., and Wrightsman, F. J: Biochemical and morphologic correlations of hepatic protein synthesis in acute ethanol intoxication in rats, Am. J. Path. 46:757, 1965.

6. Ashworth, C. T., Werner, D. J., Glass, M. D., and Arnold, N. J.: Spectrum of fine structural changes in hepatocellular injury due to thioacetamide, Am. J. Path. 47:917, 1965.

7. Baglio, C. M., and Farber, E.: Reversal by adenine of the ethionine-induced lipid accumulation in the endoplasmic reticulum of the rat liver, J. Cell Biol. 27:591, 1965.

8. Barka, T., and Popper, H.: Liver enlargement and drug toxicity, Medicine 46:103, 1967.

9. Becker, F. F., and Lane, B. P.: Regeneration of the mammalian liver. IV. Evidence on the role of cytoplasmic alterations in preparation for mitosis, Am. J. Path. 49:227, 1966.

10. ———: Regeneration of the mammalian liver. VI. Retention of phenobarbital-induced cytoplasmic alterations in dividing hepatocytes, Am. J. Path. 52:211, 1968.

11. Becker, F. F., Lane, B. P., and Teebor, G. W.: The canalicular cyst in chemical hepatectomy, Arch. Path. 83:278, 1967.

12. Benedetti, E. L., Bont, W. S. and Bloemendal, H.: Structural aspects of polyribosomes and endoplasmic reticulum fragments isolated from rat liver, Nature 210:1156, 1966.

13. Bertolini, B., and Hassan, G.: Acid phosphatase associated with the Golgi apparatus in human liver cells, J. Cell Biol. 32:216, 1967.

14. Biava, C.: Mallory's alcoholic hyalin: a heretofore unique lesion of hepatocellular ergastoplasm, Lab. Invest. 13:301, 1964.

15. ———: Studies on cholestasis: A reevaluation of the fine structure of normal human bile canaliculi, Lab. Invest. 13:840, 1964.

16. ———: Studies on cholestasis. The fine structure and morphogenesis of hepatocellular and canalicular bile pigment, Lab. Invest. 13:1099, 1964.

17. ———: Electron microscopic studies on periodic acid-Schiff-positive nonglycogenic structures in human liver cells, Am. J. Path. 46:435, 1965.

18. Biava, C., and Mukhlova-Montiel, M.: Electron microscopic observations on Councilman-like acidophilic bodies and other forms of acidophilic changes in human liver cells, Am. J. Path. 46:775, 1965.

19. Biberfeld, P., Ericsson, J. L. E., Perlmann, P., and Raftel, M.: Ultrastructural features of in vitro propagated rat liver cells, Z. Zellforsch. 71:153, 1966.

20. Biempica, L. Gutstein, S., and Arias, I. M.: Morphological and biochemical studies of benign recurrent cholestasis, Gastroenterology 52:521, 1967.

21. Bladen, H. A., Nylen, M. U., and Glenner, G. G.: The ultrastructure of human amyloid as revealed by the negative staining technique, J. Ultrastruct. Res. 14:449, 1966.

22. Boler, R. K., and Bibighaus, A. J., III: Ultrastructural alterations of the dog livers during endotoxin shock, Lab. Invest. 17:537, 1967.

23. Brewer, D. B., and Heath, D.: Electron microscopy of anoxic vacuolation in the liver cell and its comparison with sucrose vacuolation, J. Path. Bact. 90:437, 1965.

24. Bronfenmajer, S., Schaffner, F., and Popper, H.: Fat-storing cells (lipocytes) in human liver, Arch. Path. 82:447, 1966.

25. Bruni, C., and Porter, K. R.: The fine structure of the parenchymal cell of the normal rat liver. I. General consideration, Am. J. Path. 46:691, 1965.

26. Burger, P. C., and Herdson, P. B.: Phenobarbital-induced fine structural changes in rat liver, Am. J. Path. 48:793, 1966.

27. Burkel, W. E., and Low, F. N.: The fine structure of rat liver sinusoids, space of Disse and associated tissue space, Am. J. Anat. 118:769, 1966.

28. Callahan, W. P., and Lorincz, A. E.: Hepatic ultrastructure in the Hurler syndrome, Am. J. Path. 48:277, 1966.

29. Campbell, L. V., Jr., and Gilbert, E. F.: Experimental giant-cell transformation in the liver induced by E. coli endotoxin, Am. J. Path. 51:855, 1967.

30. Casley-Smith, J. R., and Reade, P. C.: An electron microscopical study of the uptake of foreign particles by the livers of foetal and adult rats, Brit. J. Exp. Path. 46:473, 1965.

31. Chiesara, E., Clementi, F., Conti, F., and Meldolesi, J.: The induction of drug-metabolizing enzymes in rat liver during growth and regeneration; a biochemical

and ultrastructural study, Lab. Invest. *16*:254, 1967.

32. Child, P. L., and Ruiz, A.: Acidophilic bodies: their chemical and physical nature in patients with Bolivian hemorrhagic fever, Arch. Path. *85*:45, 1968.

33. Confer, D. B., and Stenger, R. J.: Nodules in the liver of C3H mice after long-term carbon tetrachloride administration: a light and electron microscopic study, Cancer Res. *26*:834, 1966.

34. Cornelius, C. E., Arias, L. M., and Osburn, B. I.: Hepatic pigmentation with photosensitivity; a syndrome in Corriedale sheep resembling Dubin-Johnson syndrome in man, J. Am. Vet. Med. Assn. *146*:709, 1965.

35. Cossel, L.: Elektronenmikroskopische Befunde bei chronischer Virushepatitis und Lebercirrhose, Virchows Arch. path. Anat. *336*:354, 1963.

36. ———: Die menschlichen Leber in Elektronenmikroskop. Untersuchungen an Leberpunktaten, Jena Fisher, 1964, p. 271.

37. ———: Elektronenmikroskopische Befunde an den azidophilen Körpern bei der Virushepatitis des Menschen (Ein Beitrag zur Kenntnis der Koagulationsnekrose), J. Microscopie *4*:337, 1965.

38. ———: Elektronenmikroskopische Befunde beim intravitalen Untergang von Leberepithelzellen (Beitrag zur Kenntnis von Kolliquations und Koagulationsnekrose), Beitr. Path. Anat. *133*:156, 1966.

39. Dass, C. M. S., and Bayley, S. T.: A structural study of rat liver ribosomes, J. Cell Biol. *25*:9, 1965.

40. DeBrito, T., Borges, M. A., and DaSilva, L. C.: Electron microscopy of the liver in nonhemolytic acholuric jaundice with kernicterus (Crigler-Najjar) and in idiopathic conjugated hyperbilirubinemia (Rotor), Gastroenterologia *106*:325, 1967.

41. DeBrito, T., Marcondes Machado, M., Montans, S. D., Hoshino, G., and Freymüller, E.: Liver biopsy in human leptospirosis: a light and electron microscopic study, Virchows Arch. Exp. Path., *342*:61, 1967.

42. de Duve, C., and Baudhuin, P.: Peroxisomes (microbodies and related particles), Physiol. Rev. *46*:323, 1966.

43. De Man, J. C. H., and Blok, A. P. R.: Relationship between glycogen and agranular endoplasmic reticulum in rat hepatic cells, J. Histochem. Cytochem. *14*:135, 1966.

44. De Man, J. C. H., and Noorduyn, N. J. A.: Light and electron microscopic radioautography of hepatic cell nuclei in mice treated with actinomycin D, J. Cell Biol. *33*:489, 1967.

45. Du Boistesselin, R.: Hepatotoxicity and the ultrastructure of the liver, Excerpta Med. (Int. Congr. Series) *115*:65, 1966.

46. Edmonson, H. A., Peters, R. L., Frankel, H. H., and Borowsky, S.: The early stage of liver injury in the alcoholic, Medicine *46*:119, 1967.

47. Eliakim, M., Sadovsky, E., Stein, O., and Shenkar, Y. G.: Recurrent cholestatic jaundice of pregnancy; report of five cases and electron microscopic observations, Arch. Int. Med. *117*:696, 1966.

48. Ericsson, J. L. E., and Glinsmann, W. H.: Observations on the subcellular organization of hepatic parenchymal cells. I. Golgi apparatus, cytosomes, and cytosegresomes in normal cells, Lab. Invest. *15*:750, 1966.

49. Ericsson, J. L. E., Orrenius, S., and Holm, I.: Alterations in canine liver cells induced by protein deficiency; ultrastructural and biochemical observations, Exp. Molec. Path. *5*:329, 1966.

50. Essner, E.: Endoplasmic reticulum and the origin of microbodies in fetal mouse liver, Lab. Invest. *17*:71, 1967.

51. Franke, H., and Goetze, E.: Elektronenmikroskopische Untersuchungen über "helle" und "dunkle" Leberzellen in der regenerieren den Rattenleber, Acta biol. med. ger. *17*:99, 1966.

52. Ghidoni, J. J.: Light and electron microscopic study of primate liver 36-48 hours after high doses of 32-million-electron-volt protons, Lab. Invest. *16*:268, 1967.

53. Glinsmann, W. H., and Ericsson, J. L. E.: Observations on the subcellular organization of hepatic parenchymal cells. II. Evolution of reversible alterations induced by hypoxia, Lab. Invest. *15*:762, 1966.

54. Golberg, L.: Liver enlargement produced by drugs: its significance, Excerpta Med. (Int. Congr. Ser.) *115*:171, 1966.

55. Goldfischer, S., and Moskal, J.: Electron probe microanalysis of liver in Wilson's disease. Simultaneous assay for copper

and for lead deposited by acid phosphatase activity in lysosomes; Am. J. Path. *48*:305, 1966.

56. Hamilton, R. L., Regen, D. M., Gray, M. E., and LeQuire, V. S.: Lipid transport in liver. 1. Electron microscopic identification of very low density lipoproteins in perfused rat liver, Lab. Invest. *16*:305, 1967.

57. Heath, T., and Wissig, S. L.: Fine structure of the surface of mouse hepatic cells, Am. J. Anat. *119*:97, 1966.

58. Herdson, P. B., and Kaltenbach, J. P.: Electron microscope studies on enzyme activity and the isolation of thiohydantoin-induced myelin figures in rat liver, J. Cell Biol. *25*:485, 1965.

59. Hers, H. G.: Inborn lysosomal diseases, Gastroenterology *48*:625, 1965.

60. Hollander, M., and Schaffner, F.: Electron microscopic studies in biliary atresia. I. Bile ductular proliferation. II. Hepatocellular alterations, Am. J. Dis. Child. *116*:49, 1968.

61. Hruban, Z., Kirsten, W. H., and Slesers, A.: Fine structure of spontaneous hepatic tumors of male C3H/fGs mice, Lab. Invest. *15*:576, 1966.

62. Hruban, Z., Swift, H., and Recheigl, M., Jr.: Fine structure of transplantable hepatomas of the rat, J. Nat. Cancer Inst. *35*:459, 1965.

63. Hruban, Z., Swift, H., and Slesers, A.: Effect of triparanol and diethanolamine on the fine structure of hepatocytes and pancreatic acinar cells, Lab. Invest. *14*:1652, 1965.

64. ———: Ultrastructural alterations of hepatic microbodies, Lab. Invest. *15*:1884, 1966.

65. Huebner, G.: Direkte Tetrachlorkohlenstoffwirkung auf die Membransysteme der Zelle, Rev. int. Hépat. *15*:455, 1965.

66. ———: Zur Neubildung von dichten Körpern (sog. peribiliary bodies) in den Leberzellen der Maus, Verh. Dtsch. Ges. Path. *50*:456, 1966.

67. Hug, G., Garancis, J. C., Schubert, W. K., and Kaplan, S.: Glycogen storage disease, Types II, III, VIII and IX, Am. J. Dis. Child. *111*:457, 1966.

68. Iseri, O. A., Lieber, C. S., and Gottlieb, L. S.: The ultrastructure of fatty liver induced by prolonged ethanol ingestion, Am. J. Path. *48*:535, 1966.

69. Jatlow, P., Adams, W. R., and Hand-schumacher, R. E.: Pathogenesis of orotic acid-induced fatty change in rat liver, Am. J. Path. *47*:125, 1965.

70. Jézéquel, A.-M., Arakawa, K., and Steiner, J. W.: The fine structure of the normal neonatal mouse liver, Lab. Invest. *14*:1894, 1965.

71. Jones, A. L., and Fawcett, D. W.: Hypertrophy of the agranular endoplasmic reticulum in hamster liver induced by phenobarbital (with a review of the functions of this organelle in liver), J. Histochem. Cytochem. *14*: 215, 1966.

72. Kiessling, K. H., Pilstrom, L., Strandberg, B., and Lindgren, L.: Ethanol and the human liver; correlation between mitochondrial size and degree of ethanol abuse, Acta med. scand. *178*:533, 1965.

73. Klion, F. M., and Schaffner, F.: The ultrastructure of acidophilic "Councilman-like" bodies in the liver, Am. J. Path. *48*:755, 1966.

74. ———: Electron microscopic observations in primary biliary cirrhosis, Arch. Path. *81*:152, 1966.

75. ———: Ultrastructural features of canine hepatic auxiliary transplant rejection, Exp. Molec. Path. *6*:361, 1967.

76. ———: Ultrastructural studies in alcoholic liver disease, Digestion *1*:2, 1968.

77. Krishnan, N., and Stenger, R. J.: Effects of starvation on the hepatotoxicity of carbon tetrachloride, Am. J. Path. *49*:239, 1967.

78. Kume, F., Maruyama, S., D'Agostino, A. N., and Chiga, M.: Nucleolar change produced by mithramycin in rat hepatic cell, Exp. Molec. Path. *6*:254, 1967.

79. Kunz, F., Schaude, G., Schmid, W., and Siess, M.: Stimulation of liver growth by drugs. 1. Morphological analysis, Excerpta Med. (Int. Cong. Ser.) *115*:113, 1966.

80. Lafontaine, J. G., and Allard, C.: A light and electron microscope study of the morphologic changes induced in rat liver cells by the azo dye, 2-Me-DAB, J. Cell Biol. *22*:143, 1964.

81. Lane, B. P., and Becker, F. F.: Regeneration in the mammalian liver. V. Mitotic division in cytologically differentiated liver cells, Am. J. Path. *50*:435, 1967.

82. Lane, B. P., and Lieber, C. S.: Ultrastructural alterations in human hepatocytes following ingestion of ethanol with

adequate diets, Am. J. Path. *49*:593, 1966.

83. ————: Effects of butylated hydroxytoluene on the ultrastructure of rat hepatocytes, Lab. Invest. *16*:342, 1967.

84. Larson-Cohn, U., and Stenram, U.: Liver ultrastructure and function in icteric and nonicteric women using oral contraceptive agents, Acta med. scand. *181*:257, 1967.

85. Lundquist, R. R.: Studies on the pathogenesis of hepatolenticular degeneration. I. Acid phosphatase activity in copper-loaded rat livers. Am. J. Path. *51*:471, 1967.

86. Maruffo, C. A., Malinow, M. R., Depaoli, J. R., and Katz, S.: Pigmentary liver disease in howler monkeys, Am. J. Path. *49*:449, 1966.

87. McAdams, A. J., and Wilson, H. E.: The liver in generalized glycogen storage disease; light microscopic observations, Am. J. Path. *49*:99, 1966.

88. Meldolesi, J.: On the significance of the hypertrophy of the smooth endoplasmic reticulum in liver cells after administration of drugs, Biochem. Pharmacol. *16*:125, 1967.

89. Minio, F., and Gardiol, D.: Hépatopathie peropératoire, étude histologique, histochimique, ultrastructurale et expérimentale, Ann. Anat. Path. (Paris) *10*:301, 1965.

90. Minio, F., Gautier, A., and Magnenat, P.: L'ultrastructure du foie humain lors d'ictères idiopathiques chroniques. III. Inclusions pigmentaires dans les syndromes de Gilbert, de Rotor et de Dubin-Johnson. Z. Zellforsch. *72*:168, 1966.

91. Misugi, K., Ohajima, H., Misugi, N., and Newton, W. A., Jr.: Classification of primary malignant tumors of liver in infancy and childhood, Cancer *20*:1760, 1967.

92. Miyai, K., and Steiner, J. W.: Fine structure of interphase liver cell nuclei in acute ethionine intoxication, Lab. Invest. *16*:677, 1967.

93. Nathaniel, D. R., and Nathaniel, E. J. H.: Cytological changes in hepatic and reticuloendothelial cells in rabbit liver following gonadectomy, Am. J. Anat. *120*:537, 1966.

94. Novikoff, A. B., Essner, E., and Quintana, N.: Golgi apparatus and lysosomes, Fed. Proc. *23*:1010, 1964.

95. Novikoff, A. B.: Roheim, P. S., and Quintana, N.: Changes in rat liver cells induced by orotic acid feeding, Lab. Invest. *15*:27, 1966.

96. Ordy, J. M., Samorajski, T., Zimmerman, R. R., and Rady, P. M.: Effects of postnatal protein deficiency on weight gain, serum proteins, enzymes, cholesterol and liver ultrastructure in a subhuman primate (Macaca mulatta), Am. J. Path. *48*:769, 1966.

97. Orlandi, F., and Jézéquel, A. M.: Pathogenesis of the cholestasis induced by 17-alkylated steroids: ultrastructural and functional changes of the liver cells during treatment, Rev. int. Hépat. *16*:331, 1966.

98. Orrenius, S., and Ericsson, J. L. E.: Enzyme-membrane relationship in phenobarbital induction of synthesis of drug-metabolizing enzyme system and proliferation of endoplasmic membranes, J. Cell Biol. *28*:181, 1966.

99. Ortega, P.: Light and electron microscopy of dichlorodiphenyltrichloroethane (DDT) poisoning in the rat liver, Lab. Invest. *15*:657, 1966.

100. Palekar, S. D., and Sirsat, S. M.: Studies on the hepatocyte in azo dye carcinogenesis, Indian J. Exp. Biol. *4*:73, 1966.

101. Palmer, R. H., and Hruban, Z.: Production of bile duct hyperplasia and gallstones by lithocholic acid, J. Clin. Invest. *45*:1255, 1966.

102. Papadimitriou, J. M.: Ultrastructural features of chronic murine hepatitis after reovirus type 3 infection, Brit. J. Exp. Path. *47*:624, 1966.

103. Parks, H. F.: An experimental study of microscopic and submicroscopic lipid inclusions in hepatic cells of the mouse, Am. J. Anat. *120*:253, 1967.

104. Parry, E. W., and Ghadially, F. N.: Ultrastructural changes in the liver of tumor-bearing rats during the terminal stages of life, Cancer *19*:821, 1966.

105. Phillips, M. J., and Steiner, J. W.: Electron microscopy of liver cells in cirrhotic nodules. I. The lateral cell membranes. Am. J. Path. *46*:985, 1965.

106. ————: Electron microscopical studies on the liver cells in hyperplastic nodules of human cirrhosis, Rev. int. Hépat. *16*:307, 1966.

107. ————: Electron microscopy of cirrhotic nodules. Tubularization of the paren-

chyma by biliary hepatocytes, Lab. Invest. *15*:801, 1966.

108. Phillips, M. J., Unakar, N. J., Doornervaard, G., and Steiner, J. W.: Glycogen depletion in the newborn rat liver. An electron microscope and electron histochemical study, J. Ultrastruct. Res. *18*: 142, 1967.

109. Pollak, J. K., and Shorey, C. D.: Changes in ultrastructure of embryonic chick livers during morphogenesis, Aust. J. exp. Biol. med. Sci. *45*:393, 1967.

110. Popper, H., and Schaffner, F.: Die Mesenchymreaktion auf Parenchymschädigungen. Zum Problem der chronischen Hepatitis, Med. Welt *10*:1082, 1965.

111. ———: The problem of chronicity in liver disease, *in* Popper. H., and Schaffner, F. (eds.): Progress in Liver Diseases, vol. II, New York, Grune & Stratton, 1965, pp. 519–538.

112. Porta, E. A., Bergman, B. J., and Stein, A. A.: Acute alcoholic hepatitis, Am. J. Path. *46*:657, 1965.

113. Porta, E. A., Hartroft, W. S., and de la Iglesia, F. A: Hepatic changes associated with chronic alcoholism in rats, Lab. Invest. *14*:1437, 1965.

114. Porta, E. A., Hartroft, W. S., Gomez-Dumm, C. L. A., and Koch, O. R.: Dietary factors in the progression and regression of hepatic alterations associated with experimental chronic alcoholism, Fed. Proc. *26*:1449, 1967.

115. Remmer, H.: Liver cell damage and drug metabolizing enzymes, Excerpta Med. (Int. Congr. Ser.) *115*:154, 1966.

116. Reynolds, E. S.: Liver parenchymal cell injury. III. The nature of calcium-associated electron-opaque masses in rat liver mitochondria following poisoning with carbon tetrachloride, J. Cell Biol. *25*:53, 1965.

117. Reynolds, R. C., and Montgomery, P. O'B.: Nuclear pathology produced by acridine orange and proflavine, Am. J. Path. *57*:323, 1967.

118. Richter, G. W., and Bessis, M. C.: Commentary on hemosiderin, Blood *25*:370, 1965.

119. Rosen, S. I., Kelly, G. W., and Peters, V. B.: Glucose-6-phosphatase in tubular endoplasmic reticulum of hepatocytes, Science *152*:352, 1966.

120. Rosen, S., Roycroft, D. W., Hano, J. E., and Barry, K. G.: The liver in malaria: electron microscopic observations on a hepatic biopsy obtained 15 minutes post mortem, Arch. Path. *83*:271, 1967.

121. Rouiller, C., Colombey, N., Haenni, B., Perrelet, A., asd deTorrente, A.: Les modifications des parois des capillaires sinusoides du foie dans les intoxications aiguës expérimentales, Rev. int. Hépat. *15*:437, 1965.

122. Rubin, E., and Lieber, C. S.: Early fine structural changes in the human liver induced by alcohol, Gastroenterology *52*:1, 1967.

123. Ruebner, B. H., Gonzalez-Licea, A., and Slusser, R. J.: Electron microscopy of some human hepatomas, Gastroenterology *53*:18, 1967.

124. Ruebner, B. H., and Hirano, T.: Viral hepatitis in mice; changes in oxidative enzymes and phosphatases after murine hepatitis virus (MHV_3) infection, Lab. Invest. *14*:157, 1965.

125. Ruebner, B. H., Hirano, T., and Slusser, R. J.: Electron microscopy of the hepatocellular and Kupffer-cell lesions of mouse hepatitis, with particular reference to the effect of cortisone, Am. J. Path. *51*:163, 1967.

126. Ruffolo, P. R., Margolis, G., and Kilham, L.: The induction of hepatitis by prior partial hepatectomy in resistant adult rats injected with H-1 virus, Am. J. Path. *49*:795, 1966.

127. Ruffolo, R., and Covington, H.: Matrix inclusion bodies in the mitochondria of the human liver: Evidence of hepatocellular injury, Am. J. Path. *51*:101, 1967.

128. Safran, A. P., and Schaffner, F.: Chronic passive congestion of the liver in man, electron microscopic study of cell atrophy and intralobular fibrosis, Am. J. Path. *50*:447, 1967.

129. Sasaki, H., Schaffner, F., and Popper, H.: Bile ductules in cholestasis: morphologic evidence for secretion and absorption in man, Lab. Invest. *16*:84, 1967.

130. Schaffner, F.: Morphologic studies on bile secretion, Am. J. Dig. Dis. *10*:99, 1965.

131. ———: Electron microscopic studies in chronic hepatitis, *in* Vandenbroucke, J., and de Groote, J. (eds.): Advances in Hepatology, Tr. Int. Assoc. Study Liver Dis., Basle, S. Karger; Baltimore, Williams & Wilkins, 1965, pp. 31–38.

132. Schaffner, F.: Intralobular changes in hepatocytes and the electron microscopic mesenchymal response in acute viral hepatitis, Medicine 45:547, 1966.

133. Schaffner, F., and Felig, P.: Changes in hepatic structure in rats produced by breathing pure oxygen, J. Cell Biol. 27: 505, 1965.

134. Schaffner, F., and Javitt, N. B.: Morphologic changes in hamster liver during intrahepatic cholestasis induced by taurolithocholate. Lab. Invest. 15:1783, 1966.

135. Schaffner, F., and Popper, H.: Electron microscopy of human liver disease in Crawford T. (ed.): Modern Trends in Pathology, vol. II, London, Butterworth, 1967, pp. 252–300.

136. Schaffner, F., Roberts, D. K., Ginn, F. L., and Ulvedal, F.: Electron microscopy of monkey liver after exposure of animals to pure oxygen atmosphere, Proc. Soc. Exp. Biol. Med. 121:1200, 1966.

137. Schaffner, F., and Sasaki, H.: Ultrastructural studies on drug-induced cholestasis, Rev. int. Hépat. 15:461, 1965.

138. Schlesinger, M., and Essner, E.: Histochemical and electron microscopic studies of the liver in runt disease, Am. J. Path. 47:371, 1965.

139. Schlunk, F. F., and Lombardi, B.: Liver liposomes. I. Isolation and chemical characterization, Lab. Invest. 17:30, 1967.

140 Schnack, H., Stockinger, L., and Wewalka, W.: Die Bindegewebszelen des Disséschen Raumes in der menschlichen Leber bei Normalfällen und pathologischen Zuständen, Wien, klin. Wschr. 78: 715, 1966.

141. Shilkin, K. B., Papadimutriou, J. M., and Walters, M. N. I.: The effect of dimethylsulphoxide on hepatic cells of rats, Aust. J. Exp. Biol. Med. Sci. 44:581, 1966.

142. Skinner, M. S., Kattine, A. A., and Spurlock, B. O.: Electron microscopic observations of early amyloidosis in human liver, Gastroenterology 50:243, 1966.

143. Smuckler, E. A., and Barker, E. A.: Effect of drugs on amino acid incorporation in the liver, Excerpta Med. (Int. Congr. Ser.) 15:83, 1966.

144. Smuckler, E. A., and Benditt, E. P.: The early effects of actinomycin on rat liver. Changes in ribosomes and polysomes, Lab. Invest. 14:1699, 1965.

145. Smuckler, E. A., Ross, R., and Benditt, E. P.: Effects of carbon tetrachloride on guinea pig liver, Exp. Molec. Path. 4: 328, 1965.

146. Sparrow, W. T., and Ashworth, C. T.: Electron microscopy of nuclear glycogenosis, Arch. Path. 80:84, 1965.

147. Stein, O., and Stein, Y.: Lipid synthesis, intracellular transport, storage and secretion. I. Electron microscopic autoradiographic study of liver after injection of tritiated palmitate or glycerol in fasted and ethanol-treated rats, J. Cell Biol. 33: 319, 1967.

148. Stein, R. J., Richter, W. R., and Brynjolfsson, G.: Ultrastructural pharmacopathology. I. Comparative morphology of the livers of the normal street dog and purebred beagle; a base-line study, Exp. Molec. Path. 5:195, 1966.

149. Steiner, J. W., Jézéquel, A. M., Phillips, M. J., Miyai, K., and Arakawa, K.: Some aspects of the ultrastructural pathology of the liver, in Popper, H., and Schaffner, F. (eds.): Progress in Liver Diseases vol. II, New York, Grune & Stratton, 1965, pp. 303–372.

150. Stenger, R. J.: Fibrogenesis along the hepatic sinusoids in carbon tetrachloride-induced cirrhosis, an electron microscopic study, Exp. Molec. Path. 4:357, 1965.

151. ———: Hepatic sinusoids in carbon tetrachloride-induced cirrhosis; an electron microscopic study, Arch. Path. 81: 439, 1966.

152. ———: Concentric lamellar formations in hepatic parenchymal cells of carbon tetrachloride-treated rats, J. Ultrastruct. Res. 14:240, 1966.

153. Stenger, R. J., and Confer, D. B.: Hepatocellular ultrastructure during liver regeneration after subtotal hepatectomy, Exp. Molec. Path. 5:455, 1966.

154. Stenger, R. J., Warren, K. S., and Johnson, E. A.: An ultrastructural study of hepatic granulomas and schistosome eggshells in murine hepatosplenic schistosomiasis mansoni, Exp. Molec. Path. 7: 116, 1967.

155. Stenram, U., and Willen, R.: The effect of actinomycin D on ultrastructure and radioautographic ribonucleic acid and protein labeling in rat liver after partial hepatectomy, Cancer Res. 26:765, 1966.

156. ———: Electron microscope observations of inhibitory effect of puromycin on liver regeneration after partial hepatectomy, Exp. Cell Res. 42:457, 1967.

157. Sternlieb, I.: Electron microscopic study of intrahepatic biliary ductules, J. Microscopie 4:71, 1965.

158. ———: Perinuclear filaments and microtubules in human hepatocytes and biliary epithelial cells, J. Microscopie 4:551, 1965.

159. Sulkin, NM., and Sulkin, DF.: An electron microscopic study of the effects of chronic hypoxia on cardiac muscle, hepatic and autonomic ganglion cells, Lab. Invest. 14:1523, 1965.

160. Svoboda, D., Grady, H., and Azarnoff, D.: Microbodies in experimentally altered cells, J. Cell Biol. 35:127, 1967.

161. Svoboda, D., Grady, H. J., and Higginson, J.: Aflatoxin B₁ injury in rat and monkey liver, Am. J. Path. 49:1023, 1966.

162. ———: The effects of chronic protein deficiency in rats. II. Biochemical and ultrastructural changes, Lab. Invest. 15:731, 1966.

163. Svoboda, D., and Soga, J.: Early effects of pyrrolizidine alkaloids on the fine structure of rat liver cells, Am. J. Path. 48:347, 1966.

164. Takada, A., Porta, E. A., and Hartroft, W. S.: The recovery of experimental dietary cirrhosis. I. Functional and structural features. Am. J. Path. 51:929, 1967.

165. Tanikawa, K., and Hojiro, O.: Electron microscopic observation of the liver in kala azar, Kurume Med., J. 12:148, 1965.

166. Tanikawa, K., and Tanaka, M.: Electron microscopic observation of thioridazine-induced hepatitis, Kurume Med. J. 13:15, 1966.

167. Theron, J. J., van der Merwe, K. J., Liebenberg, N., Joubert, H. J. B., and Nel, W.: Acute liver injury in ducklings and rats as a result of ochratoxin poisoning, J. Path. Bact. 91:521, 1966.

168. Thorpe, M. E. C., and Shorey, C. D.: Long term alcohol administration; its effects on the ultrastructure and lipid content of the rat liver cell, Am. J. Path. 48:557, 1966.

169. Toker, C., and Trevino, N.: Hepatic ultrastructure in chronic idiopathic jaundice, Arch. Path. 80:453, 1965.

170. ———: Ultrastructure of human primary hepatic carcinoma, Cancer 19:1594, 1966.

171. Trump, B. F., Goldblatt, P. J., and Stowell, R. E.: Studies of necrosis in vitro of mouse hepatic parenchymal cell, Lab. Invest. 14:1946, 1969, 2000, 1965.

172. Volk, B. W., and Wallace, B. J.: The liver in lipoidosis. An electron microscopic and histochemical study, Am. J. Path. 49:203, 1966.

173. Watanabe, H.: A fine structural study of liver culture, Exp. Cell Res. 42:685, 1966.

174. Watanabe, K., and Ichida, F.: Electron microscopic studies of experimental viral hepatitis in mice, Ann. Rep. Inst. Virus Res. Kyoto Univ. 8:107, 1965.

175. Weingärtner, L., Cossel, L., and Wagner, G.: Zur Leberbeteiligung bei Säuglingstoxikosen (bioptische Untersuchungen mittels des Licht- und Elektronenmikroskopes), Arch. Kinderheilk. 174:242, 1966.

176. Wiener, J., Cottrell, T. S., Margaretten, W., and Spiro, D.: An electron microscopic study of steroid induced reticuloendothelial blockade, Am. J. Path. 50:187, 1967.

177. Wills, E. J.: Crystalline structures in the mitochondria of normal human liver parenchymal cells, J. Cell Biol. 24:511, 1965.

178. Wills, E. J., and Epstein, M. A.: Subcellular changes in surface adenosine triphosphatase activity of human liver in extrahepatic obstructive jaundice, Am. J. Path. 49:605, 1966.

179. Wood, R. L.: The fine structure of hepatic cells in chronic ethionine poisoning and during recovery, Am. J. Path. 46:307, 1965.

180. Wruble, L. D., Ladman, A. J., Britt, L. G., and Cummins, A. J.: Hepatotoxicity produced by tetracycline overdosage, J.A.M.A. 192:6, 1965.

181. Zaki, F. G.: Ultrastructure of hepatic cholestasis, Medicine 45:537, 1966.

3

Secretion of Bile

HENRY O. WHEELER, M.D.

Bile is a complex aqueous solution of organic and inorganic compounds. Its flow, composition, color, viscosity and total solid content all vary widely from time to time and from one species to another. When bile enters the duodenum a large proportion of its constituents are not irreversibly "excreted" but are destined for reabsorption and return to the liver. Thus enterohepatic circulation plays an important part in the physiology of bile formation, and the very maneuvers that are necessary for the study of the biliary system—always involving some form of biliary diversion—must necessarily disturb the normal physiology of the system. Nevertheless, information obtained from extensive human and animal investigation has provided important clues regarding the normal mechanisms of bile formation and the many factors that regulate or modify bile production.

BILE COMPOSITION

OSMOLALITY

The osmolality of bile, as measured by freezing point depression or vapor pressure, is usually close to that of plasma—that is, approximately 300 mOsm./Kg. under normal conditions of hydration.[23, 44, 119, 137] Moreover, Gilman and Cowgill showed in dogs that the osmolality of bile faithfully mirrors the plasma osmolality as the latter is varied by infusions of hypertonic or hypotonic solutions.[44] Nevertheless, some deviation from isotonicity has been observed in dogs at high bile flows, consisting of slight hypotonicity during rapid bile salt infusions

and slight hypertonicity following secretin administration.[95] This deviation rarely amounts to more than 15 per cent of total plasma osmolality and is seen only under the artificial conditions mentioned. Its significance has not been elucidated.

ORGANIC SOLUTES

The major organic solutes of bile are the bile salts, phospholipids, cholesterol and bile pigments. Other constituents including proteins are present in very low concentrations. The bile salts and phospholipids (principally lecithin), make up the major fraction of the total solids in all but the most dilute bile specimens. In the human hepatic bile specimens reported by Thureborn, for example, typical concentrations of the bile salts ranged from 3 to 45 mEq./L. (corresponding to 140 to 2230 mg.%, or 8 to 53 per cent of total solids by weight), concentrations of lecithin from 140 to 810 mg.% (or 9 to 21 per cent of solids), cholesterol concentrations from 97 to 320 mg.% (3 to 11 per cent of total solids), and bilirubin concentrations from 12 to 70 mg.% (0.4 to 2 per cent of total solids).[128] In gallbladder bile the concentrations of all these constituents are appreciably higher, owing to reabsorption of water and inorganic electrolytes by the gallbladder.[63, 65, 74, 80]

The importance of the combination of bile salts and lecithin in the solubilization of cholesterol was first recognized by Isaksson.[64] A precise picture of the physical chemistry of cholesterol solubilization has been presented recently by Bourgès, Small, and Dervichian[16] and discussed in a review by Hofmann and Small.[60] These authors em-

TABLE 3–1. HEPATIC BILE ELECTROLYTE COMPOSITION

SPECIES	NA+	K+	CA++	MG++	CL−	HCO3−	BILE SALT	REFERENCES
Man	146–165	2.7– 4.9	2.5– 4.8	1.4–3.0	88–115	27–55	3– 45	128
Dog	141–230	4.5–11.9	3.1–13.8	2.2–5.5	31–107	14–61	16–187	28, 95, 98, 100, 137
Rabbit	142–157	3.6– 6.7	2.7– 6.7	0.3–0.7	77– 89	44–49		118, 124
Sheep	154–179	6.7– 7.6			83–122			56

phasize that normal bile is a true aqueous solution in which the bile salts, lecithin and cholesterol are present as stable anionic mixed micelles—a phenomenon that accounts for the fact that biliary lecithin and cholesterol concentrations far exceed the maximal aqueous solubility of these compounds in simple solution. It is probably not a great oversimplification to say that the likelihood of cholesterol precipitation in the form of gallstones must be a predictable function of the relative concentrations of just 4 constituents: water, bile salts (regardless of type), lecithin and cholesterol.[16, 60, 74] In species that are susceptible to spontaneous gallstone formation—notably man—the relative concentrations of the 4 critical constituents in bile are frequently close to the limiting boundary for cholesterol solubilization determined *in vitro* for the pure quaternary system.[60] The problem of gallstone formation is complicated by the intriguing relationships between the constituents involved. Cholesterol is the metabolic precursor of the bile salts so that cholesterol solubilization is intimately dependent upon the concentration of its own metabolite. Moreover, Kay and Entenman[76] and Sperber[122a] have shown that biliary excretion of lecithin is intimately dependent upon the rate of bile salt excretion.

Protein concentrations in bile are very low—6 to 40 mg.% in canine bile[55] and 30 to 300 mg.% in human bile.[55, 102, 106, 128] Serum albumin is usually the most abundant protein in bile. Although nonserum proteins may also be detectable,[55, 75] the existence of a separate class of biliary proteins has been questioned.[105] The bile canaliculi and bile duct epithelium are quite impermeable to proteins.

INORGANIC SOLUTES

Whereas relatively large organic molecules—particularly bile salts and lecithin—make up the bulk of the total solid content of bile, the lighter inorganic electrolytes account for the major fraction of the total osmotic activity. The range of values reported for concentrations of the common electrolytes in bile can be appreciated from Table 3–1. In general, the relative distribution of cations is similar to that in plasma, with sodium always the most abundant cation. The bile acids in all mammalian species are conjugated with glycine or taurine, resulting in values of pK well below the physiologic range of biliary pH, and are therefore present as anions rather than undissociated acids. Thus the sum of the inorganic anion concentrations in bile equals the sum of the total cation concentrations minus the total bile salt concentration. Inorganic anions, of which chloride and bicarbonate are the most abundant, therefore often have much lower total concentrations in bile than in plasma—particularly in specimens of gallbladder bile. The bicarbonate/chloride ratio is sometimes appreciably higher in bile than in plasma. The bicarbonate concentration—both relative and absolute—may be substantially elevated under some circumstances such as secretin or gastrin stimulation (see below), and is apparently always high in certain species such as the rabbit[118, 124] and guinea pig.[118]

Table 3–1 emphasizes that the total cation concentration is often much higher in bile than in plasma (or, for that matter, in an isotonic sodium chloride solution). Sodium concentration alone may be as high as 230 mEq./L. in hepatic bile[137] and occasional sodium concentrations as high as 330 mEq./L. have been reported in gallbladder bile.[36] All of these specimens are isotonic, and the unusual electrolyte concentrations are attributable to the aggregation of individual bile salt ions into large micelles (with consequent loss of osmotic activity).

The point is illustrated in Figure 3–1, in which typical specimens of canine gallbladder bile, fasting common duct bile and plasma are compared. Hepatic bile, in which both bile salts and inorganic anions are appreciably concentrated, occupies an intermediate position between the extremes of total cation concentration illustrated in Figure 3–1. The total osmotic activity of bile has been found, empirically, to be accounted for by ignoring the bile salt anions altogether and taking the sum of the major inorganic ion concentrations (i.e., $Na^+ + K^+, + Cl^- + HCO_{-3}$).[98, 100] This is equivalent to the finding that there is, in various bile specimens, a roughly linear correlation between the total cation concentration and the bile salt concentration corresponding to the equation: $[BS^-] = 2.03 [Na^+ + K^+] - 302.$[137]

The observed relationship between bile salt concentration and total cation concentration in isotonic bile specimens need not mean, necessarily, that bile salt anions are totally inactive and other ions totally dissociated. One might expect that cations would be rendered osmotically inactive, to some extent, by attraction as "gegen ions"[59, 85] to the large polyanionic micelles, and that the bile acids, on the other hand, might not be entirely inactivated by aggregation. Diamond reports that sodium ion activity coefficients in sodium deoxycholate solutions are only 0.35 to 0.40 as measured by a sodium-sensitive glass electrode.[34] More recent studies by Moore and Dietschy, however, show that the activity coefficient of sodium in whole gallbladder bile and in bile salt solutions is 0.62 to 0.70, only slightly lower than the activity coefficient of sodium in sodium sulfate solutions of similar concentration.[86] This provides some justification for the simplified assumption that bile salt anions—in the micellar state—have little osmotic activity and that the osmolality of bile is indeed attributable, in the main, to the

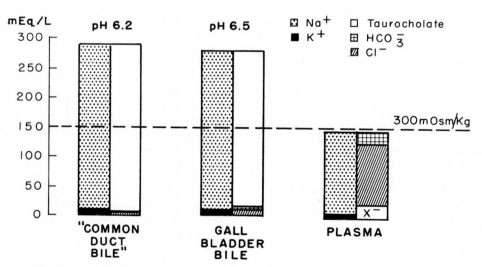

FIG. 3–1. *Composition of canine "common duct bile," gallbladder bile and plasma.* Bile withdrawn from the common bile duct of a fasting cholecystectomized dog and typical canine gallbladder bile both have very high concentrations of bile salt, total cation concentrations close to 300 mEq./L and very low concentrations of inorganic anions. The osmolality of these bile specimens, like that of plasma, is close to 300 mOsm./kg., owing to the fact that a large proportion of the bile salt is in the form of osmotically inactive micelles. (Reproduced from J. Clin. Invest.[137])

osmotic activity of its inorganic ionic constituents.

BILIARY SECRETORY MECHANISMS

ACTIVE SECRETION

Mechanisms of bile pigment excretion are discussed elsewhere in detail. The bile pigments represent but a few of the many organic compounds that are excreted into the bile in high concentration. Among the organic acids are such diverse compounds as phenolphthalein derivatives,[58, 120] certain hippuric acid derivatives,[28, 32] a number of sulfonamides,[33] penicillin,[28] erythromycin,[130] ampicillin,[8] cyanine dyes,[24, 133] phlorhizin,[68] chlorothiazide,[57] the bile salts (both natural and synthetic), and many other endogenous and exogenous organic acids.

In his review of organic anion secretion, Sperber points out the close similarity between the biliary system and the renal tubule with respect to the types of organic acids secreted.[120] However, certain differences should be mentioned. First, compounds that are firmly bound to plasma albumin (e.g., bilirubin, sulfobromophthalein, rose bengal, indocyanine green) may be rapidly excreted in bile and only sparingly excreted in urine. This does not necessarily signify a difference in renal and biliary transport capacities for these compounds but may be related to the fact that the hepatic sinusoids, unlike the peritubular capillaries, are apparently very "leaky" with respect to plasma albumin[47] so that protein-bound substances have direct access to hepatic parenchymal cells but not to renal tubular cells. Second, the bile salts do not appear to be secreted by the renal tubules. Indeed, there is evidence that they may be reabsorbed,[132] and failure of renal tubular secretion cannot be attributed to unusually firm protein binding.[104, 132] This fact, together with data from competition studies (see below), suggests that bile salt transport should be considered separately from the transport of most other organic acids.

A group of quaternary ammonium cations, of which procaine amide ethobromide (PAEB) is the best characterized, represents an entirely separate class of compounds

that are rapidly excreted into the bile.[110, 112]

Finally, there are a few compounds which are neither organic acids nor bases whose rapid biliary excretion suggests that they are actively secreted. Included among these are several cardiac glycosides[79] and low molecular weight polyethylene glycol (PEG–1500) a compound whose biliary secretion has thus far been shown only in the chicken.[121]

It is generally assumed that all of the compounds mentioned are "actively" transported from the liver cells into the bile canaliculi, but evidence for this is indirect and not entirely rigorous. The principal findings suggestive of active secretion are: concentration, saturation, and competition.

If the steady state concentration of a given compound is appreciably higher in bile than in plasma it has been assumed that an active process is responsible for its secretion.[17, 28] The fluorescence micrographs of Hanzon[54] (Fig. 3–2) and of Grafflin[50] provide striking examples of the events involved in the biliary excretion of fluorescein. Within a few seconds of intravenous injection of fluorescein in the rat there is appreciable diffuse concentration of the dye within hepatic parenchymal cells and early visualization of fluorescence in the bile canaliculi. Within 4 to 5 minutes the bile canaliculi are intensely fluorescent and thereafter the diffuse fluorescence of the liver cells gradually fades. Thus it would appear that the dye is concentrated in 2 stages (see section on kinetics below). The final biliary concentration (as judged by the intensity of fluorescence in the canaliculi) is so much higher than that observed at any time within the sinusoids or liver cells that it is reasonable to postulate the existence of a very efficient secretory mechanism located at the membrane facing the bile canaliculi. This type of evidence is intuitively satisfying and is supported by the finding that many of the other compounds in question are concentrated in the bile several hundred- or even thousandfold when compared with their plasma concentrations.

The accumulation of a particular substance in high concentration need not mean, however, that there is a specific active transport mechanism for that substance. One transport process can be coupled to another

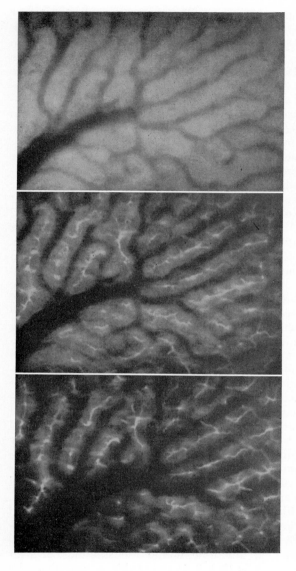

FIG. 3–2. *Fluorescence micrographs of rat liver following intravenous injection of fluorescein.*

Top: Within 55 seconds of injection the fluorescent material is no longer visible in the hepatic sinusoids (black regions) but is concentrated in hepatic parenchymal cells. *Middle:* At 4 minutes the fluorescein is seen at very high concentration in bile canaliculi and intracellular fluorescence is beginning to fade. *Bottom:* At 8 minutes intense fluorescence is seen in the canaliculi and concentration in liver cells has faded markedly. (Reproduced from the studies of V. Hanzon: Acta physiol. scand.[54])

in a variety of ways.[140] Moreover, concentration alone is not sufficient evidence for the existence of chemical disequilibrium. Charged particles may accumulate passively in response to an electrical potential gradient. For example, in the case of a monovalent ion, a gradient of approximately 60 millivolts would be associated with a tenfold concentration difference and a gradient of 180 mv. would lead to a hundredfold concentration difference at equilibrium.[131] The electrical potential difference across the canalicular membrane is unknown, but of course an electrical gradient could not account for the accumulation of neutral compounds nor for the fact that both anionic and cationic compounds have been found to accumulate in the bile. The total concentration of certain compounds may not, however, reflect true chemical activity. In particular, the total bile salt concentration in bile far exceeds the chemical activity of "free" bile salt anions, since most of this material is in the form of micelles. Thus, to some extent, the very high concentration of bile salts might be facilitated by trapping of these compounds in micelles, and it is possible that a variety of other substances could also be included in this process.

Saturation of biliary excretory capacity has been shown for several compounds. The transport maximum for conjugated bilirubin is approximately 60 μg./100 gm. body weight/minute in the rat.[7] In the case of sulfobromophthalein (BSP), an excretory transport maximum of 1.9 mg./min./10 Kg. has been found in the dog[136] and 5.7 to 14.1 mg./min. in normal man.[2, 113, 116, 136] The maximal excretory capacity for sodium taurocholate in the dog is 8.5 $\pm$ 1.6 (S.D.) μM./Kg. body weight/min.[89] and similar values have been obtained for glycocholate.[91] If a compound is toxic or if its solubility is limited, then an apparent transport maximum may be achieved when the concentration in a critical location causes impairment of function or leads to precipitation. In the cases mentioned, however, neither toxicity nor solubility appears to be limiting, and the finding of "saturation" argues strongly in favor of an association between the transported compound and some element in the transport pathway whose available binding sites are saturable. In the terminology employed by students of membrane transport, saturation implies "carrier-mediated" transport, though not necessarily primary active transport.

Competition between transported compounds has been observed in the case of the phenolphthalein derivatives[122] and between iopanoic acid and BSP.[115] Probenecid has been found to compete with the excretion of a variety of anionic compounds in the biliary system,[32, 33, 45, 57] just as it does in the kidney. Thus most of the anions that have been studied appear to share a common rate-limiting step or carrier.[120] Bile salt transport may proceed by a pathway that is separate from that involved with the other anions since bile salts do not appear to interfere with maximal sulfobromophthalein or indocyanine green excretion[135] and may, under some circumstances, actually enhance maximal biliary BSP excretion.[90] The existence of a separate biliary transport process for the bile salts could also explain the absence of renal tubular secretion of bile salts,[132] and would be consistent

with the report of Arias that mutant Corriedale sheep which have markedly depressed transport maxima for BSP (and also reduced secretion of phyllo-erythrin, conjugated bilirubin, metanephrine glucuronide and iodopanoic acid) have been found to have a perfectly normal maximal biliary excretion of taurocholate.[6] Competition studies indicate that the transport mechanism for organic cations is entirely separate from that involved in anion transport.[6, 112] Biliary excretion of the cardiac glycosides is not altered by any of the other classes of compounds and thus appears to involve still another discrete transport system.[79]

In summary, therefore, the weight of evidence based on biliary concentration, transport maxima and competition appears to favor (even if it does not prove) the existence of carrier-mediated active secretion and suggests that more or less independent transport mechanisms exist for at least 4 classes of compounds: the bulk of the organic anions, the bile salts, the organic cations, and certain neutral compounds. Additional independent transport processes may, of course, be revealed in future studies.

UPTAKE AND EXCRETORY TRANSPORT KINETICS

The foregoing comments have focused attention upon the transport of compounds from the hepatic parenchymal cells into the bile canaliculi. Under steady-state maximal loading conditions this is the process that usually appears to be rate-limiting, but all compounds that move from plasma to bile must first enter the liver cells across the sinusoidal membrane and many compounds undergo chemical modification (conjugation) prior to final transport into the bile. The kinetics of hepatic uptake, like those of excretion, appear to be saturable and to exhibit competition between similar compounds. Competition between bilirubin, BSP, and indocyanine green for hepatic uptake has been demonstrated by examination of initial disappearance rates,[62] and Goresky[48, 49] has shown that hepatic uptake of BSP exhibits saturation (i.e., Michaelis-Menton) kinetics of the form illustrated in Figure 3–3. A similar model for hepatic uptake was proposed by Winkler and Gram

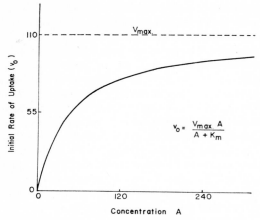

FIG. 3–3. *Illustration of the relation between approximate initial rate of hepatic uptake of sulfobromophthalein (mg./ min./10 kg. body weight) and plasma concentration (mg./100 ml.).* Hepatic uptake, like biliary secretion, exhibits saturation, but the value of V_{max} for uptake is much higher than the excretory Tm (1.9 mg./min./10 kg. body weight). (Reproduced from C. Goresky: Canad. Med. Ass. J.[49])

on the basis of their BSP disappearance studies.[141] Thus it would appear that hepatic uptake and biliary excretion *both* involve saturable carrier-mediated processes. However, the uptake step has a much higher "Tm" than the excretory step (see Fig. 3–3) and approaches saturation only during the very transient high plasma concentrations which follow a sudden large intravenous injection of a dye such as BSP.

At the intermediate plasma levels of BSP which are achieved during sustained intravenous infusions, biliary excretion may be saturated and therefore constant, but the hepatic uptake of BSP appears to operate in such a manner as to maintain a fixed ratio between the concentrations of dye in the liver cells and in the plasma.[48, 136] This has made it possible to use a multiple BSP infusion technic for the measurement of hepatic "relative storage capacity" and excretory transport maximum.[2, 113, 116, 136] The relative storage capacity (usually expressed as "S," in units of milligrams of BSP stored in the liver per milligram per cent of plasma concentration) can be viewed as a measure of

the integrity of the hepatic uptake system, but may also depend upon the binding capacity of certain intracellular constituents for the test material. The BSP excretory transport maximum, or Tm, can be estimated without bile collection by the multiple infusion technic, and the estimates agree reasonably well with direct measurements of biliary BSP output, when available.[117, 136] The use of this test has revealed that a dissociation is possible between uptake and excretory transport function in certain situations. Thus in the Dubin-Johnson syndrome,[136] or following the administration of certain steroids,[113] capacity to transport BSP into bile ("Tm") may be markedly depressed at a time when the uptake function (as measured by "S") is normal.

Intrahepatic conjugation is apparently an almost mandatory step prior to biliary excretion of bilirubin and certain other compounds. Other substances, of which indocyanine green is an example,[24, 133] are excreted without any chemical alteration. Sulfobromophthalein (BSP) is partially conjugated with glutathione prior to excretion,[26, 51, 67] and it has been postulated that conjugation is necessary for optimal transport of BSP into bile.[25] However, an analog of BSP, phenol-3,6-dibromphthalein disulfonate, is rapidly excreted without any chemical alteration,[66] which suggests that BSP conjugation may not be essential for transport. These facts are mentioned simply to emphasize the point that intrahepatic conjugation may or may not play an important role in the overall kinetics of uptake and excretion, depending upon the compound in question. While conjugation is not ordinarily rate-limiting, deficiency of bilirubin conjugation has serious consequences in the human Crigler-Najjar syndrome[29] and in the Gunn rat.[114] At the opposite extreme, conjugation need not even be considered in evaluating the kinetics of indocyanine green uptake and excretion.

MECHANISMS OF BILE FORMATION

THEORETICAL CONSIDERATIONS

Bile is normally secreted without major hydrostatic opposition. However, under experimental circumstances bile formation can proceed against opposing pressures of the order of 20 mm. Hg.[11, 12, 13, 18, 19, 101] The demonstration by Brauer, Leong, and Holloway[19] that bile secretion pressure of the isolated rat liver can greatly exceed the vascular perfusion pressure makes it clear that the energy for bile formation cannot be derived from the hydrostatic pressure of the blood. Bile formation, like the secretion processes in other exocrine glands (and unlike the formation of glomerular filtrate in the kidney), must depend upon energy supplied by local chemical sources rather than by mechanical contraction of the heart.

The possible mechanisms for translation of metabolic energy into hydraulic flow have recently come under close scrutiny in relation to studies of fluid absorption by such tissues as the intestinal epithelium, the gallbladder epithelium and the proximal renal tubule. Basically 3 mechanisms have been considered: active transport of water *per se*, active solute transport leading to local osmotic flow, and secretory vacuole formation, pinocytosis or similar mechanical phenomena.

There are certain major theoretical objections to the first mechanism, active water transport. Most cell membranes are highly permeable to water, judging by the uniformity of osmolality in all tissues except the renal medulla,[83] so that an active water "pump" would have to keep pace with an extraordinarily high rate of back-leakage. Moreover, the ratio of water molecules to solute particles in an isotonic solution is approximately 180:1, so that the theoretical capacity of a water pump would have to be far greater, in terms of moles per unit time, than that of a solute pump involved in processing the same volume of solution.

Active transport of solute into a confined region leads to the development of a local osmotic gradient which can pull water and other diffusible solutes into the same region. A model of this sort proposed by Curran,[30, 88] and further characterized by Patlak, Goldstein, and Hoffman[93] consists of 2 dissimilar membranes in series, with a nondistensible compartment between them. This model leads to predictions that are consistent with apparent active transport of an isotonic solu-

tion across the gallbladder epithelium.[77, 139] A fairly similar arrangement, in which active solute transport leads to a "standing osmotic gradient" that can pull water into a system of long, narrow channels or pores, has recently been proposed by Diamond[35, 129] to explain fluid transport by the gallbladder. Finally, the "solution pump" proposed by Frank and Mayer should be mentioned.[41] The driving osmotic force in the last model is provided by the physical alteration (polymerization and de-polymerization) of a hypothetical solute which remains confined to a double-ended compartment. The underlying mechanism in all of these models is local alteration in the solute concentration gradient across a critically located semipermeable membrane, caused by direct and specific interaction between the cell and the solute (or solutes), leading to the development of an osmotic force which in turn is responsible for fluid movement. The net result in each case is the apparent active transport of a whole solution, and each model can, theoretically, force a solution "uphill"— that is, against an opposing external hydrostatic or osmotic pressure.

Secretory vacuole formation should always be regarded as a possible mechanism in any exocrine organ. Direct morphologic evidence should be sought for such a mechanism, and the vacuoles seen around bile canaliculi[123] or some similar structural arrangement associated with the Golgi complex[103] have indeed been proposed as initial sites of bile formation. If these structures prove to be functionally important, some basic transport mechanism of the sort already mentioned must still be considered in order to explain the generation of a vacuolar fluid whose composition is decidedly different from the intracellular fluid of the hepatic parenchymal cells. In other words, the existence of a system of secretory vacuoles moves the site of bile formation "upstream" from the canaliculi, but must involve the same basic theoretical questions.

Relationship Between Solute Transport and Bile Flow

The hypothesis that active solute transport provides the driving force for bile production was first proposed by Sperber,[120,121,122]

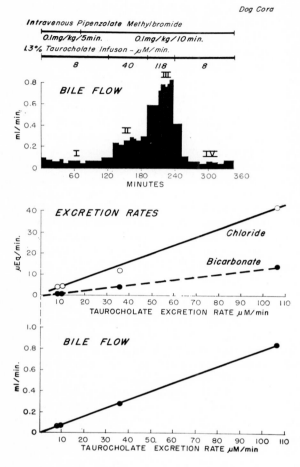

FIG. 3–4. *Effect of varying taurocholate excretion rate on bile flow and on the excretion rates of chloride and bicarbonate in a dog.* The anticholinergic drug pipenzolate methylbromide was given to minimize spontaneous variation in bile flow. The actual sequence of taurocholate infusions and the resulting bile flows are shown at the top. The excretion rates of water, as indicated by the bile flow (bottom), and of the inorganic anions chloride and bicarbonate (middle) were directly proportional to the excretion rate of taurocholate, consistent with the view that bile salt transport provides the osmotic driving force for bulk movement of water and smaller solutes into the canaliculi. (Reproduced from J. Clin. Invest.[95])

who pointed out that most actively transported organic anions are also choleretic. The idea is attractive because the vast network of bile canaliculi can be considered as an open-ended compartment with a small volume and a very large surface area appropriate for osmotic fluid transfer in response to the transport of specific solutes into the lumen. Sperber showed, in fact, that bile flow in the chicken is directly proportional to the osmotic load imposed by the secretion of a variety of dissimilar actively transported compounds.[121, 122] Normally, of course, the bile salts make up the major proportion of actively transported solute.* The study illustrated in Figure 3–4 shows that bile flow in the dog is directly proportional to the rate of sodium taurocholate excretion as the latter is varied over a wide range by intravenous

infusion of the bile salt.[95] These data support the view that bile salt excretion rate is one of the major determinants of the rate of bile production and are consistent with the hypothesis that active bile salt transport may be an important "prime mover" in the initiation of canalicular bile flow. As might be expected, interruption of enterohepatic circulation of the bile salts by acute biliary diversion results in a marked reduction in bile flow in man,[128] in the dog,[27, 43, 71, 137, 142] in the cat,[118] in the rat,[27, 82] and in sheep.[56] The rabbit[118] appears to be an exception, but

* Despite the osmotic inactivity of bile salt micelles mentioned in an earlier section, it must be recalled that the bile salt anions are always accompanied by an equivalent concentration of cation (principally sodium) so that the osmotic activity of a 100 mM. solution of sodium taurocholate, for example, is roughly 100 mOsm./Kg.

bile flow in this species is peculiarly high and may depend more upon ductal than canalicular secretion (see below).

One should not conclude, however, that canalicular bile production is attributable to bile salt secretion alone. Recent studies by Nahrwold and Grossman show that canine bile flow is independent of the rate of bile salt excretion when the latter is reduced to very low rates by acute biliary diversion,[87] and active transport of other solutes probably plays the dominant role under these conditions. Data related to "canalicular clearance" appear to support this view (see below).

CANALICULAR CLEARANCE

The use of inert solutes such as mannitol and erythritol has permitted an appraisal of the rate of fluid movement into the bile canaliculi.[40, 138] Compounds of this size equilibrate rapidly between plasma and liver cell water,[20, 40, 109, 111, 138] so that their steady state "clearance" (biliary excretion rate/ plasma concentration) is a function of the rate at which water moves from liver cells into bile canaliculi. Forker has shown that biliary erythritol clearance in the guinea pig is appreciably higher than mannitol clearance, but that both are linearly related to bile flow as the latter is varied in response to dehydrocholate administration.[40] He concludes that bile salt secretion leads to osmotic "bulk flow" of fluid into the canaliculi (consistent with the hypothesis discussed above) but that movement of mannitol across the canalicular wall (and, probably, to a lesser extent, of erythritol) is restricted. In the dog, as illustrated in Figure 3–5, mannitol clearance appears to be directly proportional to the rate of taurocholate secretion. Unlike the findings in the guinea pig, however, canine canaliculi appear to be equally permeable to mannitol, erythritol, urea and creatinine, since the clearance of each of these compounds is similar at any given rate of taurocholate secretion. Thus it would appear that the clearance of an inert molecule such as mannitol or erythritol provides a reasonable estimate of canalicular bile flow in the dog. On this basis one would conclude, from data such as that illustrated in Figure 3–5, that in a 20 Kg. dog approxi-

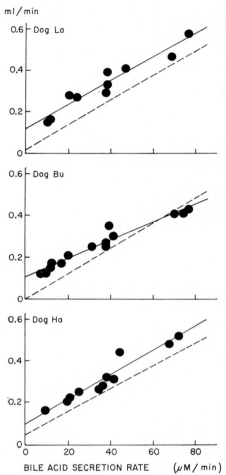

FIG. 3–5. *Biliary clearance of C^{14}-labeled mannitol in 3 dogs as a function of the secretion rate of conjugated bile acid (taurocholate).* Mannitol clearance is linearly related to bile acid secretion rate. The fact that mannitol clearance was higher than bile flow (dashed lines) in most instances suggests that an appreciable fraction of canalicular bile (up to ⅔ at low flows) is reabsorbed in the duct system. The positive intercept of mannitol clearance on the ordinate (approximately 0.1 ml./min.) suggests that mechanisms other than bile acid secretion may be responsible for a fraction of the canalicular bile production. (Reproduced from the Am. J. Physiol.[138])

mately 0.006 ml. of canalicular bile is formed for every micromole of sodium taurocholate secreted. However, the extrapolated mannitol clearance is appreciably greater than zero (roughly 0.1 ml./min.) as bile salt secretion approaches zero. This provides further evidence for the view that transport mechanisms other than those involved with bile salts play a significant role in canalicular bile formation.[87]

BILE DUCT ACTIVITY

The bile ducts may modify the canalicular bile in a number of ways and therefore have a profound influence on the flow and composition of the final product. The bile duct walls are evidently highly permeable to sodium and potassium but less permeable to inorganic anions.[22, 81] Since the composition of canalicular bile is unknown, actual changes in composition owing to activity of the ducts cannot be appraised. However a few general statements can be made about fluid transport in the bile ducts.

Clearance data of the sort illustrated in Figure 3–5 suggests that, under some circumstances at least, an appreciable fraction of canalicular bile is reabsorbed. Note that mannitol clearance, especially at lower rates of bile acid secretion, is significantly higher than the bile flow. Indeed, mannitol and erythritol are occasionally concentrated as much as threefold in canine bile as compared to plasma.[138] Similar evidence for reabsorptive activity has not been reported in other species except for a few mannitol bile-to-plasma ratios as high as 1.2 in the rats studied by Schanker and Hogben.[111] It would be important to know whether the bile ducts reabsorb fluid in normal representatives of any species, or whether the findings just cited are a result of chronic adaptation of the duct system following cholecystectomy. It is noteworthy that the bile obtained from the common duct of cholecystectomized dogs after an overnight fast (Fig. 3–1) is similar in composition to normal concentrated canine gallbladder bile.[43, 137]

The most striking example of bile duct (or ductule) secretory activity is the response to secretin. The choleretic effect of secretin has been documented in many species[37, 52, 71, 72, 73, 90, 95, 99, 118, 119, 137] and the

only exception appears to be the rabbit.[3, 119] The typical response to secretin is an increase in bile flow and a reciprocal decrease in bile salt and bile pigment concentrations. In other words, secretin apparently augments bile flow by the addition of an aqueous solution of inorganic electrolytes, and has no effect on the excretion of bile salts or other organic constituents. The magnitude of the secretin response has varied in different studies. Maximal increments in bile flow between 0.1 to 0.3 have been reported in dogs weighing 15 to 20 Kg.[71, 95, 142] and between 0.15 to 0.8 ml./min. in man.[52] Since different preparations, doses and administration rates have been used, numerical response data are not particularly important, but all workers emphasize that the biliary tract responds to secretin only about a fifth to one tenth as much as does the pancreas to similar preparations.[14] The increase in bile flow that occurs with acidification of the duodenum[56, 95, 137] is consistent with a response to endogenous secretin.

As in pancreatic stimulation, secretin causes a marked increment in biliary bicarbonate concentration. Bicarbonate concentrations as high as 70 mEq./L. have been observed in the bile of some dogs[142] following secretin administration. However, secretin leads to increased biliary excretion of both chloride and bicarbonate.[95]

Several lines of evidence suggest that secretin acts predominantly if not exclusively to stimulate fluid output by the bile duct system rather than the canaliculi. This evidence includes preferential response to hepatic arterial injection,[134] a small biliary "washout volume,"[134] lack of effect of secretin on BSP Tm[90] and lack of effect of secretin on mannitol[40, 138] or erythritol clearance.[40]

Secretin, therefore, may play a significant physiological role in the modification of bile production and it has also provided a most useful experimental tool for the demonstration of bile duct secretory activity. The demonstration that bile ducts take an active part in bile production may have considerable clinical importance, and supports the morphologists' long-standing view that these structures are not simple conduits.[4, 5, 46, 127]

OTHER FACTORS THAT INFLUENCE BILE PRODUCTION

The mechanisms whereby a number of other factors influence bile production are even less well understood than those already mentioned.

HUMORAL AND PHARMACOLOGICAL AGENTS

Cholecystokinin appears to elicit a choleresis similar to that caused by secretin. The choleresis cannot be explained by the amount of secretin in these preparations,[37, 73, 97] but could be due to some other agent present as an impurity.[31, 42] As with secretin stimulation, the biliary pH (and hence probably bicarbonate concentration) appears to rise.[97]

Histamine causes moderate choleresis in gastrectomized dogs.[142] Maximal response is elicited by an infusion of 4 mg./hr. and is approximately half that observed with secretin. Interestingly different from the secretin response, however, is the fact that histamine leads to a much greater output (and concentration) of chloride than of bicarbonate. The site of action of histamine on the biliary tree is unknown. Prior studies with histamine in animals with stomach intact[21] must be discounted because of the stimulation of gastric hydrochloric acid production leading to elaboration of endogenous secretin.[95]

Gastrin produces a moderate choleresis in gastrectomized dogs,[142] less marked than that observed with secretin but qualitatively similar in that bicarbonate output is significantly increased.

Carbonic anhydrase inhibitors have been reported to cause a consistent rise in biliary chloride concentration and fall in bicarbonate concentration in the dog.[84, 92, 137] Reports of a choleresis elicited by acetazolamide[92, 137] have not been confirmed in the recent studies of Maren et al.[84] Failure of rats to respond to large doses of acetazolamide[15] has been explained by the finding that rat liver carbonic anhydrase activity is totally unaffected by any carbonic anhydrase inhibitor tested.[84] Since respiratory alkalosis affects bile composition in the same manner as the carbonic anhydrase inhibitors, Maren suggests that a rise in intracellular pH is the common mechanism that alters chloride-bicarbonate exchange at some critical site in the biliary tract.

Antidiuretic hormone reportedly does not affect canine bile production[9] and its transient anticholeretic effect in rats has been attributed to contraction of the smooth muscle of the bile ducts.[61]

Before closing the subject of "pharmacological" agents it must be re-emphasized that any substance that is excreted in the bile in osmotically significant quantities may influence bile flow in the same manner as that discussed in connection with the bile salts. Many of the well-known choleretic agents probably act in this manner.[1, 53] If it is known (or can be reasonably assumed) that an agent is actively secreted in bile one can confidently predict that it will cause choleresis if given in sufficient quantity.[121, 122] Agents that do not form micelles (e.g., sodium dehydrocholate) have greater osmotic activity, mole for mole, than the natural bile salts and therefore are more "potent" as choleretics. Since they carry along more water they may be designated as "hydrocholeretics," a term that is somewhat misleading in the case of compounds whose mechanism of action is basically identical with that of the natural bile salts. Sperber suggests that the term "hydrocholeresis" if used at all, be reserved for phenomena comparable to secretin choleresis, in which organic solute excretion is not enhanced.[121]

NEUROGENIC FACTORS

The liver and biliary tract are richly innervated, but the role of direct neurogenic stimuli on bile production has thus far defied precise interpretation. Vagal stimulation (or insulin hypoglycemia) have been shown to cause choleresis in dogs[43, 126] and in man[10] which can be abolished by vagectomy[43] or anticholinergic drugs.[10, 43] More recent studies have suggested, however, that the effect depends on the presence of the gastric antrum[69] and that it can be reproduced by chemical stimulation of the gastric antrum.[70] Hence it may be that the previously reported effects of vagal stimulation can be attributed entirely or in large part to the release of endogenous gastrin, a known choleretic

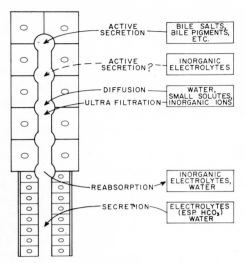

Fig. 3–6. *Summary of some of the mechanisms involved in bile formation.* Bile formed in the canaliculi in response to secretion of bile salts and other solutes is modified in the duct system either by net reabsorption or secretion of fluid.

agent.[142] Chronic vagal denervation has been reported to enhance the choleretic response to exogenous[108] and endogenous[107] secretin in dogs.

Interpretation of the anticholeretic effect of splanchnic nerve stimulation[125] is complicated by the profound effects of this maneuver on vascular perfusion.

Altered Vascular Perfusion

Acute hepatic venous congestion significantly reduces bile flow,[96, 125] but the effects of longstanding chronic congestion—which would be of considerable clinical interest—have not been appraised. Chronic occlusion of either portal vein or hepatic artery,[94] end-to-side portacaval shunt,[39] arterialization of the portal vein,[39] and acute hepatic arterial occlusion[38] reportedly have no discernible effect on canine bile flow. As might be expected, severe hepatic ischemia is associated with cessation of bile flow.[38, 78, 125] However, as Brauer's studies with perfused livers show, hypotension *per se* does not interfere with bile flow[19] and very low perfusion rates with erythrocyte-free fluid are associated, in isolated rat livers, with normal bile produc-

tion, provided hypoxemia is avoided by the use of hyperbaric oxygen.[18]

These remarks might suggest the conclusion that altered vascular perfusion has no effect on bile production (with the exception of the effect of hepatic venous congestion). However, remember that most reports deal with observations of bile flow alone. This is a relatively insensitive test of biliary tract function, as pointed out earlier in this chapter, and the subject should be re-examined in much greater detail.

SUMMARY

Bile is a complex isotonic solution containing pigments, mixed bile salt–lecithin–cholesterol micelles and inorganic electrolytes. It is produced in the bile canaliculi and modified as it passes through the bile duct system. These processes are summarized in Figure 3–6. The liver cells secrete a variety of compounds into the bile canaliculi by means of several well-characterized and evidently separate transport mechanisms. These mechanisms not only serve an excretory function but also appear to provide the osmotic driving force for the production of bile itself. The bile ducts can, under some circumstances, concentrate organic constituents by reabsorbing fluid and inorganic electrolytes. Under other circumstances, such as secretin stimulation, the ducts appear to serve a secretory function. A variety of other factors can modify bile production, but their mechanism of action and physiologic roles remain to be clarified. In the intact organism bile formation itself is but one stage in the enterohepatic circulation of the major constituents of bile.

REFERENCES

1. Acheson, E. D., McHardy, G., Dessauer, H. C., Ford, C., and Dunn, D.: Effect of florantyrone on rate of secretion of hepatic bile and on its chemical and physical properties, Gastroenterology 37:735, 1959.
2. Adams, R. H., Gordon, J., and Combes, B.: Measurements of hepatic storage and of maximal biliary transport of sulfo-

bromophthalein sodium in man. Gastroenterology 51:373, 1966.

3. Affolter, H. Von, Piller, M., and Gubler, A.: Tierexperimentelle Untersuchungen über die Wirkung von gereinigtem Sekretin und Cholecystokinin-Pankreozymin, sowie von Decholin auf die Gallensekretion. Gastroenterologia 101:247, 1964.

4. Andrews, W. H. H.: Excretory function of the liver. A re-assessment. Lancet 2: 166, 1955.

5. Andrews, W. H. H., Maegraith, B. G., and Wenzon, C. E. M.: Studies on the liver circulation. II. The micro-anatomy of the hepatic circulation. Ann. trop. Med. Parasit. 43:229, 1949.

6. Arias, I. M.: The excretion of conjugated bilirubin by the liver cell. Medicine 45: 513, 1966.

7. Arias, I. M., Johnson, L., and Wolfson, S.: Biliary excretion of injected conjugated and unconjugated bilirubin by normal and Gunn rats. Am. J. Physiol. 200: 1091, 1961.

8. Ayliffe, G. A. J., and Davies, A.: Ampicillin levels in human bile. Brit. J. Pharmacol. 24:189, 1965.

9. Baïsset, A., Montastruc, P., and Prat, J.: Recherches sur les actions extra-renales de l'hormone antidiurétique. Absence d'effet sur la sécrétion intestinale, la sécrétion biliaire et la réabsorption vésiculaire. Path. Biol. (Paris) 12:439, 1964.

10. Baldwin, J., Heer, F. W., Albo, R., Peloso, O., Ruby, L., and Silen, W.: Effect of vagus nerve stimulation on hepatic secretion of bile in human subjects. Am. J. Surg. 111:66, 1966.

11. Barber-Riley, G.: Rat biliary tree during short periods of obstruction of common duct. Am. J. Physiol. 205:1127, 1963.

12. ———: The rate of biliary secretion during flow up vertical cannulas of different bore. Experientia 20:639, 1964.

13. ———: Measurement of the capacity of the biliary tree, in Taylor, W. (ed.): The Biliary System, pp. 90-97, Oxford, Blackwell, 1965.

14. Baron, J. H., Perrier, C. V., Janowitz, H. D., and Dreiling, D. A.: Maximum alkaline (bicarbonate) output of the dog pancreas. Am. J. Physiol. 204:251, 1963.

15. Bizard, G., Vanlerenberghe, J., Guerrin, F., and Godchaux, R.: Rôle de l'anhydrase carbonique dans la formation de la bile. J. Physiol. (Paris) 50:155, 1958.

16. Bourgès, M., Small, D. M., and Dervichian, D. G.: Biophysics of lipid associations. III. The quaternary systems lecithin-bile salt-cholesterol-water. Biochim. Biophys. Acta 144:189, 1967.

17. Brauer, R. W.: Mechanisms of bile secretion. J.A.M.A. 169:1462, 1959.

18. ———: Hepatic blood supply and the secretion of bile, in Taylor, W. (ed.): The Biliary System, pp. 41-67, Oxford, Blackwell, 1965.

19. Brauer, R. W., Leong, G. F., and Holloway, R. J.: Mechanics of bile secretion: The effect of perfusion pressure and temperature on bile flow and bile secretion pressure. Am. J. Physiol. 177:103, 1954.

20. Cahill, G. F., Jr., Ashmore, J., Earle, A. S., and Zottu, S.: Glucose penetration into liver. Am. J. Physiol. 192:491, 1958.

21. Carnot, P., and Gruzewska, Z.: Variations de concentration ionique de la bile et du suc pancréatique pendant la sécrétion acide du suc gastrique, C. R. Soc. Biol. 93:240, 1925.

22. Chenderovitch, J.: Les conceptions actuelles des mécanismes de la sécrétion biliaire. Presse méd. 71:2645, 1963.

23. Chenderovitch, J., Phocas, E., and Rautureau, M.: Effects of hypertonic solutions on bile formation. Am. J. Physiol. 205:863, 1963.

24. Cherrick, G. R., Stein, S. W., Leevy, C. M., and Davidson, C. S.: Indocyanine green: observations on its physical properties, plasma decay and hepatic excretion. J. Clin. Invest. 39:592, 1960.

25. Combes, B.: The importance of conjugation with glutathione for sulfobromophthalein sodium (BSP) transfer from blood to bile. J. Clin. Invest. 44:1214, 1965.

26. Combes, B., and Stakelum, G. S.: Conjugation of sulfobromophthalein sodium with glutathione in thioether linkage by the rat. J. Clin. Invest. 39:1214, 1960.

27. Cook, D. L., Beach, D. A., Bianchi, R. G., Hambourger, W. E., and Green, D. M.: Factors influencing bile flow in the dog and rat. Am. J. Physiol. 163:688, 1950.

28. Cook, D. L., Lawler, C. A., Calvin, L. D., and Green, D. M.: Mechanisms of bile formation. Am. J. Physiol. 171:62, 1952.

29. Crigler, J. F., Jr., and Najjar, V. A.: Congenital familial nonhemolytic jaundice

with kernicterus. Pediatrics 10:169, 1952.

30. Curran, P. F., and McIntosh, J. R.: A model system for biological water transport. Nature (Lond.) 193:347, 1962.

31. Debray, C., Vaille, C., de la Tour, J., and Rozé, C.: Action sur la sécrétion biliaire de diverses sécrétines du commerce. Le problème de l'hépatocrinine. Path. Biol. (Paris) 11:1373, 1963.

32. Despopoulos, A.: Congruence of excretory functions in liver and kidney: hippurates. Am. J. Physiol. 210:760, 1966.

33. Despopoulos, A., and Sonnenberg, H.: Congruence of excretory functions of liver and kidney: sulfonamides. Am. J. Physiol. 212:1117, 1967.

34. Diamond, J. M.: The reabsorptive function of the gallbladder. J. Physiol. (Lond.) 161:442, 1962.

35. Diamond, J. M., and Bossert, W. H.: Standing-gradient osmotic flow. J. Gen. Physiol. 50:2061, 1967.

36. Dietschy, J. M., and Moore, E. W.: Diffusion potentials and potassium distribution across the gallbladder wall. J. Clin. Invest. 43:1551, 1964.

37. Edholm, P., Jonson, G., and Thulin, L.: Le débit biliaire du foie: Stimulation par la cholécystokinine, la sécrétine et l'alimentation per-orale. Path. Biol. (Paris) 10:447, 1962.

38. Engstrand, L.: Bile secretion and hepatic nitrogen metabolism in relation to variations of blood and oxygen supply to the liver. Acta chir. scand. Supp. 146:190, 1949.

39. Fisher, B., Lee, S. H., and Fedor, E. J.: Effect on permanent alteration of hepatic blood flow upon biliary secretion. A.M.A. Arch. Surg. 76:41, 1958.

40. Forker, E. L.: Two sites of bile formation as determined by mannitol and erythritol clearance in the guinea pig. J. Clin. Invest. 46:1189, 1967.

41. Franck, J., and Mayer, J. E.: An osmotic diffusion pump. Arch. Biochem. 14:297, 1947.

42. Friedman, M. H. F., and Snape, W. J.: Comparative effectiveness of extracts of intestinal mucosa in stimulating the external secretions of the pancreas and the liver. Fed. Proc. 4:21, 1945.

43. Fritz, M. E., and Brooks, F. P.: Control of bile flow in the cholecystectomized dog. Am. J. Physiol. 204:825, 1963.

44. Gilman, A., and Cowgill, G. R.: Osmotic relations between blood and body fluids. IV. Pancreatic juice, bile and lymph. Am. J. Physiol. 104:476, 1933.

45. Goetzee, A. E., Richards, T. G., and Tindall, V. R.: Experimental changes in liver function induced by probenecid. Clin. Sci. 19:63, 1960.

46. Goldfarb, S., Singer, E. J., and Popper, H.: Biliary ductules and bile secretion. J. Lab. Clin. Med. 62:608, 1963.

47. Goresky, C. A.: A linear method for determining liver sinusoidal and extravascular volumes. Am. J. Physiol. 204:626, 1963.

48. ———: Initial distribution and rate of uptake of sulfobromophthalein in the liver. Am. J. Physiol. 207:13, 1964.

49. ———: The hepatic uptake and excretion of sulfobromophthalein and bilirubin. Canad. Med. Ass. J. 92:851, 1965.

50. Grafflin, A. L., and Bagley, E. H.: Studies of hepatic structure and function by fluorescence microscopy. Bull. Johns Hopkins Hosp. 90:395, 1952.

51. Grodsky, G. M., Carbone, J. V., and Fanska, R.: Biosynthesis of a sulfobromophthalein mercaptide with glutathione. Proc. Soc. Exp. Biol. Med. 106:526, 1961.

52. Grossman, M. I., Janowitz, H. D., Ralston, H., and Kim, K. S.: The effect of secretin on bile formation in man. Gastroenterology 12:133, 1949.

53. Gunter, M. J., Kim, K. S., Magee, D. F., Ralston, H., and Ivy, A. C.: The choleretic potencies of some synthetic compounds. J. Pharmacol. Exp. Therap. 99:465, 1950.

54. Hanzon, V.: Liver cell secretion under normal and pathologic conditions studied by fluorescence microscopy on living rats. Acta physiol. scand. 28: Suppl. 101, 1-268, 1953.

55. Hardwicke, J., Rankin, J. G., Baker, K. J., and Preisig, R.: The loss of protein in human and canine hepatic bile. Clin. Sci. 26:509, 1964.

56. Harrison, F. A.: Bile secretion in the sheep. J. Physiol. (Lond.) 162:212, 1962.

57. Hart, L. G., and Schanker, L. S.: Active transport of chlorothiazide into bile. Am. J. Physiol. 211:643, 1966.

58. ———: The chemical forms in which phenol red is secreted into the bile of rats. Proc. Soc. Exp. Biol. Med. 123:433, 1966.

59. Hofmann, A. F.: Clinical implications of physiochemical studies on bile salts. Gastroenterology 48:484, 1965.

60. Hofmann, A. F., and Small, D. M.: Detergent properties of bile salts: Correlation with physiological function. Ann. Rev. Med. 18:333, 1967.

61. Homsher, E., and Cotzias, G. C.: Antidiuretic hormone and bile flow. Nature 208:687, 1965.

62. Hunton, D. B., Bollman, J. L., and Hoffman, H. N., II: The plasma removal of indocyanine green and sulfobromophthalein: Effect of dosage and blocking agents. J. Clin. Invest. 40:1648, 1961.

63. Isaksson, B.: On the lipid constituents of normal bile. Acta Soc. Med. upsalien. 56:171, 1951.

64. ———: On dissolving power of lecithin and bile salt for cholesterol in human bladder bile. Acta Soc. Med. upsalien. 59:296, 1954.

65. ———: On lipid constituents of bile from the human gallbladder containing cholesterol gallstones. Comparison with normal human bladder bile. Acta Soc. Med. upsalien. 59:277, 1954.

66. Javitt, N. B.: Phenol 3,6 dibromphthalein disulfonate, a new compound for the study of liver disease. Proc. Soc. Exp. Biol. Med. 117:254, 1964.

67. Javitt, N. B., Wheeler, H. O., Baker, K. J., Ramos, O. L. and Bradley, S. E.: The intrahepatic conjugation of sulfobromophthalein and glutathione in the dog. J. Clin. Invest. 39:1570, 1960.

68. Jenner, F. A., and Smyth, D. H.: The excretion of phlorhizin. J. Physiol. (Lond.) 146:563, 1959.

69. Jones, R. S., and Brooks, F. P.: The pyloric antrum as a mediator on insulin induced choleresis. Physiologist 8:202, 1965.

70. Jones, R. S., Powell, K. C., and Brooks, F. P.: The role of the gastric antrum in the control of bile flow. Surg. Forum 16:386, 1965.

71. Jonson, G., Sundman, L., and Thulin, L.: The influence of chemically pure secretin on hepatic bile output. Acta physiol. scand. 62:287, 1964.

72. Jorpes, J. E., Mutt, V., Jonson, G., Thulin, L. and Sundman, L.: The effect of secretin on bile flow. Gastroenterology 45:786, 1963.

73. ———: The influence of secretin and cholecystokinin on bile flow, in Taylor,

W. (ed.): The Biliary System, pp. 293-301, Oxford, Blackwell, 1965.

74. Juniper, K.: Physiochemical characteristics of bile and their relation to gallstone formation. Am. J. Med. 39:98, 1965.

75. Katsuki, T., Shimura, H., Johnston, C. G., and Miyake, H.: Constitution of bile proteins. Proc. Soc. Exp. Biol. 103:272, 1960.

76. Kay, R. E., and Entenman, C.: Stimulation of taurocholic acid synthesis and biliary excretion of lipids. Am. J. Physiol. 200:855, 1961.

77. Kaye, G., Wheeler, H. O., Whitlock, R. T., and Lane, N.: Fluid transport in the rabbit gallbladder. A combined physiological and electron microscopic study. J. Cell Biol. 30:237, 1967.

78. Kjellgren, K.: Biliary secretion in relation to the liver temperature and the blood pressure. Acta Soc. Med. upsalien. 60:172, 1955.

79. Kupferberg, H. J., and Schanker, L. S.: Biliary secretion of ouabain-H^3 and its uptake by liver slices in the rat. Am. J. Physiol. 214:1048, 1968.

80. Large, A. M., Johnston, C. G., Katsuki, T., and Fachnie, H. L.: Gallstones and pregnancy. The composition of gallbladder bile in the pregnant woman at term. Am. J. Med. Sci. 239:713, 1960.

81. Leong, G. F., Holloway, R. J., and Brauer, R. W.: Mechanics of bile formation. Transfer of potassium, sodium, chloride, phosphate and sulfate ions from perfusion medium to bile. Fed. Proc. 14:363, 1955.

82. Light, H. G., Witmer, C., and Vars, H. M.: Interruption of the enterohepatic circulation and its effect on rat bile. Am. J. Physiol. 197:1330, 1959.

83. Maffly, R. H., and Leaf, A.: The potential of water in mammalian tissues. J. Gen. Physiol. 42:1257, 1959.

84. Maren, T. H., Ellison, A. C., Fellner, S. K., and Graham, W. B.: A study of hepatic carbonic anhydrase. Molecular Pharmacol. 2:144, 1966.

85. McBain, E. L., and Hutchinson, E.: Solubilization and Related Phenomena. p. 147, New York, Academic Press, 1955.

86. Moore, E. W., and Dietschy, J. M.: Na and K activity coefficients in bile and bile salts determined by glass electrodes. Am. J. Physiol. 206:1111, 1964.

87. Nahrwold, D. L., and Grossman, M. I.:

Secretion of bile in response to food with and without bile in the intestine. Gastroenterology 53:11, 1967.

88. Ogilvie, J. T., McIntosh, J. R., and Curran, P. F.: Volume flow in a series membrane system. Biochim. Biophys. Acta 66:441, 1963.

89. Ó'Máille, E. R. L., Richards, T. G., and Short, A. H.: Acute taurine depletion and maximal rates of hepatic conjugation and secretion of cholic acid in the dog. J. Physiol. (Lond.) 180:67, 1965.

90. ————: Factors determining the maximal rate of organic anion secretion by the liver and further evidence on the hepatic site of action of the hormone secretin. J. Physiol. (Lond.) 186:424, 1966.

91. Ó'Máille, E. R. L., Richards, T. G., and Short, A. H.: The influence of conjugation of cholic acid on its uptake and secretion: hepatic extraction of taurocholate and cholate in the dog. J. Physiol. (Lond.) 189:337, 1967.

92. Pak, B. H., Hong, S. S., Pak, H. K., and Hong, S. K.: Effects of acetazolamide and acid-base changes on biliary and pancreatic secretion. Am. J. Physiol. 210:624, 1966.

93. Patlak, C. S., Goldstein, D. A., and Hoffman, J. F.: The flow of solute and solvent across a two-membrane system. J. Theor. Biol. 5:426, 1963.

94. Popper, H. L., Jefferson, N. C., Wulkan, E., and Necheles, H.: Bile secretion and blood supply of the liver. Am. J. Physiol. 181:435, 1955.

95. Preisig, R., Cooper, H. L., and Wheeler, H. O.: The relationship between taurocholate secretion rate and bile production in the unanesthetized dog during cholinergic blockade and during secretin administration. J. Clin. Invest. 41:1152, 1962.

96. Preisig, R., Rankin, J. G., Sweeting, J. G., Williams, R., and Bradley, S. E.: Bile formation during hepatic ischemia. J. Clin. Invest. 42:966, 1963 (Abstract).

97. Ramorino, M. L., Luzietti, L., and Campioni, N.: Effetti della colecistocinina su l'attivita' biligentica del fegato. Folia endocr. 14:266, 1961.

98. Ravdin, I. S., Johnston, C. G., Riegel, C., and Wright, S. L., Jr.: Studies of gallbladder function. VII. The anion-cation content of hepatic and gall-bladder bile. Am. J. Physiol. 100:317, 1932.

99. Razin, E., Feldman, M. G., and Dreiling, D. A.: Studies on biliary flow and composition in man and dog. J. Mt. Sinai Hosp. 32:42, 1965.

100. Reinhold, J. G., and Wilson, D. W.: The acid-base composition of hepatic bile. Am. J. Physiol. 107:378, 1934.

101. Richards, T. G., and Thomson, J. Y.: The secretion of bile against pressure. Gastroenterology 40:705, 1961.

102. Rosenthal, W. S., Kubo, K., Dolinski, M., Marino, J., Mersheimer, W. L., and Jerzy Glass, G. B.: The passage of serum albumin into bile in man. Am. J. Dig. Dis. 10:271, 1965.

103. Rouiller, C., and Jézéquel, A.-M.: Electron microscopy of the liver, in Rouiller, C. (ed.): The Liver. Morphology, Biochemistry, Physiology, vol. 1, pp. 195-264, New York, Academic Press, 1963.

104. Rudman, D., and Kendall, F. E.: Bile acid content of human serum. II. The binding of cholanic acids by human plasma proteins. J. Clin. Invest. 36:538, 1957.

105. Russell, I. S., and Burnett, W.: The proteins of human bile. Gastroenterology 45:730, 1963.

106. Russell, I. S., Fleck, A., and Burnett, W.: The protein content of human bile. Clin. Chim. Acta 10:210, 1964.

107. Saburov, G. E.: The effect of vagotomy on the bile-secreting function of the liver, Sechenov Physiol. J., U.S.S.R. 47:685, 1961. (English translation, New York, Pergamon, 1962.)

108. ————: Effect of secretin on bile secretion under conditions of partial denervation of the liver. Bull. Exp. Biol. Med. 59:45, 1965. (English translation, Consultants Bureau, N. Y., 1965.)

109. Sacks, J., and Bakshy, S.: Insulin and tissue distribution of pentose in nephrectomized cats. Am. J. Physiol. 189:339, 1957.

110. Schanker, L. S.: Hepatic transport of organic cations, in Taylor, W. (ed.): The Biliary System, pp. 469-480, Oxford, Blackwell, 1965.

111. Schanker, L. S., and Hogben, C. A. M.: Biliary excretion of inulin, sucrose, and mannitol: analysis of bile formation. Am. J. Physiol. 200:1087, 1961.

112. Schanker, L. S., and Solomon, H. M.: Active transport of quaternary ammonium compounds into bile. Am. J. Physiol. 204:829, 1963.

113. Scherb, J., Kirschner, M., and Arias, I.: Studies of hepatic excretory function. The effect of 17α-ethyl-19-nortestosterone on sulfobromophthalein sodium (BSP) metabolism in man. J. Clin. Invest. 42:404, 1963.

114. Schmid, R., Axelrod, J., Hammaker. L., and Swarm, R. L.: Congenital jaundice in rats, due to a defect in glucuronide formation. J. Clin. Invest. 37:1123, 1958.

115. Schoenfield, L. J., and Foulk, W. T.: Studies of sulfobromophthalein sodium (BSP) metabolism in man. II. The effect of artificially induced fever, norethandrolone (Nilevar) and iopanoic acid (Telepaque). J. Clin. Invest. 43:1419, 1964.

116. Schoenfield, L. J., Foulk, W. T., and Butt, H. R.: Studies of sulfobromophthalein sodium (BSP) metabolism in man. I. In normal subjects and patients with hepatic disease. J. Clin. Invest. 43:1409, 1964.

117. Schoenfield, L. J., McGill, D. B., and Foulk, W. T.: Studies of sulfobromophthalein sodium (BSP) metabolism in man. III. Demonstration of a transport maximum (Tm) for biliary excretion of BSP. J. Clin. Invest. 43:1424, 1964.

118. Scratcherd, T.: Electrolyte composition and control of biliary secretion in the cat and rabbit, in Taylor, W. (ed.): The Biliary System, pp. 515-529, Oxford, Blackwell, 1965.

119. Sobotka, H.: Physiological Chemistry of the Bile. Baltimore, Williams and Wilkins, 1937.

120. Sperber, I.: Secretion of organic anions in the formation of urine and bile. Pharm. Rev. 11:109, 1959.

121. ———: Biliary excretion and choleresis in Proc. 1st Internat'l Pharm. Meeting, Stockholm, 1961, 4:137, Oxford, Pergamon Press, 1963.

122. ———: Biliary secretion of organic anions and its influence on bile flow, in Taylor, W. (ed.): The Biliary System, pp. 457-467, Oxford, Blackwell, 1965.

122a. ———: Personal communication.

123. Steiner, J. W., and Carruthers, J. S.: Studies on the fine structure of the terminal branches of the biliary tree. I. The morphology of normal bile canaliculi, bile preductules (ducts of Hering) and bile ductules. Am. J. Path. 38:639, 1961.

124. Stransky, E.: Untersuchungen über die Pharmakologie der Gallensekretion, IV. Mitteilung. Ausscheidung von stoffen durch die Galle, Z. ges. exp. Med. 77:807, 1931.

125. Tanturi. C. A., and Ivy, A. C.: A study of the effect of vascular changes in the liver and the excitation of its nerve supply on the formation of bile. Am. J. Physiol. 121:61, 1938.

126. ———: On the existence of secretory nerves in the vagi for, and the reflex excitation and inhibition of, bile secretion. Am. J. Physiol. 121:270, 1938.

127. Theiler, K.: Do bile ducts act solely as biliary channels? German Med. Monthly 8:202, 1963.

128. Thureborn, E.: Human hepatic bile. Composition changes due to altered enterohepatic circulation. Acta chir. scand. Suppl. 303:1-63, 1962.

129. Tormey, J. McD., and Diamond, J. M.: The ultrastructural route of fluid transport in rabbit gallbladder. J. Gen. Physiol. 50:2031, 1967.

130. Twiss, J. R., Berger, W. V., Gillette, L., Aronson, A. R., and Siegel, L.: The biliary excretion of erythromycin (Ilotycin) Surg. Gynec. Obstet. 102:355, 1956.

131. Ussing, H. H.: The distinction by means of tracers between active transport and diffusion. Acta physiol. scand. 19:43, 1949.

132. Weiner, I. M., Glasser, J. E., and Lack, L.: Renal excretion of bile: taurocholic, glycocholic, and cholic acids. Am. J. Physiol. 207:964, 1964.

133. Wheeler, H. O., Cranston, W. I., and Meltzer, J. I.: Hepatic uptake and biliary excretion of indocyanine green in the dog. Proc. Soc. Exp. Biol. Med. 99:11, 1958.

134. Wheeler, H. O., and Mancusi-Ungaro, P. L.: Role of bile ducts during secretin choleresis in dogs. Am. J. Physiol. 210:1153, 1966.

135. Wheeler, H. O., Mancusi-Ungaro, P. L., and Whitlock, R. T.: Bile salt transport in the dog. J. Clin. Invest. 39:1039, 1960 (abstract).

136. Wheeler, H. O., Meltzer, J. I., and Bradley, S. E.: Biliary transport and hepatic storage of sulfobromophthalein sodium in the unanesthetized dog, in normal man, and in patients with hepatic disease. J. Clin. Invest. 39:1131, 1960.

137. Wheeler, H. O., and Ramos, O. L.: Determinants of the flow and composition in the unanesthetized dog during con-

stant infusions of sodium taurocholate. J. Clin. Invest. *39:*161, 1960.

138. Wheeler, H. O., Ross, E. D., and Bradley, S. E.: Canalicular bile production in dogs, Am. J. Physiol. *214:*866, 1968.

139. Whitlock, R. T., and Wheeler, H. O.: Coupled transport of solute and water across rabbit gallbladder epithelium. J. Clin. Invest. *43:*2249, 1964.

140. Wilbrandt, W., and Rosenberg, T.: The concept of carrier transport and its corol-laries in pharmacology. Pharmacol. Rev. *13:*109, 1961.

141. Winkler, K., and Gram, C.: Models for description of bromsulfalein elimination curves in man after single intravenous injection. Acta. med. scand. *169:*263, 1961.

142. Zaterka, S., and Grossman, M. I.: The effect of gastrin and histamine on secretion of bile. Gastroenterology *50:*500, 1966.

4

Bile Salts and Hepatobiliary Disease

JAMES B. CAREY, JR., M.D., PH.D.

Bile salts are white, crystalline, steroid compounds derived from cholesterol and are not to be confused with pyrrole pigments in bile. They are the chief solid constituent of bile and have numerous interesting properties. From a functional standpoint they are of chief importance as detergents and micelle formers at low concentrations. Thus many otherwise insoluble constituents of bile and intestinal content are held in solution by mixed bile salt micelles which facilitate transport and absorption.[147]

Bile salts are also the chief oxidative products of cholesterol catabolism and therefore their formation, metabolism and excretion are of fundamental importance to the whole problem of the relationship of cholesterol to arterial disease.[11, 250] Because bile salts are synthesized from cholesterol exclusively in the liver, they provide specific and important biochemical information about the liver, especially when it is diseased.[39, 55]

A large number of special properties in addition to micelle formation and their role as end products of cholesterol oxidation have been discovered. A naturally occurring bile salt in man, lithocholate, is a potent pyrogenic and inflammatory agent[217] and produces hepatic cirrhosis when fed to animals,[20] a finding that may be of significance in the perpetuation of human liver injury.[55, 56] It shares with other bile salts strong hemolytic properties for red cells.[213] Deoxycholate, another bile salt in man, forms choleic acid enteroliths,[103] disrupts membranes of most cells including many bacteria[140] and strongly inhibits most membrane-associated metabolic processes thus far studied,[222] including intestinal cholesterol synthesis as does free or unconjugated cholic acid.[75, 76] Bile salts are also antiviral agents.[130]

Conjugated bile salts facilitate the absorption of vitamins A,[211] D[117] and K,[226] calcium,[282] iron,[283] and cholesterol.[266, 277] They also facilitate cholesterol esterification,[276] cleavage of β-carotene to retinal,[116] the action of pancreatic lipase[74] and synthesis of long chain fatty acids.[75]

The micellar aggregates of bile salts, cholesterol and lecithin in bile are of basic importance to the problem of gallstone formation.[162, 255] And, finally, bile salts that occur throughout the vertebrate kingdom reflect evolutionary history, including that of man.[135]

These and other bile salt subjects have been reviewed recently by Haslewood,[134] Hofmann and Small,[147] Kappas and Palmer,[163] and Taylor.[270]

This chapter is confined mainly to the subject of bile salts in human liver disease. Structure, synthesis and metabolism are discussed briefly, for they relate to the alterations that occur in liver disease. Comments on altered bile salt metabolism in certain intestinal disorders and gallstone disease are also included because the liver is integrally involved in these processes as well.

DEFINITIONS

The principal type of bile acid in man, as shown in Figure 4–1, is a 24-carbon compound having a nucleus with the cyclopentanoperhydrophenanthrene configuration

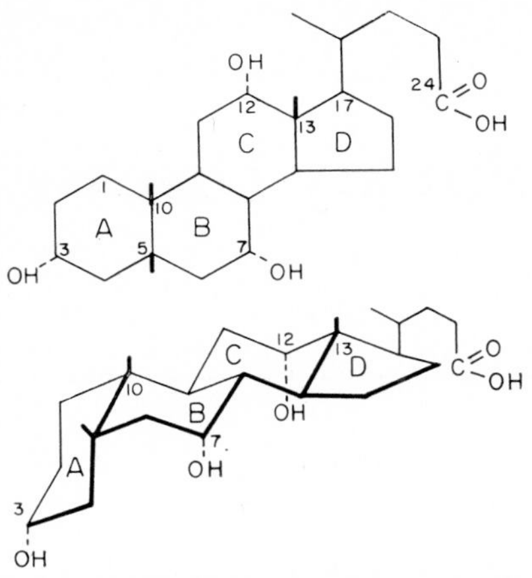

FIG. 4–1. Structural formulas for cholic acid. *Above*, a conventional "flat" diagram. *Below*, diagram illustrating three-dimensional steric relationships on a two-dimensional surface. (Cf. Fig. 4–2.)

common to the other steroids and sterols such as cholesterol (from which bile acids are derived), testosterone, estradiol and adrenal steroids. The side chain contains 5 carbon atoms terminating in a carboxyl group which behaves as an organic acid and thus the name bile acid. Most naturally occurring bile acids have one or more hydroxyl groups ($-OH$) or keto groups ($=O$) at-

tached to the ring. The hydroxyl groups project above (β) or below (α) the plane of the ring.

The shape of a bile acid molecule determines its chemical behavior, especially its detergent properties. A model of a cholic acid molecule is shown in Figure 4–2 and a two-dimensional representation is shown in Figure 4–1. The junction of the A and B rings is such that the hydrogen at the C-5 position projects above the plane of the rings (β position) and is on the same side (*cis*) of the rings as the methyl group at C-10. Thus 24-carbon bile acids with this configuration are designated as 5β-cholanoic acids and cholic acid with its 3 hydroxyl groups is written as 3α, 7α, 12α-trihydroxy-5β-cholanoic acid. More than 90 per cent of the bile acids in man and most other mammals are of the 5β-cholanoic acid type. The 5α epimer of cholic acid, allocholic acid (3α, 7α, 12α trihydroxy-5α-cholanoic acid), has been isolated from human bile in very small amounts but is the chief bile acid in certain lizards such as the iguana.[134]

Bile acids in man are conjugated by peptide linkage with either taurine or glycine. This amino acid conjugation is accomplished in the hepatic cell via CoA intermediates and enhances solubility in aqueous systems by

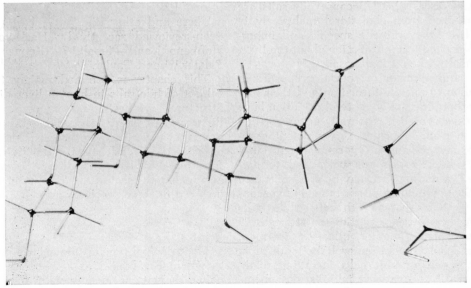

FIG. 4–2. Photograph of a molecular model of cholic acid.

lowering the dissociation constant for free (unconjugated) bile acids from a pKa of about 6 to about 4 for glycine conjugates and about 2 for taurine conjugates. Practically all bile acids in human bile normally occur as amino acid conjugates.

At pH values normally present almost everywhere in the body except the stomach and first portion of the duodenum, conjugated bile acids are in the form of salts, usually of sodium. The same is true of unconjugated (free bile acids) except that with their higher pKa of about 6, they may be un-ionized and more readily precipitated in urine and gastric juice.

The terms *bile acids* and *bile salts* are often used interchangeably because, although usually in the form of salts, these compounds are frequently converted to their acid form for extraction, separation and quantitation. It is probably preferable, however, to use the term bile salt unless the term bile acid is specifically required.

The terms *trihydroxy* and *dihydroxy* bile salts or bile acids are frequently used and refer to the number of hydroxyl groups on the nucleus. Cholic acid shown in Figure 4–1 has 3 hydroxy groups and is therefore a trihydroxy bile acid.

The terms *primary* and *secondary* bile acids or salts are also frequently used. Primary bile salts are formed in the liver from cholesterol. Secondary bile salts are formed from bacterial alteration of a primary bile salt. The 2 primary bile salts in man are cholate and chenodeoxycholate. The 2 secondary bile salts usually formed in greatest amounts in man are deoxycholate and lithocholate, each formed by bacterial 7α-dehydroxylation of their respective primary bile salts, cholate and chenodeoxycholate. See Figure 4–4.

Two 27-carbon bile salts isolated from human bile are intermediates in the transformation of cholesterol to bile salts. Both compounds are 5β-coprostanoic acids and have the formulas, 3α, 7α, 12α-trihydroxy-5β-coprostan-26 (or 27)-oic acid and 3α, 7α-dihydroxy-5β-coprostan-26 (or 27)-oic acid.[46, 55] Both compounds are the chief bile salts of alligators and crocodiles,[71, 133] and therefore end products in the conversion of cholesterol to bile salts in primitive animals

serve as intermediates in this conversion in more recently evolved vertebrates who have 24-carbon bile salts.[43]

BILE SALT SYNTHESIS IN MAN

METABOLIC PATHWAYS

The two 24-carbon primary bile salts in man, cholate and chenodeoxycholate, are formed from cholesterol in the liver. The identity and proper sequence of all intermediate compounds involved in primary bile salt synthesis in man are unknown. The process has been studied extensively in other animals, especially the rat.

The pathways shown in Figure 4–3 are based on observations in man, animals, liver homogenates and subcellular fractions of liver. Only a few of the intermediates shown in the figure have been identified or isolated from human bile. Those that have been identified in human bile are: cholesterol, *I*; 3α, 7α, 12α-trihydroxy-5β-coprostan-26 (or 27)-oic acid, *IX*[46, 261]; 5β-cholestane-3α, 7α-diol, *XII*[228]; 3α, 7α-dihydroxy-5β-coprostan-26 (or 27)-oic acid, *XIV*[55]; and, of course, cholic acid, *X*, and chenodeoxycholic acid, *XV*. Compound *IX* has been crystallized from human fistula bile[46] and shown to be derived from cholesterol[43, 261] and converted to cholic acid in man.[43] Compound *XII* has been identified in human bile as a metabolite of cholesterol.[228] Elucidation of these pathways and characterization of the enzyme systems along these pathways ought to help to explain why bile salt synthesis is sometimes altered extensively in liver disease, often resulting in almost complete inhibition of cholic acid synthesis.

It has been observed in the rat at least that oxidation of the cholesterol side chain inhibits 12α-hydroxylation[12] and that the 12α-hydroxylase enzyme has a high substrate specificity for 7α-hydroxycholest-4-en-3-one, *IV*.[64] The routes for conversion of cholesterol to cholic acid appear to be more restricted and possibly confined to a single major pathway and consequently more easily suppressed, whereas the formation of chenodeoxycholate (which does not require 12α-hydroxylation) apparently may proceed efficiently along several pathways. One pathway

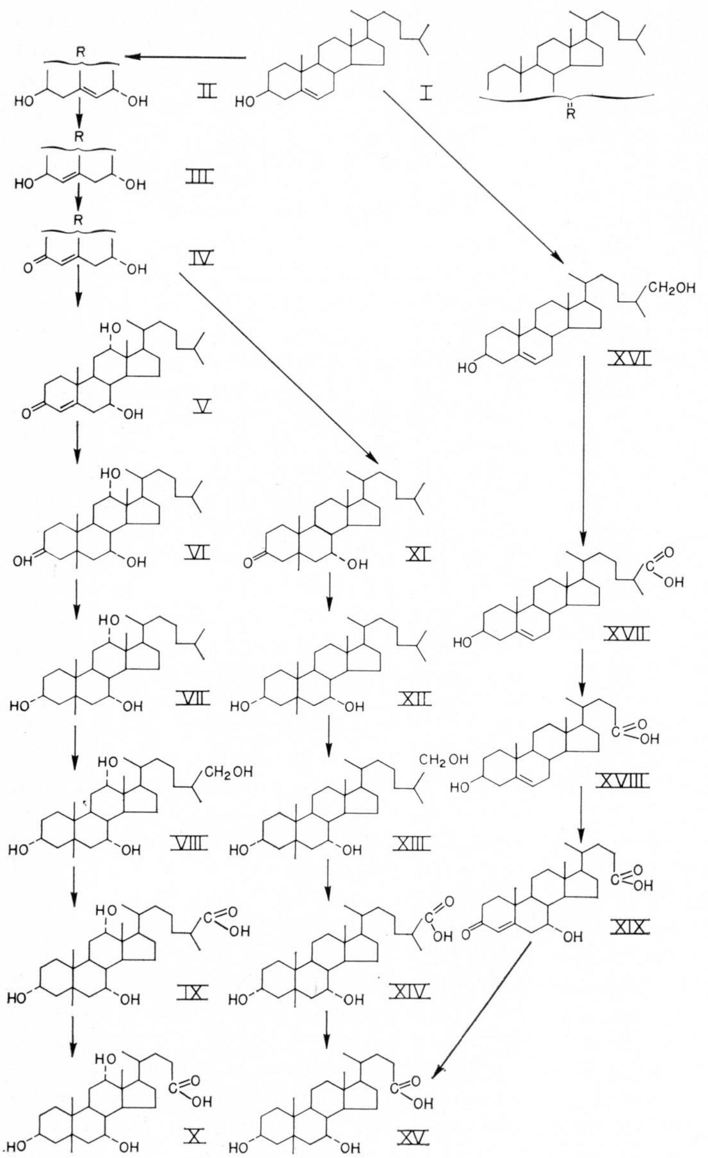

Fig. 4–3. Possible pathways for the formation of cholic and chenodeoxycholic acids in man. (Compiled from various sources including Danielsson and co-workers,[12, 16, 17, 62–66] Staple and co-workers,[31, 32, 188, 190, 191, 228, 261] Dean and Whitehouse,[70–72] and Mitropoulos and Myant.[194–196])

is similar to the cholic acid pathway in which all ring alterations are completed before side chain oxidation. In a second pathway oxidation of a terminal methyl group on the cholesterol side chain yields 26-hydroxycholesterol, *XVI*, which is readily converted to chenodeoxycholic acid but not cholic acid in the rat.[195, 196]

SYNTHESIS RATES

The rate at which cholic acid is synthesized in man is about 200 to 300 mg./day as measured by isotope dilution studies. The rate for chenodeoxycholic acid is similar, so that about 400 to 600 mg. of bile salt is synthesized each day in a healthy adult, and when a steady state exists, synthesis equals excretion and thus an equal amount is excreted in the feces each day.

Table 4–1 gives values for turnover time, pool size and half-life of cholate and chenodeoxycholate and the excretion rates for

TABLE 4-1. VALUES FOR BILE SALT TURNOVER, HALF-LIFE AND POOL SIZE IN MAN

Subjects and Conditions (Number of Subjects)	Total Formation or Excretion mg./day	Cholate Turnover mg./day	Cholate ½ Life days	Cholate Pool Size grams	Chenodeoxycholate Turnover mg./day	Chenodeoxycholate ½ Life days	Chenodeoxycholate Pool Size grams	Authors and Reference Numbers
Normal subjects (2)	490	190–200	2–4	0.54–1.19	290–390	4.3–6.0	2.42–2.52	Danielsson[66]
Normal subjects (3) fat free	130–650							Ali[3]
Normal subjects (8)		360	2.8	1.38			1.45	Lindstedt[180]
Patients (2)	290							Rosenfeld[231]
Normal (5) Butter	473							Moore[198]
Normal (5) Safflower oil	564							Moore[198]
Normal (9) Butter		295	3.2	1.120				Hellström[138]
Normal—Corn oil		314	3.2	1.294				Hellström[138]
Hypercholesterolemia (4) Butter		191	4.2	1.036				Hellström[138]
Hypercholesterolemia— Corn oil		161	5.3	1.238				Hellström[138]
Hypercholesterolemia (5)	272	137	1.1–3.7	0.32–0.65	134	1.4–5	0.30–0.78	Kottke[167]
Mixed Hyperlipidemia (3)	1,172	766			397			Kottke[167]
Hypercholesterolemia (1)	330							Moore[199]
Hypercholesterolemia (1) Cholestyramine	1,076							Moore[199]
Hypercholesterolemia— Cocoanut oil	790							Avigan[7]
Hypercholesterolemia— Safflower oil	540							Avigan[7]
Normal—High cholesterol feed	280–1,070							Wilson[289]
Normal—Low cholesterol feed	230–830							Wilson[289]

both as measured by various investigators using either isotope dilution or isotope balance studies. In one study[3] excretion rates are calculated from direct quantitation of fecal bile acids by gas-liquid chromatography and the total bile acid excretion rate obtained in this way compares favorably with those obtained by isotope balance methods.[197, 198]

CONDITIONS THAT INFLUENCE SYNTHESIS RATES AND POOL SIZE

More factors affect synthesis rates than pool size. If a T tube diverts most or all of the bile outside the body, synthesis of chenodeoxycholic acid increases to about 768 mg./day and cholic acid to about 2,068 mg./day.[51] This represents roughly a four- to sixfold increase, which may be the maximum for man (for rats, ten- to twentyfold).[12] The pool size under these circumstances is probably small and confined largely to the liver and biliary tree. In patients in whom the ileum has been removed, is severely diseased (ileitis) or is bypassed, the bile acid half-life and pool size is greatly reduced and the daily bile acid fractional excretion rate increases from 0.12 to values of 0.5 to 1.5.[260] Cholestyramine may also be expected to accelerate bile salt synthesis rates in man, since it produces a 3.2 fold increase in fecal bile salt excretion.[199] Intestinal cholesterol synthesis rates increase when rats are fed cholestyramine, and this has been attributed to the binding of bile salts in the gut lumen so that they cannot inhibit intestinal cholesterol synthesis as they normally do.[76]

Measurements in patients with hypercholesterolemia have not shown significant changes in bile salt synthesis nor has feeding of nicotinic acid in patients in whom this agent lowered blood cholesterol. In hypercholesterolemia associated with hyperlipidemia (mixed type), synthesis rates for both cholic and chenodeoxycholic acids increase significantly[167] (Table 4–1).

Manipulation of dietary fats to alter serum cholesterol concentrations has relatively little effect on the metabolism of bile acids in man,[7, 181] and the lowering of serum cholesterol concentrations associated with feeding unsaturated fat is not accompanied by significantly increased formation of cholic

acid in man as measured by isotope dilution.[138] In isotope balance studies, however, in which fecal excretion of bile acids and neutral sterols are calculated, bile acid excretion increases significantly when unsaturated fats are fed, sufficient to account for the lowered plasma cholesterol concentrations.[58, 198]

Ingestion of high or low amounts of cholesterol in man is not associated with corresponding changes in bile acid output, according to the studies of Wilson.[289]

CONJUGATION

Bile salt conjugates are synthesized in at least 2 steps: bile acid coenzyme A (CoA) derivatives are formed which in turn combine with taurine or glycine to yield the conjugates.[28, 251] The most active subcellular fractions are microsomes which can be strongly stimulated by the addition of a lysosome fraction (which may contain some peroxisome particles).[241]

The conjugation is apparently complete, for unconjugated (free) bile salts are found only in trace amounts in human bile from healthy subjects or in that examined from patients with various types of liver disease. Conjugation may be required for bile salt excretion, but under experimental conditions small amounts of ^{14}C-labeled free bile acids (1 to 2 per cent) appear in fistula bile following intravenous administration.[51]

Numerous species of bacteria hydrolyze conjugated bile salts.[104, 204] Under normal circumstances this takes place mainly in the colon so that bile salts excreted in the feces are almost entirely unconjugated. If antibiotics are administered, conjugated bile salts are excreted in the feces.[203] Absorption of unconjugated bile salts from the colon may account for the high concentrations of free bile salts in the serum in cirrhosis,[21] a condition in which removal of bile salts from the blood by the liver is delayed.[159]

In healthy adults glycine conjugation predominates and average glycine/taurine ratios are 2.0 to 3.2. (Values of 4 to 6 are observed sometimes.[36, 253]) Bile salts in the human fetus and first few days of life are almost entirely taurine conjugates.[22, 89, 220]

The capacity to synthesize bile salt conjugates is altered in hepatobiliary disorders. This is discussed in a subsequent section.

ENTEROHEPATIC CIRCULATION

Bile salts are formed from cholesterol and conjugated with amino acids in the liver (details of this synthesis are discussed in the preceding section). They are excreted via the bile into the small intestine where they assist with the digestion and absorption of lipids. They are absorbed from the small bowel, mainly by the ileal segment, into the portal circulation and returned to the liver to be excreted again into the bile, thus undergoing enterohepatic circulation (Figure 4–4). It has been estimated that the bile salt pool, which is about 3.5 Gm. in man,[180] undergoes enterohepatic circulation about 10

times daily[25] so that approximately 35 Gm. of bile salt perfuse the liver, biliary tree and small bowel each day, a quantity usually adequate to help "solubilize" the major lipids and pigments in bile and intestinal content.

Most of the bile salt pool is normally confined to the enterohepatic circulation and probably largely to the gallbladder in the fasting state. About 0.5 to 0.6 Gm. of bile salts are synthesized each day and added to the pool, and a similar amount is excreted daily in the feces (Table 4–1).

Bile salts that escape absorption in the small intestine pass into the colon where bacteria remove or alter substituted nuclear groups at the 3, 7 and 12 positions and remove the amino acid conjugate. Bile salts that result from such bacterial action are

Formation of Primary and Secondary Bile Acids from Cholesterol

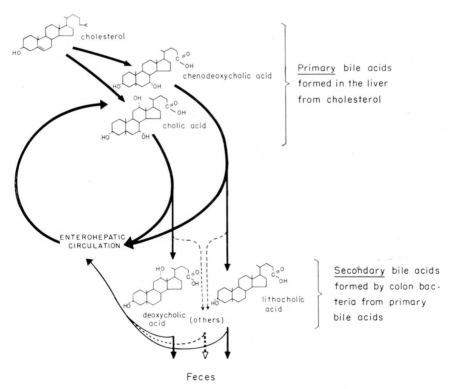

FIG. 4–4. Formation of primary and secondary bile acids from cholesterol, and the enterohepatic circulation of bile salts. See Table 4–2 for a list of secondary bile acids in feces.

called secondary bile salts, whereas bile salts produced from cholesterol in the liver are called primary bile salts. Secondary bile acids are largely excreted in the feces but some are absorbed from the colon and returned to the liver, where they are again conjugated with amino acids and excreted into the bile. Bile salts of normal human bile and serum thus consist of a mixture of primary and secondary types. When bile is excluded from the intestine as occurs with a total external bile fistula, only primary bile salts are found in the bile and no bile salts are found in the feces. The conversion of primary to secondary bile salts by bacteria in the colon is nearly complete so that usually only very small amounts of primary bile salts are found in the feces in healthy sub-

jects. One common reaction performed by colon bacteria is 7α-dehydroxylation of the 2 primary bile salts cholate and chenodeoxycholate, yielding deoxycholic and lithocholic acids, respectively, as shown in Figure 4–4. These are often the 2 major bile salts found in human feces and together usually account for well over half of the bile acids in the feces. Sometimes, however, other secondary bile salts predominate such as the 3β-OH epimer of lithocholic acid, isolithocholic acid.[205]

A partial list of 24 bile acids found in human feces is presented in Table 4–2 and emphasizes the wide variety of secondary bile acids produced by colon bacteria from the 2 primary bile acids (cholic and chenodeoxycholic acids) synthesized in the liver.

TABLE 4–2. 5β-CHOLANOIC ACIDS IDENTIFIED IN HUMAN FECES

POSITION AND NATURE OF SUBSTITUTED GROUPS ON RING NUCLEUS			COMMON NAME	PRIMARY ACID DERIVED FROM*
3	7	12		
αOH	αOH	Keto		Cholic
αOH	Keto	αOH		Cholic
αOH	βOH	αOH		Cholic
βOH	βOH	αOH		Cholic
βOH	αOH	αOH		Cholic
αOH	αOH	αOH	Cholic	
αOH		αOH	Deoxycholic	Cholic
Keto		Keto	Dehydrodeoxycholic	Cholic
αOH		Keto		Cholic
βOH		Keto	12 Keto lithocholic	Cholic
Keto		αOH		Cholic
αOH		βOH		Cholic
βOH		αOH		Cholic
βOH		βOH		Cholic
αOH	αOH		Chenodeoxycholic	
Keto	αOH			Chenodeoxycholic
βOH	αOH			Chenodeoxycholic
αOH	Keto		7 Keto lithocholic	Chenodeoxycholic
αOH	βOH		Ursodeoxycholic	Chenodeoxycholic
βOH	βOH			—
αOH			Lithocholic	Chenodeoxycholic
βOH			Isolithocholic	Chenodeoxycholic
Keto				Chenodeoxycholic
—			Cholanic	—

(Compiled from Eneroth, P., Gordon, B., and Sjövall, J.; J. Lipid Res. 7:524, 1966 and Ali, S. S., Kuksis, A., and Beveridge, J. M. R.; Canad. J. Biochem. 44:957, 1966. Allocholic acid, unsaturated compounds and those with substitutions at positions other than C-3, C-7 or C-12 are not listed.)

* Hill and Drasar[141] have isolated bacterial strains that possess 12α-dehydroxylase, and it is thus possible that some lithocholic acid in feces is derived from cholic acid via 12α-dehydroxylation of deoxycholic acid.

This circumstance makes the quantitation of bile acids considerably more difficult in feces than in either blood or bile. Apparently, none of the proteolytic enzymes in the small bowel deconjugates or otherwise alters bile salts, for in germ-free animals and in those treated with antibiotics, primary conjugated bile acids are excreted in the feces.[122, 123]

ROLE OF BILE SALTS IN DIGESTION AND ABSORPTION

PHYSICOCHEMICAL BEHAVIOR

As discussed in the section on structure, the bile salt molecule has hydroxyl groups and a carboxyl group on one side which are polar and have an affinity for water (hydrophilic). The other side of the molecule does not possess any polar groups and is hydrophobic with 2 neutral, nonpolar angular methyl groups at C-10 and C-13 (Figs. 4–1 and 4–2). The molecule may thus be considered amphipathic and orients itself at an oil/water interface with its polar side toward the aqueous phase and its nonpolar side toward the oil phase. When these amphipathic molecules are brought into solution and their concentration is increased to a certain critical value, some molecules clump together into polymolecular aggregates called micelles. The single molecules in the solution constantly exchange with those in the micelles so that the monomolecular and polymolecular states of dispersion are in stable equilibrium.

The concentration at which micelles form is called the critical micellar concentration (CMC). The CMC for bile salts is about 2 mM.; thus, concentrations normally found in bile and intestinal content exceed the CMC and the bile salts are therefore in micellar solution. The micelles are small; their radius is about 16 to 24 Å assuming near spherical shape,[23, 175] so that such solutions do not scatter light and appear clear as does a tube of normal bile when held up to the light, despite the fact that it contains water-insoluble compounds such as cholesterol.

Bile salt micelles can incorporate other less soluble or insoluble molecules into their structure such as lecithin, cholesterol, mono-glycerides and fatty acids. Such aggregates are called mixed micelles. They are slightly larger than simple bile salt micelles but small enough to give clear solutions. The chief micelles in bile are mixed, containing conjugated bile salts, lecithin and cholesterol in molecular ratios of about 6:2:1 respectively, according to Small.[255] This mixed micellar system permits cholesterol, which is insoluble in water, to be "solubilized" in bile. Its role in gallstone disease is discussed in a later section.

Following a meal containing fat, the jejunal content may be separated by centrifugation into an emulsified oil phase and a micellar phase. The oil phase contains mainly triglycerides, diglycerides and unionized fatty acids. The micellar phase contains mixed micelles of partially ionized fatty acids, monoglycerides and bile salts.[24, 100, 145] Pancreatic lipase hydrolyzes triglycerides, liberating fatty acids and monoglycerides which are neutralized (ionized) by bicarbonate which favors their incorporation into mixed micelles. Such molecular dispersion of the fatty acids and monoglycerides presumably favors their transfer into mucosal cells so that the mixed bile salt–monoglyceride–fatty acid micelle serves as an important transport phase for the passage of water-insoluble products of pancreatic lipolysis into the mucosal cell. The absorption of lipolytic products by the mucosal cell balances the equilibrium of these reactions in the direction of continued lipolysis.

The role of bile salts in fat absorption is thus shifted from the traditional concept of emulsion formation to one of micelle formation, and the chief function of bile salts in fat absorption is considered to be molecular dispersion of the products of pancreatic lipolysis into a micellar phase.

EFFECTS ON METABOLIC PROCESSES

Bile salts have important inhibiting effects on a number of metabolic processes in the small bowel. Highly purified conjugated bile salts inhibited adenosine triphosphatase activity of jejunal mucosal homogenates and brush border preparations in rats in the studies of Pope et al.[222] but Faust and Wu found increased ATPase activity and decreased ATP in rat mucosal tissues.[99] Conjugated bile salts also inhibit cholesterol synthesis in the small bowel, and the site of this inhibition is the conversion of hydroxy-methylglutarate to mevalonic acid.[76]

Unconjugated bile salts, especially deoxycholate, inhibit all metabolic processes in the small bowel thus far examined except sorbose transport[222] and synthesis of long chain fatty acids.[75] Dietschy draws attention to the well-established observation that low concentrations of deoxycholate quickly damage biologic membranes, which may account for its inhibitory effects on enzymes bound to mitochondrial or endoplasmic reticular membranes, whereas soluble enzyme systems are not inhibited by deoxycholate. The extent of inhibition by deoxycholate is modified and sometimes reduced by the presence of conjugated bile salts.[75]

Conjugated bile salts enhance the activity of pancreatic lipase in triglyceride hydrolysis.[74] But they do not affect activities of certain nonlipolytic digestive enzymes such as trypsin, chymotrypsin, amylase and ribonuclease.[183] Apparently they also do not affect transport of glucose or the incorporation of glucose into triglyceride or acetate into lipid.[222]

Conjugated bile salts enhance the intestinal uptake and esterification of palmitate[69] and oleate.[236] A specific cholic acid enzyme complex appears to exist for cholesterol esterification and absorption in which the esterase requires cholic acid or its conjugates not only for significant activity but also to protect itself against the action of proteolytic enzymes.[277] This is regarded as a property of the cholate-esterase complex since conjugated cholate, as mentioned, has, by itself, no effect on the activities of proteolytic enzymes.[183] Cytochrome oxidase activity is inhibited by deoxycholate.[60]

The uptake and central cleavage of carotene into 2 molecules of retinal (vitamin A aldehyde) requires bile salts,[116, 211] as does absorption of vitamins D[117] and K.[226]

Bile salts increase the solubility of calcium salts in lipid solvents in approximately the same proportion as they increase calcium absorption from the gut, possibly by forming a calcium complex which diffuses more rapidly through the cell wall.[282] Bile is not required for absorption of soluble ferrous iron but absorption of sparingly soluble iron phosphate salts is enhanced by bile salts.[283]

The deconjugation of bile salts and the conversion of cholate to deoxycholate by bacterial proliferation in the small bowel (blind loop syndrome) leads to decreased amounts of conjugated bile salts and relatively increased amounts of free bile acids including deoxycholate in the gut lumen.[230] Since unconjugated bile salts are more readily absorbed from the proximal small bowel than conjugated bile salts,[77] bacterial deconjugation of bile salts may lead to a lower total bile salt concentration in the small bowel content and the formation of an adequate micellar phase may be impaired. This circumstance together with the inhibiting effects of deoxycholate on membrane-bound enzymes may well account for the steatorrhea of the blind loop syndrome.

Intestinal Absorption of Bile Salts

The old concept that the ileum is the major site for bile salt absorption[106, 229, 269] has now become well established by many recent studies in a variety of animals[8, 113, 171] and it has been shown that ^{14}C-taurocholate has a half-life of less than 1 day (normally about 3 days) when the ileum is removed or bypassed in man, because it is poorly absorbed and rapidly excreted in the feces.[6, 189] The major role of the ileum in bile salt absorption did not account, however, for the observation that 80 per cent of ^{14}C-cholate given orally to a patient with a bile fistula and ileal bypass was recovered in the fistula bile in less than 12 hours,[44] which demonstrates that other segments of the intestine could absorb bile salt efficiently.

This difference in absorption of conjugated and unconjugated bile salt has been elucidated by Dietschy,[77] who has shown that there are at least 3 transport processes by which bile salts may be absorbed by the small bowel in the rat: (1) ionic diffusion at the rate of 400 moles/min./cm./1.0 mM. activity, (2) nonionic diffusion at 2,000 moles/min./cm./1.0 mM. activity and (3) active transport at a maximum velocity of approximately 2,000 moles/min./cm. in the terminal ileum. Both conjugated and unconjugated bile salts may be absorbed by ionic diffusion in any segment of the small bowel.

Un-ionized bile salts may also pass into mucosal cells at any level of the small intestine at a rate 5 times greater than ionized bile salts. Active transport is apparently limited to the terminal ileum, and both conjugated and unconjugated bile salts are absorbed efficiently by this process.

Under normal circumstances almost all of the bile salts in the small bowel content are conjugated. Conjugated bile salts have pKa values of about 1.8-3.7[80a] and are thus largely ionized at the pH of luminal content which is approximately 6 to 8.[25] Bile salts are absorbed in the jejunum normally by ionic diffusion of conjugated bile salts at rates proportional to their intraluminal concentration and activity. This process is relatively slow and does not keep pace with the absorption rates required to maintain fecal excretion rates, and the bile salt fractional fecal excretion rate increases four- to twelve-fold in patients who have ileal disease, ilectomy or ileal bypass and who must depend mainly on jejunal bile salt absorption.

Both ionic diffusion and active transport take place in the ileum so that this becomes the major site for bile salt absorption, especially its terminal segments.

Bacterial proliferation in the small bowel content leads to bile salt deconjugation. The resulting free bile acids have a higher pKa, about 6, and at the pH of intestinal content are not as fully ionized as conjugated bile salts. Under these conditions the more rapid process of nonionic diffusion, which approaches ileal active transport rates, occurs throughout the small bowel, and luminal bile salt concentrations are lowered if the bacteria deconjugate the bile salts extensively. Bile salt conjugation with taurine or glycine by the liver provides detergent compounds with a sufficiently low pKa to prevent them from being absorbed prematurely by nonionic diffusion and thus they remain for the most part in the lumen of the small intestine to assist with the micellar phase of fat digestion until they are finally absorbed mainly by active transport in the terminal ileum.[75, 172]

The concentrations of bile salts in the intestinal content rise to values of 13 to 46 mEq./L. as the gallbladder empties and then decline rapidly to 2.5 to 10 mEq./L.

during the remaining period of digestion and absorption.[252] The concentrations remain fairly uniform throughout the human small intestine until the terminal segment is reached, which is additional evidence that bile salts are absorbed mainly in the terminal ileum.

Less is known regarding bile salt transport in the colon. Deoxycholate and lithocholate are formed in the colon and regularly occur in human bile when the enterohepatic circulation is intact (Table 4–3). Thus bile salts are absorbed in the colon. Deoxycholic acid is almost always present in amounts that exceed the quantities of lithocholate, yet the 2 acids occur in about equal amounts in feces and this may be related to the less polar nature of lithocholate, differences in ionization constants or both.

BILE SALT ALTERATIONS IN HEPATOBILIARY DISORDERS

SOURCES FOR BILE SALT DETERMINATIONS

Information concerning alterations in bile salt metabolism in various hepatobiliary disorders has been derived from measurement of bile salt concentrations in blood serum, bile, intestinal content, urine, feces and skin. The advantages and limitations of bile salt determinations from these 6 sources should be considered briefly.

From a methodological standpoint bile salts are most easily quantitated in bile where they are the chief solid constituent. But bile and duodenal contents are cumbersome to obtain in a routine way and their composition is variable, especially that of duodenal content unless collected under standardized conditions. Despite these difficulties, there are some excellent studies of bile salt alterations in bile and duodenal content in hepatobiliary disease, and these will be discussed.

Quantitation of bile salts in serum is complicated by its meager bile salt content and high protein concentration (which is why methods for bile are often unsuitable for blood) but is relatively uniform in composition and conveniently obtained. Possibly for these reasons most of the information concerning bile salt alterations in hepatobiliary disease discussed in these sections is based on measurements in blood and compared when possible with duodenal content. Studies on bile, urine, skin and feces are included where appropriate.

The healthy liver efficiently extracts bile salts from portal blood so that under normal circumstances the bile salt pool is confined largely to the enterohepatic cycle (liver → bile → intestine → portal blood → liver). In hepatobiliary disease the liver is often rendered less efficient in clearing bile salts from the blood,[159] which results in a slight shift in the distribution of the bile salt pool so that bile salts are more concentrated in systemic blood, urine and skin. Even with such a shift, however, serum bile salt concentrations remain in the microgram/ml. range whereas the concentrations in bile are in the milligram/ml. range (1 mg. = 1000 μg.).

Numerous methods have been devised for serum bile salt analysis, and "normal" values depend on the methods used. (For reviews of these methods, see MacIntyre and Wootton[186] and Sandberg et al.[235]) Briefly, most modern methods involve bile salt quantitation by spectrophotometry or gas-liquid chromatography in a protein-free extract of serum which has been hydrolyzed with strong alkali (4N NaOH) to obtain free (unconjugated) bile acids. Enzymatic cleavage of the amino acid–bile acid peptide bond[200] may greatly facilitate bile salt analysis in serum as it has in bile and avoid losses incurred by hydrolysis with strong alkali. Sandberg and Sjövall have successfully employed an Amberlyst anion exchange resin followed by chromatography on alumina to provide a serum fraction suitable for gas-liquid chromatography.[235] Conventional extraction procedures and celite column chromatography are also satisfactory for gas-liquid chromatography and permit estimation of lithocholic acid concentrations.[52] Serum bile salt analysis by gas-liquid chromatography permits separation and quantitation of individual primary and secondary bile salts, whereas spectrophotometric methods often quantitate bile salts as trihydroxy and dihydroxy fractions. The trihydroxy fraction is mainly cholate and the dihydroxy fraction is largely chenodeoxycholate with lesser amounts of deoxycholate.

When serum bile salt concentrations are elevated well above the normal range the increase is accounted for almost entirely by the 2 primary bile salts cholate and chenodeoxycholate (concentrations of secondary bile salts seldom exceed 2 to 3 μg./ml.), and consequently the spectrophotometric method quantitates all but a few micrograms of the bile salts in serum specifically as cholate and chenodeoxycholate when the concentrations are elevated. This is apparent from comparison of trihydroxy/dihydroxy ratios with cholate/chenodeoxycholate for individuals listed in Table 4–5. They are virtually identical.

Normal Bile Salt Concentrations and Ratios in Blood and Bile

A range of values for bile salt concentrations and their ratios in serum, duodenal content, hepatic bile, gallbladder bile and fistula bile, compiled from various sources is presented in Table 4–3. As expected, bile salt concentrations are highest in gallbladder bile and lowest in serum, and the difference is large, by factors of approximately 10^3 to 10^4. Bile salt concentrations in hepatic bile are in the range of 18 mg./ml. and in the duodenum, about 2 mg./ml. Fistula bile (usually T tube drainage of the common bile duct) represents a circumstance in which the enterohepatic cycle is partially or totally interrupted and bile salt concentrations are reduced from those found in hepatic bile to about 4 mg./ml.

The relative quantities (concentration ratios) of the 2 primary bile salts, cholate and chenodeoxycholate, are in general similar in bile and blood with a tendency for predominance of cholate in bile and chenodeoxycholate in serum, especially when measured in serum by gas-liquid chromatography.

The 2 secondary bile salts most often measured in bile and blood, deoxycholate and lithocholate usually occur in lower concentrations and concentration ratios when compared with primary bile salts, especially lithocholate.

Concentration ratios in duodenal content reflect fairly accurately those found in hepatic and gallbladder bile.[253] Also, in general concentration ratios for blood and duodenal

TABLE 4-3. NORMAL BILE SALT CONCENTRATIONS AND CONCENTRATION RATIOS IN BLOOD AND BILE

SOURCE AND METHOD	CHOLATE	CHENODE-OXYCHOLATE	DEOXY-CHOLATE	LITHO-CHOLATE	TOTAL	TRI-HYDROXY	DI-HYDROXY	REFERENCES
Concentrations								
Serum G.L.C. (Sandberg) µg./ml.	0.03–0.65	0.05–1.30	0.05–0.45	–	0.3 –2.3			235
Serum G.L.C. (Carey) µg./ml.	0–0.95	0.22–0.95	0.01–0.27	0–0.11	0.33–2.11			52
Serum U.V. spectrum µg./ml.					0–5.3	0–3.4	0–1.9	39
Duodenal content G.L.C. mg./ml.	0.98	0.59	0.50	0.01	2.08	0.98	1.1	a.l.*
Fistula bile U.V. spec. mg./ml.					4.4	3.1	1.3	a.l.
Hepatic bile mg./ml.					18.0			36
Gallbladder bile G.L.C. mg./ml.	18.3	11.5	6.7	1.5	7–64			202
Ratio of Average Values								
Serum	0.45	1	0.38	0.09		1.9	1	
Duodenal content	1.6	1	0.8	0.01		0.9	1	
Fistula bile						2.4	1	
Gallbladder bile	1.6	1	0.6	0.1				

* *a.l.*, results obtained in the author's laboratory.

TABLE 4–4. SIMULTANEOUS MEASUREMENT OF BILE SALT CONCENTRATIONS AND CONCENTRATION RATIOS IN BLOOD AND DUODENAL CONTENT

	CHOLATE	CHENODEOXY-CHOLATE	DEOXY-CHOLATE	LITHO-CHOLATE
Patient with Portal Cirrhosis				
Concentrations (μg./ml) in:				
Serum	4.5	8.6	2.2	0.27
Duodenal content	1,425	2,610	714	44
Ratios in:				
Serum	0.52	1	0.26	0.03
Duodenal content	0.55	1	0.27	0.02
Patient with Carcinoma, Common				
bile duct				
Concentrations (μg./ml) in:				
Serum	19.8	16.9	0	0
Duodenal content	2,180	1,550	31.7	0.39
Ratios in:				
Serum	1.2	1	—	—
Duodenal content	1.4	1	0.02	0.0003

content correlate well when measured simultaneously (Table 4–4). In other words, if chenodeoxycholate predominates in blood it also predominates in bile and duodenal content. But this is true in blood only if the concentration of at least one of the bile salts is increased above the normal range. This is so because the normal concentrations for cholate and chenodeoxycholate usually differ by less than 1 μg./ml. in serum and are so small that they are close to the error of the method, which may be 0.05 to 0.8 μg./ml., and hence the ratio may change from > 1 to < 1 simply by error alone. When the concentration of one of the bile salts is elevated above the normal range, however, with the error of the method remaining the same, the ratio is not altered significantly by error and thus becomes valid. Serum bile salt concentration ratios in healthy subjects are valid if expressed as the average of multiple determinations in an individual or single determinations in a group. The values presented in Table 4–3 represent averages for a group of healthy subjects.

SERUM BILE SALTS IN HEPATOBILIARY DISORDERS

The liver is the only organ known to synthesize the 2 primary bile salts, cholate and chenodeoxycholate. Measurement of their concentrations in serum is thus specific for the liver and the biochemical processes of bile salt metabolism in the liver and enterohepatic circulation, and therefore may be expected to provide useful information concerning hepatobiliary disease. Determining the individual primary bile salt concentrations and comparing these by means of a concentration ratio is vastly more informative than measuring total serum bile salt concentrations. For this reason, this section emphasizes the bile salt concentration ratio and how it is altered with disease.

The cholate/chenodeoxycholate ratio rises with cholestasis and biliary tract obstruction and declines with liver injury. The cholate/chenodeoxycholate ratio is similar to the trihydroxy/dihydroxy bile salt ratio when serum bile salt concentrations are elevated because the increase is due almost entirely to cholate (trihydroxy) and chenodeoxycholate (dihydroxy). The concentration of the other major dihydroxy bile salt in blood, deoxycholate, rarely exceeds 2 to 3 μg./ml. When serum bile salt concentrations are increased above the normal range, therefore, the trihydroxy/dihydroxy concentration ratio may be regarded for all practical purposes as equivalent to the cholate/chenodeoxycholate primary bile salt ratio and may be used interchangeably. (See Table 4–5 for a comparison of trihydroxy/

diyhdroxy ratios with cholate/chenodeoxy-cholate ratios.)

Bile Duct Obstruction and Cholestasis

In bile duct obstruction serum bile salt concentrations commonly increase and cholate usually predominates so that the cholate/chenodeoxycholate ratio and therefore the trihydroxy/dihydroxy ratio is usually greater than one. The range of values for the trihydroxy/dihydroxy ratio in 79 patients is plotted in Figure 4–5. In 82 per cent of these patients the ratio is greater than one, which is of interest compared with the portal cirrhosis group in which 81 per cent had a ratio less than one. The values for the trihydroxy/dihydroxy ratio are 0.001 to 28 with a median value of 3.0 and an average of 3.1.

Concentrations for trihydroxy bile salts range up to 110.7 µg./ml. and for the dihydroxy fraction up to 60.3 µg./ml. These increases are probably accounted for almost exclusively by cholic and chenodeoxycholic acids, for when the individual bile salts are quantitated by gas-liquid chromatography, as shown in Table 4–5, deoxycholate and lithocholate are frequently absent, a circumstance noted more often with bile duct obstruction or during the obstructive (cholestatic) phase of viral hepatitis than with portal cirrhosis in which secondary bile acids are more commonly present in normal or increased concentrations. Diminished concentrations or absence of deoxycholic acid in duodenal contents in bile duct obstruction[253] is compatible with the findings in serum. Low concentrations or absence of secondary bile salts in blood and duodenal content in bile duct obstruction or cholestasis may be accounted for by the fact that smaller quantities of primary bile salts enter

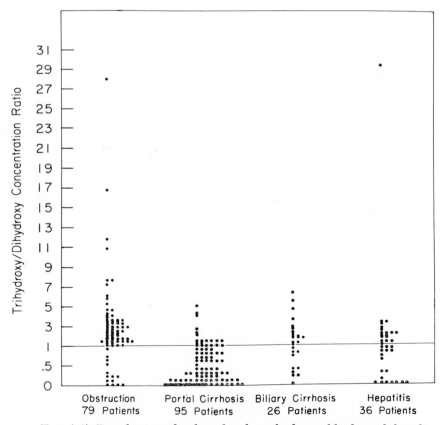

Fig. 4–5. Distribution of values for the trihydroxy/dihydroxy bile salt concentration ratios in serum for 4 major types of hepatobiliary disease.

TABLE 4–5. REPRESENTATIVE VALUES FOR SERUM BILE SALT CONCENTRATIONS AND CONCENTRATION RATIOS IN SOME COMMON DISEASES

PATIENT AND DISEASE	SERUM CONCENTRATIONS μG./ML.				CONCENTRATION RATIOS				
	Cholate	Chenodeoxy-cholate	Deoxy-cholate	Litho-cholate	Tri-hydroxy-Dihydroxy	Cholate	Chenodeoxy-cholate	Deoxy-cholate	Litho-cholate
1. Carcinoma, pancreas	65.0	16.3	0	0	4.0	4.0	1.0	—	—
2. Carcinoma, pancreas	34.3	12.8	0	0	2.7	2.7	1.0	—	—
3. Portal cirrhosis	9.3	16.0	0	0.02	0.6	0.6	1.0	—	0.001
4. Portal cirrhosis	2.2	3.6	0.5	0.02	0.5	0.6	1.0	0.14	0.005
5. Portal cirrhosis	5.6	11.8	0.8	0.13	0.4	0.47	1.0	0.07	0.01
6. Portal cirrhosis	1.1	16.7	0.7	0.47	0.06	0.07	1.0	0.04	0.03
7. Portal cirrhosis	3.2	15.6	1.1	0.97	0.2	0.2	1.0	0.07	0.06
8. Hepatitis, viral	79.4	23.1	0	0	3.4	3.4	1.0	—	—
9. Hepatitis, viral	30.9	20.9	0	0	1.4	1.4	1.0	—	—
10. Hepatitis, inf. mono.*	75.0	25.0	0	0.04	3.0	3.0	1.0	—	0.002
11. Biliary cirrhosis	19.0	8.0	0	0.03	2.0	2.0	1.0	—	0.004
12. Biliary cirrhosis	100.0	37.0	0	0	2.7	2.7	1.0	—	—

* Infectious mononucleosis.

tients the concentrations were observed to decrease tenfold in 5 days or less. This rapid fall is, of course, observed with other measurements such as the serum bilirubin, alkaline phosphatase and serum transaminase enzymes, but tends to occur more rapidly with bile salt concentrations, especially when compared with the rate of decline in bilirubin concentrations.

An example of the rapid decline of serum bile salt concentrations in hepatitis is shown in Figure 4–6. These observations are in contrast to those of Frosch, who observed that serum bile salt concentrations remained elevated after bilirubin concentrations and enzyme activities returned to normal, and therefore regarded serum bile salt measurements as superior to other tests in revealing abnormal liver cell function.[107, 108]

The concentration ratios of primary bile salts may change during the course of the disease, being higher during the early stages and then falling to values approaching 1. The average ratio for this group was 1.9, and thus similar to the biliary cirrhosis group. The ratio frequently becomes less than 1 as the bile salt concentrations fall rapidly, possibly because cholate may have a shorter half-life than chenodeoxycholate (cf. Table 4–1). Under these conditions, the less than 1 ratio probably does not reflect severe liver injury nor does it indicate a poor prognosis, especially when other tests show improvement such as lowering of alkaline phosphatase, bilirubin and transaminase enzymes. Such a low ratio is transient and only briefly present as the concentrations fall rapidly. If the ratio remains less than 1 for a week or more, however, it may indicate more serious liver injury, often reflected by a rise in bilirubin concentration.

Post-transfusion Hepatitis. Serum bile salt concentrations and concentration ratios appear to behave in a fashion very similar to the changes encountered in infectious hepatitis, except that the rapid changes are less often seen in the post-transfusion group.

Cholangiolytic hepatitis described by Watson and Hoffbauer[281] and regarded by some as a form of chronic active hepatitis in which cholestasis is a predominant feature, is accompanied by increased serum bile salt concentrations and the ratio is usually

greater than 1, a finding compatible with the elevated alkaline phosphatase values and relatively little change in serum proteins, cephalin flocculation or thymol turbidity found in these patients.

Infectious Mononucleosis. In the type of hepatitis frequently associated with infectious mononucleosis, serum bile salt concentrations may be very high just as in infectious (viral) hepatitis, but the trihydroxy/dihydroxy ratio seldom falls below 1, which is in keeping with the relatively benign and self-limited course of this disease (Table 4–5).

Chronic Types of Hepatitis. With chronic forms of hepatitis, such as plasma cell hepatitis, granulomatous hepatitis, lupoid hepatitis, and chronic active hepatitis in which the disease undergoes repeated exacerbations and remissions, serum bile salt concentrations tend to parallel the rise and fall of other laboratory tests used to follow the course of these conditions, such as serum bilirubin, transaminase enzymes and serum immunoglobulin concentrations. During exacerbations when serum bile salt concentrations are often increased, chenodeoxycholate often predominates and the trihydroxy/dihydroxy ratio is less than 1. In remissions brought about by immunosuppressive agents, serum bile salt concentrations are lowered as are the concentrations of bilirubin, immunoglobulins and transaminase enzymes, despite the fact that certain of these agents, such as 6-mercaptopurine, are known to induce hepatic injury when used in larger doses.

Drug-Induced Jaundice

The 8 patients listed in Table 4–6 had jaundice associated with ingestion of an agent that was regarded as having induced the jaundice. The drugs ingested by most of this group are well-known icterogenic agents such as chlorpromazine, 5-fluorouracil, carbarsone and Nilevar. In all patients who took these agents the serum bile salt concentrations were elevated and the trihydroxy/dihydroxy ratio was greater than 1, a finding that is consistent with the cholestatic type of jaundice induced by these agents in which serum alkaline phosphatase activities increase also.

TABLE 4–6. SERUM BILE SALT CONCENTRATIONS AND CONCENTRATION
RATIOS IN DRUG-INDUCED JAUNDICE

PATIENT AND DRUG	TRIHYDROXY μg./ml.	DIHYDROXY μg./ml.	TRI/DI RATIO	TOTAL BILIRUBIN mg.%	ALKALINE PHOSPHATASE K.A. units
1. Chlorpromazine	47.6	17.0	2.8	4.4	64.6
2. 5-Fluorouracil	24.9	14.3	1.7	11.4	62.4
3. Nilevar	20.6	7.4	2.7	—	47.8
4. Carbarsone	76.1	31.5	2.4	7.9	55.6
5. Tolbutamide°	137.4	19.5	7.0	15.7	64.0
6. Dilantin	75.9	38.6	1.9	—	—
7. Isoniazide	5.0	8.4	0.6	6.0	27.0
8. Mestranol†	112.0	28.0	4.3	—	—

° Case reported by Gregory, Zaki, Sarosi, and Carey, Arch. Path. *84*:194, 1967.
† Mestranol is the estrogen component of Enovid. Case reported by Urban, Frank and Kern, Ann. Int. Med. *68*:598, 1968.

In one patient receiving isoniazid (INH), (Patient 7, Table 4–6), the primary bile salt ratio was less than 1, which is compatible with the more severe type of hepatocellular injury induced by this group of compounds.

Various sulfonurea hypoglycemic agents occasionally induce jaundice but tolbutamide apparently does so only rarely. Patient 5 had jaundice with the eventual development of biliary cirrhosis, having continued to take tolbutamide for over 1 year after the onset of jaundice. It appears that mestranol, the estrogen component of Enovid, is responsible for cholestatic jaundice and pruritus sometimes associated with Enovid ingestion,[274] and this steroid can also produce high serum bile salt concentrations (Patient 8, Table 4–6).

Other Liver Disorders

Table 4–7 lists serum bile salt concentrations for a group of less common liver diseases. In 2 patients with *Gilbert's disease*, serum bile salt concentrations were not elevated during periods of jaundice, a finding that is consistent with the benign course of the syndrome and the usually normal values obtained for other laboratory studies. Serum

TABLE 4–7. SERUM BILE SALT CONCENTRATIONS AND CONCENTRATION
RATIOS IN LESS COMMON DISEASES INVOLVING THE LIVER

PATIENT AND CONDITION	TRIHY- DROXY μg./ml.	DIHYDROXY μg./ml.	TRI/DI RATIO	TOTAL BILIRUBIN mg.%	ALKALINE PHOSPHATASE K.A. units
1. Gilbert's disease	0	0	—	2.8	—
2. Gilbert's disease	0	1.3	—	2.6	12.0
3. Polycystic-liver	0.3	0.9	0.33	0.3	—
4. Polycystic-liver	0	1.4	—	—	56.6
5. Dubin-Johnson syndrome	0	1.2	—	1.8	4.2
6. Dubin-Johnson syndrome	6.7	2.3	2.9	3.2	—
7. Gaucher's disease	3.3	2.9	1.1	0.5	33.0
Gaucher's pregnant	27.1	6.0	4.5	0.8	37
Gaucher's cholestyramine	4.3	2.2	2.0	0.9	—
8. Portal vein thrombosis	3.1	1.3	2.3	—	—
9. Wilson's disease	0.2	17.8	0.01	2.4	9.0
10. Wilson's disease	0	23.7	—	1.0	11.0
11. Hemochromatosis	0	0.9	—	0.3	4.8
12. Hepatic cholesterol storage (Schiff et al.[242])	4.7	7.1	0.67	normal	elevated

TABLE 4–8. SERUM BILE SALT CONCENTRATIONS AND CONCENTRATION
RATIOS IN ACUTE ALCOHOLIC LIVER INJURY

PATIENT	ADMISSION			10 DAYS AFTER ADMISSION		
	Trihydroxy μg./ml.	Dihydroxy μg./ml.	Ratio	Trihydroxy μg./ml.	Dihydroxy μg./ml.	Ratio
1	10.8	23.4	0.5	1.1	11.0	0.1
2	2.5	15.1	0.2	1.1	3.8	0.3
3	4.1	53.6	0.1	1.0	1.4	0.7
4	0.8	32.4	0.02	5.4	3.7	1.5
5	0.4	19.2	0.02	1.6	5.9	0.3
6	10.1	9.2	1.1	6.5	13.5	0.5
7	1.1	28.8	0.04	2.2	34.5	0.06

bile salt concentrations were also normal in 2 patients with *polycystic disease* involving the liver; one had esophageal varices and died from hemorrhage, the other died from carcinoma of the breast (no hepatic metastasis). In one of the jaundiced patients with *Dubin-Johnson syndrome*, bile salt concentrations were slightly elevated in the serum and the trihydroxy/dihydroxy ratio was 2.9. Other routine blood studies were normal in this patient except for BSP retention of 21 per cent.

An adult female with *Gaucher's disease* suffered intense pruritus during each of 2 pregnancies and was found to have elevated serum bile salt concentration (tri/di = 27.1/6.0 μg./ml.) repeatedly. The serum bilirubin concentrations remained normal and the serum bile salt concentrations were lowered with cholestyramine which relieved the pruritus.

A patient with *portal vein thrombosis* and a normal liver biopsy had normal serum bile salt concentrations and BSP retention of 22 per cent, but the serum bilirubin remained normal.

Two patients with *Wilson's disease* had little or no detectable cholic acid in their serum with appreciable concentrations of chenodeoxycholate thus yielding very low cholate/chenodeoxycholate ratios. The first patient listed died 23 days after the serum bile salts were measured.

In a patient with *hemochromatosis* serum bile salt concentrations were not elevated in keeping with the usually normal liver function tests encountered in this disease. (See Chap. 21.)

In *hepatic cholesterol ester storage disease*[242] serum bile salt concentrations are increased with a trihydroxy/dihydroxy ratio of less than 1 so that chenodeoxycholate predominates in the serum of the patients and their siblings but liver function tests are normal and the patients do not appear especially ill with severe liver disease, as the primary bile acid ratio of less than 1 would imply.

Alcoholic Liver Injury

Changes in serum bile salt concentrations and concentration ratios are pronounced in alcoholic liver disease, especially during the stages of acute alcoholism.[39] Table 4–8 lists a group of 7 patients with alcoholic liver disease admitted following a period of excessive alcoholic consumption, a familiar circumstance in large public hospitals. Serum bile salt concentrations were elevated in all and the ratio was less than 1 in all but one. Ten days following admission, serum bile salt concentrations declined in the first 5 patients and the ratio increased in all but the first of these 5. For the last 2 patients represented in the table the bile salt concentrations worsened. The changes in serum bile salts may be interpreted as compatible with acute liver injury associated with excessive ethanol consumption and further support the view that ethanol itself may be directly toxic to the liver.[177, 232]

Pruritus and Jaundice in Pregnancy

In a group of 28 pregnant women studied by Sjövall and Sjövall[254] 22 were healthy. Their serum bile salt concentrations were normal and did not vary appreciably with the week of gestation. In 6 patients with pruritus in the third trimester the mean serum cholate concentration was 19.9 μg./ml. and for chenodeoxycholate 4.4 μg./ml., giving a primary bile salt ratio of 4.5, a value similar to those found in the bile duct obstruction–cholestasis group. Only one of the 6 patients was jaundiced, and pruritus disappeared in all shortly after delivery. Serum bile salt concentrations measured in 2 subjects following delivery fell toward normal values.

Three pregnant patients from our group with pruritus and jaundice also had increased serum bile salt concentrations. The ratios were greater than 1 in 2 patients but was 0.9 in the third who had eclampsia. Estrogens appear to play a role in idiopathic jaundice of pregnancy and pruritus gravidarum. Estrogens with phenolic A rings impair hepatic BSP disposal.[110] In patients who were jaundiced or pruritic during pregnancy, ethinyl estradiol produced similar symptoms and impaired liver function.[168] A carefully studied patient had increased serum bile salt concentrations when given mestranol, the estrogen component of Enovid (Table 4–6) and other evidence of liver dysfunction but was not so affected when given the progestational component norethynodrel.[274]

The pruritus is readily relieved with cholestyramine, as is discussed in the section on therapeutic agents.

SERUM BILE SALTS IN OTHER DISEASES

A wide variety of diseases not generally regarded as primary hepatobiliary disorders may be accompanied by jaundice, hepatomegaly or both. Examples of a few such conditions are presented in this section but too few patients are studied in any category to permit any general conclusions.

Two patients with *sickle cell disease* (one with hepatic micro infarcts) had small elevations in serum chenodeoxycholate concentrations.[235] A patient with *hyperlipidemia*[235] and one with *hypercholesterolemia* had normal serum bile salt concentrations. In 5 jaundiced patients with various types of *hemolytic anemias* studied in the author's laboratory, 4 had normal serum bile salt con-

centrations, one had 10.7 μg./ml. of cholate, cephalin flocculation 4+, BSP retention 3 per cent. Because the liver is the chief excretory organ for lipids and pigments, when presented with excessive quantities of these substances, hepatic transport of bile salts could be impaired, especially if common pathways for organic anions are involved as proposed by Sperber[259] and discussed by Lathe.[174]

Two patients with *sprue* and no evidence of liver disease had normal serum bile salt concentrations. In 6 jaundiced patients with various types of *myeloid and lymphatic leukemia* and hepatomegaly, serum bile salt concentrations were elevated and leukemic infiltrations were found in the liver at autopsy. No consistent change was noted in the primary bile salt ratio, but this feature was undoubtedly influenced by the variety of chemotherapeutic agents given to many of these patients. Such agents alone influence bile salt concentrations and concentration ratios as discussed in the section on drug-induced jaundice. One of these patients not receiving chemotherapy, however, had a relatively high serum chenodeoxycholate concentration (15 μg./ml.) with no detectable cholate and at autopsy 9 days later the liver was found to be small and composed largely of fat. Another of these patients with acute myeloid leukemia had severe pruritus sometimes associated with this condition but serum bile salt concentrations were not sufficiently high to account for this (trihydroxy 1.0 μg./ml., dihydroxy, 2.3 μg./ml.). Similarly serum bile salt concentrations were normal in 2 patients with severe pruritus associated with *Hodgkin's disease* but without hepatic involvement. When Hodgkin's disease does involve the liver, serum bile salt concentrations increase.

In 2 jaundiced patients with *congestive heart failure* serum bile salt concentrations were normal.

In a patient with chronic glomerulonephritis undergoing a course of *malaria* therapy, serum bile salt concentrations increased slightly (trihydroxy 4.9 μg./ml., dihydroxy 1.0 μg./ml.), but serum bilirubin concentrations remained normal.

A patient with *thyrotoxicosis* had normal serum bile salt concentrations. Of 7 patients with *hypothyroidism, myxedema* or both, 4 had serum cholate concentrations of 4.1 to 25.6 μg./ml., but chenodeoxycholate concentrations remained normal. Administration of thyroxine to rats stimulates bile salt synthesis[263] with a relatively greater effect on chenodeoxycholate formation possibly by stimulating side chain cleavage.[194]

Serum bile salt concentrations were studied in 3 patients with *regional enteritis* and in 4 patients with *ulcerative colitis*.[54] Concentrations of chenodeoxycholate were moderately elevated in one of the patients with regional enteritis and in 2 with ulcerative colitis; all 3 had other evidence of liver disease. Only trace amounts of lithocholate were found in the serum of the 2 ulcerative colitis patients with increased serum chenodeoxycholate concentrations and none could be detected in the remaining 5 patients. It thus does not appear plausible, on the basis of this limited survey, that in chronic inflammatory bowel disease the mucosa is more permeable to secondary bile salts which may possibly be toxic to the liver, such as lithocholic acid, thus either inducing or perpetuating liver disease. If anything, the reverse is more likely, that the circumstances accompanying chronic inflammatory bowel disease (damaged mucosa, increased volume of intestinal content and diarrhea) render such intestinal tracts less permeable to bile salts.

PRURITUS OF JAUNDICE

Bile salts are the only compounds that have been regularly shown to occur in increased concentrations in the blood and skin of patients with the type of pruritus associated with jaundice. Conditions in which other substances, such as bilirubin, cholesterol, phospholipids, neutral lipids or free fatty acids reach their highest concentrations in the blood or skin without increased bile salt concentrations are not associated with pruritus.

Despite some conflicting observations, the bulk of recent evidence supports the hypothesis that increased concentrations of bile salts in the skin, resulting from sustained elevations in serum concentrations, are responsible for the pruritus of jaundice. The evidence for and against this hypothesis has been reviewed with welcomed succinctness

by Schoenfield, Sjövall and Perman,[244] who demonstrated higher concentrations of bile salts in the skin of patients who itched than in those who did not. They also demonstrated a reduction in high skin bile salt concentrations in a jaundiced patient with pancreatic carcinoma and pruritus following cholecystojejunostomy which relieved the pruritus and lowered the serum bile salt concentrations. Since skin itches and not blood, these studies provide the best evidence to date for the role of bile salts in pruritic jaundice.

Serum bile salt concentrations can be lowered with cholestyramine feeding,[49, 278] and when serial serum bile salt determinations are done at frequent intervals the concentrations reach near normal levels before pruritus stops; when cholestyramine is withheld, high serum concentrations are reached before pruritus starts. This lag period, which may be a day or more, may represent the period of time required for concentrations of bile salts sufficient to induce pruritus to accumulate in or leave the skin.[49]

Such a lag period might sometimes account for the discrepancy between skin and serum bile salt concentrations and for the occasional instance in which an isolated measurement of serum bile salt concentration bears no apparent relationship to the presence or absence of pruritus in jaundiced patients. Therefore, serial determinations of serum or skin bile salt concentrations must be done when studying their relationship to pruritus, for, when serum bile salt concentrations are falling, low values can be obtained before itching stops and when concentrations are rising high values can be obtained before itching starts.[49]

Treatment of pruritic jaundice is discussed in the section on therapeutic agents.

CHANGES IN BILE AND DUODENAL CONTENT

As mentioned, the concentration ratios of cholate, chenodeoxycholate and deoxycholate in duodenal content are similar to those in bile. They also correspond to those in serum except that the ratios for cholate and deoxycholate tend to be slightly lower in serum (Table 4–3). Changes in these ratios with hepatobiliary disease are the same as those found in serum as discussed in the preceding sections.

Sjövall studied bile salt concentration ratios in duodenal content of patients with gallstones, obstructive jaundice and portal cirrhosis and found that the chief alteration in *cholelithiasis* was a relative increase in the amounts of deoxycholate, sometimes exceeding the concentrations of cholate and chenodeoxycholate.[253] In *obstructive jaundice*, cholate increased (ratio, 2.3) and deoxycholate declined (ratio, 0.25), the same type of ratio alteration found in serum in this condition in which the average cholate/chenodeoxycholate ratio was 3.1 (Fig. 4–5). In *portal cirrhosis*, chenodeoxycholate predominates in most patients, giving a lower cholate ratio (0.58) and deoxycholate ratio (0.11), a change again similar to that found in serum, in which the average cholate ratio was 0.6.

Duodenal contents of infants do not contain deoxycholic acid and the cholate/chenodeoxycholate ratio is 2.5.[89] Taurine conjugates predominate at birth but glycine conjugates gradually increase, approaching the proportions found in adults at 7 to 12 months.[22, 220]

EXCRETION IN URINE AND FECES

Urine. Bile salts have not been detected in the urine of healthy subjects when examined by conventional methods[233, 275] but trace amounts may be present when other technics are employed. Grundy found in the urine 2 per cent of the radioactivity from orally administered ^{14}C-cholic acid in a study in which 100 per cent of the radioactivity was accounted for.[119] Of 13 patients with Laennec's cirrhosis examined by Rudman and Kendall,[233] 2 had dihydroxy bile acid concentrations of 4.0 and 7.3 mg./24 hours. No trihydroxy acids were found, and in these 2 patients dihydroxy acids also predominated in the blood. In patients with bile duct disease and serum trihydroxy/dihydroxy bile salt ratios greater than 1, considerable quantities of trihydroxy (up to 121 mg./24 hours) and dihydroxy (up to 28 mg./24 hours) bile salts were found in the urine. The relationship, however, between the concentration ratios in serum and urine was inconsistent.

In a more recent study, Gregg found urinary bile salts in all of the 22 jaundiced patients studied.[118a] The highest 24-hour excretion rates were found in patients with common bile duct obstruction (58 mg.) and drug-induced cholestasis (40 mg.). The cholate/chenodeoxycholate ratio was > 0.59 in this group, whereas the ratio was < 0.50 in patients with cirrhosis or hepatitis. Alterations of the primary bile acid ratio produced by various hepatobiliary disorders in blood and urine are therefore similar in that the ratio tends to be higher with bile duct obstruction or cholestasis and lower with cirrhosis or hepatitis. Bile acids excreted in the urine in Gregg's study were mainly conjugated.

Feces. Fecal bile acids have been studied intensively with respect to alterations induced by the type and quantity of dietary fat. These studies are discussed briefly in the section on bile salt synthesis. Studies on fecal bile acids in hepatobiliary disorders or in intestinal disease are limited. In diarrhea the amounts of cholic and chenodeoxycholic acids are often greatly increased in feces (an observation made in 1844 by Pettenkofer who found fecal cholic acid in patients with diarrhea but none in the feces of healthy subjects), especially in diarrhea associated with a diseased, bypassed or removed ileum. Patients with total bile fistulas have no bile salts in the feces.[51]

DISSOCIATED JAUNDICE

In the early part of this century a number of French authors[34, 178, 185] were proponents of a concept termed dissociated jaundice (dissociations de la sécrétion biliare, ictère dissociée). The term refers to a dissociation of bilirubin and bile salt excretion in which bilirubin is retained, leading to jaundice, but bile salts are excreted in a normal manner so that the patients are icteric but no bile salts are detected in blood or urine. This dissociation was often observed in hepatitis, benign infections or cirrhosis but seldom seen in common bile duct obstruction. The concept held that only the hepatic cells could selectively retain pigment but secrete bile salts and that the bile ducts or gallbladder could not. The phenomenon was therefore regarded as useful in distinguish-

Fig. 4–7. Simultaneous comparison of serum *trihydroxy* bile salt and bilirubin concentrations measured in the same sample of blood. Dotted lines indicate upper limit of normal values.

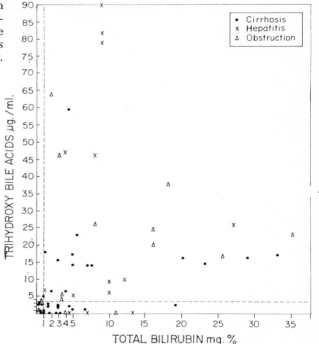

Fig. 4–7. Simultaneous comparison of serum *trihydroxy* bile salt and bilirubin concentrations measured in the same sample of blood. Dotted lines indicate upper limit of normal values.

ing jaundice due to hepatitis or cirrhosis from that caused by common duct obstruction. The concept has now been largely abandoned in favor of more suitable methods for making this distinction, but it is of interest to re-examine it using more specific methods.

Comparison of the serum concentrations of total bilirubin with trihydroxy bile salts (Fig. 4–7) and dihydroxy bile salts (Fig. 4–8) in a group of patients having hepatitis, cirrhosis or bile duct obstruction reveals that 35 per cent of the cirrhosis group had jaundice but normal serum bile salt concentrations, whereas 12 per cent of the bile duct obstruction group had jaundice but normal serum trihydroxy bile salt concentrations. In the hepatitis group 21 per cent had this combination. When the cirrhosis and hepatitis groups are combined and compared with the bile duct obstruction group, it is found that jaundice in the presence of normal serum trihydroxy bile salt concentrations occurred in 31 per cent of the cirrhosis-hepatitis group and in 12 per cent of the bile duct obstruction group.

The reverse situation in which serum bile salt concentrations are increased in the absence of jaundice is less commonly seen, occurring in only 3 per cent of the total group, the numbers in each group being too small for valid comparison.

Thus the early observations of the French investigators were correct to some extent in that dissociated jaundice is more commonly seen in patients with cirrhosis or hepatitis than in those with bile duct obstruction when these comparisons are made with more accurate methods. However, 52 to 79 per cent of jaundiced patients have increased serum bile salt concentrations regardless of the type of disease involved, and hence the observation of dissociated jaundice is of some differential diagnostic value only when it is present, and of no value when not.

The Primary Bile Salt Ratio

A primary bile salt ratio (cholate/cheno-deoxycholate) or trihydroxy/dihydroxy ratio of less than 1 relates well to the extent of liver injury as judged by concentrations of albumin, prothrombin, retained BSP, and immunoglobulins in the serum and other

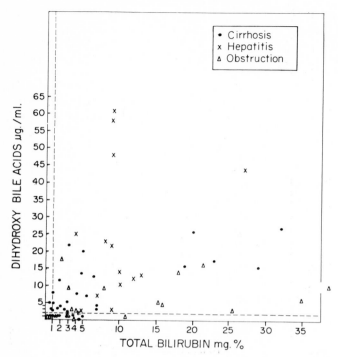

FIG. 4–8. Simultaneous comparison of serum *dihydroxy* bile salt and bilirubin concentrations measured in the same sample of blood. Dotted lines indicate upper limit of normal values.

signs of advanced liver disease such as impending hepatic coma.

A ratio of less than 1, sometimes referred to as a reversed ratio, may therefore be regarded as biochemical evidence of hepatic injury, and a sustained reversed ratio indicates fairly intensive hepatic damage. The reversed primary bile acid ratio therefore has prognostic significance.

The factors that lead to increased amounts of chenodeoxycholate relative to cholate in bile and blood in liver injury are not fully understood. It is possible that the change results from a relative decrease in the synthesis of cholate with respect to chenodeoxycholate rather than a change in the size or distribution of the cholate or chenodeoxycholate pool. The preliminary evidence for this is that in a few patients examined, the metabolites of chenodeoxycholate (mainly lithocholate) were present in greater quantities than the cholate metabolites in the feces, and increased amounts of lithocholate appeared in the blood. If these observations hold for a larger number of patients with a reversed bile acid ratio, it would support the view that relatively less cholate is being formed in these patients. A second observation that supports this view is that in an occasional patient with severe liver injury, no cholate can be detected in the blood in the presence of large amounts of chenodeoxycholate.

If the reversed ratio is actually due to the formation of relatively less cholate, then the problem arises as to what point or points in the pathway for cholate synthesis this relative suppression occurs.

The only structural difference between cholate and chenodeoxycholate is the absence of a 12α-hydroxyl group in the latter. If these 2 compounds have in man a common synthetic pathway or at least the same sequence of ring changes preceding side-chain oxidation, then possibly suppression of the 12α-hydroxylase enzyme(s) would account for the relative reduction in cholate formation. The isolation of 3α-7α-dihydroxycoprostane (a compound with the chenodeoxycholate nucleus and an unoxidized cholesterol side chain) from human bile[228] may be interpreted as evidence for a common pathway. On the other hand, a second pathway for chenodeoxycholate synthesis as shown in Figure 4–3, in which side-chain oxidation precedes ring alterations or at least 12α-hydroxylation, may predominate with liver injury to account for the reversed ratio. In speculating about these possibilities emphasis has been given to relative rates of formation of cholate and chenodeoxycholate. It is possible that the synthesis rates may be increased for both. Blum and Spritz have demonstrated an increase in cholic acid turnover rate which exceeded normal values in 4 of 7 patients with advanced cirrhosis.[21] Further studies are needed to explain the means by which chenodeoxycholate predominates in blood and bile in liver injury.

LITHOCHOLIC ACID IN LIVER DISEASE

The toxicity of bile has been recognized since ancient times; early observations have been reviewed by Horrall.[152] Experimental evidence that a specific bile salt, lithocholate, produces cirrhosis of the liver when fed to rabbits was obtained by Holsti[148, 149] who also demonstrated that its precursor, chenodeoxycholate, has the same effect.[150] Lithocholate is also cirrhotogenic when fed to a variety of other mammals,[154] birds[83, 153] and a primitive lizard, the iguana.[262] In acute experiments, intravenously administered sodium taurocholate produces cholestasis in rats[156] and hamsters.[238]

These observations naturally lead to a consideration of its possible harmful effects on the human liver since lithocholate is a normally occurring bile salt in man. The definitive experiment, the ingestion of large amounts of lithocholate by man, cannot of course be performed and therefore the problem must be studied indirectly.

In certain patients with portal cirrhosis in whom chenodeoxycholate (the lithocholate precursor) predominates in the blood, serum concentrations of lithocholate tend to be higher than in patients with mainly cholate in their serum.[53] This observation raises the possibility that the predominance of chenodeoxycholate in cirrhosis perpetuates liver injury because of the increased amounts of its metabolite, lithocholate, perfusing the liver.[56] Reduction of serum lithocholate concentrations to normal or zero values by feeding cholestyramine or neomycin is associated with a decline in serum concentra-

tions of chenodeoxycholate, bilirubin, SGOT and alkaline phosphatase. Such changes did not occur in untreated but otherwise similar control patients during the 10 day study period.[53]

The quantity of lithocholate that must be fed to rats (about 625 mg./kg.) to produce hepatic damage exceeds by approximately 100 times the quantity normally found in man. The concentration of lithocholic acid in human gallbladder bile is 0.2 to 5 mg./ml. (mean 1.5 mg./ml.),[202] whereas that in serum rarely exceeds 1 μg./ml. In rats, however, lithocholic acid is readily converted to a variety of other less toxic bile acids,[272] the chief one being 3α-6β-dihydroxy-5β-cholanic acid in feeding experiments.[293] Human liver on the other hand, does not convert intravenously administered lithocholate to other compounds to any appreciable extent.[51] Therefore, on a mg./kg. basis, lithocholate may be more toxic for man than for the rat. Rabbits are much more sensitive than rats because, as in man, lithocholate is not converted to other compounds[157] and the liver is injured at the 0.25 per cent dietary level (about 0.17 mg./kg./day). An estimate of lithocholic acid synthesis is 3 to 4 mg./kg./day in man.

The major question regarding possible toxic effects of lithocholate is whether the quantities that perfuse the human liver are ever large enough to produce hepatic injury. The role of lithocholic acid sulfate formation in liver injury is of interest.[215]

CONJUGATION IN HEPATOBILIARY DISORDERS

A significant reduction in the capacity to conjugate bile salts has been demonstrated in liver homogenates obtained from jaundiced patients with stone or cancer occluding the common bile duct.[240] A relative reduction in the capability to conjugate with glycine was found in liver biopsy homogenates from patients with toxic or infectious hepatitis, cirrhosis and obstructive jaundice.[84] This finding is reflected in duodenal content in which the bile salt glycine/taurine ratio was found to be lowered in 4 of 7 patients with obstructive jaundice.[253] Glycine/taurine ratios are variable in patients with cirrhosis, hepatitis and other liver disorders but the change is usually in the direction of reduced glycine conjugation. In myxedema, however, glycine/taurine ratios were very high in 2 patients, exceeding values found in any condition mentioned above.[253]

TARGET CELLS AND BILE SALTS

The studies of Cooper and Jandl[59] show that the physical properties of red blood cell membranes, such as shape and fragility, are greatly affected by their free cholesterol content. Bile salts affect the free cholesterol content of red cell membranes in at least 2 ways. First, they inhibit serum cholesterol transesterase activity which in turn inhibits removal of free cholesterol from the red cell membrane. Secondly, bile salts induce a shift in the cell/serum free cholesterol partition ratio in favor of the cell so that the concentrations of cholesterol in the cells are supranormal. Such cells are flat and osmotically resistant and are recognized on stained smears as target cells. These cells are especially numerous in obstructive jaundice in which serum bile salt concentrations are high. It is therefore believed that increased serum concentrations of bile salts are responsible for target cell formation by virtue of the alterations they induce in the cholesterol content of the red cell membrane which in turn determines the shape of the membrane and its appearance as a target cell.

INTESTINAL DISEASE AND BILE SALT METABOLISM

STEROID WASTING ENTEROPATHY

A group of disorders that have in common a failure of the ileum to absorb conjugated bile salts are designated by Stanley and Nemchausky as steroid wasting enteropathies.[260] This includes regional enteritis involving the distal ileum, ileal bypass or resection; conditions associated with osmotic diarrhea such as that produced experimentally by Meihoff and Kern, Jr.,[189] with mannitol in which cholate absorption was impaired, and possibly other examples such as mucosal disaccharidase deficiencies, Zollinger-Ellison syndrome, radiation ileitis and viral or bacterial enteritis. Celiac sprue, if it includes the terminal ileum, and other

disorders yet to be studied may eventually be included in this group.

In patients with steroid wasting enteropathy studied by Stanley and Nemchausky, the first 50 per cent of an intravenously administered dose of carboxyl ^{14}C-sodium cholate was excreted in the feces in 0.46 to 1.38 days whereas in healthy subjects the average time was 7.4 ± 0.97 days. The amount excreted per day (fractional fecal excretion rate) in steroid wasting enteropathy was 0.50 to 1.50, whereas the normal fractional excretion rate was 0.12 ± 0.015 per day. Similar rapid turnover rates in steroid wasting enteropathy have been demonstrated by Meihoff and Kern.[189] These values indicate that loss of bile salts from the body is greatly increased and in some patients the excretion rate (which should equal synthesis rate in the steady state) may well exceed the maximum capacity of the liver to synthesize bile salts. Under these circumstances the bile salt pool becomes depleted and a state of uncompensated bile salt deficiency exists in which the intraluminal concentration of bile salts in the small bowel is reduced to the point of impaired micelle formation, which has been demonstrated in several patients.[129] Bile salt deficiency resulting in reduced micelle formation of the products of lipolysis is believed to account for the steatorrhea seen in these subjects.

Hofmann[143] draws attention to a serious paradox in steroid wasting enteropathy in which failure of the ileum to absorb bile salts produces concentrations in the jejunum that are too low, resulting in steatorrhea, and concentrations in the colon that are too high, thus causing watery diarrhea by virtue of their cathartic action. Hofmann calls this condition cholerheic enteropathy in which steatorrhea and watery diarrhea may occur together when the enterohepatic circulation is virtually or nearly interrupted. The therapeutic dilemma presented by this paradoxical situation is discussed in the section on therapy.

THE BLIND LOOP SYNDROME

The blind loop syndrome may be broadly defined as a condition in which stasis and bacterial proliferation in the small bowel content are associated with steatorrhea, vitamin B_{12} deficiency or both. The vitamin B_{12} deficiency appears to result from successful competition for the vitamin by the bacteria that bind most of orally administered radioactive cyanocobalamine.[80] Steatorrhea of the blind loop syndrome has a somewhat more complicated pathogenesis. Donaldson originally provided evidence[80] that bacteria in the small bowel content converted cholate to deoxycholate and that deoxycholate inhibited intestinal uptake and esterification of oleic acid. The bacteria did not damage the mucosa as judged by histologic appearance and did not impair lipolysis nor take up sufficient lipid to account for the steatorrhea. The steatorrhea could be abolished by antibiotics.

Rosenberg, Hardison and Bull[230] extend these observations by showing that bacteria deconjugate bile salts in the small bowel lumen, and have identified free cholate, chenodeoxycholate and deoxycholate in the small bowel content of 2 patients with bacterial proliferation in the small bowel. They attributed the steatorrhea to the toxic and inhibitory effects of unconjugated bile salts on the intestine. Others found that if jejunal bacterial counts are less than 4×10^7/ml, no free bile acids are in the jejunal content and steatorrhea is only slight, whereas persons with counts of more than 10^8/ml. have free bile salts and pronounced steatorrhea.[267] Careful culture technics have disclosed 15 strains of bacteroides isolated from jejunal content that can deconjugate bile salts.[81] The inhibitory effects of unconjugated bile salts (cholate and especially deoxycholate) on a variety of metabolic processes in the intestine have been demonstrated.[75, 222]

THERAPEUTIC AGENTS

BILE SALTS

Bile salts have been employed as general digestive aids and as cathartics for centuries. Recently their use has become more limited and perhaps wisely so. Most commercial bile salt preparations consist of desiccated or crude extracts of cattle bile that contain mainly conjugated bile salts. These preparations usually have small amounts of pigment and fatty acids and are generally supplied as 0.2 or 0.3 Gm. tablets. The usual dose is 0.4 to 0.6 Gm. 3 times daily with meals. Dehydrocholic acid is oxidized cholic acid (3,7,12-triketo-5β-cholanoic acid, triketocholanic acid) and is pure but does not form micelles and hence does not assist fat absorption significantly and would be of little value for replacement therapy. Sodium dehydrocholate is supplied as a 20 per cent solution in ampules and is widely used to measure blood circulation times.

The most common situations in which bile salts are deficient in the small intestine are (1) T tube drainage of the common bile duct or total external bile fistula and (2) partial or complete interruption of ileal absorption as in regional enteritis or ileal resection or bypass. In the former group, common bile duct drainage is usually temporary and most patients tolerate this period well without administration of bile salts. If near total drainage is maintained for more than a few weeks, however, oral bile salts are indicated since they aid fat absorption and are essential for the absorption of the fat-soluble vitamins A, D and K. The customary dose of bile salts (0.2 to 0.6 Gm.) is probably too small for patients in whom all bile is being drained from the common bile duct. The bile salt pool (about 3.5 Gm.) is largely in the gallbladder in normal fasting subjects and is estimated to circulate at least twice during a meal (7 Gm.) so that theoretically a dose approximating this quantity should be given with each meal. Such large amounts, however, often cause diarrhea and thus a compromise of 3 to 4 Gm. with meals is preferable. Animals, including growing puppies, with chronic total bile fistulas may survive for years without impaired growth or other apparent ill effects provided vitamins A, D and K are supplied parenterally.[226, 227]

In post-ileectomy steatorrhea, administration of 3.6 Gm. bile salts with meals is therapeutic.[129] Administration of bile salts in this condition may aggravate diarrhea, however, and the use of medium chain triglyceride as the chief source of fat and cholestyramine to "bind" bile salts has been recommended as a means of dealing with steatorrhea in the presence of cholerheic diarrhea.[143, 294]

Administration of bile salts in jaundice due to hepatobiliary disease is contraindicated, especially if pruritus is present, for bile salts only serve to aggravate this.

Some bile salt preparations contain hog bile rather than cow bile. The hog has little if any 12α-hydroxylating enzyme activity and an active 6α-hydroxylating enzyme so that hog bile contains mainly hyocholic (3α, 6α, 7α-trihydroxy-5β-cholanoic acid), hyodeoxycholic (3α, 6α-trihydroxy-5β-cholanoic acid), the bacterially produced secondary bile acid of hyocholic, chenodeoxycholate, and possibly small amounts of cholate.[134] The human liver does not appear to hydroxylate the nucleus of 24-carbon bile acids to any appreciable extent,[51] and it is unlikely that pig bile salts are altered by the human liver.

There is a need for preparations of pure conjugated bile salts of the human type for bile salt therapy or at least better standards of purity for those now used, especially with respect to the presence of potentially harmful bile salts or their precursors. The bile salts used by Holsti to produce cirrhosis in rabbits were supplied for human use and were obtained from a pharmaceutical house.[148] This is not to imply that U.S.P. oxgall or similar preparations are unsafe for human use, for the rabbit is unusual in that it utilizes a secondary bile salt, deoxycholate, as its major bile salt (rabbit bile contains mainly deoxycholate), and thus the secondary bile salt of chenodeoxycholate, lithocholate, probably reaches much higher concentrations in the rabbit than it would or does in man. (Rabbit liver does not convert lithocholate to other compounds.[157]) However, the composition of bile salt preparations must be known if they are to be used safely.

ANION EXCHANGE RESINS

Cholestyramine is a strongly basic anion exchange resin and is highly useful in certain disorders of bile salt metabolism. It is a polystyrene polymer with a 2 per cent divinyl benzene cross linkage and quarternary ammonium groups in the chloride form. The polymer is not absorbed by the intestine[112] because of its high molecular weight, and exchanges a chloride ion for an ionized bile salt molecule which it carries out in the feces. In spite of a close affinity of the resin for bile salt, bacteria remove the amino acid conjugate and convert primary to secondary bile salts so that the feces of patients fed cholestyramine contain unconjugated secondary bile salts[49] as do normal feces, but the fecal excretion of bile salts is increased about 3 times.[199] Use of cholestyramine may thus be regarded as a means for producing a partial medical bile fistula and for removing bile salts from the enterohepatic circulation. It has been used chiefly in pruritic jaundice,[49] especially that accompanied by biliary cirrhosis.[67, 239, 278] The usual starting dose is 10 Gm./day (3.3 Gm. 3 times daily with meals), best taken as a suspension in water followed by fruit juice or other suitable beverage. Five to 10 days may be required to relieve pruritus, for reasons discussed in the section on pruritus. Warn the patient about this so that the resin is not abandoned before it has a chance to become effective. As originally provided, the resin had a strong amine odor and gritty consistency but more palatable products are now being provided.

Cholestyramine, 10 Gm./day, usually relieves the pruritus of jaundice, and this is associated with a fall in serum bile acid concentrations.[49, 278] The resin does not relieve pruritus in patients with complete common bile duct obstruction such as that which sometimes occurs with pancreatic carcinoma in which the quantity of bile salt that enters the intestine is so small or nonexistent that there is nothing for the resin to remove. Under these circumstances fecal urobilinogen excretion is less than 5 mg./day.[280] A fecal Ehrlich determination is thus a practical guide for predicting the effectiveness of cholestyramine therapy because it is a much simpler test than quantitation of fecal bile salts. Of course, patients with extrahepatic bile duct obstruction require surgical treatment, even if an external bile fistula (bile duct catheter) is required for drainage as is sometimes necessary with extensive abdominal tumors in which choledochojejunostomy or removal may be precluded.

When the 10 Gm./day dose relieves some pruritic patients with biliary cirrhosis and those with pruritic jaundice accompanying metastatic carcinoma of the liver, pruritus is often relieved with a smaller maintenance dose of 6 or even 3 Gm./day.

In other patients with biliary cirrhosis and in many children with bile duct atresia or absence of intrahepatic bile ducts it is often necessary to use up to 20 or 30 Gm./day.[247] Since such quantities often produce moderate steatorrhea,[132] supply parenteral vitamin K.

Children with intrahepatic bile duct atresia or "ductopenia" in whom growth is retarded sometimes return toward a normal growth curve when serum bile salt concentrations are lowered by effective cholestyramine treatment.[247]

The pruritus that sometimes occurs for a few days early in the course of acute infectious hepatitis is usually so transient that cholestyramine is probably not effective quickly enough to shorten this already brief period of pruritus.

The effects of cholestyramine on hepatic and intestinal bile salt and cholesterol synthesis is discussed in the section on bile salt synthesis. Calcification in the biliary tree after cholestyramine feeding has been reported.[239, 285] Gallstone formation has been induced[243] and prevented[10] with cholestyramine in animals.

ANTIBIOTICS

Norman[203] has shown that antibiotics administered to rats abolish deconjugation and secondary bile acid formation by intestinal bacteria. The rat feces under these conditions contained the same primary conjugated bile salts found in rat bile.

The most common indication for antibiotic treatment of altered bile salt metabolism in man is the blind loop syndrome[80] in which bacteria proliferate in the small bowel content, producing deconjugation of primary bile salts and formation of secondary bile salts with resulting interference in fat absorption and steatorrhea. This condition has been treated successfully with tetracycline[80] and erythromycin[230] which suppress bacterial growth and thus restore conjugated and predominantly primary bile salts to the content of the small intestine with disappearance of steatorrhea.

Neomycin is a polybasic, poorly absorbed antibiotic which forms insoluble precipitates with bile salts.[93] It has been shown to lower serum cholesterol concentrations in man[114, 115, 234] and chickens[93] while increasing fecal bile acid excretion. It inhibits the hepatotoxic effects of lithocholic acid ingestion in chickens[93] and prevents the bacterial conversion of cholate to deoxycholate.[125] Six to 12 Gm./day induces a malabsorption syndrome and mucosal changes similar to those seen in sprue.[155] Neomycin therefore has at least 3 properties that directly affect bile salt metabolism: (1) It is polybasic, so that it forms insoluble compounds with bile salts and thus has an effect similar to cholestyramine. (2) It has antimicrobial properties that suppress or prevent secondary bile salt formation. (3) It is directly toxic to intestinal mucosa, and thus possibly impairs bile salt absorption. Of these properties, bile salt binding probably accounts for most of the increased fecal excretion of bile salts and hypocholesterolemic effects and also protection against hepatic toxicity from lithocholic acid ingestion. Serum lithocholate concentrations in human subjects can be lowered with either cholestyramine or neomycin.[53] Perhaps neomycin acts by its combined effects of bile salt binding and antimicrobial properties, the latter suppressing lithocholate formation.

EFFECTS OF CHOLESTYRAMINE AND NEOMYCIN ON THE LIVER

Administration of neomycin or cholestyramine to patients with elevated serum bile salt concentrations is usually associated with a lowering of these concentrations and often other laboratory tests improve such as serum bilirubin concentrations, alkaline phosphatase activity and BSP retention.[53, 55, 184, 247] This response has been interpreted as at least one piece of evidence that high serum bile salt concentrations, especially lithocholate, may be injurious to the liver. The toxicity of lithocholate for the mammalian liver is well established as is the observation that unconjugated deoxycholate (which may be present in serum)[21] damages biologic membranes in even small concentrations. Improved liver function is especially prominent in children with a paucity of intrahepatic ducts but without cirrhosis or inflammatory changes in the liver. In 3 such patients all previous abnormal liver function studies became normal except alkaline phosphatase, and the patients' growth curves returned to normal rates when serum bile salt concentrations were maintained at normal values.[247] This is in contrast to studies in adults[68, 239] in which no significant changes were noted in liver function studies with prolonged cholestyramine feeding but it was not determined if normal serum bile salt concentrations were obtained. It appears that sufficiently large doses of cholestyramine must be given to produce normal or near normal serum bile salt concentrations, if beneficial effects for the liver are to be achieved.

GALLSTONE FORMATION

The commonest type of gallstone in Western countries is composed chiefly of cholesterol. As discussed in the section on digestion and absorption, cholesterol is held in "solution" in bile in micellar form. The micelles consist of bile salts, lecithin and cholesterol in proportion of about 6:2:1.[255] When the concentration of cholesterol exceeds the capacity of the micelles to "solubilize" it, the excess cholesterol exists in crystalline form in the bile because of the high water content of bile (about 90 per cent), in which cholesterol is insoluble.

The presence of a suitable nidus, such as bacteria, calcium bilirubinate or calcium carbonate, may act as a nucleation point for aggregation of the cholesterol crystals, resulting in the formation of macroscopic stones which may grow in size and be aggregated in the gallbladder by mucin of high viscosity. This accounts for the radiolucent line sometimes seen in cholecystograms in which the small gallstones are held in a layer of tenacious mucin in the bile[29] (Fig. 4–9). The adhesive properties of mucin may also account for the retention of multiple small stones in the gallbladder which would otherwise be expelled with the bile as the gallbladder contracts.[29]

The finding of small quantities of unconjugated and secondary bile salts at the centers of gallstones may be interpreted as evidence that bacteria proliferate in the bile at the onset of crystalline cholesterol aggregation.[245]

When the relative concentrations of cholesterol, lecithin, bile salt and water are plotted as moles per cent in a 4 component phase diagram[147] the concentrations of lecithin and bile salts can vary over a wide range (10 to 60 per cent for lecithin and 40 to 95 per cent for bile salts) and still form micelles in 90 per cent water. Cholesterol, on the other hand, can vary no more than about 10 per cent before its concentration exceeds the amount solubilized in micellar form. The excess cholesterol is in crystalline form outside the micelle. The range of concentrations for lecithin and bile salt within the micellar zone is so great that they are almost never, if ever, exceeded and therefore it is unlikely that the relatively small differences in concentrations of these substances found in patients with gallstones is of critical importance. The comparatively small range for cholesterol concentration (5 to 10 per cent) is close to the limit of the micellar zone even in normal subjects and on the borderline during pregnancy. In 4 groups of patients studied with cholesterol gallstones, all had bile cholesterol concentrations outside the micellar zone.[147] Thus it appears that cholesterol concentration rather than lecithin or bile salt concentration is the critical factor for initiating the formation of cholesterol gallstones.

The same considerations probably apply to calcium bilirubinate which, like cholesterol, is virtually insoluble in water and is produced when bacterial glucuronidase deconjugates bilirubin glucuronide in an infected biliary system.[187] Pigment stones (calcium bilirubinate) are more common in Asian countries; this is apparently related to environmental factors, for Asians living in America or Europe have mainly cholesterol stones.

The foregoing paragraphs briefly summarize the complicated problem of gallstone formation in man which is far from being resolved. The literature dealing with this

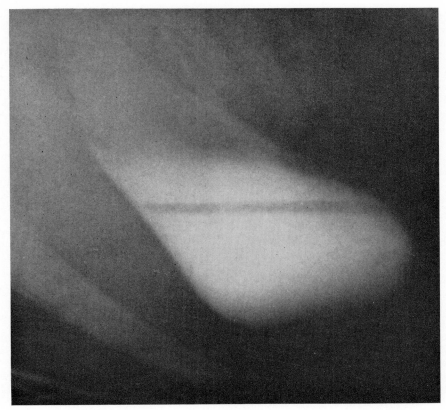

Fig. 4–9. Cholecystogram, decubitus position, showing small gallstones within a radiolucent line. Examination of the gallbladder content following cholecystectomy revealed this line to consist of clear tenacious mucin which bound the small stones in a cohesive web. (Brenckman et al.[29])

problem is enormous. For illuminating discussions and quick access to important references see Juniper[162] and Small.[255, 257]

ENTEROLITHS

Primary bile acid enteroliths are rare and usually consist of choleic acid which is a molecular coordinate complex of deoxycholic acid and another organic compound, frequently a fatty acid in enteroliths. The size of the fatty acid molecule determines the number of deoxycholic acid molecules which form around it in a cylindrical fashion. For stearic and oleic acids, the deoxycholic–fatty acid ratio is 8:1. Deoxycholic acid is the only naturally occurring bile acid that forms choleic acids. Methyl esters, diformate and

glycine or taurine conjugates of deoxycholic acid do not form these molecular inclusion compounds.

Enteroliths may consist of mixtures of unconjugated primary bile acids (cholic and chenodeoxycholic) as was found in the afferent loop of a patient with a gastroenterostomy[101] and in a diverticulum of the second part of the duodenum in another patient.[95]

It is probable that bacterial proliferation in the small bowel is common to all examples of enterolith formation in man. Bacterial enzymes deconjugate the bile salts in the intestinal lumen which raises their pKa to a value of about 6 so that a good deal of the free bile acid is un-ionized and precipitates at the pH of intestinal content. The presence of a suitable nidus such as vegetable matter[15] promotes aggregation of the precipitated crystals and enterolith formation. Bacterial enzymes also convert primary to secondary bile salts (cholic → deoxycholic), which combine with fatty acids to form choleic acids which have an even higher pKa (about 7) so that they are more readily precipitated than free deoxycholic acid. This feature may account for the more frequent occurrence of choleic acid enteroliths than primary bile acid enteroliths, of which only 2 have been described.[95, 101]

The major difference in the formation of gallstones and enteroliths is the nature of their insoluble constituents: cholesterol or calcium bilirubinate in gallstones and choleic acids or free primary bile acids in enteroliths.

REFERENCES

1. Ahrens, E. H., Jr., Payne, M. A., Kunkel, H. G., Eisenmenger, W. J., and Blondheim, S. H.: Primary biliary cirrhosis, Medicine 29:299, 1950.
2. Akita, H., Kuck, J. F. R., Walker, G. L., and Johnston, C. G.: The application of the enterohepatic circulation of bile acid to a study of the patency of portacaval shunts, Surgery 36:941, 1954.
3. Ali, S. S., Kuksis, A., and Beveridge, J. M. R.: Excretion of bile acids by three men on a fat-free diet, Canad. Biochem. 44:957, 1966.
4. Anfinsen, C. B., and Horning, M. G.: Enzymatic degradation of the cholesterol side chain in cell-free preparations, J. Am. Chem. Soc. 75:1511, 1953.
5. Archambeau, J. O., Maetz, M., Jesseph, J. E., and Brenneis, H. J.: Production of diarrhea in dogs prepared with a gallbladder-colon fistula, Arch. Surg. 95:230, 1967.
6. Austad, W. I., Lack, L., and Tyor, M. P.: Importance of bile acids and of an intact distal small intestine for fat absorption, Gastroenterology 52:638, 1967.
7. Avigan, J., and Steinberg, D.: Sterol and bile acid excretion in man and the effects of dietary fat, J. Clin. Invest. 44:1845, 1965.
8. Baker, R. D., and Searle, G. W.: Bile salt absorption at various levels of rat small intestine, Proc. Soc. Exp. Biol. Med. 105:521, 1960.

9. Beher, W. T., Rao, B., Beher, M. E., and Bertasius, J.: Bile acid synthesis in normal and hypophysectomized rats: a rate study using cholestyramine, Proc. Soc. Exp. Biol. Med. 124:1193, 1967.
10. Bergman, F., and van der Linden, W.: Diet-induced cholesterol gallstones in hamsters: prevention and dissolution by cholestyramine, Gastroenterology 53:418, 1967.
11. Bergstrom, S.: Metabolism of bile acids, Fed. Proc. 21: Supp. 11, 28, 1962.
12. Bergstrom, S., Danielsson, H., and Samuelsson, B.: The formation and metabolism of bile acids, in Bloch, K. E. (ed.): Lipid Metabolism, New York, Wiley, 1960.
13. Berseus, O.: On the stereospecificity of 26-hydroxylation of cholesterol, Acta Chem. Scand. 19:325, 1965.
14. Berseus, O., Danielsson, H., and Einarsson, K.: Synthesis and metabolism of cholest-5-ene-3β, 7α, 12α-triol, J. Biol. Chem. 242:1211, 1967.   .
15. Bewes, P. C., Haslewood, G. A. D., and Roxburgh, R. A.: Bile-acid enteroliths and jejunal diverticulosis, Brit. J. Surg. 53:709, 1966.
16. Bjorkhem, I., and Danielsson, H.: On the formation of cholic acid from cholest-4-ene-3α, 7α, 12α-triol and cholest-4-ene-3β, 7α, 12α-triol, Acta Chem. Scand. 19:2298, 1965.
17. Bjorkhem, I., Danielsson, H., and Einarsson, K.: On the conversion of cholesterol to 5β-cholestane-3α, 7α-diol in guinea pig liver homogenates, Europ. J. Biochem. 2:294, 1967.
18. Bjorkhem, I., Danielsson, H., Einarsson, K., and Johansson, G.: Formation of bile acids in man: conversion of cholesterol into 5β-cholestane-3α, 7α, 12α-triol in liver homogenates, J. Clin. Invest. 47:1573, 1968.
19. Bloch, K., Berg, B. N., and Rittenberg, D.: The biological conversion of cholesterol to cholic acid, J. Biol. Chem. 149:511, 1943.
20. Blomquist, H. E., Setala, K., Holsti, P., and Wangel, G.: Experimental liver cirrhosis induced in rabbits fed with 9,10-dimethyl-1,2-benzanthracene, heated fats and bile constituents, alone and in combination with the injection of a sclerosing agent, Ann. med. exper. et biol. Fenniae 32:101, 1954.
21. Blum, M., and Spritz, N.: The metabo-

lism of intravenously injected isotopic cholic acid in Laennec's cirrhosis, J. Clin. Invest. *45*:187, 1966.

22. Bongiovanni, A. M.: Bile acid content of gallbladder of infants, children and adults, J. Clin. Endocrinol. *25*:678, 1965.

23. Borgström, B.: The dimensions of the bile salt micelle; measurements by gel filtration, Biochim. Biophys. Acta *106*: 171, 1965.

24. ————: Partition of lipids between emulsified oil and micellar phases of glyceride-bile salt dispersions, J. Lipid Res. 8:598, 1967.

25. Borgström., B., Dahlqvist, A., Lundh, G., and Sjövall, J.: Studies of intestinal digestion and absorption in the human, J. Clin. Invest. *36*:1521, 1957.

26. Bourges, M., Small, D. M., and Dervichian, D. G.: Biophysics of lipid associations. III. The quaternary systems lecithin-bile salt-cholesterol-water, Biochim. Biophys. Acta *144*:189, 1967.

27. Boyd, G. S., Eastwood, M. A., and Mac-Lean, N.: Bile acids in the rat: studies in experimental occlusion of the bile duct, J. Lipid Res. 7:83, 1966.

28. Bremer, J.: Choly-CoA as an intermediate in taurocholic acid formation by rat liver microsomes, Acta Chem. Scand. 9: 1036, 1955.

29. Brenckman, W., Grage, T., Gedgaudes, E., and Carey, J.: The role of mucin in gallstone formation (In press.)

30. Bridgwater, R. J., and Lindstedt, S.: On the metabolism of 3α, 7α, 12α-trihydroxycoprostanic acid in the rat, Acta Chem. Scand. *11*:409, 1957.

31. Briggs, T., Whitehouse, M. W., and Staple, E.: Formation of bile acids from cholesterol in the alligator, Arch. Biochem. Biophys. *85*:275, 1959.

32. ————: Metabolism of trihydroxycoprostanic acid: formation from cholesterol in the alligator and conversion to cholic acid and carbon dioxide *in vitro* by rat liver mitochondria, J. Biol. Chem. *236*:688, 1961.

33. Brown, D. F., Porta, E. A., and Reder, J.: Idiopathic jaundice of pregnancy, Arch. Int. Med. *111*:592, 1963.

34. Brulé, M.: Recherches sur les Ictères, ed. 3, Paris, Masson, 1922.

35. Buchwald, H., Gebhard, R. L., and Carey, J. B., Jr.: Bile salt absorption following intestinal bypass, Surg. Forum *17*:27, 1966.

36. Burnett, W.: The pathogenesis of gallstones, *in* Taylor, W. (ed.): The Biliary System, p. 601, Philadelphia, Davis, 1965.

37. Carey, J. B., Jr.: Chenodeoxycholic acid in human blood serum, Science *123*:892, 1956.

38. ————: Serum dihydroxy-trihydroxy bile acid ratio in liver and biliary tract disease, J. Clin. Invest. *35*:695, 1956 (Abstract).

39. ————: Serum trihydroxy-dihydroxy bile acid ratio in liver and biliary tract disease, J. Clin. Invest. *37*:1494, 1958.

40. ————: Lowering of serum bile acid concentrations and relief of pruritus in jaundiced patients fed a bile acid sequestering resin, J. Lab. Clin. Med. *56*:797, 1960.

41. ————: Identification of a "primitive" bile acid in man as an intermediate in the transformation of cholesterol to cholic acid; a biochemical sign of human evolution, J. Clin. Invest. *42*:921, 1963.

42. ————: Bile acids, cirrhosis and human evolution, Gastroenterology *46*:490, 1964 (Editorial).

43. ————: Conversion of cholesterol to trihydroxycoprostanic acid and cholic acid in man, J. Clin. Invest. *43*:1443, 1964.

44. Carey, J. B., Jr., Buchwald, H., and Varco, R. L.: Intestinal absorption of bile salts in man and rabbits with ileal bypass, J. Clin. Invest. *44*:1033, 1965 (Abstract).

45. Carey, J. B., Jr., Figen, J., and Watson, C. J.: The bile acids in normal human serum with comparative observations in patients with jaundice, J. Lab. Clin. Med. *46*:802, 1955 (Abstract).

46. Carey, J. B., Jr., and Haslewood, G. A. D.: Crystallization of trihydroxycoprostanic acid from human bile, J. Biol. Chem. *238*:855, 1963.

47. Carey, J. B., Jr., Hoffbauer, F. W., Zaki, F. G., and Nwokolo, C.: Choledocholithiasis and hepatic ductular proliferation induced in rats by lithocholic acid (a bile acid occurring naturally in man), Gastroenterology *48*:809, 1965.

48. Carey. J. B., Jr., and Watson, C. J.: Isolation of deoxycholic acid from normal human feces, J. Biol. Chem. *216*:847, 1955.

49. Carey, J. B. Jr., and Williams, G.: Relief of the pruritus of jaundice with a bile acid sequestering resin, J.A.M.A. *176*: 432, 1961.

50. ————: Pathways of secondary bile acid formation as excretory metabolites of

cholesterol: Conversion of primary to secondary bile acids in man, J. Lab. Clin. Med. 60:865, 1962.

51. ———: Metabolism of lithocholic acid in bile fistula patients, J. Clin. Invest. 42: 450, 1963.

52. ———: Lithocholic acid in human blood serum, Science 150:620, 1965.

53. Carey, J. B., Jr., Wilson, I. D., Onstad, G., and Zaki, F. G.: Role of 12α hydroxylase deficiency in continuing liver injury, J. Clin. Invest. 46:1042, 1967.

54. Carey, J. B., Jr., Wilson, I. D., and Williams, G.: Serum lithocholic acid concentrations in patients with ulcerative colitis and regional enteritis, Gastroenterology 52:315, 1967 (Abstract).

55. Carey, J. B., Jr., Wilson, I. D., Zaki, F. G., and Hanson, R. F.: The metabolism of bile acids with special reference to liver injury, Medicine 45:461, 1966.

56. Carey, J. B., Jr., Wilson, I. D., Zaki, F. G., and Williams, G.: Predominance of the dihydroxy primary bile acid pathway in cholesterol catabolism in liver cirrhosis: a potential source of liver injury, J. Lab. Clin. Med. 68:862, 1966 (Abstract).

57. Chaikoff, I. L., Siperstein, M. D., Dauben, W. G., Bradlow, H. L., Eastham, J. F., Tomkins, G. M., Meier, J. R., Chen, R. W., Hotta, S., and Srere, P. A.: C^{14} cholesterol. II. Oxidation of carbons 4 and 26 to carbon dioxide by the intact rat, J. Biol. Chem. 194:413, 1952.

58. Conner, W. E., Witiak, D. T., Stone, D. B., and Armstrong, M. L.: Cholesterol balance in normal men fed dietary fats of different fatty acid composition, Circulation 36: Supp. 2, 7, 1967.

59. Cooper, R. A., and Jandl, J. H.: Bile salts and cholesterol in the pathogenesis of target cells in obstructive jaundice, J. Clin. Invest. 47:809, 1968.

60. Cooperstein, S. J.: The effect of deoxycholate on cytochrome oxidase, J. Biol. Chem. 238:3750, 1963.

61. Cronholm, T., and Sjövall, J.: Bile acids in portal blood of rats fed different diets and cholestyramine, Europ. J. Biochem. 2:375, 1967.

62. Danielsson, H.: On the oxidation of 3α, 7α, 12α-trihydroxycoprostane by mouse and rat liver homogenates, Acta Chem. Scand. 14:348, 1960.

63. ———: Present status of research on catabolism and excretion of cholesterol, Advances in Lipid Research, 1:335, 1963.

64. Danielsson, H., and Einarsson, K.: On the conversion of cholesterol to 7α,12α-dihydroxycholest-4-en-3-one, J. Biol. Chem. 241:1449, 1966.

65. Danielsson, H., Einarsson, K., and Johansson, G.: Effect of biliary drainage on individual reactions in the conversion of cholesterol to taurocholic acid, Europ. J. Biochem. 2:44, 1967.

66. Danielsson, H., Eneroth, P., Hellström, K., Lindstedt, S., and Sjövall, J.: On the turnover and excretory products of cholic and chenodeoxycholic acid in man, J. Biol. Chem. 238:2299, 1963.

67. Datta, D. V., and Sherlock, S.: Treatment of pruritus of obstructive jaundice with cholestyramine, Brit. Med. J. 1:216, 1963.

68. ———: Cholestyramine for long term relief of the pruritus complicating intrahepatic cholestasis, Gastroenterology 50: 323, 1966.

69. Dawson, A. M., and Isselbacher, K. J.: Studies on lipid metabolism in the small intestine with observations on the role of bile salts, J. Clin. Invest. 39:730, 1960.

70. Dean, P. D. G., and Alpin, R. T.: Mass spectrometric studies on bile acids: the differentiation between chenodeoxycholic and deoxycholic acid and the identification of 3α,7α-dihydroxy-5β-cholestanoic acid in alligator bile, Steroids 8:565, 1966.

71. Dean, P. D. G., and Whitehouse, M. W.: The identification of 3α,7α-dihydroxy-5β-cholestanoic (coprochenodeoxycholic) acid in alligator bile, Biochem. J. 99:9p, 1966.

72. ———: Inhibition of hepatic sterol oxidation by cholanic (bile) acids and their conjugates, Biochim. Biophys. Acta 137: 328, 1967.

73. DePalma, R. G., Levey, S., Hartman, P. H., and Hubay, C. A.: Bile acids and serum cholesterol following T-tube drainage, Arch. Surg. 94:271, 1967.

74. Desnuelle, P.: Pancreatic lipase, in Nord, F. F. (ed.): Advances in Enzymology, vol. 23, p. 129, New York, Interscience, 1961.

75. Dietschy, J. M.: Effects of bile salts on intermediate metabolism of the intestinal mucosa, Fed. Proc. 26:1589, 1967.

76. ———: The role of bile salts in controlling the rate of intestinal cholesterogenesis, J. Clin. Invest. 47:286, 1968.

77. Dietschy, J. M., Saloman, H. S., and

Siperstein, M. D.: Bile acid metabolism. I. Studies on the mechanisms of intestinal transport, J. Clin. Invest. *45*:832, 1966.

78. Dietschy, J. M., and Siperstein, M. D.: Cholesterol synthesis by the gastrointestinal tract: localization and mechanisms of control, J. Clin. Invest. *44*:1311, 1965.

79. Dietschy, J. M., and Wilson, J. D.: Cholesterol synthesis in the squirrel monkey: Relative rates of synthesis in various tissues and mechanisms of control, J. Clin. Invest. *47*:166, 1968.

80. Donaldson, R. M., Jr.: Studies on the pathogenesis of steatorrhea in the blind loop syndrome, J. Clin. Invest. *44*:1815, 1965.

80a. Dowling, H. R., and Small, D. M.: Personal communication.

81. Drasar, B. S., Hill, M. J., and Shiner, M.: The deconjugation of the bile salts by human intestinal bacteria, Lancet *1*:1237, 1966.

82. Eastwood, M. A., and Boyd, G. S.: The distribution of bile salts along the small intestine of rats, Biochim. Biophys. Acta *137*:393, 1967.

83. Edwards, H. M., and Boyd, F. M.: Action of lithocholic acid in the germ-free chick, Proc. Soc. Exp. Biol. Med. *113*:294, 1963.

84. Ekdahl, P.-H., and Bennike, T.: On the conjugation of bile acids in the human liver, Acta Chir. Scand. *115*:203, 1958.

85. Ekdahl, P.-H., and Sjövall, J.: Metabolism of deoxycholic acid in the rabbit, Acta Physiol. Scand. *34*:287, 1955.

86. Ekwall, P., Lindstrom, E. V., and Setala, K.: Stability of micelles in bile acid salt solutions of different acidities, Acta Chem. Scand. *5*:990, 1951.

87. Ellin, R. I., Mendeloff, A. I., and Turner, D. A.: Quantitative determination of 3α, 7α,12α-triketocholanic acid in biological fluids by gas liquid chromatography, Analyt. Biochem. *4*:198, 1962.

88. Emerman, S., and Javitt, N. B.: Metabolism of taurolithocholic acid in the hamster, J. Biol. Chem. *242*:661, 1967.

89. Encrantz, J. C., and Sjövall, J.: On the bile acids in duodenal contents of infants and children, Clin. Chim. Acta *4*:793, 1959.

90. Eneroth, P., Gordon, B., and Sjövall, J.: Characterization of trisubstituted cholanoic acids in human feces, J. Lipid Res. *7*:524, 1966.

91. Eriksson, S.: Biliary excretion of bile acids and cholesterol in bile fistula rats, Proc. Soc. Exp. Biol. Med. *94*:578, 1957.

92. Evrard, E., and Janssen, G.: Gas-liquid chromatographic determination of human fecal bile acids, J. Lipid Res. *9*:226, 1968.

93. Eyssen, H., Evrard, E., and Vanderhaeghe, H.: Cholesterol-lowering effects of N-methylated neomycin and basic antibiotics, J. Lab. Clin. Med. *68*:753, 1966.

94. Failey, R. B., Jr., and Childress, R. H.: The effect of para-aminobenzoic acid on the serum cholesterol level in man, Am. J. Clin. Nut. *10*:158, 1962.

95. Fantl, P., Rollo, A. J., and Strosberg, H.: Chemical analysis of an enterolith, Gut *6*:384, 1965.

96. Fast, B. B., and Roulston, T. M.: Idiopathic jaundice of pregnancy, Am. J. Obstet. Gynec. *88*:314, 1964.

97. Faust, R. G., and Wu, S. L.: The action of bile salts on fluid and glucose movement by rat and hamster jejunum *in vitro*, J. Cell. Comp. Physiol. *65*:435, 1965.

98. ———: The effects of bile salts on tissue ATP levels of everted sacs of rat and hamster ileum, J. Cell. Comp. Physiol. *65*:449, 1965.

99. ———: Observations on the active transport of bile salts by rat and hamster ileum in vitro, Biochim. Biophys. Acta *120*:299, 1966.

100. Feldman, E. B., and Borgström, B.: Phase distribution of sterols: studies by gel filtration, Biochim. Biophys. Acta *125*:136, 1966.

101. Fisher, J. C., Bernstein, E. F., and Carey, J. B., Jr.: Primary bile acid enterolith, Gastroenterology, *49*:272, 1965.

102. Forth, W., Doenecke, P., and Glasner, H.: Zur spektrofluorometrischen Bestimmung von Gallensäuren nach Trennung mit Hilfe von Dünnschichtchromatographie, Klin. Wschr. *43*:1102, 1965.

103. Fowweather, F. S.: Bile acid enteroliths: With an account of a recent case, Biochem. J. *44*:607, 1949.

104. Frankel, M.: The biological splitting of conjugated bile acids, Biochem. J. *30*:2111, 1936.

105. Frantz, I. D., Jr., Carey, J. B., Jr., Moss, R., Eckert, J. F., Goldfarb, M., and Katz, H. I.: Observations on the turnover of cholesterol in a human subject, Minn. Med. *41*:157, 1958.

106. Frö   licher, E.: Die Resorption von Gallensäuren aus verschiedenen Dünndarmab-
schnitten, Biochem. Zeitschr. 283:273,
1936.

107. Frosch, B.: Das Verhalten der konjugier-
ten Serumgallensauren, Dtsch. Gesell-
schaft für Innere Medizin 72:697, 1966.

108. Frosch, B., and Wagener, H.: Quantitative determination of conjugated bile
acids in serum in acute hepatitis, Nature
213:404, 1967.

109. Gagnon, M., and Dawson, A. M.: The
effect of bile on vitamin A absorption in
the rat, Proc. Soc. Exp. Biol. Med. 127:
99, 1968.

110. Gallagher, T. F., Jr., Mueller, M. N., and
Kappas, A.: Estrogen pharmacology. IV.
Studies on the structural basis for estro-
gen-induced impairment of liver function,
Medicine 45:471, 1966.

111. Gallo, D. G., Bailey, K. R., and Sheffner,
A. L.: The interaction between choles-
tyramine and drugs, Proc. Soc. Exp. Biol.
Med. 120:60, 1965.

112. Gallo, D. G., and Sheffner, A. L.: The
disposition of orally administered choles-
tyramine-C^{14}, Proc. Soc. Exp. Biol. Med.
120:91, 1965.

113. Glasser, J. E., Weiner, I. M., and Lack,
L.: Comparative physiology of intestinal
taurocholate transport, Am. J. Physiol.
208:359, 1965.

114. Goldsmith, G. A., Hamilton, J. G., and
Miller, O. N.: Investigation of mechanisms by which unsaturated fats, nicotinic
acid and neomycin lower serum lipid
concentrations: excretion of sterols and
bile acids, Tr. Ass. Am. Phycns 72:207,
1959.

115. ———: Lowering of serum lipid concentrations, Arch. Int. Med. 105:512, 1960.

116. Goodman, D. S., and Huang, H. S.: Biosynthesis of vitamin A with rat intestinal
enzymes, Science 149:879, 1965.

117. Greaves, J. D., and Schmidt, C. L. A.:
The role played by bile in the absorption
of vitamin D in the rat, J. Biol. Chem.
102:101, 1933.

118. Gregg, J. A.: Presence of bile acids in
jaundiced human urine, Nature 214:29,
1967.

118a. ———: Urinary excretion of bile acids
in patients with obstructive jaundice and
hepatocellular disease, Am. J. Clin. Path.
49:404, 1968.

119. Grundy, S. M., Ahrens, E. H., Jr., and
Miettinen, T. A.: Quantitative isolation

and gas-liquid chromatographic analysis
of total fecal bile acids, J. Lipid Res. 6:
397, 1965.

120. Grundy, S. M., and Sjövall, J.: Studies
on bile acids in rat systemic blood, Proc.
Soc. Exp. Biol. Med. 107:306, 1961.

121. Guckian, J. C., and Perry, J. E.: Granulomatous hepatitis of unknown etiology,
Am. J. Med. 44:207, 1968.

122. Gustafsson, B. E., Gustafsson, J. A., and
Sjövall, J.: Intestinal and fecal sterols in
germ-free and conventional rats, Acta
Chem. Scand. 20:1827, 1966.

123. Gustafsson, B. E., and Midtvedt, T., and
Norman, A.: Isolated fecal microorganisms capable of 7α-dehydroxylating bile
acids, J. Exp. Med. 123:413, 1966.

124. Gustafsson, B. E., Norman, A., and
Sjövall, J.: Influence of E. coli infection
on turnover and metabolism of cholic
acid in germ-free rats, Arch. Biochem.
Biophys. 91:93, 1960.

125. Hamilton, J. G.: The effect of oral neomycin on the conversion of cholic acid to
deoxycholic in man, Arch. Biochem.
Biophys. 101:7, 1963.

126. Hardison, W. G., and Norman, J. C.:
Effect of bile salt and secretion upon bile
flow from the isolated perfused pig liver,
Gastroenterology 53:412, 1967.

127. ———: Ex vivo pig liver perfusion for
acute hepatic failure: bile salt composition of pig bile during perfusion, Medicine 46:97, 1967.

128. Hardison, W. G., and Rosenberg, I. H.:
Bile salt therapy in post-ileectomy steatorrhea, Clin. Res. 13:536, 1965 (Abstract).

129. ———: Bile-salt deficiency in the steatorrhea following resection of the ileum
and proximal colon, New Engl. J. Med.
277:337, 1967.

130. Hardy, J. L., Scherer, W. F., and Carey,
J. B., Jr.: Differential inactivation of arth-
ropod-borne animal viruses by bile and
bile salts in plasma or serum, Am. J. Epidemiol. 82:73, 1965.

131. Harinasuta, U., and Zimmerman, H. J.:
Diphenylhydantoin sodium hepatitis,
J.A.M.A. 203:1015, 1968.

132. Hashim, S. A., Bergen, S. S., Jr., and Van
Italle, T. B.: Experimental steatorrhea
induced in man by bile acid sequestrant,
Proc. Soc. Exp. Biol. Med. 106:173,
1961.

133. Haslewood, G. A. D.: Comparative studies of "bile salts". 5 Bile salts of Croc-
odylidae, Biochem. J. 52:583, 1952.

134. Haslewood, G. A. D.: Bile Salts, New York, Barnes & Noble; London, Methuen, 1967.

135. ———: Bile salt evolution, J. Lipid Res. 8:535, 1967.

136. Hayakawa, S., Kanematsu, Y., and Fujiwara, T.: New dehydroxylation reaction observed in the microbiological degradation pathway of cholic acid, Nature 214:520, 1967.

137. Hayakawa, S., and Samuelsson, B.: Transformation of cholic acid in vitro by Corynebacterium simplex, J. Biol. Chem. 239:94, 1964.

138. Hellström, K., and Lindstedt, S.: Studies on the formation of cholic acid in subjects given standardized diet with butter or corn oil as dietary fat, Am. J. Clin. Nut. 18:46, 1966.

139. Hellström, K., and Sjövall, J.: On the origin of lithocholic acid and ursodeoxycholic acids in man, Acta Physiol. Scand. 51:218, 1961.

140. Hill, M. J.: Action of bile salts on cell walls, Nature 214:1152, 1967.

141. Hill, M. J., and Drasar, B. S.: Bacterial degradation of bile salts, Biochem. J. 104:55P, 1967.

142. Hofmann, A. F.: Clinical implications of physicochemical studies on bile salts, Gastroenterology 48:484, 1965.

143. ———: The syndrome of ileal disease and the broken enterohepatic circulation: Cholerheic enteropathy, Gastroenterology 52:752, 1967.

144. Hofmann, A. F., and Borgström, B.: Physico-chemical state of lipids in intestinal content during their digestion and absorption, Fed. Proc. 21:43, 1962.

145. ———: The intraluminal phase of fat digestion in man: the lipid content of the micellar and oil phases of intestinal content obtained during fat digestion and absorption, J. Clin. Invest. 43:247, 1964.

146. Hofmann, A. F., and Grundy, S. M.: Abnormal bile salt metabolism in a patient with extensive lower intestinal resection, Clin. Res. 13:254, 1965 (Abstract).

147. Hofmann, A. F., and Small, D. M.: Detergent properties of bile salts: correlation with physiological function, Ann. Rev. Med. 18:333, 1967.

148. Holsti, P.: Experimental cirrhosis of the liver in rabbits induced by gastric instillation of desiccated whole bile, Acta Path. Microbiol. Scand., Supp. 113:1, 1956.

149. ———: Cirrhosis of the liver induced in rabbits by gastric instillation of 3-monohydroxycholanic acid, Nature 186:250, 1960.

150. ———: Bile acids as a cause of liver injury—cirrhogenic effect of chenodeoxycholic acid in rabbits, Acta Path. Microbiol. Scand. 54:479, 1962.

151. Holt, P. R.: Competitive inhibition of intestinal bile salt absorption in the rat, Am. J. Physiol. 210:635, 1966.

152. Horrall, O. H.: Bile: Its Toxicity and Relation to Disease, Chicago, Univ. Chicago Press, 1938.

153. Hunt, R. D., Leveille, G. A., and Sauberlich, H. E.: Dietary bile acids and lipid metabolism. II. The ductular cell reaction induced by lithocholic acid, Proc. Soc. Exp. Biol. Med. 113:139, 1963.

154. ———: Dietary bile acids and lipid metabolism. III. Effects of lithocholic acid in mammalian species, Proc. Soc. Exp. Biol. Med. 115:277, 1964.

155. Jacobson, E. D., Chodos, R. B., and Faloon, W. W.: An experimental malabsorption syndrome induced by neomycin, Am. J. Med. 28:524, 1960.

156. Javitt, N. B.: An experimental model for the study of cholestasis, Gastroenterology 50:394, 1966.

157. Johansson, G.: On the metabolism of lithocholic acid in chicken and rabbit, Acta Chem. Scand. 20:240, 1966.

158. Josephson, B.: Die Dissoziationskonstanten der Gallensäuren, Biochem. Zeitschr. 263:428, 1933.

159. Josephson, B.: Elimination of cholic acids. IV. In patients with liver disease, J. Clin. Invest. 18:343, 1939.

160. ———: The circulation of the bile acids in connection with their production, conjugation and excretion, Physiol. Rev. 21:463, 1941.

161. Josephson, B., and Rydin, A.: The resorption of bile acids from the intestines, Biochem. J. 30:2224, 1936.

162. Juniper, K., Jr.: Physicochemical characteristics of bile and their relation to gallstone formation, Am. J. Med. 39:98, 1965.

163. Kappas, A., and Palmer, R. H.: Selected aspects of steroid pharmacology, Pharm. Rev. 15:123, 1963.

164. Kim, S. K., and Bollman, J. L.: Absorption of fat in the absence of both bile and pancreatic juice, A.M.A. Arch. Surg. 69:247, 1954.

165. Kim, Y. S., Spritz, N., Blum, M., Terz, J., and Sherlock, P.: The role of altered bile acid metabolism in the steatorrhea of experimental blind loop, J. Clin. Invest. 45: 956, 1966.

166. Knoebel, L. K., and Ryan, J. M.: Digestion and mucosal absorption of fat in normal and bile-deficient dogs, Am. J. Physiol. 204:509, 1963.

167. Kottke, B. A.: Differences in bile acid kinetics as a means of distinguishing two types of hyperlipidemia, J. Lab. Clin. Med. 70:990, 1967 (Abstract).

168. Kreek, M. J., Weser, E., Sleisenger, M. H., and Jeffries, G. H.: Idiopathic cholestasis of pregnancy, New Engl. J. Med. 277:1391, 1967.

169. Krone, C. L., Theodore, E., and Jeffries, G. H.: Intraluminal phase of lipid digestion in malabsorptive disorders, J. Clin. Invest. 46:1080, 1967.

170. Kumler, W. D., and Halverstadt, I. F.: The acid strength of bile acids, J. Biol. Chem. 137:765, 1941.

171. Lack, L., and Weiner, I. M.: In vitro absorption of bile salts by small intestine of rats and guinea pigs, Am. J. Physiol. 200:313, 1961.

172. ———: Intestinal bile salt transport: structure-activity relationships and other properties, Am. J. Physiol. 210:1142, 1966.

173. ———: The ileal bile salt transport system: effect of the charged state of the substrate on activity, Biochim. Biophys. Acta 135:1065, 1967.

174. Lathe, G. H.: Transport aspects of bile secretion, Proc. Royal Soc. Med. 60:335, 1967.

175. Laurent, T. C., and Persson, H.: A study of micelles of sodium taurodeoxycholate in the ultracentrifuge, Biochim. Biophys. Acta 106:616, 1965.

176. Lee, H., and Richards, V.: Possible new approach to the evaluation of radiation injury of bone marrow, Nature 212:1593, 1966.

177. Lelbach, W. K.: Relation between alcohol ingestion and liver damage, Gastroenterology 53:670, 1967.

178. Lemierre, A., Brulé, M., and Garban, H.: Les rétentions biliaires par lésion de la cellule hépatique, Semaine méd. 34:301, 1914.

179. Lewis, B.: Effect of certain dietary oils on bile-acid secretion and serum cholesterol, Lancet 1:1090, 1958.

180. Lindstedt, S.: The turnover of cholic acid in man, Acta Physiol. Scand. 40:1, 1957.

181. Lindstedt, S., Avigan, J., Goodman, D. S., Sjövall, J., and Steinberg, D.: The effect of dietary fat on the turnover of cholic acid and on the composition of the biliary bile acids in man, J. Clin. Invest. 44:1754, 1965.

182. Linscheer, W. G., Patterson, J. F., Moore, E. W., Clermont, R. J., Robins, S. J., and Chalmers, T. C.: Medium and long chain fat absorption in patients with cirrhosis, J. Clin. Invest. 45:1317, 1966.

183. Lippel, K., and Olson, J. A.: The activity of nonlipolytic digestive enzymes of the pancreas in the presence of conjugated bile salts, Biochim. Biophys. Acta 127: 243, 1966.

184. Lottsfeldt, F. L., Krivit, W., Aust, J. B., and Carey, J. B., Jr.: Cholestyramine therapy in intrahepatic biliary atresia, New Engl. J. Med. 269:186, 1963.

185. Lyon-Caen, L.: Recherches expérimentales sur la tension superficielle des urines; applications à la differenciation des ictères, J. physiol. path. gén. 12:758, 1910.

186. MacIntyre, I., and Wootton, I. D. P.: Clinical Biochemistry, I. Bile acids in blood, Ann. Rev. Biochem. 29:635, 1960.

187. Maki, T.: Pathogenesis of calcium bilirubinate gallstones; role of E. coli, β-glucuronidase and coagulation by inorganic ions, polyelectrolytes and agitation, Ann. Surg. 164:90, 1966.

188. Masui, T., and Staple, E.: The formation of cholic acid from 3α, 7α, 12α-24ε-tetrahydroxycoprostanic acid by rat liver, Biochim. Biophys. Acta 104:305, 1965.

189. Meihoff, W. E., and Kern, F., Jr.; Bile salt malabsorption in regional ileitis, ileal resection and mannitol-induced diarrhea, J. Clin. Invest. 47:261, 1968.

190. Mendelsohn, D., Mendelsohn, L., and Staple, E.: The in vitro catabolism of cholesterol: A comparison of the formation of cholest-4-en-7α-ol-3-one and 5β-cholestan-7α-ol-3-one from cholesterol in rat liver, Biochemistry 5:1286, 1966.

191. ———: The in vitro catabolism of cholesterol. Formation of cholic acid from cholesterol in rat liver, Biochemistry 5: 3194, 1966.

192. Miettinen, T. A., Pelkonen, R., Nikkila, E. A., and Heinonen, O.: Low excretion of fecal bile acids in a family with hyper-

cholesterolemia, Acta Med. Scand. *182*: 645, 1967.

193. Mirvish, S. S.: Bile acids and other lipids in the gallbladder biles of Africans with primary cancer of the liver, Brit. J. Cancer *18*:478, 1964.

194. Mitropoulos, K. A., and Myant, N. B.: The metabolism of cholesterol in the presence of liver mitochondria from normal and thyroxin-treated rats, Biochem. J. *94*:594, 1965.

195. ————: The formation of lithocholic acid, chenodeoxycholic acid and α- and β-muricholic acids from cholesterol incubated with rat-liver mitochondria, Biochem. J. *103*:472, 1967.

196. ————: The formation of lithocholic and chenodeoxycholic acid and other bile acids from 3β-hydroxychol-5-enoic acid *in vitro* and *in vivo*, Biochim. Biophys. Acta *144*:430, 1967.

197. Moore. R. B.. Anderson, J. T., Keys, A., and Frantz, I. D., Jr.: Effect of dietary fat on the fecal excretion of cholesterol and its degradation products in human subjects, J. Lab. Clin. Med. *60*:1000, 1962 (Abstract).

198. Moore, R. B., Anderson, J. T., Taylor, H. L., Keys, A.. and Frantz. I. D., Jr.: The effect of dietary fat on the fecal excretion of cholesterol and its degradation products in man, J. Clin. Invest. *47*:1517, 1968.

199. Moore, R. B., Crane, C. A., and Frantz, I. D., Jr.: The effect of cholestyramine on the fecal excretion of intravenously administered cholesterol-4-14C and its degradation products in a hypercholesterolemic patient, J. Clin. Invest. *47*:1664, 1968.

200. Nair, P. P., Cordon, M., and Reback, J.: The enzymatic cleavage of the carbon-nitrogen bond in 3α, 7α, 12α-trihydroxy-5β-cholan-24-oylglycine, J. Biol. Chem. *242*:7, 1967.

201. Nakayama, F.: Cholesterol-holding capacity of bile in relation to gallstone formation, Clin. Chim. Acta *14*:171, 1966.

202. ————: Quantitative microanalysis of bile, J. Lab. Clin. Med. *69*:594, 1967.

203. Norman, A.: Influence of chemotherapeutics in the metabolism of bile acids in the intestine of rats, Acta Physiol Scand. *33*:99, 1955.

204. Norman, A., and Grubb, R.: Hydrolysis of conjugated bile acids by clostridia and enterococci, Acta Path. Microbiol. Scand. *36*:537, 1955.

205. Norman, A., and Palmer, R. H.: Metabolites of lithocholic acid-24-C14 in human bile and feces, J. Lab. Clin. Med. *63*:986, 1964.

206. Norman. A.. and Shorb, M. S.: *In vitro* formation of deoxycholic and lithocholic acid by human intestinal microorganisms, Proc. Soc. Exp. Biol. Med. *110*:552, 1962.

207. Norman, A., and Widström, O. A.: Hydrolysis of conjugated bile acids by extracellular enzymes present in rat intestinal contents, Proc. Soc. Exp. Biol. Med. *117*: 442, 1964.

208. Okishio, T., and Nair, P. P.: Studies on bile acids. Some observations on the intracellular localization of major bile acids in rat liver, Biochemistry *5*:3662, 1966.

209. Okishio. T., Nair, P. P.. and Gordon, M.: Studies on bile acids; the microquantitative separation of cellular bile acids by gas-liquid chromatography, Biochem. J. *102*:654, 1967.

210. Okuda, K., and Danielsson, H.: Synthesis and metabolism of 5β-cholestane 3α, 7α, 12α-triol-26-al., Acta Chem. Scand. *19*: 2160, 1965.

211. Olson. J. A.: The effect of bile and bile salts on the uptake and cleavage of β-carotene into retinol ester (vitamin A ester) bv intestinal slices, J. Lipid Res. *5*:402, 1964.

212. Osborn, E. C., Wooton, I. D. P., Da Silva, L. C., and Sherlock, S.: Serum bile-acid levels in liver disease, Lancet *2*:1049, 1959.

213. Palmer, R. H.: Haemolytic effects of steroids, Nature *201*:1134, 1964.

214. ————: Gallstones produced experimentally bv lithocholic acid in rats, Science *148*:1339, 1965.

215. ————: The formation of bile acid sulfates: A new pathway of bile acid metabolism in humans, Proc. Nat. Acad. Sci. *58*:1047, 1967.

216. Palmer, R. H., and Bolt, M. G.: Sulfate esters of lithocholic acid and its conjugates: a new pathway of bile acid metabolism in humans, J. Lab. Clin. Med. *70*: 873, 1967.

217. Palmer, R. H., Glickman, P. B., and Kappas, A.: Pyrogenic and inflammatory properties of certain bile acids in man, J. Clin. Invest. *41*:1573, 1962.

218. Palmer, R. H., and Hruban, Z.: Production of bile duct hyperplasia and gallstones by lithocholic acid, J. Clin. Invest. 45:1255, 1966.

219. Playoust, M. R., Lack, L., and Weiner, I. M.: Effect of intestinal resection on bile salt absorption in dogs, Am. J. Physiol. 208:363, 1965.

220. Poley, J. R., Dower, J. C., Owen, C. A., Jr., and Stickler, G. B.: Bile acids in infants and children, J. Lab. Clin. Med. 63:838, 1964.

221. Poley, J. R., and Hofmann, A. F.: Effective treatment of the diarrhea of cholerheic enteropathy with cholestyramine, J. Lab. Clin. Med. 70:1024, 1967.

222. Pope, J. L., Parkinson, T. M., and Olson, J. A.: Action of bile salts on the metabolism and transport of water-soluble nutrients by perfused rat jejunum in vitro, Biochim. Biophys. Acta 130:218, 1966.

223. Portman, O. W.: Nutritional influences on the metabolism of bile acids, Am. J. Clin. Nut. 8:462, 1960.

224. Portman, O. W., and Murphy, P.: Bile acid-lipoprotein relationships using cholic acid-24-C¹⁴, Am. J. Physiol. 195:189, 1958.

225. Portman, O. W., Shah, S., Antonis, A., and Jorgensen, B.: Alteration of bile salts by bacteria, Proc. Soc. Exp. Biol. Med. 109:959, 1962.

226. Quick, A. J., Hussey, C. V., and Collentine, G. E., Jr.: Vitamin K requirements of adult dogs and the influence of bile on its absorption from the intestine, Am. J. Physiol. 176:239, 1954.

227. ———: The effect of bile deprivation in the growing puppy, J. Lab. Clin. Med. 44:909, 1954.

228. Rabinowitz, J. L., Herman, R. H., Weinstein, D., and Staple, E.: Isolation of 3α 7α-dihydroxycoprostane derived from cholesterol in human bile, Arch. Biochem. Biophys. 114:233, 1966.

229. Rohrig, A.: Ueber den Einfluss der Galle auf die Herzthatigkeit, Archiv Heilkunde, 4:385, 1863.

230. Rosenberg, I. H., Hardison, W. G., and Bull, D. M.: Abnormal bile-salt patterns and intestinal bacterial overgrowth associated with malabsorption, New Engl. J. Med. 276:1391, 1967.

231. Rosenfeld, R. S., and Hellman, L.: Excretion of steroid acids in man, Arch. Biochem. Biophys. 97:406, 1962.

232. Rubin, E., and Lieber, C. S.: Early fine structural changes in the human liver induced by alcohol, Gastroenterology 52:1, 1967.

233. Rudman, D., and Kendall, F. E.: Bile acid content of human serum. I. Serum bile acids in patients with hepatic disease, J. Clin. Invest. 36:530, 1957.

234. Samuel, P., and Steiner, A.: The effect of neomycin on serum cholesterol level in man, Proc. Soc. Exp. Biol. Med. 100:193, 1959.

235. Sandberg, D. H., Sjövall, J., Sjövall, K., and Turner, D. A.: Measurement of human serum bile acids by gas-liquid chromatography, J. Lipid Res. 6:182, 1965.

236. Saunders, D. R., and Dawson, A. M.: The absorption of oleic acid in the bile fistula rat, Gut 4:254, 1963.

237. Savary, P.: Sur la solubilisation micellaire des acides palmitique, stéarique et oléique dans les solutions d'acides biliaires conjugués, Biochim. Biophys. Acta 125:328, 1966.

238. Schaffner, F., and Javitt, N. B.: Morphologic changes in hamster liver during intrahepatic cholestasis induced by taurolithocholate, Lab. Invest. 15:1783, 1966.

239. Schaffner, F., Klion, F. M., and Latuff, A. J.: The long term use of cholestyramine in the treatment of primary biliary cirrhosis, Gastroenterology 48:293, 1965.

240. Schersten, T.: The synthesis of taurocholic and glycocholic acids by preparations of human liver, I. Distribution of activity between subcellular fractions, Biochim. Biophys. Acta 141:144, 1967.

241. Schersten, T., Björntorp, P., Ekdahl, P. H., and Björkerud, S.: The synthesis of taurocholic and glycocholic acids by preparations of human liver. II. An analysis of the stimulating effect of the L fraction, Biochim. Biophys. Acta 141:155, 1967.

242. Schiff, L., Schubert, W. K., McAdams, A. J., Spiegel, E. L., and O'Donnell, J. F.: Hepatic cholesterol ester storage disease, a familial disorder. I. Clinical aspects, Am. J. Med. 44:538, 1968.

243. Schoenfield, L. J., and Sjövall, J.: Bile acids and cholesterol in guinea pigs with induced gallstones, Am. J. Physiol. 211:1069, 1966.

244. Schoenfield, L. J., Sjövall, J., and Perman, E.: Bile acids on the skin of patients with pruritic hepatobiliary disease, Nature 213:93, 1967.

245. Schoenfield, L. J., Sjövall, J., and Sjövall, K.: Bile acid composition of gallstones from man, J. Lab. Clin. Med. 68:186, 1966.

246. Senior, J. R.: Intestinal absorption of fats, J. Lipid Res. 5:495, 1964.

247. Sharp, H. L., Carey, J. B., Jr., White, J. G., and Krivit, W.: Cholestyramine therapy in patients with a paucity of intrahepatic bile ducts, J. Pediat. 71:723, 1967.

248. Sherlock, S., and Walshe, V.: Blood cholates in normal subjects and liver disease, Clin. Sci. 6:223, 1948.

249. Simmonds, W. J., Hofmann, A. F., and Theodor, E.: Absorption of cholesterol from a micellar solution: intestinal perfusion studies in man, J. Clin. Invest. 46:874, 1967.

250. Siperstein, M. D., and Murray, A. W.: Cholesterol metabolism in man, J. Clin. Invest. 34:1449, 1955.

251. ———: Enzymatic synthesis of cholyl CoA and taurocholic acid, Science 123:377, 1956.

252. Sjövall, J.: On the concentration of bile acids in the human intestine during absorption, Acta Physiol. Scand. 46:339, 1959.

253. ———: Bile acids in man under normal and pathological conditions. Bile acids and steroids 73, Clin. Chim. Acta 5:30, 1960.

254. Sjövall, K., and Sjövall, J.: Serum bile acid levels in pregnancy with pruritus (bile acids and steroids 158), Clin. Chim. Acta 13:207, 1966.

255. Small, D. M.: Physicochemical studies of cholesterol gallstone formation, Gastroenterology 52:607, 1967.

256. Small, D. M., and Bourges, M.: Lyotropic paracrystalline phases obtained with ternary and quaternary systems of amphiphilic substances in water: Studies on aqueous systems of lecithin, bile salt and cholesterol, Molecular Crystals 1:541, 1966.

257. Small, D. M., Bourges, M., and Dervichian, D. G.: Ternary and quarternary aqueous systems containing bile salt lecithin and cholesterol, Nature 211:816, 1966.

258. Sobotka, H., and Goldberg, A.: Choleic acids, Biochem. J. 26:555, 1932.

259. Sperber, I.: Biliary secretion of organic anions and its influence on bile flow, in Taylor, W. (ed.): The Biliary System, p. 457, Philadelphia, Davis, 1965.

260. Stanley, M. M., and Nemchausky, B.: Fecal C14-bile acid excretion in normal subjects and patients with steroid-wasting syndromes secondary to ileal dysfunction, J. Lab. Clin. Med. 70:627, 1967.

261. Staple, E., and Rabinowitz, J. L.: Formation of trihydroxycoprostanic acid from cholesterol in man, Biochim. Biophys. Acta 59:735, 1962.

262. Stolk, A.: Induction of hepatic cirrhosis in iguana by 3-monohydroxycholanic acid treatment, Experientia 16:507, 1960.

263. Strand, O.: Effects of D- and L-triiodothyromine and of propylthiouracil on the production of bile acids in the rat, J. Lipid Res. 4:305, 1963.

264. Sullivan, M. F.: Dependence of radiation diarrhea on the presence of bile in the intestine, Nature 195:1217, 1962.

265. Sullivan, M. F., Hulse, E. V., and Mole, R. H.: The mucus-depleting action of bile in the small intestine of the irradiated rat, Brit. J. Exp. Path. 46:235, 1965.

266. Swell, L., Trout, E. C., Jr., Hopper, J. R., Field, H., Jr., and Treadwell, C. R.: Specific function of bile salts in cholesterol absorption, Proc. Soc. Exp. Biol. Med. 98:174, 1958.

267. Tabaqchali, S., and Booth, C. C.: Jejunal bacteriology and bile salt metabolism in patients with intestinal malabsorption, Lancet 2:12, 1966.

268. Tamesue, N., and Juniper, K., Jr.: Concentrations of bile salts at the critical micellar concentration of human gallbladder bile, Gastroenterology 52:473, 1967.

269. Tappeiner, H.: Über die Aufsaugung der Gallensauren Alkalien im Dunndarme. Sitzungsberichte der mathematisch naturwissenschaftlichen Classe. Der Kaiserlichen Akademie der Wissenschaften 77:281, 1878.

270. Taylor, W. (ed.): The Biliary System, Philadelphia, Davis, 1965.

271. Tennent, D. M., Siegel, H., Zanetti, M. E., Kuron, G. W., Ott, W. H., and Wolf, F. J.: Plasma cholesterol lowering action of bile acid binding polymers in experimental animals, J. Lipid Res. 1:469, 1960.

272. Thomas, P. J., Hsia, S. L., Matschiner, J. T., Doisy, E. A., Jr., Elliott, W. H., Thayer, S. H., and Doisy, E. A.: Bile

acids. XIX. Metabolism of lithocholic acid-24-^{14}C in the rat, J. Biol. Chem. *239*:102, 1964.

273. Truswell, A. S., Mitchell, W. D., and McVeigh, S.: The effect of chlorphenoxyisobutyrate (Atromid S) on the pattern of bile acids in human bile, J. Atheroscler. Res. *6*:591, 1966.

274. Urban, E., Frank, B. W., and Kern, F.: Liver dysfunction with mestranol but not with norethynodrel in a patient with Enovid-induced jaundice, Ann. Int. Med. *68*:598, 1968.

275. Usui, T., Nakasone, S., and Kawamoto, M.: Bile acids in human urine, Yonago Acta Medica *10*:250, 1966.

276. Vahouny, G. V., Kothari, H., and Treadwell, C. R.: Specificity of bile salt protection of cholesterol ester hydrolase from proteolytic inactivation, Arch. Biochem. Biophys. *121*:242, 1967.

277. Vahouny, G. V., Weersing, S., and Treadwell, C. R.: Function of specific bile acids in cholesterol esterase activity *in vitro*, Biochim. Biophys. Acta *98*:607, 1965.

278. Van Itallie, T. B., Hashim, S. A., Cramptom, R. S., and Tennent, D. M.: The treatment of pruritus and hypercholesteremia of primary biliary cirrhosis with cholestyramine, New Engl. J. Med. *265*: 469, 1961.

279. Visintine, R. E., Michaels, G. D., Fukayama, G., Conklin, J., and Kinsell, L. W.: Xanthomatous biliary cirrhosis treated with cholestyramine, Lancet 2:341, 1961.

280. Watson, C. J.: Studies of urobilinogen. III. Per diem excretion of urobilinogen in common forms of jaundice and disease of the liver, Arch. Int. Med. *59*:206, 1937.

281. Watson, C. J., and Hoffbauer, F. W.: The problem of prolonged hepatitis with particular reference to the cholangiolytic type and to the development of cholangiolytic cirrhosis of the liver, Ann. Int. Med. *25*:195, 1946.

282. Webling, D. A., and Holdsworth, E. S.: Bile salts and calcium absorption, Biochem. J. *100*:652, 1966.

283. ———: Bile and the absorption of strontium and iron, Biochem. J. *100*:661, 1966.

284. Weiner, I. M., and Lack, L.: Absorption of bile salts from the small intestine in vivo, Am. J. Physiol. *202*:155, 1962.

285. Wells, R. F., Knepshield, J. H., and Davis, C.: Right upper quadrant calcification in a patient receiving long-term cholestyramine therapy for primary biliary cirrhosis, Am. J. Digest. Dis. *13*:86, 1968.

286. Whiteside, C. H., Fluckiger, H. B., and Sarett, H. P.: Comparison of *in vitro* bile acid binding capacity and *in vivo* hypocholesteremic activity of cholestyramine, Proc. Soc. Exp. Biol. Med. *121*:153, 1966.

287. Wilson, I. D., Onstad, G. R., Williams, R. C., Jr., Carey, J. B., Jr., and Yount, W. J.: Changes in serum immunoglobulin class and subgroup concentrations in patients with alcoholic cirrhosis, J. Lab. Clin. Med. *70*:879, 1967.

288. Wilson, J. D.: Biosynthetic origin of serum cholesterol in the squirrel monkey: Evidence for a contribution by the intestinal wall, J. Clin. Invest. *47*:175, 1968.

289. Wilson, J. D., and Lindsey, C. A., Jr.: Studies on the influence of dietary cholesterol on cholesterol metabolism in the isotopic steady state in man, J. Clin. Invest. *44*:1805, 1965.

290. Wollenweber, J., Kottke, B. A., and Owen, C. A., Jr.: Pool size and turnover of bile acids in six hypercholesteremic patients with and without administration of nicotinic acid, J. Lab. Clin. Med. *69*:584, 1967.

291. Wood, P. D. S., Shioda, R., and Kinsell, L. W.: Dietary regulations of cholesterol metabolism, Lancet 2:604, 1966.

292. Yamane, I., Nakamura, T., and Takani, S.: On the hemolytic action of keto bile acids. Yonago Acta Medica 2:1957, 1957.

293. Zaki, F. G., Carey, J. B., Jr., Hoffbauer, F. W., and Nwokolo, C.: Biliary reaction and choledocholithiasis induced in the rat by lithocholic acid, J. Lab. Clin. Med. *69*:737, 1967.

294. Zurier, R. B., Hashim, S. A., and Van Itallie, T. B.: Effect of medium-chain triglyceride on cholestyramine-induced steatorrhea in man, Gastroenterology *49*: 490, 1965.

5

Disordered Hemostasis in Hepatic Disease

OSCAR D. RATNOFF, M.D.

A characteristic and troublesome feature of many disorders of the liver or biliary tree is the appearance of generalized hemorrhagic phenomena. The association was recognized early. In 1846, Budd wrote, "There is . . . a tendency to hemorrhage from the nose and other parts in which there is no particular stress on the vessels. Small purpuric spots often appear on the face or forehead, sometimes on the distended belly; and, if the patient be cupped, ecchymosis is apt to take place about the puncture."[16]

Since Budd's day, innumerable careful clinical descriptions of the hemorrhagic phenomena associated with hepatic or biliary tract disease have been published. Although the usual case of infectious hepatitis is not complicated by a bleeding tendency,[145] severely affected patients may bleed from the skin and mucous membranes, an event which may presage a fatal outcome.[40, 117] Other acute disorders that involve the liver, such as leptospirosis, may be complicated by cutaneous or mucosal bleeding, but these symptoms are not necessarily related to hepatic dysfunction. Patients with chronic hepatic disease are more likely to have clinical evidences of a bleeding tendency. In one series, a fourth of patients with Laennec's cirrhosis had epistaxis, cutaneous purpura, gingival bleeding or menometrorrhagia[106]; similar phenomena are common in postnecrotic cirrhosis.[107] Bleeding into the skin or from the mucous membranes is also a concomitant of untreated chronic obstruction of the biliary tree,[89] and the danger of surgery under these conditions was commented upon as early as 1878.[115]

As one might expect from the central metabolic role of the liver, the pathogenesis of bleeding is often complex. In hepatic disorders the plasma may be deficient in clotting factors, the platelets may be qualitatively or quantitatively defective, endogenous anticoagulant substances may be present and the plasma fibrinolytic systems may behave abnormally. These laboratory abnormalities presumably reflect defective hemostasis. Among patients with cirrhosis, those who sustain episodes of gastrointestinal, vaginal or postoperative hemorrhage severe enough to require transfusion are more likely to have laboratory evidences of a bleeding tendency than those who do not bleed.[120] Admittedly, it is difficult to prove that the prognosis after bleeding from esophageal varices is related to hemostatic function. Nonetheless, patients in whom the normal mechanisms of hemostasis are impaired may bleed excessively at surgery, and in such individuals, punch biopsy of the liver may be dangerous. The care of patients with hepatic disease is often influenced by the physician's assessment of the degree to which the hemostatic mechanisms are deranged, and by his awareness of the measures which can be used to treat or prevent hemorrhage.

PHYSIOLOGY OF HEMOSTASIS

Several interrelated mechanisms stanch the flow of blood from injured blood vessels. In the smallest vessels, the earliest discernible event is the rapid accumulation of platelets at the site of the damage. Vasodilatation, which may follow injury to small vessels, slows the flow of blood, diverting platelets from the center of the stream to the periphery. There, clumps of platelets accumulate, probably attracted by collagen-like protein exposed by the endothelial damage. Aggregation of platelets may also be fostered by adenosine diphosphate (ADP), released by damaged endothelial cells and by the platelets themselves. At first, the mass of platelets is unstable and may break off. After a brief interval, thrombin forms in the vicinity of the platelet mass, and, under its influence, the platelets undergo morphologic changes in which their individual identity is lost, fibrin fibers appear and a more stable plug forms, which can seal the gap in the blood vessel.

Although platelets undoubtedly participate in the control of bleeding from defects in larger blood vessels, hemostasis under these conditions is largely a function of the clotting mechanism. The final stage in the events leading to blood coagulation is the formation of a network of insoluble fibrin, in the meshes of which serum and the cellular elements of blood are trapped. The clot nearly always plugs the hole in the vessel. If this is unsuccessful, exsanguination ensues or, if bleeding has occurred in a confined area, the pressure of the extravasated blood may slow hemorrhage until treatment is possible. The exposed anatomic situation of esophageal varices is such that when they rupture, hemorrhage is unopposed by the back pressure of distended tissues.

Fibrin is formed through the action of a proteolytic enzyme, thrombin, which splits off 4 small fragments, the fibrinopeptides, from each molecule of fibrinogen, the precursor of fibrin. The molecules of fibrinogen from which the fibrinopeptides have been separated, now called fibrin monomers, polymerize to form insoluble threads of fibrin. In purified systems, this fibrin is held together loosely, and can be dissolved by agents such as 5M urea or 1 per cent monochloracetic acid. In normal blood, on the other hand, the fibrin molecules are bound by firm chemical bonds, induced by a second enzyme, fibrin stabilizing factor (factor XIII). This enzyme, probably inactive in circulating blood and activated by thrombin during clotting, unites the adjacent fibrin monomers by transamidation. Fibrin formation is fostered by calcium ions and by a poorly defined accelerator in plasma.

Thrombin, the agent responsible for the formation of fibrin, cannot be detected in freshly drawn blood, but evolves during coagulation from its precursor, prothrombin. How this comes about is disputed. The following is but one of several contemporary views. At least 2 mechanisms have been discerned. In one, clotting is initiated by contact of blood with injured tissue; this process is therefore described as the *extrinsic pathway*. The active principle of injured tissue, tissue thromboplastin, interreacts with a plasma protein, factor VII, to form a complex which, in the presence of calcium ions, activates another plasma protein, Stuart factor (factor X). Activated Stuart factor then reacts with proaccelerin (factor V), calcium ions and phospholipid to form a prothrombin converting principle which changes prothrombin to thrombin via an enzymatic process. The phospholipid for this reaction is furnished by the injured tissue, by the plasma itself, and by platelets. The effectiveness of proaccelerin appears to be greatly increased if it is first altered by thrombin, a process misnamed autocatalysis.

The second sequence through which thrombin generates in shed blood does not involve the intervention of tissue thromboplastin and has therefore been called the *intrinsic pathway*. The waterfall[25] or cascade[69] hypothesis of blood coagulation envisions the successive participation of a number of plasma proteins. When blood comes into contact with glass or similar insoluble agents, Hageman factor (factor XII), a plasma protein, is activated, a process which, in purified systems, seems to involve the polymerization of its molecules. The biological counterpart of glass is not known. Activated Hageman factor changes PTA (plasma thromboplastin antecedent, factor XI) to a hydrolytic enzyme which, in the presence of calcium ions, activates Christmas factor (factor IX). Next, activated Christmas factor reacts with AHF (antihemophilic factor, factor VIII) to yield activated AHF; this step is accelerated if

AHF is first altered by thrombin. Activated AHF then activates Stuart factor. The subsequent steps in the intrinsic pathway are apparently identical with those of the extrinsic route. AHF and Stuart factor are activated only if calcium and phospholipids are present, the latter furnished both by the plasma itself and by the disintegration of platelets.

Platelets, essential for normal hemostasis, are derived from the cytoplasm of megakaryocytes, located principally, in the adult, in the bone marrow. Besides their capacity to plug small vascular defects and to furnish phospholipids for clotting, platelets promote clot retraction, a process in which the clot shrinks, expelling the serum contained within. Retraction is initiated by thrombin and depends on the presence in platelets of a contractile protein, thrombasthenin, which, like muscle actomyosin, is an adenosine triphosphatase. Perhaps this enzyme helps to provide the energy required for retraction. Although the utility of retraction is not known, individuals in whom this function is impaired have a bleeding tendency. Platelets also contain proteins identical with or closely similar to proaccelerin, AHF, PTA, fibrinogen and fibrin stabilizing factor; how these agents aid in hemostasis is also conjectural.

Besides its various clot-promoting properties, plasma contains *inhibitors* of the clotting process, of which those that interfere with the function of activated PTA, tissue thromboplastin (or its complex with factor VII) and thrombin have been characterized most fully. Activated Stuart factor, and probably other activated clotting factors which may form inadvertently within the circulating blood, can also be inactivated by passage through the liver or reticuloendothelial system. Plasma also possesses a potentially powerful enzyme system which can digest fibrin and other procoagulant proteins; *fibrinolysis* is discussed in detail in a subsequent section.

TESTS OF HEMOSTATIC FUNCTION

For the most part, defects in hemostasis are diagnosed in the laboratory. Many excellent texts describe in detail the technics used.[14, 18, 75, 95, 123, 133] Certain tests are particularly helpful in the clinical care of patients with hepatic disease.

The *clotting time* of whole blood is a function of the concentration of factors that participate in the intrinsic pathway of blood clotting. Measured in glass tubes, the clotting time is prolonged only when the deficiency of these factors is profound; it is unaltered by thrombocytopenia or by deficiencies of factor VII or fibrin stabilizing factor. An abnormally long clotting time may also reflect the presence of intrinsic or extrinsic inhibitors of blood clotting, of which heparin, administered therapeutically, is the commonest. In patients with catastrophic fibrinolytic purpura, whole blood may seem to be incoagulable because the fibrin strands dissolve as rapidly as they form. The sensitivity of the clotting time may be enhanced by using silicone-coated or polystyrene tubes, but the tedium of this modification makes it impractical for routine use.

Both in obstructive jaundice and in parenchymal hepatic disease, particularly cirrhosis of the liver, the clotting time is occasionally prolonged when measured in glass tubes[33] and, more often, when tested in silicone-coated or plastic tubes.[51]

The insensitivity of the clotting time of whole blood may be circumvented to some extent by measuring, instead, the *partial thromboplastin time,* that is, the clotting time of a mixture of citrated plasma, calcium ions and crude phospholipid derived from brain tissue or soy beans; the test is sometimes modified by the addition of kaolin or glass to activate Hageman factor as completely as possible. Like the clotting time of whole blood, the partial thromboplastin time is prolonged if factors of the intrinsic pathways are deficient or if inhibitors are present. Although more sensitive than the clotting time of whole blood, the partial thromboplastin time may be normal in mild coagulative disorders. In hepatic disease or obstructive jaundice, the partial thromboplastin time is often moderately prolonged.

Several simple tests help to localize the coagulative defects of patients with hepatic disease. The *thrombin time,* that is, the clotting time of a mixture of citrated plasma and bovine thrombin, measures the formation of fibrin. The thrombin time may be prolonged if the concentration of fibrinogen is excessively low or high, or if this protein is qualitatively abnormal. It is also long if intrinsic or extrinsic inhibitors of fibrin formation are present, or if the plasma accelerator of this step is deficient. The thrombin time is not affected by the concentration of fibrin stabilizing factor, a deficiency of which is detected by noting the solubility of clotted plasma in 5M urea or in 1 per cent monochloracetic acid.

The *one-stage prothrombin time* assesses the extrinsic pathway of thrombin formation. The test is performed by measuring the clotting time of a mixture of citrated plasma, tissue thromboplastin and calcium ions. A long one-stage prothrombin time, a common finding in obstructive jaundice or hepatic disease,[97] may reflect deficiencies of factor VII, Stuart factor, proaccelerin, prothrombin or fibrinogen, or the presence of inhibitors of the formation of the prothrombin converting principle or fibrin. Among patients with cirrhosis, those who have had a major episode of bleeding are more likely to have a prolonged one-stage prothrombin time than those who have escaped this symptom.[120]

When the one-stage prothrombin time is normal, an abnormally long partial thromboplastin time suggests deficiencies of Hageman factor, PTA, Christmas factor or antihemophilic factor, or the presence of inhibitors of these substances.

The *platelets* may be counted by a variety of means; the normal range is 150,000 to 350,000/cu.mm. Platelet function may be tested by observing *clot retraction* grossly or by measuring it semi-quantitatively. Clot retraction is usually impaired only if the platelet count is less than about 100,000/cu.mm. Qualitative abnormalities of platelets can impair retraction, and are also suggested when their aggregation by ADP or collagen suspensions is impaired, but such tests are ordinarily not available.

Thrombocytopenia and qualitative abnormalities of platelets are usually accompanied by prolongation of the *bleeding time*. I prefer to measure the bleeding time by a modification of Duke's method, in which the ball of the finger is punctured with a scalpel blade. In thrombocytopenic states, this test gives abnormal results only when the platelet count is less than 100,000/cu.mm., a level not often reached in hepatic disease. A long bleeding time is also found in thrombocythemia, in which the platelet count is above about 800,000/cu.mm., in von Willebrand's disease, a hereditary disorder in which the concentration of antihemophilic factor is often decreased, and in one or another of the dysproteinemias. In some patients with abnormal bleeding, no obvious cause for a prolonged bleeding time can be found.

Further investigation of the hemostatic mechanisms requires procedures not generally available. Quantitative or semi-quantitative assays can be performed for each plasma clotting factor, as well as tests that detect and localize circulating anticoagulants in plasma, that is, abnormal inhibitory substances. Abnormal fibrinolytic activity can be measured, with increasing sensitivity, in clots of whole blood, plasma or the euglobulin fraction of plasma. The components of the fibrinolytic system can be assayed with more or less confidence. The tourniquet test, widely used to demonstrate increased capillary fragility, is unreliable and provides little useful information.

DEFICIENCIES OF VITAMIN K–DEPENDENT CLOTTING FACTORS

Four clotting factors in mammalian plasma—Christmas factor, factor VII, Stuart factor and prothrombin—are synthesized only if vitamin K is available. The properties of these 4 factors are extraordinarily similar, which raises many questions not yet answerable. Their synthesis is impaired in obstructive jaundice or liver disease, contributing in an important way to the bleeding tendency in these conditions.

A wide variety of compounds, all derivatives of naphthoquinone, exhibit vitamin K–like activity. These agents cannot be synthesized by mammals, but are furnished by the ingestion of plant foods, particularly leafy green vegetables, and by intestinal flora. Naturally occurring compounds with vitamin K–like activity are lipid-soluble, and as a consequence their optimal absorption from the gastrointestinal tract requires the presence of bile salts and, probably, pancreatic lipase as well.[73, 94, 116]

Once absorbed, vitamin K is utilized by the parenchymal cells of the liver to synthesize the 4 clotting factors that depend upon this agent.[10, 92] The vitamin is not incorporated into the structure of the clotting factors. Olson, Miller and Troup[88] and Suttie[128] have demonstrated that puromycin, which blocks the protein synthetic function of ribosomes, inhibits the formation of vitamin K–dependent clotting factors. Olson's experiments[88] suggest that vitamin K acts only after the formation of a protein precursor of the clotting factors, a view supported on other grounds by Hemker and his associates.[52] Presumably, vitamin K acts only to impart some special structural configuration to the factors, but how this is done is not known. Martius[73] champions the concept that vitamin K is required for normal cellular respiration and oxidative phosphorylation. In this view, the effect upon the synthesis of the 4 clotting factors reflects the peculiar needs of this process.

Why vitamin K is needed for the synthesis of 4 apparently separable clotting factors is unsolved; as far as I know, no other proteins have this requirement. The 4 factors have many characteristics which, superficially at least, suggest that their essential chemical structure is similar. For example, the administration of coumarin-like compounds or the presence of hepatic disease depresses the synthesis of all 4 substances, whereas the concentrations of all increase during pregnancy. All are readily adsorbed from plasma by calcium phosphate, aluminum hydroxide or barium sulfate. All have similar heat stabilities and are stable for long periods at −20° C., unlike antihemophilic factor and proaccelerin. All are present in fresh serum, either in native form or activated; the activated form of prothrombin, thrombin, is unstable, so that aged serum is deficient in this substance. Each factor is readily inhibited by exposure to sulfhydryl compounds. Their chemical similarities are such that for a long time it was difficult to obtain purified preparations of any one totally deficient in the other 3; present-day chromatographic techniques have made such separations possible.

One exciting way to explain the similarities of the vitamin K–dependent factors is proposed by Seegers.[111] He offers the view that the 4 factors are part of a complex, to which he gives the name prothrombin. In his opinion, the apparent separability of the 4 compounds by chromatography is artifactual. The observation that carboxypeptidase and the first component of complement are similar complexes fortifies this hypothesis.

Three major difficulties weaken the theory that the vitamin K–dependent clotting factors are part of a single entity. The separate hereditary deficiencies of these factors are at least superficially incompatible with their being part of the same molecule. Moreover, each factor has distinctive functions in the clotting mechanism. And each also has a different biological half-life, and is therefore regenerated at a different rate. Although these criticisms are valid, they are by no means crucial. An hypothesis to explain the peculiar similarities of the vitamin K–dependent clotting factors is sorely needed and experiments in this direction should be profitable.

The physiologic role of vitamin K in the synthesis of clotting factors is put to practical use in the management of patients with obstructive jaundice or hepatic disease. In obstructive jaundice vitamin K is absorbed poorly, because bile salts are prevented from entering the duodenum. As a result, such individuals may be deficient in each vitamin K–dependent clotting factor, a change reflected by an abnormally long one-stage prothrombin time.[97] These deficiencies are apparently responsible for the susceptibility to hemorrhage in obstructive jaundice.[95] Bleeding, once a common and dangerous complication of surgery in obstructive jaundice,[140] can usually be prevented by daily parenteral administration of vitamin K[17]; small amounts of a water-soluble analogue—for example, 5 mg. of menadione sodium bisulfite—are usually sufficient. The effects of therapy can be assessed by measuring the one-stage prothrombin time. If this is abnormally long because the absorption of vitamin K is impaired, it will shorten within a few days. A more rapid response follows the intramuscular or intravenous injection of lipid-soluble vitamin K_1. The response to vitamin K is useful not only therapeutically, but diagnostically[67] for, as noted shortly, patients with hepatic disease usually do not benefit from the injection of small amounts of this substance. The revolution in the care of patients with obstructive jaundice brought about by therapy with vitamin K is epitomized by the statement of one contemporary writer that, "in patients with calculus obstruction of the common duct, the defect in hemostasis is rarely so severe as to cause spontaneous bruising and bleeding."[62]

Vitamin K–dependent clotting factors may be deficient in both acute and chronic parenchymal hepatic disease.[8] Deficiencies of prothrombin,[72, 78, 110] factor VII, Stuart factor and Christmas factor[35, 99, 120] are usually found together. Other abnormalities in hepatic disease also prolong the one-stage prothrombin time, notably, a deficiency of proaccelerin or, much less commonly, fibrinogen. As mentioned, an abnormally low concentration of Christmas factor is not detected by the one-stage prothrombin time.[99] In some patients with parenchymal disease, particularly those with severe jaundice, the prothrombin time is shortened by the administration of vitamin K, for example, the intramuscular injection of vitamin K_1.[112, 113, 124] In such cases, this response to vitamin K may suggest a component of intrahepatic obstruction of the biliary tree, indistinguishable physiologically from extrahepatic obstruction. This explanation is probably too simple, for the dose of vitamin K needed to shorten the prothrombin time in parenchymal hepatic disease is often much larger than that needed in obstructive jaundice, for example, 25 or 50 mg. of vitamin K_1.

In the majority of patients in whom an abnormally long one-stage prothrombin time is associated with parenchymal hepatic disease, the administration of vitamin K is without obvious benefit. Spector and Corn[120] found that patients who had had a major hemorrhage never responded to therapy with this vitamin. Presumably, in these individuals, vitamin K cannot be utilized for the synthesis of the deficient clotting factors. As a result, in hepatic disease, therapy of the hemorrhagic state associated with deficiency of the vitamin K–dependent factors is diffi-

cult. If the patient does not respond to vitamin K, its use is not continued, since this vitamin may be toxic in large amounts.[4] Transfusion of normal blood or plasma may tide the patient over an acute crisis.[95] Since the vitamin K–dependent clotting factors are stable during storage at 4° C., there is no particular necessity to use fresh blood or plasma. But other defects in the plasma of patients with liver disease, such as proaccelerin deficiency, are not corrected by the use of ordinary stored plasma. Thus the use of fresh frozen plasma, which contains adequate amounts of proaccelerin, or fresh blood, which contains viable platelets as well, is preferable.[121]

When an adult with hepatic disease is thought to be bleeding because of a deficiency of the vitamin K–dependent clotting factors, the transfusion of 1,000 ml. of fresh frozen plasma provides adequate concentrations of these substances; proportionately smaller amounts are used in children. Unfortunately, the transfused factors, particularly factor VII, disappear rapidly from the circulation, so that the patients must be transfused repeatedly; 200 ml. of plasma every 4 hours is a minimal amount. But greater volumes may so overload the circulation as to pose the danger of rupture from esophageal varices, unless at the same time blood is being lost from active hemorrhage. Experimentally, concentrates of the vitamin K–dependent factors help to sustain the level of these agents without overloading the circulation, but such preparations are not generally available.[13, 119] If the bleeding is sufficient to reduce the hematocrit, as in esophageal varices, blood transfusions are needed to sustain the blood volume; fresh blood, if available, is more efficacious than that stored in the blood bank.

Anticoagulant therapy is seldom indicated in hepatocellular disease. If the need arises, however, treatment with coumarin-like anticoagulants should be approached with caution. Experimentally, liver damage prolongs the effect of these drugs,[96] and in hepatic disease, the response to the administration of coumarin-like compounds is exaggerated compared to that of individuals without hepatic damage.[108, 113] Heparin therapy, too, has its dangers, for patients with thrombocytopenia may be peculiarly sensitive to this agent.

PROACCELERIN DEFICIENCY

Besides deficiencies of the vitamin K–dependent clotting factors, the commonest coagulative defect in acute or chronic hepatic disease is probably a decrease in the concentration of proaccelerin in plasma.[15, 90, 99] Proaccelerin is probably synthesized largely or exclusively in the liver. Evidence of this has been provided by experiments in which proaccelerin was elaborated by the perfused rat liver; synthesis was suppressed by the administration of puromycin.[88] Further, the concentration of proaccelerin is depressed in experimental animals subjected to hepatectomy[71, 80] or chloroform intoxication.[129] Perhaps, then, in hepatic disease, the decreased concentration of proaccelerin is the result of impaired synthesis of this protein. Another possibility is that excessive plasma proteolytic activity, common in chronic hepatic disease, is responsible for the decreased concentration of proaccelerin, for this substance is readily inactivated by plasmin.[2, 30, 65] It is doubtful, however, that this abnormality can be attributed to plasmin in most cases, for in other situations similar degrees of excessive plasma proteolytic activity do not affect the concentration of proaccelerin.[48] Perhaps, in the rare cirrhotic with fibrinolytic purpura, plasmin contributes to the deficiency of proaccelerin.[11] Rarely, too, proaccelerin deficiency may be a concomitant of intravascular coagulation.

An isolated deficiency of proaccelerin is reflected by an abnormality of the one-stage prothrombin time. Since this test is sensitive to deficiencies of other factors, specific procedures are needed for its measurement. That a deficiency of proaccelerin contributes to the bleeding tendency of patients with hepatic disease is known only by analogy; patients with hereditary deficiencies of proaccelerin, similar in degree to those of patients with cirrhosis, may have a slight tendency to bleed, usually after an injury.

In hepatic disease an isolated deficiency of proaccelerin does not usually need to be corrected. The only available measure is the transfusion of fresh blood or fresh frozen plasma. Proaccelerin survives storage at 4° C. in the blood bank only erratically. Since the half-life of proaccelerin after transfusion is only a matter of hours,[54] such therapy is suitable only for an acute episode of bleeding. The schedule of transfusion is similar to that used for the vitamin K–dependent clotting factors. Vitamin K therapy is useless, since this vitamin is not utilized in the synthesis of proaccelerin.

FIBRINOGEN AND FIBRIN FORMATION

A commonly mentioned but relatively unusual defect in hepatic disorders is a decrease in the concentration of fibrinogen in circulating plasma. This protein is synthesized largely or exclusively in the liver. Direct evidence of hepatic synthesis was first obtained by Miller,[76, 77] who demonstrated that the isolated liver, unlike the liverless animal, incorporated radioactive amino acids into fibrinogen. These observations have been confirmed repeatedly in the perfused liver[44, 88] or in hepatic slices.[125] Fluorescent antibody technics have localized the site of synthesis to the parenchymal cells.[39]

Hypofibrinogenemia, usually of moderate degree, is found in an occasional patient with acute or chronic hepatic disease, in whom it suggests a poor prognosis.[35, 43, 51, 64, 66] More often, the concentration of fibrinogen is normal or even elevated.[48] Patients with cirrhosis may not respond to stimuli, such as infection, which, in other individuals, would induce an increased concentration of fibrinogen in plasma.[49]

Hypofibrinogenemia may result from decreased synthesis of fibrinogen, from its consumption during intravascular coagulation, from unreplaced loss during massive hemorrhage, or from its destruction by abnormal plasma fibrinolytic activity. Decreased synthesis is probably an important element in the rare case of hypofibrinogenemia accompanying catastrophic acute hepatitis. Several cases of hepatic disease have been described in which hypofibrinogenemia, along with other coagulative defects, has been attributed to the consumption of clotting factors during intravascular coagulation[12, 58, 138]; in one of these, the site of thrombosis may have been the splenic vein.[138] Hypofibrinogenemia attributed to fibrinolysis is discussed in subsequent paragraphs. Suffice it to say, the pathogenesis of hypofibrinogenemia in hepatic disorders is usually not known.

In clinical situations in which hypofibrinogenemia is an isolated finding, abnormal bleeding does not occur if the concentration of fibrinogen is above about 100 mg./100 ml. plasma. Below this point, bleeding is excessive from the site of injury or surgical procedures, but spontaneous bleeding is uncommon. In liver disease, hypofibrinogenemia is invariably only one of many hemostatic defects, and can therefore be expected to be of much greater moment. If hypofibrinogenemia is thought to be contributing to a bleeding tendency, attempts should be made to correct this defect at least temporarily. Hypofibrinogenemia due to decreased synthesis or to intravascular coagulation is probably best treated by the intravenous injection of concentrated human fibrinogen. The usual initial dose is 4 Gm. of Cohn fraction I.

The effect of an injection of fibrinogen is relatively short-lived; after an initial period during which it disappears from the circulation relatively more rapidly, about 15 per cent of an injected dose disappears each day. Since the infusion of fibrinogen is often followed by homologous serum jaundice, one should be circumspect about its use. Fractions of plasma rich in antihemophilic factor, prepared by Pool's cryoprecipitation technic, can be used as a source of fibrinogen. Since fewer donors are needed than are used to supply the pools from which Cohn fraction I is prepared, the risk of hepatitis is proportionately less. Unfortunately, cryoprecipitates are still in short supply. Although heparin has been proposed in the treatment of the syndrome of intravascular coagulation in cirrhosis, evidence for its value is still insecure, and this anticoagulant is, of course, potentially dangerous.

A different anomaly of the final stages of clotting is common in hepatic disease. When oxalated or citrated plasma is mixed with thrombin, the clotting time of the mixture, that is, the thrombin time, is often prolonged.[15, 19, 27, 51, 57, 102, 121] Many different changes may contribute to this delay in the formation of thrombin. Excessively high or low concentrations of plasma fibrinogen lengthen the thrombin time.[48] Occasionally, too, the fibrinogen molecule itself is abnormal, so that it reacts more slowly than normally to the addition of thrombin.[102] In other cases, there seems to be a qualitative or quantitative deficiency of that property of plasma responsible for accelerating the conversion of fibrinogen to fibrin by thrombin.[57, 102] In support of this view, Spector noted that the transfusion of fresh frozen plasma shortened the abnormally long thrombin time of patients with cirrhosis.[121] In still other cases, circulating anticoagulants, whose nature is not always clear, may be present.[22] Perhaps, in some instances, these anticoagulants are the products of digestion of fibrinogen or fibrin by plasmin (vide infra). But treatment of patients with cirrhosis with epsilon aminocaproic acid, a potent antifibrinolytic agent, does not shorten an abnormally long thrombin time.[12]

The abnormally long thrombin time of plasma obtained from patients with hepatic disease cannot be attributed to an alteration in its antithrombic properties. Normally, plasma inactivates thrombin, but at a rate too slow to affect the thrombin time. In any event, the antithrombic properties are usually diminished, rather than increased, in cirrhosis or acute yellow atrophy.[56, 118] In hepatitis or obstructive jaundice, on the other hand, plasma antithrombic activity is ordinarily normal.[48, 118]

The degree to which prolongation of the thrombin time contributes to a bleeding tendency is uncertain. The modest prolongation usually found in cirrhosis is of the same order of magnitude as that observed in preeclampsia, unassociated with evidences of a hemorrhagic tendency. Possibly, abnormalities in fibrin formation augment defective hemostasis when other defects are present.

In normal blood clotting, the fibrin strands are bonded chemically by fibrin stabilizing factor. Individuals with a hereditary deficiency of this substance have a severe bleeding diathesis, and wounds may break down, delaying healing. In hepatic disorders, particularly severe cirrhosis or metastatic disease of the liver, the plasma behaves as if it is deficient in fibrin stabilizing factor.[86] Interestingly, in almost all these cases, full activity is restored to the plasma by the addition of cysteine, as if the fibrin stabilizing factor is in an unusual, inactive state. Perhaps the defect in fibrin stabilizing factor explains the report that the tensile strength of fibrin, measured by thromboelastography, is impaired in cirrhosis.[15]

ABNORMAL PLASMA FIBRINOLYTIC ACTIVITY

In 1914, Goodpasture[45] described an extraordinary phenomenon in patients with cirrhosis of the liver, namely, that their clotted blood reliquefied upon incubation at 37° C. He ascribed the liquefaction to the digestion of fibrin by the plasma's intrinsic proteolytic activity. Goodpasture's studies have been confirmed many times.[11, 28, 34, 61, 101, 122] When normal plasma is clotted by the addition of calcium or thrombin, the fibrin which forms may dissolve after an interval of several days. In contrast, in cirrhosis, fibrinolysis may occur within a day or 2. Rapid clot lysis is, however, unusual in acute hepatic disease or carcinoma of the liver.

The mechanisms that underlie rapid fibrinolysis in the plasma of patients with cirrhosis are not yet clarified. Human plasma's potentiality for digesting fibrin resides in one or more plasma proteases known collectively as plasmin or fibrinolysin. Plasmin is a protease with broad specificity. Besides digesting fibrin, it hydrolyzes fibrinogen; inactivates proaccelerin, antihemophilic factor, Christmas factor and prothrombin[65]; and digests gamma globulin, ACTH, glucagon and somatotropin. Plasmin also converts the first component of complement into its active form, C'1 esterase, and releases biologically active kinins from their precursor in plasma, thus contributing to the events of inflammation. Besides substrates that might be met in nature, casein, gelatin, denatured hemoglobin, beta lactoglobulin and various synthetic amino acid esters are hydrolyzed by plasmin.

Not surprisingly, in normal blood plasmin is largely or completely in the form of its inert precursor, plasminogen (profibrinolysin). Plasminogen can be activated in the test tube in many ways, for example, by incubating plasma or its euglobulin fraction with chloroform, with streptokinase (a product of certain hemolytic streptococci), with urokinase (a proteolytic enzyme in urine), or with tissue particles. Streptokinase is thought by some to activate plasminogen only after it combines with a proactivator in plasma; the bulk of evidence suggests that the proactivator is plasminogen itself.

Equally to be expected, plasma is rich in inhibitory activity directed against plasmin. Two, and probably 3 entities have been detected in human plasma which can block the action of this enzyme, and the possibility exists that there are also inhibitors against its activation from plasminogen.[64]

In the test tube, plasmin may become active "spontaneously," without the participation of extrinsic activators. Although clots formed from normal plasma may not lyse for many days, those formed from its euglobulin fraction often dissolve within 6 or 8 hours. More rapid lysis may be observed not only in cirrhosis of the liver, but also after a variety of stresses, such as exercise, anxiety, childbirth or surgical procedures. Rapid fibrinolysis, as measured in the test tube, may also follow the intravenous injection of nicotinic acid or the subcutaneous injection of epinephrine.

The rapid fibrinolysis that occurs in these various stressful situations has been attributed to the presence in plasma of one or more activators of plasmin. In some experimental situations, such an activator appears to be derived from vascular endothelium, but there is no reason to suppose that this is the only source of plasminogen activator. Nor should this activator be confused with the component of plasma with which streptokinase reacts, although the literature is often unclear about this distinction.

Rapid fibrinolysis, as I have described it, is a test tube phenomenon. It has been known since Goodpasture's time that the proteolytic agent responsible for the lysis of a clot is relatively inert in *unclotted* plasma. The fibrin of clotted plasma may dissolve at a time when the fibrinogen content of its unclotted mate is essentially unchanged, as if the development of fibrinolytic activity is accelerated by the presence of fibrin or by the clotting process itself. In different situations, one or the other of these mechanisms may operate. Thus, streptokinase induces the solution of fibrin more readily than the digestion of fibrinogen, as if plasminogen adsorbed to fibrin is separated from its inhibitors in plasma, and therefore more accessible to activation. Moreover, at least one clotting factor may serve an as yet undefined function in the evolution of fibrinolytic activity. Niewiarowski[84] and Iatridis[55] found that fibrinolytic properties evolved more slowly than normally in the euglobulin fraction of plasma deficient in Hageman factor. In unpublished experiments, Derek Ogston and I have obtained evidence that Hageman factor does not activate plasminogen directly, but rather through an effect upon an as yet unidentified agent in plasma. In any event, the frequency with which fibrinolysis accompanies diffuse intravascular coagulation emphasizes the importance of the relationship between the clotting and lytic mechanisms.

Were plasmin to become excessively active in the body, one would anticipate that clots, formed to seal wounds, might dissolve before healing was complete. In fibrinolytic states, hemostasis may be impaired through other mechanisms as well. Products of the digestion of fibrin impede coagulation by inhibiting the generation of prothrombin converting activity and by interfering with the reaction between fibrinogen and thrombin, prolonging the thrombin time.[82, 83, 134] Moreover, when digestion products of fibrinolysis are present in plasma, polymerization of fibrin is defective.[3, 9] The digestion products of fibrinolysis can be demonstrated immunologically in the plasma of individuals in whom this process has been induced by the therapeutic administration of urokinase, as well as in the serum of individuals with spontaneous fibrinolytic states.[36, 74]

The pathogenesis of the increased rate of fibrinolysis in the plasma in cirrhosis is unknown. Whatever the mechanism, it does not seem to be operative in most acute forms of liver disease. Experimentally, total hepatectomy need not be associated with increased fibrinolytic activity,[20, 31] although

this is not universally agreed to,[41, 139] and in the totally hepatectomized human being, clot lysis is greatly accelerated.[139]

In cirrhosis or hepatitis, the concentration of plasminogen, the precursor of the fibrinolytic enzyme, is not excessive and may even be below normal.[12, 93, 100, 137, 142] Nor is the concentration of the inhibitors depressed,[37, 64, 100] although this is disputed.[11, 61, 87, 93] In the test tube, plasma inhibitors of plasmin appear to be less stable in cirrhotics than in normal individuals, their potency decreasing sharply at the same time that fibrinolysis occurs.[142] The nature of this instability is unknown, nor, indeed, whether it merely reflects an artifact of measurement.

Experiments of Fletcher and his associates[38] further illuminate this problem. In essence, they confirm Weiner's[141] observation that enhanced fibrinolysis, induced by the intravenous injection of nicotinic acid, is exaggerated in cirrhosis. They attribute this response to reduced clearance of a plasminogen activator by the diseased liver. In agreement with this interpretation, injection of nicotinic acid induces significant decreases in plasma plasminogen and fibrinogen, and a rise in the thrombin time in patients with cirrhosis but not in normal subjects. Perhaps this explains the fibrinolytic state noted in human subjects after total hepatectomy.[139] Further, Beaumont demonstrated that extracts of normal liver prevent fibrinolysis[11]; he reported no studies with abnormal hepatic tissue, but Astrup and his colleagues found that the cirrhotic liver itself is rich in an activator of plasminogen.[7] Were this agent to enter the blood stream, it might contribute to plasma fibrinolytic activity.

Determination of the "clot lysis time" in cirrhosis has interest as a laboratory oddity. It is doubtful whether the observation of fibrinolytic phenomena serves either as a diagnostic aid or as an explanation for the hemorrhagic tendency of most patients with cirrhosis of the liver. A short clot lysis time, of the degree found in cirrhosis, is found after many stresses, unaccompanied by a bleeding tendency. Were the fibrinolysis to occur *in vivo* in cirrhosis, the impairment of coagulation by the products of digestion might aggravate a pre-existing bleeding tendency. Such products have been demonstrated in the plasma or serum of cirrhotics,[36, 74, 85, 131] although this is disputed.[64]

The question must be raised whether bleeding from esophageal varices is exaggerated by lysis of clots which form within the ruptured vessels. Data concerning this possibility are not available, yet were fibrinolysis of importance in this situation, therapy with epsilon aminocaproic acid, which inhibits the activation and action of plasmin,[1, 114] might seem in order. But Lewis and Doyle noted no improvement in hemostatic function in patients treated with 10 Gm. of this drug daily, and one of their patients died of gastrointestinal hemorrhage after a day of therapy.[64]

Fibrinolytic purpura, that is, a bleeding state induced by excessive fibrinolysis, has been described in a few patients with hepatic disease[11, 130, 136] but it is rare and, when it occurs, may be secondary to intravascular coagulation.[11] If fibrinolysis is thought to be the primary process, epsilon aminocaproic acid may be beneficial, but if secondary to intravascular coagulation, attempts to inhibit fibrinolysis are probably contraindicated.

Grossi, Rousselot and Panke[46] were impressed with the frequency with which portasystemic shunts led to increased fibrinolytic activity in patients with cirrhosis. Excessive fibrinolysis was usually detectable more readily in portal than systemic venous blood. These investigators believed that the intravenous injection of 4 Gm. of epsilon aminocaproic acid reduced capillary bleeding during surgery, and also helped to control systemic hemorrhage in the weeks after surgery.[47]

OTHER COAGULATIVE PROBLEMS IN HEPATIC DISEASE

Naeye[81] and Rapaport[98] observed a decrease in the concentration of plasma thromboplastin antecedent (PTA) in the plasma of patients with cirrhosis of the liver. In congenital PTA deficiency the bleeding tendency varies considerably from patient to patient; to what extent a deficiency of this factor contributes to the hemostatic defect in hepatic disease is not known. The only known therapy for PTA deficiency is the transfusion of blood or plasma, but there is no evidence that this is needed in hepatic disease.

Originally patients with cirrhosis were thought to be deficient in Hageman factor,[59, 103] but this has not been confirmed.[105] The methods originally used to detect Hageman factor were not sufficiently specific.

Chloroform intoxication is said to depress the concentration of antihemophilic factor (AHF) in dogs.[91] AHF is usually present in normal or even elevated concentrations in the plasma in hepatitis, cirrhosis or metastatic hepatic disease.[35, 99, 126, 144] A slight depression in the concentration of AHF was noted in 2 of 20 patients with cirrhosis studied by Hallén and Nilsson,[48] but the degree of the defect was not clinically significant. The sites of synthesis of PTA, Hageman factor and AHF are unknown, but Gardikas[42] found that the concentration of AHF in hepatic venous blood is twice that in peripheral blood. Claims that the spleen is a principal site of AHF synthesis have not been substantiated.

PLATELET ABNORMALITIES

Portal hypertension is a common result of cirrhosis of the liver, and may sometimes accompany other forms of hepatic disease as well. Patients in whom the portal pressure is elevated may bleed as the result of rupture of distended collateral veins, particularly esophageal varices. In these individuals, the immediate cause of bleeding is the mechanical break in the vascular wall. The extent to which defects in hemostatic mechanisms contribute to the bleeding tendency has not been clarified, but presumably varies from patient to patient. Portal hypertension itself, however, may result in thrombocytopenia, an association emphasized by Rosenthal in 1928.[109]

A significantly low platelet count is a commonplace in cirrhosis. In one series, for example, in 43 of 119 patients with alcoholic cirrhosis the platelet counts were below 100,000/cu.mm.[63] In these patients, thrombocytopenia is probably directly related to the congestive splenomegaly secondary to portal hypertension.[132] But gastrointestinal hemorrhage is probably much more the result of increased portal pressure than of the coincident thrombocytopenia. In none of the cirrhotic patients studied by Desforges, Bigelow and Chalmers did thrombocytopenia appear to be responsible for the continuation of massive gastrointestinal bleeding.[29]

The pathogenesis of thrombocytopenia in portal hypertension has been disputed. Megakaryocytes are in the marrow in normal or increased numbers.[68] One hypothesis proposed is that the diseased spleen removes platelets from the circulation at an excessive rate or so alters them that they are removed from the circulation prematurely. This view is in accord with data suggesting that the life span of platelets in congestive splenomegaly is shortened.[21, 32] Aster, on the other hand, attributes thrombocytopenia in splenomegaly secondary to cirrhosis to sequestration of platelets within the spleen,[6] an opinion supported by Davey.[24] Cohen, Gardner and Barnett believe that platelet production may also be diminished.[21] Agglutinins directed against platelets have been described in patients with cirrhosis, whether or not thrombocytopenia is present.[50, 135] No evidence exists that these agglutinins are antibodies directed against platelets. Perhaps they react with plasma proteins adsorbed to the platelets. There is no evidence that the agglutinins contribute to the development of thrombocytopenia.

The thrombocytopenia of portal hypertension is seldom severe enough to be the sole cause of a generalized bleeding tendency. When, however, the platelet count is less than 100,000/cu.mm., the question of whether splenectomy should be performed is sure to arise.[132] Unquestionably, splenectomy is often followed by a rise in the platelet count and amelioration of hemorrhagic phenomena. A proper concern, however, is whether such a procedure should not be combined with splenorenal anastomosis, in an attempt to relieve the underlying portal hypertension. Interestingly, portacaval anastomosis without splenectomy is sometimes followed by a rise in the platelet count.[127]

A rare complication of splenectomy in portal hypertension is worth noting because of its perplexing nature. I have observed the development of thrombocythemia following splenectomy, once in a patient with cirrhosis and once in a patient with extrahepatic portal hypertension. The pathogenesis of the thrombocythemia is unknown, and even more puzzling is the fact that serious bleeding phenomena, notably epistaxes, may occur. The proper course of treatment in the thrombocythemia observed in this situation is not clear; in other situations, marrow depressants have been given.

Other causes of thrombocytopenia in cirrhosis of the liver must be considered. Treatment of severe bleeding from esophageal varices may entail the transfusion of many liters of blood over a short period of time. Under these circumstances, a generalized bleeding tendency may supervene. Although the pathogenesis of this complication is complex, a major element is the appearance of thrombocytopenia.[60] Presumably, in such cases, platelets lost through bleeding are not restored by the transfused blood which, under ordinary conditions of storage, is depleted of viable platelets. Antihemophilic factor and proaccelerin are also deficient in stored blood, compounding the difficulty. The only known prophylaxis for the hemorrhagic state that arises from massive transfusion is the use of blood drawn with minimal trauma and transfused as soon as possible.[32, 35] Unfortunately, the volume needed too often necessitates the use of stored blood.

In some patients with Laennec's cirrhosis, thrombocytopenia may be due to a concomitant deficiency of folic acid rather than portal hypertension.[53] In such individuals, the thrombocytopenia may respond to folic acid therapy. A dosage as small as 0.2 mg./day, administered orally or intramuscularly, is probably adequate to correct the deficiency. Whether the deficiency of folic acid is due to an inadequate dietary supply of this substance or to a defect in its metabolism is not certain.

Thrombocytopenia is occasionally seen in acute infectious hepatitis,[5, 143] in which its pathogenesis is obscure. In one case, congestive splenomegaly appeared to be a factor,[79] whereas in another, thrombocytopenia was part of a pancytopenia.[26] No therapy is available for correcting the thrombocytopenia of infectious hepatitis; the efficacy of steroids is not known.

The suggestion has been made that platelets are qualitatively defective in hepatic disease.[15, 23, 27, 70, 102] Thomas and his colleagues[131] found that in patients with Laennec's cirrhosis the aggregation of platelets, normally induced *in vitro* by the addition of ADP or thrombin, was delayed in those patients in whom the thrombin time was prolonged. These investigators attributed the delay to the presence in plasma of abnormal fibrinogen breakdown products, secondary to excessive fibrinolysis. Although this may well be true, it must be recalled that the long thrombin time in cirrhosis has many possible causes.

• • • • •

This chapter has stressed the complex origin of the hemorrhagic tendency seen in some patients with hepatic disease. Not all the defects described are susceptible to treatment, but effective therapy, to the extent that it is available, is based upon a rational analysis of the pathogenesis of bleeding in each individual patient.

REFERENCES

1. Ablondi, F. B., Hagan, J. J., Philips, M., and De Renzo, E. C.: Inhibition of plasmin, trypsin and the streptokinase-activated fibrinolytic system by 6-amino-caproic acid, Arch. Biochem. Biophys. 82:153, 1959.
2. Alagille, D., and Soulier, J. P.: Action des enzymes protéolytiques sur le sang total "in vitro"; modifications des facteurs de coagulation et du complément, Sem. hôp. Paris 32:355, 1956.
3. Alkjaersig, N., Fletcher, A. P., and Sherry, S.: Pathogenesis of the coagulation defect developing during pathological plasma proteolytic ("fibrinolytic") states. II. The significance, mechanism and consequences of defective fibrin polymerization, J. Clin. Invest. 41:917, 1962.
4. Allison, A. C.: Danger of vitamin K to newborn, Lancet 1:669, 1955.
5. Alt, H. L., and Swank, R. L.: Thrombocytopenic purpura associated with catarrhal jaundice: report of a case, Ann. Int. Med. 10:1049, 1937.
6. Aster, R. H.: Pooling of platelets in the spleen: role in the pathogenesis of "hypersplenic" thrombocytopenia, J. Clin. Invest. 45:645, 1966.
7. Astrup, T., Rasmussen, J., Amery, A., and Poulsen, H. E.: Fibrinolytic activity of cirrhotic liver, Nature 185:619, 1960.
8. Bancroft, F. W., Stanley-Brown, M., and Quick, A. J.: Postoperative thrombosis and embolism, Am. J. Surg. 28:648, 1935.
9. Bang, N. U.: Ultrastructure of the fibrin clot, *in* Seegers, W. H. (ed.): Blood Clotting Enzymology, New York, Academic Press, 1967.
10. Barnhart, M. I.: Cellular site for prothrombin synthesis, Am. J. Physiol. 199:360, 1960.
11. Beaumont, J. L., Beaumont, V., and Domart, A.: Research on the spontaneous fibrinolytic activity of the plasma in liver cirrhosis, Rev. franç. Étud. clin. biol. 1:667, 1956.
12. Bergström, K., Blombäck, B., and Kleen, G.: Studies on the plasma fibrinolytic activity in a case of liver cirrhosis, Acta med. scand. 168:291, 1960.
13. Bidwell, E., Booth, J. M., Dike, G. W. R., and Denson, K. W. E.: The preparation for therapeutic use of a concentrate of Factor IX containing also Factors II, VII and X, Brit. J. Haemat. 13:568, 1967.
14. Biggs, R., and Macfarlane, R. G.: Human Blood Coagulation and its Disorders, ed. 3, Oxford, Blackwell; Philadelphia, Davis, 1962.
15. Breddin, K.: Hämorrhagische Diathesen bei Lebererkrankungen unter besonderer Berücksichtigung der Thrombocytenfunktion, Acta haemat. 27:1, 1962.
16. Budd, G.: On Diseases of the Liver, Philadelphia, Lea & Blanchard, 1846.
17. Butt, H. R., Snell, A. M., and Osterberg, A. E.: The use of vitamin K and bile in treatment of the hemorrhagic diathesis in cases of jaundice, Proc. Staff Mayo Clin. 13:74, 1938.
18. Cartwright, G. E.: Diagnostic Laboratory Hematology, ed. 3, New York, Grune & Stratton, 1963.
19. Chalmers, T. C., Bigelow, F. S., and Desforges, J. F.: The effects of massive gastrointestinal hemorrhage on hemostasis. II. Coagulation factors, J. Lab. Clin. Med. 43:511, 1954.
20. Clay, R. C., and Ratnoff, O. D.: Modified one-stage hepatectomy in the dog, with some notes on the effect of hepatectomy

on the coagulability and proteolytic activity of the blood, Bull. Johns Hopkins Hosp. *88*:457, 1951.

21. Cohen, P., Gardner, F. H., and Barnett, G. O.: Reclassification of the thrombocytopenias by the Cr^{51}-labeling method for measuring platelet life span, New Engl. J. Med. *264*:1294, 1961.

22. Conley, C. L., Hartmann, R. C., and Morse, W. I., II: Circulating anticoagulants: technique for their detection and clinical studies, Bull. Johns Hopkins Hosp. *84*:255, 1949.

23. Cortet, P., Klepping, C., Devant, J., Lebel, J.-P., and Jacquot, B.: Le facteur plaquettaire au cours des cirrhoses alcooliques. Etude de l'adhésivité *in vivo* par le test de Borchgrevink, Arch. Mal. Appar. dig. *53*:1041, 1964.

24. Davey, M. G.: The Survival and Destruction of Human Platelets, Basle, S. Karger, 1966.

25. Davie, E. W., and Ratnoff, O. D.: Waterfall sequence for intrinsic blood clotting, Science *145*:1310, 1964.

26. Deller, J. J., Jr., Cirksena, W. J., and Marcarelli, J.: Fatal pancytopenia associated with viral hepatitis, New Engl. J. Med. *266*:297, 1962.

27. De Nicola, P.: Liver and blood coagulation. Changes in blood coagulation factors in experimental liver injuries and hepatopathies, Acta hepato-splenol. (Stuttg.) *7*:86, 1960.

28. De Nicola, P., and Soardi, F.: Fibrinolysis in liver diseases: study of 109 cases by means of the fibrin plate method, Thrombos. Diathes. Haemorrh. *2*:290, 1958.

29. Desforges, J. F., Bigelow, F. S., and Chalmers, T. C.: The effects of massive gastrointestinal hemorrhage on hemostasis. I. The blood platelets, J. Lab. Clin. Med. *43*:501, 1954.

30. Donaldson, V. H.: Effect of plasmin *in vitro* on clotting factors in plasma, J. Lab. Clin. Med. *56*:644, 1960.

31. Drapanas, T., Shim, W. K. T., and Stewart, J. D.: Studies of fibrinolytic activity after hepatectomy, Arch. Surg. *87*:64, 1963.

32. Ebeling, W. C., Bunker, J. P., Ellis, D. S., French, A. B., Linton, R. R., and Jones, C. M.: Management of patients with portal hypertension undergoing venous-shunt surgery, New Engl. J. Med. *254*·141, 1956.

33. Eisenmenger, W. J., Slater, R. J., and Bongiovanni, A. M.: Hypercoagulability of the blood of patients with hepatic cirrhosis following administration of ACTH, Am. J. Med. *13*:27, 1952.

34. Fearnley, G. R.: Fibrinolysis, London, E. Arnold & Co., Ltd., 1965.

35. Finkbiner, R. B., McGovern, J. J., Goldstein, R, and Bunker, J. P.: Coagulation defects in liver disease and response to transfusion during surgery, Am. J. Med. *26*:199, 1959.

36. Fisher, S., Fletcher, A. P., Alkjaersig, N., and Sherry, S.: Immunoelectrophoretic characterization of plasma fibrinogen derivatives in patients with pathological plasma proteolysis, J. Lab. Clin. Med. *70*:903, 1967.

37. Fletcher, A. P., Alkjaersig, N., and Sherry, S.: Pathogenesis of the coagulation defect developing during pathological plasma proteolytic ("fibrinolytic") states. I. The significance of fibrinogen proteolysis and circulating fibrinogen breakdown products, J. Clin. Invest. *41*:896, 1962.

38. Fletcher, A. P., Biederman, O., Moore, D., Alkjaersig, N., and Sherry, S.: Abnormal plasminogen-plasmin system activity (fibrinolysis) in patients with hepatic cirrhosis: its cause and consequences, J. Clin. Invest. *43*:681, 1964.

39. Forman, W. B., and Barnhart, M. I.: Cellular site for fibrinogen synthesis, J.A.M.A. *187*:128, 1964.

40. Frerichs, F. T.: A Clinical Treatise on Diseases of the Liver, translated by Murchison, C., Baltimore, Wood, 1860.

41. Gans, H.: Study of fibrinogen turnover rates after total hepatectomy in dogs, Surgery *55*:544, 1964.

42. Gardikas, C., Bakaloudis, P., Hatzioannou, J., and Kokkinos, D.: The Factor-VIII concentration of the hepatic venous blood, Brit. J. Haemat. *11*:380, 1965.

43. Geill, T.: Die differentialdiagnostische Bedeutung des Fibringehaltes im Blut bei Leber und Gallenwegsleiden, Acta med. scand. Suppl. *78*:243, 1936.

44. Goldsworthy, P. D., Peppers, J., and Volwiler, W.: Pacific Slope Bioch. Conf., Abstr., p. 6, 1963.

45. Goodpasture, E. W.: Fibrinolysis in chronic hepatic insufficiency, Bull. Johns Hopkins Hosp. *25*:330, 1914.

46. Grossi, C. E., Rousselot, L. M., and Panke, W. F.: Coagulation defects in

patients with cirrhosis of the liver under-going portasystemic shunts, Am. J. Surg. *104*:512, 1962.

47. ———: Hemorrhagic diatheses during and after portacaval shunts in patients with cirrhosis of the liver; their recognition and management, Am. J. Gastroent. *41*:117, 1964.

48. Hallén, A., and Nilsson, I. M.: Coagulation studies in liver disease, Thrombos. Diathes. Haemorrh. (Stuttg.) *11*:51, 1964.

49. Ham, T. H., and Curtis, F. C.: Plasma fibrinogen response in man. Influence of the nutritional state, induced hyperpyrexia, infectious disease and liver damage, Medicine *17*:413, 1938.

50. Harrington, W. J., and Arimura, G.: Immune reactions of platelets *in* Johnson, S. A., et al. (eds.): Blood Platelets, Boston, Little, 1961, pp. 659-670.

51. Harrington, W. J., Manheimer, R. H., Desforges, J. F., Minkel, H. P., Crow, C. B., and Stohlman, F.: Bleeding tendency in hepatocellular and obstructive jaundice, Bull. New Engl. Med. Cent. *12*:121, 1950.

52. Hemker, H. C., Veltkamp, J. J., Hensen, A., and Loeliger, E. A.: Nature of prothrombin biosynthesis: preprothrombinaemia in vitamin-κ-deficiency, Nature *200*:589, 1963.

53. Herbert, V.: Hematopoietic factors in liver diseases, *in* Popper, H., and Schaffner, F. (eds.): Progress in Liver Disease, New York, Grune & Stratton, 1965, p. 257.

54. Hjort, P. F., and Hasselback, R.: A critical review of the evidence for a continuous hemostasis in vivo, Thrombos. Diathes. Haemorrh. (Stuttg.) *6*:580, 1961.

55. Iatridis, S. G., and Ferguson, J. H.: Effect of surface and Hageman factor on the endogenous or spontaneous activation of the fibrinolytic system, Thrombos. Diathes. Haemorrh. (Stuttg.) *6*:411, 1961.

56. Innerfield, I., Angrist, A., and Boyd, L. J.: Plasma antithrombin titer in incipient and advanced liver failure, Gastroenterology *20*:417, 1952.

57. Jim, R. T. S.: A study of the plasma thrombin time, J. Lab. Clin. Med. *50*:45, 1957.

58. Johannson, S.-A.: Studies on blood co-agulation factors in a case of liver cirrhosis; remission of the hemorrhagic tendency on treatment with heparin, Acta med. scand. *175*:177, 1964.

59. Jürgens, J.: Significance of the Hageman factor for the effect of wettable surface on thrombocytes, Thrombos. Diathes. Haemorrh. (Stuttg.) 7:48, 1962.

60. Krevans, J. R., and Jackson, D. P.: Hemorrhagic disorder following massive whole blood transfusions, J.A.M.A. *159*: 171, 1955.

61. Kwaan, H. C., McFadzean, A. J. S., and Cook, J.: Plasma fibrinolytic activity in cirrhosis of the liver, Lancet *1*:132, 1956.

62. LeQuesne, L. P.: Choledocholithiasis *in* Smith, R., and Sherlock, S. (eds.): Surgery of the Gall Bladder and Bile Ducts, Washington, London, Butterworth, 1964.

63. Levrat M., and Truchot, R.: Le role de la thrombopénie dans les hémorragies des cirrhoses du foie, Arch. Mal Appar. dig. *51*:1394, 1962.

64. Lewis, J. H., and Doyle, A. P.: Effects of epsilon aminocaproic acid on coagulation and fibrinolytic mechanisms, J.A.M.A. *188*:56, 1964.

65. Lewis, J. H., Howe, A. C., and Ferguson, J. H.: Thrombin formation. II. Effects of lysin (fibrinolysin, plasmin) on prothrombin, Ac-globulin and tissue thromboplastin, J. Clin. Invest. *28*:1507, 1949.

66. Lian, C., Sassier, Facquet, J., and Frumusan, P.: Valeur séméiologique du dosage pondéral de la fibrinémie dans les affections hépatiques, Bull. Soc. Méd. Paris *52*:603, 1936.

67. Lord, J. W., Jr., and Andrus, W. deW.: Differentiation of intrahepatic and extrahepatic jaundice. Response of the plasma prothrombin to intramuscular injection of menadione (2-methyl-1,4-naphthoquinone) as a diagnostic aid, Arch. Int. Med. *68*:199, 1941.

68. Lozner, E. L.: Differential diagnosis, pathogenesis and treatment of thrombocytopenic purpuras, Am. J. Med. *14*:459, 1953.

69. Macfarlane, R. G.: An enzyme cascade in the blood clotting mechanism, and its function as a biochemical amplifier, Nature *202*:498, 1964.

70. Mandel, E. E., and Lazerson, J.: Thrombasthenia in liver disease, New Engl. J. Med. *265*:56, 1961.

71. Mann, F. D., Shonyo, E. S., and Mann,

F. C.: Effect of removal of the liver on blood coagulation, Am. J. Physiol. *164*: 111, 1951.

72. Mann, J. D.: Plasma prothrombin in viral hepatitis and hepatic cirrhosis; evaluation of the two-stage method in 75 cases, Gastroenterology *21*:263, 1952.

73. Martius, C.: Chemistry and function of vitamin K, *in* Seegers, W. H. (ed.): Blood Clotting Enzymology, New York, Academic Press, 1967.

74. Merskey, C., Kleiner, G. J., and Johnson, A. J.: Quantitative estimation of split products of fibrinogen in human serum, relation to diagnosis and treatment, Blood *28*:1, 1966.

75. Miale, J. B.: Laboratory Medicine Hematology, St. Louis, Mosby, 1967.

76. Miller, L. L., and Bale, W. F.: Synthesis of all plasma protein fractions except gamma globulins by the liver. The use of zone electrophoresis and lysine-ϵ-C^{14} to define the plasma proteins synthesized by the isolated perfused liver, J. Exp. Med. *99*:125, 1954.

77. Miller, L. L., Bly, C. G., Watson, M. L., and Bale, W. F.: The dominant role of the liver in plasma protein synthesis. A direct study of the isolated perfused rat liver with the aid of lysine-ϵ-C^{14}, J. Exp. Med. *94*:431, 1951.

78. Mindrum, G., and Glueck, H. I.: Plasma prothrombin in liver disease: its clinical and prognostic significance, Ann. Int. Med. *50*:1370, 1959.

79. Monteil, R., Vigne, J., Bourdet, P., Raby, C., and Cantegrit, M.: Purpura thrombocytopénique au cours d'une hepatité virale, Hémostase *1*:267, 1961.

80. Munro, F. L., Hart, E. R., Munro, M. P., and Walkling, A. A.: Changes in components A and B of prothrombin in dog following hepatectomy, Am. J. Physiol. *145*: 206, 1945.

81. Naeye, R. L.: Hemophilioid factors: acquired deficiencies in several hemorrhagic states, Proc. Soc. Exp. Biol. Med. *94*:623, 1957.

82. Niewiarowski, S., and Kowalski, E.: Un nouvel anticoagulant dérivé du fibrinogène, Rev. d'hémat. *13*:320, 1958.

83. Niewiarowski, S., Latallo, Z., and Stachurska, J.: Apparition d'un inhibiteur de la thromboplastinoformation au cours de la protéolyse du fibrinogène, Rev. Hémat. *14*:118, 1959.

84. Niewiarowski, S., and Prou-Wartelle, O.: Rôle du Facteur Contact (Facteur Hageman) dans la fibrinolyse, Thrombos. Diathes. Haemorrh. (Stuttg.) *3*:593, 1961.

85. Niléhn, J.-E., and Nilsson, I. M.: Demonstration of fibrinolytic split products in human serum by an immunologic method in spontaneous and induced fibrinolytic states, Scand. J. Haemat. *1*:313, 1964.

86. Nussbaum, M., and Morse, B. S.: Plasma fibrin stabilizing factor activity in various diseases, Blood *23*:669, 1964.

87. O'Connell, R. A., Grossi, C. E., and Rousselot, L. M.: Role of inhibitors of fibrinolysis in hepatic cirrhosis, Lancet *2*: 990, 1964.

88. Olson, J. P., Miller, L. L., and Troup, S. B.: Synthesis of clotting factors by the isolated perfused rat liver, J. Clin. Invest. *45*:690, 1966.

89. Osler, W.: Principles and Practice of Medicine, ed. 2, New York, Appleton. 1896.

90. Owren, P. A.: Diagnostic and prognostic significance of plasma prothrombin and Factor V levels in parenchymatous hepatitic and obstructive jaundice, Scand. J. Clin. Lab. Invest. *1*:131, 1949.

91. Penick, G. D., Roberts, H. R., Webster, W. P., and Brinkhous, K. M.: Hemorrhagic states secondary to intravascular clotting; an experimental study of their evolution and prevention, A.M.A. Arch. Path. *66*:708, 1958.

92. Pool, J. G., and Robinson, J.: In vitro synthesis of coagulation factors by rat liver slices, Am. J. Physiol. *196*:423, 1959.

93. Purcell, G., Jr., and Phillips, L. L.: Fibrinolytic activity in cirrhosis of the liver, Surg. Gynec. Obstet. *117*:139, 1963.

94. Quick, A. J.: The coagulation defect in sweet clover disease and in the hemorrhagic chick disease of dietary origins; a consideration of the source of prothrombin, Am. J. Physiol. *118*:260, 1937.

95. ———: The Hemorrhagic Diseases and the Physiology of Hemostasis, Springfield, Thomas, 1942.

96. ———: Hemorrhagic Diseases and Thrombosis, ed. 2. Philadelphia, Lea & Febiger, 1966.

97. Quick, A. J., Stanley-Brown, M., and Bancroft, F. W.: Study of the coagulation defect in hemophilia and in jaundice, Am. J. Med. Sci. *190*:501, 1935.

98. Rapaport, S. I.: Plasma thromboplastin antecedent levels in patients receiving coumarin anticoagulants and in patients

with Laennec's cirrhosis, Proc. Soc. Exp. Biol. Med. *108*:115, 1961.

99. Rapaport, S. I., Ames, S. B., Mikkelsen, S., and Goodman, J. R.: Plasma clotting factors in chronic hepatocellular disease, New Engl. J. Med. *263*:278, 1960.

100. Ratnoff, O. D.: Studies on proteolytic enzyme in human plasma. III. Some factors controlling rate of fibrinolysis, J. Exp. Med. *88*:401, 1948.

101. ———: Studies on proteolytic enzyme in human plasma; rate of lysis of plasma clots in normal and diseased individuals, with particular reference to hepatic disease, Bull. Johns Hopkins Hosp. *84*:29, 1949.

102. ———: An accelerating property of plasma for the coagulation of fibrinogen by thrombin, J. Clin. Invest. *33*:1175, 1954.

103. Ratnoff, O. D., and Donaldson, V. H.: The liver; three aspects of hepatic failure: cholemia, ascites, and hemorrhagic phenomena, *in* Mellors, R. C. (ed.): Analytic Pathology, New York, McGraw-Hill, 1957.

104. ———: Physiologic and pathologic effects of increased fibrinolytic activity in man, Am. J. Cardiol. *6*:378, 1960.

105. ———: The biology and pathology of the initial stages of blood coagulation, Progr. Hemat. *5*:204, 1966.

106. Ratnoff, O. D., and Patek, A. J., Jr.: The natural history of Laennec's cirrhosis of the liver; an analysis of 386 cases, Medicine *21*:207, 1942.

107. ———: Postnecrotic cirrhosis of the liver, J. Chron. Dis. *1*:266, 1955.

108. Reisner, E. H., Jr., Norman, J., Field, W. W., and Brown, R.: The effect of liver dysfunction on the response to Dicumarol, Am. J. Med. Sci. *217*:445, 1949.

109. Rosenthal, N.: The blood picture in purpura, J. Lab. Clin. Med. *13*:303, 1927-28.

110. Scanlon, G. H., Brinkhous, K. M., Warner, E. D., Smith, H. P., and Flynn, J. E.: Plasma prothrombin and the bleeding tendency; with special reference to jaundiced patients and vitamin K therapy, J.A.M.A. *112*:1898, 1939.

111. Seegers, W. H.: Prothrombin in Enzymology, Thrombosis and Hemophilia, Springfield, Thomas, 1967.

112. Sherlock, S., and Alpert, L.: Bleeding in surgery in relation to liver disease, Proc. Royal Soc. Med. *58*:257, 1965.

113. Sherlock, S. P. V., Barber, K. M., Bell, J. L., and Watt, P. J.: Anticoagulants

and the liver, *in* Pickering, G. W. (ed.): Proc. Symp. on Anticoagulants, London, Harvey, 1960.

114. Sherry, S., Fletcher, A. P., and Alkjaersig, N., and Sawyer, W. D.: ε-Aminocaproic acid, "a potent anti-fibrinolytic agent," Tr. Ass. Am. Phycns 72:62, 1959.

115. Sims, J. M.: Remarks on cholecystotomy in dropsy of the gall-bladder, Brit. Med. J. *1*:811, 1878.

116. Smith, H. P., Warner, E. D., Brinkhous, K. M., and Seegers, W. H.: Bleeding tendency and prothrombin deficiency in biliary fistula dogs: effect of feeding bile and vitamin K, J. Exp. Med. *67*:911, 1938.

117. Snavely, J. R.: Fatal hepatitis, Am. J. Med. Sci. *219*:89, 1950.

118. Sokal, G., Schmid, F., and Hörder, M. H.: Die Antithrombinaktivitäten des Plasmas bei Lebererkrankungen und Verschlussikterus, Klin. Wschr. *33*:934, 1955.

119. Soulier, J. P.: Nouvelles fractions coagulantes à usage thérapeutique, *in* Proc. 8th Congr. Europ. Soc. Haemat., #388, 1961.

120. Spector, I., and Corn, M.: Laboratory tests of hemostasis; the relation to hemorrhage in liver disease, Arch. Int. Med. *119*:577, 1967.

121. Spector, I., Corn, M., and Ticktin, H. E.: Effect of plasma transfusions on the prothrombin time and clotting factors in liver disease, New Engl. J. Med. *275*: 1032, 1966.

122. Stefanini, M.: Hemorrhagic diathesis of liver dysfunction and obstructive jaundice, Proc. 3rd Internat. Congr., Internat. Soc. Haemat., 1951, p. 484.

123. Stefanini, M., and Dameshek, W.: The Hemorrhagic Disorders: A Clinical and Therapeutic Approach, ed. 2, New York, Grune & Stratton, 1962.

124. Steigmann, F., Schrifter, H., Yiotsas, Z. D., and Pamukcu, F.: Vitamin K therapy in liver disease: need for a reevaluation, Am. J. Gastroent. *31*:369, 1959.

125. Straub, P. W.: A study of fibrinogen production by human liver slices *in vitro* by an immunoprecipitin method, J. Clin. Invest. *42*:130, 1963.

126. Straub, P. W., Riedler, G., and Meile, E. O.: Erhöhung des antihämophilen γ-globulins (Factor VIII) bei letaler Lebernekrose, Schweiz. med. Wschr. *96*: 1199, 1966.

127. Sullivan B. H., Jr., and Tumen, H. J.: Effect of portacaval shunt on thrombocytopenia associated with portal hypertension, Ann. Int. Med. 55:598, 1961.

128. Suttie, J. W.: Control of prothrombin and Factor VII biosynthesis by vitamin K, Arch. Biochem. Biophys. 118:166, 1967.

129. Sykes, E. M., Jr., Seegers, W. H., and Ware, A. G.: Effect of acute liver damage on ac-globulin activity of plasma, Proc. Soc. Exp. Biol. Med. 67:506, 1948.

130. Tagnon, H. J., Levenson, S. M., Davidson, C. S., and Taylor, F. H. L.: Occurrence of fibrinolysis in shock, with observations on prothrombin time and plasma fibrinogen during hemorrhagic shock, Am. J. Med. Sci. 211:88, 1946.

131. Thomas, D. P., Ream, V. J., and Stuart, R. K.: Platelet aggregation in patients with Laennec's cirrhosis of the liver, New Engl. J. Med. 276:1344, 1967.

132. Tocantins, L. M.: The hemorrhagic tendency in congestive splenomegaly (Banti's syndrome); its mechanism and management, J.A.M.A. 136:616, 1948.

133. Tocantins, L. M., and Kazal, L. A.: Blood Coagulation, Hemorrhage and Thrombosis; Methods of Study, New York, Grune & Stratton, 1964.

134. Triantaphyllopoulos, D. C.: Anticoagulant effect of incubated fibrinogen, Canad. J. Biochem. Physiol. 36:249, 1958.

135. Tullis, J. L.: Identification and significance of platelet antibodies, New Engl. J. Med. 255:541, 1956.

136. Vachon, A., Favre-Gilly, J., and Potton, F.: Fibrinolyse hémorragique mortelle au cours d'une cirrhose avec ictère, Lyon méd. 187:165, 1952.

137. Van de Loo, J., and Schmiesing, G.: Faktoren des fibrinolytischen Systems bei Leberkrankheiten, Thrombos. Diathes. Haemorrh. (Stuttg.) 14:580, 1965.

138. Verstraete, M., Vermylen, C., Vermylen, J., and Vandenbroucke, J.:Excessive consumption of blood coagulation components as cause of hemorrhagic diathesis, Am. J. Med. 38:899, 1965.

139. von Kaulla, K. N., Kaye, H., von Kaulla, E., Marchioro, T. L., and Starzl, T. E.: Changes in blood coagulation before and after hepatectomy or transplantation in dogs and man, Arch. Surg. 92:71, 1966.

140. Wangensteen, O. H.: Hemorrhagic diathesis of obstructive jaundice and its treatment, Ann. Surg. 88:845, 1928.

141. Weiner, M.: The fibrinolytic response to nicotinic acid in abnormal liver states, Am. J. Med. Sci. 246:294, 1963.

142. Witte, S., and Dirnberger, P.: Über die Verlängerung der Profibrinolysinzeit bei Leberkrankheiten, Klin. Wschr. 33:931, 1955.

143. Woodward, T. E.: Thrombocytopenic purpura complicating acute catarrhal jaundice: report of a case, review of the literature and review of 48 cases of purpura at University Hospital, Ann. Int. Med. 18:799, 1943.

144. Zetterqvist, E., and von Francken, I. Koagulationsfaktoren vid levers-jukdom, Nord. Med. 69:81, 1963.

145. Zimmerman, H. J., Lowry, C. F., Uyeyama, K., and Reiser, R.: Infectious hepatitis: clinical and laboratory features of 295 cases, Am. J. Med. Sci. 213:395, 1947.

6

Laboratory Tests

BURTON COMBES, M.D., AND *STEVEN SCHENKER*, M.D.

Laboratory tests play an important role in the clinical assessment of hepatic dysfunction. First, they are of value in detecting abnormalities in the liver. This is particularly important in the nonjaundiced patient. For example, abnormal tests may be the only indication of liver involvement in anicteric patients with viral hepatitis, drug toxicity, infiltrative lesions of the liver such as tumor and granuloma, and some phases of cirrhosis, to name but a few. Second, once an abnormality is demonstrated, the pattern of abnormal test results may confirm or suggest the nature of the underlying liver disorder—in both jaundiced and nonjaundiced patients. Third, some tests provide an index of the extent of hepatic disease and thus offer some prognostic information. Finally, the evaluation of test results serves as a valuable means of following the course of hepatic dysfunction and its management.

Many tests have been proposed for assessment of liver disease. No single laboratory procedure fulfills the objectives outlined above. The combination of a number of tests, some that appraise hepatic function, others that reflect liver cell damage and necrosis, still others that detect infiltrative processes in liver or reflect intra- or extrahepatic obstruction have been used effectively, however. The present discussion is oriented to an analysis of tests that we feel are of most value in the clinical appraisal of liver diseases, and therefore is not encyclopedic in scope. An effort is made to indicate for each test its (a) sensitivity in detecting liver abnormalities, (b) specificity for liver dysfunction, (c) selectivity in differentiating

hepatocellular diseases one from another and from obstructive liver disorders, and (d) role in indicating the severity of liver damage.

TESTS BASED ON BILE PIGMENT METABOLISM

Bilirubin metabolism is analyzed in detail in Chapter 8 (Jaundice). The following discussion includes brief background information about the various tests used most commonly to assess alterations in bile pigment metabolism.

SERUM BILIRUBIN

Bilirubin is a tetrapyrrole pigment derived in normal man principally from the catabolism of hemoglobin of senescent erythrocytes.[76, 107, 118] Ten to 30 per cent of bilirubin may originate from so-called shunt pathways, i.e., processes linked to hemoglobin synthesis within the bone marrow, from heme precursors within the liver and bone marrow, and from myoglobin and other nonhemoglobin heme proteins.[118] Bilirubin formed in extrahepatic sites is released into plasma and is carried in the circulation attached primarily to albumin,[107, 118] a bond which makes possible the transport in plasma of the virtually water-insoluble pigment. Bilirubin is taken up by the parenchymal cells of the liver and is rendered water soluble by intrahepatic conjugation before elimination into bile. Conjugation involves a complex series of steps which result in the transfer of glucuronic acid derived from uridine diphosphate glucuronic acid to the carboxyl groups

165

of bilirubin.[76, 107] The process is catalyzed by the microsomal enzyme glucuronyl transferase.[76, 107] Most of the conjugated bilirubin excreted into bile contains a glucuronide attached to each of the 2 propionic acid carboxyl groups and is thus a diglucuronide. The rest is excreted as the "monoglucuronide" (1 mole of glucuronic acid per mole of bilirubin), and as other water-soluble compounds.[76, 118]

The bilirubin normally present in serum represents a balance between input from production and hepatic removal of the pigment. Hyperbilirubinemia, therefore, may result from (a) overproduction of bile pigment, (b) impaired uptake, conjugation or excretion of bilirubin, or (c) leak back of unconjugated or conjugated pigment from damaged cells or bile ducts. One may anticipate that an increase in unconjugated bilirubin in serum results from overproduction or impairment of uptake or conjugation, whereas an increase in the conjugated moiety would be due to decreased excretion or backward leakage of the pigment.

Bilirubin in serum is measured, as a rule, by the diazo (van den Bergh) reaction. In this assay, bilirubin couples with diazotized sulfanilic acid, the bilirubin molecule splitting into 2 relatively stable dipyrryl azopigments which exhibit a maximal spectral absorption at 540 mμ. The reaction is specific for bilirubin, and only mesobilirubin (bilirubin with vinyl groups reduced to ethyl)

and monopyrroles react similarly.[76] Unconjugated bilirubin gives an indirect van den Bergh reaction (requiring the solubilizing effect of alcohol for the coupling reaction), whereas conjugated bilirubin reacts directly (without alcohol). For measurement of total serum bilirubin, the diazo reaction is carried out in the presence of alcohol which allows coupling to occur with both types of pigment. In addition, the conjugated moiety may be estimated in the absence of alcohol, and the difference represents the approximate quantity of unconjugated bilirubin present. The differential behavior of these 2 types of bilirubin with the diazo reagent probably depends on their different solubilities in aqueous solutions, although more complex organic chemical explanations have been suggested.[118]

Some differences in properties of unconjugated and conjugated bilirubin are listed in Table 6–1. The chemical formulas for unconjugated and conjugated bilirubin, their chromatographic separation into the various pigments and the basis for the diazo reaction are shown in Figure 6–1. The "monoglucuronide" may be separated from both unconjugated bilirubin and bilirubin diglucuronide by column chromatography and the distinct band called Pigment I (Fig. 6–1) has been considered a chemical entity.[183] The most recent evidence, however, suggests that this compound represents a labile equimolar complex of unconjugated

TABLE 6–1. DIFFERENCES BETWEEN UNCONJUGATED AND CONJUGATED BILE PIGMENTS

PROPERTY	UNCONJUGATED BILIRUBIN	CONJUGATED BILIRUBIN
van den Bergh reaction	Indirect (+ alcohol)	Direct
Solubility in aqueous solution	−	+
Solubility in lipid solvents	+	−
Attachment to plasma albumin	+	+
Presence in icteric urine	−	+
Presence in bile	−*	+
Affinity for brain tissue	+	−
Association with hemolytic jaundice	++	±
Association with obstructive and hepatocellular jaundice	+	+++

* A small quantity of unconjugated bilirubin may be present in common duct bile in the form of bilirubin monoglucuronide. It is unknown whether some unconjugated bilirubin is excreted as such into canalicular bile and subsequently is reabsorbed by the biliary ducts.

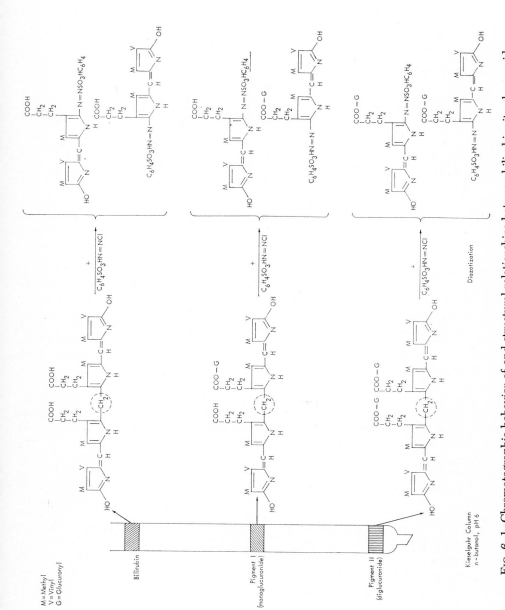

FIG. 6–1. Chromatographic behavior of and structural relationships between bilirubin, its glucuronides and their respective azopigment derivatives. (Adapted from Klatskin, G.: Bile pigment metabolism, Ann. Rev. Med. 12:211.)

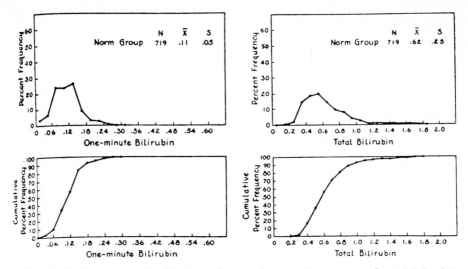

FIG. 6–2. Frequency distributions of normal serum 1-minute and total bilirubin concentrations in mg.%. N, number of individuals studied; $\bar{X}$, the mean; S, standard deviation. (Zieve, L., and Hill, E.: Gastroenterology 28:766.)

bilirubin and bilirubin diglucuronide.[78, 208]

Total Serum Bilirubin. In healthy individuals, the total serum bilirubin concentration (diazo-reactive material measured 30 minutes after addition of alcohol) usually is 0.3 to 1.0 mg./100 ml. (Fig. 6–2). From statistical analysis of a large group of determinations, the upper limit of normal has been designated as 1.5 mg./100 ml.[221] This value, however, is difficult to define precisely since the distribution curve of values obtained from presumably normal individuals is skewed to the right and may include a number of persons with an actual disturbance of pigment metabolism. Virtually all of the bilirubin normally present in serum is unconjugated.

A major value of the total serum bilirubin measurement is its specificity for liver dysfunction. A documented increase in serum bilirubin concentration indicates hepatobiliary disease, or some cause of overproduction of bilirubin such as intravascular hemolysis or "shunt" hyperbilirubinemia. Since the diazo test for measuring serum bilirubin is easily performed and reliable, there seems to be little use for the nonspecific and inaccurate method of estimating bilirubin by the icterus index test.

Total serum bilirubin is not a sensitive indicator of hepatic dysfunction and may not accurately reflect the degree of liver damage. Hyperbilirubinemia may not be detected in instances of moderate or severe hepatic parenchymal damage or in the rare case of an obstructed hepatic duct. This lack of sensitivity is partly explained by observations obtained in normal individuals infused with unconjugated bilirubin[199] and in patients with uncomplicated hemolysis,[158] which suggest that the capacity of the human liver to remove bilirubin from serum before hyperbilirubinemia ensues is at least twofold greater than the daily pigment load (250 to 300 mg.) normally presented to this organ. Furthermore, although in a steady state the height of serum bilirubin usually accurately reflects the intensity of jaundice and the increase in total body bile pigment, on occasion the serum bilirubin concentration may be lowered transiently by the presence in serum of substances (such as salicylates, sulfonamides, free fatty acids) that displace bilirubin from its attachment to plasma albumin and enhance transfer of the pigment into tissues. Conversely, an increase in serum albumin concentration may induce a temporary shift of bilirubin from tissue sites into the circulation.[51, 101]

The height of total serum bilirubin is seldom of value in specifying the cause of jaundice in the individual patient because

TABLE 6–2. CAUSES OF UNCONJUGATED HYPERBILIRUBINEMIA

Pediatric	Mechanism
Physiologic	
Crigler-Najjar[42]	Immaturity or inborn or acquired impairment of hepatic glucuronide-conjugating system
Breast milk[6]	
Lucey-Driscoll[7]	
Pediatric and Adult	
Intravascular hemolysis	Overproduction of bilirubin
"Shunt" hyperbilirubinemia	
Constitutional hepatic dysfunction (Gilbert's)	Impaired uptake and/or conjugation
Posthepatitic	Unknown ? Impaired uptake
Post portacaval shunt	? Overproduction from hemolysis
Miscellaneous (cardiac, hepatobiliary, etc.)[119]	Unspecified

values among the various types of jaundice overlap considerably.[92] On the average, however, uncomplicated hemolysis seldom causes a serum bilirubin in excess of 5 mg./100 ml.,[107] and parenchymal liver disease or incomplete extrahepatic obstruction due to biliary calculi gives lower serum bilirubin values than those seen with malignant obstruction of the common bile duct.

Few controlled studies critically assess the prognostic value of height and duration of hyperbilirubinemia in liver disease. In general, the higher the serum bilirubin concentration is in viral hepatitis, the greater is the histologic evidence of hepatocellular damage and the longer is the course of the disease.[185] Nevertheless, patients may die of fulminant hepatitis with only modest elevation of serum bilirubin. The presence of concomitant hemolysis with overproduction of bilirubin may also confuse the issue by causing higher serum bilirubin values than would be expected for any degree of hepatocellular damage present. In acute alcoholic hepatitis, hyperbilirubinemia in excess of 5 mg./100 ml. is one of the findings that connotes a graver prognosis.[87, 88]

Fractional Serum Bilirubin Determinations. Separation of serum bilirubin into unconjugated and conjugated fractions has definite differential diagnostic value in contrast to the total serum bilirubin determination by itself. The conjugated moiety is usually estimated by the direct diazo reaction (without alcohol), and the unconjugated fraction is considered to be the difference between total and direct-reacting diazo pigments. Coupling times of 1, 15 and 30 minutes have been used to estimate direct-reacting bilirubin. Most of the color develops within 1 minute and the bulk of clinical data, both in normal individuals and those with liver disease, has been compiled for the 1-minute reaction.[221] In normal persons, a small fraction of serum bilirubin, usually up to 0.25 mg./100 ml., reacts directly with the diazo reagent within 1 minute (Fig. 6–2). However, it has not been established whether this represents conjugated pigment or a fraction of unconjugated bilirubin rendered soluble by substances such as bile salts, urea and citrate which are normally present in serum.[107] The direct-reacting pigment in hyperbilirubinemic serum is largely conjugated bilirubin, however.

A major value of fractionating total serum bilirubin into unconjugated and direct-reacting moieties is in detecting states characterized by unconjugated hyperbilirubinemia (Table 6–2). Such a diagnosis appears warranted when the serum indirect-reacting bilirubin is in excess of 1.2 mg./100 ml. and the direct reacting fraction constitutes less than 20 per cent of total serum bilirubin. Whereas differential diagnosis of unconjugated hyperbilirubinemia from hyperbilirubinemia occurring in cirrhosis, hepatitis and obstructive jaundice based on the above criteria is good (Fig. 6–3), the 2 groups overlap somewhat, especially when total serum bilirubin is low and the measurement of direct-reacting bilirubin is technically less accurate.

When conjugated bilirubin accounts for more than 30 per cent of the total serum bilirubin, fractionation, whether by the diazo test[142] (Fig. 6–3) or the solvent-partition method of Weber and Schalm,

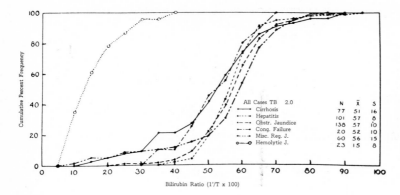

Fig. 6–3. Direct-reacting/total bilirubin ratio in various types of jaundice. TB, total bilirubin in serum. Other abbreviations as in Fig. 6-2. (Modified from Zieve et al.: J. Lab. Clin. Med. 38:446.)

does not allow one to differentiate accurately parenchymal (intrahepatic) jaundice from obstructive (extrahepatic) jaundice because of considerable overlap of values,[58] although in parenchymal jaundice the fraction of serum bilirubin that is conjugated may be somewhat lower on the average. It has been suggested that Pigment I ("monoglucuronide") is disproportionately increased in serum of patients with hepatocellular damage, presumably because of impaired hepatic synthesis of the diglucuronide. However, estimation of Pigment I as well as Pigment II (bilirubin diglucuronide) and free bilirubin in the serum of patients with obstructive and hepatocellular jaundice by reverse phase column partition chromatography or by the solvent-partition methods of Eberlein or Schachter, has failed to differentiate consistently between these 2 groups.[9, 181] This difficulty likely is due to inability of current methods to accurately measure the individual serum bile pigments, lack of knowledge concerning the structure and origin of "monoglucuronide" and the complex disturbance of hepatic bilirubin transport in these various disease states.[181]

The prompt-reacting bilirubin measurement also serves as a more sensitive test than total bilirubin for detecting early or mild liver injury.[139] In various series of patients with liver dysfunction due to cirrhosis, hepatitis, congestive heart failure, metastatic liver disease and other disorders, 30 to 50 per cent of patients manifested an increase in the 1-minute direct-reacting serum bilirubin whereas total bilirubin was normal.[68, 176, 205] Elevation of direct reacting bilirubin persisted in some instances even after values

for total serum bilirubin returned to normal.[68] Nevertheless, the direct-reacting serum bilirubin determination lacks popularity, probably because of lack of confidence in the low optical density or galvanometer readings of the direct-reacting-diazo complex in normal serum or with slight elevation of direct-reacting bilirubin concentration. While this criticism seems reasonable, in a series of 719 healthy individuals only 1 per cent had a 1-minute direct bilirubin value in excess of the normal limit of 0.24 mg./100 ml. (Fig. 6–2). A recent modification promises to enhance the accuracy of the test.[68] The direct-reacting bilirubin assay seems to add sensitivity to the serum bilirubin test and deserves a more prominent place in the detection of early or mild liver disease.

URINE BILIRUBIN

Detection of bilirubin in the urine immediately implies the presence of hepatobiliary disease since normal urine is free of bile pigment. The optimal routine methods currently in use can detect bilirubin concentrations as low as 0.05 mg./100 ml. of urine,[108] and the test is specific for this pigment. A urine bilirubin determination is of value in the following clinical situations. First, the test rapidly detects clinically suspected jaundice. Second, the presence of bilirubin in urine may antedate overt icterus or a rise in total or even direct-reacting serum bilirubin and hence may serve as an early clue to the presence of hepatobiliary dysfunction. Early detection of viral hepatitis by this test before the onset of hyperbilirubinemia has been well documented[69, 139] (Table 6–3).

TABLE 6–3. RELATIVE SENSITIVITY OF URINE BILIRUBIN AND SERUM BILIRUBIN IN DETECTING EARLY VIRAL HEPATITIS (34 CASES)

Total serum bilirubin mg.%	Patients with positive urine bilirubin test
< 1.0	59%
< 1.5	70%
One-minute direct-reacting bilirubin	
< 0.15	43%
< 0.25	75%

(Neefe, J. R., and Reinhold, J. G.: Gastroenterology 7:393.)

Similar findings have been reported in other types of liver disease.[98] Third, the absence of bilirubin in urine in the presence of jaundice (acholuric jaundice) suggests the presence of unconjugated hyperbilirubinemia since only conjugated bilirubin is excreted into urine. However, in some types of unconjugated hyperbilirubinemia (i.e., hemolysis) a small fraction of serum bilirubin is conjugated and may appear in urine.[201]

Although current data suggest that conjugated bilirubin passes into urine primarily by glomerular filtration of a small dialyzable serum fraction,[67] much remains to be learned about factors that influence the renal clearance of bilirubin. The quantity of bilirubin excreted is not a simple function of the concentration of conjugated bilirubin in serum. For example, no bilirubin may be detected in urine in phases of viral hepatitis despite significant elevation of serum direct-reacting bilirubin.[207] This is particularly evident late in the course when serum bilirubin is falling. Variable excretion of bilirubin into urine at comparable serum bilirubin levels is also observed in jaundiced patients with other hepatic disorders. These findings may reflect differences in serum concentrations of bile salts, substances that displace conjugated bilirubin from serum proteins and make the pigment more readily ultrafilterable.[66] Some instances undoubtedly are also due to concomitant renal insufficiency, the loss of bilirubin from urine allowed to stand unrefrigerated in light, or the use of nonspecific methods for measuring urine bilirubin. Despite these considerations, the simplicity, specificity and inexpensiveness of the urine bilirubin determination indicate that

the test be retained as a routine screening and diagnostic procedure.

URINARY UROBILINOGEN

Conjugated bilirubin is transformed by bacterial action in the intestinal lumen to colorless urobilinogens and their colored oxidation products, the urobilins. In normal individuals, the major part of these substances is excreted in the feces in an amount varying from 40 to 250 mg./day (average 100 mg.).[189] Approximately 10 to 15 per cent of the urobilinogens are absorbed into the portal circulation. Most of this undergoes enterohepatic circulation with only 0.2 to 3.3 mg. excreted in the urine per day.[189, 218] In a study of 676 normal subjects, only 5 per cent excreted more than 3.3 mg., and 1 per cent 5.5 mg./day.[218] Early studies and those recently carried out with radioactive-labeled urobilinogen[117] have established that urinary urobilinogen is increased when (1) excessive bile pigment forms, as in hemolysis, (2) intestinal transit time is prolonged, as in constipation, allowing increased contact of urobilinogen with the intestinal wall and possibly augmenting the duration of bacterial action, (3) bacteria invade the small intestine, allowing increased formation and reabsorption of urobilinogen at the site, and, most importantly, (4) hepatic dysfunction interferes with normal enterohepatic disposition of urobilinogen. Conversely, urobilinogen excretion in urine is decreased when (1) entry of bilirubin into the intestinal tract diminishes (intra- or extrahepatic obstruction), (2) intestinal bacterial flora is reduced, (3) intestinal transit time is shortened, (4) bilirubin production decreases due to severe aregenerative anemia, or (5) renal insufficiency is present.

Urinary output of urobilinogen is also influenced by urine pH, the time of urine collection, and the conditions of the assay.[19] (a) Urine pH is an important determinant of urinary urobilinogen output (Fig. 6–4). According to current concepts, urobilinogen is excreted into urine by a combination of glomerular filtration, proximal tubular secretion and pH-dependent back diffusion in the distal tubules.[19] Since urobilinogen is a weak organic acid with a pKa of 5.45, formation

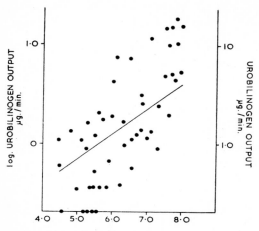

FIG. 6–4. Urobilinogen output in a normal subject related to urinary pH. There is a positive linear correlation between log. urobilinogen output and pH. The calculated regression line is given. (Bourke, E., Milne, M. D., and Stokes, G. S.: Brit. Med. J. 2:1510.)

of the un-ionized lipid soluble fraction increases as urine pH falls, and nonionic diffusion results in a greater absorption of urobilinogen from an acid than an alkaline urine. The urine pH should be alkaline, therefore, to minimize back diffusion and assure an accurate estimate of the quantity of urobilinogen entering the urine. If necessary, this can be accomplished by oral administration of sodium bicarbonate.[19]

(b) There is a normal diurnal variation in urine urobilinogen output. Recent studies have confirmed the fact that urine urobilinogen output usually is highest between noon and 4 P.M.[19] This probably reflects the observations that plasma concentration of urobilinogen is high, and urine pH is usually high during this period. While this establishes the conventional 2 to 4 P.M. period as the usual optimal time for a fractional urine collection, peak excretion occurs at other times in some persons. This should be considered when the data obtained from fractional 2-hour urine samples do not fit the clinical impression and should be checked with a 24-hour urine collection.[204] For a truly quantitative analysis, a 24-hour urine analysis is optimal.

(c) Urobilinogen is not stable in acid urine, and the Ehrlich aldehyde reaction which is used most commonly for its estimation is not specific for urobilinogen.[84] The combination of factors discussed above, therefore, tends to result in low estimates of urine urobilinogen excretion. Technical details of tests for urinary urobilinogen and urobilin are discussed elsewhere.[84, 154, 206]

A urinary urobilinogen determination is of major value as a liver function test when chromogen is absent from urine (or only traces are present) in jaundice. This indicates virtually complete cessation of bilirubin delivery into the intestine without specifying the precise cause of the obstruction. On a statistical basis, however, such complete biliary obstruction, especially if persistent, suggests malignant involvement of the biliary tree.[204] On the other hand, an increase in urinary urobilinogen may confirm excess bilirubin production (hemolysis) when the absence of liver disease can otherwise be ascertained. Other than this, increased urinary urobilinogen merely indicates the presence of liver damage; it does not elucidate the cause of the dysfunction. The sensitivity of the test is difficult to determine since most reported studies do not take urinary pH into account. It would appear that urinary urobilinogen increases prior to overt icterus in viral hepatitis and thus may be of value as a screening test in suspected cases or in an endemic setting.[139] Increased urobilinogen excretion may also be observed in other febrile illnesses,[43, 102] however, and its specificity for viral hepatitis in the anicteric febrile patient is therefore of limited value. Its relative value as compared with the SGOT determination in detecting early hepatic dysfunction in hepatitis remains to be established. A urinary urobilinogen also may be of help in following the course of an overt case of viral hepatitis by providing early evidence of a decrease in intrahepatic obstruction.[186] Reappearance of urobilinogen in the urine after temporary absence usually precedes or accompanies other evidence of improvement.

FECAL UROBILINOGEN

The interpretation of a fecal urobilinogen determination is influenced by some of the same factors that affect urinary urobilinogen, i.e., bilirubin entry into the gut, intestinal bacterial flora and intestinal transit time. The assay is more arduous, and results are less consistent from day to day in the same individual, however. A meaningful analysis, therefore, ideally requires several consecutive daily stool collections or a pooled 4-day one.[206]

A fecal urobilinogen determination is useful in 2 types of clinical situations. First, a striking decrease of fecal urobilinogen, usually to less than 5 or 6 mg./day, is believed to indicate complete biliary obstruction and thus statistically to suggest the presence of malignant extrahepatic obstruction of the common bile duct. However, a number of patients with extrahepatic malignancy excrete more than 6 and sometimes greater than 10 mg. of fecal urobilinogen per day,[214] and some patients with biliary calculi and cholestatic hepatitis excrete less than 5 mg./day.[70] A fecal urobilinogen determination, therefore, has some limitations in determining the nature of obstructive jaundice. The absence of urinary urobilinogen in jaundice as a rule offers the same information with a much lesser expenditure of effort.[204] In a small number of cases, however, the fecal urobilinogen determination may be the more sensitive test for demonstrating complete biliary obstruction.[204]

The second and more important value of a fecal urobilinogen determination is in the documentation of overproduction of bile pigment, as in hemolysis, in which case excretion of urobilinogen in stool is increased. This is of special importance in clinical situations characterized by shunt hyperbilirubinemia (i.e., overproduction of bilirubin through enhanced ineffective erythropoiesis or from other hemes or their precursors) wherein overt evidence of intravascular hemolysis is lacking. Furthermore, increased urinary urobilinogen excretion in liver disease does not permit any conclusions as to the presence of hemolysis, whereas a consistent and significant increase in fecal urobilinogen (i.e., > 400 mg./day) always signifies overproduction of bile pigments (excluding recent release of biliary obstruction).[206] Fecal urobilinogen, therefore, provides a better index of the presence of hemolysis than a urinary urobilinogen assay.

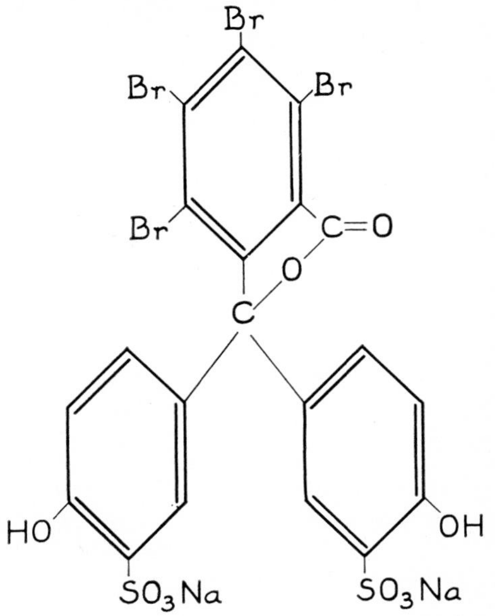

FIG. 6–5. Structural formula for sulfobromophthalein sodium (sodium phenoltetrabromphthalein disulfonate).

DYE TESTS

SULFOBROMOPHTHALEIN SODIUM

Sulfobromophthalein sodium, BSP, introduced by Rosenthal and White in 1924,[171] is a brominated phthalein dye, sodium phenoltetrabromphthalein disulfonate (Fig. 6–5), that is used extensively in the detection of hepatic dysfunction. Following intravenous administration, the dye is removed rapidly from the blood, primarily by the liver, and subsequently is excreted more slowly into bile.[26] A number of tests that utilize BSP are based on the observations that dye removal from blood is delayed in hepatic dysfunction. In the tests used most frequently the BSP concentration in plasma is determined at a specific time after a standard dose of dye per unit body weight has been administered intravenously.[129] Abnormal retention of BSP in plasma is noted in a large proportion of patients with hepatic disease and is generally considered to be one of the most sensitive indices of hepatic dysfunction. The test can be refined by obtaining blood samples at frequent intervals after a single intravenous injection, and determining the initial rate at which BSP dis-

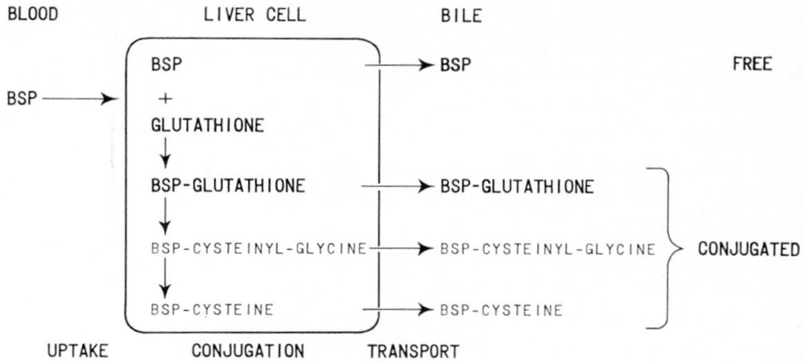

Fig. 6–6. Movement of BSP from blood to bile.

appears from plasma.[73, 97] Continuation of sampling for up to 60 minutes usually reveals a plasma disappearance curve for dye characterized by 2 exponential components. By analyzing these curves, one can calculate the transfer rates of dye from plasma to liver, from liver back to plasma, and from liver into bile.[13]

BSP is also used in a prolonged infusion method devised by Wheeler and associates to quantitatively assess hepatic uptake and storage and maximal biliary excretion of dye.[211, 212] The single sample test is of particular value in detecting abnormal removal of BSP from plasma. It provides no insight, however, into the mechanisms that delay the disappearance of dye. The prolonged infusion method[212] and the analysis of plasma disappearance curves,[13, 131] although more involved, may be even more sensitive in detecting abnormalities in hepatic BSP removal mechanisms. They are of major value, however, in delineating the principal factors that account for abnormal removal of BSP from plasma.

An examination of the hepatic disposition of injected BSP indicates that the dye undergoes transport across the sinusoidal membrane, metabolic transformation in the liver cell, and transport of unchanged as well as of metabolically transformed dye across the canalicular membrane into the biliary system (Fig. 6–6). Movement of BSP from blood to bile is susceptible to interference at many sites, which undoubtedly accounts for the frequency with which hepatic disease and dysfunction result in abnormal dye removal from plasma. Injected dye is rapidly bound to serum proteins, primarily to albumin and α_1-lipoprotein.[10] The quantity of

protein-bound dye carried to the liver per unit time is obviously a function of hepatic blood flow. Once presented to this organ, BSP is rapidly taken up by liver cells from the space of Disse across the sinusoidal membrane by an unknown mechanism that apparently does not involve entry of protein-BSP into the hepatic cells. It is not clear whether the substrate for uptake is the small quantity of unbound BSP in plasma, continuously supplied by dissociation of dye from plasma protein as uptake proceeds, or also includes protein-bound BSP, thus requiring an uncoupling mechanism for uptake to occur. The latter is suggested in a recent report.[11]

The uptake process appears to be saturable,[74] and competition for uptake between BSP and bilirubin, indocyanine green, rose bengal and Bunamiodyl has been demonstrated.[95] These features suggest that uptake of BSP is carrier mediated, but since there is no information about relative concentrations of unbound dye on either side of the sinusoidal membrane, it is not known whether uptake involves an active transport process or is an example of facilitated transport. BSP contained in the liver cell is also largely protein-bound. Unpublished observations (Mizuta and Combes) have demonstrated that dye is bound to most of the electrophoretically separated liver proteins of the rat which have an affinity for BSP similar to that of the mixture of proteins in rat serum, but less than that of serum albumin. No specific hepatic binding protein has yet been demonstrated.

Much of the BSP within liver cells conjugates with glutathione.[38, 79, 100] The sulfhydryl group of glutathione interacts with the dye compound liberating HBr, a hydrogen ion from the tripeptide and a bromine, presumably from position 4 or 5 (possibly both, thus forming isomers) from the dye, and forms a thio-ether compound.[38, 99, 100] Conjugation, which is catalyzed by a liver enzyme, takes place in the soluble cytoplasm of the cell where virtually all of the enzyme and most of the glutathione is contained.[37, 72] A number of other conjugates including BSP-cysteinyl glycine and BSP-cysteine are also formed, presumably by cleavage of glutamic acid and glycine from the glutathione moiety. Both conjugated and free BSP are then excreted across canalicular membranes into the biliary tract. Conjugation is not required for uptake, nor does it appear to determine the extent of hepatic uptake of BSP.[34, 150] Likewise, conjugation is not obligatory for biliary excretion of the dye. However, it does appear to be advantageous for the latter process since conjugated BSP compounds are preferentially excreted into bile.[34, 150] The reason for their preferential excretion is not known, but one likely possibility is based on the observation that conjugated dye is less tightly bound to intracellular proteins (Mizuta and Combes, unpublished observation). It may thus become more easily available to the carrier mechanisms involved in BSP transport into bile.

BSP compounds are transported into bile in high concentration, and when compared to intracellular concentration, against large concentration gradients. There is also evidence that other organic anions compete with BSP for biliary excretion, and thus presumably for a common canalicular transport system.[33] Finally, biliary excretion appears to have many of the characteristics of a rate-limited transport process,[39, 211, 212] although recent data indicate that apparent maximal biliary excretion of BSP is altered significantly, and in the same direction, by changes in canalicular bile flow.[80, 144, 170] Excretion against high concentration gradients, competition with other compounds for excretion, and characteristics of a rate-limited process all suggest that BSP transport is active, thus carrier mediated and intimately linked to an energy source.

Observations in mutant sheep with congenital transport defects, Corriedale sheep with a hepatic excretory defect,[5] and Southdown sheep with a hepatic uptake defect[41] for many organic anions including BSP, indicate that carrier activity may be determined genetically. This further suggests that function of the sinusoidal and canalicular carrier mechanisms depends on genetically determined proteins which may be required either as components of or for synthesis of components of the postulated carrier compounds. Such genetic factors may also determine the sensitivity of carriers to other compounds, for example, the probable sensitivity of the canalicular transport system in cholestatic jaundice of pregnancy to various steroids including oral contraceptive agents.

Impairment of BSP removal from blood may be due to interference predominantly with one or some combination of the factors described above. Generally accepted or suspected clinical conditions that may affect the various steps in BSP transfer from blood to bile are listed in Table 6–4.

In the most commonly used BSP tests, BSP retention in blood is measured 30 or 45 minutes after the single intravenous injection of 5 mg. BSP/kg. body weight. (The weight of any ascites is ignored since virtually no dye enters ascitic fluid.[97]) It is assumed that dye is injected into a plasma volume of 50 ml./kg. body weight, and that with instantaneous mixing, a concentration of 10 mg./100 ml. of plasma is achieved. This value is considered to represent 100 per cent retention. Concentrations of BSP measured in plasma are compared to this value and reported as per cent retention. Ten per cent retention (1 mg./100 ml.) at 30 minutes, and 5 per cent at 45 minutes are frequently considered to be the upper limits of normal for this test. The data of Zieve and Hill demonstrate that this is an oversimplification, however.[218] Forty-five minute BSP tests performed in 718 normal men revealed that approximately 50 per cent had BSP retention values below 4 per cent, 90 per cent below 8 per cent, and 99 per cent below 14 per cent (Fig. 6–7).

The selection of a value for definite abnormality in a general population is complicated by the observations that values for BSP retention are higher as body weight

176   Laboratory Tests

TABLE 6–4. CAUSES OF IMPAIRMENT OF BSP REMOVAL FROM BLOOD

PROCESS AFFECTED	CONDITION RESULTING IN IMPAIRMENT
Delivery of dye to liver	Decreased hepatic blood flow
	Heart failure
	Hemorrhage
	Collapse of the circulation
	Cirrhosis
Hepatic uptake	Impaired function of carrier mechanism
	Congenital — Mutant Southdown sheep
	Acquired — Hepatic diseases
	Drug toxicity
	Toxins
	Competition for carrier
	Bilirubin
	Bile salts
	Compounds used to visualize gallbladder
	X-5709 C (other drugs)
Conjugation	Delayed maturation in premature and newborn infants
	Malnutrition
	Hepatic diseases?
Biliary excretion	Impaired function of carrier mechanism
	Congenital — Dubin-Johnson syndrome
	Mutant Corriedale sheep
	Delayed maturation in premature and newborn infants
	Acquired — Hepatic diseases
	Drug toxicity
	Toxins
	Pregnancy
	Estrogens
	Anabolic steroids
	Oral contraceptive agents
	Panhypopituitarism
	Anoxia
	Competition for carrier
	Bilirubin
	Bile salts
	Other anionic dyes
	Extrahepatic obstruction

increases,[218] and are particularly evident in the obese patient.[64, 217] This is undoubtedly related to a number of factors, including: (a) BSP dose is based on body weight, (b) plasma volume in the obese patient is less than the idealized 50 ml./kg., (c) hepatic functional mass and perfusion probably do not increase proportionately to increases in body weight of the obese patient. Attempts to correct BSP retention values for weight,[64, 217] or to adjust dosage to surface area or fat-free weight,[24] or to yield initial plasma dye concentrations comparable to non-obese patients[64] may have

merit. Nevertheless, these procedures have not yet been demonstrated to separate obese patients with liver disease from those without it. At present, therefore, the test appears to be of limited value as a sensitive index of hepatic function in the obese person.

BSP retention is also increased in older persons, particularly those over the age of 60.[64, 197] However, age affects overall BSP results[64] less than obesity. Tests may be abnormal in febrile patients. It is not clear whether this is related to increased temperature *per se* or represents hepatic damage occurring in the course of the disease in

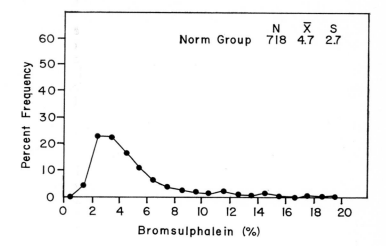

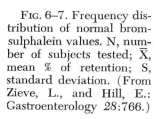

FIG. 6–7. Frequency distribution of normal bromsulphalein values. N, number of subjects tested; $\overline{X}$, mean % of retention; S, standard deviation. (From Zieve, L., and Hill, E.: Gastroenterology 28:766.)

question. The test should be performed before or several days after gallbladder dyes are administered, since these compounds compete with BSP for hepatic transport mechanisms.[132, 187]

Local tissue damage may ensue if dye is injected into the perivascular tissues. Anaphylactic reactions, sometimes fatal, have been reported, but fortunately these are rare.[96] Care should be taken to insure that the dye is administered intravenously, and slowly over a period of a few minutes. Despite the limitations enumerated above, the BSP test clearly has a wide margin of safety and offers a sensitive means of detecting hepatic dysfunction. However, BSP retention is abnormal in all types of liver abnormalities (Table 6–4) and therefore the test is not selective for the type of hepatic disturbance.

Occasionally, results are normal with properly performed tests (correct dose of dye, accurate sampling time) in obvious liver disease. Analysis of plasma disappearance curves may disclose that removal of BSP is delayed in such patients.[131] Routine performance of a multiple sampling test probably offers little advantage over the standard single sample technic, however.

A BSP test is seldom justified in jaundice since hepatic disease is evident, and no new useful information is likely to be provided. However, continued sampling of blood beyond 45 to 60 minutes may be of value in

characterizing some patients with congenital conjugated hyperbilirubinemia. An initial fall in plasma BSP concentration followed by a late rise, attributed to appearance in plasma of conjugated dye, has been observed thus far only in a few patients with the Dubin-Johnson syndrome.[25, 52, 126] By contrast, a progressive although delayed disappearance of BSP from plasma without a secondary rise has been described in patients with the apparently related Rotor syndrome.[52, 179] Most of the BSP in plasma was unconjugated in the latter patients. Whether these differences in BSP disposal are demonstrated consistently in such patients, however, is not clear and must await additional observations.

Once increased retention of BSP is demonstrated with a standard test, a number of technics further characterize the abnormality. Analysis of plasma for BSP metabolites when combined with a 45 or a 60 minute dye retention test differentiates most patients with hepatitis and cirrhosis from those with intra- or extrahepatic obstruction; a larger fraction of retained BSP is conjugated in the latter groups.[27] By contrast, determination of metabolites excreted in urine did not differentiate the various disorders.[27, 44] Analysis of plasma disappearance curves of BSP may indicate whether hepatic uptake or transport is altered, or both.[13]

We have had considerable experience

TABLE 6–5. RESULTS OF BSP S AND TM MEASUREMENTS

	S mg./mg.%	Tm mg./min.
Normal[36, 160, 212]		
Males	64	9.1
Females	53	7.6
Increasing age[197]	↓	N
Hepatitis[36]	↓	↓
Cirrhosis[182, 212]	↓	↓
Obstruction[182]		
extrahepatic		
intrahepatic	↓	↓
Dubin-Johnson syndrome[212]	N	↓
Normal pregnancy[36]		
First half	N,↑	N
Second half	↑	↓
Hyperemesis gravidarum[35]	N,↓	↓
Estrogens[137]	N,↑	↓
17-α-ethyl-19 nortestosterone[178]	N	↓
Panhypopituitarism[180]	N	↓
Acromegaly[159]	N	↑
Portal vein thrombosis[198]	↓	N

with the prolonged infusion method of Wheeler and associates.[2, 212] Values are obtained for S, a proportionality factor, defined as the number of milligrams of BSP taken up into storage in the liver for each increment of plasma concentration of 1 mg.%, and for the maximal rate at which dye is excreted into bile in milligrams per minute, the BSP Tm. Results obtained with the procedure by various investigators are summarized in Table 6–5. Selective changes in S or Tm are observed in some conditions, whereas in others, both S and Tm are altered, either in the same or divergent directions. As these findings indicate, BSP is an important tool for examining alterations in hepatic function.

The definition of factors that account for these changes should provide valuable information about hepatic function in health and disease. In many ways, the dye is handled by liver in a manner similar to that of bilirubin. Therefore, information derived from studies with BSP frequently may be applied to bilirubin, a compound that is much more difficult to work with.

INDOCYANINE GREEN

This tricarbocyanine dye (Fig. 6–8) also has characteristics suitable for appraisal of hepatic transport function. The dye in plasma is bound to albumin and α_1-lipoproteins.[10] Uptake into liver cells accounts for rapid disappearance from plasma. There is no evidence of extrahepatic removal.[28, 210] The dye is stored in parenchymal cells from which it is gradually secreted into bile. There is evidence that indocyanine green and BSP utilize the same sinusoidal transport system,[95] and suggestive evidence that they share a common canalicular secretory process.[210]

Indocyanine green is not conjugated,[25, 28] and virtually all of the injected dye is recovered in bile.[210] In tests that appraise hepatic function, plasma concentration of the dye is measured at some fixed time after a single intravenous injection of a dose based on body weight, and the rate at which the dye disappears from plasma is determined.[25, 28, 40, 116] Experience with the compound is still limited. Optimal doses for injection, and sampling times that best differentiate patients with and without liver damage have to be determined. Similar sensitivity in detecting liver dysfunction is inferred from studies in which retention of indocyanine green and BSP have been compared. Toxic reactions similar to those observed with BSP have not yet been reported with indocyanine green.

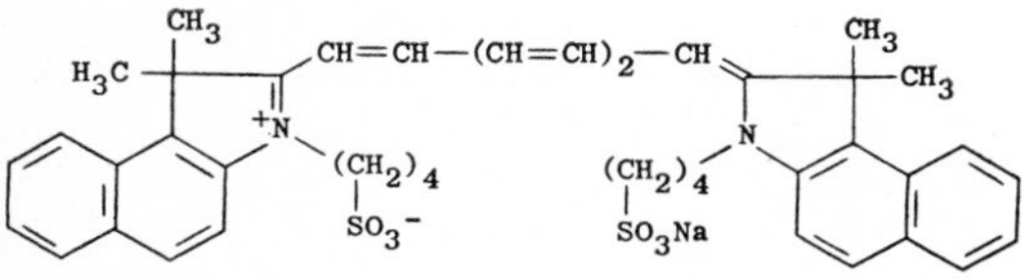

FIG. 6–8. Structural formula for indocyanine green.

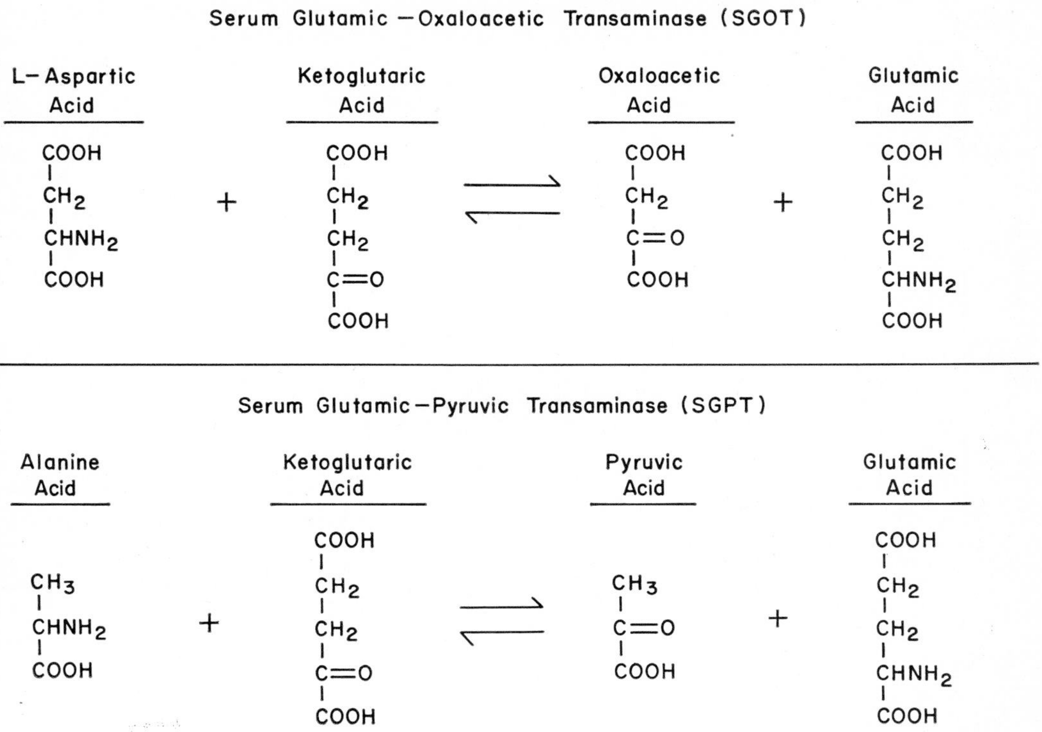

Serum Glutamic –Oxaloacetic Transaminase (SGOT)

L–Aspartic Acid		Ketoglutaric Acid			Oxaloacetic Acid		Glutamic Acid

$$\begin{array}{c} \text{COOH} \\ | \\ \text{CH}_2 \\ | \\ \text{CHNH}_2 \\ | \\ \text{COOH} \end{array} \;+\; \begin{array}{c} \text{COOH} \\ | \\ \text{CH}_2 \\ | \\ \text{CH}_2 \\ | \\ \text{C}=\text{O} \\ | \\ \text{COOH} \end{array} \;\rightleftharpoons\; \begin{array}{c} \text{COOH} \\ | \\ \text{CH}_2 \\ | \\ \text{C}=\text{O} \\ | \\ \text{COOH} \end{array} \;+\; \begin{array}{c} \text{COOH} \\ | \\ \text{CH}_2 \\ | \\ \text{CH}_2 \\ | \\ \text{CHNH}_2 \\ | \\ \text{COOH} \end{array}$$

Serum Glutamic–Pyruvic Transaminase (SGPT)

Alanine Acid		Ketoglutaric Acid			Pyruvic Acid		Glutamic Acid

$$\begin{array}{c} \text{CH}_3 \\ | \\ \text{CHNH}_2 \\ | \\ \text{COOH} \end{array} \;+\; \begin{array}{c} \text{COOH} \\ | \\ \text{CH}_2 \\ | \\ \text{CH}_2 \\ | \\ \text{C}=\text{O} \\ | \\ \text{COOH} \end{array} \;\rightleftharpoons\; \begin{array}{c} \text{CH}_3 \\ | \\ \text{C}=\text{O} \\ | \\ \text{COOH} \end{array} \;+\; \begin{array}{c} \text{COOH} \\ | \\ \text{CH}_2 \\ | \\ \text{CH}_2 \\ | \\ \text{CHNH}_2 \\ | \\ \text{COOH} \end{array}$$

FIG. 6–9. Reactions catalyzed by transaminases. (Maclagan, N. F.: *in* Schiff, L. (ed.): Diseases of the Liver, ed. 2, p. 154, Philadelphia, J. B. Lippincott, 1963.)

SERUM ENZYMES

SERUM TRANSAMINASES

The transaminases are a group of enzymes that catalyze the transfer of an amino group from an alpha amino acid to an α-keto acid. In the clinical literature, the enzymes are designated by a term that describes the favored products of the reaction at equilibrium. Measurement of the activity in serum of the 2 enzymes glutamic oxalacetic transaminase (SGOT) and glutamic pyruvic transaminase (SGPT) has been used extensively in the diagnosis of liver diseases. The reactions catalyzed by these enzymes are illustrated in Figure 6–9.

Both transaminases are detected normally in serum (Fig. 6–10). The source of these enzymes is unknown, however. If tissues rich in transaminases are damaged or destroyed, the enzymes are released into the circulation. The increment in serum activities under these circumstances reflects the relative rates at which the enzymes enter and leave the circulation. Injected transaminase is distributed in interstitial fluid as well as in the plasma volume from which

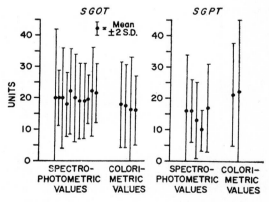

FIG. 6–10. Normal values of spectrophotometric and colorimetric methods in different laboratories. (Clermont, R. J., and Chalmers, T. C.: Medicine *46*:197.)

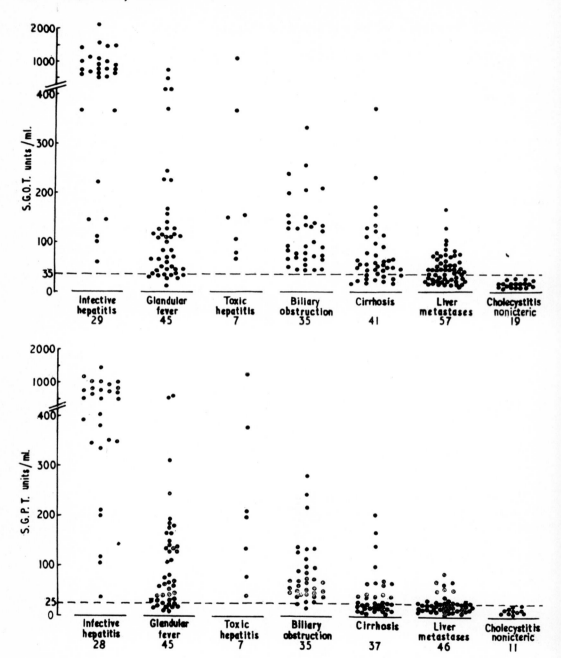

FIG. 6–11. Serum SGOT and SGPT levels in different types of liver disease. (From J. H. Wilkinson.[213])

it gradually disappears.[54] Virtually none is lost in the urine, and renal metabolism is insignificant.[54] Although transaminases are normally present in bile, biliary excretion does not represent a major means of dis-

posing of serum transaminase.[54, 61] Presumably metabolism of the enzymes, which constitute part of the protein pool of the body, largely accounts for the disappearance from blood, although the sites and factors determining the rates of metabolism are unknown.

Serum transaminase activity increases in most disorders that produce hepatic dysfunction[213, 215, 222] (Fig. 6–11). Moreover, the tests are sensitive indicators of liver cell damage. Elevated transaminase values are among the first laboratory abnormalities detected in the preicteric phase of hepatitis (Figs. 6–12, 6–13).[111] The transaminase values return to normal as jaundice subsides (Fig. 6–13). Rebounds of transaminase values, or persistent elevations, usually indicate recrudescences or chronic hepatic inflammation and necrosis. Thus, these tests provide one of the important means of following the clinical activity of hepatic disease. High results are also noted frequently in anicteric patients with liver cell injury produced by drugs and hepatotoxins or occurring in the course of heart failure, infectious mononucleosis, various infections, metastatic carcinoma, granulomatous and alcoholic liver diseases as well as other hepatic disorders. In the jaundiced patient,

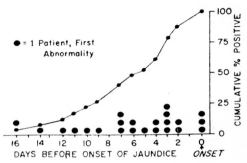

FIG. 6–12. Diagnostic usefulness of the SGOT in the earliest stages of acute viral hepatitis. Relation of first abnormality to onset of jaundice among 23 patients or volunteers being followed closely during the incubation period. (Clermont, R. J., and Chalmers, T. C.: Medicine 46:197.)

transaminase tests have differential diagnostic significance since values in excess of 300 to 400 units usually indicate acute hepatocellular disease (Fig. 6–11, Table 6–6). Similar values may occur with extrahepatic

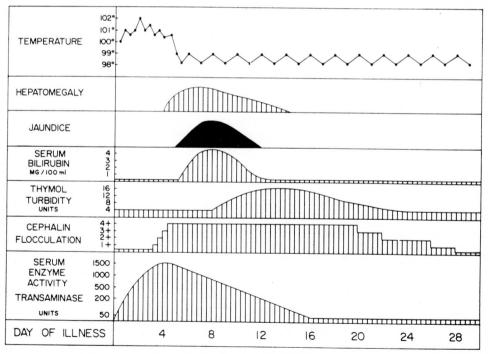

FIG. 6–13. Schematic diagram of the clinical course of a typical case of infectious hepatitis; correlation of liver function tests with clinical manifestations. Note that jaundice is first detected when serum transaminase activity has reached peak levels. (Krugman, S., and Ward, R.: Infectious Diseases of Children, ed. 2, St. Louis, Mosby, 1960.)

TABLE 6–6. TRANSAMINASE VALUES REPORTED IN 28 PAPERS WITH DATA ON PATIENTS WITH INFECTIOUS HEPATITIS AND IN 14 WITH DATA ON PATIENTS WITH OBSTRUCTIVE JAUNDICE*

	SGOT		SGPT	
	INFEC-TIOUS HEPATITIS	OBSTRUC-TIVE JAUNDICE	INFEC-TIOUS HEPATITIS	OBSTRUC-TIVE JAUNDICE
UNITS	Cumulative %		Cumulative %	
"Normal"	1	10	1	20
34(46)†–200	27	81	27	60
201–400	43	98	39	93
401–600	50	99	43	97
601–800	64	99	48	99
801–1000	72	100	53	100
1001–2000	95	—	83	—
2001–3000	99	—	91	—
3000	100	—	100	—
Total pts.	274	181	177	97

* Either initial or maximal values are used because they were the same in 44 of the 49 instances in which both were presented; the maximal were recorded in the 5 exceptions.
† 33 units for SGOT and 45 units for SGPT being the upper limit of normality.
(Clermont, R. J., and Chalmers, T. C.: Medicine 46:197.)

obstruction, but are distinctly uncommon (Table 6–6). The largest elevations, frequently in excess of 1,000 units, are observed early in the course of hepatitis (Fig. 6–14),[31] during acute toxic injury produced by carbon tetrachloride and in collapse of the circulation. Transaminase values less than 300 units in jaundice have no selective function since they occur in a significant number of patients with acute and chronic hepatocellular diseases as well as with obstructive jaundice (Fig. 6–11, Table 6–6).

The SGOT/SGPT ratio has been proposed as an additional means of detecting

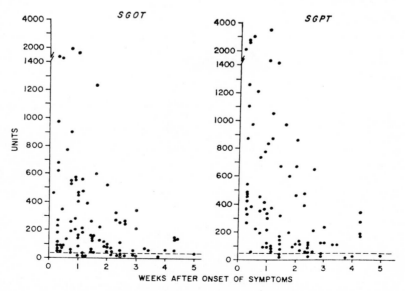

FIG. 6–14. Relation of admission transaminase value to onset of symptoms. (Clermont, R. J., and Chalmers, T. C.: Medicine 46:197.)

hepatitis regardless of the absolute transaminase values, since the ratio is less than 1 in the majority of cases.[48] The value of the ratio in differential diagnosis of jaundice in a single patient has important limitations, however, since ratios greater than 1 have been reported in (a) one fourth to a third of patients with hepatitis[31, 222] (Table 6–7) and in (b) a majority of chronic hepatocellular diseases; and (c) ratios less than 1 are not restricted to hepatocellular diseases, being recorded in a significant number of patients with acute extrahepatic obstruction[31, 222] (Table 6–7).

Although increases in serum transaminase activity reflect liver cell damage, the degree of elevation is of little prognostic value. Thus, in acute hepatitis, fulminant necrosis may ensue when the enzymatic activity of serum is increased only modestly, whereas rapid recovery may be observed when transaminase values are 3,000 units or greater. Moreover, transaminase values are usually less than 300 units in the majority of cirrhotic patients and frequently are elevated only slightly in periods of terminal hepatic failure.

Elevated SGOT and SGPT values are not specific for hepatic diseases since they may also be observed in patients with severe cardiac and skeletal muscle damage.[215, 222] SGOT increases with greater frequency than SGPT in myocardial infarction and is undoubtedly of cardiac origin in most. Rises in SGPT in cardiac disease may be of hepatic origin however, since they are usually seen in the setting of large infarcts, heart failure and circulatory collapse—in all of which hepatic ischemia is likely to occur. Increased SGPT in muscle disease is probably derived from muscle, however.[53, 215] The extent of enzyme elevation with muscle disease is almost invariably less than 300 units and does not reach the very high value observed in acute hepatocellular damage.[215]

SERUM ALKALINE PHOSPHATASE

The term alkaline phosphatase is applied to a group of enzymes that catalyze the hydrolysis of a number of organic phosphate esters optimally at an alkaline pH with liberation of inorganic phosphate and the organic radical.[82, 155] The enzyme is identified

TABLE 6–7. RATIO OF SGOT TO SGPT IN PATIENTS DIVIDED INTO THOSE WITH HIGH AND LOW VALUES (<500 OR ≥500 UNITS)

Highest value of either test	<500 Ratio <1.0	≥1.0	≥500 Ratio <1.0	≥1.0	Total pts.
Infectious hepatitis					
No. pts.	66	37	61	7	171
%	64	36	90	10	
Infectious mononucleosis					
No. pts.	43	7	4	0	54
%	86	14			
Obstructive jaundice					
No. pts.	33	22	6	1	62
%	60	40	86	14	
Cirrhosis					
No. pts.	4	64	1	1	70
%	6	94			
Total pts.	146	130	72	9	357

(Clermont, R. J., and Chalmers, T. C.: Medicine 46:197.)

in many tissues, but its function is unknown. Alkaline phosphatase activity is normally demonstrable in serum. There is good evidence that serum enzyme in the normal adult is derived primarily from 3 sources, the skeleton, hepatobiliary system and the intestinal tract, and it is estimated that bone phosphatase accounts for 40 to 75 per cent of serum activity.[155] Contribution from the intestines is of importance primarily in persons with blood groups O and B who are secretors, and is enhanced by prior consumption of a fatty meal.[155, 156] Circulating enzyme, like other proteins, is disposed of mainly by catabolism in the body, although the sites of degradation are not known.[32, 57, 155]

Some details of 3 of the more popular procedures used to measure alkaline phosphatase activity (Bodansky, King-Armstrong, and Bessey-Lowry) including substrates used, end products measured, and the usual range of normal values for adults aged 17 to 55 are contained in Table 6–8. Results obtained with these methods appear to be

TABLE 6–8. RANGE OF NORMAL VALUES FOR SERUM ALKALINE PHOSPHATASE
ACTIVITY IN *Adult* MAN[82, 200]

METHOD	SUBSTRATE	UNIT	NORMAL RANGE
Bodansky	β-Glycerophosphate	1 mg. P/100 ml./60′	1.5–4.0
King-Armstrong	Phenylphosphate	1 mg. phenol/100 ml./30′	3–13
Bessey-Lowry	p-Nitrophenylphosphate	1 mM. p-Nitrophenol/100 ml./30′	0.8–3.0

equally effective in detecting a wide variety of clinical diseases.[49] Conversion factors permit interchange of values obtained by the different methods (Table 6–9). However, these factors are based on average values, and individual converted results show a wide scatter and imperfect correlation with results obtained by the method to whose units the values are being changed.[49, 200] Our knowledge of the effect of normal and abnormal constituents of serum as inhibitors and activators of the various enzyme fractions which comprise serum alkaline phosphatase is still rudimentary.[82, 155] Factors such as phosphate, citrate and urea concentration and perhaps even the duration of freezing of serum prior to assay, may modify serum alkaline phosphatase activity.[121, 155]

In the 17 to 55 age group, the mean serum alkaline phosphatase activity is somewhat higher in men than in women.[48] By contrast, for persons past age 60 that of women equals or exceeds that of men, and both sexes tend to have somewhat higher values than younger adults.[89, 106] The reasons for these differences are not known. In children, serum alkaline phosphatase activity is considerably elevated in both sexes, correlates well with the rate of bone growth (Fig. 6–15) and appears to be accounted for by influx of enzyme from osteoid tissue.[30]

Serum alkaline phosphatase in normal adolescent males may reach mean levels of 7 to 8 Bessey-Lowry units, without implying the presence of hepatobiliary disease. Enzyme activity in serum may double late in normal pregnancy because of influx of placental phosphatase.[18, 130]

Although elevation of serum alkaline phosphatase activity is observed frequently in various hepatobiliary diseases, similar elevations are observed in various disorders of bone characterized by increased osteoblastic activity, and as indicated, occur normally during growth and pregnancy. Occasionally, the intestinal tract may be the source of an elevated serum enzyme value. Three major approaches have been utilized to increase the specificity of an alkaline phosphatase determination.

First, attempts have been made to differentiate the phosphatases derived from liver, bone and placenta on the basis of differences in their electrophoretic mobility.[16, 21, 29, 140, 196] Good separation of protein bands with alkaline phosphatase activity (isoenzymes) has been reported. Although patterns emerge that favor origin from one tissue, the procedures used have the following limitations: (1) patterns overlap between patients with elevated alkaline phosphatases attributable to diseases of different organ systems,

TABLE 6–9. APPROXIMATE CONVERSION FACTORS FOR ALKALINE PHOSPHATASE*

CONVERSION FROM	CONVERSION TO BESSEY-LOWRY	CONVERSION TO BODANSKY	CONVERSION TO KING-ARMSTRONG
Bessey-Lowry	—	X 1.3	X 3.5
Bodansky	X 0.79	—	X 2.8
King-Armstrong	X 0.29	X 0.34	—

* Conversion factors based on 215 specimens in various disease states. However, they must be considered as only *approximations*, since 95 per cent confidence limits of duplicate determinations on any specimen show much scatter.

(Deren, J. J., et al.: New Engl. J. Med. 270:1277.)

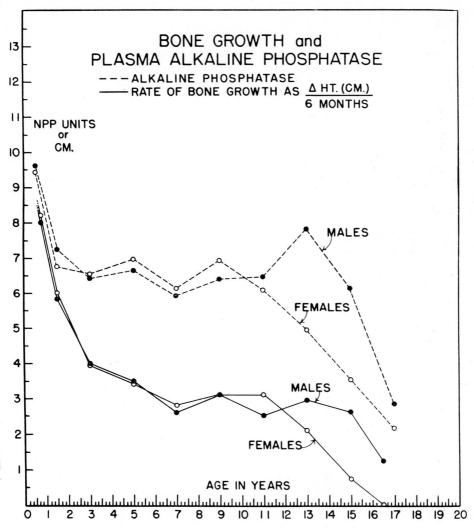

Fig. 6–15. Normative data for growing children. NPP, nitrophenyl phosphate units; CM, centimeters. (Clarke, L. C., and Beck, E.: J. Pediat. 36:335.)

(2) results of various investigators often disagree, which possibly reflects differences in technics used to separate the isoenzymes, and (3) the electrophoretic technics are complicated and are not yet suitable for routine use. Future refinements in methodology may resolve these problems, but at present, serum electrophoresis is not a satisfactory practical method for increasing the specificity of the serum alkaline phosphatase determination.

The second approach is based on the observation that alkaline phosphatases from

individual tissues differ in susceptibility to inactivation by heat.[130, 157] Placental alkaline phosphatase is fully "heat stable" after exposure to 56° C. for 30 minutes, whereas the enzymes derived from bone and liver are partly inactivated. Accordingly, finding of an elevated serum alkaline phosphatase in a pregnant patient with all of the excess enzyme "heat stable," strongly suggests that the placenta is the sole source of the elevated enzyme in serum.

For phosphatase from bile, liver and bone susceptibility to heat increases respec-

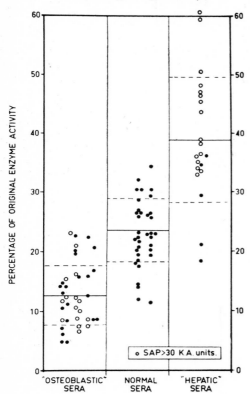

SERUM ALKALINE PHOSPHATASE ACTIVITY REMAINING
AFTER HEATING SERA FOR 15 MINUTES AT 56°C.
(as percentage of original activity.)

Fig. 6–16. Serum alkaline phosphatase activity (as percentage of activity in each unheated sample) in 94 sera heated at 56° C. for 15 minutes. The solid lines represent the means, the broken lines one standard deviation. (Posen, S., Neale, F. C., and Clubb, J. S.: Ann. Int. Med. 62:1234.)

tively. When sera from patients with increased osteoblastic activity or hepatobiliary disease were heated at 56° C. for 15 minutes, alkaline phosphatase activity fell to a much greater extent in the osteoblastic group, and these groups of patients were separated strikingly (Fig. 6–16). For all sera in the "osteoblastic" group, alkaline phosphatase was inactivated to less than 25 per cent of original activity, whereas for all but 2 of the "hepatic" sera residual activity was more than 25 per cent of that measured prior to heating. The serum phosphatase in

the first group thus resembled bone phosphatase, whereas that of the hepatic group resembled bile phosphatase. Additional experience with this technic is needed, but current findings suggest that it may provide a valuable means of increasing the specificity of the serum alkaline phosphatase determination in clinical diagnosis.

In the third and at present the best substantiated approach, serum leucine aminopeptidase and 5′-nucleotidase activity are measured. These enzymes, discussed below, are not elevated by bone disorders, and are elevated only with liver dysfunction or in pregnancy. Increase of these enzymes in serum in nonpregnant patients indicates, therefore, that an elevated serum alkaline phosphatase is due at least in part to hepatobiliary disease.

The mechanism by which hepatobiliary disease leads to an elevation of serum alkaline phosphatase is controversial. Most evidence suggests that this occurs primarily because of regurgitation of enzyme formed in the liver from the intrahepatic biliary tree into the circulation. Retention of phosphatase of osseous origin due to impaired biliary excretion does not seem to be an important mechanism of this hyperphosphatasia.[32, 57, 151, 155] The contribution of the biliary tree in excreting hepatic phosphatase and also in serving as a major source of the enzyme in liver may explain the very early elevation of serum alkaline phosphatase in intrahepatic and extrahepatic bile duct obstruction. In these disorders serum phosphatase often is elevated before jaundice develops, and may persist after icterus disappears as the only clue to continued biliary obstruction. By contrast, in hepatocellular diseases that primarily affect the liver parenchyma (cirrhosis, hepatitis), in which the phosphatase concentration is relatively low,[82, 155] the serum phosphatase may never rise, or, if elevated, may follow other evidence of liver damage. In addition to serving as a sensitive index of biliary obstruction, serum alkaline phosphatase is helpful in the early diagnosis of infiltrative diseases of the liver due to granulomas (tuberculosis, sarcoidosis, fungal disorders, etc.) and space-occupying lesions (abscesses and neoplasms). In hepatomegaly due to metastatic carcinoma, for example, serum alkaline phosphatase increases in over 90 per cent of cases.[23] The mechanism of increased serum alkaline phosphatase in these disorders is unknown but the small obstructive element present suggests hepatic overproduction of the enzyme.

The major value of the serum alkaline phosphatase in specifying the cause of liver disease is in differentiating hepatocellular from obstructive jaundice.[83, 209] When obstruction is complete and prolonged, as in carcinomatous involvement of the common bile duct, the serum enzyme activity is usually above 10 (about 80 per cent) and often over 25 Bodansky units. Levels below 10 units may be noted in obstructive jaundice of brief duration or in incomplete occlusion as in choledocholithiasis or ampullary carcinoma. Normal values in either group, however, are rare and strongly argue against obstructive jaundice. By contrast, in portal cirrhosis serum alkaline phosphatase rarely exceeds 15 Bodansky units, whereas in only about a third or less of patients with viral hepatitis is phosphatase over 10, and in only 5 per cent are values in excess of 15 Bodansky units. These incidence figures differ somewhat depending on the series of patients considered. Nevertheless, although incidence figures overlap somewhat for obstructive and parenchymal liver disease, a low serum alkaline phosphatase activity strongly argues against obstructive jaundice.[17, 177] A low value is more significant than a high one (greater than 15 Bodansky units), since the enzyme may be elevated substantially not only in extrahepatic obstructive jaundice but also in infiltrative or space-occupying lesions of the liver, cholangiolitic (viral or drug-induced) hepatitis, biliary cirrhosis and even portal cirrhosis accompanied by a fatty-obstructive syndrome.

In some series of cirrhotics, a serum alkaline phosphatase of over 15[47] and even of over 7 Bodansky units[77] favored a diagnosis of concomitant hepatoma. However, in 56 per cent of a series of 80 individuals with hepatoma the serum phosphatase was below 15 Bodansky units,[47] and in our own experience the overlap in phosphatase among cirrhotics with and without hepatoma renders the phosphatase of limited diagnostic value in the individual patient.

SERUM 5'-NUCLEOTIDASE

This phosphatase specifically catalyzes hydrolysis of nucleotides such as adenosine-5'-phosphate and inosine-5'-phosphate in which the phosphate is attached to the 5 position of the pentose moiety. Assay of the enzyme in serum is complicated since nonspecific alkaline phosphatase also catalyzes hydrolysis of a substrate such as adenosine-5'-phosphate. This has been circumvented by preliminary incubation of the serum with EDTA, which in appropriate concentrations inactivates only the alkaline phosphatase. Subsequently, the rate of hydrolysis of adenosine-5'-phosphate, at pH 7.5 and in the presence of 0.05 M Mg^{++} is determined, and a unit of 5'-nucleotidase activity is designated as equivalent to 1 mg. of phosphate liberated per hour per 100 ml. of serum. These units are analogous to Bodansky units of phosphatase activity and are expressed as such.[216] In most series of normal adult patients, the serum 5'-nucleotidase ranges from 0.3 to 3.2 Bodansky units, and apparently is not influenced by age, sex or race.[14, 91, 109, 216] Extensive data for children are not available, however.[91] The metabolism of serum 5'-nucleotidase has not been investigated and its physiologic function, if any, is unknown. In liver, the enzyme is located primarily in the canaliculi and sinusoidal membranes.

Serum values of this enzyme are elevated primarily in (1) normal pregnancy (presumably derived from placenta) and (2) hepatobiliary diseases with a spectrum of abnormality similar to that found for alkaline phosphatase. The major advantage of 5'-nucleotidase over the nonspecific alkaline phosphatase measurement in serum therefore is enhancement of specificity. Most studies show that serum 5'-nucleotidase does not rise in bone disease[91, 109, 216] (Fig. 6–17), and in the few instances in which an increase was observed it was of low magnitude.[55, 91] This is in striking contrast to alkaline phosphatase.

There is controversy concerning the relative sensitivity of 5'-nucleotidase and alkaline phosphatase in detecting hepatobiliary disease. Most studies indicate that on an average the 2 enzymes are equally valuable in demonstrating biliary obstruction or hepatic infiltrative and space-occupying lesions.[91, 109, 177, 216] In selected instances, however, either enzyme is elevated and the other is normal.[14, 55, 91, 202] While the coefficient of correlation between the 2 enzymes is high,[177] the values may not rise proportionately in individual patients.[14, 55]

As regards the relative value of 5'-nucleotidase and serum alkaline phosphatase in differentiating obstructive from parenchymal liver disease, there is considerable difference of opinion. All investigators have shown some overlap in 5'-nucleotidase values in obstructive and hepatocellular jaundice. Some have found this overlap to be small, and have concluded that this assay is equal to or better than the measurement of serum alkaline phosphatase for differentiating between these 2 types of jaundice,[14, 216] whereas in the studies of others,[55] the alkaline phosphatase had greater selective value.

Further experience is required to assess adequately the relative sensitivity and selectivity of serum 5'-nucleotidase and alkaline phosphatase determinations. The major value of the nucleotidase assay is its specificity for hepatobiliary disease. An increased serum 5'-nucleotidase level in a nonpregnant individual suggests, therefore, that concomitantly increased serum alkaline phosphatase is at least in part of hepatic origin. A normal nucleotidase in the presence of an elevated serum alkaline phosphatase, however, does not necessarily indicate that the phosphatase is not of hepatic origin since, as indicated above, occasionally either enzyme is normal and the other elevated in liver disease.[91]

SERUM LEUCINE AMINOPEPTIDASE

Leucine aminopeptidase, a proteolytic enzyme, can hydrolyze amino acids from the N-terminal end of a number of proteins and polypeptides. The enzyme is called leucine aminopeptidase since it reacts most rapidly with leucine compounds. Leucine aminopeptidase has been demonstrated in all human tissues assayed, with high activity in the liver where it is localized primarily in

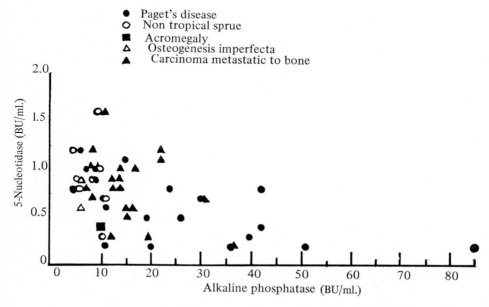

FIG. 6–17. 5'-Nucleotidase versus alkaline phosphatase in diseases affecting bone. Note that 5'-nucleotidase is normal in all instances. Cross-hatched area represents the normal range. *BU*, Bodansky unit. (Kowlessar, O. D., Haeffner, L. J., Riley, E. M., and Sleisenger, M. H.: Am. J. Med. *31*:231.)

biliary epithelium.[109] The intracellular function of this enzyme is not known but possibly involves hydrolysis of a peptide bond near an L-leucine residue or the transfer of L-leucine from one peptide to another.[173] The leucine aminopeptidase of normal serum as a rule is electrophoretically homogeneous and probably originates in liver, but in hepatobiliary disease several peaks of activity are detected and probably represent isoenzymes.[110]

The prevalent method for measuring serum leucine aminopeptidase involves α-leucyl-β-naphthyl-amide hydrochloride as a substrate with the liberated β-naphthylamine assayed colorimetrically by a modified Bratton-Marshall reaction.[71] There is some evidence that the peptidase responsible for this reaction differs from those that hydrolyze other leucine compounds.[147] Accordingly, in extrapolating data from one study to another one should carefully consider the substrate employed. Normal values, using α-leucyl-β-naphthylamine, usually range from 50 to 220 units without significant difference due to sex, age (from 18 to 75), or fasting.[12, 161]

The major advantage of the leucine aminopeptidase determination over serum alkaline phosphatase as for that of serum 5′-nucleotidase, is in its specificity. Leucine aminopeptidase is not elevated in patients with bone disease[12, 109, 172] and values of the enzyme in children, although based on a small number of determinations, are comparable to those of adults.[174] The only condition other than hepatobiliary disease known to result in an increase in this enzyme is pregnancy.[22, 23] Serum leucine aminopeptidase reaches an average value of 308 units at 2 months of gestation, rises to 382 units by 3 to 5 months and to 694 units at term. After delivery, the enzyme level falls, decreasing by about 35 per cent in 4 days. Electrophoresis of serum leucine aminopeptidase from pregnant individuals and those with liver disease shows much overlap between the various isoenzymes, and this procedure is probably of no practical value in differentiating between these 2 sources of the enzyme.[16]

There is general agreement that serum leucine aminopeptidase is at least as sensitive as alkaline phosphatase and 5′-nucleotidase in detecting obstructive, infiltrative or space-occupying lesions of the liver.[12, 14, 23, 109] Some consider leucine aminopeptidase superior in this respect, however, especially when compared to alkaline phosphatase and in the absence of icterus.[172] Contrary to original reports, pancreatic malignancy in the absence of hepatobiliary disease does not cause an elevation in serum leucine aminopeptidase.[23]

There is disagreement as to the value of leucine aminopeptidase in differentiating parenchymal hepatic involvement from obstructive and infiltrative liver disease. Banks and associates find values of more than 450 units only rarely (5 to 6 per cent) in patients with jaundice due to cirrhosis and hepatitis, but frequently in those with jaundice due to extrahepatic biliary obstruction caused by pancreatic carcinoma (85 per cent) or due to hepatic metastases (54 per cent).[12] In patients without overt jaundice, a less marked but similar difference among the various groups was found by these investigators.[172] Others observed a considerable overlap in values among the various patient groups and concluded that alkaline phosphatase is more selective in establishing the diagnosis.[23, 109] Further studies with emphasis on serial determinations may resolve these differences. Electrophoretic analysis of serum leucine aminopeptidase has demonstrated several isoenzymes in various forms of liver disease. The precise origin of these heterogeneous enzyme peaks is not established. Analysis of available data suggests that partition of serum into leucine aminopeptidase isoenzymes by current methods will not enhance the selectivity of this assay.[110]

The major confirmed value for serum leucine aminopeptidase is its specificity for liver disease. In this regard, both it and the 5′-nucleotidase seem to have equal merit, though more data are available for aminopeptidase.

SERUM PROTEINS

Serum contains a complex mixture of proteins which have been studied extensively by a variety of technics.[162] A schematic representation of the results of some of the methods in current use are shown in Figure 6–18. The liver is the major source of most of these serum proteins; the parenchymal cells are responsible for synthesis of albumin, fibrinogen and other coagulation factors, and most of the α and β-globulins.[60, 112, 127, 133] Gamma globulins are an important exception, being synthesized in the reticuloendothelial system.[133]

Of the various methods for assessing serum proteins, fractionation into major constituents by a fractional salting out method[81] or by paper electrophoresis,[145] is used most frequently in the clinical appraisal of hepatobiliary disease. Salting out methods provide values for albumin and globulins whereas electrophoretic technics give values for albumin, α_1, α_2, β and γ-globulins. Salting out technics do not separate the protein

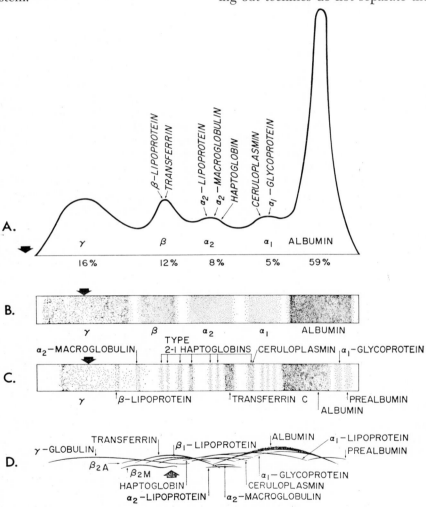

Fig. 6–18. Schematic representation of the electrophoretic pattern of normal human serum in pH 8.6 buffer as obtained by 4 methods: (A) Tiselius or free boundary electrophoresis, (B) paper electrophoresis, (C) starch-gel electrophoresis and (D) immunoelectrophoresis. The broad, vertical arrow indicates the starting point in each case. β_{2M}-Globulin remains in the starting slot in starch-gel electrophoresis but moves in the γ- to β-range in other methods. (Putnam, F. W.: Structure and function of the plasma proteins, in Neurath, H., ed.: The proteins, vol. III, ed. 2, New York, Academic Press, 1965.)

TABLE 6–10. DISTRIBUTION OF PROTEINS IN NORMAL SERUM

TOTAL PROTEIN	ALBUMIN	GLOBULINS				
		Total	α_1	α_2	β	γ
1. Howe's method—gm.%						
Mean 7.2[1]	5.2	2.0				
Range (6.5–7.9)	(4.7–5.7)	(1.3–2.5)				
2. Paper electrophoresis,[2] pH 8.6						
a. Per cent of total protein						
Mean	60		4	8	12	16
Range	(52–68)		(2–6)	(5–11)	(8–16)	(10–22)
b. gm.% 7.2 X mean % for each fraction	4.3	2.9	0.3	0.6	0.9	1.1

1. Data of Gutman, A. B., et al.: J. Clin. Invest. *20*:765.
2. Adapted from Owen, J. A., *in* Sobotka, H., and Stewart, C. P., eds.: Advance in Clinical Chemistry, vol. I, p. 237. New York, Academic Press, 1958.

fractions completely. Thus, with the commonly used Howe's method,[93, 94] the fraction called globulins and which precipitates in 21.5% sodium sulfate solution contains all the γ-globulins, approximately three-fourths of the β-globulins, and one-fourth of the α-globulins, whereas the "albumin" filtrate contains albumin plus most of the α-globulins and a portion of the β-globulins.[81, 149] The relationships between the results of Howe's and electrophoretic methods are less predictable in diseases states.[149] Therefore, higher values for albumin are usually obtained by a salting out than by an electrophoretic method, and the reverse is true for values for total globulins.

Results for albumin and globulins obtained by Howe's method and by paper electrophoresis are compared in Table 6–10. The range of normal values varies from those presented, depending on the specific technics used in any laboratory, and the data recorded in Table 6–10 should be considered as illustrative. Electrophoretic methods permit a more detailed fractionation of serum proteins (Fig. 6–18). These procedures separate proteins by an electric field in which the extent to which a protein migrates is determined primarily by its net charge. Of the various technics, filter paper electrophoresis is used most extensively at present. Results are reported as the proportion of the total protein migrating as albumin, α_1, α_2, β

and γ-globulins. Absolute concentrations for each electrophoretic fraction may be obtained by multiplying values for total protein, measured separately, by the proportion of protein in each fraction. Absolute values provide little additional information above proportions, however, since the level of total protein usually remains within the normal range in the majority of patients with hepatobiliary disease.[146, 153]

A fall in the concentration of serum albumin and a rise in globulins, primarily due to an increase in γ-globulin, are the changes found most commonly in most forms of hepatobiliary disease[62, 63, 81, 128, 138, 146, 148, 169, 175, 193, 194] (Fig. 6–19, Table 6–11). The extent of these protein alterations appears to depend on both the severity and the duration of the underlying hepatic disease, and is reflected equally well in results obtained by the salting out or electrophoretic methods. In mild cases of acute viral hepatitis the serum proteins are usually normal. With more severe hepatic involvement, albumin concentration falls and globulins rise. Elevations of γ-globulin to 40 per cent or more of the total proteins, and of total globulins to 4 gm.% or higher, frequently, although not invariably, indicate that the disease is progressing to a chronic active stage.[146] This impression is supported more strongly when the concentration of albumin falls simultaneously to less than 3 gm.%. These protein

TABLE 6–11. SERUM-PROTEIN LEVELS IN PATIENTS WITH HEPATOBILIARY DISEASE

DIAGNOSIS	No. OF CASES	TOTAL PROTEIN (Gm. per 100 ml.)	ALBUMIN (%)	GLOBULIN (%)			
				α_1	α_2	β	γ
Normal	34	7.0 (5.6–8.4)	65 (57–72)	5 (2–8)	6 (3–9)	9 (5–14)	15-(10–21)
Infective hepatitis	21	7.1	53	5	7	13	22
Extrahepatic neoplasm	13	6.3	43	6	11	16	23
Stone in common bile-duct	22	6.4	46	6	10	12	25
Cholecystitis	9	6.7	50	6	10	12	23
Diffuse hepatic fibrosis	12	6.3	31	6	6	9	47
Precirrhotic hepatitis	4	7.3	56	5	9	11	20
Cardiac cirrhosis	7	6.1	49	7	10	15	20
Secondary neoplasm in liver	5	5.8	46	7	12	12	23
Reticulosis in liver	3	5.3	51	8	10	11	20
Acute hepatic necrosis	2	6.7	49	3	3	6	41
"Cholangiolitic cirrhosis"	2	6.8	40	6	9	12	34

(Results are expressed as means to the nearest whole number, with the range (±2 S.D.) for normals only; the ranges in each diagnostic category were never less than the corresponding value in normals)
(Owen, J. A., and Robertson, R. F.: Lancet 2:1125, 1956.)

changes may be observed even in the absence of jaundice. By contrast, maintenance of albumin near normal, and only modest elevation of total and γ-globulins usually

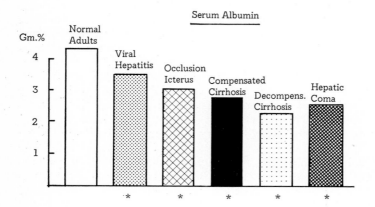

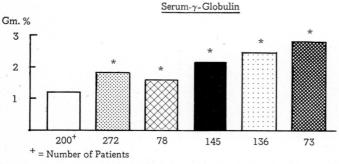

+ = Number of Patients

* = p <0.001 in comparison with the Normal Values

FIG. 6–19. Serum protein levels in 704 patients with liver disease. (Müting, D., and Reikowski, H., in Popper, H., and Schaffner, F. (eds.): Progress in Liver Disease, vol. II, p. 84, New York, Grune & Stratton, 1965.)

indicate a good outcome, even when hepatitis is judged to be severe symptomatically.[146] An exception is the occasional patient in whom fulminant hepatic necrosis supervenes so quickly that serum proteins are not altered much.

Hypoalbuminemia and hyperglobulinemia are also characteristic findings in the various cirrhoses and tend to be more marked than in acute hepatocellular disease. In advanced cases albumin values are frequently reduced to 2 to 3 gm.% and total globulins exceed 3.5 gm.%. Very high globulins, in excess of 5 gm.%, are found in some patients with active postnecrotic cirrhosis, particularly in the early stages. Persistent hyperglobulinemia with normal serum albumin may be seen in well-compensated cirrhotics of the alcoholic-nutritional and postnecrotic types. Progression of alcoholic liver disease from a noncirrhotic to a cirrhotic stage is frequently indicated by a progressive rise in globulins.

Alpha-globulins may increase slightly, remain unchanged or even fall in hepatic disorders, and their alterations are seldom of diagnostic value. In some cases of extrahepatic obstruction and of metastatic tumor, the α_2-globulins are increased considerably and γ-globulins are normal. This may be of some diagnostic assistance. β-Globulins tend to rise in most hepatic diseases. Marked rises are observed in many cases with extrahepatic obstruction, primary biliary cirrhosis and the "obstructive" phase of viral hepatitis with the Tiselius electrophoretic method,[153, 193] and largely reflect the increase in serum lipoproteins in these disorders. Such changes are usually not recorded by paper electrophoresis, however.[146]

Information obtained from protein fractionation indicates the extent of hepatocellular damage and has prognostic significance. As indicated, a serum albumin value of less than 3 gm.% and globulins greater than 4 gm.% usually connote a chronic or progressive form of liver disease or both. An albumin value of 2 to 3 gm.% in a malnourished cirrhotic that increases to or toward normal with treatment indicates a reasonable improvement in hepatocellular function, and obviously implies a more favorable prognosis than if albumin remains low, or falls even further despite abstinence from alcohol and good intake of food. In the latter instance, usually various complications intercede during the course of chronic liver disease. The importance of the protein changes in hepatitis are referred to above.

Protein analysis is limited in 3 main spheres. First, it is not a sensitive indicator of liver disease. Second, it has little value in differential diagnosis, because frequently serum proteins are altered similarly in all types of liver disease. Experience with immunoglobulin determinations is still too limited to know if they will be of much assistance in diagnosis. Third, even marked protein changes are not specific for liver disease. Hypoalbuminemia and hyperglobulinemia primarily due to hypergammaglobulinemia are observed in many disorders that are not primarily hepatic.

FLOCCULATION TESTS

In a number of semi-empirical tests the addition of reagents to sera from patients with diffuse liver cell injury usually produces a precipitate, turbidity or flocculation. By contrast, little or no effect is detected with sera from normal persons or the majority of patients with obstructive jaundice.

Most of the tests depend on an imbalance of factors in sera: some produce and others inhibit the particular reaction.[8, 103, 115, 124, 125, 136, 167, 168] For example, normal γ-globulin contains flocculating activity. Gamma globulin from patients with hepatitis and cirrhosis has greater activity. Antiflocculating or stabilizing activity is attributable to the serum albumin–α_1-globulin fraction. The inhibitory potency of these latter proteins is decreased in sera obtained from patients with diffuse parenchymal disease. Thus, qualitative and/or quantitative changes in the serum protein fractions resulting in enhanced flocculating or diminished inhibitory activity, or both, account for the flocculation reactions. Alterations in other protein components of serum such as the α- and β-globulins may also contribute to flocculation, and mucoproteins are considered to be inhibitory. The cephalin-cholesterol flocculation[86] and thymol turbidity tests,[122] probably the most widely used in this group, are largely based on the interaction of the

TABLE 6–12. CHEMISTRY OF FLOCCULATION TESTS

TEST	PRECIPITATING AGENT	pH	IONIC STRENGTH	SERUM DILUTION FACTOR	PROTEIN FRACTION ACTIVE Precipitating	Inhibitory
Takata-Ara	$HgCl_2$	ca 10	0.15	2–16	α, β, γ	Albumin
Formol gel	HCH:O	ca 8	0.15	1	α, β, γ	Albumin
Cephalin-cholesterol	CC Emulsion	ca 8	0.12	26	$(\alpha, \beta), \gamma$	Albumin
$CdSO_4$	$CdSO_4$	ca 8	0.10	1	$(\alpha, \beta), \gamma$	Albumin
Sharlach red	Sharlach red	ca 8	0.075	2–8	?	?
Weltmann	$CaCl_2$	ca 8	0.02–0.002	51	$(\alpha, \beta), \gamma$	Albumin
Colloidal gold	Colloidal gold	7.8	0.01	61	γ	Albumin α, β
Thymol	Thymol	7.8	0.01	61	$\gamma (\beta)$	Albumin
$ZnSO_4$	$ZnSO_4$	7.5	0.002	61	γ	—
$(NH_4)_2SO_4$	$(NH_4)_2SO_4$	5.5	4.8	51	γ	—

(Maclagan, N. F., *in* Schiff, L., ed.: Diseases of the Liver, ed. 2, p. 157, Philadelphia, Lippincott, 1963.)

protein factors enumerated above. The zinc sulfate[113] and ammonium sulfate turbidity tests[45] more closely reflect the concentration of γ-globulin in serum.[125] Alterations in other protein components of serum have comparatively little or no influence on these reactions. Lipids in serum also exert an important influence on some tests, particularly in the thymol turbidity test.[115] Phospholipids provide an essential ingredient of the latter reaction in which a protein-lipid-thymol precipitate forms. Moreover, the extent of turbidity in the thymol test is significantly affected by the degree of lipemia.[115]

A considerable number of flocculation tests have been introduced for the study of liver diseases (Table 6–12). These are described and discussed in detail in excellent reviews by Maclagan et al.[125] and Reinhold.[168] Selection of tests for laboratory appraisal of patients is undoubtedly influenced by local experience.

In general, the cephalin-cholesterol flocculation, thymol turbidity and zinc turbidity tests are used most frequently. Most importantly, these tests differentiate hepatocellular from obstructive liver diseases since they are sensitive indicators of active liver cell damage.[83, 86, 90, 92, 114, 123, 139, 190, 219, 220] Results are abnormal in approximately 80 to 90 per cent of patients with acute hepatitis. The incidence of abnormal thymol tests is somewhat lower in homologous serum hepatitis. These tests are likewise abnormal in a high

proportion of patients with cirrhosis in the presence of continuing liver cell damage, although the results tend to be more variable than in hepatitis. Cephalin flocculation is abnormal more frequently than thymol turbidity in cirrhosis of the alcoholic, whereas in active postnecrotic cirrhosis, both tests are positive with approximately equal frequency. The percentage of abnormal results falls in inactive cirrhosis. Zinc turbidity is abnormal less frequently in acute hepatitis, but is positive in a high proportion of cirrhotics, undoubtedly reflecting quantitative alterations in γ-globulin in these conditions. By contrast to the results observed in hepatocellular diseases, cephalin flocculation and thymol turbidity tests are abnormal in approximately 25 per cent of patients with obstructive jaundice of short duration, and zinc turbidity is elevated in an even smaller proportion, although there is less published experience with the latter test. Nevertheless, the cephalin-cholesterol flocculation was considered to be the most discriminative test in distinguishing between hepatocellular and obstructive jaundice.[90] The frequency of abnormal results increases with long-standing obstruction, and in the presence of superimposed infection, thus decreasing the differential diagnostic value of these tests.

Sensitivity of the flocculation tests in indicating hepatocellular disease is of value in a number of other circumstances. The cephalin-cholesterol flocculation test becomes positive early in acute hepatitis.[139] Soon thereafter, the thymol test becomes elevated.[114, 139] These changes commonly precede the appearance of hyperbilirubinemia and jaundice, thus providing early evidence of liver cell dysfunction. In this regard, they are not as sensitive as the transaminases which become abnormal even earlier than the flocculation tests[111] (Fig. 6–13). Abnormal results also serve as a sensitive means of detecting anicteric cases of hepatitis. They also are very helpful in differentiating the hepatic dysfunction of severe hyperemesis gravidarum from that of hepatitis in pregnancy. Whereas modest hyperbilirubinemia and transaminase elevations may occur in hyperemesis, flocculation tests are almost always normal.[3] By contrast, flocculation tests are abnormal in over 90 per cent of pregnant women with hepatitis.[1] These tests are of little value in assessing the course of hepatitis, because their return to normal may be delayed for months in a patient whose hepatitis has subsided by other criteria. In the jaundiced patient, negative flocculation as well as other liver tests indicate various types of congenital hyperbilirubinemia.

The alterations in serum proteins that account for abnormal flocculation tests are found in mild and severe forms of liver disease. Thus, the tests provide no index of the severity of liver cell damage. Moreover, serum proteins are changed similarly in a number of disorders that are not primarily hepatic. Abnormal flocculation tests in these conditions do not reflect hepatic cell damage and may be considered as false positive. Occasionally, false positive reactions in which turbidity results from an interaction of lipids and thymol may be found with grossly lipemic sera. Raising the ionic strength of the thymol buffer is said to detect such reactions since turbidity due to γ-globulin is abolished, whereas the false positive reaction due to lipemia persists.[115]

PROTHROMBIN TIME
(See Chap. 5)

Clotting is the end result of a complex series of chemical reactions involving some

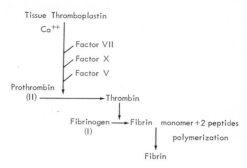

FIG. 6–20. Factors involved in Quick, one-stage prothrombin time.

13 factors (as of this writing).[163] Factors I—fibrinogen[60, 85, 135, 143]; II—prothrombin[3, 4, 15]; VII—serum prothrombin conversion accelerator (SPCA), stable factor[143, 152]; and X—Stuart-Prower factor[143] are synthesized in liver. Indirect evidence suggests the same for factors V—proaccelerin, labile factor; and IX—Christmas factor, plasma thromboplastin component.[166] Components of the clotting mechanism are frequently abnormal in the course of hepatic diseases.[50, 59, 141, 164, 166, 188] These abnormalities can be assessed by tests that measure one factor or the interplay of a number of factors. The one-stage prothrombin time of Quick[163] is one of the most useful tests available. It measures the rate at which available prothrombin is converted to thrombin in the presence of a tissue extract (thromboplastin), calcium ions, and a series of activated coagulation factors, followed by the polymerization of fibrinogen by thrombin to fibrin (Fig. 6–20). It is influenced by factors I, II, V, VII and X. The results may be expressed in (1) time in seconds; or, in an effort to standardize the procedure, as (2) a percentage read from a curve constructed from serial dilution in saline of commercial or pooled human plasma; or (3) as a ratio of the plasma prothrombin time to a control plasma time.[184] The second method of reporting is used most widely. A normal control is usually in the range of 11.5 to 12.5 seconds. In general, activity less than 75 per cent is considered abnormal, and values less than 50 per cent indicate a group at risk from bleeding.[188] The prothrombin time is prolonged if any of the involved factors is deficient,

TABLE 6–13. Number of Patients with Various Liver Diseases Showing Abnormal Results of Tests for Individual Blood Clotting Factors

Disease	Hepatitis (67 Cases)		Early Cirrhosis (60 Cases)		Postnecrotic Cirrhosis (29 Cases)		Severe Cirrhosis (67 Cases)		Biliary Obstruction (18 Cases)		Cancer (16 Cases)		Misc. Liver Diseases† (34 Cases)	
Test (method)	No. abnormal	No. less than 50% normal	No. abnormal	No. less than 50% normal	No. abnormal	No. less than 50% normal	No. abnormal	No. less than 50% normal	No. abnormal	No. less than 50% normal	No. abnormal	No. less than 50% normal	No. abnormal	No. less than 50% normal
Prothrombin time (Quick)	41	11	28	5	25	7	57	22	10	6	9	1	22	6
Factor II	41	14	26	7	27	10	56	31	11	6	7	1	26	9
Factor V	19	5	18	3	18	6	39	21	*	–	*	2	16	6
Factor VII	43	16	27	7	26	16	53	34	14	8	11	3	24	12
Factor X	17	4	21	6	20	3	38	26	7	5	6	1	16	6

* Frequently increased.

† Includes porphyria cutanea tarda, hemochromatosis, Wilson's disease, steatosis and primary biliary cirrhosis.

(Compiled from Deutsch, E.: Blood coagulation changes in liver diseases, in Popper, H., and Schaffner, F., eds.: Progress in Liver Diseases, vol. II. New York, Grune & Stratton, 1965.)

singly or in combination. Table 6–13 shows the frequency with which the test and the contributing factors are abnormal in various types of liver disease.

A prolonged prothrombin time is not specific for liver disease, being observed in various congenital deficiencies of coagulation factors[165, 166] and in acquired conditions including ingestion of drugs that affect the prothrombin complex.[163, 166] In these instances, the underlying cause can usually be elucidated. When the above are excluded, therefore, a prolonged prothrombin time may be the consequence of either (a) hypovitaminosis K as observed with prolonged obstructive jaundice, steatorrhea[20] or, much less commonly, dietary deficiency,[65, 104] or intake of antibiotics that alter the gut flora,[65] or of (b) poor utilization of vitamin K due to parenchymal liver disease. These 2 situations can usually be differentiated by parenteral administration of vitamin K_1.[20, 50, 191, 192] If the prothrombin time returns to normal, or rises by at least 30 per cent within 24 hours after a single parenteral injection of vitamin K_1 (doses of 5 to 10 mg. are usually used), one may surmise that parenchymal function is good and that hypovitaminosis K was responsible for the original prothrombin time. By contrast, no or a slight improvement is observed in the majority of patients with parenchymal liver disease. Most patients with extrahepatic obstruction respond promptly to vitamin K, and one would hesitate to make such a diagnosis if the prothrombin time did not respond. In jaundice, the type of response to vitamin K_1 is of some value in differential diagnosis, therefore. Observations of sluggish responses to vitamin K_1, with low values still recorded at 24 hours before normalization at 48 hours in some patients with obstructive jaundice, and of good responses in some patients with hepatocellular disease complicate interpretation, however.

The prothrombin test is not a sensitive index of liver disease, for even in severe cirrhosis results may be normal or the prothrombin time prolonged only slightly. On the other hand, the test has valuable prognostic value particularly in acute hepatocellular disease. In our experience, an abnormal prothrombin time with confirmed activity of less than 40 per cent of control is the single laboratory test that draws attention early to the likelihood of fulminant hepatic necrosis developing in the course of acute parenchymal damage, as seen with acute viral hepatitis, for example. Such a prolonged prothrombin time often precedes by days the manifestations of liver failure. Nevertheless, not all patients with abnormal prothrombin times of this extent develop evidence of fulminant hepatic necrosis.[56] Progressive shortening of the prothrombin time to normal usually precedes or accompanies other evidence of clinical improvement in this latter group, however. The degree of prolongation of the prothrombin time also is prognostic in alcoholic steatonecrosis. A prothrombin time greater than 4 seconds above control values occurred 6 times as often in a group of patients who died (60 per cent) as in a group who survived (10 per cent).[88] In chronic hepatocellular disease, an abnormal prothrombin time, particularly less than 50 per cent of normal, that does not respond to parenteral vitamin K_1 indicates extensive parenchymal damage and carries a poor long-term prognosis.[105, 188]

The prothrombin test is particularly important in the management of the patient with liver disease. It permits an assessment of the tendency to bleed before any contemplated surgical or diagnostic procedure such as closed liver biopsy, splenic puncture and transhepatic cholangiography. When the prothrombin time is prolonged, vitamin K_1 should be administered routinely in doses of 5 to 10 mg./day parenterally for up to 3 doses. It is difficult to indicate at what level of prothrombin time diagnostic procedures such as needle biopsy of the liver are contraindicated, since the risks of bleeding have not been well correlated with the values of this test. Furthermore, vascular reactivity and coagulation factors such as platelets exert an important contributory role. In our hospital, we do not perform closed needle biopsies if the prothrombin time is below 50 per cent; other hospitals are more restrictive.[186] For patients with prothrombin activity of less than 50 per cent of normal that does not respond to vitamin K_1, mortality is high after surgery such as portacaval shunt.[120] Obviously the performance of any open surgical procedure is determined by the urgency of the situation. The more pressing the need, the lower the prothrombin time that is accepted. Laparotomy without undue bleeding has been successful in several of our patients with liver disease in the face of prothrombin activity of 25 to 35 per cent of normal.

USE OF TESTS

We routinely perform the following group of tests at least once in patients in whom hepatic dysfunction is obvious or suspected:
1. Serum bilirubin: 1-minute direct-reacting and total.
2. SGOT.
3. Cephalin-cholesterol flocculation.
4. Thymol turbidity.
5. Serum alkaline phosphatase.
6. Total proteins with albumin and globulin partition.
7. Prothrombin time (Quick).
8. Urine for bilirubin.

These usually are sufficient to detect and characterize abnormalities in nonicteric and icteric patients. At times, a BSP test is included, usually in the patient with suspected liver disease when other tests are normal or the results do not clearly indicate hepatic dysfunction. An abnormal BSP test may be the only or earliest indication of liver disorder in patients with cirrhosis, hepatic metastases, granulomatous disease, amyloidosis, and drug reactions, to name but a few.

Occasionally, an elevated value for alkaline phosphatase is the only abnormal finding, or is accompanied by abnormal flocculation tests and by hyperglobulinemia. In the latter case, it may be difficult to determine whether the protein disturbances are due to liver disease or not. Measurements of leucine aminopeptidase or 5'-nucleotidase activity is then helpful in deciding whether the alkaline phosphatase abnormality is due to hepatic or extrahepatic disease. This is of definite value in the adult, and should be in children and adolescents, although information is sparse in persons with hepatic disease in the latter age group. These latter tests do not provide the same assistance in the latter half of pregnancy, during which activity is normally elevated. The extent to

which serum alkaline phosphatase is inactivated by heating may also indicate organ specificity, but additional experience with this technic is required before it can be recommended for routine use. When abnormal alkaline phosphatase results are accompanied by the presence of bilirubin in the urine, hyperbilirubinemia or elevations in transaminase activity, hepatic dysfunction can be inferred safely, and leucine aminopeptidase or 5'-nucleotidase activity is of little additional value.

DETECTION OF ABNORMALITIES

The SGOT and BSP tests are probably the most sensitive tests for detecting hepatic dysfunction. Other tests of value in this regard are the urine bilirubin, serum direct-reacting bilirubin, cephalin flocculation, thymol turbidity and alkaline phosphatase determinations. Urine bilirubin and serum direct-reacting bilirubin are the most specific for hepatic disease. This group of tests is of considerable value for screening purposes, particularly for detecting adverse reactions to drugs, preicteric or anicteric hepatitis, and infiltrative lesions of the liver.

PATTERN OF ABNORMALITIES

Differential Diagnosis of Jaundice. The partition of an elevated serum bilirubin into 1-minute direct-reacting and total divides most jaundiced patients into an unconjugated or conjugated group each with its respective diagnostic possibilities. Additional tests are required to determine whether or not unconjugated hyperbilirubinemia is characterized by overproduction of bile pigment (hemolysis, shunt hyperbilirubinemia). Bilirubin is absent as a rule from the urine in uncomplicated (no liver damage) unconjugated hyperbilirubinemia, but is usually present in conjugated hyperbilirubinemia.

When conjugated hyperbilirubinemia is present, the results of the initial group of tests aid in discriminating between hepatocellular and obstructive jaundice. An alkaline phosphatase greater than 10 Bodansky or 30 King-Armstrong units is found in the majority of patients with obstructive jaundice and supports the diagnosis, but may also be observed with hepatocellular disease. Alkaline phosphatase values that are normal should make one doubt the possibility of obstructive jaundice. Elevated transaminases in excess of 300 SGOT or 400 SGPT units indicate hepatocellular disease (the higher the value, the greater the support for acute hepatocellular disease). Values less than these are also consistent with hepatocellular disease but they are of little differential diagnostic assistance since frequently transaminase is elevated up to 300 or 400 units in hepatocellular and obstructive jaundice. Abnormal flocculation tests also indicate hepatocellular damage. Some feel that performance of these tests has become unnecessary with the introduction of transaminase tests. As indicated above, when transaminase values are very high, little additional information is provided by flocculation tests. However, we have found them to be of considerable diagnostic assistance in the jaundiced patient with transaminase results in the range that is not differentially diagnostic. For example, our initial appraisal of the jaundiced patient with the following findings: serum bilirubin, 1-minute direct-reacting 4 mg.%, total 6 mg.%, alkaline phosphatase 15 Bodansky units, SGOT 200 units, SGPT 250 units, is suggestive of obstructive jaundice when the cephalin-cholesterol flocculation is negative and thymol turbidity is less than 4 units, but is geared to hepatocellular disease when the cephalin-cholesterol flocculation is 4+ and the thymol turbidity 10 units. Normal transaminases and negative flocculation tests strongly suggest that conjugated hyperbilirubinemia is of congenital type.

Results of transaminase, flocculation and alkaline phosphatase tests usually overlap in acute and chronic hepatocellular diseases (hepatitis and cirrhosis are by far the major considerations). Transaminases in excess of 300 to 400 units favor acute hepatocellular disease whereas hyperglobulinemia, particularly when accompanied by hypoalbuminemia, favors chronic hepatocellular disease.

Even when hepatic diseases can be classified by laboratory tests into obstructive, hepatocellular (acute or chronic), hemolytic, etc., additional information is required to make a more precise diagnosis. For example,

obstructive jaundice chemically is not synonymous with surgical jaundice. Extrahepatic obstruction may be mimicked by disorders such as primary biliary cirrhosis, cholestatic drug reactions and certain types of viral hepatitis. The recently described immunofluorescent test[75, 203] that detects anticytoplasmic antibodies in the serum of patients with primary biliary cirrhosis but not with extrahepatic obstruction may provide an additional means of selecting patients with obstructive chemistries for surgery.

Laboratory tests commonly yield mixed results, with features of both hepatocellular and obstructive disease. History, physical examination, other laboratory tests, liver biopsy, radiologic studies as well as the course of the disease are some of the factors utilized in the overall assessment of each clinical problem that is bound to be influenced by the experience and judgment of the physician.

Early Recognition of Infiltrative Lesions. Elevated serum alkaline phosphatase by itself, or when accompanied by bilirubin in the urine, with or without a slight increase in direct-reacting or total serum bilirubin, may be the first indication of infiltrative lesions of the liver such as carcinoma, granuloma or amyloidosis. The same applies to leucine aminopeptidase and 5′-nucleotidase, although there is less experience with these latter enzymes. Abnormal BSP retention is also common. However, this constellation of findings may also be observed with incomplete obstruction of the biliary tract produced by common duct stone or stricture, with unilateral duct obstruction, and in the early stages of primary biliary cirrhosis.

EXTENT OF HEPATIC DYSFUNCTION—PROGNOSIS

Most of the tests discussed previously provide little prognostic information. The prothrombin time and serum albumin concentration are of most value in this regard. Serum bilirubin values are useful in alcoholic steatonecrosis.

The prothrombin time is probably the most valuable single test for early detection of acute hepatocellular disease (viral and toxic hepatitis) in which the syndrome of fulminant massive necrosis is likely to supervene. Prolongation of the prothrombin time to greater than 40 per cent, without improvement after parenteral administration of vitamin K, is frequently a grave finding in such a patient. Similar findings in cirrhosis also indicate severe parenchymal disease. If the prothrombin time does not improve with therapy, the overall prognosis is poor, but the course may be prolonged for many months or even longer. A similar connotation is inherent in the finding of a serum albumin concentration of less than 3 gm.% on the basis of parenchymal liver disease, when there is no response to therapy and particularly when progressive lowering of the albumin level ensues. Hyperbilirubinemia in excess of 5 mg./100 ml. is a poor prognostic finding in alcoholic steatonecrosis.

REFERENCES

1. Adams, R. H., and Combes, B.: Viral hepatitis during pregnancy, J.A.M.A. *192*:195, 1965.
2. Adams, R. H., Gordon, J., and Combes, B.: Measurements of hepatic storage and of maximal biliary transport of sulfobromophthalein sodium in man, Gastroenterology *51*:373, 1966.
3. ———: Hyperemesis gravidarum. I. Evidence of hepatic dysfunction, Obstet. & Gynecol. *31*:659, 1968.
3a. Anderson, G. F., and Barnhart, M. I.: Intracellular localization of prothrombin, Proc. Soc. Exp. Biol. Med. *116*:1, 1964.
4. ———: Prothrombin synthesis in the dog, Am. J. Physiol. *206*:929, 1964.
5. Arias, I., Bernstein, L., Toffler, R., Cornelius, C., Novikoff, A. B., and Essner, E.: Black liver disease in Corriedale sheep; a new mutation affecting hepatic excretory function, J. Clin. Invest. *43*:1249, 1964 (Abstract).
6. Arias, I. M., Gartner, L. M., Seifter, S., and Furman, M.: Prolonged neonatal unconjugated hyperbilirubinemia associated with breast feeding and a steroid, pregnane-3(α),20(β)-diol, in maternal milk that inhibits glucuronide formation *in vitro*, J. Clin. Invest. *43*:2037, 1964.
7. Arias, I. M., Wolfson, S., Lucey, J. F., and McKay, R. J., Jr.: Transient familial neonatal hyperbilirubinemia, J. Clin. Invest. *44*:1442, 1965.
8. Armas-Cruz, R., Lobo-Parga, G., Madrid, M., and Velasco, C.: Normal and pathologic proteins and flocculation tests; a contribution to the study of the mechanism of flocculation tests, Gastroenterology *35*:298, 1958.
9. Baikie, A. G.: The chromatographic separation of the serum bile pigments in jaundice, Scot. Med. J. *2*:359, 1957.
10. Baker, K. J.: Binding of sulfobromophthalein (BSP) sodium and indocyanine green (ICG) by plasma α_1 lipoproteins, Proc. Soc. Exp. Biol. Med. *122*:957, 1966.
11. Baker, K. J., and Bradley, S. E.: Binding of sulfobromophthalein (BSP) sodium by plasma albumin. Its role in hepatic BSP extraction, J. Clin Invest. *45*:281, 1966.
12. Banks, B. M., Pineda, E. P.. Goldbarg, J. A., and Rutenberg, A. M.: Clinical value of serum leucine aminopeptidase determinations, New Engl. J. Med. *263*:1277, 1960.
13. Barber-Riley, G., Goetzee, A. E., Richards, T. G., and Thomson, J. Y.: The transfer of Bromsulphthalein from the plasma to the bile in man, Clin. Sci. *20*:149, 1961.
14. Bardawill, C., and Chang, C.: Serum lactic dehydrogenase, leucine aminopeptidase and 5-nucleotidase activities: observations in patients with carcinoma of the pancreas and hepatobiliary disease, Canad. Med. Ass. J. *89*:755, 1963.
15. Barnhart, M. I.: Prothrombin synthesis: an example of hepatic function, J. Histochem. Cytochem. *13*:740, 1965.
16. Bechman, L.: Monographs in Human Genetics. I. Isozyme Variations in Man, Basel, New York, S. Karger, 1966.
17. Becker, K. L., and Stauffer, M. H.: Evaluation of concentrations of serum alkaline phosphatase in hepatitis and obstructive jaundice, Am. J. Med. Sci. *243*:222, 1962.
18. Birkett, D. J., Done, J., Neale, F. C., and Posen, S.: Serum alkaline phosphatase in pregnancy: an immunological study, Brit. Med. J. *1*:1210, 1966.
19. Bourke, E., Milne, M. D., and Stokes, G. S.: Mechanisms of renal excretion of urobilinogen, Brit. Med. J. *2*:1510, 1965.
20. Bouvier, C. A., and Maurice, P. A.: Liver and blood coagulation *in* Rouiller, C.

(ed.): The Liver, vol. II, pp. 177-213, New York, Academic Press, 1964.

21. Boyer, S. H.: Alkaline phosphatase in human sera and placentae, Science *134*: 1002, 1961.

22. Bressler, R., and Forsyth, B. R.: Serum leucine aminopeptidase activity in normal pregnancy and in patients with hydatidiform mole, New Engl. J. Med. *261*:746, 1959.

23. Bressler, R., Forsyth, B. R., and Klatskin, G.: Serum leucine aminopeptidase activity in hepatobiliary and pancreatic disease, J. Lab. Clin. Med. *56*:417, 1960.

24. Brohult, J.: Standardization of the Bromsulphalein test with respect to body composition, Scand. J. Clin. Lab. Invest. *19*: 67, 1967.

25. Caesar, J., Shaldon, S., Chiandussi, L., Guevara, L., and Sherlock, S.: The use of indocyanine green in the measurement of hepatic blood flow and as a test of hepatic function, Clin. Sci. *21*:43, 1961.

26. Cantarow, A., and Wirts, C. W.: Excretion of Bromsulphalein in the bile, Proc. Soc. Exp. Biol. Med. *47*:252, 1941.

27. Carbone, J. V., Grodsky, G. M., and Hjelte, V.: Effect of hepatic dysfunction on circulating level of sulfobromophthalein and its metabolites, J. Clin. Invest. *38*:1989, 1959.

28. Cherrick, G. R., Stein, S. W., Leevy, C. M., and Davidson, C. S.: Indocyanine green: observations on its physical properties, plasma decay, and hepatic extraction, J. Clin. Invest. *39*:592, 1960.

29. Chiandussi, L., Greene, S. F., and Sherlock, S.: Serum alkaline phosphatase fractions in hepatobiliary and bone diseases, Clin. Sci. *22*:425, 1962.

30. Clark, L. C., and Beck, E.: Plasma "alkaline" phosphatase activity. I. Normative data for growing children, J. Pediat. *36*:335, 1950.

31. Clermont, R. J., and Chalmers, T. C.: The transaminase tests in liver disease, Medicine *46*:197, 1967.

32. Clubb, J. S., Neale, F. C., and Posen, S.: The behavior of infused human placental alkaline phosphatase in human subjects, J. Lab. Clin. Med. *66*:493, 1965.

33. Combes, B.: Excretory function of the liver *in* Rouiller, C. (Ed.): The Liver. Vol. II, Chap. 12, New York, Academic Press, 1964.

34. ———: The importance of conjugation with glutathione for sulfobromophthalein sodium (BSP) transfer from blood to bile, J. Clin. Invest. *44*:1214, 1965.

35. Combes, B., Adams, R. H., Gordon, J., Trammell, V., and Shibata, H.: Hyperemesis gravidarum. II. Alterations in sulfobromophthalein sodium-removal mechanisms from blood, Obstet. & Gynec. *31*:665, 1968.

36. Combes, B., Shibata, H., Adams, R., Mitchell, B. D., and Trammell, V.: Alterations in sulfobromophthalein sodium-removal mechanism from blood during normal pregnancy, J. Clin. Invest. *42*: 1431, 1963.

37. Combes, B., and Stakelum, G. S.: A liver enzyme that conjugates sulfobromophthalein sodium with glutathione, J. Clin. Invest. *40*:981, 1961.

38. ———: Conjugation of sulfobromophthalein sodium with glutathione in thioether linkage by the rat, J. Clin. Invest. *39*:1214, 1960.

39. Combes, B., Wheeler, H. O., Childs, A. W., and Bradley, S. E.: The mechanisms of Bromsulphalein removal from the blood, Trans. Assoc. Am. Phycns. *69*: 276, 1956.

40. Cooke, A. R., Harrison, D. D., and Skyring, A. P.: Use of indocyanine green as a test of liver function, Am. J. Digest. Dis. *8*:244, 1963.

41. Cornelius, C. E., and Gronwall, R. R.: A mutation in Southdown sheep affecting the hepatic uptake of sulfobromophthalein (BSP), indocyanine green, rose bengal, sodium cholate, and phylloerythrin from blood, Fed. Proc. *24*:144, 1965 (Abstract).

42. Crigler, J. F., and Najjar, V. A.: Congenital familial nonhemolytic jaundice with kernicterus, Pediatrics *10*:169, 1952.

43. Curphey, T. J., and Solomon, S: Studies on liver function in pneumococcus pneumonia, Am J. Med. Sci. *196*:348, 1938.

44. de Fraiture, W. H., Heemstra, H., Vegter, J. J. M., and Mandema, E.: Chromatographic separation of different Bromsulphalein metabolites in urine and bile, Acta Med. Scand. *165*:153, 1959.

45. de la Huerga, J., and Popper, H.: Estimation of serum gamma globulin concentration by turbidimetry, J. Lab. Clin. Med. *35*:459, 1950.

46. De Ritis, F., Giusti, G., Piccinino, F., and Cacciatore, L.: Biochemical laboratory

tests in viral hepatitis and other hepatic diseases, Bull. Wld. Hlth. Org. 32:59, 1965.

47. Delores, S. J., Cady, A., West, M., Chomet, B., and Zimmerman, H. J.: Primary carcinoma of the liver. Analysis of clinical and biochemical features of 80 cases, Am. J. Digest. Dis. 10:657, 1965.

48. Dent, C. E., and Harper, C. M.: Plasma-alkaline-phosphatase in normal adults and in patients with primary hyper-parathyroidism, Lancet 1:559, 1962.

49. Deren, J. J., Williams, L. A., Muench, H., Chalmers, T., and Zamcheck, N.: Comparative study of four methods of determining alkaline phosphatase, New Engl. J. Med. 270:1277, 1964.

50. Deutsch, E.: Blood coagulation changes in liver diseases in Popper, H., and Schaffner, F. (Eds.): Progress in Liver Diseases, New York, Grune & Stratton, 1965, Vol. 2, pp. 69-83.

51. Diamond, I., and Schmid, R.: Experimental bilirubin encephalopathy; the mode of entry of bilirubin-^{14}C into the central nervous system, J. Clin. Invest. 45:678, 1966.

52. Dollinger, M. R., and Brandborg, L. L.: Late elevation in serum Bromsulfalein in Dubin-Johnson Syndrome, Am. J. Digest. Dis. 12:413, 1967.

53. Dreyfus, J.-C., Schapira, G., and Schapira, F.: Serum enzymes in the physiopathology of muscle, Ann. N. Y. Acad. Sci. 75:235, 1959.

54. Dunn, M., Martins, J., and Reissmann, K. R.: The disappearance rate of glutamic oxalacetic transaminase from the circulation and its distribution in the body's fluid compartments and secretions, J. Lab. Clin. Med. 51:259, 1958.

55. Eshchar, J., Rudzki, C., and Zimmerman, H. J.: Serum levels of 5′-nucleotidase in disease, Am. J. Clin. Path. 47:598, 1967.

56. Fenster, L. F.: Viral hepatitis in the elderly; an analysis of 23 patients over 65 years of age, Gastroenterology 49:262, 1965.

57. Fenster, L. F., and Simon, F. R.: Studies on biliary excretion of alkaline phosphatase in the rat, Yale J. Biol. Med. 40:57, 1967.

58. Fevery, J., Claes, J., Heirwegh, K., and De Groote, J.: Hyperbilirubinemia: significance of the ratio between direct-reacting and total bilirubin, Clin. Chim. Acta 17:73, 1967.

59. Finkbiner, R. B., McGovern, J. J., Goldstein, R., and Bunker, J. P.: Coagulation defects in liver disease and response to transfusion during surgery, Am. J. Med. 26:199, 1959.

60. Forman, W. B., and Barnhart, M. I.: Cellular site for fibrinogen synthesis, J.A.M.A. 187:168, 1964.

61. Frankl, H. D., and Merritt, J. H.: Enzyme activity in the serum and common duct bile of dogs, Am. J. Gastroent. 31:166, 1959.

62. Franklin, M., Bean, W. B., Paul, W. D., Routh, J. I., de la Huerga, J., and Popper, H.: Electrophoretic studies in liver disease. I. Comparison of serum and plasma electrophoretic patterns in liver disease, with special reference to fibrinogen and gamma globulin patterns, J. Clin. Invest. 30:718, 1951.

63. ————: Electrophoretic studies in liver disease. II. Gamma$_1$ globulin in chronic liver disease, J. Clin. Invest. 30:729, 1951.

64. Freston, J. W., and Englert, E.: The influence of age and excessive body weight on the distribution and metabolism of Bromsulphalein, Clin. Sci. 33:301, 1967.

65. Frick, P. G., Riedler, G., and Brogli, H.: Dose response and minimal daily requirement for vitamin K in man, J. Appl. Physiol. 23:387, 1967.

66. Fulop, M., and Sandson, J.: The role of bile salts in urinary bilirubin excretion in Bouchier, I. A. D., and Billing, B. H. (Eds.): Bilirubin Metabolism, Oxford and Edinburgh, Blackwell, 1967, pp. 253-262.

67. Fulop, M., Sandson, J., and Brazeau, P.: Dialyzability, protein binding, and renal excretion of plasma conjugated bilirubin, J. Clin. Invest. 44:666, 1965.

68. Gambino, S. R., Other, A., and Burns, W.: Direct serum bilirubin and sulfobromophthalein test in occult liver disease, J.A.M.A. 201:1047, 1967.

69. Gellis, S. S., and Stokes, J., Jr.: The methylene blue test in infectious (epidemic) hepatitis, J.A.M.A. 128:782, 1945.

70. Gliedman, M. L., Popowitz, L., and Dennis, C.: The preoperative diagnosis of cancerous obstructive jaundice—the quantitative fecal urobilinogen test in

Ariel, I. M. (Ed.): Progress in Clinical Cancer, Vol. II, p. 68, New York, Grune & Stratton, 1966.

71. Goldbarg, J. A., and Rutenburg, A. M.: Colorimetric determination of leucine aminopeptidase in urine and serum of normal subjects and patients with cancer and other diseases, Cancer *11*:283, 1958.

72. Goldstein, J., and Combes, B.: Spectrophotometric assay of the liver enzyme that catalyzes glutathione conjugation, J. Lab. Clin. Med. *67*:863, 1966.

73. Goodman, R. D., and Kingsley, G. R.: Sulfobromophthalein clearance test, J.A.M.A. *153*:462, 1953.

74. Goresky, C. A.: Initial distribution and rate of uptake of sulfobromophthalein in the liver, Am. J. Physiol. *207*:13, 1964.

75. Goudie, R. B., MacSween, R. N. M., and Goldberg, D. M.: Serological and histological diagnosis of primary biliary cirrhosis, J. Clin. Path. *19*:527, 1966.

76. Gray, C. H.: Bile Pigments in Health and Disease, Springfield, Ill., C. C Thomas, 1961.

77. Greene, L. S., and Schiff, L.: Primary carcinoma of the liver—a plea for earlier diagnosis with emphasis on the serum alkaline phosphatase values, Gastroenterology *40*:219, 1961.

78. Gregory, C. H.: Studies of conjugated bilirubin. III. Pigment I, a complex of conjugated and free bilirubin, J. Lab. Clin. Med. *61*:917, 1963.

79. Grodsky, G. M., Carbone, J. V., and Fanska, R.: Biosynthesis of a sulfobromophthalein mercaptide with glutathione, Proc. Soc. Exp. Biol. Med. *106*:526, 1961.

80. Gronwall, R., and Cornelius, C. E.: Biliary excretion of sulfobromophthalein in sheep, Fed. Proc. *25*:576, 1966 (Abstract).

81. Gutman, A. B.: The plasma proteins in disease *in* Anson, M. L., and Edsall, J. T. (Eds.): Advances in Protein Chemistry, Vol. IV, p. 155, New York, Academic Press, 1948.

82. ————: Serum alkaline phosphatase activity in diseases of the skeletal and hepatobiliary systems, Am. J. Med. *27*:875, 1959.

83. Gutman, A. B., and Hanger, F. M., Jr.: Differential diagnosis of jaundice; by combined serum phosphatase determination and cephalin flocculation test, Med. Clin. N. Amer. *25*:837, 1941.

84. Ham, T. H.: A syllabus of laboratory examinations in clinical diagnosis; critical evaluation of laboratory procedures in the study of the patient, Cambridge, Mass., Harvard U. Press, 1950, pp. 327-333.

85. Hamashima, Y., Harter, J. G., and Coons, A. H.: The localization of albumin and fibrinogen in human liver cells, J. Cell Biol. *20*:271, 1964.

86. Hanger, F. M.: Serological differentiation of obstructive from hepatogenous jaundice by flocculation of cephalin-cholesterol emulsions, J. Clin. Invest. *18*:261, 1939.

87. Hardison, W. G., and Lee, F. I.; Prognosis in acute liver disease of the alcoholic patient, New Engl. J. Med. *275*:61, 1966.

88. Harinasuta, U., Chomet, B., Ishak, K., and Zimmerman, H. J.: Steatonecrosis— Mallory body type, Medicine *46*:141, 1967.

89. Heino, A. E., and Jokipii, S. G.: Serum alkaline phosphatase levels in the aged, Ann. Med. Intern. Fenn. *51*:105, 1962.

90. Hill, E., and Zieve, L.: Discrimination between obstructive and hepatocellular jaundice by means of the commonly used serum tests, Am. J. Clin. Path. *27*:6, 1957.

91. Hill, P. G., and Sammons, H. G.: An assessment of 5′-nucleotidase as a liver-function test, Quart. J. Med. *36*:457, 1967.

92. Hoffbauer, F. W., Rames, E. D., and Meinert, J. K.: Limitations and merits of a single serum sample analysis in differential diagnosis of jaundice, J. Lab. Clin. Med. *34*:1259, 1949.

93. Howe, P. E.: The determination of proteins in blood—a micro method, J. Biol. Chem. *49*:109, 1921.

94. ————: The use of sodium sulfate as the globulin precipitant in the determination of proteins in blood, J. Biol. Chem. *49*:93, 1921.

95. Hunton, D. B., Bollman, J. L., and Hoffman, H. N., II: The plasma removal of indocyanine green and sulfobromophthalein: effect of dosage and blocking agents, J. Clin. Invest. *40*:1648, 1961.

96. Iber, F. L.: Reactions to sulfobromophthalein sodium injection, USP, Bull. Johns Hopkins Hosp. *116*:132, 1965.

97. Ingelfinger, F. J., Bradley, S. E., Mendeloff, A. I., and Kramer, P.: Studies with Bromsulphalein. I. Its disappearance from the blood after a single intravenous injection, Gastroenterology *11*: 646, 1948.

98. Ivy, J. H., and Hurley, J. W.: Routine urine bilirubin determinations, J.A.M.A. *176*:689, 1961

99. Javitt, N. B.: Phenol 3,6 dibromphthalein disulfonate, a new compound for the study of liver disease, Proc. Soc. Exp. Biol. Med. *117*:254, 1964.

100. Javitt, N. B., Wheeler, H. O., Baker, K. J., Ramos, O. L., and Bradley, S. E.: The intrahepatic conjugation of sulfobromophthalein and glutathione in the dog, J. Clin. Invest. *39*:1570, 1960.

101. Johnson, L. M.: The effect of certain substances on bilirubin levels and occurrence of kernicterus in genetically jaundiced rats, *in* Sass-Kortsak, A. (ed.): Kernicterus, Toronto, U. Toronto Press, 1961.

102. Jordan, W. S., Jr., and Albright, R. W.: Liver function tests in infectious mononucleosis, J. Lab. Clin. Med. *35*:688, 1950.

103. Kabat, E. A., Hanger, F. M., Moore, D. H., and Landow, H.: The relation of cephalin flocculation and colloidal gold reactions to the serum proteins, J. Clin. Invest. *22*:563, 1943.

104. Kark, R., and Lozner, E. L.: Nutritional deficiency of vitamin K in man: Study of 4 non-jaundiced patients with dietary deficiency, Lancet *2*:1162, 1939.

105. Katz, R., Velasco, M., Klinger, J., and Alessandri, H.: Corticosteroids in the treatment of acute hepatitis in coma, Gastroenterology *42*:258, 1962.

106. Klaassen, C. H. L.: Age and serum-alkaline-phosphatase, Lancet *2*:1361, 1966.

107. Klatskin, G.: Bile pigment metabolism, Ann. Rev. Med. *12*:211, 1961.

108. Klatskin, G., and Bungards, L.: An improved test for bilirubin in urine, New Engl. J. Med. *248*:712, 1953.

109. Kowlessar, O. D., Haeffner, L. J., Riley, E. M., and Sleisenger, M. H.: Comparative study of serum leucine aminopeptidase, 5-nucleotidase and non-specific alkaline phosphatase in diseases affecting the pancreas, hepatobiliary tree and bone, Am. J. Med. *31*:231, 1961.

110. Kowlessar, O. D., Haeffner, L. J., and Sleisenger, M. H.: Localization of leucine aminopeptidase in serum and body fluids by starch gel electrophoresis, J. Clin. Invest. *39*:671, 1960.

111. Krugman, S., and Ward, R.: Infectious Diseases of Children, ed. 2, St. Louis, Mosby, 1960.

112. Kukral, J. C., Sporn, J., Louch, J., and Winzler, R. J.: Synthesis of α- and β-globulins in normal and liverless dog, Am. J. Physiol. *204*:262, 1963.

113. Kunkel, H. G.: Estimation of alterations of serum gamma globulin by a turbidimetric technique, Proc. Soc. Exp. Biol. Med. *66*:217, 1947.

114. ———: Value and limitations of the thymol turbidity test as an index of liver disease, Am. J. Med. *4*:201, 1948.

115. Kunkel, H. G., and Hoagland, C. L.: Mechanism and significance of the thymol turbidity test for liver disease, J. Clin. Invest. *26*:1060, 1947.

116. Leevy, C. M., Smith, F., Longueville, J., Paumgartner, G., and Howard, M. M.: Indocyanine green clearance as a test for hepatic function, J.A.M.A. *200*:236, 1967.

117. Lester, R.: The intestinal phase of bile pigment excretion (editorial), Gastroenterology *47*:424, 1964.

118. Lester, R., and Schmid, R.: Bilirubin metabolism, New Engl. J. Med. *270*: 779, 1964.

119. Levine, R. A., and Klatskin, G.: Unconjugated hyperbilirubinemia in the absence of overt hemolysis; importance of acquired disease as an etiologic factor in 366 adolescent and adult subjects, Am. J. Med. *36*:541, 1964.

120. Liebowitz, H. R., and Rousselot, L. M.: Bleeding Esophageal Varices; Portal Hypertension, Springfield, Ill., Charles C Thomas, 1959.

121. Long, C. H., Ullrey, D. E., and Miller, E. R.: Serum alkaline phosphatase in the post-natal pig and effect of serum storage on enzyme activity, Proc. Soc. Exp. Biol. Med. *119*:412, 1965.

122. Maclagan, N. F.: Thymol turbidity test as an indicator of liver dysfunction, Brit. J. Exp. Path. *25*:234, 1944.

123. ———: Liver function tests in the diagnosis of jaundice; a review of 200 cases, Brit. Med. J. *2*:197, 1947.

124. Maclagan, N. F., and Bunn, D.: Flocculation tests with electrophoretically separated serum proteins, Biochem. J. *41*:580, 1947.

125. Maclagan, N. F., Martin, N. H., and Lunnon, J. B.: The mechanism and inter-relationships of the flocculation tests, J. Clin. Path. 5:1, 1952.

126. Mandema, E., de Fraiture, W. H., Nieweg, H. O., and Arends, A.: Familial chronic idiopathic jaundice (Dubin-Sprinz disease), with a note on Bromsulphalein metabolism in this disease, Am. J. Med. 28:42, 1960.

127. Marsh, J. B., and Whereat, A. F.: The synthesis of plasma lipoprotein by rat liver, J. Biol. Chem. 234:3196, 1959.

128. Martin, N. H.: An electrophoretic study of the components of the serum proteins in cirrhosis of the liver, Brit. J. Exp. Path. 30:231, 1949.

129. Mateer, J. G., Baltz, J. I., Marion, D. F., and MacMillan, J. M.: Liver function tests, J.A.M.A. 121:723, 1943.

130. McMaster, Y., Tennant, R., Clubb, J. S., Neale, F. C., and Posen, S.: The mechanism of the elevation of serum alkaline phosphatase in pregnancy, J. Obstet. Gynaec. Brit. Emp. 71:735, 1964.

131. Mendenhall, C. L., and Leevy, C. M.: False-negative Bromsulphalein tests, New Engl. J. Med. 264:431, 1961.

132. Meyer, R. R.: Effect of iopanoic acid on the sulfobromophthalein test, J.A.M.A. 194:343, 1964.

133. Miller, L. L., and Bale, W. F.: Synthesis of all plasma protein fractions except gamma globulin by the liver, J. Exp. Med. 99:125, 1954.

134. Miller, L. L., Bly, C. G., and Bale, W. F.: Plasma and tissue proteins produced by non-hepatic rat organs as studied with lysine-ϵ-C^{14}; gamma globulins, the chief plasma protein fraction produced by non-hepatic tissues, J. Exp. Med. 99:133, 1954.

135. Miller, L. L., Bly, C. G., Watson, M. L., and Bale, W. F.: The dominant role of the liver in plasma protein synthesis; a direct study of isolated perfused rat liver with the aid of lysine-ϵ-C^{14}, J. Exp. Med. 94:431, 1951.

136. Moore, D. B., Pierson, P. S., Hanger, F. M., and Moore, D. H.: Mechanism of the positive cephalin-cholesterol flocculation reaction in hepatitis, J. Clin. Invest. 24:292, 1945.

137. Mueller, M. N., and Kappas, A.: Estrogen pharmacology. I. The influence of estradiol and estriol on hepatic disposal of sulfobromophthalein (BSP) in man, J. Clin. Invest. 43:1905, 1964.

138. Müting, D., and Reikowski, H.: Protein metabolism in liver disease, in Popper, H., and Schaffner, F. (eds): Progress in Liver Diseases, vol. II, p. 84. New York, Grune & Stratton, 1965.

139. Neefe, J. R., and Reinhold, J. G.: Laboratory aids in the diagnosis and management of infectious (epidemic) hepatitis. Analysis of results obtained by studies on 34 volunteers during the early and convalescent stages of induced hepatitis, Gastroenterology 7:393, 1946.

140. Newton, M. A.: The clinical application of alkaline phosphatase electrophoresis, Quart. J. Med. 36:17, 1967.

141. Norcross, J. W.: The anemia of liver disease, Med. Clin. N. Amer. 50:543, 1966.

142. Nosslin, B.: The direct diazo reaction of bile pigments in serum: experimental and clinical studies, Scand. J. Clin. Lab. Invest. 12 (Suppl. 49), pp. 1-176, 1960.

143. Olson, J. P., Miller, L. L., and Troup, S. B.: Synthesis of coagulation factors by the in vitro perfused liver, Blood 22:828, 1963.

144. O'Máille, E. R. L., Richards, T. G., and Short, A. H.: Factors determining the maximal rate of organic anion secretion by the liver and further evidence on the hepatic site of action of the hormone secretin, J. Physiol. 186:424, 1966.

145. Owen, J. A.: Paper electrophoresis of proteins and protein-bound substances in clinical investigations, in Sobotka, H., and Stewart, C. P. (eds.): Advances in Clinical Chemistry, vol. I, p. 237, New York, Academic Press, 1958.

146. Owen, J. A., and Robertson, R. F.: Paper electrophoresis of serum proteins in hepatobiliary disease, Lancet 2:1125, 1956.

147. Patterson, E. K., Keppel, A., and Hsiao, S.: Evidence from purification procedures that the enzyme which hydrolyzes L-leucyl-β-naphthylamide is not the classical leucine aminopeptidase, J. Histochem. Cytochem. 9:609, 1961 (Abstract).

148. Petermann, M. L.: Alterations in plasma protein patterns in disease, in Putnam, F. W. (ed.): The Plasma Proteins, vol. II, p. 309. New York, Academic Press, 1960.

149. Petermann, M. L., Young, N. F., and Hogness, K. R.: A comparison of the Howe and the electrophoretic methods

for the determination of plasma albumin, J. Biol. Chem. *169*:379, 1947.

150. Philp, J. R., Grodsky, G. M., and Carbone, J. V.: Mercaptide conjugation in the uptake and secretion of sulfobromophthalein, Am. J. Physiol. *200*:545, 1961.

151. Polin, S. G., Spellberg, M. A., Teitelman, L., and Okumura, M.: The origin of elevation of serum alkaline phosphatase in hepatic disease. An experimental study, Gastroenterology *42*:431, 1962.

152. Pool, J. G., and Robinson, J.: In vitro synthesis of coagulation fraction by rat liver slices, Am. J. Physiol. *196*:423, 1959.

153. Popper, H., Bean, W. B., de la Huerga, J., Franklin, M., Tsumagari, Y., Routh, J. I., and Steigmann, F.: Electrophoretic serum protein fractions in hepatobiliary disease, Gastroenterology *17*:138, 1951.

154. Popper, H., and Schaffner, F.: Liver: Structure and Function, New York, McGraw-Hill, 1957, pp. 359-364.

155. Posen, S.: Alkaline phosphatase, Ann. Int. Med. *67*:183, 1967.

156. Posen, S., Neale, F. C., Birkett, D. J., and Brudenell-Woods, J.: Intestinal alkaline phosphatase in human serum, Am. J. Clin. Path. *48*:81, 1967.

157. Posen, S., Neale, F. C., and Clubb, J. S.: Heat inactivation in the study of human alkaline phosphatase, Ann. Int. Med. *62*:1234, 1965.

158. Powell, L. W., Billing, B. H., and Williams, H. S.: An assessment of red cell survival in idiopathic unconjugated hyperbilirubinaemia (Gilbert's syndrome) by the use of radioactive diisopropylfluorophosphate and chromium, Aust. Ann. Med. *16*:221, 1967.

159. Preisig, R., Morris, T. Q., Shaver, J. C., and Christy, N. P.: Volumetric, hemodynamic, and excretory characteristics of the liver in acromegaly, J. Clin. Invest. *45*:1379, 1966.

160. Preisig, R., Williams, R., Sweeting, J., and Bradley, S. E.: Changes in sulfobromophthalein transport and storage by the liver during viral hepatitis in man, Am. J. Med. *40*:170, 1966.

161. Pruzanski, W., and Fischl, J.: The evaluation of serum leucine-aminopeptidase estimation; the influence of the administration of steroids on S-LAP activity in obstructive disease of the biliary tract (preliminary report), Am. J. Med. Sci. *248*:581, 1964.

162. Putnam, F. W.: Structure and function of the plasma proteins, in Neurath, H. (ed.): The Proteins, vol. III, p. 153. New York and London, Academic Press, 1965.

163. Quick, A. J.: Hemorrhagic Diseases and Thrombosis, ed. 2, p. 391, Philadelphia, Lea and Febiger, 1966.

164. Rapaport, S. I., Ames, S. B., Mikkelsen, S., and Goodman, J. R.: Plasma clotting factors in chronic hepatocellular disease, New Engl. J. Med. *263*:278, 1960.

165. Ratnoff, O. D.: Bleeding Syndromes: A Clinical Manual, Springfield, Ill., Charles C Thomas, 1960.

166. ———: Hemostatic mechanisms in liver disease, Med. Clin. N. Amer. *47*:721, 1963.

167. Recant, L., Chargaff, E., and Hanger, F. M.: Comparison of the cephalin-cholesterol flocculation with the thymol turbidity test, Proc. Soc. Exp. Biol. Med. *60*:245, 1945.

168. Reinhold, J. G.: Flocculation tests and their application to the study of liver disease, in Sobotka, H., and Stewart, C. P. (eds.): Advances in Clinical Chemistry, vol. III, p. 83, New York, Academic Press, 1960.

169. Ricketts, W. E., and Sterling, K.: Electrophoretic studies of the serum proteins in virus hepatitis, J. Clin. Invest. *28*:1477, 1949.

170. Ritt, D. J., and Combes, B.: Enhancement of apparent excretory maximum of sulphobromophthalein sodium (BSP) by taurocholate and dehydrocholate, J. Clin. Invest. *46*:1108, 1967 (Abstract).

171. Rosenthal, S. M., and White, E. C.: Studies in hepatic function. VI. A. The pharmacological behavior of certain phthalein dyes; B. The value of selected phthalein compounds in the estimation of hepatic function, J. Pharmacol. Exp. Ther. *24*:265, 1924.

172. Rutenberg, A. M., Banks, B. M., Pineda, E. P., and Goldbarg, J. A.: A comparison of serum aminopeptidase and alkaline phophatase in the detection of hepatobiliary disease in anicteric patients, Ann. Int. Med. *61*:50, 1964.

173. Rutenberg, A. M., Goldbarg, J. A., and Pineda, E. P.: Leucine aminopeptidase activity; observations in patients with cancer of the pancreas and other diseases, New Engl. J. Med. *259*:469, 1958.

174. Rutenberg, A. M., Pineda, E. P., Gold-

barg, J. A., Levitan, R., Gellis, S. S., and Silverberg, M.: Serum leucine aminopeptidase activity: in normal infants, in biliary atresia, and in other diseases, Am. J. Dis. Child. *103*:47, 1962.

175. Satoskar, R. S., Lewis, R. A., and Gaitonde, B. B.: Electrophoretic studies of the plasma proteins in virus hepatitis, J. Lab. Clin. Med. *44*:349, 1954.

176. Schaefer, J., and Schiff, L.: Liver function tests in metastatic tumor of the liver: study of 100 cases, Gastroenterology *49*: 360, 1965.

177. Schenker, S., Balint, J., and Schiff, L.: Differential diagnosis of jaundice: Report of a prospective study of 61 proved cases, Am. J. Dig. Dis. *7*:449, 1962.

178. Scherb, J., Kirschner, M., and Arias, I. M.: Studies of hepatic excretory function: The effect of 17-α-19-nortestosterone on sulfobromophthalein sodium (BSP) metabolism in man, J. Clin. Invest. *42*:404, 1963.

179. Schiff, L., Billing, B. H., and Oikawa, Y.: Familial nonhemolytic jaundice with conjugated bilirubin in the serum; a case study, New Engl. J. Med. *260*:1315, 1959.

180. Schmidt, M. L., Gartner, L. M., and Arias, I. M.: Studies of hepatic excretory function. III. Effect of hypopituitarism on the hepatic excretion of sulfobromophthalein sodium in man, Gastroenterology *52*:998, 1967.

181. Schoenfield, L. J., Foulk, W. T., and Bollman, J. L.: Bile pigment partition in hepatic disease, Gastroenterology *47*:35, 1964.

182. Schoenfield, L. J., Foulk, W. T., and Butt, H. R.: Studies of sulfobromophthalein sodium (BSP) metabolism in man. I. In normal subjects and patients with hepatic disease, J. Clin. Invest. *43*: 1409, 1964.

183. Schoenfield, L. J., Grindlay, J. H., Foulk, W. T., and Bollman, J. L.: Identification of extrahepatic bilirubin monoglucuronide and its conversion to Pigment 2 by isolated liver, Proc. Soc. Exp. Med. Biol. *106*:438, 1961.

184. Seide, M. J.: Laboratory control of coumarin therapy: the clinician's dilemma, Ann. Int. Med. *57*:572, 1962.

185. Sherlock, S.: Biochemical investigations in liver disease; some correlations with hepatic histology, J. Path. Bact. *58*:523, 1946.

186. ———: Diseases of the Liver and Biliary System, Oxford, Blackwell Scientific Pub.; Philadelphia, Davis, 1963, p. 271.

187. Shotton, D., Carpenter, M., and Rinehart, W. B.: Bromsulphalein retention due to administration of a gall-bladder dye (Bunamiodyl), New Engl. J. Med. *264*:550, 1961.

188. Spector, I., and Corn, M.: Laboratory tests of hemostasis. The relation to hemorrhage in liver disease, Arch. Int. Med. *119*:577, 1967.

189. Steigmann, F., and Dyniewicz, J. M.: Studies of urobilinogen. I. The daily urobilinogen excretion in urine and feces in health and disease; an evaluation of Watson's and Sparkman's methods, Gastroenterology *1*:743, 1943.

190. Steigmann, F., Popper, H., Hernandez, R., and Shulman, B.: Flocculation tests in the diagnosis of hepatobiliary disease, Gastroenterology *13*:9, 1949.

191. Stein, H. B.: Effect of 2-methyl-1,4-naphthoquinone on clotting factors of blood of jaundiced patients with hypoprothrombinaemia, S. Afr. J. Med. Sci. *7*:72, 1942.

192. ———: "Prothrombin response to vitamin K test" in the differentiation between intra- and extrahepatic jaundice, S. Afr. J. Med. Sci. *9*:111, 1944.

193. Sterling, K., and Ricketts, W. E.: Electrophoretic studies of the serum proteins in biliary cirrhosis, J. Clin. Invest. *28*:1469, 1949.

194. Sterling, K., Ricketts, W. E., Kirsner, J. R., and Palmer, W. L.: The serum proteins in portal cirrhosis under medical management; electrophoretic studies, J. Clin. Invest. *28*:1236, 1949.

195. Straub, P. W.: A study of fibrinogen production by human liver slices in vitro by an immunoprecipitin method, J. Clin. Invest. *42*:130, 1963.

196. Taswell, H. F., and Jeffers, D. M.: Isoenzymes of serum alkaline phosphatase in hepatobiliary and skeletal disease, Am. J. Clin. Path. *40*:349, 1963.

197. Thompson, E. N., and Williams, R.: Effect of age on liver function with particular reference to Bromsulphalein excretion, Gut *6*:266, 1965.

198. Thompson, E. N., Williams, R., and Sherlock, S.: Liver function in extrahepatic portal hypertension, Lancet, *2*:1352, 1964.

199. Thompson, H. E., and Wyatt, B. L.: Ex-

perimentally induced jaundice (hyper-bilirubinemia); report of animal experimentation and of physiologic effect of jaundice in patients with atrophic arthritis, Arch. Int. Med. 61:481, 1938.

200. Tietz, N. W., Woodrow, D., and Woodrow, B.: A comparative study of the Bodansky and the Bessey-Lowry and Brock methods for alkaline phosphatase in serum, Clin. Chim. Acta 15:365, 1967.

201. Tisdale, W. A., Klatskin, G., and Kinsella, E. D.: The significance of the direct-reacting fraction of serum bilirubin in hemolytic jaundice, Am. J. Med. 26:214, 1959.

202. Vinnik, I. E., Kern, F., Jr., and Corley, W. D.: Serum 5-nucleotidase and pericholangitis in patients with chronic ulcerative colitis, Gastroenterology 45:492, 1963.

203. Walker, J. G., Doniach, D., Roitt, I. M., and Sherlock, S.: Serological tests in diagnosis of primary biliary cirrhosis, Lancet 1:827, 1965.

204. Watson, C. J.: Regurgitation jaundice: clinical differentiation of the common forms, with particular reference to the degree of biliary obstruction, J.A.M.A. 114:2427, 1940.

205. ———: The importance of the fractional serum bilirubin determination in clinical medicine, Ann. Int. Med. 45:351, 1956.

206. Watson, C. J., and Hawkinson, V.: Studies of urobilinogen. VI. Further experience with the simple quantitative Ehrlich reaction. Corrected calibration of Evelyn colorimeter with a pontacyl dye mixture in terms of urobilinogen, Am. J. Clin. Path. 17:108, 1947.

207. Watson, C. J., and Hoffbauer, F. W.: Liver function in hepatitis, Ann. Int. Med. 26:813, 1947.

208. Weber, A. P., Schalm, L., and Witmans, J.: Bilirubin monoglucuronide (Pigment I): a complex, Acta Med. Scand. 173:19, 1963.

209. West, M., and Zimmerman, H. J.: Serum enzymes in hepatic disease, Med. Clin. N. Amer. 43:371, 1959.

210. Wheeler, H. O., Cranston, W. I., and Meltzer, J. I.: Hepatic uptake and biliary excretion of indocyanine green in the dog, Proc. Soc. Exp. Biol. Med. 99:11, 1958.

211. Wheeler, H. O., Epstein, R. M., Robinson, R. R., and Snell, E. S.: Hepatic storage and excretion of sulfobromophthalein sodium in the dog, J. Clin. Invest. 39:236, 1960.

212. Wheeler, H. O., Meltzer, J. I., and Bradley, S. E.: Biliary transport and hepatic storage of sulfobromophthalein sodium in unanesthetiezd dog, in normal man, and in patients with hepatic disease, J. Clin. Invest. 39:1131, 1960.

213. Wilkinson, J. H.: Blood enzymes in diagnosis, in London University (Brit. Postgrad. Med. Fed.): Lectures on the Scientific Basis of Medicine, London, Athlone Press, 1958.

214. Wollaeger, E. E., and Gross, J. B.: Complete obstruction of the extrahepatic biliary tract due to carcinoma as determined by the fecal urobilinogen test: incidence and effect on serum bilirubin concentrations, Medicine 45:529, 1966.

215. Wroblewski, F.: The clinical significance of transaminase activities of serum, Am. J. Med. 27:911, 1959.

216. Young, I. I.: Serum 5-nucleotidase: characterization and evaluation in disease states, Ann. N. Y. Acad. Sci. 75:357, 1958.

217. Zelman, S.: The liver in obesity, Arch. Int. Med. 90:141, 1952.

218. Zieve, L., and Hill, E.: An evaluation of factors influencing the discriminative effectiveness of a group of liver function tests. II. Normal limits of 11 representative hepatic tests, Gastroenterology 28:766, 1955.

219. ———: An evaluation of factors influencing the discriminative effectiveness of a group of liver function tests. III. Relative effectiveness of hepatic tests in cirrhosis, Gastroenterology 28:785, 1955.

220. Zieve, L., Hill, E., and Hanson, M.: An evaluation of factors influencing the discriminative effectiveness of a group of liver function tests. V. Relative effectiveness of hepatic tests in viral hepatitis, Gastroenterology 28:927, 1955.

221. Zieve, L., Hill, E., Hanson, M., Falcone, A. B., and Watson, C. J.: Normal and abnormal variations and clinical significance of the one-minute and total serum bilirubin determinations, J. Lab. Clin. Med. 38:446, 1951.

222. Zimmerman, H. J., and West, M.: Serum enzyme levels in the diagnosis of hepatic disease, Am. J. Gastroent. 40:387, 1963.

7

Needle Biopsy of the Liver

LEON SCHIFF, m.d., ph.d., and *EDWARD A. GALL*, m.d.

Although puncture of the liver has been practiced for many years in the diagnosis and the treatment of hepatic abscess, the first attempt at diagnostic aspiration of liver tissue by means of a syringe and a trocar is said to have been made by Lucatello in 1895.[32] Scattered reports on the aspiration of liver tissue fragments for diagnostic purposes between 1907 and 1928 are recorded by Roholm, Krarup, and Iversen.

In 1939 Baron published his experience with 48 hepatic aspirations performed on 35 patients.[4] He used a 20-cc Luer-Lok or "Record" syringe and a 13-gauge needle about 9 cm. long. The intercostal route was employed in several cases, but he preferred the subcostal approach, presuming this to offer less hazard of hemorrhage. He appended a note to his report indicating that he had one death from hemorrhage directly attributable to the procedure in a case of extensive metastatic carcinoma of the liver. He found the method of value in the recognition of metastatic carcinoma of the liver and in the differential diagnosis of jaundice. In the same year (1939) Iversen and Roholm[25] published their paper on aspiration biopsy of the liver and their studies in acute epidemic hepatitis.

These reports served as an important impetus to the use of the method. Needle biopsy is now employed throughout the world and is an important factor in the clinical appraisal of hepatic disorders.

METHOD

While various needles and procedural modifications have been proposed,[5, 11, 20, 21,] [25, 35–37, 40, 51, 53, 60, 61, 73, 76, 78, 84] the technic most commonly used in this country is essentially the transthoracic approach of Iversen and Roholm. The Vim-Silverman needle, a cutting mechanism originally utilized by Tripoli and Fader[73] for hepatic biopsy via the subcostal route, has proved to be an instrument of wide choice, although it has been replaced in many areas by the Menghini and other needles.

At the Cincinnati General Hospital, needle biopsy of the liver is carried out on the wards, and the intercostal approach is used almost exclusively. It provides the whole transverse depth of the right lobe for puncture, and intra-abdominal viscera are avoided. It does, however, involve puncture of the pleural cavity. The subcostal approach is applicable only if the liver is enlarged to at least 6 cm. below the right costal margin. It has the theoretical advantage of selecting for puncture a specific area on the surface of the liver. We have not used the subxiphoid approach.

The technic employing the Vim-Silverman needle (Fig. 7–1) is still the one of choice at the Cincinnati General Hospital and is carried out as follows:

The upper limit of liver dullness at the end of expiration is suitably marked, and the point of biopsy selected one interspace below, between the anterior and the midaxillary lines. The point of entry is usually the eighth or ninth intercostal space. The area chosen is sterilized with thimerosal tincture, N.F., followed by 70 per cent alcohol, and is draped with sterile towels. The operator wears sterile rubber gloves.

It is advisable to test the patient's ability to

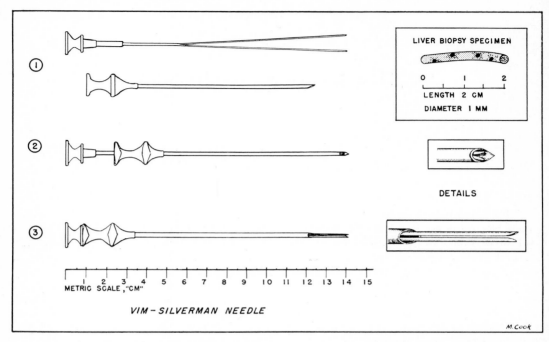

FIG. 7–1. Vim-Silverman needle and average size of biopsy specimen. (1) Forked obturator removed from outer cannula; (2) position of the obturator as the needle is introduced into the liver; and (3) position of the obturator as it cuts a tissue specimen. (McGregor Instrument Co., Needham, Mass.) (Schiff, L.: Clinical Approach to Jaundice, Springfield, Ill., Charles C Thomas)

hold his breath after inhaling and exhaling deeply 3 times. The skin, subcutaneous tissue, intercostal muscle, pleura, diaphragm, Glisson's capsule, and hepatic substance are infiltrated with 2 per cent procaine hydrochloride solution, care being taken to penetrate beyond the intercostal space only while the patient is holding his breath at the end of full expiration. Approximately 8 cc. of procaine hydrochloride solution is used. A small incision is made in the skin over the procaine bleb with a No. 11 Bard-Parker blade to permit easy entry of the biopsy needle. *The needle must be sharp.*

The Vim-Silverman needle is introduced into the incision, with the forked obturator retracted back of the tip, as first suggested by Hoffbauer. After the patient has inhaled and exhaled deeply 2 or 3 times, he is instructed to hold his breath at the end of complete expiration. The needle assembly is inserted promptly a distance of approximately 6 cm. (2 to 3 cm. into the substance of the liver) in a slightly downward direction. Then the obturator is pushed firmly until the final 1.5 cm. enters into the needle, while the latter is held steady. At this point *the obturator tip is held steady while the carrier needle is advanced over it with a*

rotating motion, bringing the assembly back to its original relations but advanced 1.5 cm. farther into the liver. This bores a cylinder of hepatic tissue which is usually 1 mm. in diameter and 1 to 2 cm. in length and grasps it tightly in the obturator fork. The entire assembly is rotated approximately 90°, breaking the terminal attachment of the liver fragment, and then is withdrawn. (The average time elapsing between entry of the Vim-Silverman needle into the substance of the liver and its removal is 5 to 10 seconds.)

A simple dressing is applied. The patient is kept in bed on his back for 24 hours and observed carefully for evidences of hemorrhage. This is particularly important during the first 8 to 12 hours when hourly pulse and blood pressure readings are desirable. Often a synthetic vitamin K preparation (10 mg.) is administered parenterally a day before and for 2 or 3 days after the procedure. Nelson has described his method in detail,[40] in which he uses a modified Vim-Silverman needle.

MENGHINI TECHNIC

Stressing the fact that the greatest risk of needle biopsy of the liver occurs while the needle is in the liver substance, Menghini[35-38] has introduced a technic in which the needle remains in the liver only about 1 second, instead of the usual 5 to 10 seconds with the Vim-Silverman needle. He accomplishes this with the aid of suction and a specially designed needle that does not require rotation to cut loose the tissue specimen.

Since it is generally accepted that the risk of hemorrhage increases with increase in the diameter of the needle, the walls of the needle are ultrathin (90 μ) to allow for a relatively wider specimen. The cannula is 7 cm. long. The tip is oblique and slightly convex toward the outside. A needle 3.5 cm. long is recommended for pediatric use. Menghini has abandoned the wide (2 mm.) gauge and employs 1.4, 1.2 and 1 mm. needles only; he recommends the 1.2 mm. needle for routine clinical practice and the 1 mm. bore for beginners.[39]

The needle without stylet is provided with a short stopping point in the shape of a nail with a blunted end 3 cm. long (Fig. 7–2). This prevents the tissue specimen from being sucked up into the syringe end and thus fragmented.

Although the technic was originally designed for one operator and is most commonly so used,[36] Menghini has modified it by employing 2 operators.[37] He found that beginners had difficulty in co-ordinating the quick movement of the plunging-extraction while maintaining the syringe in the operating position. In the new technic the syringe (5 to 10 cc. of any type) is no longer connected rigidly to the needle but is secured to a rubber tube about 35 cm. in length.[37]

After the Record syringe is filled with sterile isotonic solution, the flexible tube is attached to the syringe and the biopsy needle at its other extremity. The tube is held vertically with the needle upward, and the piston of the syringe is pushed until the solution flows from the needle. About 2 ml. of solution should remain in the syringe; this serves in part to expel possible fragments of cutaneous and adipose tissue from the needle and in part to permit, at the end of the operation, recovery of the hepatic tissue.

The patient is placed in the supine position, the head turned to the left, and the right arm raised and adducted so that the right hand may grasp the border of the bed at the height of the left shoulder.

The biopsy is performed in the intercostal space corresponding to the point of maximum hepatic dullness between the anterior and the posterior axillary lines. After preliminary sterilization of the skin, 2 or 3 ml. of a 1 to 2 per cent procaine solution is infiltrated into the

FIG. 7–2. Menghini needle. *Top, left,* profile of tip; *right,* diagram of longitudinal section of needle. *Bottom,* diagrammatic representation of the working of the internal blockage point at (A) moment of insertion, (B) beginning of extraction, and (C) completion of extraction. The long arrow indicates direction of movement, the short one shows the aspiration. (Menghini, G.: Gastroenterology *35:* 190.)

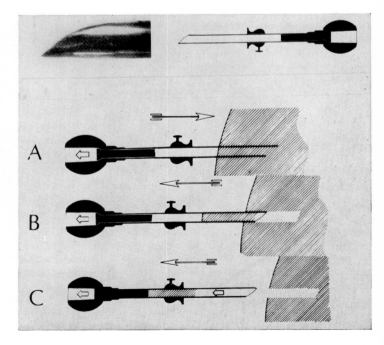

skin and the intercostal space with a short, thin anesthesia needle (20 x 0.45 mm.) The skin is perforated by the stylet to a depth of 2 to 4 mm. The operator, on the right side of the patient, holds the needle firmly with the right hand, while with the thumb of the left hand he controls the intercostal space adjoining the selected site. The assistant, to the right of the operator, holds the cylinder in his left hand; in his right hand he holds the piston of the syringe. The different tasks in the successive phases are as follows:

Step 1.   The operator pushes the needle into the subcutaneous tissue to a depth of about 4 mm., in the opening made by the stylet, and orients it perpendicular to the thoracic wall and inclined slightly medially and downward.

Step 2.   The assistant injects about half of the physiologic solution contained in the syringe in order to expel from the needle any cutaneous and adipose tissue; then the patient is requested to stop breathing after an expiration.

Step 3.   The operator brings the syringe into aspirating position and holds the piston at the 5-ml. line until the procedure is finished.

Steps 4 and 5.   The operator performs the actual biopsy with a rapid plunging rectilinear movement and immediate withdrawal. The plunge-extraction movements must be made perfectly without change of direction and without any rotation, so that the force of aspiration will not be lost or weakened. There must be no delay between the plunge and withdrawal.

The biopsy having been performed, the assistant must keep the syringe in aspirating position until the operator immerses the tip of the needle into a glass capsule containing 10 to 20 cc. of saline solution, or into the fixative directly, at which moment the assistant gradually releases the aspiration and expels from the syringe the residual solution and with it the tissue from the cannula into the capsule.

Then the patient is made to lie on the right side, with the arm flexed under the hypochondrium for 1 hour, and is kept in bed 24 hours.

Obviously, the Menghini technic has the virtue of simplicity, and, because of the short interval the needle remains in the liver and the lesser overall diameter of the needle, a greater factor of safety. Furthermore, it lends itself to use in the less cooperative patients, particularly children. A disadvantage is the occurrence of fragmentation of cirrhosis specimens, the smaller samples, and a higher failure rate in obtaining them.

OTHER TECHNICS

Klatskin uses a needle made by the Becton-Dickman Company. Both sides of the edge are beveled and it comes to a sharp point; it does not contain an internal plug as in the Menghini needle.

This needle is attached to a 10 cc. syringe filled with 8 cc. of saline. After the skin and the liver capsule have been anesthetized in the usual manner with 1 per cent procaine, a small hole is made with a punch provided with the biopsy set (instead of a scalpel). The needle is then inserted just under the skin far enough to avoid the entrance of air. This is necessary in order to maintain adequate suction. The patient now holds his breath in expiration. One cc. of saline is injected subcutaneously to clear the needle, the left hand is placed on the needle at the depth one wishes to penetrate, the right hand retracts the barrel of the syringe to the 9 cc. mark (thus creating 2 cc. of suction), and the needle is rapidly inserted into the liver and withdrawn.

The specimen is found in the syringe barrel and is removed by removing the plunger. When one anticipates a cirrhosis, as much as 3 cc. of suction may be used. If the specimen is badly fragmented, less suction should be used.

Klatskin believes that there is less fragmentation of the needle specimen with this than with the Menghini technic.[26]

Reynolds uses an aspiration needle obtained from the Hub Company of Boston. He finds that it produces a more fragmented specimen in cirrhosis than the Vim-Silverman needle, but is much less painful for the patient. It is sturdier than the Menghini needle and less costly.[45]

Liver biopsy should not be attempted unless adequate facilities for blood transfusion are available. Some physicians type and cross-match the blood of all patients prior to the biopsy, but this has not been our practice. Gillman and Gillman recommend that these biopsy procedures be carried out under basal conditions in the morning.[20] They prefer a preparatory 12-hour fast in order to avoid the possibility of penetrating a distended stomach. Obviously, this is not a problem if the transthoracic route is employed.

For a long time we gave no preliminary

medication. At present we administer a hypodermic injection of 50 mg. of meperidine (Demerol) about 30 minutes before the biopsy is made, and, frequently, 100 mg. of pentobarbital sodium (Nembutal) orally.

About 1 in 5 patients require medication for pain following the procedure, but it is most unusual for an analgesic to be required after 24 hours. The patient is permitted to leave the hospital after 24 to 48 hours.

Failure to obtain adequate tissue for proper interpretation may be a problem in unpracticed hands. However, with experience, failures of this type should be minimized. We do not hesitate in making an immediate second effort to procure a suitable specimen if the original yield appears to be grossly unsuitable.

Terry[69] emphasized the diagnostic value of gross inspection of the biopsy specimen. Sherlock previously pointed out that specimens obtained from fatty livers appear to be greasy; those removed from cirrhotic livers tend to crumble into fragments with a lobulated contour; and those obtained from malignant neoplasm appear dull and white. The tissue may be placed upon nonglossy paper or upon a cover slip, a medium that facilitates transillumination.

The specimen must be examined without delay and before fixation in order to avoid opacification. According to Terry, the fragment of normal liver has:

. . . a mild chocolate hue, which varies in depth with the concentration of glycogen and which on closer inspection is seen to be slightly mottled, the darker areas corresponding to the central zones. The specimen is opaque to transillumination and no vascularity is visible within the tissue. In obstructive jaundice the specimen has a speckled appearance . . . against a background paler than normal, the central zones appear as dark green irregular spots up to 1 mm. in diameter. . . . This green speckling . . . is occasionally observed in hepatitis with marked biliary stasis, especially the cholangiolitic type. . . . In viral and toxic hepatitis and in jaundice complicating cirrhosis, the specimen is pale and uniformly icteric, without any green speckling. . . . In hemochromatosis the biopsy specimen is unusually brown in color. . . .[69]

Needle specimens obtained from the livers

of patients with the Dubin-Johnson syndrome have a greenish-black hue.

In Boeck's sarcoid and in miliary tuberculosis the tubercles are not apparent on superficial examination, but if the specimen is transilluminated the rounded granulomas usually are detected, for they are brightly translucent and contrast sharply with the opaque normal tissue. It was Terry's contention that the gross demonstration of these translucent foci may be as helpful as the microscopic examination for correlation with clinical findings. He points out that detection of the lesions also indicates at once a successful biopsy.

CONTRAINDICATIONS

The following should be considered to be contraindications to needle biopsy of the liver.

An Uncooperative Patient. This was first emphasized by Sherlock. There must be a certain ability and willingness to follow instructions. This is particularly pertinent to the avoidance of breathing at the time the specimen is actually cut during transthoracic biopsy. Stuporous, delirious, psychotic, or comatose patients should be excluded.

Nevertheless, Foulk et al.[17] advocate the performance of transthoracic biopsy during a brief period of apnea (20 to 30 seconds) induced by the rapid intravenous administration of 4 to 6 cc. of freshly prepared 2.5 per cent solution of thiopental sodium (Pentothal Sodium) in uncooperative psychotic patients. They procured specimens in this manner in 96 cases with only one minor complication—transient pleural pain. Equipment to provide the usual precautionary measures during anesthesia was immediately available, and the patient was observed carefully.

Depleted Prothrombin Content. A blood prothrombin level of less than 50 per cent of normal value or the presence of a blood dyscrasia with hemorrhagic tendency constitutes a serious hazard. On occasion the procedure may be carried out safely with a prothrombin level of 40 per cent.

Local Infection. Infectious organisms in the lower lobe of the right lung or the pleural cavity may be carried into the liver or the peritoneum. The presence of perito-

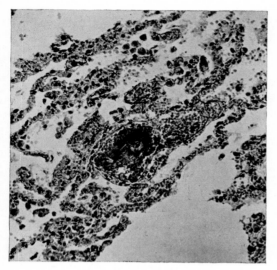

FIG. 7–3. Lung, bile embolism. A small pulmonary vascular channel is occluded and distended by a dark-staining, somewhat refractile bile coagulum. Intermixed with the pigmented substance is thrombotic material containing neutrophils.

nitis is also a contraindication for similar reasons.

Ascites. This increases the difficulty of obtaining a satisfactory tissue specimen, particularly in cases of hepatic cirrhosis. Paracentesis with reduction in the amount of abdominal fluid should be done before the biopsy is attempted.

High-Grade Extrahepatic Obstructive Jaundice. This is especially hazardous in the elderly patient with an enlarged palpable gallbladder. Intrahepatic biliary pressure is apt to be high under such circumstances.[22] In rare instances pulmonary bile embolism has been induced (Fig. 7–3). Bile leakage from the puncture wound in the liver or from a penetrated bile duct may result in bile peritonitis. Moreover, examination of the biopsy specimen, though establishing the presence of obstruction, rarely indicates its cause.

Marked Anemia.

Prolonged Bleeding From the Skin Incision at the Time of Biopsy. Terry advises postponing the biopsy if cutaneous bleeding lasts more than 10 minutes. He believes that

this precaution has avoided carrying out biopsy in patients with abnormal bleeding tendencies in association with uremia, thrombocytopenia, and low prothrombin levels which were reported incorrectly as normal or became abnormal unexpectedly. Zamcheck and Klausenstock have abandoned the performance of biopsy when bleeding from the preliminary nick of the skin is prolonged unduly. We, too, have adopted this practice, although on occasion a second attempt on the following day may be unaccompanied by significant bleeding and thus permit completion of the procedure.

REACTIONS AND COMPLICATIONS

Pain at the site of entry may be referred to the right shoulder at the time of the biopsy procedure and persist thereafter. In our experience this occurs in about a fourth of the patients and usually is mild and transient. Pain has been reported variously in 5 to 50 per cent of patients.[21] The right shoulder pain probably is due to the presence of a small amount of blood on the undersurface of the diaphragm.[13] Pain in the right hypochondrium may indicate a subcapsular accumulation of blood or bile.[24] One of our patients felt pain over the entire right chest shortly after the specimen was removed. Exaggerated by respiration, the pain was present for more than an hour after the biopsy was completed; no abnormalities were detected on physical or x-ray examination of the chest.

Epigastric discomfort or pain may be experienced during the time the needle is in the liver substance or for a period afterward, and sometimes is described as a feeling of having one's "wind knocked out." A friction rub occasionally develops in the region of the biopsy site. While usually of short duration, the rub may last for several weeks.

Hemorrhage Into the Peritoneum. Although uncommon, this is the chief fatal complication of liver biopsy. Most cases of fatal hemorrhage have resulted from perforation of distended portal or hepatic veins or aberrant arteries.[85] In some cases a tear in the liver occurs when the patient breathes deeply while the needle lies in the liver. Hemorrhage usually is manifest within 24 hours after performance of the biopsy. Fortunately, it ordinarily ceases spontaneously and should be controlled by blood transfusions.

Through the peritoneoscope, post-biopsy bleeding has been observed to consist of a thin trickle from the puncture wound in the liver. It lasts only 10 to 20 seconds and totals 5 to 10 cc.[23] In 2 patients who died of unrelated causes 13 and 24 hours after biopsy, Roholm, Krarup and Iversen[50] noted in each a small punctate wound in the liver and a tablespoonful of blood in the peritoneal cavity. After longer intervals in other cases there was no stigma of the needle puncture, and no blood was visible in the abdominal cavity. In a patient with hepatic metastases from a carcinoma of the gallbladder, these observers found a "palm-sized" coagulum over the upper surface of the liver at necropsy done 24 hours after the biopsy.

Terry[68] found serious significant hemorrhage recorded in 16 (0.2 per cent) of 7,532 reported biopsy cases which he reviewed. Laparotomy was required in 4 patients, transfusion alone in 3 and expectant treatment sufficed in 9. We have encountered serious hemorrhage 6 times in over 2,500 patients who have had liver biopsy. Repeated blood transfusions were required in all 6 patients, and laparotomy was necessary in one. All recovered. Reynolds has encountered significant post-biopsy bleeding in about 1 patient in 100.

Bile Peritonitis. This complication apparently occurs only in the presence of obstructive jaundice and probably reflects the accompanying biliary tract infection. Terry reported 11 cases in his survey of the literature.[68] Laparotomy was required in 3 of 7 cases in one series. One fatality was reported among 4 other recorded instances. Hoffbauer[22] has stressed the importance of early recognition in order to initiate prompt surgical decompression of the bile duct system if necessary. The complication proved fatal in one of our patients—a woman 79 years of age with common duct stone, and represents our sole fatality directly attributable to liver biopsy. In another instance, a rigid and tender abdomen noted 2 days after needle biopsy and thought to be due to bile peritonitis proved to be caused by an unrelated perforated duodenal ulcer with generalized peritonitis![58]

Hemorrhage into the pleural cavity or pleural effusion has been reported to result from injury to the pleura or penetration of an intercostal vessel. Arterial injury can be avoided by keeping the needle close to the lower border of the intercostal space. Passage of ascitic fluid into the thorax through a needle perforation of the right leaf of the diaphragm with mild respiratory embarrassment has been reported in 3 instances.[85]

Pneumothorax has occurred twice in our experience, and in both instances the symptoms were mild, and the pulmonary collapse did not exceed 10 per cent.

Severe apprehension associated with various nervous and hysterical manifestations may be observed on rare occasions. When these become evident as the procedure is begun, biopsy should be postponed.

Shock may occur uncommonly after the procedure. Kleckner and associates reported 2 cases of transient pleural shock lasting 1 to 2 hours after biopsy. Fatal shock, not explainable on the basis of blood loss, has been described in 2 instances.[85] Roholm, Krarup and Iversen encountered mild shocklike states 3 times in performing 297 biopsies. These authors considered these to be similar to episodes exhibited by nervous and apprehensive patients following venipuncture. Kleckner[28] reported "pleural shock" in 8 cases among a total of 145 consecutive liver biopsy procedures, some of which were carried out transabdominally. We know of 2 other instances of shock, one of which occurred in our own series. Both subjects were elderly males with obstructive jaundice. One of our patients had common duct stone with suppurative cholangitis and multiple liver abscesses, while the other had a carcinoma of the ampulla of Vater.

Procaine reactions have been reported by Nelson[40] but have not been encountered in our own experience.

Fatal pulmonary bile embolism has been reported following aspiration needle biopsy in a patient with carcinoma of the ampulla

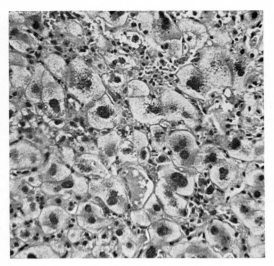

Fig. 7–4. Acute viral hepatitis. A high-power view, demonstrating swollen parenchymal elements ("balloon cells") with ground-glass cytoplasm and amitotic nuclear division. Focal inflammatory aggregates are evident, but the liver cells exhibit no fatty vacuolization.

of Vater.[9] This need not necessarily be considered a complication of needling, since we have observed 2 instances in which it occurred spontaneously in patients with high-grade biliary obstruction and infection.

Tumor Seeding. Implantation of tumor cells in the needle tract has been reported.[43, 63, 64, 72] We have not observed this phenomenon and do not consider it a serious deterrent.

Penetration of Abdominal Viscera. Theoretically, this is apt to occur less frequently following transthoracic biopsy than with utilization of the anterior route. Hoffbauer[21] noted a case of perforation of the colon with fatal peritonitis following needling by the subcostal approach. Baron recovered a piece of colonic mucosa without serious consequence.[4] Reynolds had a similar experience; in his case there was no evidence of peritonitis at laparotomy 3 days after biopsy.[46] Perforation of the gallbladder is also rare. Gamble and Sullivan report 2 cases of accidental gallbladder biopsy using the intercostal approach.[19] There were no serious consequences.

CLINICAL APPLICATION

The needle method has proved to have considerable application in the clinical evaluation of hepatic disease.[57] Indeed, many misconceptions of long standing have been clarified, and the understanding of liver ailments has attained a high level in a relatively short period. The following represent some of the many avenues that have been opened.

Exclusion of Hepatic Disease in Apparent Hepatomegaly. An incorrect presumption of hepatic disease is common when the liver is palpable, particularly in a patient with a prolonged history of alcoholism or one who is known to have a malignant tumor which may have metastasized to this organ. Normally, the liver may extend 1 to 2 fingerbreadths below the costal margin and may be displaced downward in individuals with pulmonary emphysema or right pleural effusion, or may extend below this level in hyposthenic individuals (see "Physical Examination" of the liver, Chap. 8). When possible, the determination of the upper border of liver dullness is helpful in assessing the size of the organ.

Exclusion of Hepatic Disease in the Presence of Abnormal Liver-Function Tests. Abnormalities of one or more liver function tests are encountered not infrequently in the absence of liver disease. This may result from alterations in blood proteins which affect the cephalin-cholesterol flocculation and the thymol and zinc turbidity tests. Abnormal Bromsulphalein retention is encountered in the presence of fever, shocklike states, or in older persons without demonstrable liver disorders. The advent of many tests for liver malfunction has not lessened the usefulness of the biopsy method.

Distinction Between Medical and Surgical Jaundice. The histologic changes that characterize viral hepatitis[2, 12, 33, 49, 62, 82] and those related to obstructive jaundice[34, 44, 48, 82] have been well described by many authors. Morphologic differentiation between the conditions is almost always possible (Figs. 7–4 and 7–5). Certain histologic changes in the needle biopsy specimen invariably indicate the presence of extrahepatic obstructive jaundice, but are observed

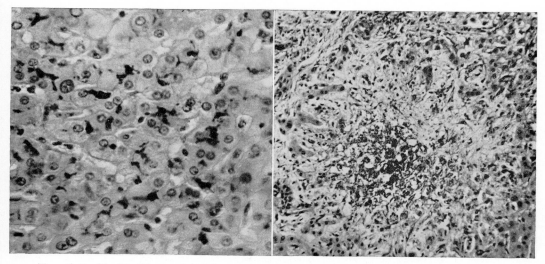

FIG. 7–5. (*Left*) Obstructive bile stasis, carcinoma of the head of the pancreas. Intercellular bile capillaries are brought into prominence by dark-staining inspissated plugs of static bile. Liver cells appear essentially normal and exhibit none of the features observed in viral hepatitis. (These findings may be simulated in intrahepatic cholestasis.)

(*Right*) Extrahepatic obstructive jaundice; carcinoma of the hepatic duct at the liver hilum. A central pool of coagulated bile (bile-lake) is surrounded by a pale-staining radial zone of disintegrating liver cells ("feathery degeneration").

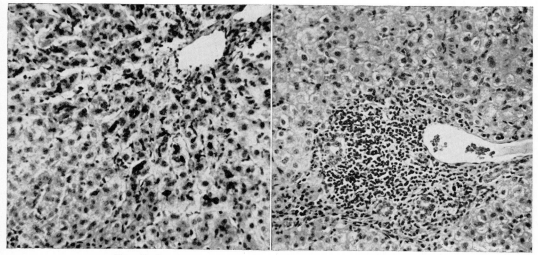

FIG. 7–6   FIG. 7–7

FIG. 7–6. Chlorpromazine jaundice. Severe centrilobular canalicular bile stasis is accompanied by minimal parenchymal cell alteration. The portal areas in this specimen exhibited mild lymphocytic infiltration only. No eosinophils were encountered.

FIG 7–7. Prolonged viral hepatitis; clinical duration, 9 weeks. Portal area exhibits heavy lymphocytic infiltration and reduplication of interlobular bile ducts. Parenchymal cells are moderately disarranged and swollen, and occasionally contain double nuclei.

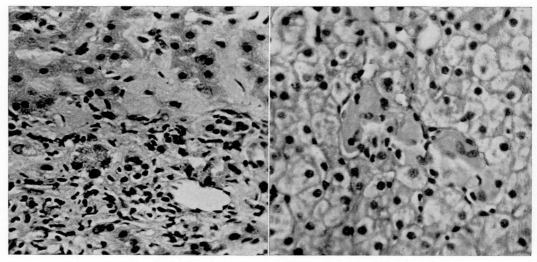

FIG. 7–8. (*Left*) Amyloidosis; patient with severe longstanding rheumatoid arthritis. Liver cells were attenuated and surrounded by a homogeneous deposit of hyaline substance which proved to be metachromatic when stained with crystal violet.

(*Right*) Gaucher's disease; young man, asymptomatic; liver and spleen not palpable. Several Kupffer cells are markedly enlarged by reason of a palely eosinophilic homogeneous cytoplasmic content. The substance proved to be strongly PAS positive.

in only a small proportion of cases. These changes have recently been discussed by Gall and Dobrogorski.[18] These authors conclude that no single histologic feature has regular significance, but combinations of these are of considerable differential value.

In recent years the utilization of a number of pharmaceutical agents (certain steroid compounds, chlorpromazine, and related substances) has led to the sporadic occurrence of jaundice with varying intensity. Although distinguishable, in the main, on clinical and laboratory grounds, an occasional instance requires liver biopsy for clarification, since obstructive icterus may be mimicked. In most of these, parenchymal and inflammatory lesions are negligible, but evidence of centrilobular bile capillary stasis (Fig. 7–6) may create difficulty in distinction from extrahepatic biliary obstruction, particularly during the first week or 10 days of jaundice.

Observations of the Natural Course of Liver Disease. The disappearance or persistence of manifestations of viral hepatitis or the development of cirrhosis are ascertained best by means of liver biopsy.[55] Clarification of the so-called posthepatitis syndrome

and its differentiation from chronic or relapsing hepatitis is approached best by this means (Fig. 7–7). The evaluation of the fatty liver and the determination of its relation to cirrhosis can be investigated only by biopsy.

Evaluation of Effectiveness of Therapy. Several authors have remarked about the value of the liver biopsy in determining the effects of various forms of therapy.[66, 78, 79] Notable among the conditions that may be investigated in this manner are the fatty liver, hemochromatosis, and even tuberculosis.

Elucidation of the Cause of Hepatomegaly. The liver may be enlarged as the result of many different lesions—a number of which may remain obscure without recourse to histologic study. Among these are amyloid disease (Fig. 7–8, *left*), genetic metabolic disorders (Fig. 7–8, *right*), fatty liver, toxic hepatitis of the alcoholic (Fig. 7–9), anicteric hepatitis, cirrhosis, granulomatous disease, hemochromatosis, aleukemic leukemia, extramedullary hematopoiesis, and fungus disease (Fig. 7–10), to mention some of those which have come to light among our own cases. In our experience the needle

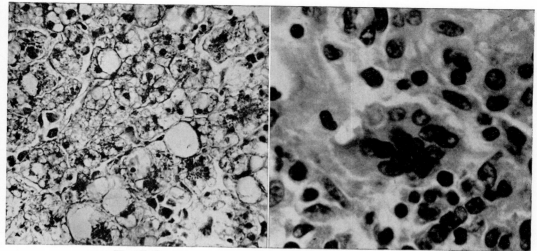

Fig. 7-9   Fig. 7-10

Fig. 7-9. Toxic ("alcoholic") hepatitis. Liver cells are swollen, misshapen and disarranged. The lipid-filled cytoplasm has a finely vacuolated foamy appearance and often contains dark-staining eosinophilic "alcoholic hyalin." Kupffer cells are made prominent by eosinophilia and bile pigment content.

Fig. 7-10. Margin of a necrotizing tubercular granuloma. A multinucleated giant cell contains a fungus spore (subsequently proved by culture to be *Candida albicans*). Periodic acid-Schiff stain.

specimen has pinpointed repeatedly the nature of an ailment, or, equally important, has served to exclude one that was incorrectly believed to be present.

Distinction Between Intrahepatic and Extrahepatic Portal Vein Obstruction. This has attained a level of considerable importance since the advent of vascular shunt procedures in the relief of portal hypertension and collateral venous abnormalities. The practical value of determining the desirability and the potential risk of operation in relation to the presence or the absence and the nature of underlying hepatic disease is obvious.[18] Naturally, the biopsy cannot indicate the character or the location of the vascular occlusion in those instances in which the liver is not the site of venous obstruction. In a few instances pylephlebitis associated with alimentary tract infections has been demonstrated in needle specimens (Fig. 7-11).

Recognition of Granulomatous and Other Systemic Inflammatory Disorders. The liver is often involved in a wide variety of infectious diseases of systemic character. Liver

biopsy may bring one or another of these to light when it has not been suspected clinically (Fig. 7-12, *left*). Notable among these ailments are the tubercular granulomatous processes of which tuberculosis, brucellosis, sarcoidosis, syphilis and fungus disease are important and common examples.[3, 10, 15, 27, 54, 65, 74, 75] Usually the nature of the lesion is such that a definitive etiologic basis cannot be established from the specimen alone, although in a few instances the causative agent may be demonstrated by stain or culture. On the other hand, the detection of a tubercular process may serve to initiate pertinent clinical tests that lead to clarification (Fig. 7-12, *right*).

Detection of Intrahepatic Neoplasm. Needle biopsy has been surprisingly fruitful in detecting neoplasm (Fig. 7-13). In our original report,[52] tumor was detected in 41 of 53 cases (77 per cent) of proved neoplasm. In a later study,[80] tumor was demonstrated in 82 of 111 patients (74 per cent), and at a still later date,[42] in 115 of 164 cases (70 per cent). These figures are in gen-

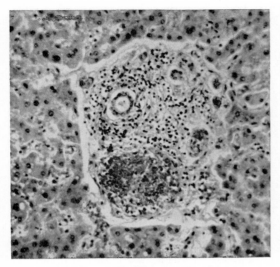

FIG. 7–11. Pylephlebitis. Venular component in the portal area is distended by a septic thrombus. Surrounding connective tissue is edematous and contains a moderate leukocytic exudate. Patient with perforated suppurative appendicitis.

eral agreement with the experience of others.[7, 14, 43, 85]

In our experience and that of others[7, 14, 43, 77, 85] the incidence of complications follow-ing needle biopsy is not necessarily greater in cases of malignant neoplasm. For example, we noted no serious complications following needle biopsy of the liver among 164 patients with proved hepatic neoplasm. Parets reported that among 76 patients, with biopsy showing malignant tumor of the liver, there was one instance of severe intraperitoneal hemorrhage requiring operation and one of mild peritonitis following biopsy.[43] Both patients recovered.

Fisher and Faloon reported 4 deaths among 33 patients with liver metastases following needle biopsy.[16] While the association of post-biopsy hemorrhage and death may or may not have been fortuitous, one of their patients was moribund at the time of the procedure. Certainly, their experience has not paralleled that of others.

Occasionally, biopsy affords a clue as to the primary site of the tumor or may, of itself, establish the presence of a primary hepatoma of the liver (Fig. 7–14).

Clinical Research. The potential value of transcutaneous biopsy in the investigation of both the normal and the disordered liver appears to be vast.[85] Metabolic activities in normal and disease states, the progress of

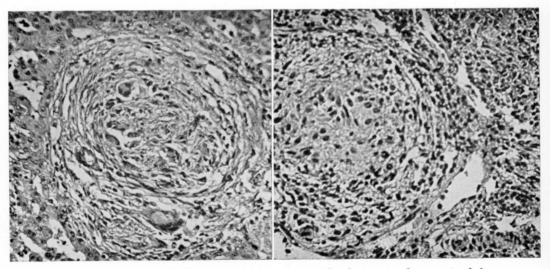

FIG. 7–12. (*Left*) Miliary tubercle. Sarcoidosis. The lesion is characterized by concentrically arranged epithelioid cells interspersed among which may be seen inflammatory giant cells. There is little peritubercular inflammatory cell reaction.

(*Right*) Miliary tubercle. Tuberculosis. Early caseation appears in the center of the tubercle. Surrounding it is a pronounced lymphocytic exudate. The lesion is nondiagnostic but consistent with tuberculosis.

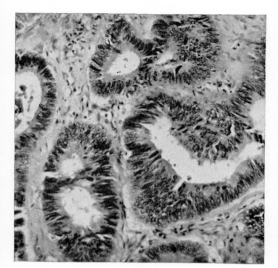

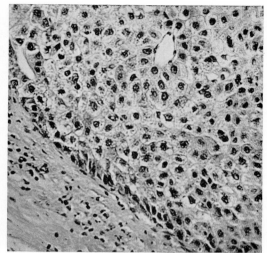

FIG. 7–13. Metastatic adenocarcinoma. Liver parenchyma is replaced by neoplastic acini exhibiting secondary gland formation. Nuclei are hyperchromatic and pseudostratified; mucus secretion is minimal. Primary lesion, sigmoid colon.

FIG. 7–14. Hepatoma. Neoplastic cells resemble hepatic parenchymal elements but lack radial arrangement and are not accompanied by portal area structures. Pseudoacinar and sinusoid-like patterns are manifest.

disease and the effect of therapeutic agents are all susceptible to study by this means. The method has been employed in the investigation of hepatic enzyme activity,[1, 81] and the biochemistry of liver lipids.[6, 60]

Chemical studies have also included estimation of nucleic acids and protein, water content and glycogen.[67] A micromethod has been described that determines vitamin A content in the liver in human subjects.[83] The effect of antibiotic therapy on active tuberculosis also has been evaluated.[47] The adaptation of biopsy to electron microscopy has opened an entirely new vista.[41, 56]

Clinical Value. During a 14-year period (1944–58), covering 1,455 needle specimens obtained from 1,324 patients, the biopsy specimens proved to be of significant aid in establishing a diagnosis in 72 to 85 per cent of cases. The specimens confirmed the pre-biopsy clinical diagnosis in 49.8 to 55.7 per cent and altered the clinical impression in 22 to 29.3 per cent (Fig. 7–15). The specimen proved to be noncontributory in 9.4 to 18.4 per cent (Fig. 7–16). In these instances normal liver tissue or specimens with negligible alterations were obtained. In 3 to 4.4 per cent of cases the biopsy study failed to

establish the correct diagnosis as shown at necropsy or surgical exploration or by subsequent clinical developments. The specimen obtained proved to be inadequate in 1.2 to 6.8 per cent of cases (Fig. 7–15). The needle specimens were particularly valuable in detecting unsuspected fatty degeneration and systemic granulomatous diseases and, in addition, often aided in establishing the presence or the absence of cirrhosis and neoplasm of the liver, in distinguishing between hepatitis and obstructive jaundice and in revealing hepatitis alone in alcoholics suspected of cirrhosis.

Obviously, the needle biopsy method is not without limitations. The procedure is relatively safe, but deaths have followed its use. In a survey of the literature comprising over 10,000 needle biopsies, Terry listed a mortality of 0.12 per cent and an incidence of major complications of 0.32 per cent.[69]

In a review of 20,016 needle biopsies of the liver, in which the large majority was carried out presumably with the Vim-Silverman needle, Zamcheck and Klausenstock reported a mortality of 0.17 per cent.[84] Thaler reported a mortality rate of 0.017 per cent among 23,382 percutaneous needle biopsies in which the Menghini needle was used.[70, 71] Lindner reported a mortality rate of 0.013 per cent among 77,721 (and later a mortality of 0.015 per cent among a total of 79,381[30]) percutaneous needle biopsies based on a questionnaire to which 97 replies were obtained.[31] He points out that those questioned had heard of a further 16 deaths, but these were not included in his statistics. It appears likely that the true mortality rate following percutaneous needle biopsy of the liver is not known, but is higher than the figures indicate. The evidence suggests that the risk may be less with the use of the Menghini needle.

With selective observance of the contraindications enumerated, serious complications should constitute a negligible risk. We have found that the experienced individual is much less prone to encounter difficulty or to provide an unsuitable specimen. Therefore, in our own institution only adequately trained and responsible persons carry out the needle biopsy.

The smallness of the specimen has been claimed by some to limit its value. However, we and others[8] have found the narrow core of tissue to be representative in diffuse liver disorders. Indeed, we have come to prefer the Vim-Silverman instrument in procuring specimens during surgical exploration, except in suspected cases of primary biliary cirrhosis in which a wedge biopsy is preferred. The ordinary wedge section removed by the surgeon has the disadvantage of reflecting, on the one hand, the nonspecific distortions common to the subcapsular regions and, on the other, acute inflammatory reactions to the immediate surgical manipulations. A better appraisal of the status of the

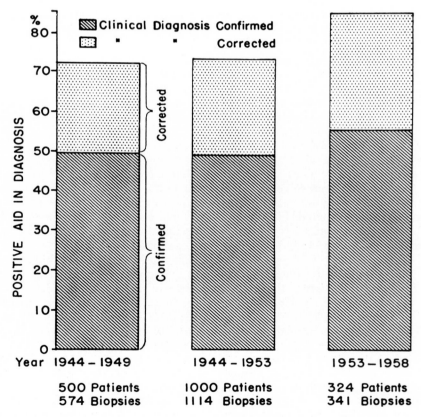

FIG. 7–15. Clinical evaluation of liver biopsy, showing analysis of positive aid in diagnosis. (Schiff, L., Gall, E., and Oikawa, Y.: Proc. World Congr. Gastroenterology, 1958; Baltimore, Williams & Wilkins.)

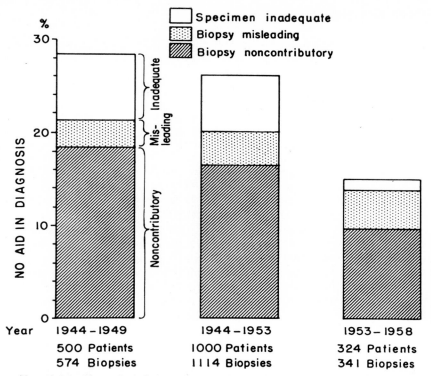

FIG. 7–16. Clinical evaluation of liver biopsy, showing analysis of cases in which no aid in diagnosis resulted. (Schiff, L., Gall, E., and Oikawa, Y.: Proc. World Congr. Gastroenterology, 1958; Baltimore, Williams & Wilkins.)

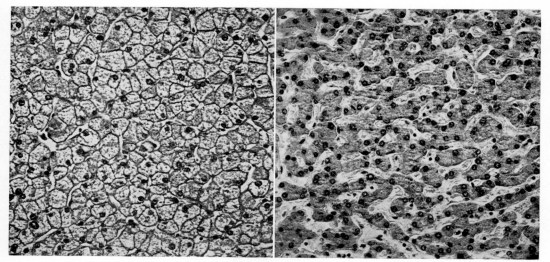

FIG. 7–17. (*Left*) Normal liver—needle biopsy specimen. A high-power photomicrograph, revealing narrow sinusoids, sharply demarcated parenchymal cells and characteristic ground-glass clarity of cytoplasm. Hematoxylin and eosin stains.

(*Right*) Normal liver—autopsy specimen. The contrast with the biopsy specimen is readily apparent (magnification is identical). Sinusoids are wide, and a space is perceived between endothelium and liver cells. The latter appear shrunken and contain a smudgy opaque cytoplasm. Cell margins are inapparent. Specimen procured 5 hours postmortem; death due to malignant hypertension and acute pyelonephritis. Hematoxylin and eosin stains.

liver can be obtained from a specimen removed from its depths.

A minor problem in the histologic interpretation of biopsy specimens derives from the rather impressive difference in appearance of tissues promptly fixed in the living state from those procured at necropsy in which postmortem alterations usually are advanced. Occasionally individuals accustomed to autopsy material have interpreted the normal biopsy specimen as an abnormal one. In the biopsy section, parenchymal cells are outlined sharply and lack the smudgy opacity evident in most postmortem tissues. Indeed, the normal clarity of staining has been misinterpreted as indicative of vacuolization. However, it is believed to indicate preservation of glycogen and an absence of "cloudy swelling" that commonly occurs during the agonal state. Sinusoids are not as readily apparent as in the autopsy specimen, and the cordlike quality of the liver plates is obscured (Fig. 7–17). Familiarity with these and other characteristics of biopsy tissue is readily attained.

While liver biopsy obtained at peritoneoscopy offers the advantage of visualization of the liver surface and thus choice of a biopsy site, specimens so obtained rarely gather tissue more than 3 to 4 mm. deep to the capsule unless a specially designed Vim-Silverman needle is employed. Peritoneoscopic examination is a much more formidable procedure. It must be performed in an operating room; it requires the creation of a tense pneumoperitoneum; and usually it is followed by much more discomfort than transmural needle biopsy.[21] Furthermore, it entails a greater risk to the patient.

For a long time disorders of the liver have been beclouded by inexact clinical pronouncements, by retrospective speculations derived from study of advanced lesions in a postmortem state, and by overly zealous faith in the results of so-called liver-function tests. The contribution that has been made to the modern dynamic concept of liver disease by the transcutaneous biopsy method is incalculable. One may not gainsay the value of intelligent clinical appraisal and the proper interpretation of accurately performed laboratory tests. Nonetheless, liver biopsy constitutes a keystone in the arch of the understanding of liver disease. Volwiler, Jones and Mallory aptly remarked:

> The most careful clinical scrutiny of a patient with any chronic hepatitis may not permit one to predict with even moderate accuracy the histologic phase of the liver disease present. Neither do any laboratory tests, even when repeated serially, always correctly reflect the true histologic state of the liver at a given time, or the changes taking place during clinical observation; frequently the only means of determining this is microscopic examination of actual liver tissue.[79]

We are convinced that the procedure should be carried out only in institutions in which 1 or 2 physicians are experienced with the technic, are aware of the risk entailed, and will follow the patients closely for at least 24 hours after the procedure is completed.

REFERENCES

1. Arias, I. M., and London, I. M.: Bilirubin glucuronide formation in vitro: demonstration of a defect in Gilbert's disease, Science *126*:563, 1957.
2. Axenfeld, H., and Brass, K.: Klinische und bioptische Untersuchungen über den sogenannten Icterus catarrhalis, Frankfurt. Z. Path. *57*:147, 1942.
3. Baird, M. M., Bogoch, A., and Fenwick, J. B.: Liver biopsy in sarcoidosis, Canad. Med. Ass. *62*:562, 1950.
4. Baron, E.: Aspiration for removal of biopsy material from the liver, Arch. Int. Med. *62*:276, 1939.
5. Beierwaltes, W. H., and Mallery, O. T., Jr.: Liver biopsy: clinical evaluation of a trephine needle, Univ. Hosp. Bull., Ann Arbor *12*:13, 1946.
6. Billing, B. H., Conlon, H. J., Hein, D. E., and Schiff, L.: The value of needle biopsy in the chemical estimation of liver lipids in man, J. Clin. Invest. *32*:214, 1953.
7. Bowden, L., and Kravitz, S.: Needle biopsy of the liver: a diagnostic aid in the treatment of cancer, Cancer *6*:1010, 1953.
8. Braunstein, H.: Needle biopsy of the liver in cirrhosis: diagnostic efficiency as determined by postmortem sampling, A.M.A. Arch. Path. *62*:87, 1956.
9. Brown, C. Y., and Walsh, G. C.: Fatal bile embolism following liver biopsy, Ann. Int. Med. *36*:1529, 1952.

10. Cazal, P.: Les lésions de l'hépatite brucellienne, Sem. hôp. Paris 25:1351, 1949.
11. Davis, W. D., Scott, R. W., and Lund, H. Z.: Needle biopsy of the liver, Am. J. Med. Sci. 212:449, 1946.
12. Dible, J. H., McMichael, J., and Sherlock, S. P. V.: Pathology of acute hepatitis: aspiration biopsy studies of epidemic, arsenotherapy and serum jaundice, Lancet 2:402, 1943.
13. Dieulafoy, G.: Kystes hydatiques, Gaz. d. hôp. 45:586, 1872 (quoted by Baron[4]).
14. Fenster, L. F., and Klatskin, G.: Manifestations of metastatic tumors of the liver; a study of 81 patients subjected to needle biopsy, Am. J. Med. 31:238, 1961.
15. Finckh, E. S., Baker, S. J., and Ryan, M. M. P.: The value of liver biopsy in the diagnosis of tuberculosis and sarcoidosis, Med. J. Aus. 2:369, 1953.
16. Fisher, C. J., and Faloon, W. W.: Needle biopsy of the liver: comparison of initial clinical and histologic diagnoses, with a note on postbiopsy mortality in patients with metastatic neoplasm, Am. J. Med. 25:368, 1958.
17. Foulk, W. T., Frazier, S. H., Cain, J. C., and Bartholomew, L. G.: A technic for liver biopsy applicable to uncooperative psychotic patients, Proc. Mayo Clinic 34:8, 1959.
18. Gall, E. A., and Dobrogorski, O.: Hepatic alterations in obstructive jaundice, Am. J. Clin. Path. 41:126, 1964.
18a. Gall, E. A., and Keirle, A. M.: Portal systemic venous shunt. Pathological factors contributing to postoperative survival, Gastroenterology 49:656, 1965.
19. Gamble, R. D., and Sullivan, B. H., Jr.: Needle biopsy of the liver. Clinical evaluation of 323 biopsies; report of two cases of accidental biopsy of the gallbladder, Gastroenterology 24:394, 1953.
20. Gillman, T., and Gillman, J.: A modified liver aspiration biopsy apparatus and technique, with special reference to its clinical application as assessed by 500 biopsies, S. Afr. J. Med. Sci. 10:53, 1945.
21. Hoffbauer, F. W.: Needle biopsy of the liver, J.A.M.A. 134:666, 1947.
22. ———: Needle biopsy of the liver (editorial), Surg. Gynec. Obstet. 92:113, 1951.
23. Hoffbauer, F. W., Evans, G. T., and Watson, C. J.: Cirrhosis of the liver, with particular reference to correlation of composite liver function studies with liver biopsy, Med. Clin. N. Amer. 29:363, 1945.
24. Iversen, P., Bjørnboe, M., and Krarup, N. B.: Biopsy studies of the liver and kidney, Adv. Int. Med. 6:161, 1954.
25. Iversen, P., and Roholm, K.: On aspiration biopsy of the liver, with remarks on its diagnostic significance, Acta med. scand. 102:1, 1939.
26. Klatskin, G.: Personal communication.
27. Klatskin, G., and Yesner, R.: Hepatic manifestations of sarcoidosis and other granulomatous diseases: a study based on histological examination of tissue obtained by needle biopsy of the liver, Yale J. Biol. Med. 23:207, 1950.
28. Kleckner, M. S., Jr.: Needle biopsy of the liver; an appraisal of its diagnostic indications and limitations, Ann. Int. Med. 40:1177, 1954.
29. Kleckner, M. S., Jr., Stauffer, M. H., Bargen, J. A., and Dockerty, M. B.: Hepatic lesions in the living patient with chronic ulcerative colitis as demonstrated by needle biopsy, Gastroenterology 22:13, 1952.
30. Lindner, H.: Limitations and dangers in percutaneous liver biopsies with the Menghini needle, Proc. Third World Congress of Gastroenterology 3:373, 1966.
31. ———: Grenzen und Gefahren der perkutanen Leberbiopsie mit der Menghini-Nadel; erfahrungen bei 80,000 leberbiopsien, Dtsch. Med. Wschr. 92:1751, 1967.
32. Lucatello, L.: Sulla puncture del fegato a scopo diagnostico in Lavori del congressi di medicina interna, p. 327, Rome, 1895 (quoted by Hoffbauer[21]).
33. Mallory, T. B.: Liver biopsy in the diagnosis and investigation of cirrhosis of the liver in man, Bull. Acad. Med., Toronto 23:9, 1949.
34. McMichael, J.: Disease of the liver. A review of some clinical and biochemical problems as revealed by systematic biopsy studies, J.A.M.A. 137:234, 1948.
35. Menghini, G.: Biopsia y microbiopsia del higado: un effectivo progreso methodologico, Scientia med. ital. 6:212, 1957.
36. ———: One-second needle biopsy of the liver, Gastroenterology 35:190, 1958.
37. ———: Two-operator needle biopsy of the liver; a new, easier and safer version of the one-second technic, Am. J. Dig. Dis. 4:682, 1959.
38. ———: Probleme der Leberbiopsie, in Wildhirt, E. (ed.): Fortschritte der Gastroenterologie, Muenchen, Urban & Schwarzenberg, 1960, pp. 222-230.

39. Menghini, G.: Personal communication.
40. Nelson, R. S.: The development and function of a liver biopsy program: training of personnel, description of a modified Vim-Silverman needle and clinical value of 500 biopsies, Am. J. Med. Sci. 227:152, 1954.
41. Novikoff, A. B., and Essner, E.: The liver cell: some new approaches to its study, Am. J. Med. 29:102, 1960.
42. Oikawa, Y., and Schiff, L.: Unpublished observations.
43. Parets, A. D.: Detection of intrahepatic metastases by blind needle liver biopsy, Am. J. Med. Sci. 237:335, 1959.
44. Popper, H., and Franklin, M.: Diagnosis of hepatitis by histologic and functional laboratory methods, J.A.M.A. 137:230, 1948.
45. Reynolds, T. B.: Personal communication.
46. Reynolds, W. S.: Discussion of Stone, C. T., Jr., and Graber, W. C.: Needle biopsy of liver (critical appraisal), Texas J. Med. 46:825, 1950.
47. Ringleb, O.: Über Retsthelknötchen der Leber bei Tuberkulösen, Arch. path. Anat. 324:357, 1953.
48. Roholm, K., and Iversen, P.: Changes in the liver in acute epidemic hepatitis (catarrhal jaundice) based on 38 aspiration biopsies, Acta path. microbiol. scand. 16:427, 1939.
49. Roholm, K., and Krarup, N. B.: Histopathology of the liver in obstructive jaundice, examined by aspiration biopsy, Acta med. scand. 108:48, 1941.
50. Roholm, K., Krarup, N. B., and Iversen, P.: Aspirationsbiopsie der Leber. Mit einer ubersicht über die Ergebnisse bei 297 Biopsien, Ergebn. inn. Med. Kinderh. 61:635, 1942.
51. Roth, A. A., and Turkel, H.: A technique of prostatic biopsy, J. Urol. 51:66, 1944.
52. Safdi, S. A., Gall, E. A., Kumpe, C. W., and Schiff, L.: Needle biopsy of the liver. II. Experiences with malignant neoplasm, Gastroenterology 11:93, 1948.
53. Sborov, V. M.: Simple guard for Vim-Silverman needle, J. Lab. Clin. Med. 36:773, 1950.
54. Scadding, J. G., and Sherlock, S.: Liver biopsy in sarcoidosis, Thorax 3:79, 1948.
55. Schaefer, J. W., Schiff, L., Gall, E. A., and Oikawa, Y.: Progression of acute hepatitis to postnecrotic cirrhosis, Am. J. Med. 42:348, 1967.
56. Schaffner, F., and Popper, H.: Electron microscopic study of human cholestasis, Proc. Soc. Exp. Biol. Med. 101:777, 1959.
57. Schiff, L.: The clinical value of needle biopsy of the liver, Ann. Int. Med. 34:948, 1951.
58. Schiff, L., Gall, E. A., and Oikawa, Y.: The clinical value of needle biopsy of the liver; selected case experiences, Proc. World Congr. Gastroenterology, Washington; Baltimore, Williams & Wilkins, 1958.
59. Schiff, L., Schubert, W. K., McAdams, A. J., Spiegel, E. L., and O'Donnell, J. F.: Hepatic cholesterol ester storage disease, a familial disorder. I. Clinical aspects. Am. J. Med. 44:538, 1968.
60. Sherlock, S.: Aspiration liver biopsy; technique and diagnostic application, Lancet 2:397, 1945.
61. Silverman, I.: Improved Vim-Silverman biopsy needle, J.A.M.A. 155:1060, 1954.
62. Smetana, H. F.: The histologic diagnosis of viral hepatitis by needle biopsy, Gastroenterology 26:612, 1954.
63. Snapper, I.: Discussion of Rappaport, E. M.: Liver biopsy, Rev. Gastroenterol. 18:649, 1951.
64. Sommerfelt, S. C.: Malignant hepatoma with implantation metastasis following liver puncture, Nord. med. Tidskr. 46:1492, 1951.
65. Spink, W. W., Hoffbauer, F. W., Walker, W. W., and Green, R. A.: Histopathology of the liver in human brucellosis, J. Lab. Clin. Med. 34:40, 1949.
66. Steigmann, F.: Efficacy of lipotropic substances in the treatment of cirrhosis of the liver, J.A.M.A. 137:239, 1948.
67. Stuart, K. L., Bras, G., Patrick, S. J., and Waterlow, J. C.: Further clinical and investigative use of the liver biopsy; an analysis of 527 biopsies, A.M.A. Arch. Int. Med. 101:67, 1958.
68. Terry, R.: Risks of needle biopsy of the liver, Brit. M. J. 1:1102, 1952.
69. ———: Macroscopic diagnosis in liver biopsy, J.A.M.A. 154:990, 1954.
70. Thaler, H.: Erfahrungen mit der leberbiopsiemethode nach Menghini, Wien. klin. Wschr. 70:622, 1958.
71. ———: Ueber Vorteil und Risiko der Leberbiopsiemethode nach Menghini, Wien. Klin. Wschr. 76:533, 1964.
72. Topp, J. H., Lindert, M. C. F., and Murphy, F. D.: Needle biopsy of the liver, Arch. Int. Med. 81:832, 1948.
73. Tripoli, C. J., and Fader, D. E.: The dif-

ferential diagnosis of certain diseases of the liver by means of punch biopsy, Am. J. Clin. Path. *11*:516, 1941.

74. Van Beek, C., and Haex, A. J. C.: Aspiration-biopsy of the liver in mononucleosis infectiosa and Besnier-Boeck-Schaumann's disease, Acta med. scand. *113*:125, 1943.

75. Van Buchem, F. S. P.: On morbid conditions of the liver and the diagnosis of the disease of Besnier-Boeck-Schaumann, Acta med. scand. *124*:168, 1946.

76. Voegtlin, W. L.: An improved liver biopsy needle, Gastroenterology *11*:56, 1948.

77. Volwiler, W.: Personal communication.

78. Volwiler, W., and Jones, C. M.: The diagnostic and therapeutic value of liver biopsies with particular reference to trocar biopsy, New Engl. J. Med. *237*:651, 1947.

79. Volwiler, W., Jones, C. M., and Mallory, T. B.: Criteria for the measurement of results of treatment in fatty cirrhosis, Gastroenterology *11*:164, 1948.

80. Ward, J., Schiff, L., Young, P., and Gall, E. A.: Needle biopsy of the liver. IX. Further experiences with malignant neoplasm, Gastroenterology *27*:300, 1954.

81. Waterlow, J.: Enzyme activity in human liver, p. 72, Tr. 11th Liver Injury Conf., New York, Macy, 1952.

82. Weisbrod, F. G., Schiff, L., Gall, E. A., Cleveland, F. P., and Berman, J. R.: Needle biopsy of the liver. III. Experiences in the differential diagnosis of jaundice, Gastroenterology *14*:56, 1950.

83. With, T. K.: Micromethod for the determination of vitamin A in liver biopsies in man and larger animals, Biochem. J. *40*:249, 1946.

84. Zamcheck, N., and Klausenstock, O.: Needle biopsy of the liver. II. The risk of needle biopsy, New Engl. J. Med. *249*:1062, 1953.

85. Zamcheck, N., and Sidman, R. L.: Needle biopsy of the liver. I. Its use in clinical and investigative medicine, New Engl. J. Med. *249*:1020, 1953.

8

Jaundice

LEON SCHIFF, M.D., PH.D., AND *BARBARA H. BILLING*, PH.D.

Jaundice, or icterus, is the condition recognized clinically by a yellowish discoloration of the plasma, the skin and the mucous membranes, caused by staining by bile pigment. It is often the first and sometimes the sole manifestation of liver disease. Frequently it is detected best in the peripheral portions of the ocular conjunctivae; it can also be observed in the mucous membrane of the hard palate or in the lips when compressed with a glass slide. It may be overlooked in poor or artificial light. It may be preceded for a day or more by the passage of dark urine or light-colored stools. Occasionally, attention is first directed to it by a laboratory report of "serum icteric." Icterus may be detected by the skilled observer when the concentration of serum bilirubin reaches 2 mg./100 cc., and is obvious to the most unobservant when the concentration exceeds 7 or 8 mg.%.

BILIRUBIN METABOLISM

STRUCTURE OF BILE PIGMENTS

Bile pigments may be defined as compounds that consist of a chain of four pyrrole rings linked together at their α positions by methene ($-CH_2$) or methyne ($-CH=$) groups. The naturally occurring pigments are derived from protoporphyrin IX, the iron complex of which constitutes heme, the prosthetic group of hemoglobin. They are formed as the result of oxidative scission at the α linkage (i.e., between the two pyrrole rings bearing the vinyl groups) and therefore possess a IXα structure.[81] It is probable that the two hydroxyl groups in the two terminal pyrroles tautomerize to give a lactam structure.[81]

Biliverdin is the bile pigment most nearly related to protoporphyrin, since its four pyrrole groups are joined through three of the original methyne bridges, and the side chains are unaltered. When the central methyne group is reduced to a methene group, bilirubin is formed. Bilirubin is the only common bile pigment to give the well-known van den Bergh reaction.

The urobilinoids are formed as the result of chemical or bacterial hydrogenation of bilirubin. Numerous compounds have been described, the commonest found in human feces being urobilin IXα, stercobilin and d-urobilin; these have a characteristic absorption spectra at 490 to 500 mμ and form intense green fluorescing zinc complexes with ethanolic zinc acetate after oxidation with iodine (Jaffe-Schlesinger reaction). They can be distinguished by their optical rotation, infrared spectra, melting point, and behavior in the mesobiliviolin and dioxane reactions. Their fully hydrogenated precursors, the urobilinogens, react with Ehrlich's aldehyde reagent to form characteristic red pigments; this reaction is, however, not specific for urobilinogen and a positive result is given by porphobilinogen, as well as other compounds. The relation between the different bile pigments is shown in Figure 8–1. An excellent account of the structure and chemical properties of the bile pigments is given by T. K. With.[238]

FORMATION OF BILE PIGMENTS

From Hemoglobin. It is generally accepted that the formation of bilirubin from hemoglobin from effete red cells occurs mainly in the cells of the reticuloendothelial system (RES). Studies with erythrocytes labeled with ^{51}Cr and ^{59}Fe have shown that the principal sites of hemoglobin catabolism are the bone marrow, the spleen and the liver,[101] while the kidneys, the lungs and the intestines play a minor role.[238] Recent experiments with hemoglobin labeled with iron emphasize that the liver is the main site of hemoglobin degradation and suggest that the parenchymal cells as well as the Kupffer cells (RES) play an important role in the process.[238]

The intermediate steps in hemoglobin catabolism have been much discussed but are poorly understood. The early workers considered that first the globin is split off to form hematin and then the iron is removed to give protoporphyrin and that finally the porphyrin ring is opened and biliverdin is formed.[79] Alternatively, in vitro studies by Lemberg, Kench and many Japanese investigators[104, 117, 129] have suggested that the heme moiety of hemoglobin is oxidized while still linked to the globin to give choleglobin, and that the protein and iron are subsequently removed during its conversion to biliverdin. Although choleglobin has not been detected in vivo in man (only in the red cells of rabbit[129]), present evidence indicates that the porphyrin iron is probably not removed until after the ring is opened.

Although experiments involving the intravenous administration of hematin into animals with bile fistula have provided inconclusive results, studies with tracer doses of ^{15}N-hematin[137] and ^{14}C-hematin[208] have shown that hematin can be readily converted into bilirubin. This does not, however, prove that hematin is necessarily an intermediate, since there is always the theoretical possibility that it first becomes hemoglobin and then is catabolized in the normal way. Similar results have been obtained with protoporphyrin.[103, 140]

Renewed interest in this problem has resulted from the reports of Nakajima and colleagues[148] that liver and kidney contain an enzyme "heme α-methenyl oxygenase" which catalyzes the transformation of the hemoglobin bound to haptoglobin to formyl biliverdin, a possible precursor of biliverdin IXα.[149] Hematin and protoporphyrin are not substrates for this enzyme, which has not been located in effective concentrations in the spleen or bone marrow. Furthermore, hemoglobin, in excess of that bound to haptoglobin,[157] can be readily converted to bilirubin, so that it seems unlikely that the formation and subsequent degradation of the haptoglobin complex will prove to be of importance in the catabolism of hemoglobin

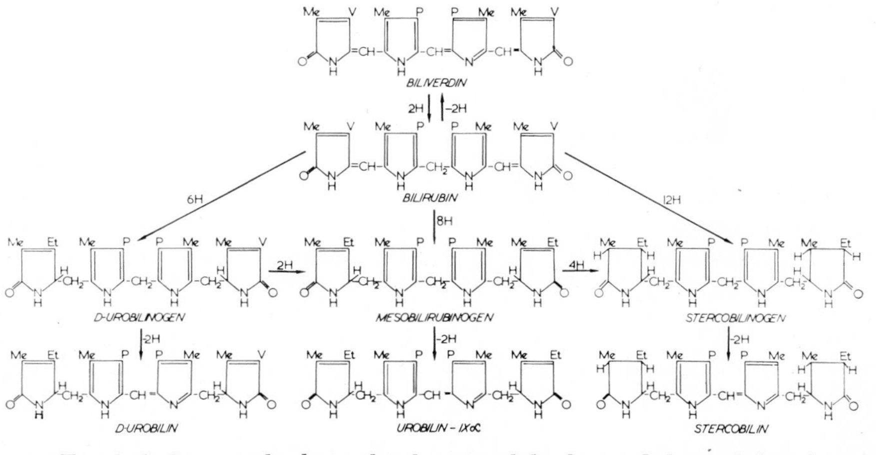

Fig. 8–1. Structural relationship between bilirubin and the urobilinoids. (Gray, C. H.: Bile Pigments in Health and Disease, Springfield, Ill., Thomas, 1961.)

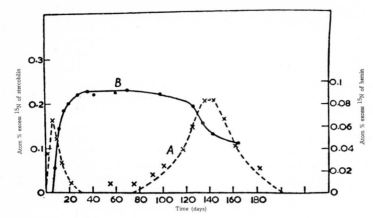

Fig. 8–2. [15]N contents of hemin samples (full line) and of stercobilin (dotted line) at various times after administration of glycine (12 Gm.) containing 31.65 atoms per cent excess ^{15}N to a normal subject. (Gray, C. H., Neuberger, A., and Sneath, P. H. A.: Biochem. J. 47:87.)

in vivo. The above findings have not yet been confirmed by other investigators,[118] so that the importance of heme α-methenyl oxygenase in this process has still to be established.

There seems little doubt that biliverdin is the immediate precursor of bilirubin, and a NAD (or NADP) dependent enzyme "biliverdin reductase" has been isolated from guinea pig liver and spleen as well as human liver, which will catalyze this reaction.[207] It has also been demonstrated *in vivo* that biliverdin can be converted to bilirubin.[78, 177]

From Other Heme Compounds. Studies in which human subjects were given a labeled precursor of heme, such as [15]N- or ^{14}C-glycine, have shown that a large peak of labeled bile pigment was present in the feces between 90 and 150 days after isotope administration, which is the average erythrocyte life span.[80, 85, 138] A smaller peak, accounting for 10 to 20 per cent of the total labeled pigment in the normal subject, was found during the first few days. (Fig. 8–2). Marked increases in this early pigment formation have been found in diseases associated with "ineffective erythropoiesis" such as pernicious anemia, thalassemia and sideroblastic anemia as well as in porphyria and after bleeding.[82, 86, 139, 173] Therefore, it was postulated that the early labeled peak (ELP) of bile pigment originated from the degradation of hemoglobin, formed in the bone marrow during erythroid cell development, which never reached the circulation.

Subsequently it has been shown that there is a second component of ELP, which is derived from sources which are independent of either the production or the destruction of erythrocytes. This was first demonstrated by administering isotopic δ-amino levulinic acid (ALA) which preferentially labels bilirubin from extra-erythroid sites.[108, 172, 202] Maximal formation of ELP occurs within 1 to 2 hours, which indicates that this bilirubin is derived from heme compounds with a rapid rate of turnover. It has been postulated that the microsomal heme enzymes cytochrome-P_{450} and cytochrome-b_5 are possible precursors.[198] Isolated rat liver perfusion experiments[171] have indicated that the liver is probably the main organ involved in this process but such tissues as the kidney may also play a role.[201] The work of Petryka has raised the possibility that some of this early labeled bilirubin may not have a IXα structure[161]; the significance of this finding has to be established.

Studies of Israels and co-workers strongly suggest that in normal man ELP has both nonerythropoietic and erythropoietic components.[245] Robinson and associates[170] did not, however, find any evidence for the latter component in a child with congenital nonhemolytic hyperbilirubinemia, whose ELP pattern closely resembled that found in the Gunn rat. Differences in methodology could account for the lack of agreement between these two groups of investigators and further work is obviously required to determine to what extent the bone marrow is important in the production of ELP and whether in certain disease conditions the nonerythropoietic component is increased.

Animal experiments have shown that the hepatic component of ELP is increased after surgery[106] and so may contribute to the rise in serum bilirubin frequently observed in the immediate postoperative period; Israels has suggested that this increased production of ELP is an index of hepatic dysfunction. In the newborn, Vest[223] has reported an increase in the early labeled bilirubin compared with the normal adult, but its origin has not yet been established.

The degradation of heme is associated with the production of carbon monoxide. When ^{14}C-glycine is administered to man, the labeling of the carbon monoxide occurs before that of heme, which suggests that it originates from sources other than that of the circulating hemoglobin. *In vitro* studies[235a] have shown that the production of ^{14}C-carbon monoxide is associated with concomitant production of hepatic ELP, which supports the concept that they both originate from hepatic heme. It has therefore been proposed that measurements of ^{14}C-carbon monoxide formation following the administration of labeled bilirubin precursors could be used to give assessment of nonerythropoietic bilirubin formation.

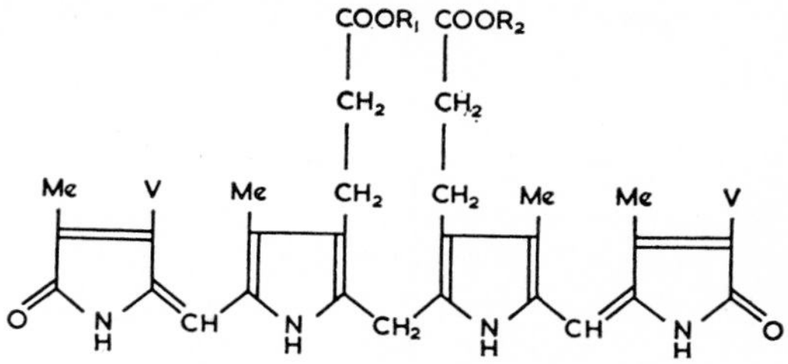

FATE OF BILE PIGMENTS

Transport in the Blood. Since unconjugated bilirubin is almost insoluble at a physiologic pH, it is transported in the blood bound tightly to albumin. The maximum binding capacity is 2 moles bilirubin/1 mole albumin,[157a] which is equivalent in the normal adult to a plasma unconjugated bilirubin concentration of 60 to 80 mg./100 ml. There is therefore little likelihood that the binding capacity of the plasma would become saturated in the jaundiced patient. An equilibrium is established between the pigments in the plasma and the tissues, and the studies of Schmid and Hammaker[196] using ^{14}C-bilirubin in a case of idiopathic unconjugated hyperbilirubinemia, have indicated that the size of the extravascular pool for unconjugated bilirubin is approximately twice that of the plasma pool.

Organic anions such as sulfonamides,[110] salicylates,[110] thyroxine[110] and free fatty acids[110] compete with bilirubin for protein binding in the plasma and in this way influ-

Fig. 8–3. Structure of bile pigments. (Bilirubin, R_1 and R_2 = H; Pigment I, R_1 = glucuronyl and R_2 = H; Pigment II, R_1 and R_2 = glucuronyl; in all, Me = methyl and V = vinyl.)

ence the distribution of bilirubin between the plasma and tissues, including the brain. Metabolic and respiratory acidosis[59] have also been shown to increase the deposition of bilirubin in the brain. The danger of giving the drugs mentioned above to the newborn who are not able to excrete bilirubin, due to a deficiency of glucuronyl transferase, is obvious, since kernicterus could develop.

In spite of the strong binding of bilirubin to plasma albumin, it can cross biological membranes in an unbound form. This has been shown in the placenta,[131, 184] liver,[4, 39] intestine[75, 132] and gallbladder[156] but not in the kidney.

Hepatic Uptake of Bilirubin. Under normal conditions, bilirubin is removed almost completely from the circulation by the liver, so that the serum bilirubin level remains below 1 mg./100 ml. (see Gilbert's Syndrome). Isotope studies have shown that this is an extremely rapid process involving first the detachment of the albumin at the cell surface.[39] The pigment is then accepted by one or more specific intracellular proteins present in the cell sap. The nature of these binding sites is under active investigation by many groups of workers,[87] and at present it can only be concluded that the protein is not albumin. A preliminary report by Arias and associates[134] indicates that competition for one of the binding sites probably explains why the drugs bunamiodyl (Orabilix)[24, 33] and flavaspidic acid (male fern oil)[90, 154] cause unconjugated hyperbilirubinemia; previous studies had suggested that there was interference in hepatic uptake, but had not defined the mechanism.

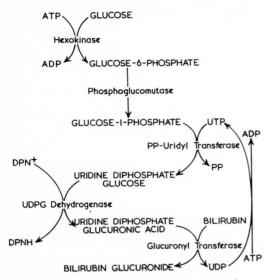

ATP · GLUCOSE

Hexokinase

ADP · GLUCOSE-6-PHOSPHATE

Phosphoglucomutase

GLUCOSE-1-PHOSPHATE · UTP
ADP

PP-Uridyl Transferase

DPN⁺

URIDINE DIPHOSPHATE · PP
GLUCOSE

UDPG Dehydrogenase

URIDINE DIPHOSPHATE   BILIRUBIN
GLUCURONIC ACID

DPNH

Glucuronyl Transferase
ATP

BILIRUBIN GLUCURONIDE · UDP

FIG. 8–4. Possible mechanism for the conjugation of bilirubin with glucuronic acid. (Billing, B. H., and Lathe, G. H.: Am. J. Med. 24:111.)

There is indirect evidence from bilirubin loading tests that a defect in the mechanism of hepatic uptake is one of the reasons for the mild jaundice observed in Gilbert's syndrome.[18, 29] Electron microscopy has demonstrated a lesion in the cell membrane,[74, 126] and it remains to be seen whether a deficiency of the intrahepatic binding protein is responsible for the increased reflux of bilirubin from liver to plasma, which has been reported in these patients.

Conjugation. Bilirubin is a lipid soluble, nonpolar pigment, which gives an "indirect" reaction with diazotized sulfanilic acid in the van den Bergh test at an acid pH. The pigment which is excreted in the bile differs from bilirubin in that it is water soluble at physiologic pHs and gives a "direct" van den Bergh reaction; it has an affinity for denatured plasma proteins, is more easily oxidized and is also present in icteric urine. Serum from patients with hepatocellular and obstructive jaundice contains both "direct" and "indirect" bilirubin, and a knowledge of the relative amounts of these two pigments may be of diagnostic value in clinical practice, particularly if all the pigment is in the "indirect" (unconjugated) form.

The difference in properties exhibited by the pigment in bile compared with that of bilirubin is due to a change in its chemical structure during passage through the liver. This reaction involves the esterification of the carboxyl groups of bilirubin with glucuronic acid to form an alkali-labile acyl diglucuronide[28, 181, 194, 216] (Fig. 8–3). It is catalyzed by a microsomal enzyme, bilirubin UDP-glucuronyl transferase,[88, 127, 197] which is located predominantly in the smooth and also in the rough portions of the endoplasmic reticulum[235]; uridine diphosphate glucuronic acid (UDPGA) serves as the glucuronyl donor (Fig. 8–4). There is increasing evidence that bilirubin conjugation requires a specific enzyme[89, 220] for this reaction, and it is therefore not justifiable to study rates of glucuronide formation using other acceptor molecules (i.e., menthol, 4-methyl umbelliferone and salicylamide) either *in vitro* or *in vivo* and assume that they necessarily reflect the capacity of the liver to conjugate bilirubin.

Although bilirubin UDP-glucuronyl transferase is present in tissues other than the liver there is at present no conclusive evidence to indicate that the extrahepatic conjugation of bilirubin plays an important role in man; it has been demonstrated only in the hepatectomized animal.[99]

Chromatographic analysis of both bile and sera from patients with obstructive jaundice and hepatocellular disease has suggested that small quantities of bilirubin monoglucuronide (Pigment I) as well as bilirubin diglucuronide (Pigment II) may be formed.[53] The evidence in favor of a monoglucuronide structure for Pigment I is, however, also compatible with the pigment being a complex of bilirubin and bilirubin diglucuronide[28, 84, 153, 232]; the solution of this problem must await isolation of pure preparations of both pigments.

In man, more than 90 per cent of the bilirubin excreted in bile is in the form of bilirubin diglucuronide. Other conjugates of bilirubin, such as the sulfate,[151, 152] have been detected but there have been no reports of increases in alternative types of conjugation to compensate for a reduction in glucuronide formation.

A deficiency of UDPGA or of bilirubin

UDP-glucuronyl transferase causes an unconjugated hyperbilirubinemia. In the newborn the enzyme may be slow to develop so that "physiologic jaundice" results. In rare instances this deficiency may continue into adult life. If it is only a relative deficiency then administration of phenobarbital will cause a marked reduction in the serum bilirubin level, probably as the result of enzyme induction.[55, 170, 234, 244]; this effect will not be observed if there is an absolute deficiency of glucuronyl transferase (see *chronic nonhemolytic unconjugated hyperbilirubinemia*).[14] Animal experiments have suggested that bilirubin may itself have induction properties[16]; if this is so then it will be possible to account for the presence of conjugated bilirubin in cases of severe hemolytic disease in the newborn, in spite of an immature liver.

Disposal of Bile Pigments. *In the Normal Adult.* Although very small quantities of unconjugated bilirubin may be excreted in bile,[156] the main biliary pigment is bilirubin glucuronide. It is concentrated in the liver cell prior to excretion. This latter process involves an active transport mechanism, the necessary energy for which is derived from the metabolism of glucose.[30] Recent studies have suggested that the excretion of bilirubin glucuronide may be under hormonal control since hypophysectomized animals have a decreased ability to excrete conjugated bilirubin, which can be corrected by treatment with pituitary hormone and thyroxine.[73] Organic anions as well as such drugs as the anabolic steroids[10] will compete with bilirubin glucuronide for excretion, and may thus cause jaundice.

Conjugated bilirubin forms a large molecular complex with cholesterol, phospholipids and bile salts, so that it appears in bile as a mixed micelle.[35] In the adult subject intestinal bacteria will cause the conjugated bilirubin to undergo deconjugation and hydrogenation, so that urobilinoids are formed. It is not known which of these processes occurs first and whether unconjugated bilirubin is formed in sufficient amounts for the enterohepatic circulation of bilirubin to be of physiological significance.[75, 132] The nature of the final pigment in the feces will depend on the type of

bacterial flora present, and is not related to the state of health or disease of the subject[230]; it will consist of a mixture of stercobilin, urobilin IXα and d-urobilin and their respective precursors, all of which will be estimated in the standard procedure for "fecal urobilinogen." Although recent isotopic studies have confirmed that there is an enterohepatic circulation for urobilinogen,[133] this does not appear to be of importance in the disposal of bile pigments in the normal subject, since only about 1 per cent of the total amount of pigment formed reaches the systemic circulation after absorption and appears in the urine.[36]

Fecal urobilinogen excretion varies between 50 and 250 mg./day. In general this is markedly less than the 300 mg./day which would be expected from determination of direct biliary drainage and from calculations based on the turnover rates of the red cell and other heme-containing compounds [231] and ^{14}C-bilirubin turnover studies.[18]

It has been suggested that this deficit is due to the existence of other pathways for hemoglobin catabolism than its conversion to bilirubin or to unknown mechanisms for the disposal of bilirubin or urobilinogen; the present evidence available suggests that the dipyrrole mesobilifuscin is not a breakdown product and is more likely to be anabolic in origin.[76]

In Chronic Unconjugated Hyperbilirubinemia. A deficiency of glucuronyl transferase results in impaired excretion of pigment into the bile. In chronic nonhemolytic idiopathic hyperbilirubinemia, bilirubin must be removed by alternate metabolic pathways, if the plasma level of bilirubin is to remain constant while pigment is being produced continuously. Since unconjugated bilirubin cannot be excreted directly into the urine, two alternatives exist: First, bilirubin could be excreted across the intestinal wall as bilirubin and then be excreted unchanged, or be converted to fecal urobilinogen. Secondly, the pigment could be converted to water-soluble derivatives of bilirubin which appear in the feces and to a lesser extent in the urine. Studies in which ^{14}C-bilirubin was given to a child with the Crigler-Najjar syndrome,[196] have demonstrated that the catabolism of

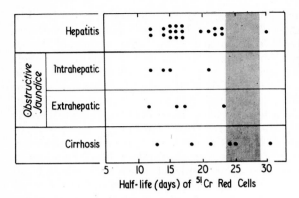

FIG. 8–5. Survival of ^{51}Cr-labeled red cells in 36 patients with liver disease. The shaded area shows the normal range for the half-chromium time. (Pitcher, C. S., and Williams, R.: Clin. Sci. 24:239.)

bilirubin is probably its main method of disposal; the origin of the small amount of fecal urobilinogen which was excreted has not been established.

The rare condition of chronic nonhemolytic unconjugated hyperbilirubinemia is known to be associated with a deficiency of hepatic glucuronyl transferase activity. Arias et al. have reviewed 16 such cases and have presented evidence that this disorder can occur in two forms which appear to be genetically heterogeneous. [14] The patients in their first group were more severely jaundiced (18 to 43 mg./100 ml.) and four out of five had kernicterus. Their bile was essentially colorless and the only pigment present was a trace of unconjugated bilirubin. Their hyperbilirubinemia was unaffected by phenobarbital administration. The eleven patients in the second group were less severely jaundiced (16 to 22 mg./100 ml.) and had pigmented bile which contained bilirubin glucuronide; their response to phenobarbital was dramatic in spite of the fact that only small amounts of bilirubin glucuronyl transferase were apparently detected in liver biopsy specimens. The two groups could not be differentiated by their abnormal response to the menthol tolerance test or by their marked reduction in hepatic glucuronyl transferase activity assayed in biopsy specimens *in vitro* using 4-methyl umbelliferone as the glucuronide receptor. Using the menthol tolerance test it appeared that in group 1 the conjugation defect is transmitted as an autosomal recessive, whereas in group 2 it is an autosomal dominant character. The fundamental

difference between the two groups is unknown, but it would appear that in the group 1 patients the bilirubin glucuronyl transferase deficiency is absolute, whereas in group 2 patients it is probably relative.

In hemolytic disease, production of bilirubin is increased which results, in the presence of a normal liver, in an increased excretion of fecal urobilinogen. This is reflected in an increased urinary excretion of urobilinogen. Only in severe cases is the excretory capacity of the liver exceeded so that hyperbilirubinemia results.[163] The capacity of the liver to excrete bilirubin is greatly in excess of that normally required, so that even if the rate of red cell destruction were increased six-fold, the serum bile pigment concentration would be unlikely to rise above 5 mg./100 ml. Unconjugated bilirubin is the main pigment found in the serum of these patients; therefore, bilirubinuria is not usually observed. Occasionally, if there is also hepatic dysfunction, conjugated bilirubin appears in the plasma.[219] On the other hand, very marked hemolysis can be accompanied by the presence of considerable quantities of conjugated bilirubin in the blood and with bilirubinuria.[182] This is not necessarily based on liver damage *per se*, but rather on overloading of the excretory capacity of an otherwise normal liver.

In Obstructive Jaundice and Hepatocellular Disease. In the majority of patients with liver disease, red cell survival is reduced,[162] and therefore the amount of bilirubin to be disposed of is greater than in the normal subject (Fig. 8–5). In bile duct obstruction, whether intra- or extrahepatic in origin, the serum pigment rises and then, if the obstruction is complete, the level plateaus and values of 10 to 30 mg./100 ml. may be recorded.[242] This value is unrelated to the duration of the obstruction, and an adequate explanation for the individual variation has not yet been given. Isotopic studies in biliary atresia[43] and in experimental animals with bile duct ligation[1, 4, 44] suggest that urine excretion is the major factor in controlling bilirubin homeostasis in these conditions; catabolism of the bile pigments also occurs.

The rise in serum bile pigment concentration is due almost entirely to conjugated bilirubin; recent studies, using extraction rather than diazo technics, indeed suggest that the apparent rises in unconjugated bilirubin may be technical artifacts.[222] There is, therefore, evidence that conjugation is rarely impaired in liver disease (except in cases of unconjugated hyperbilirubinemia). Assays of bilirubin-UDP glucuronyl transferase[31] on liver biopsy specimens have con-

firmed this impression and have indicated that in many instances the values of the enzyme are raised; in interpreting these results, however, consideration must be given to the therapy the patient is receiving, since drugs such as phenobarbital cause induction of the enzyme.

Chromatographic technics have indicated that in hepatocellular disease, the dominant pigment is Pigment I, whereas in obstructive jaundice it is Pigment II.[99] It is, however, impossible to attach any real significance to these findings until the nature of Pigment I is established and the technics for separating the different forms of bilirubin are improved.

The presence of ether-soluble bilirubin[50, 100, 217] in the plasma of many patients with malignant disease has been noted, but has not been found to be diagnostic. The extracted pigment appears to be a stable complex of either unconjugated or conjugated bilirubin with phospholipid and is bound mainly to plasma albumin.

Analytical difficulties have prevented satis-

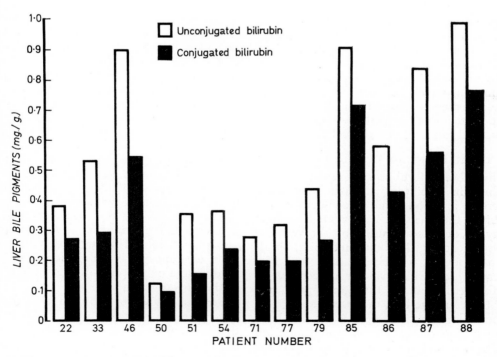

FIG. 8–6. Concentrations of conjugated and unconjugated bilirubin in livers from 13 patients with large duct biliary obstruction. (Raia, S.: Gastroenterology. In Press)

factory determinations of the pool sizes and turnover rates of unconjugated and conjugated bilirubin in obstructive jaundice. Studies in which ^{14}C-bilirubin was given to animals[4] whose bile ducts had been ligated do, however, suggest that the extravascular pool of conjugated bilirubin is considerably greater than that of unconjugated bilirubin, so that, apparently, the protein binding of the two types of bilirubin is different.

Histochemical and chemical determinations of bile pigments in the cholestatic liver have demonstrated that approximately 50 per cent of the bilirubin present is unconjugated[166] (Fig. 8–6), which suggests that bilirubin glucuronide has been deconjugated. A close association between the lysosomes and the granules of the unconjugated bilirubin in both the Kupffer and hepatic cells has been noted by Raia, so that it is tempting to speculate that lysosomal β-glucuronidase plays a role in the intracellular hydrolysis of bilirubin glucuronide.[166] Experiments in which ^{14}C conjugated bilirubin has been administered to Gunn rats show that bilirubin glucuronide can be deconjugated *in vivo*, but it has yet to be established that this necessarily takes place in the liver, or that this process is of importance in the normal subject.[3]

Studies with ^{3}H-urobilinogen[23] have established that in hepatic insufficiency, urobilinogen, which has been absorbed from the intestine, escapes from the enterohepatic circulation into the systemic circulation, and can then be excreted in the urine.

RENAL EXCRETION OF BILE PIGMENTS

Bilirubin. Bilirubin is excreted by the kidney in significant amounts only when there is a raised level of conjugated bilirubin in the plasma. Unconjugated bilirubin may be detected in urine by the van den Bergh reaction, if conjugated bilirubin is also present; it is probably present as Pigment I.[53] Many observations are compatible with the hypothesis that conjugated bilirubin is excreted in the urine mainly by glomerular filtration.[4, 68, 97, 226] It has been shown that whereas unconjugated bilirubin is firmly bound to plasma albumin and cannot be separated from it by ultrafiltration, approximately 0.6 per cent of human plasma

conjugated bilirubin is dialyzable[70] and it is generally believed that it is this fraction which is available for glomerular filtration. Although bilirubin glucuronide can be shown histochemically to accumulate in the renal tubules, most investigators now consider that bile pigments are probably not secreted by the tubules.[6, 68] The role of tubular absorption is not clearly understood, but indirect evidence suggests that the increased excretion of bile pigments observed in systemic alkalosis is due to decreased absorption, while acidosis causes an increase.[4]

Compounds such as salicylate, sulfisoxazole and bile salts, which compete with bilirubin glucuronide for protein binding and thus increase the amount of dialyzable conjugated bilirubin available, will augment the renal excretion of bile pigments.[6] Unfortunately, neither these substances nor sodium bicarbonate can be used as therapeutic agents for the reduction of cholestatic jaundice, for the dose required to get a significant effect would be too great.

The threshold level of serum conjugated bilirubin at which bilirubinuria occurs varies greatly and may alter during the course of the disease. Thus, in the acute phase of hepatitis, bile pigments may be detected in the urine before clinical icterus occurs, whereas during recovery urinary bile pigments may be absent, even though the serum level is as high as 10 mg./100 ml. Factors that influence the binding of conjugated bilirubin to plasma albumin may be important, and it has been postulated that conjugated bile salts have a controlling influence.[69] However, bilirubinuria occurs in hemolytic disease, if there is a conjugated hyperbilirubinemia, and since in this condition it is unlikely that bile salts will be detected in the urine, other factors must also play a role. The suggestion that the renal clearance of bilirubin depends upon binding to a polypeptide carrier[70] also needs further investigation.

Renal clearance of bilirubin glucuronide is very low[238]; compared with biliary excretion it is an inefficient method of disposing of bilirubin. Values of 0.07 to 0.82 ml./min. have been recorded; according to most investigators these measurements of renal clearance have no diagnostic value. The diversity in the results reported in the literature is due mainly to the use of nonspecific analytical methods for the estimation of the pigment in urine and its chemical instability. If attention is paid to these points[64] it is possible to show that in parenchymatous liver disease the renal clearance is independent of the urine output and the serum bilirubin concentration, slightly higher values being recorded in cirrhosis than in hepatitis. Significantly higher values have been found in cholestatic jaundice where there is a positive correlation between the clearance value and the bilirubin concentration; it has been postulated that it is due to the increased bile salt concentration in the blood of these patients.

Urobilinogen. Urobilinogen is approximately 80 per cent bound to plasma protein, so that only a small fraction of the total plasma content is filtered by the glomerulus. There is some suggestive evidence that urobilinogen is also secreted by the proximal tubules. In addition, Milne and co-workers

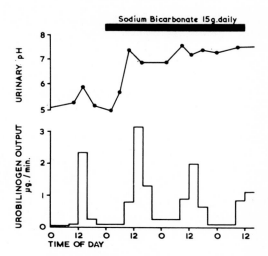

FIG. 8–8. Diurnal variation in urinary urobilinogen in a normal subject with and without sodium bicarbonate ingestion. (Bourke, E., Milne, M. D., and Stokes, G. S.: Brit. Med. J. 2:1510, 1965.)

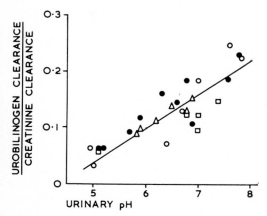

FIG. 8–7. Urobilinogen clearance (expressed as a fraction of the simultaneous endogenous creatinine clearance) related to urinary pH in four patients with hemolytic anemia or hepatocellular jaundice. There is a positive correlation between the two variables. The calculated regression line is given. Closed circles: hereditary spherocytosis. Open circles: sickle cell anemia. Triangles: cholangiolitic hepatitis. Squares: infectious hepatitis. (Bourke, E., Milne, M.D., and Stokes, G. S.: Brit. Med. J. 2:1510, 1965.)

have shown that distal tubular pH-dependent back diffusion takes place.[36] Urobilinogen excretion correlates well with urinary pH both in normal subjects and in patients with hepatic dysfunction or hemolytic disease, higher values being recorded in alkaline than in acid urines (Fig. 8–7). The significance of urinary urobilinogen determinations in these conditions can be assessed only if allowance is made for urinary pH.

It has been known for over 70 years that diurnal variation in urobilinogen excretion occurs. Two of the possible causes for this phenomenon are variations in renal clearance due to diurnal changes in urinary pH, and alterations in plasma urobinogen concentration. The relationship of diurnal variation in urinary urobilinogen to ingestion of sodium bicarbonate in a normal subject is shown in Figure 8–8. For analysis a 2- or 4-hour specimen collected between noon and 4 P.M. appears to be the best.

Normal subjects excrete 0 to 4 mg. urobilinogen/day. This amount is increased in parenchymal liver damage, hemolytic disease and partial bile duct obstruction, and is decreased or absent in neoplastic bile duct obstruction; in hepatitis, fluctuations occur. It is generally accepted that only "free" urobilinogen appears in the urine, although it is not possible to establish this with present-day technics. The fact that its mode of excretion differs from that of bilirubin glucuronide, which does not involve nonionic diffusion, and that it is readily absorbed from the intestine, is in keeping with this hypothesis.

CLASSIFICATION AND MECHANISMS

The fact that through the years various classifications of jaundice have been proposed would indicate the lack of an ideal one. (Refer to the second edition of Diseases of the Liver for a discussion of these.) One of us (L. S.) prefers the following clinical classification of jaundice (although admittedly not ideal): (1) hemolytic, (2) hepatocellular (a, without features of biliary obstruction; b, cholestatic; and c, congenital) and (3) obstructive types. The hepatocellular type is composed chiefly of the various forms of hepatitis and hepatic cirrhosis and includes the intrahepatic cholestatic forms due to the hepatitis virus or viruses, various drugs, including particularly chlorpromazine, methyl testosterone, anabolic steroids, oral contraceptives, and the recurrent idiopathic form[214] and the intrahepatic cholestasis of pregnancy (the last two are considered in Chapter 30). The obstructive form includes biliary obstruction due to neoplasm, gallstones, stricture, cholangitis or contiguous inflammatory processes (pancreatitis) or, uncommonly, cysts.

With advances in knowledge of cellular structure and increasing interest in cellular physiology and cell transport and the discovery of the conjugation of bilirubin, more attention is being focused on the liver cell

itself in the pathogenesis of icterus. Thus jaundice may result from decreased uptake of bilirubin by the liver cell, defective conjugation by the cell or impaired excretion into the bile canaliculi (or blockage to the flow of bile through the ductal system) (Fig. 8–9).

A classification of hyperbilirubinemia related to the type of defect involved is given in Table 8–1.

HEREDITARY HYPERBILIRUBINEMIAS (IN THE ADULT)

Gilbert's Syndrome (Constitutional Hepatic Dysfunction, Idiopathic Unconjugated Hyperbilirubinemia). Caution must be exercised in the diagnosis of Gilbert's syndrome, for chronic unconjugated hyperbilirubinemia in the absence of overt hemolysis may accompany a number of diseased states such as cardiac disease, fatty liver and alcoholism, biliary tract disease, cirrhosis, malignant tumors and infections.[135] Unconjugated hyperbilirubinemia may follow a bout of viral hepatitis[102, 114] and may occasionally represent a compensated hemolytic state.[66] It has been reported as a variant of other hereditary hyperbilirubinemias (see below). It may also appear in patients who have undergone portacaval shunt with hemolysis playing an important role in pathogenesis.[57] It may occur in thyrotoxicosis even in the absence of congestive failure.[83] Unconjugated hyperbilirubinemia may also occur at high altitudes.[22]

True Gilbert's syndrome is probably inherited as an autosomal dominant and the patients are heterozygous for a single mutant gene.[164] Unconjugated hyperbilirubinemia has been detected in 16.1 per cent of

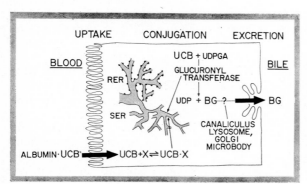

FIG. 8–9. Schematic representation of current concept of the hepatic metabolism of bilirubin. *BG*, bilirubin glucuronide; *RER*, rough endoplasmic reticulum; *SER*, smooth endoplasmic reticulum; *UCB*, unconjugated bilirubin; *UDP*, uridine diphosphate; *UDPGA*, uridine diphosphate glucuronic acid; *X*, cytoplasmic acceptor of UCB. (Arias, I. M.: Postgrad. Med. *41*:15.)

TABLE 8–1. CLASSIFICATION OF HYPERBILIRUBINEMIA RELATED TO TYPE OF DEFECT INVOLVED

HYPERBILIRUBINEMIA	MECHANISM	CONDITION
	Overproduction	Hemolytic disease Shunt hyperbilirubinemia Postsurgery
	Uptake Defect	Idiopathic unconjugated hyperbilirubinemia (Gilbert's syndrome) Drugs, e.g., cholecystographic agents
UNCONJUGATED	Glucuronyl transferase a) deficiency	"Physiologic jaundice in newborn" Crigler-Najjar syndrome ?Idiopathic unconjugated hyperbilirubinemia
	b) inhibition	Drugs, e.g., novobiocin Steroids—breast milk maternal plasma
	Excretion Defect a) metabolic	Conjugated hyperbilirubinemia in newborn Dubin-Johnson and Rotor syndromes Jaundice of pregnancy Anabolic steroids
CONJUGATED	b) obstruction	Cirrhosis Hepatitis Extrahepatic obstruction Drug jaundice

healthy parents and 27.5 per cent of healthy siblings of patients with this disorder.[164] The distribution of values of serum bilirubin in normal controls, probands and healthy first-degree relatives is shown in Figure 8–10. Gilbert's syndrome is most commonly seen in young males, and jaundice may be present from birth or may be first noted in adult life and persist into old age, but tends to lessen with age. The icterus fluctuates in degree and may be increased by fatigue, emotional tension, excessive intake of alcohol, intercurrent infection, or menstruation. Neither hepatomegaly nor splenomegaly is present. Hepatic function is usually normal, except for an impaired bilirubin tolerance, and histologic examination of the liver is usually normal, although fatty infiltration has been reported. The mode of presentation of 42 patients with Gilbert's syndrome is listed in Table 8–2,

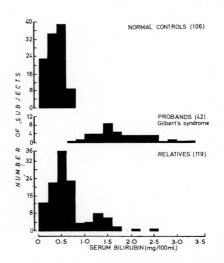

FIG. 8–10. Serum bilirubin in Gilbert's syndrome. (Powell, Hemingway, Billing, and Sherlock: New Engl. J. Med. 277: 1108.)

240   Jaundice

TABLE 8–2. MODE OF PRESENTATION OF 42
PATIENTS WITH IDIOPATHIC, UNCONJUGATED
HYPERBILIRUBINEMIA

PRESENTATION	NO. OF PATIENTS	PER-CENT-AGE
Gastrointestinal complaints:		
Nausea	2	
Abdominal pain:		
Mild	6	
Severe	3	
X-ray examination negative:		
Dyspepsia	2	
Constipation or diarrhea	3	
	16	38.1
Fatigue or malaise or both	13	30.9
Asymptomatic jaundice	7	16.7
Jaundice apparently precipitated by:		
Influenzal illness	3	
Exercise	1	
Migraine	1	
Epilepsy	1	
	6	14.3

From Powell, Hemingway, Billing and Sherlock: New Engl. J. Med. 277:1108.

The majority of patients have an unconjugated bilirubinemia of 1 to 4 mg./100 ml. In 33 per cent of a series of cases, there was at least one estimation of serum bilirubin in the normal range. It has been postulated that a defect in the uptake of bilirubin by the liver cell is responsible for the jaundice in these patients; and analysis of plasma bilirubin disappearance curves, following an injection of bilirubin, tends to substantiate this hypothesis.[29] In vivo and in vitro studies of glucuronide synthesis using ether-forming glucuronide receptors[17, 66, 195, 224] have given results within the normal range so that it has been postulated that the glucuronyl activity with respect to bilirubin is also normal. However, Black and Billing have recently obtained evidence of impairment in bilirubin conjugation when they used bilirubin as the substrate in the assay of UDP glucuronyl transferase activity in needle specimens of liver.[31] This finding requires explanation in

view of the fact that the pigment composition of the bile of these patients is apparently normal, as is their fecal urobilinogen excretion.

Patients with a hyperbilirubinemia greater than 5 mg./100 ml. are rare, and it seems likely that in these subjects there is a defect in glucuronide formation such as is seen in infants with the Crigler-Najjar syndrome but to a varying extent.[8] Fecal urobilinogen excretion is usually decreased, and it would be of interest to know whether other routes of bilirubin breakdown are employed in these enzyme-deficient people to keep the plasma level constant. The administration of ACTH or prednisolone does not appear to affect the degree of jaundice in these patients.[145] Phenobarbital administration will lower the serum bilirubin concentration in these cases.[234]

Chronic Idiopathic Jaundice (Dubin-Johnson Syndrome). This disorder, which was first described independently by two groups—Dubin and Johnson[60a] and Sprinz and Nelson[212]—is a chronic or intermittent form of jaundice with both free and unconjugated bilirubin in the plasma. It is characterized by the presence of large amounts of a yellow-brown or black pigment in the otherwise normal liver cells. This gross discoloration may be detected in a needle biopsy specimen and prove to be of diagnostic value. The pigment has the physical and chemical characteristics of melanin (Fig. 8–11). For a distribution of the pigment in the liver and other appearances on electron microscopy, refer to Chapter 2.

Corriedale sheep have been found to have both morphologic and functional defects similar to those of patients with the Dubin-Johnson syndrome.[54] They exhibit impairment in biliary excretion of bilirubin and dyes, which are organic anions, but excrete bile acids and cations normally, which indicates that different mechanisms are involved in the excretion of these two groups of compounds.[13]

Accumulation of a similar appearing pigment—but thought to be lipofuscin—has been reported in howler monkeys.[144]

As in Gilbert's syndrome this disorder manifests itself as a form of chronic or intermittent jaundice most commonly seen in young people and frequently familial in occurrence. Unlike Gilbert's syndrome, there is an increase in both the conjugated and the free bilirubin levels in the serum. According to Dubin, most patients complain of abdominal pain in the region of the liver, and the liver is palpable and tender in about one half of the cases.[60] A striking feature is the failure of the gallbladder, although normal, to visualize on oral cholecystography.

Jaundice may be precipitated or aggravated by many factors, including pregnancy, surgical operations, severe physical strain, alcoholism and infectious diseases.[60, 60a] The icterus may be mistaken for the obstructive variety because of abdominal pain, dark urine, pale stools, increase in direct-reacting bilirubin, and a nonvisualizing gallbladder. Prognosis is excellent, as indicated by the long duration of the disease and the absence of progressive hepatic damage in long-standing cases.[60, 60a]

Such tests as determination of serum proteins, transaminases, bile acids, alkaline phosphatase as well as the flocculation tests are usually within normal limits but may be raised slightly. On the other hand, all patients show a marked retention of such dyes as Bromsulphalein,[49, 142] rose bengal,[239] and methylene blue[42] which appears to be due to a defect in excretion by hepatic cells. Marked retention of indocyanine green has also been reported.[203] During the first 30 minutes after the injection, Bromsulphalein is cleared from the plasma at a rate similar to or slightly reduced from that seen in the normal subject; the level of the dye in the plasma then rises again and remains elevated for many hours so that it can still be detected after 48 to 72 hours, although exceptions to this may occur.[10] With Bromsulphalein the proportion of dye conjugated with glutathione in the plasma gradually rises and an appreciable amount of the injected dye can be recovered from the urine.

Measurements of serum bilirubin show elevation in both the conjugated (direct) and the total levels. These levels tend to fluctuate under the influence of the factors mentioned above and range from normal

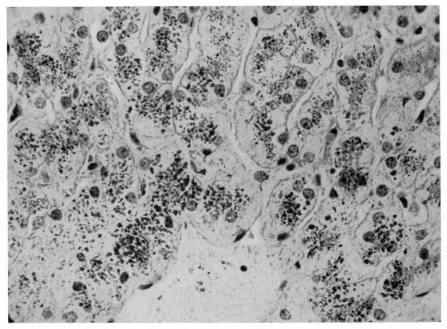

Fig. 8–11. Dubin-Johnson syndrome. Photomicrograph showing pigmentation in liver cells. (Courtesy of the American Forces Institute of Pathology.)

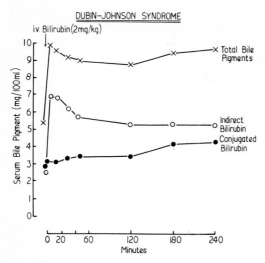

FIG. 8–12. Effect of intravenous bilirubin (2 mg./kg.) on the serum bile pigment concentration of a patient with chronic idiopathic jaundice. (Billing, B. H., et al.: Clin. Sci. 27:245.)

to 19 mg./100 ml. of plasma. Approximately 60 per cent of the cases have total bile pigment concentrations under 6 mg./100 ml. of plasma. Values for conjugated bilirubin have been quoted as ranging from 26 to 86 per cent of the total bilirubin, with a mean value of 60 per cent.[60, 60a]

Of considerable interest is the occurrence of unconjugated hyperbilirubinemia in some instances of the Dubin-Johnson syndrome[179, 200] and even alternating increases in the conjugated and unconjugated serum bilirubin.[180] Slight elevations of serum concentrations of unconjugated but not conjugated bilirubin have been reported in 20 per cent of members of a family of two sisters with the Dubin-Johnson syndrome.[41]

The response of these patients to an injection of bilirubin gives further evidence of impairment in hepatic excretion. Unlike the normal subject, or patients with Gilbert's syndrome, the amount of conjugated bilirubin in the plasma increases and is only removed slowly, mainly by the kidneys[27] (Fig. 8–12). In 4 patients studied, 2 had an impaired hepatic uptake of bilirubin, while the other 2 were normal in this respect.[29] There is no indication of any defect in glucuronide conjugation.

Bile pigments will be detected in the urine if the serum level of conjugated bilirubin is sufficiently high and in some cases urobilinogen is also present. Urinary porphyrin excretion has been reported increased in one case, and melanuria has been noted in another. Fecal stercobilinogen is normal.

Rotor's Syndrome.[174, 192] Possibly this syndrome is a variant of the Dubin-Johnson syndrome as originally suggested by the case studied by Arias[9] and by the demonstration of only a borderline increase in pigment in some members of families with chronic idiopathic jaundice.[239]

The disease appears to be familial in occurrence, with both sexes probably equally represented, and is characterized by a chronic, relatively mild jaundice, fluctuating in degree. As in Gilbert's syndrome, the icterus may increase with fatigue, emotional upsets, or respiratory infections.[95] In one patient the icterus was said to diminish during each of 3 pregnancies,[95] in direct contrast with behavior of cases of the Dubin-Johnson syndrome.[60, 60a] In one of Rotor's cases, ingestion of fatty foods was said to deepen the jaundice. Abdominal pain is usually absent, and the liver and the spleen are not enlarged.

The disorder is chronic, not incapacitating, requires no treatment and appears to be compatible with a normal life. In contrast with the Dubin-Johnson syndrome, the oral cholecystogram is normal, and no pigment is present in the liver cells. However, the bile ducts may fail to visualize roentgenologically following the intravenous injection of iodipamide,[159, 192] though shown to be patent and otherwise normal at peritoneoscopy and laparotomy.[48, 58] Davis and Young have observed coincidental gallbladder calculi. The liver biopsy specimen is essentially normal on light microscopy and fluorescence microscopy.[192] In the case studied by Arias[9] the pericanalicular lysosomes appeared to be increased in numbers and in dispersion throughout the cell as examined with the electron microscope.

Information based on the few cases studied would indicate that the cephalin flocculation test is sometimes abnormal, but the thymol turbidity, zinc sulfate turbidity, total lipids, serum proteins and serum transaminases are within normal limits. The serum alkaline phosphatase activities may tend toward the low side of normal; the level of the serum trihydroxy and dihydroxy bile acids may be within normal range.

There is abnormal retention of Bromsulphalein in the plasma, and the appearance of the dye in the bile following intravenous injection may be somewhat delayed. The retained Bromsulphalein has been found to be almost entirely in the unconjugated form[159, 192] at 45 minutes after injection of the dye.

The serum bilirubin levels fluctuate and are usually less than 10 mg.%, with the free and conjugated pigments present in about equal proportion. Bile pigments can be detected in the urine, provided that the level of conjugated pigments is sufficiently high. Abnormal amounts of urinary urobilinogen are usually not present, although they have been reported; the fecal urobilinogen is not increased.

The response of a patient to a single intravenous injection of bilirubin (2 mg./kilo) shows that the removal of both bilirubin and conjugated bilirubin is considerably delayed as compared with a normal subject. This suggests a diminished uptake of bilirubin by the hepatic cell as well as a specific defect in the secretion of conjugated bilirubin, the mechanism of which is not known.

The available genealogical data, as reported by Rotor and associates,[174] Haverback and Wirtschafter[95] and Arias[11] suggest that familial Rotor's syndrome is transmitted as a dominant (Fig. 8–13).

Idiopathic Dyserythropoietic Jaundice[22a] (Shunt Hyperbilirubinemia). It has been mentioned previously that not all the bilirubin that is formed originates from the breakdown of mature red blood cells. There is, therefore, the possibility that an overproduction of bilirubin unrelated to hemolysis may occur. Israels and colleagues[107] have suggested that such a mechanism is responsible for an unconjugated bilirubinemia that they have observed in four individuals from two Mennonite families. The disorder appears to be very similar to congenital spherocytic anemia except for the fact that after splenectomy the patients remained slightly jaundiced and, in spite of a normal ^{51}Cr red cell survival time, they had a considerable increase in the excretion of fecal urobilinogen, amounting in one case

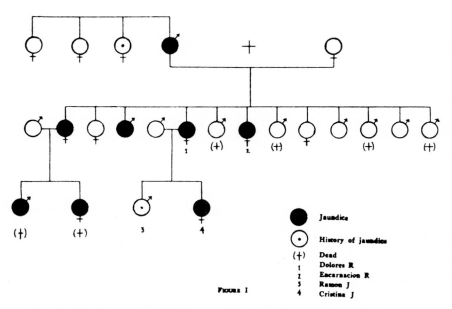

FIGURE I

● Jaundice
⊙ History of jaundice
(+) Dead
1 Dolores R
2 Encarnacion R
3 Ramon J
4 Cristina J

FIG. 8–13. Genealogy of the R Family. (From Rotor, A. B., Manahan, L., and Florentin, A., Acta Medica Philippina, p. 49, 1948.)

to 978 mg./24 hrs. It has now been shown that this excessive pigment excretion was due to an increase in the erythropoietic component of the "early labeled" bilirubin and resulted from hemoglobin released from erythroid cells or their precursors in the bone marrow.[245] The term "shunt hyperbilirubinemia" which was originally used for this condition is therefore inappropriate since it suggests an alternative pathway of bilirubin production direct from porphyrin precursors without the formation of heme.

Similar findings have been described in patients without spherocytosis.[11a, 22a, 122b] It would appear that this condition has the following characteristics: (1) chronic unconjugated hyperbilirubinemia with serum bilirubin concentrations up to 7 mg./100 ml.; (2) normal liver function tests; (3) a reticulocytosis in the peripheral blood; (4) erythroid hyperplasia of the bone marrow; (5) an increased plasma iron turnover, increased serum-iron and percentage saturation of the total iron-binding capacity; (6) normal red cell survival time; (7) increased fecal and urinary urobilinogen excretion; (8) normal autohemolysis, red cell osmotic fragility and red cell enzyme[122a]; and (9) normal red cell protoporphyrin and coproporphyrin concentrations.[22a]

CLINICAL APPROACH

As a rule, the clinician has little difficulty in distinguishing hemolytic from hepatocellular and obstructive jaundice. His usual task is to determine whether jaundice is due to primary liver disease or dysfunction or to obstruction of the extrahepatic bile ducts. In the differentiation of the various forms of jaundice, he has available 6 methods of approach, short of surgical intervention: (1) the history and the physical examination, (2) laboratory tests, (3) response of the serum bilirubin to steroid administration, (4) duodenal drainage, (5) x-ray examination, including percutaneous transhepatic cholangiography and (6) needle biopsy of the liver in selected cases.

We are aware of the extensive use of peritoneoscopy in patients with liver disease (both with and without jaundice) by Caroli,[45, 45a] Kalk,[113] Royer,[175, 176] Ruddock,[178] and Benedict[21] and would therefore refer the reader to their writings.

HISTORY

Family History. The familial occurrence of icterus should suggest the possibilities of hereditary spherocytosis (congenital hemolytic jaundice), Gilbert's syndrome, the Dubin-Johnson or the Rotor syndrome and recurrent intrahepatic cholestasis. A history of consanguinity of parents should arouse suspicion of Wilson's disease.

Occupation. The importance of inquiring into the occupation and environment of a patient with jaundice is evident, with particular reference to exposure to hepatotoxic agents. The increased likelihood of hepatic cirrhosis in bartenders and brewery workers and the predisposition to Weil's disease among workers in rat-infested premises are well known.

Recent contact with a jaundiced individual should suggest the possibility of infectious hepatitis, as should a history of recent travel or ingestion of raw oysters or steamed clams.[123, 124] A bout of painless jaundice in childhood or early adulthood is due most commonly to infectious hepatitis which usually confers permanent immunity. Therefore, another episode of jaundice in later years is likely to be due to some other cause. However, the possibility that the original bout of jaundice may have been due to infectious mononucleosis or homologous serum hepatitis or to another strain of the virus of infectious hepatitis must be considered.

The exposure to or ingestion of hepatotoxic drugs, particularly carbon tetrachloride, Thorazine, methyl testosterone, norethandrolone, oral contraceptives, and mono-amine-oxidase inhibitors, may be of etiologic importance. (See Chap. 14, Toxic and Drug-Induced Hepatitis.) Confronting the patient with a Thorazine tablet as advocated by Brick[37] occasionally helps in the etiologic diagnosis of jaundice. Any drug the patient has been taking should be scrutinized with reference to possible hepatotoxic effects.

Needle puncture from 6 weeks to 6

months prior to the onset of jaundice should lead to suspicion of serum hepatitis (although incubation periods of only 2 weeks may be seen in parenterally transmitted infectious hepatitis). This applies not only to the administration of blood plasma and convalescent serum but also to the use of improperly sterilized needles and syringes for drawing blood, administering parenteral therapy or injecting local anesthetics during dental operations, and to stylettes for puncturing the finger or the ear lobe.

A history of a recent gallbladder operation should lead to suspicion of a residual common duct stone or stricture as the cause of icterus, but careful inquiry should be made as to the transfusion of blood or plasma at the time of surgery in order to exclude serum hepatitis.[185] If multiple transfusions were given, the likelihood of a serum hepatitis becomes proportionately increased, as it does in the case of pooled plasma. Injury to any of the major bile ducts at the time of operation would predispose to the development of a stricture.

History of Resection of a Malignant Tumor. If the interval between resection of the tumor and the appearance of icterus is more than 6 months, homologous serum hepatitis may be excluded. If the interval is greater than 3 or 4 years, an unrelated cause of the icterus should be considered. While metastatic tumor of the liver may make its appearance after so long an interval, it is much more apt to do so within 2 or 3 years.[187]

While **chills and fever** in a jaundiced patient are usually indicative of cholangitis, it is well to remember that they may be prominent during the preicteric phase of infectious hepatitis or in Thorazine jaundice and may recur in some cases of active chronic hepatitis.

Pruritus. As George Budd pointed out over 100 years ago, pruritus is most pronounced in cases of occlusion of the common bile duct, particularly by tumor. According to Schoenfield,[199] pruritus occurs with extrahepatic obstruction in 75 per cent of patients with malignant lesions and in 50 per cent of those with benign conditions. He believes that the itching that occurs in

20 per cent of patients with hepatitis and 10 per cent of those with cirrhosis is often associated with clinical and laboratory evidence of intrahepatic cholestasis, and finds that about 75 per cent of patients with bile duct stricture or primary biliary cirrhosis have pruritus. Itching is very prominent in recurrent intrahepatic cholestasis and in the recurrent jaundice of pregnancy. In the experience of the senior author, the pruritus of the jaundiced patient is often most pronounced on the palms and soles and, like itching in general, more prominent at night and in a warm environment.

While an increase in serum bile acids has long been suspected as the cause of the pruritus, clinicians have long known that itching of the skin not infrequently precedes or follows the appearance or disappearance of icterus. It is not surprising, therefore, that pruritus may occur with low serum bile acid concentrations[199, 211] or may not occur with very high serum bile acid values[155, 199] and that relief of itching may follow the use of norethandrolone without concomitant decrease in serum bile acids.[155, 199]

Of much interest is the observation that the concentration of bile acids on the skin is greater in patients with hepatobiliary disease and associated pruritus than in similar patients without pruritus, and that the proportion of free bile acids and deoxycholic acid on their skin is greater than in their serum.[199]

Abdominal pain is usually inconspicuous in patients with viral hepatitis who are much more apt to complain of an uncomfortable dragging or aching sensation in the epigastrium or the right upper abdomen. It is likewise a minor feature in hepatic cirrhosis. In common duct stone the pain generally is colicky and is accompanied by nausea and vomiting; usually it requires an opiate for relief. It need not be confined to the right upper quadrant; frequently, it is located in the epigastrium and occasionally in other parts of the abdomen. It may be absent, particularly in older individuals.

It is well recognized that pain occurs in most cases of pancreatic carcinoma. While the nature of the pain is not pathognomonic, it is usually located in the epigastrium and is often described as boring in nature. It frequently radiates to the back. As pointed out by Chauffard,[51] it is worse when the patient lies on his back and is lessened by turning on one side and drawing up the knees, by changing to the prone position, or by sitting up and bending forward.[51] Frequently, it is so severe as to require an opiate. While the pain usually precedes the onset of icterus in cases of pancreatic cancer, occasionally it may follow the appearance of jaundice. An "atypical" pain pattern may be produced by peritoneal tumor implants. The senior author has observed one patient with a proved carcinoma of the body of the pancreas who told him that walking with the trunk flexed afforded him relief. Another patient with this disease said that he had obtained relief of pain by the use of 2 aspirin tablets every 4 hours, day and night, for 1 year.

Abdominal pain is usually prominent and may be the presenting symptom in cases of malignant tumor of the liver, primary more than metastatic. It is usually localized to the right hypochondrium and may be dull or sharp and intermittent in character. It may radiate to the right infrascapular area or right flank and may be increased by deep breathing, coughing, exertion or changes in posture. It is presumably due to invasion or stretching of the liver capsule by the neoplasm.

Preicteric Period. It is important to ask the patient how he felt *before the onset of icterus.* If he experienced anorexia, malaise, nausea, diarrhea, epigastric discomfort, weakness, aches and pains, and fever and chills for about a week or so preceding jaundice, viral hepatitis should be strongly suspected. If the preicteric period has extended over several weeks or months, subacute hepatic necrosis should be suspected.[218] The presence of symptoms of an abdominal disorder for several months, accompanied by weight loss, should suggest a neoplastic process. A story of upper abdominal discomfort and digestive symptoms of many years' standing, aggravated by the ingestion of fried or fatty foods and accompanied by bloating, belching, heartburn and constipation, should suggest common duct stone.

A rapidly developing icterus is usually indicative of hepatocellular or hemolytic jaundice.

Color of Urine and Stools. The appearance of dark urine is the best criterion of the onset of jaundice and is apt to precede the yellowish discoloration of the skin or sclerae by one to several days. Reliable information regarding the color of the urine and the stools may be of diagnostic value. In cases of infectious hepatitis the stools are usually clay-colored for a few days to a week or so. In common duct stone they may be alternately acholic and cholic. Occasionally, a seemingly acholic stool may be due to admixture of barium ingested during an upper G.I. x-ray study made to elucidate the basis of the icterus. In neoplastic jaundice they usually remain acholic. The occurrence of brown stools in the presence of deep jaundice is usually indicative of hepatocellular jaundice,[236] but may rarely occur in jaundice due to carcinoma of the pancreas.[191] Although it may prove to be caused by an unsuspected bleeding peptic ulcer, the passage of tarry stools by an icteric patient should suggest carcinoma of the ampulla of Vater or cancer of the pancreas invading the duodenum or the stomach in the absence of marked hypoprothrombinemia.

PHYSICAL EXAMINATION

Age and Sex. The age and the sex of the patient are of diagnostic help. Infectious hepatitis and active chronic hepatitis are seen most commonly in young adults, while common duct stone and neoplastic jaundice usually occur in middle-aged or older individuals. Weil's disease, at least in this country, is said to be rare in females and in children.[15] Portal cirrhosis, hepatoma, pancreatic cancer and primary hemochromatosis predominate in the male, whereas common duct stone, primary biliary cirrhosis and carcinoma of the gallbladder are more prevalent in the female.

Vascular Spiders.[20] These structures should be looked for carefully with the aid of a good light. Inspection with a hand lens may be necessary to distinguish them from small papular lesions. They may pulsate and can be obliterated by pressing on their central point with the end of a pencil. They usually indicate the presence of hepatic cirrhosis, and have been linked with the presence of esophageal varices.[38]

Breath. A peculiar sickly sweetish breath (*hepatic fetor*) is characteristic of severe hepatic disease with necrosis.[228] According to Hoffbauer,[98] hepatic fetor is detected sometimes on the breath of patients with well-compensated hepatic cirrhosis, or it may follow the therapeutic use of large quantities of pure methionine. Methyl mercaptan has been isolated from the urine of patients with hepatic fetor,[46] and this, coupled with a high plasma level of methionine, suggests that the mercaptan arises by hydrolytic or reductive fission of the sulfur-carbon bond in methionine.

Cervical Lymphadenopathy should suggest the presence of viral hepatitis, infectious mononucleosis or Hodgkin's disease.

Prominent Superficial Abdominal Veins are observed most often in patients with hepatic cirrhosis but may occur in the presence of peritoneal tumor implants, obstruction of the portal vein by tumor or in cases of inferior caval obstruction. Normal veins may be made more prominent by stretching and thinning of the overlying skin as a result of abdominal distention in the absence of portal hypertension. (See Chapter 9, Portal Hypertension.) In portal hypertension the blood flow in the abdominal veins is radially away from the umbilicus, whereas in inferior caval obstruction it is always upward over the abdominal wall.[206]

Liver. "One good feel of the liver is worth any two liver function tests" (F. M. Hanger, Jr.). We have been so much impressed with the truth of this dictum that we would strongly emphasize the necessity for a painstaking palpation of the liver in the detection of hepatic disease. To obtain a good "feel" of the liver, the examiner's hand should be warm and the patient should lie on his back, with head slightly raised, arms at his sides and knees flexed. After the examiner has placed his hand below the right rib margin, the patient may be asked to breathe deeply. The first "feel" is often the best be-cause flipping the liver edge at the end of inspiration may be painful and cause the patient to restrict subsequent inspirations. The normal liver is soft, smooth and frequently tender. It has a sharp edge which may not be palpable or may extend 1 to 2 fingerbreadths below the right costal margin.

While a reliable method for estimating liver size is not available—and it has been shown that a direct relationship between the position of lower liver borders and liver weight does not exist—it is safe to assume that a liver which extends 3 fingerbreadths or more below the right costal margin is probably enlarged (and hence the seat of disease), provided that one may exclude downward displacement by right pleural cavity fluid or marked pulmonary emphysema, or the presence of marked visceroptosis. Variations in the shape and the position of the liver appear to accompany body types. In a stocky person, the liver may often extend to the left lateral abdominal wall with its lower edge lying relatively high; it may not be palpable beneath the costal margin. In a lanky individual, the normal liver, including the left lobe, may lie entirely in the right abdomen and may extend 5 fingerbreadths below the costal margin. Here the slant of the liver edge may be steep and may approach an angle of 60°, according to Fleischner and Sayegh.[65] The senior author recalls a patient with a marked hyposthenic habitus whose liver extended down to the level of the navel over the years and was found to be normal at laparotomy and surgical biopsy.

The liver should be palpated on more than one visit, since variations in the degree of abdominal relaxation, in the examiner's own perceptivity and in the time he devotes to the examination will explain the ability to palpate the organ on one day and failure to do so on another. Our own approach is to begin palpation with one hand and to follow with bimanual examination. Before concluding that the liver is impalpable, it is well to feel the abdomen in the lateral decubitus position.

A liver that is unduly firm is apt to be diseased, as is one with a blunted edge or an irregular contour. Lesser degrees of surface irregularity may not be detectable clinically. A very irregular, firm, nodular liver is most commonly indicative of intrahepatic malignant neoplasm. However, the large regenerating nodules of postnecrotic cirrhosis may produce an irregularity of contour which may closely simulate that produced by tumor. The same may hold true in the fatty liver and in congenital cystic disease of the liver.

The examiner should palpate and listen for a friction rub over the liver. Occasionally, the rub may be detected in the right lower chest, anteriorly or anterolaterally. A hepatic friction rub is most commonly indicative of malignant tumor[67] (invading or breaking through the liver capsule). It may also be found in hepatic syphilis, hepatic abscess and in gonococcal perihepatitis associated with acute salpingitis. It may follow percutaneous needle biopsy of the liver. Rarely a friction rub produced by fibrinous exudate localized to an area of pericolic extension of a neoplasm of the ascending colon proves confusing.

The examiner should auscultate the abdomen for the presence of a bruit. The detection of a harsh (arterial) murmur over the liver either with systolic accentuation or purely systolic in character should suggest the presence of hepatoma or alcoholic hepatitis.[52] This type of murmur is not affected by posture, respiration or local pressure with the stethoscope. It is apparently due to locally increased arterial blood flow and should be contrasted with the venous hum of portal hypertension, which arises from collateral venous channels. The venous hum is lower in pitch than the arterial murmur and is altered by posture and by respiration and is frequently obliterated by pressure with the stethoscope. (See Chapter 9, Portal Hypertension.) A systolic murmur over the liver has been described in cases of anemia and may decrease after appropriate blood transfusions.[125]

The liver may not extend below the right costal margin in cases of hepatitis or cirrhosis. Usually it is found 1 to 2 (or 2 to 3) fingerbreadths below the right costal margin in viral hepatitis and is frequently tender in this disease. A *very large liver* (one extending 4 to 5 fingerbreadths or more below the right costal margin) is usually indicative of fatty vacuolization, cirrhosis, tumor, amyloidosis or congestive failure. Enlargement of the left lobe of the liver should suggest hepatic syphilis but may be caused by primary or metastatic tumor or by abscess.

The absence of a palpable liver in a patient who has had jaundice for 2 to 3 weeks or more would tend to exclude neoplastic obstruction of the bile ducts, since sufficient bile stasis should result, by this time, to produce detectable hepatic enlargement.[186]

Gallbladder. The presence of a smooth, nontender, *distended gallbladder* in a patient with jaundice is almost always indicative of neoplastic obstruction of the common bile duct in accordance with Courvoisier's law, but is occasionally encountered in common duct stone. A distended gallbladder is found much more frequently at operation or necropsy than at the bedside. This discrepancy is produced by the overlying right lobe of the liver or, less frequently, by a thick abdominal wall. Failure to detect the presence of a distended gallbladder clinically therefore is of no value in excluding the diagnosis of obstruction or invasion of the common bile duct by tumor. Painless distention of the gallbladder may be encountered in patients who have been vomiting and not ingesting fats.[111]

Where there has been a difference of clinical opinion regarding the presence of a distended gallbladder or an enlarged liver, on occasions the author has summoned an anesthetist to administer a small dose of Pentothal Sodium intravenously in order to produce satisfactory abdominal relaxation. Generally speaking, when there is some doubt at the bedside as to the presence of a palpable gallbladder, the gallbladder will prove to be distended.

Exceptionally, a distended gallbladder may be more visible than palpable. At times it may be found in the right lower abdominal quadrant. Sometimes its long axis lies transversely. As in the case of a palpable liver, a distended gallbladder may be detected on one examination and not on another, for the same reasons.

Spleen. Usually, the spleen is palpated best with the patient on his right side, with

Fig. 8–14. Abdominal findings in various forms of jaundice.

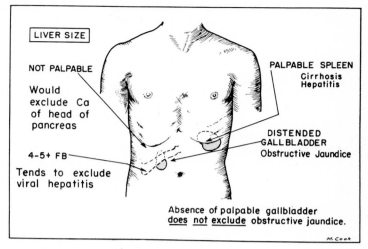

knees bent and left arm extended above the head. One of the examiner's hands should be placed below the left costal margin and the other behind in order to displace the spleen forward. The patient is instructed to breathe deeply, the spleen being felt best at the end of inspiration. In some instances it may be palpated with the patient lying supine with or without his left arm extending across the back.

Increase in splenic size may be determined also by percussion. Nixon [150] advises that the patient be placed in the right lateral recumbent position with the left arm extended forward and upward, and that percussion be initiated at the lower level of pulmonary resonance in approximately the posterior axillary line and carried downward obliquely toward the lower mid-anterior costal margin. He finds that the upper border of dullness extends 6 to 8 cm. above the costal margin, and that dullness increased over 8 cm. is indicative of an enlarged spleen in the adult.

In the absence of hemolytic jaundice a palpable spleen usually is indicative of hepatocellular jaundice. The spleen is palpable in about one half of patients with hepatic cirrhosis, in about 10 to 15 per cent of patients with viral hepatitis and about 20 per cent of cases of hepatic neoplasm.[63] It is well to bear in mind that in obstructive jaundice of long standing splenomegaly may be a manifestation of obstructive cirrhosis. In cancer of the body and the tail of the

pancreas splenic enlargement may result from encroachment of the tumor on the splenic vein.[61] Splenomegaly is also encountered occasionally in periampullary tumor. (The diagnostic value of the physical findings obtained on examination of the liver, the gallbladder and the spleen is depicted in Fig. 8–14.)

Ascites. The presence of ascites in a jaundiced patient usually is indicative of hepatic cirrhosis but may also be observed in massive hepatic necrosis, subacute hepatic necrosis, in the presence of peritoneal tumor implants or following invasion of the portal vein by tumor.

Lesser amounts of fluid may accumulate without producing the conventional signs of a fluid wave or shifting dullness in the flanks. We have been impressed with the frequency with which these signs are lacking in patients with very definite fluid accumulations as proved by transabdominal paracentesis, laparotomy or necropsy.

Ascitic fluid may conceal an enlarged liver, even if the examiner palpates by "dipping" or ballotting, which should always be done in the face of peritoneal fluid accumulation. The senior author recalls instances in which he was no longer able to palpate a considerably enlarged tumorous liver following the accumulation of ascitic fluid, only to palpate it again following paracentesis. Hemorrhagic ascitic fluid should suggest hepatoma, peritoneal tumor implants or tuberculous peritonitis.

Palmar Erythema. Patek[158] and Perera[160] have pointed out the frequency of a symmetric erythema—so-called palmar erythema—involving the eminences of the palms and the digits of the hands in patients with hepatic cirrhosis.

Miscellaneous findings include the presence of an abdominal mass, usually indicative of intra-abdominal tumor. *Absence of axillary or pectoral hair* is suggestive of cirrhosis of the liver, as are *testicular atrophy* and *gynecomastia*, although the last two have been reported in hepatitis.[122] Parotid enlargement[34, 241] and Dupuytren's[240] contracture have also been reported in cases of cirrhosis. The presence of multiple venous thrombi in a jaundiced patient should suggest cancer of the body or the tail of the pancreas.[119]

"Routine" Tests

Blood Count. According to Havens,[93] the white cell count usually is reduced during the preicteric and normal during the icteric phase of infectious hepatitis, although Jones and Minot[112] reported leukocytosis within the first few days of the disease. The chief value of a white cell count in a patient with jaundice is in ruling out uncomplicated viral hepatitis by the presence of leukocytosis which is found frequently in toxic hepatitis, amebic hepatitis, metastatic hepatic neoplasm, common duct stone (with cholangitis) and Weil's disease. The white cell count is apt to rise in fulminant hepatitis. The presence of eosinophilia should suggest toxic hepatitis. In the absence of blood loss the presence of anemia should suggest a hemolytic process, as should the finding of reticulocytosis and spherocytosis.

Blood Urea Nitrogen. Elevation of the blood urea nitrogen in a patient with jaundice should suggest the possibility of Weil's disease or exposure to a hepatotoxic agent which is also injurious to the kidney, such as carbon tetrachloride. Renal failure complicating liver disease must also be considered.

Urine Analysis. The presence of albuminuria should suggest the possibility of Weil's disease, although it may occur in the preicteric and the early icteric phases of viral hepatitis. Since jaundice may occur in amyloidosis, the simultaneous occurrence of marked albuminuria should also arouse suspicion of this disorder.

Stool Examination. Strongly positive tests for occult blood in the stools should arouse suspicion of an ulcerating periampullary lesion or a pancreatic cancer eroding the stomach or the duodenum.

Serum Lipids. Increase in serum lipids should suggest biliary cirrhosis, fatty liver, carcinoma of the bile ducts or Zieve's syndrome.[246]

Liver "Profile"

Refer to Chapter 6 for a discussion of laboratory tests as applied to the differential diagnosis of jaundice. Figure 8–15 reveals the differences in the results in hepatocellular versus obstructive jaundice.

The "liver profile" may be of aid in differentiating cases of common duct stone from neoplastic obstruction. The concentration of prompt-reacting serum bilirubin usually is less than 10 mg. % in patients with common duct stone but usually exceeds this level in patients with neoplastic jaundice. Likewise, the serum alkaline phosphatase is increased relatively less in cases of common duct stone. The cephalin flocculation is more frequently negative, and the thymol turbidity more frequently normal in neoplastic jaundice. The higher levels of serum bilirubin and serum alkaline phosphatase in neoplastic jaundice, as compared with common duct stone, can be explained by the more nearly complete and more persistent biliary obstruction in the cases with tumor. The more frequent occurrence of a positive cephalin flocculation and increased thymol turbidity in patients with common duct stone is a reflection of the higher incidence of cholangitis with secondary hepatitis. The total serum bilirubin may reach any value—high or low—in cases of hepatitis. Values of less than 5 mg. % would tend to exclude extrahepatic biliary obstruction of any variety.[183] In some clinics it is believed that when jaundice is due to liver disease the proportion of prompt to total bilirubin is less than 50 per cent, and that the reverse occurs in extrahepatic biliary obstruction,[229] but this has not been our general experience.

The application of immunologic technics to the differentiation of obstructive jaundice from other forms of icterus warrants further trial. A recent study would indicate the value of elevation of the serum IgM in distinguishing some patients with intrahepatic cholestasis from those with extrahepatic obstructive jaundice.[25, 62] Sera of patients with primary biliary cirrhosis produce granular cytoplasmic staining in unfixed tissue sections using fluorescein conjugates of anti-human gamma-globulin and anticompliment in the double layer immunofluorescent technic. This test appears to be consistently positive in primary biliary cirrhosis and consistently negative in extrahepatic obstructive jaundice and should prove of inestimable value if this is borne out by further experience.[115, 225]

It is well recognized that most of the individual laboratory tests constituting the so-called "liver profile" are not specific liver function tests and hence may be positive in the absence of liver disease. The importance of the clinical examination in the interpretation of the results of these liver function tests becomes evident. As Himsworth has stated so well, "There is yet no test which approaches in value a careful clinical assessment of the patient and none which can be interpreted without it."[96] This is well exemplified by increases in the serum alkaline phosphatase which occur in the presence of osseous lesions such as Paget's disease and hyperparathyroidism and by positive cephalin flocculation tests observed in infectious mononucleosis, hemolytic jaundice, disseminated lupus erythematosus, pernicious anemia, acute leukemia, chronic malaria and diffuse diseases of the reticuloendothelial system.[92]

PROTHROMBIN RESPONSE[141, 221]

Four of the clotting factors in plasma appear to be synthesized exclusively in the liver, namely, prothrombin, factor VII (pro-SPCA or proconvertin), factor X (Stuart-Prower factor) and Christmas factor (plasma thromboplastin component). (See Chapter 5.) Their formation depends on the normal absorption of vitamin K from the intestine and the functional integrity of the liver cells.

LIVER PROFILE IN JAUNDICE

	A. Hepatocellular	B. Obstructive
ceph. floc.	3-4 + (24 hrs.)	neg.
thymol turb.	> 5 units	< 5 units
zinc sulph. turb.	normal or sl. +	normal or ↓
S. A. P.	< 10 B.U. % < 30 K.A. units %	> 10 B.U. % > 30 K.A. units %
S. Transaminase	> 500 units (1000 +)	< 400 units

FIGURE 8–15.

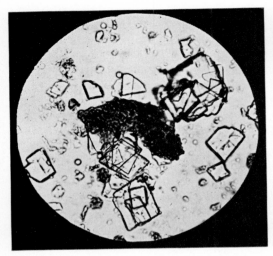

FIG. 8–16. Combination of cholesterin and calcium bilirubinate crystals is pathognomonic for stones ($\times$ 360). (Lyon, B. B. V.: Atlas on Biliary Drainage Microscopy, privately printed.)

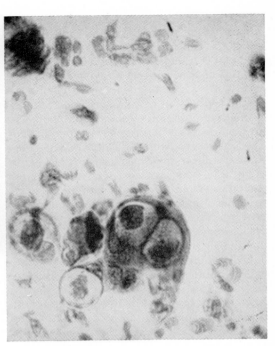

FIG. 8–17. One of many clumps of neoplastic cells surrounded by tall columnar normal epithelial cells, found in duodenal sediment of patient with carcinoma of head of pancreas, pathologically reported as resembling hepatoma ($\times$ 800). (Lemon, H. M., and Byrnes, W. W.: J.A.M.A. *141*:254.)

Three of these factors—prothrombin, factor VII and factor X—influence the one-stage prothrombin time. Thus a long prothrombin time may be due to the exclusion of bile from the intestine and/or severe liver injury. If the prothrombin time of the blood of an icteric patient is markedly prolonged (that is, "prothrombin activity" under 40 per cent of normal) and returns to normal within 24 hours after parenteral administration of vitamin K, it is probable that liver cell function is reasonably good and that the jaundice is due to extrahepatic obstruction. The failure of the prothrombin time to shorten under these circumstances would indicate the presence of parenchymal liver disease. An adequate amount of vitamin K is provided by 10 mg. of menadione sodium bisulfite (Hykinone) given subcutaneously. In order to exclude intrinsic errors in the test itself, it is best to determine the blood prothrombin time on two separate days both before and after the administration of the vitamin K.

RESPONSE TO STEROIDS

When patients with hepatocellular jaundice are given 40 to 60 mg. of prednisone (or prednisolone) daily for 4 to 6 days, the serum bilirubin frequently drops by 50 per cent or more, the greatest decrease occurring during the first 24 to 48 hours.[237a] This is then followed by a more gradual decline which is apt to continue even after steroid withdrawal. In cases that respond to prednisolone, Williams and Billing found a mean fall in serum bilirubin of 32 per cent per day for the short early period, and 7.4 per cent per day for the later and longer phase. In control patients recovering without steroid therapy, they observed a single rate of clearance, with a mean of 21.9 per cent fall per day. They noted that in some cases of infectious hepatitis the rate of bilirubin clearance did not seem to be affected by prednisolone.

Lesser or no decreases in serum bilirubin concentration are obtained with similar doses of steroids in most cases of extrahepatic obstructive jaundice and, if a decrease occurs, a rebound or no further change is apt to follow discontinuation of the drug. The effect of steroids, therefore, has been advocated as useful in the differentiation of hepatocellular from obstructive jaundice.[109, 116, 190, 210, 213, 237, 237a, 243] Unfortunately, variations in response and overlapping of effects make the test unreliable in individual cases.[47] Nevertheless, a definite response to the initial test, followed by continued improvement with (or without) further therapy would argue strongly for hepatitis.

The mechanism of the resulting decrease in serum bilirubin is not known. It is not that of increased biliary excretion, increased renal clearance of bile pigments or decrease in the rate of red cell breakdown. An additional metabolic pathway for bilirubin[237a] has been suggested, as has inhibition of hepatic bilirubinogenesis.[116] The latter would appear unlikely, since if steroids affected "early bilirubin" production, then this should presumably be apparent in obstructive jaundice as well as in hepatitis.

DUODENAL DRAINAGE

Although rarely employed nowadays, duodenal drainage may be valuable in the differential diagnosis of jaundice (1) by helping to confirm or disprove the presence of biliary obstruction, (2) by furnishing

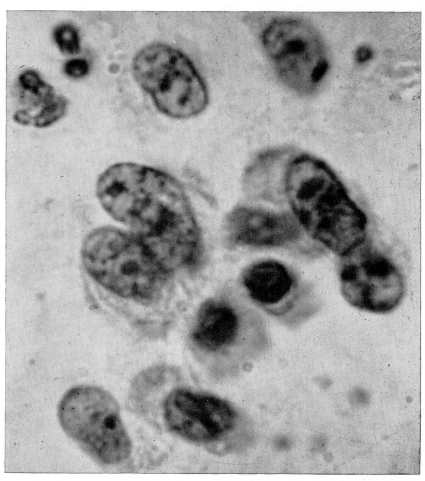

FIG. 8–18. Increase in nuclear clumping, thickening of the nuclear border and over-all enlargement of the nucleus in carcinoma of head of pancreas × 900. (From Dr. Howard Raskin.)

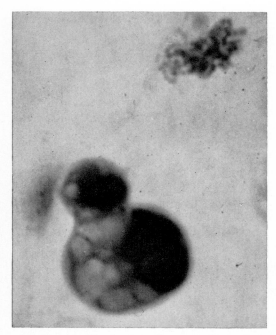

FIG. 8–19. Group of two cells with lobulated nucleus and irregularly vacuolated cytoplasm in carcinoma of head of pancreas × 900. (From Dr. Howard Raskin.)

material that can be tested for its content of pancreatic enzymes, (3) by yielding material for cytologic examination, (4) by demonstrating the presence of gross blood in the duodenal contents, which is strongly suggestive of ulcerating tumor of the ampulla of Vater,[56] and (5) by furnishing evidence of cholelithiasis in the form of calcium bilirubinate and cholesterol crystals (Fig. 8–16).[32, 105, 204, 215] Opinion differs on the diagnostic value of the presence of calcium bilirubinate and cholesterol crystals in duodenal contents. Admittedly, they are looked for much less frequently than formerly, due largely to advances in the roentgen diagnosis of gallstones.

Cytologic examination of the sediments of duodenal aspiration is of value in the diagnosis of tumors of the gallbladder, the extrahepatic bile ducts and the pancreas.[77, 130, 146, 167, 168] The following method has been used by Raskin et al., who report a 60 per cent overall accuracy of correct diagnosis in proved cases of pancreatic, bile duct,

gallbladder and primary duodenal carcinoma[168] (Figs. 8–17 to 8–19).

Patient Preparation. The patient is fasted overnight but is permitted to drink water. One hundred and sixty mg. of sodium pentobarbital is given intramuscularly an hour before the test.

Intubation. The patient sits on a cot, elevated 16 in. at one end. A double lumen gastroduodenal radiopaque tube (Diamond tube), with a 3 to 5 Gm. weight at the tip, is passed through the mouth to a position just below the cardioesophageal junction (45 cm.). The patient is placed on his left side, with head elevated, and fed an additional 15 cm. of tubing so that the tip of the tube will be lying just proximal to the antrum along the greater curvature. The patient then sits up and bends forward, taking a few deep breaths. The tip of the tube slips into the antrum as the anterior wall of the stomach falls away from the posterior wall. Next, the patient is placed on his right side (feet elevated), and 10 more cm. of tubing is slowly introduced, which should send the tube into the first part of the duodenum. Finally, the patient lies on his back for 2 minutes and swallows an additional 15 cm. of tube. A check of the tube's position fluoroscopically will reveal the tip of the tube between the second and third portions of the duodenum. The complete intubation usually requires about 15 minutes.

Duodenal Drainage. Tape the tube to the side of the patient's face. Before the actual collection is started, the stomach is aspirated to remove the residuum. Connect the gastric and duodenal segments to a Gomco vacuum pump (120 mm. Hg pressure). The gastric secretion is drained directly into a large collecting jar; the duodenal aspirate is trapped in 50-cc. plastic tubes immersed in an ice-water bath. Secretin may be injected intravenously after a 20-minute control period has shown duodenal juice to be consistently alkaline to litmus paper and the gastric juice to be acid. (The dose of secretin is 1 unit per kilogram.)

Three 10-minute samples are collected, and the gastric and the duodenal secretions are checked frequently with litmus paper in order to ensure independent collection.

Record the volume of the 30-minute postsecretin pancreatic secretion and then centrifuge the fluid for 5 minutes. Decant the supernatant, which is saved for bicarbonate determination, and smear the sediment on glass slides for cytologic study.

ROENTGEN EXAMINATION

X-ray examination has been of limited value in the differential diagnosis of jaundice, due largely to: (1) inability to furnish direct evidence of hepatitis, (2) inadequacies of present-day technics in the demonstration of tumors producing jaundice, (3) limitations of cholecystography and intravenous cholangiography, and (4) lack of proof that gallstones are the cause of jaundice by their mere demonstration.

X-ray changes caused by tumors producing icterus depend largely on effects on contiguous structures resulting from expansion of the neoplasm and may not be present during the early stages of tumor growth. A carcinoma of the head of the pancreas producing jaundice may not be large enough to bulge appreciably on the surface of the gland and therefore may escape detection on roentgen examination.

Despite its limitations, the roentgen examination may contribute importantly to the diagnosis of the cause of jaundice. (See Chap. 29.)

NEEDLE BIOPSY OF THE LIVER

Jaundice *per se* is not a contraindication to needle biopsy of the liver, nor is the presence of metastatic neoplasm of the liver. On the other hand, obstructive jaundice is a contraindication because of the risk of bile peritonitis.

The use of needle biopsy of the liver should be confined to selected cases of jaundice. In the first place, the cause of jaundice can be diagnosed in 85 to 90 per cent of cases on the basis of the clinical examination and the results of laboratory tests.[91, 183, 193, 227] Furthermore, the diagnostic use of steroids may occasionally decrease the need for needle biopsy in the jaundiced patient, particularly when marked lessening of the icterus results, and the steroids are then continued therapeutically. In addition, marked increases of the serum glutamic transaminases (of an order of 1,000 units or more) justify deferment of the biopsy because of their strong likelihood in indicating the presence of hepatitis.

The microscopic changes in viral hepatitis are well known (Councilman-like acidophilic bodies, universal triaditis, focal necrosis not confined to areas of bile stasis, pseudoacinus formation, etc.). These changes may, however, be mimicked by drug-induced hepatitis. The diagnosis of drug-induced hepatitis is favored over viral hepatitis if cholestasis (centrilobular bile stasis), portal inflammation and hepatic eosinophilia are present, in contrast with acidophilic bodies and focal necrosis not related to bile stasis. The characteristic histologic changes in alcoholic hepatitis include necrosis, lobular disarray, polymorphonuclear cellular infiltration, fatty vacuolization, and the characteristic Mallory bodies with their coarsely acidophilic cytoplasm. Certain histologic changes in the needle biopsy specimens almost always indicate the presence of extrahepatic obstructive jaundice but are observed in only a very small proportion of cases. These changes have recently been discussed by Gall and Dobrogorski.[71] Contrary to our earlier beliefs, needle biopsy of the liver has proved to be of very limited value in differentiating between intrahepatic cholestasis and extrahepatic obstructive jaundice.

For the technic of the procedure and for the changes revealed in the various disorders causing jaundice, refer to Chapter 7 by Schiff and Gall, Needle Biopsy of the Liver.

PITFALLS IN DIAGNOSIS

A number of factors may mislead the clinician in his quest for the cause of jaundice.

The pre-icteric period of infectious hepatitis may be mistaken for a primary flu-like infection and drugs thus administered may be erroneously suspected of inducing the subsequent icterus.

A *history of alcoholism* may lead him to suspect hepatic cirrhosis in a patient whose liver proves to be normal or the seat of some other disorder.[189] In a reported study, the highest percentage of errors in the initial clinical diagnosis of the cause of jaundice occurred in patients with hepatitis who were thought to have cirrhosis because of their alcoholism.[183]

The age of the patient may be misleading.

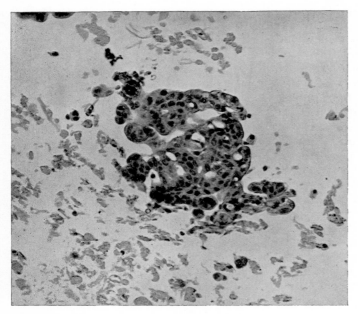

FIG. 8–20. Bile duct carcinoma, T.F. Section of the sediment of fluid aspirated from the common duct at laparotomy. The photograph demonstrates an isolated cluster of neoplastic epithelium in which abortive acino formation can be detected. Nuclei are hyperchromatic and vary considerably in size and configuration.

Viral hepatitis, particularly serum hepatitis, is not uncommon in the older age group, and young adulthood does not necessarily exclude neoplasm. We have seen a number of proved cases of carcinoma of the bile ducts in individuals in their early thirties and recall a case of carcinoma of the periampullary region in an individual aged 28 and one of carcinoma of the pancreas at 24.

Prominent weight loss strongly suggests neoplasm as the cause of jaundice, but may occur in severe cases of hepatitis as a result of marked anorexia and in cases of common duct stone because of nausea and vomiting.

A *history of tumor resection* preceding jaundice may wrongly suggest the presence of metastatic neoplasm of the liver. In some instances the clinician may be surprised to find that he is dealing with serum hepatitis secondary to blood or plasma administered at the time of operation.

Jaundice occurring shortly after major surgery may wrongly implicate the operation (especially if multiple transfusions have been given) *or if halothane anesthesia has been used.* A case of icterus recently observed that developed within a few days after surgery proved to be due to a common duct stone which had previously been silent.

Painless jaundice in elderly individuals suffering with common duct stone may *prove misleading.* Variations in the color of the urine and stools over a period of time may be an important diagnostic clue.

Obstructive cirrhosis may be mistaken for hepatitis or portal cirrhosis. Laboratory tests in keeping with obstructive jaundice, the prolonged duration of jaundice, and the results of x-ray studies may put the clinician on the right track. Duff has pointed out that splenomegaly may be produced by encroachment of carcinoma of the body of the pancreas on the splenic vein.[61] The senior author has observed a patient with obstructive cirrhosis secondary to a carcinoma of the ampulla of Vater in whom splenomegaly and hepatomegaly preceded marked icterus by many months.

Focusing too much attention on the icterus may be responsible for *overlooking the pallor* of hemolytic jaundice.

Exposure to a known hepatotoxic agent does not indicate that the ensuing jaundice is due to a toxic hepatitis, although such an assumption is justifiable and usually will prove to be correct. The inability to demonstrate specific circulating antibodies or skin sensitivity adds to the uncertainty of diagnosis.

Unusually prolonged jaundice does not necessarily exclude neoplasm as the cause. The senior author has seen a patient with proved carcinoma of the ampulla of Vater with icterus of 18 months' duration and one with carcinoma of the bile ducts in whom jaundice lasted for 3 years.

Carcinoma at the hepatic duct bifurcation may be overlooked at surgery and even at repeated operation.[121] Its malignant nature may not be suspected since the lesion may resemble a scar in its gross appearance. The surprisingly long duration of jaundice of even up to 5½ years[7] may further detract from suspicion of its malignant character. Direct exploration and even cholangiography may fail to reveal any evidence of obstruction. Percutaneous transhepatic cholangiography may reveal the lesion[147] and might prove worthwhile at the time of surgery when difficulty is encountered in identifying the common bile duct.[121]

In some cases the ducts may not be adequately filled with x-ray contrast medium because most of the dye may escape into the duodenum when it is introduced through a T-tube. Jaundice may temporarily clear after a catheter is forced above the lesion.[120] Microscopic examination of bile aspirated from a major bile duct at laparotomy may reveal the presence of tumor cells and perhaps should be practiced oftener (Fig. 8–20). The triad of (1) marked microscopic changes of obstructive jaundice in the needle specimen of the liver, particularly the presence of bile lakes, (2) mild clinical jaundice and (3) a negative surgical exploration should suggest the diagnosis.[120, 188]

The lymphocytosis of infectious hepatitis may suggest infectious mononucleosis. The atypical lymphocytes may resemble closely those seen in infectious mononucleosis, as may the physical findings of lymphadenopathy, a tender liver and splenomegaly, and the occurrence of positive flocculation tests. Differentiation may be made only by means of the heterophile agglutination test. In order to avoid error, remember that this test is frequently negative in the first 3 weeks of infectious mononucleosis[72] and may not become positive until 8 weeks after onset.[2] Occasionally, heterophile tests are positive in viral hepatitis,[94, 128] but the antibodies are apt to be absorbed by guinea pig kidney and not by beef red cells, the

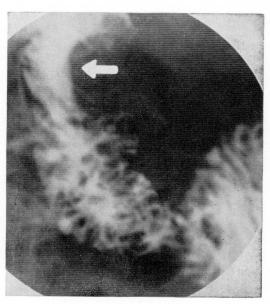

Fig. 8–21. A.T. 22038. Duodenal defect from multiple common duct stones.

reverse of the pattern of absorption that occurs in infectious mononucleosis.

The mere roentgen demonstration of gallstones does not necessarily implicate them as the cause of jaundice in a given case. Calculous cholecystitis may notoriously be asymptomatic.

Roentgen changes suggesting periampullary tumor may occur rarely in infectious hepatitis.[143] Presumably, they are due to edema or inflammation in the periampullary region. It is conceivable that they may be caused by aberrant pancreatic tissue in some cases. Sometimes a duodenal defect simulating that produced by periampullary tumor occurs in cases of common duct stone (Fig. 8–21).

THE TIME FACTOR

Today, with our greater array of laboratory tests, the cause of jaundice is usually diagnosed earlier than formerly when clinicians were more wont to assess the influence of time on the icteric state. A spontaneous decrease in jaundice argued for a benign process such as common duct stone or subsiding hepatitis, whereas a persistent or increasing icterus favored obstructive jaundice due to tumor. While this reasoning still holds in the absence of persistent or progressive hepatitis, it is well to note that the concentration of serum bilirubin may reach a horizontal plateau after about 3 weeks of jaundice due to carcinoma of the head of the pancreas or the bile ducts. This leveling off of the serum bilirubin concentration is probably explained by a balance between bilirubin formation and excretion (albeit by alternate routes, such as the kidneys).[242] Years ago, one of us (L.S.) observed a decrease in the serum bilirubin concentration of an icteric patient with carcinoma of the head of the pancreas due presumably to decreased bilirubin production associated with a concomitant drop in hemoglobin concentration.

GLIMPSE INTO THE FUTURE

In spite of advances in knowledge and methodology—both basic and clinical—elucidation of the cause of jaundice still offers a challenge to the clinician. This challenge will lose much of its impetus when the virus or viruses of infectious and serum hepatitis are isolated and specific immunologic tests are developed. Increased production of bilirubin by the liver from nonhemoglobin heme may prove an important factor in selected cases of jaundice. Furthermore, the demonstration of specific circulating antibodies to hepatotoxic drugs or the development of reliable and practical methods of confirming drug toxicity will replace the "post hoc, ergo propter hoc" type of reasoning which presently obtains. Measures may be discovered for correcting presently harmless—though annoying—congenital hyperbilirubinemias. The search should continue for means of confirming or excluding the presence of extrahepatic obstructive jaundice, for this would avoid delay in invoking surgical treatment and, on the other hand, would help to eliminate unnecessary surgery. When these goals are attained, the clinician will lose much of the thrill and satisfaction he presently derives in tracking down the basis of so major a clinical finding as jaundice.

REFERENCES

1. Abei, T., and Iber, F. L.: The distribution and kinetics of removal of C[14] labeled bilirubin in the dog with ligation of the common bile duct, Johns Hopkins Med. J. *122*:112, 1968.
2. Abrams, H. L.: Infectious mononucleosis with intense jaundice of long duration, New Engl. J. Med. *238*:295, 1948.
3. Acocella, G., Tenconi, L. T., Armas-Merino, R., Raia, S., and Billing, B. H.: Does deconjugation of bilirubin glucuronide occur in obstructive jaundice? Lancet *1*:68, 1968.
4. Ali, M. A. M., and Billing, B. H.: Effect of acid-base changes in renal clearance of bile pigments, Clin. Sci. *30*:543, 1966.
5. ———: Plasma disappearance of conjugated and unconjugated C[14] bilirubin in the rat with obstructive jaundice, Proc. Soc. Exp. Biol. Med. *124*:339, 1967.
6. ———: Renal excretion of bilirubin by the rat, Am. J. Physiol. *214*:1340, 1968.
7. Altemeier, W. A., Gall, E. A., Zinninger, M. M., and Hoxworth, P. I.: Sclerosing carcinoma of the major intrahepatic bile ducts, A.M.A. Arch. Surg. *75*:450, 1957.
8. Arias, I. M.: Panel: Bilirubin metabolism, Gastroenterology *36*:166, 1959.
9. ———: Studies of chronic familial nonhemolytic jaundice with conjugated bilirubin in the serum and without an unidentified pigment in the liver cells, Am. J. Med. *31*:510, 1961.
10. ———: Personal communication.
11. ———: Effects of a plant acid (icterogenin) and certain anabolic steroids on the hepatic metabolism of bilirubin and sulfobromophthalein (B.S.P.), Ann. N. Y. Acad. Sci. *104*:1014, 1963.
11a. ———: Chronic unconjugated hyperbilirubinemia with increased production of bile pigment not derived from the hemoglobin of mature circulating erythrocytes, J. Clin. Invest. *41*:1341, 1962 (Abstract).
12. Arias, I. M., Bernstein, L., Toffler, R., and Ben Ezzer, J.: Biliary and urinary excretion of metabolites of 7-H[3]-epinephrine in mutant Corriedale sheep with hepatic pigmentation, Gastroenterology *48*:495, 1965 (Abstract).
13. Arias, I. M., Bernstein, L., Toffler, R., Cornelius, C., Novikoff, A. B., and Essner, E.: Black liver disease in Corriedale sheep: a new mutation affecting hepatic

excretory function, J. Clin. Invest. *43*: 1249, 1964.

14. Arias, I. M., Gartner, L. M., Cohen, M., Ben Ezzer, J. and Levi, A. J.: Chronic non-hemolytic unconjugated hyperbilirubinemia with glucuronyl transferase deficiency: evidence for genetic heterogeneity. Presented at AGA meeting, Philadelphia, 1968.

15. Ashe, W. F., Pratt-Thomas, H. R., and Kumpe, C. W.: Weil's disease: a complete review of American literature and abstract of the world literature; 7 case reports, Medicine *20*:145, 1941.

16. Bakken, A. F., and Fog, J.: Bilirubin conjugation in newborn rats, Lancet *2*: 309, 1967

17. Barniville, H. T. F., and Misk, R.: Urinary glucuronic acid excretion in liver disease and the effect of a salicylamide load, Brit. Med. J. *1*:337, 1959.

18. Barrett, P. V. D., Berk, P. D., Menken, M., and Berlin, N. I.: Bilirubin turnover studies in normal and pathologic states using bilirubin C^{14}, Ann. Int. Med. *68*: 355, 1968.

19. Barrett, P. V. D., Cline, M. J., and Berlin, N. I.: The association of urobilin "early peak" and erythropoiesis in man, J. Clin. Invest. *45*:1657, 1966.

20. Bean, W. B.: The cutaneous arterial spider: a survey, Medicine *24*:243, 1945.

21. Benedict, E. B.: Endoscopy, Baltimore, Williams & Wilkins, 1951.

22. Berendsohn, S.: Hepatic function at high altitudes, Arch. Int. Med. *109*:256, 1962.

22a. Berendsohn, S., Lowman, J., Sunberg, D., and Watson, C. J.: Idiopathic dyserythropoietic jaundice, Blood *24*:1, 1964.

23. Bernstein, R. B., Troxler, R. F., and Lester, R.: The effect of hepatobiliary disease on urobilinogen excretion, Gastroenterology *54*:150, 1968.

24. Berthelot, P., and Billing, B. H.: Effect of bunamiodyl on hepatic uptake of sulfobromophthalein in the rat, Am. J. Physiol. *211*:395, 1966.

25. Bevan, G.: Personal communication.

26. Bevan, G., Baldus, W. P., and Gleich, G. J.: Serum immunoglobulin (Ig) levels in the differential diagnosis of cholestasis. Presented before the meeting of the Am. Assoc. for the Study of Liver Diseases, Chicago, Ill., Nov. 2, 1967.

27. Billing, B. H.: The role of conjugation in the excretion of bilirubin, Elsevier Monograph, Amsterdam, 1961.

28. Billing, B. H., Cole, P. G., and Lathe, G. H.: The excretion of bilirubin as a diglucuronide giving the direct van den Bergh reaction, Biochem. J. *65*:774, 1957.

29. Billing, B. H., Williams, R., and Richards, T. G.: Defects in hepatic transport of bilirubin in congenital hyperbilirubinemia: an analysis of plasma bilirubin disappearance curves, Clin. Sci. *27*:245, 1964.

30. Bizard, G.: Enzyme inhibitors and biliary excretion *in* Taylor, W. (ed.): The Biliary System (NATO Advanced Study Inst. Symposium), Oxford, Blackwell Scientific Pub., p. 315, 1965.

31. Black, M., and Billing, B. H.: Unpublished observations.

32. Bockus, H. L.: Personal communication.

33. Bolt, R. J., Dillon, R. S., and Pollard, H. M.: Interference with bilirubin excretion by a gallbladder dye (bunamiodyl), New Engl. J. Med. *265*:1043, 1961.

34. Bonnin, H., Moretti, G., and Geyer, A.: Les grosses parotides des cirrhoses alcoholiques, Presse méd. *62*:1449, 1954.

35. Bouchier, I. A. D., and Cooperband, S. R.: Isolation and characterisation of a macromolecular aggregate associated with bilirubin, Clin. Chim. Acta *15*:291, 1967.

36. Bourke, E., Milne, M. D., and Stokes, G. S.: Mechanisms of renal excretion of urobilinogen, Brit. Med. *2*:1510, 1965.

37. Brick, I. B.: Prolonged jaundice (over 3 months) occurring during chlorpromazine administration, Gastroenterology *33*:192, 1957.

38. Brick, I. B., and Palmer, E. D.: Esophageal varices and vascular spiders (nevi araneosi) in cirrhosis of the liver, J.A.M.A. *155*:8, 1954.

39. Brown, W. R., Grodsky, G. M., and Carbone, J. V.: Intracellular distribution of tritiated bilirubin during hepatic uptake and excretion, Am. J. Physiol. *207*: 1237, 1964.

40. Budd, G.: On Diseases of the Liver, Philadelphia, Lea & Blanchard, 1846.

41. Butt, H. R., Anderson, V. E., Foulk, W. T., Baggenstoss, A. H., Schoenfield, L. J., and Dickson, E. R.: Studies of chronic idiopathic jaundice (Dubin-John-

son syndrome): evaluation of a large family with trait, Gastroenterology 51: 619, 1966.

42. Calderon, A., and Goldgraber, M. B.: Chronic idiopathic jaundice: a case report, Gastroenterology 40:244, 1961.

43. Cameron, J. L., Filler, R. M., Iber, F. L., and Randolph, J. G.: Metabolism and excretion of C14-labelled bilirubin in children with biliary atresia, New Engl. J. Med. 274:231, 1966.

44. Cameron, J. L., Pulaski, E. J., Abei, T., and Iber, F. L.: Metabolism and excretion of bilirubin C14 in experimental obstructive jaundice, Ann. Surg. 163:330, 1966.

45. Caroli, J.: Les Ictères par Rétention, Paris, Masson, 1956.

45a. Caroli, J., and Ricordeau, P.: Value of peritoneoscopy and peritoneoscopic photography in color and of scintillography in the diagnosis of liver disease in Popper, H., and Schaffner, F. (eds.): Progress in Liver Disease, p. 296, New York, Grune & Stratton, 1961.

46. Challenger, F., and Walshe, J. M.: Fetor hepaticus, Lancet 1:1239, 1955.

47. Chalmers, T. C., Gill, R. J., Jernigan, T. P., Svec, F. A., Jordan, R. S., Waldstein, S. S. and Knowlton, M.: Evaluation of a 4-day ACTH test in the differential diagnosis of jaundice, Gastroenterology, 30:894, 1956.

48. Charbonnier, A.: Personal communication.

49. Charbonnier, A., and Brisbois, P.: Notes on Bromsulphalein clearance in Dubin-Johnson's jaundice, Rev. méd. mal. foie 35:75, 1960.

50. Charbonnier, A., and Poungouras, P.: Les éther-solubilités de la bilirubine, Rev. Hépat. Int. Hépat. 9:589, 1959.

51. Chauffard, M. A.: Le cancer du corps de pancréas, Bull. Acad. méd. 60:242, 1908.

52. Clain, H., Wartuoby, K., and Sherlock, S.: Abdominal arterial murmurs in liver disease, Lancet 2:516, 1966.

53. Cole, P. G., Lathe, G. H., and Billing, B. H.: Separation of the bile pigments of serum, bile and urine, Biochem. J. 57:514, 1954.

54. Cornelius, C. E., Arias, I. M., and Osburn, B. I.: Hepatic pigmentation with photosensitivity: a syndrome in Corriedale sheep resembling Dubin-Johnson

syndrome in man, J. Am. Vet. Assoc. 146: 709, 1965.

55. Crigler, J. F., Jr., and Gould, N. I.: Effects of phenobarbital on metabolism of bilirubin-H3 and -C14 in infant with congenital non-hemolytic jaundice and kernicterus, J. Clin. Invest. 46:1047, 1967 (Abstract).

56. Crohn, B. B.: New growths involving the terminal bile and pancreatic ducts: their early recognition by means of duodenal content analyses, Am. J. Med. Sci. 148:839, 1914.

57. de Silva, L. C., Jamra, M. A., Maspes, V., Pontes, J. F., Pieroni, R. R., and de Ulhóa Cintra, A. B.: Pathogenesis of indirect reacting hyperbilirubinemia after portacaval anastomosis, Gastroenterology 44:117, 1963.

58. Davis, W. D., and Young, P. C.: An unusual type of hyperbilirubinemia with Bromsulphalein retention and microscopically normal liver, Gastroenterology 37:206, 1959.

59. Diamond, I., and Schmid, R.: Experimental bilirubin encephalopathy; the mode of entry of bilirubin C14 in the central nervous system, J. Clin. Invest. 45:678, 1966.

60. Dubin, I. N.: Chronic idiopathic jaundice: a review of 50 cases, Am. J. Med. 24:268, 1958.

60a. Dubin, I. N., and Johnson, F. B.: Chronic idiopathic jaundice with unidentified pigment in liver cells: new clinico-pathologic entity with report of 12 cases, Medicine 33:155, 1954.

61. Duff, G. L.: The clinical and pathological features of carcinoma of the body and tail of the pancreas, Bull. Johns Hopkins Hosp. 65:69, 1939.

62. Fahey, J. L., and McKelvey, E. M.: Quantitative determination of serum immunoglobin in antibody-agar plates, J. Immunol. 94:84, 1965.

63. Fenster, L. F., and Klatskin, G.: Manifestations of metastatic tumors of the liver: a study of 81 patients subjected to needle biopsy, Ann. Med. 31:238, 1961.

64. Fevery, J., Heirwegh, K., and de Groote, J.: Renal bilirubin clearance in liver patients, Clin. Chim. Acta 17:63, 1967.

65. Fleischner, F. G., and Sayegh, V.: Assessment of the size of the liver; roentgenologic considerations, New Engl. J. Med. 259:271, 1958.

66. Foulk, W. T., Butt, H. R., Owen, C. A., Jr., and Whitcomb, F. F., Jr.: Constitutional hepatic dysfunction (Gilbert's disease): its natural history and related syndromes, Medicine 38:25, 1959.

67. Fred, H. L., and Brown, G. R.: The hepatic friction rub, New Engl. J. Med. 266:554, 1962.

68. Fulop, M., and Brazeau, P.: The renal excretion of bilirubin in dogs with obstructive jaundice, J. Clin. Invest. 43: 1192, 1964.

69. Fulop, M., and Sandson, J.: The effect of bile salts on the binding of bilirubin by plasma proteins, Clin. Sci. 33:459, 1967.

70. Fulop, M., Sandson, J. B., and Brazeau, P.: Dialysability, protein binding acid and renal excretion of plasma conjugated bilirubin, J. Clin. Invest. 44:666, 1965.

71. Gall, E. A., and Dobrogorski, O.: Hepatic alterations in obstructive jaundice, Am. J. Clin. Path. 41:126, 1964.

72. Gardner, H. T., and Paul, J. R.: Infectious mononucleosis at the New Haven Hospital, 1921 to 1946, Yale J. Biol. Med. 19:839, 1947.

73. Gartner, L. M., and Arias, I. M.: Pituitary regulation of bilirubin excretion by the liver, J. Clin. Invest. 45:1011, 1966.

74. Gentilini, P., Mallegni, V., and Milli, G.: Electron microscopic study of 3 cases of Gilbert's syndrome, Arch. Ital. Mal. Appar. Dig. 32:267, 1965.

75. Gilbertsen, A. S., Bossenmaier, I., and Cardinal R.: Enterohepatic circulation of unconjugated bilirubin in man, Nature 196:141, 1962.

76. Gilbertsen, A. S., Hawkinson, V., and Watson, C. J.: Studies of the dipyrrylmethene ("fuscin") pigments. II. The contrasting ratios and significance of the fecal urobilinogen and mesobilifuscin in certain anemias, J. Clin. Invest. 38:1175, 1959.

77. Goldgraber, M. B., Rubin, C. E., and Owens, F. J.: The cytologic diagnosis of duodenal sarcoma (polymorphic reticulosarcoma), Ann. Int. Med. 39:1316, 1953.

78. Goldstein, G. W., and Lester, R.: Reduction of biliverdin-14 to bilirubin C14 in vivo, Proc. Soc. Exp. Biol. Med. 117: 681, 1964.

79. Gray, C. H.: Bile Pigments in Health and Disease, Am. Lecture Series No. 422, Springfield, Ill., Thomas, 1961.

80. Gray, C. H., Neuberger, A. and Sneath, P. H. A.: Studies in congenital porphyria. II. Incorporation of N^{15} in the stercobilin in the normal and in the porphyric, Biochem. J. 47:87, 1950.

81. Gray, C. H., Nicholson, D. C., and Nicolaus, R. A.: The IX-α structure of the common bile pigments, Nature 181:183, 1958.

82. Gray, C. H., and Scott, J. J.: The effect of hemorrhage on the incorporation of (α- C^{14}) glycine into stercobilin, Biochem. J. 71:38, 1959.

83. Greenberger, N. J., Milligan, F. D., De Groote, L. V., and Isselbacher, K. J.: Jaundice and thyrotoxicosis in the absence of congestive heart failure, Am. J. Med. 36:840, 1964.

84. Gregory, C. H.: Studies of conjugated bilirubin. III. "Pigment I," a complex of conjugated and free bilirubin, J. Lab. Clin. Med. 61:917, 1963.

85. Grinstein, M., Aldrich, R. A., Hawkinson, V., and Watson C. J.: An isotopic study of porphyrin and hemoglobin metabolism in a case of porphyria, J. Biol. Chem. 179:983, 1949.

86. Grinstein, M., Bannerman, R. M., Vavra, J. D., and Moore, C. V.: Hemoglobin metabolism in thalassemia; in vivo studies, Am. J. Med. 29:18, 1960.

87. Grodsky, G.: Studies in the uptake and intrahepatic transport of H^3 bilirubin in Bouchier, I. A. D., and Billing, B. H. (eds.): Bilirubin Metabolism, Oxford, Blackwell Scientific Pub., p. 99, 1967.

88. Grodsky, G. M., and Carbone, J. V.: The synthesis of bilirubin glucuronide by tissue homogenates, J. Biol. Chem. 226: 449, 1957.

89. Halac, E., Jr., and Reff, A.: Studies in bilirubin UDP-glucuronyl transferase, Biochim. Biophys. Acta 139:328, 1967.

90. Hammaker, L., and Schmid, R.: Interference with bile pigment uptake in the liver by flavaspidic acid, Gastroenterology 53:31, 1967.

91. Hanger, F. M.: Diagnostic problems of jaundice, Arch. Int. Med. 86:169, 1950.

92. ———: The meaning of liver function tests, Am. J. Med. 16:565, 1954.

93. Havens, W. P., Jr.: Infectious hepatitis, Medicine 27:279, 1948.

94. Havens, W. P., Jr., Gambescia, J. M., and Knowlton, M.: Results of hetero-

phile antibody agglutination and Kahn tests in patients with viral hepatitis, Proc. Soc. Exp. Biol. Med. 67:437, 1948.

95. Haverback, B. J., and Wirtschafter, S. K.: Familial non-hemolytic jaundice with normal liver histology and conjugated bilirubin, New Engl. J. Med. 262:113, 1960.

96. Himsworth, H. P.: Lectures on the Liver and Its Diseases, ed. 2, Cambridge, Mass., Harvard, 1950.

97. Hoenig, V., and Schück, O.: Dialysability of conjugated bilirubin from plasma of jaundiced dogs and patients, Lancet 2:1297, 1964.

98. Hoffbauer, F. W.: Bedside diagnosis of jaundice, Northwest Med. 48:757, 1949.

99. Hoffman, H. N., II, Whitcomb, F. F., Jr., Butt, H. R., and Bollman, J. L.: Bile pigments of jaundice, J. Clin. Invest. 39: 132, 1960.

100. Howe, R. B., and Pinto, S. de T.: Ether-soluble bilirubin, Medicine 45:523, 1966.

101. Hughes-Jones, N. C., and Cheney, B.: The use of Cr^{51} and Fe^{59} as red cell labels to determine the fate of normal erythrocytes in the rat, Clin. Sci. 20:323, 1961.

102. Hult, H.: Cholemic simple familial (Gilbert) and posthepatitic states without fibrosis of the liver, Acta med. scand. 138: Suppl. 244, pp. 1-96, 1950.

103. Ibrahim, G. W., Schwartz, S., and Watson, C. J.: The conversion of protoporphyrin C^{14} heme compound and bilirubin in dogs, Metabolism 15:1120, 1966.

104. Imai, K.: Formation of verdohemochromogen induced by pyridine hemin and tissues of various organs, Igaku Kenkyu (Acta Medica) 24:1388, 1954.

105. Ingelfinger, F.: Differential diagnosis of jaundice, DM, Nov. 1958, Chicago, Year Book Pub., 1958.

106. Israels, L. G., Levitt, M., Novak, W., and Zipursky, A.: The early bilirubin, Medicine 45:517, 1966.

107. Israels, L. G., Suderman, H. J., and Ritzman, S. E.: Hyperbilirubinemia due to an alternate path of bilirubin production, Am. J. Med. 27:693, 1959.

108. Israels, L. G., Yamamoto, T., Skanderbeg, J., and Zipursky, A.: Shunt bilirubin; evidence for 2 components, Science 139: 1054, 1963.

109. Johnson, H. C., and Doenges, J. P.: Intrahepatic obstructive jaundice (primary cholestasis), a clinicopathologic syndrome of varied etiology: a review with observations of the use of corticotropin as a diagnostic tool, Ann. Int. Med. 44:589, 1956.

110. Johnson, L., Sarmiento, F., Blanc, W. A., and Day, R.: Kernicterus in rats with an inherited deficiency of glucuronyl transferase, Am. J. Dis. Child. 97:591, 1959.

111. Jones, C. M.: Personal communication.

112. Jones, C. M., and Minot, G. R.: Infectious (catarrhal) jaundice, an attempt to established a clinical entity; observations on excretion and retention of bile pigments and on blood, Boston M. & S. J. 189: 531, 1923.

113. Kalk, H.: Laparoskopie und Gastroskopie, Stuttgart, Thieme, 1951.

114. Kalk, H., and Wildhirt, E.: Die posthepatitische hyperbilirubinamie, Z. Klin. Med. 155:547, 1959.

115. Kantor, F. S., and Klatskin, G.: Serological diagnosis of primary biliary cirrhosis: a potential clue to pathogenesis, Trans. Ass. Am. Phycns. 80:267, 1967.

116. Katz, R., Ducci, H., and Allesandri, H.: Influence of cortisone and prednisolone on hyperbilirubinemia, J. Clin. Invest. 36:1370, 1957.

117. Kench, J. E.: Bile pigment formation in vitro from haematin and haem derivatives, Biochem. J. 56:669, 1954.

118. Kench, J. E., Du Toit, F. E., and Green, M.: Some observations on the breakdown of hemoglobin, S. African J. Lab. Clin. Med. 9:272, 1963.

119. Kenney, W. E.: The association of carcinoma of the body and tail of the pancreas with multiple venous thrombi, Surgery 14:600, 1943.

120. Klatskin, G.: Personal communication.

121. ————: Adenocarcinoma of the hepatic duct at its bifurcation within the porta hepatis, Am. J. Med. 38:241, 1965.

122. Klatskin, G., and Rappaport, E. M.: Gynecomastia due to infectious hepatitis of the homologous serum type, Am. J. Med. Sci. 214:121, 1947.

122a. Klaus, D.: Primary shunt hyperbilirubinemia, Germ. Med. Month. 9:509, 1964.

122b. Klaus, D., and Feine, U.: Primary shunt hyperbilirubinemia, Germ. Med. Month. 10:89, 1965.

123. Koff, R. S., Grady, G. F., Chalmers, T. C., Mosley, J. W., Swartz, B. L., and the Boston Inter-Hospital Group: Viral hepatitis in a group of Boston hospitals. III. Importance of exposure to shellfish in a

non-epidemic area, New Engl. J. Med. *276*:703, 1967.

124. Koff, R. S., and Sear, H. S.: Internal temperature of steamed clams, New Engl. J. Med. *276*:737, 1967.

125. Konar, N. R., Datta, S. K., Nag, A., and Konar, A.: Murmur over liver in cases of severe anemia, Brit. Med. J. *4*:154, 1967.

126. Krustev, B. *in* Read, A. E. (ed): The Liver (Colston Papers), London, Butterworth's Scientific Pub., No. 19, 1967.

127. Lathe, G. H., and Walker, M.: The synthesis of bilirubin glucuronide in animal and human liver, Biochem. J. *70*:705, 1958.

128. Leibowitz, S.: Heterophile antibody in normal adults and in patients with virus hepatitis, Am. J. Clin. Path. *21*:201, 1951.

129. Lemberg, R.: The chemical mechanism of the bile pigment formation, Rev. Pure Appl. Chem. *6*:1, 1956.

130. Lemon, H. M., and Byrnes, W. W.: Cancer of the biliary tract and pancreas. Diagnosis from cytology of duodenal aspirations, J.A.M.A. *141*:254, 1949.

131. Lester, R., Behrman, R. E., and Lucey, J. F.: Transfer of bilirubin-C^{14} across the monkey placenta, Pediatrics *32*:416, 1963.

132. Lester, R., and Schmid, R.: Intestinal absorption of bile pigments. II. Bilirubin absorption in men, New Engl. J. Med. *269*:178, 1963.

133. Lester, R., Schumer, W., and Schmid, R.: Intestinal absorption of bile pigments. IV. Urobilinogen absorption in man, New Engl. J. Med. *272*:939, 1965.

134. Levi, A. J., Gatmaitain, Z., and Arias, I. M.: Two cytoplasmic proteins from rat liver and their role in hepatic uptake of sulfobromophthalein (BSP) and bilirubin, J. Clin. Invest. *47*:61a, 1968 (Abstract).

135. Levine, R. A., and Klatskin, G.: Unconjugated hyperbilirubinemia in absence of overt hemolysis, Am. J. Med. *36*:541, 1964.

136. Levitan, R., Diamond, H. D., and Craver, L. F.: Jaundice in Hodgkin's disease, Am. J. Med. *30*:99, 1961.

137. London, I. M.: The conversion of hematin to bile pigment, J. Biol. Chem. *184*:373, 1950.

138. London, I. M., Shemin, D., West, R., and Rittenberg, D.: Heme synthesis and red blood cell dynamics in normal humans and in subjects with polycythemia vera, sickle-cell anemia and pernicious anemia, J. Biol. Chem. *179*:463, 1949.

139. London, I. M., and West, R.: The formation of bile pigment in pernicious anemia, J. Biol. Chem. *184*:359, 1950.

140. London, I. M., Yamasaki, M., and Sabella, G.: Conversion of protoporphyrin to bile pigment, Fed. Proc. *10*:217, 1951.

141. Lord, J. W., Jr., and Andrus, W. DeW.: Differentiation of intrahepatic and extrahepatic jaundice: response of the plasma prothrombin to intramuscular injection of menadione (2 methyl-1, 4-naphthoquinone) as a diagnostic aid, Arch. Int. Med. *68*:199, 1941.

142. Mandema, E., de Fraiture, W. H., Nieweg, H. O., and Arends, A.: Familial chronic idiopathic jaundice (Dubin-Sprinz disease) with a note on Bromsulphalein metabolism in this disease, Am. J. Med. *28*:42, 1960.

143. Markoff, N.: Dünndarmveränderungen bei Hepatitis epidemica, Gastroenterologia *70*:24, 1945.

144. Maruffo, C. A., Malinow, M. R., Depaoli, J. R., and Katz, S.: Pigmentary liver disease in howler monkeys, Am. J. Path. *49*:445, 1966.

145. McMahon, F. G.: Effect of prednisolone, physical activity, fat intake and chloretic agents on the serum bilirubin level in a case of constitutional hepatic dysfunction (Gilbert's disease), Gastroenterology *32*:325, 1957.

146. McNeer, G., and Ewing, J. H.: Exfoliated pancreatic cancer cells in duodenal drainage; a case report, Cancer *2*:643, 1949.

147. Mistilis, S., and Schiff, L.: A case of jaundice due to unilateral hepatic duct obstruction with relief after hepatic lobectomy, Gut *4*:13, 1963.

148. Nakajima, H., Takemura, T., Nakajima, O., and Yamaoka, K.: Studies on heme-α-methenyl oxygenase. I. Enzymatic conversion of pyridine hemichromogen and hemoglobin-haptoglobin into possible precursor of biliverdin, J. Biol. Chem. *238*:3784, 1963.

149. Nakajima, O., and Gray, C. H.: Studies in haem α-methenyl oxygenase; isomeric structure of formylbiliverdin, a possible precursor of biliverdin, Biochem. J. *104*:20, 1967.

150. Nixon, R. K., Jr.: Detection of spleno-

megaly by percussion, New Engl. J. Med. *250*:166, 1954.

151. Noir, B. A., Groszman, R. J., and de Walz, A. T.: Studies on bilirubin sulphate, Biochim. Biophys. Acta *117*:297, 1966.

152. Noir, B. A., de Walz, A. T., and Rodriguez Garay, E.: Studies on bilirubin sulphate in human bile *in* Bouchier, I. A. D., and Billing, B. H. (eds.): Bilirubin Metabolism, Oxford, Blackwell Scientific Pub., p. 99, 1967.

153. Nosslin, B.: The direct diazo-reaction of bile pigments in serum, Scand. J. Clin. Lab. Invest., vol. 12, Supp. 49, 1960.

154. Nosslin, B.: Bromsulphalein retention and jaundice due to unconjugated bilirubin following treatment with male fern extract, Scand. J. Clin. Lab. Invest. *15*:206, 1963.

155. Osborn, E. C., Wooton, I. D. P., da Silva, L. C., and Sherlock, S.: Serum bile acid levels in liver disease, Lancet *2*:1049, 1959.

156. Ostrow, J. D.: Absorption of bile pigments by the gall bladder, J. Clin. Invest. *46*:2035, 1967.

157. Ostrow, J. D., Jandl, J. H., and Schmid, R.: The formation of bilirubin from hemoglobin *in vivo*, J. Clin. Invest. *41*:1628, 1962.

157a. Ostrow, J. D., Schmid, R., and Samuelson, D.: The protein binding of C^{14}-bilirubin in human and murine serum, J. Clin. Invest. *42*:1286, 1963.

158. Patek, A. J., Jr.: Quoted by Perera.[160]

159. Peck, O. C., Rey, D. F., and Snell, A.: Familial jaundice with free and conjugated bilirubin in the serum and without liver pigmentation, Gastroenterology *39*:625, 1960.

160. Perera, G. A.: A note on palmar erythema (so-called liver palms), J.A.M.A. *119*:1417, 1942.

161. Petryka, Z. J.: The identification of non-IX α isomers in bilirubin, Proc. Soc. Exp. Biol. Med. *123*:464, 1966.

162. Pitcher, C. S., and Williams, R.: Reduced red cell survival in jaundice and its relation to abnormal glutathione metabolism, Clin. Sci. *24*:239, 1963.

163. Powell, L. W., Billing, B. H., and Williams, H. S.: The assessment of red cell survival in idiopathic unconjugated hyperbilirubinaemia (Gilbert's syndrome) by the use of radioactive diisopropyl-

fluorophosphate and chromium, Aust. Ann. Med. *16*:221, 1967.

164. Powell, L. W., Hemingway, E., Billing, B. H., and Sherlock, S.: Idiopathic unconjugated hyperbilirubinemia (Gilbert's syndrome), New Engl. J. Med. *277*:1108, 1967.

165. Pruzanski, W.: Evaluation of the influence of steroids on the level of serum bilirubin in viral hepatitis, Gastroenterologia *104*:225, 1965.

166. Raia, S.: Personal communication.

167. Raskin, H. F., Kirsner, J. B., and Palmer, W. L.: Exfoliative cytology of the gastrointestinal tract *in* Jones, F. A. (ed.): Modern Trends in Gastroenterology, 2nd series, London, Butterworth, 1958.

168. Raskin, H. F., Kirsner, J. B., Palmer, W. L., Pleticka, S., and Yarema, W. A.: Gastrointestinal cancer: definitive diagnosis by exfoliative cytology, A.M.A. Arch. Surg. *76*:507, 1958.

169. *Idem:* Dept. of Med., University of Chicago, 1957.

170. Robinson, S. H., Lester, R., Crigler, J. F., and Tsong, M.: Early-labeled peak of bile pigment in man; studies with glycine-C^{14} and delta-aminolevulinic acid-H^3, New Engl. J. Med. *277*:1323, 1967.

171. Robinson, S. H., Owen, C. A., Jr., Flock, E. V., and Schmid, R.: Bilirubin formation in liver from non hemoglobin sources; experiments with isolated, perfused rat liver, Blood *26*:823, 1965.

172. Robinson, S. H., Tsong, M., Brown, B. W., and Schmid, R.: The sources of bile pigment in the rat; studies of the "early labelled" fraction, J. Clin. Invest. *45*:1569, 1966.

173. Robinson, S., Vanier, T., Desforges, J. F., and Schmid, R.: Jaundice in thalassemia minor: a consequence of "ineffective erythropoiesis," New Engl. J. Med. *267*:523, 1962.

174. Rotor, A. B., Manahan, L., and Florentin, A.: Familial non-hemolytic jaundice with direct van den Bergh reaction, Acta med. Philipp. 5:37, 1948.

175. Royer, M.: La colangiografia Laparascopia, Buenos Aires, El Ateneo, 1952.

176. ———: Cholangiography *in* Popper, H., and Schaffner, F. (eds.): Progress in Liver Disease, p. 262, New York, Grune & Stratton, 1961.

177. Royer, M., Rodriguez Garay, E., and Argerich, T.: Action of biliverdin in the

rat, Acta Physiol. Lat. Amer. *12*:84, 1962.

178. Ruddock, J. C.: Peritoneoscopy, West. J. Med. *42*:392, 1934.

179. Sageld, W., Dolgaard, O. Z., and Tygstrup, N.: Constitutional hyperbilirubinemia with unconjugated bilirubin in the serum and lipochrome-like pigment granules in the liver, Ann. Int. Med., *56*:308, 1962.

180. Satler, J.: Another variant of constitutional familial hepatic dysfunction with permanent jaundice and with alternating serum bilirubin relations, Acta Hepatosplen. *13*:38, 1966.

181. Schachter, D.: Nature of the glucuronide in direct-reacting bilirubin, Science *126*: 507, 1957.

182. Schalm, L., and Weber, A. P.: Jaundice with conjugated bilirubin in hyperhaemolysis, Acta med. scand. *176*:549, 1964.

183. Schenker, S., Balint, J., and Schiff, L.: Differential diagnosis of jaundice: a report of a prospective study of 61 proved cases, Am. J. Dig. Dis., *7*:449, 1962.

184. Schenker, S., Dowber, N. H., and Schmid, R.: Bilirubin metabolism in the fetus, J. Clin. Invest. *43*:32, 1964.

185. Schiff, L.: Homologous serum hepatitis: clinical implications, New Orleans M. S. J. *99*:611, 1947.

186. ———: Absence of a palpable liver: a sign of value in excluding obstructive jaundice due to pancreatic cancer, Gastroenterology *32*:1143, 1957.

187. ———: Diagnostic significance of the time interval between resection of a malignant tumor and the appearance of jaundice, Am. J. Dig. Dis. *5*:573, 1960.

188. ———: Unpublished observations.

189. ———: Jaundice in the alcoholic, Arch. Int. Med. *110*:824, 1962.

190. ———: The use of steroids in liver disease, Medicine *45*:565, 1966.

191. ———: The differential diagnosis of jaundice, Postgrad. Med. *41*:39, 1967.

192. Schiff, L., Billing, B. H., and Oikawa, Y.: Familial nonhemolytic jaundice with conjugated bilirubin in the serum; a case study, New Engl. J. Med. *260*:1315, 1959.

193. Schiff, L., and Frank, H.: Unpublished observations.

194. Schmid, R.: The identification of "direct-reacting" bilirubin as bilirubin glucuronide, J. Biol. Chem. *229*:881, 1957.

195. Schmid, R., and Hammaker, L.: Glucuronide formation in patients with constitutional hepatic dysfunction (Gilbert's disease), New Engl. J. Med. *260*:1310, 1959.

196. ———: Metabolism and disposition of C^{14}-bilirubin in congenital nonhemolytic jaundice, J. Clin. Invest. *42*:1720, 1963.

197. Schmid, R., Hammaker, L., and Axelrod, J.: The enzymic formation of bilirubin glucuronide, Arch. Biochem. Biophys. *70*:285, 1957.

198. Schmid, R., Marver, H. S., and Hammaker, L.: Enhanced formation of rapidly labelled bilirubin by phenobarbital; hepatic microsomal cytochromes as possible source, Biochem. Biophys. Res. Commun. *24*:319, 1966.

199. Schoenfield, L. J.: The relationship of bile acids to pruritus in hepatobiliary disease. Presented at a conference on bile salt metabolism sponsored by the U. of Cincinnati Med. Center, Cincinnati, Sept. 28 and 29, 1967. (To be published)

200. Schoenfield, L. J., McGill, D. B., Hunton, D. B., Foulk, W. T., and Butt, H. R.: Studies of chronic idiopathic jaundice (Dubin-Johnson syndrome). I. Demonstration of hepatic excretory defect, Gastroenterology *44*:101, 1963.

201. Schwartz, S., and Cardinal, R.: Nonhemoglobin heme intermediates in the biosynthesis of bile pigments, Medicine *46*:73, 1967.

202. Schwartz, S., Ibrahim, G., and Watson, C. J.: The contribution of nonhemoglobin hemes to the early labelling of bile bilirubin, J. Lab. Clin. Med. *64*:1003, 1964.

203. Shaldon, S., and Caeser, J. J.: Personal communication.

204. Shay, H.: Personal communication.

205. Shemin, D., and Rittenberg, D.: The life span of the human red blood cell, J. Biol. Chem. *166*:627, 1946.

206. Sherlock, S.: Cirrhosis of the liver, Postgrad. M. J. *26*:472, 1950.

207. Singleton, J. W., and Laster, L.: Biliverdin reductase of guinea pig liver, J. Biol. Chem. *240*:4780, 1965.

208. Snyder, A. L., and Schmid, R.: The conversion of hematin to bile pigment, J. Lab. Clin. Med. *65*:817, 1965.

209. Solem, J. H.: The value of ACTH administration in the differential diagnosis of jaundice, Gastroenterologia *87*:23, 1957.

210. Solem, J. H., and Olsen, A.: The course of icterus index and prothrombin value during corticotropin treatment of acute hepatitis and obstructive jaundice, Acta med. scand. *146*:281, 1953.

211. Spiegel, E. L., Schubert, W., Perrin, E., and Schiff, L.: Benign recurrent intrahepatic cholestasis, with response to cholestyramine, Am. J. Med. *39*:682, 1965.

212. Sprinz, H., and Nelson, R. S.: Persistent nonhemolytic hyperbilirubinemia associated with lipochrome-like pigment, Ann. Int. Med. *41*:952, 1954.

213. Summerskill, W. H. J., and Jones, F. A.: Corticotrophin and steroids in the diagnosis and management of "obstructive" jaundice, Brit. Med. J. *2*: 1499, 1958.

214. Summerskill, W. H. J., and Walshe, J. M.: Benign recurrent intrahepatic "obstructive" jaundice, Lancet *2*:686, 1959.

215. Sun, D.: Personal communication.

216. Talafant, E.: Properties and composition of bile pigment giving a direct diazo reaction, Nature *178*:312, 1956.

217. Talafant, E., and Applelt, G.: Complexing bilirubin-diglucuronide with phospholipids to form "ether extractible" bilirubin, Clin. Chim. Acta *19*:383, 1963.

218. Tisdale, W. A.: Subacute hepatitis, New Engl. J. Med. *268*:85 & 138, 1963.

219. Tisdale, W. A., Klatskin, G., and Kinsella, E. D.: The significance of direct-reacting fraction of serum bilirubin in hemolytic jaundice, Am. J. Med. *26*:214, 1959.

220. Tomlinson, G. A., and Yaffe, S. J.: Formation of bilirubin and p-nitrophenyl glucuronides by rabbit liver, Biochem. J. *99*:507, 1966.

221. Turner, R. H.: Quoted by Schiff, L.: Differential Diagnosis of Jaundice, p. 250, Chicago, Year Book Pub., 1946.

222. Tygstrup, N., and Brodersen, R.: The diagnostic use of specific determination of unconjugated bilirubin, Scand. J. Clin. Lab. Invest. *21*:62, 1968.

223. Vest, M. F., Strebel, L., and Hauenstein, D.: The extent of "shunt" bilirubin and erythrocyte survival in the newborn infant measured by the administration of N^{15} glycine, Biochem. J. *95*:11C, 1965.

224. Wakisaka, G., and others: Clinical and enzymological observations on cases with Gilbert's disease, Jap. Arch. Int. Med. *8*:634, 1961.

225. Walker, J. G., Doniach, D., Roitt, I. M., and Sherlock, S.: Serological tests in the diagnosis of primary biliary cirrhosis, Lancet, *1*:827, 1965.

226. Wallace, D. K., and Owen, E. E.: An evaluation of the mechanism of bilirubin excretion by the human kidney, J. Lab. Clin. Med. *64*:741, 1964.

227. Watson, C. J.: An approach to the distinction of medical and surgical jaundice, Minn. Med. *32*:973, 1949.

228. ———: The prognosis and treatment of hepatic insufficiency, Ann. Int. Med. *31*:405, 1949.

229. ———: The importance of the fractional serum bilirubin determination in clinical medicine, Ann. Int. Med. *45*: 351, 1956.

230. ———: Composition of the urobilin group in urine, bile, and feces and the significance of variations in health and disease, J. Lab. Clin. Med. *54*:1, 1959.

231. ———: Recent studies of the urobilin problem, J. Clin. Path. *16*:1, 1963.

232. Weber, A. R., Schalm, L., and Witmans, J.: Bilirubin monoglucuronide (pigment I): a complex, Acta med. scand. *173*:19, 1963.

233. Wheeler, H. O., Meltzer, J. I., and Bradley, S. E.: Biliary transport and hepatic storage of sulfobromphthalein sodium in the unanesthetized dog, in normal man, and in patients with hepatic disease, J. Clin. Invest. *39*:1131, 1960.

234. Whelton, M. J., Krustev, L. P., and Billing, B. H.: Reduction in serum bilirubin by phenobarbital in adult unconjugated hyperbilirubinaemia: is enzyme induction responsible? Am. J. Med. *45*: 160, 1968.

235. White, A. E.: The distribution of glucuronyl transferase in cell membranes *in* Bouchier, I. A. D., and Billing, B. H. (eds.): Bilirubin Metabolism, Oxford, Blackwell Scientific Pub., p. 183, 1967.

235a. White, P. Silvers, A. H., Rother, M. L., Shafer, B. C., and Williams, W. J.: Hepatic production of bilirubin and carbon monoxide "in vitro," J. Clin. Invest. *45*: 1085, 1966.

236. White, F. W.: A study of errors in the diagnosis of jaundice, New Engl. J. Med. *229*:997, 1943.

237. Williams, R.: The place of steroid therapy in the treatment of liver disease, Med. Clin. N. Amer. *47*:801, 1963.

237a. Williams, R., and Billing, B. H.: Action of steroid therapy in jaundice, Lancet 2:392, 1961.

238. With, T. K.: Bile Pigments: Chemical, Biological and Clinical Aspects, New York, Academic Press, 1968.

239. Wolf, R. L., Pizette, M., Richman, A., Dreiling, D. A., Jacobs, W., Fernandez, O., and Popper, H.: Chronic idiopathic jaundice; a study of 2 afflicted families, Am. J. Med. 28:32, 1960.

240. Wolfe, S. J., Summerskill, W. H. J., and Davidson, C. S.: Thickening and contraction of the palmar fascia (Dupuytren's contracture) associated with alcoholism and hepatic cirrhosis, New Engl. J. Med. 255:559, 1956.

241. ———: Parotid swelling, alcoholism and cirrhosis, New Engl. J. Med. 256:491, 1957.

242. Wollaeger, E. E., and Gross, J. B.: Complete obstruction of the extrahepatic biliary tract due to carcinoma as determined by the fecal urobilinogen test: incidence and effect on serum bilirubin concentrations, Medicine 45:529, 1966.

243. Wruble, L. D., Kalser, M. H., Jones, R. H., Vloedman, D., and Bachorik, P.: Jaundice; value of five-day steroid test in differential diagnosis of jaundice, J.A.M.A. 195:184, 1966.

244. Yaffe, S. J., Levy, G., Matsuzawa, T., and Baliah, T.: Enhancement of glucuronide conjugation capacity in hyperbilirubinaemic infant due to apparent enzyme induction by phenobarbital, New Engl. J. Med. 275:1461, 1966.

245. Yamamoto, T., Skanderbeg, J., Zipursky, A., and Israels, L. G.: The early appearing bilirubin; evidence for two components, J. Clin. Invest. 43:31, 1965.

246. Zieve, L.: Jaundice, hyperlipemia and hemolytic anemia: a heretofore unrecognized syndrome associated with alcoholic fatty liver and cirrhosis, Ann. Int. Med. 48:471, 1958.

9

Portal Hypertension

TELFER B. REYNOLDS, M.D.

ANATOMY OF THE PORTAL VENOUS SYSTEM*

The portal vein collects blood from the splanchnic area—which includes the abdominal portion of the digestive tube, the pancreas and the spleen—and transports it to the liver. The arteries supplying this blood are the nonhepatic branches of the celiac axis and the superior and inferior mesenteric arteries. There are frequent variations in the anatomy of the branches of the portal venous system but the portal vein itself begins rather constantly at the level of the second lumbar vertebra, posterior to the head of the pancreas, at the junction of the splenic and superior mesenteric veins (Fig. 9–1). It is about 6 to 8 cm. long and 1.2 cm. in diameter and contains no valves. At the liver hilum it separates into a right branch that supplies the right lobe and a left branch that supplies the left, caudate and quadrate lobes. The ligamentum teres joins the left branch of the portal vein and contains within it one or more potential lumens (umbilical or para-umbilical veins) that are remnants of the fetal circulation running from the umbilicus to the left portal vein. The most frequent variations in portal system anatomy are in the inferior mesenteric vein, which may join the superior mesenteric instead of the splenic, and in the left gastric (coronary) vein, which may join the splenic instead of the portal.

Portal venous blood passes through one capillary system in the splanchnic viscera and leads to another capillary system, the hepatic sinusoids. Portal venous blood differs from most other venous blood in being under slightly higher pressure in order to overcome the resistance of the hepatic sinusoids, in being less depleted in oxygen because of the relatively high blood flow through the splanchnic area, and in containing many nutrients and bacterial waste products from the digestive tube that are en route to the liver.

Normal fasting hepatic blood flow approximates 1,500 ml./minute. The high pressure hepatic arterial and low pressure portal venous streams unite at the level of the hepatic sinusoid. The best estimates available indicate that about two-thirds of the hepatic blood flow and about half of the total oxygen consumption is supplied by the portal vein while the hepatic artery contributes the remainder.[127, 151, 152]

DEFINITION OF PORTAL HYPERTENSION

Normal portal vein pressure is said to be 5 to 10 mm. Hg. It is difficult to be certain of this value, however, since indirect pressure measurements are only approximate, and for direct measurements the subject must be anesthetized. Though the resistance to the flow of the portal blood through the

* The opinions expressed in this chapter inevitably reflect those of a group of the author's associates at the University of Southern California with long-standing interest in portal hypertension. This group includes internists Alan Redeker, Oliver Kuzma and Fred Lieberman; pathologists Hugh Edmondson and Robert Peters; and surgeons William Mikkelsen, Fred Turrill and Arthur Donovan.

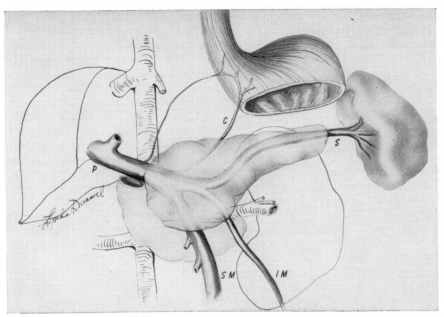

FIG. 9–1. Portal vein and its major tributaries. *C*, coronary (left gastric);
IM, inferior mesenteric; *P*, portal; *S*, splenic; *SM*, superior mesenteric.

hepatic sinusoids is low, some pressure head in the portal vein is required to overcome it. By definition, portal hypertension implies a persistent increase above normal in portal vein pressure. Barring technical errors in measurement, direct portal system pressures at surgery over 30 cm. of saline, intrasplenic pressures over 17 mm. Hg, and wedged hepatic vein pressures more than 4 mm. Hg above inferior vena caval pressure are reliable indications of portal hypertension. In most instances this appears to be due to a primary increase in vascular resistance somewhere in the portal circuit and is accompanied by dilatation of the venous bed behind the obstruction with stasis and a decrease in rate of blood flow. There is a decrease in the amount of blood flowing through the normal vascular channels with a reciprocal increase in collateral blood flow around the liver. The final level of pressure in the portal bed depends on the degree of vascular obstruction, the resistance in the collateral vessels, and the rate of inflow of blood into the splanchnic bed. Since the stimulus for collateral blood flow is the in-

crease in portal tension, the latter can never be entirely relieved by the collateral flow.

HISTORY OF PORTAL HYPERTENSION

Portal hypertension was probably recognized in the early decades of the twentieth century. Investigators such as McIndoe[74] and McMichael[76] used the term "portal hypertension" in their publications. The first manometric measurements in the portal circulation were reported by Thompson, Caughey, Whipple and Rousselot from the Presbyterian Hospital in New York in 1937.[145] In America, surgical therapy for portal hypertension was initiated in 1945 by Blakemore and Whipple working with this same group.[11] Whipple divided portal hypertension into intrahepatic and extrahepatic types.[164] Hemodynamic studies of the portal circulation followed the introduction of hepatic vein catheterization by Warren and Brannon in 1944,[160] the development of a method for measuring hepatic blood flow by Bradley and co-workers in 1945,[14] and the method for measuring hepatic wedge pressure by Friedman and Weiner,[46] Myers and Taylor,[86] Krook[61] and Sherlock and co-workers[98] in the early 1950's.

CAUSE OF PORTAL HYPERTENSION

According to available evidence, most types of portal hypertension result from increased resistance to blood flow in the portal vein, liver or hepatic vein. That hepatic blood flow in portal hypertension is normal or reduced indicates abnormal resistance to blood flow. In all varieties of portal hypertension except 2, it seems that the primary cause is an anatomical lesion which increases the resistance to blood flow through the portal bed. The 2 forms in which increased vascular resistance may not be the primary cause are: (1) Portal hypertension associated with arteriovenous fistulae in the splanchnic bed, in which an increased splanchnic arterial inflow is probably the primary problem, with a secondary increase in portal vascular resistance. (2) "Idiopathic portal hypertension" in which only minor anatomical changes are evident and are possibly secondary to an increase in splanchnic blood flow.

METHODS FOR INVESTIGATION OF THE PORTAL SYSTEM

Portal Venography and Manometry

The most commonly used procedures for visualizing and measuring pressure in the portal system are described in detail in Chapter 10. Two additional technics are available. *Umbilical portography* can be performed through the umbilical vein remnant.[6, 63] This vein is often enlarged in portal hypertension and carries collateral blood flow from the left branch of the portal vein to the anterior abdominal wall. When enlarged, it can be found easily by surgical dissection in the preperitoneal fat, cephalad to the umbilicus. Even when not enlarged it is usually identifiable as a cord-like structure with a lumen that can be dilated sufficiently to hold a catheter. The catheter can then be threaded into the portal vein. When the vein is small and does not contain blood, a narrowed area near the portal vein has to be forcibly dilated with the catheter or with a probe. If the catheter can be placed in the portal vein, pressure can be measured, venography performed and portal blood obtained for metabolic studies. Experience and technical skill are necessary for optimum results with this technic. It is often difficult to fill the main body of the portal vein with contrast media. Ideally, the approach will remain extraperitoneal but sometimes the peritoneal cavity is entered inadvertently, which may mean the loss of any ascitic fluid present. Some groups employ epidural anesthesia for the procedure.

Portal venography can sometimes be performed at *peritoneoscopy*. A skillful operator may be able to withdraw a small piece of omentum through the peritoneoscopy incision with forceps and cannulate a small omental vein for pressure measurement and venography. Excellent venograms of the portal system are obtainable by this technic.[167]

Barium Esophagram

For unknown reasons the lower esophagus is often dilated and has reduced peristalsis in portal hypertension. Varices appear as nodular filling defects in the partially barium-filled lower esophageal lumen. Esophageal relaxation after a peristaltic wave allows the varices to distend for visualization, which is usually achieved best with thick barium paste, swallowed in the prone position. The Valsalva maneuver may be helpful.

Multiple films are important since varices may be evident in one but not in several other exposures. Cineradiography improves visualization moderately.[1] Balloon tamponade of the upper esophagus has been recommended to distend varices for better visualization, but this was not found helpful in a controlled trial by Conn and associates.[32]

In our clinic about half of the patients with varices seen at esophagoscopy have normal barium esophagrams. False positive reports of varices on x-ray are not infrequent. Gastric varices are more difficult to demonstrate since they are usually limited to the fundus. Occasionally they resemble a small tumor mass.

Esophagoscopy

Most clinics use a flexible tipped instrument which is passed into the esophagus after the posterior pharynx has been anesthetized by a topical agent. In portal hypertension, varices are demonstrated at esophagoscopy much more often than by barium meal. Large varices bulge into the lower esophageal lumen like hemorrhoids; moderate size varices appear as blue, tortuous channels under the mucosa. The blue color is not always detectable, however, in which case it may be difficult to differentiate varices and esophageal folds. There is considerable opportunity for observer "variation" in the latter circumstance, especially with limited experience.[34] According to Conn, Binder and Brodoff, the newer flexible fiberoptic esophagoscope has not reduced observer "variation," though it is tolerated better by the patient.[30]

Hepatic Vein Catheterization

The venous system can be catheterized by exposure of an arm or neck vein or by the Seldinger approach to a femoral vein. Because of the direction taken by the main hepatic veins, it may be difficult to force a catheter into the wedged position from the femoral vein approach, so we prefer to use an arm or neck vein. Hepatic vein catheterization may be difficult in the patient with advanced liver disease and ascites, possibly because of a change in the normal angle that the hepatic vein makes with the vena cava. However, with suitable image-amplifying x-ray equipment, failure to enter an hepatic vein is rare. There is virtually no morbidity from the procedure.

Wedged hepatic vein pressure (WHVP) is obtained by wedging the catheter into a peripheral hepatic venule. The catheter tip is, in effect, extended into the hepatic parenchyma by this maneuver insofar as an area of vascular stasis is achieved. For a zero reference point for WHVP, one can use the externally estimated right atrial position (5 cm. below the sternal angle with the patient supine), or one can use the pressure measurement in the inferior vena cava. Our group prefers the latter since we often find small pressure gradients between the vena

cava and the right atrium that we feel have no relationship to portal hypertension and, therefore, should not be included in the WHVP measurement. If the right atrial zero reference point is used, pressures up to 10 mm. Hg are considered normal for WHVP, whereas with vena caval pressure as a baseline we consider anything over 4 mm. Hg as abnormal.

Regardless of which zero point is used, the pressure must be recorded during withdrawal of the catheter from the wedged position. Any abrupt fall in pressure under these circumstances is abnormal. Since the catheter fails to advance on occasion when it is not wedged, it is a useful precaution to confirm wedging by injection of a small amount of contrast media. Wedged pressures in different areas of the liver, including the left lobe, often vary a few mm. Hg but are seldom widely divergent.

It has been assumed that a catheter wedged in an hepatic venule produces stasis in the vasculature only as far into the liver as the hepatic sinusoid, where multiple intersinusoidal anastomoses are present. Any elevation of WHVP has been ascribed to increased resistance in this area of vascular stasis, which has been assumed to be "post-sinusoidal." It seems evident, however, that wedging of a catheter into an hepatic venule obstructs blood flow in a relatively large segment of the hepatic vasculature. In Figure 9–2, contrast media has been allowed to flow into a wedged catheter, by gravity, at a pressure that is just sufficient to allow for slow flow. It is clear that stasis extends well back into the sinusoidal bed of the segment drained by the blocked hepatic vein. Anastomoses with unblocked hepatic sinusoids are around the periphery of the stagnant area, tending to decompress it, but it seems likely that the catheter will record a pressure close to that of the portal blood entering the sinusoidal bed. Increased sinusoidal as well as post-sinusoidal resistance will, then, be reflected by WHVP increase. It is correct to speak of portal hypertension accompanied by normal wedge pressure as "pre-sinusoidal." We think it is incorrect, however, to assume that elevation of wedged pressure indicates only "post-sinusoidal" resistance increase. Either sinusoidal *or* post-

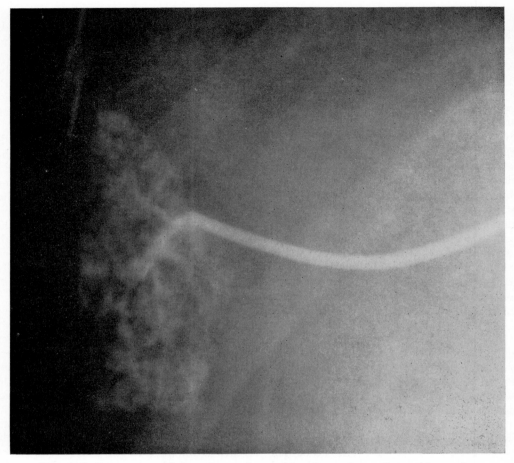

Fig. 9–2. Large area of vascular stasis resulting from the wedging of a catheter into a small hepatic vein; 8 ml. of 50 per cent Hypaque was administered over a 2-minute period by gravity drip at a pressure just sufficient to allow flow into the liver. (Popper, H., and Schaffner, F., eds.: Progress in Liver Disease, New York, Grune & Stratton, 1965.)

sinusoidal resistance increases or both cause elevation of wedge pressure.

Hepatic blood flow is usually measured by the Fick principle after the catheter has been withdrawn to one of the larger hepatic veins. Hepatic extraction of the test substance is measured during a continuous infusion or after a single injection. Substances used include Bromsulphalein, indocyanine green, various radioactive colloids, radioactive rose bengal and ethyl alcohol. The first 3 are most commonly utilized. Calculations of hepatic blood flow from arterial levels of test substances, assuming a constant hepatic extraction, are not reliable since hepatic extraction of all of these materials decreases considerably with liver disease. There are inherent sources of error in all of the methods used for calculating hepatic blood flow. These sources of error become proportionally much larger when hepatic extraction of the test substance is reduced as it is in states of poor hepatic function. Measurement of hepatic blood flow then becomes progressively less reliable as liver disease increases.

Splanchnic oxygen consumption can be calculated as the product of hepatic blood flow and the arterial-hepatic venous oxygen difference. Hepatic oxygen consumption cannot be calculated; there is no way to separate intestinal and hepatic oxygen uptake because portal vein blood cannot be sampled.

Hepatic Venography

Interesting x-rays can be obtained by injecting contrast media into a wedged hepatic vein catheter. Small injections fill a small portion of the hepatic venous tree, whereas larger injections may opacify large areas of the liver and may show reflux into the portal venous tree. The major hepatic veins and upper portion of the inferior vena cava can be outlined by rapid injections into the free hepatic vein. Several investigators claim that hepatic venography is clinically useful,[128, 162] but it is not employed widely.

Direct Measurement of Intrahepatic Pressure

A large bore needle, such as a Silverman liver biopsy needle, or a Teflon catheter over a needle, is inserted into the liver substance and filled with saline. "Tissue pressure" is then recorded with a strain gauge. A limited number of investigators have had experience with this technic and claim that the tissue pressure correlates closely with portal vein pressure and with wedged hepatic vein pressure.[9, 64, 90, 153] More experience is needed with this relatively simple technic to see if the "tissue pressure" is a consistent and meaningful parameter.

Injection of Isotopes or Other Tracer Substances into the Spleen

By monitoring over the heart and over the hilum of the liver after intrasplenic injection of ^{131}I-albumin, one can detect abnormal collateral circulation from the portal system by early arrival of the isotope at the heart.[130] Two scintillation-type gamma detectors are needed, similar to those used for the radioactive renogram.

Several investigators have attempted to quantitate the collateral flow from the portal circulation by measuring the proportion of splenic injectate that appears in the hepatic vein.[19] This calculation has limited useful-

ness because the isotope may escape through splenic vein collaterals before mixing with the entire portal blood stream and thus may provide an index of only splenic collateral flow.

Ammonium Tolerance

Many investigators have demonstrated an abnormal rise in blood ammonium after patients with chronic liver disease ingest an ammonium salt. As shown by hepatic vein catheterization, the rise may be due to either poor hepatic function and failure to metabolize portal blood ammonium or to portal hypertension with portal-systemic collateral flow.[165] There is general agreement that the latter mechanism is the most common reason for a marked blood ammonium rise; consequently ammonium tolerance may be used as a screening test for portal hypertension. One method of performing the test is to give 3 Gm. of ammonium chloride orally and to consider a rise of arterial ammonium above 150 μg.% at 45 minutes as an abnormal result.[29]

DISEASES ASSOCIATED WITH PORTAL HYPERTENSION

Traditionally portal hypertension is divided into 3 major types—suprahepatic, intrahepatic and extrahepatic—based on the location of the presumed increase in vascular resistance. Recently Imanaga and co-workers[54] and Sherlock[135] proposed new classifications that incorporate both the site of the vascular block and the findings at hepatic vein catheterization. Intrahepatic portal hypertension is divided into types with normal wedged hepatic vein pressure (pre-sinusoidal, portal vein obstruction) and with raised wedged hepatic vein pressure (post-sinusoidal, hepatic vein obstruction). As mentioned, we object to the use of the word "post-sinusoidal" (see "Hepatic Vein Catheterization.") Since in many of the syndromes accompanied by portal hypertension there is insufficient hemodynamic data available to be certain of the precise location of the increased vascular resistance, we have not attempted a classification in this chapter.

Portal Hypertension Due to Block of the Hepatic Veins or Inferior Vena Cava (Budd-Chiari Syndrome)

When the major hepatic veins or the vena cava above the orifice of the hepatic veins is occluded, the liver becomes swollen and congested and develops sinusoidal hypertension and often hemorrhagic infarction of the areas around the central veins. Arterial blood must leave the liver via the portal vein and collateral veins, and pressure in the portal vein rises.

The cause of hepatic vein or vena caval occlusion is usually unknown. Venous thrombosis is found in a minority of cases, often when there is some predisposing disease such as polycythemia vera or paroxysmal nocturnal hemoglobinuria or a neighboring tumor, cyst or abscess. Tumors, particularly hypernephromas and hepatomas, may directly invade the vena cava or hepatic veins and occlude them. In most instances of the Budd-Chiari syndrome, however, there is simply narrowing and fibrous obliteration of the ostia of the major hepatic veins and/or the intrahepatic portion of the vena cava, and it is uncertain whether or not this is the consequence of a previous venous thrombosis.

In a review of the literature in 1959, Parker pointed out the failure to find a definite cause for vein obliteration in 115 of 164 reported cases.[96] In Japan, in the great majority of patients a fibrous diaphragm occludes or narrows the upper portion of the vena cava and the orifices of the left and middle hepatic veins. The right hepatic vein is usually open.[60, 168] It has been postulated that this is a congenital anomaly related to closure of the ductus venosus, though most patients do not demonstrate clinical disease until adult life. In Egypt, relatively large numbers of children are reported with the Budd-Chiari syndrome due to fibrous occlusion of the orifices of the main hepatic veins, usually without vena caval involvement.[123]

The clinical consequences of obstruction of the vena cava or major hepatic veins include hepatomegaly (sometimes painful if the occlusion is acute), ascites, esophageal varices with hematemesis, and, if the vena cava is occluded, the appearance of vena caval collateral vessels on the abdominal wall. Unless the vena cava is closed, diagnosis is difficult and is usually achieved only by recognizing the characteristic histologic changes on liver biopsy. If a patient survives the acute phase, the liver may show only diffuse scarring that is misinterpreted as cirrhosis. There may be marked caudate lobe hypertrophy because this lobe has veins that drain directly into the vena cava. Splenoportography usually fails to opacify the portal vein because of reverse blood flow. Failure to enter the hepatic veins with the catheter is not diagnostic since it is sometimes impossible to do this in a patient with cirrhosis and an open hepatic vein.

If the vena cava is occluded, as it is in the majority of cases in Japan and about one-third of cases in this country, the diagnosis is much easier. Femoral vein pressure is above normal. Vena caval catheterization from below should demonstrate both the site of occlusion and marked collateral flow on venography. Characteristic vena caval collaterals appear on the anterior abdominal wall and can be differentiated from portal collaterals by the sugar test (see p. 285).

Portal Hypertension Due to Veno-Occlusive Disease

Bras, Brooks and Watler have pointed out that approximately one-third of the "cirrhosis" seen at autopsy in their department in Jamaica is a nonportal type of fibrosis with occlusion of centrolobular hepatic veins and subsequent centrolobular fibrosis.[17] Most patients with this lesion are under 20 years of age. Ascites and severe portal hypertension with bleeding from esophageal varices are prominent clinical manifestations. These investigators believe that the acute form of the disease is due to occlusion of small branches of the hepatic veins with resulting severe centrolobular congestion and loss of hepatocytes in the center of the lobule. Various pyrrolozidine alkaloids from *Crotalaria* and *Senecio* plants are suspected as etiologic agents because they are used in native "bush-tea" and they produce somewhat similar lesions in experimental animals.[16, 75]

We know of no hepatic vein catheterization studies in this syndrome. One would expect the wedged hepatic vein pressure to be high since the blood flow seems to be obstructed in the outflow tract of the liver. There are certain similarities between "VOD" and "Indian childhood cirrhosis,"[56] and it is possible that different toxins in various parts of the world affect the hepatic vasculature.

PORTAL HYPERTENSION IN PARENCHYMAL LIVER DISEASE

Cirrhosis

Distortion of the intrahepatic vasculature is a constant accompaniment of cirrhosis. Corrosion casts of the liver show a decrease in volume of both the portal venous and hepatic venous trees.[49] Portography usually shows a "winter tree" appearance of the portal vessels. Serial sections demonstrate that the regenerative nodule compresses and distorts the hepatic veins.[58] Portal fibrosis and scarring may cause narrowing of the peripheral portal venules. Though these features seem to provide an adequate anatomic basis for increased vascular resistance in the cirrhotic liver, some investigators argue that increased flow from the hepatic artery into the portal vein may be the primary cause of portal hypertension. Postmortem perfusions and corrosion casts show a relative increase in hepatic artery mass in cirrhosis[49, 52] and abnormal communications can be seen between the smaller ramifications of the hepatic artery and the portal vein.[103] It would seem more logical to regard these as compensatory phenomena for reduced portal vein flow rather than a primary cause of portal hypertension. However, any increase in hepatic arterial inflow is bound to contribute to portal hypertension if the principal resistance to blood flow is in the hepatic sinusoids or hepatic venules.

Many investigators have studied hepatic hemodynamics in cirrhosis by hepatic vein catheterization. Results from many publications are summarized in a review by Lacroix and Leusen in 1965.[62] Most values for hepatic blood flow have been normal or decreased. The inherent errors in the standard Bromsulphalein method for measuring liver blood flow tend to give an artefactually high result when hepatic extraction of BSP is poor, as it often is in liver disease. This prob-

ably explains the relatively few high values reported for hepatic blood flow. If portal hypertension were primarily due to increased splanchnic inflow, then hepatic blood flow measurements should tend to be high in cirrhosis, whereas if vascular obstruction is the major problem they should tend to be low, as they appear to be.

Wedged hepatic vein pressure (WHVP) is elevated in cirrhosis, roughly proportional to the stage of the disease. In alcoholic cirrhosis, WHVP is nearly as high as simultaneously measured portal vein pressure.[112, 154] This suggests that most of the increased vascular resistance in alcoholic cirrhosis is sinusoidal or post-sinusoidal, rather than pre-sinusoidal. We have not compared WHVP and portal vein pressure simultaneously in nonalcoholic cirrhosis, however, nor have we seen reports of this in the literature. With admittedly only limited data to draw on, it is our impression that wedge pressure levels are somewhat lower in nonalcoholic than in alcoholic cirrhosis which, if true, may indicate a larger component of pre-sinusoidal portal venous resistance increase in nonalcoholic cirrhosis.

In other types of cirrhosis (hemochromatosis, Wilson's disease, primary biliary cirrhosis, secondary biliary cirrhosis), portal hypertension is usually a late manifestation, and uncommonly causes death from bleeding varices. WHVP is elevated in most of these conditions when portal hypertension is present, but again there are no direct comparisons available between WHVP and portal vein pressure to allow any speculation regarding the relative importance of portal venous, sinusoidal and post-sinusoidal resistance increase. An interesting exception is Wilson's disease; a careful hemodynamic investigation of 4 patients by Taylor, Jackson and Jensen[142] showed very small elevations of wedge pressure in 3 of the patients in spite of severe portal hypertension—which implies a marked pre-sinusoidal resistance increase. This is not a universal finding in Wilson's disease as indicated by one of their 4 patients and 2 patients of our own with considerable wedge pressure elevation. More measurements are needed in Wilson's disease as well as in other types of nonalcoholic cirrhosis to determine the frequency of predominant "pre-sinusoidal" vascular resistance increase.

Alcoholic Liver Disease Without Cirrhosis

Severe acute liver damage may develop in the alcoholic in the absence of cirrhosis. Histologically there is usually fatty infiltration, liver cell injury with "ballooning," necrosis, alcoholic hyaline and polymorphonuclear infiltration. This lesion has been variously called "alcoholic hepatitis,"[7] "florid cirrhosis"[104] and "sclerosing hyaline necrosis."[39] Our pathologists have drawn our attention to the predominantly centrilobular location of the cellular injury and the collagen formation that accompanies it. Extensive centrilobular collagen deposition may greatly distort the hepatic architecture without the development of any regenerative nodules (Fig. 9–3).

We have found, by wedged hepatic vein pressure measurements, that portal hypertension develops early in this lesion. Ascites often accompanies the acute stage. In the subacute and chronic stages of the lesion, collagen formation in the liver is diffuse, predominantly in the central areas, being somewhat reminiscent of the "centrilobular cirrhosis" described by Bras and colleagues in veno-occlusive disease.[17] Many of our alcoholic patients in Los Angeles die in the subacute stages of this lesion, with a smooth liver surface, with all of the clinical features of portal hypertension including ruptured esophageal varices, and without regenerative nodules microscopically. Acute sclerosing hyaline necrosis may resolve, leaving minimal hepatic scarring, or it may progress to cirrhosis, with regenerative nodules. Prior to the development of cirrhotic nodules, this type of lesion is ideally located in the liver lobule to produce a primarily "outflow block" and would be expected to cause a wedge pressure elevation that closely approaches portal vein pressure level. Elements of this lesion in many patients with alcoholic liver disease may help explain why WHVP levels are so close to those measured in the portal system.

Sarcoidosis

Scattered in the literature are reports of hepatic sarcoidosis with manifest ascites and esophageal varices. The cause of the portal

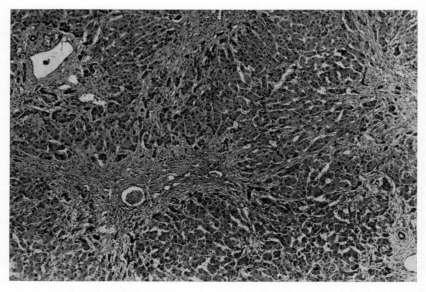

Fig. 9–3. Predominantly centrilobular fibrosis without regenerative nodules as seen in chronic sclerosing hyaline disease due to alcoholism. This patient had a smooth liver surface and elevated wedged hepatic vein pressure. (Sommers, S. C., ed.: Pathology Annual: 1967, New York, Appleton-Century-Crofts, 1967.)

hypertension has not been determined. Hunt considered it to be a manifestation of increased inflow through the large spleen.[53] It has been postulated that the granulomas obstruct the portal venules, hepatic venules or sinusoids.[82] Alternatively, periportal fibrosis and disruption of lobular architecture caused by the healing phase of the granulomatous lesions could cause portal hypertension. Our own experience includes only 3 patients with ascites, all of whom had moderate elevation of wedge pressure. From histologic examination in 2 of them we were unable to decide the cause of portal hypertension.

Cystic Disease of the Liver

The liver lesion commonly called "congenital hepatic fibrosis"[59] is likely a form of cystic disease and we prefer the term "microcystic disease of the liver." The liver surface does not have a cystic appearance; microscopic sections show marked bile duct hyperplasia in broad fibrous bands in the portal areas. Liver function is good and portal hypertension is prominent, often causing variceal bleeding in childhood. The disorder is hereditary with a pattern resembling that of an autosomal recessive trait. There is frequent association with some form of renal cystic disease. Kerr and colleagues found a considerable gradient (11 mm. Hg) between portal vein and wedged hepatic vein pressure in one patient, and postulated that portal hypertension is due to compression or reduction of the portal venous radicles in the fibrous portal bands.[59] However, hepatic vein catheterization data from 6 additional patients, summarized by Fauvert, Benhamou and Meyer, do not favor a predominantly pre-sinusoidal vascular obstruction.[44]

The usual type of polycystic disease of the liver is probably rarely, if ever, associated with portal hypertension. Three patients with "polycystic disease" and portal hypertension reported by Campbell and associates in 1958 are probably examples of microcystic disease.[21]

"Partial Nodular Transformation" of the Liver

Sherlock, Feldman, Moran and Scheuer have described 4 patients with portal hypertension apparently due to an unexplained nodular transformation of the perihilar portion of the liver, without appreciable fibrosis.[137] Hemodynamic studies in one patient demonstrated a high wedge pressure. Whether the portal hypertension is due to compression of the hepatic outflow by the nodules or to disease of the hepatic veins is unknown.

PORTAL HYPERTENSION WITH HEMATOLOGIC DISORDERS

Portal hypertension with ascites, esophageal varices and an open portal vein has been reported in occasional patients with the myeloproliferative syndrome, Hodgkin's disease, leukemia or Gaucher's disease. Some authorities have held that increased splenic arterial inflow is the cause of portal hypertension in these situations.[76, 97, 99] Considerably increased values for hepatic blood flow have been recorded by Benhamou and colleagues in one patient with Gaucher's disease[8] and by Rosenbaum and co-workers in 5 patients with the myeloproliferative syndrome.[119]

An alternate view is that portal hypertension is caused by vascular obstruction from the portal or intrasinusoidal infiltrate of the hematologic disease. In support of this, a normal hepatic blood flow with portal hypertension was found by Shaldon and Sherlock in 2 patients, one with Hodgkin's disease and one with myelosclerosis,[134] and by Dal Palu in one patient with leukemia.[36] The increased vascular resistance seemed to be pre-sinusoidal in Shaldon and Sherlock's patients and sinusoidal or post-sinusoidal in Dal Palu's patient.

The mechanism for portal hypertension in hematologic disorders is unknown. Hemodynamic studies before and after splenectomy would be most useful; this should cure portal hypertension due to increased splenic artery inflow and only moderately affect portal hypertension due to vascular obstruction in the liver.

PORTAL HYPERTENSION WITH METASTATIC CARCINOMA

Ascites not due to peritoneal implants, together with splenomegaly and esophageal varices, may complicate metastatic carcinoma in the liver.[122] Portal hypertension in this situation seems to be due to tumor emboli in the portal or hepatic venules or both. Hepatic vein catheterization measurements have been performed on a number of patients with metastatic liver carcinoma, but none had evidence of portal hypertension. Presumably, wedge hepatic vein pressure is high if the predominant obstruction is in the hepatic venules and low if it is in the portal venules.

INTRAHEPATIC PORTAL VEIN OBSTRUCTION DUE TO SCHISTOSOMIASIS

The ova of *Schistosoma mansoni* and *S. japonicum* are laid in the submucosa of the colon and rectum. Some pass into the portal blood stream and lodge as emboli in the intrahepatic portal venules. A foreign body "pseudotubercle" tissue reaction with granulomatous change and eosinophilic infiltrate develops in the portal area with eventual healing and scarring. Portal hypertension follows, with splenomegaly and esophageal varices and relatively good preservation of liver function. The site of obstruction to blood flow appears to be the portal venules. On hepatic vein catheterization one would predict a relatively normal wedge pressure level with this type of pre-sinusoidal obstruction; several studies have recorded such findings.[2, 84, 106] When wedge pressure is moderately elevated it usually accompanies greater distortion of hepatic architecture due to either a more advanced stage of the disease or to complicating liver cirrhosis of other cause.

PORTAL HYPERTENSION WITH ARTERIOVENOUS FISTULAE IN THE SPLANCHNIC BED

In 1965 Stone and co-workers reviewed 38 examples of splanchnic arteriovenous fistulae from the literature.[140] Many patients demonstrated ascites, esophageal varices and gastrointestinal bleeding. Portal hypertension was often documented by operative manometry.

The usual causes for acquired splanchnic arteriovenous fistulae are trauma or rupture of aneurysms of the splenic or hepatic artery. Congenital arteriovenous fistulae occur in hereditary hemorrhagic telangiectasia. It seems logical to ascribe the portal hypertension to increased flow of blood into the portal system. The hepatic vasculature must resist the increased flow sufficiently so that portal hypertension develops and thus prevents the onset of high-output heart failure which seems to be a rare finding in this disorder. One would expect a moderate or marked increase in hepatic blood flow, depending upon how much compensatory increase in hepatic vascular resistance developed. Unfortunately, hepatic hemodynamic data in this important prototype of portal hypertension is sparse.

A recent patient of ours with clinical portal hypertension, esophageal varices and a right hepatic artery–portal vein fistula due to an old gunshot wound had a portal vein pressure of 57 cm. of saline at laparotomy. At hepatic vein catheterization, hepatic blood flow was within normal limits (1,650 ml./min. by the indocyanine green technic) and wedged hepatic vein pressure was only mildly elevated (9 mm. Hg above inferior vena cava pressure). Liver biopsy showed definite changes in the portal areas similar to what we have called "hepatoportal sclerosis,"[80] with sclerosis of the portal radicles and increased portal collagen. If these hemodynamic findings are typical for this type of portal hypertension, we can no longer exclude increased portal inflow as a cause of portal hypertension simply because of a failure to find increased hepatic blood flow. Perhaps our patient did have increased hepatic blood flow prior to the development of portal venous thickening and sclerosis. It is also possible that a "functional" increase in portal venous resistance could keep hepatic blood flow within the broad range of normal prior to the development of organic vascular pathology.

In dogs, portal vein arterialization can cause anatomical changes in portal venules that include thickening of the wall, hypertrophy of the muscularis and fibrinoid necrosis.[45, 107] Hemodynamic data in this type of animal preparation is limited. Siderys and his co-workers found a marked increase in hepatic blood flow and moderate portal hypertension in 6 dogs 6 weeks after constructing a fistula between the aorta and splenic vein.[138] These findings are quite different from those in our patient referred to above. Further hemodynamic studies in this type of portal hypertension should be of great interest.

IDIOPATHIC PORTAL HYPERTENSION

Portal hypertension without any apparent cause is a relatively uncommon but vexing problem. In reports in the United States, such patients are characterized as having normal or near normal hepatic function, a smooth liver surface, little or no histologic abnormality and, of course, an open portal vein.[50, 102, 147] Imanaga and colleagues in Nagoya state that approximately one-third of their patients with portal hypertension do not have cirrhosis but rather have varying degrees, often minor, of portal fibrosis.[54] Boyer and colleagues report 16 patients from Calcutta with "idiopathic portal hypertension," who had excellent liver function, a smooth liver surface and mild to moderate portal fibrosis without cirrhotic nodules.[13]

It is uncertain whether all of these patients from different geographic areas have the same disorder. We have used the term "hepatoportal sclerosis" to describe this condition because of the consistent finding of scattered portal areas enlarged by deposition of perivascular and periductular collagen and with intimal thickening and eccentric sclerosis of the portal vein walls.[80] Imanaga uses the term "intrahepatic pre-sinusoidal (portal vein) obstruction," because of normal hepatic vein catheterization findings. Boyer and colleagues use the term "idiopathic portal hypertension," though emphasizing the presence of varying degrees of portal fibrosis and portal phlebosclerosis. Some may prefer the term "Banti's syndrome." Until the pathogenesis of this condition is better understood, "idiopathic portal hypertension" is probably the best designation.

Hemodynamic studies in the Nagoya patients consistently show nearly normal or normal wedged hepatic vein pressure and hepatic blood flow.[54] In the Calcutta patients, WHVP was usually elevated, though to a lesser extent than in cirrhotic patients studied by the same investigators.[13] Hepatic blood flow was slightly decreased. One patient investigated by Benhamou and colleagues had normal hepatic blood flow and slight elevation of wedge pressure.[10]

We could obtain only limited hemodynamic data in our own patients. WHVP was normal in 3 and hepatic blood flow was moderately decreased in 2.[80] This hemodynamic pattern is similar to that found in schistosomiasis with portal hypertension, which suggests that the intrahepatic radicles of the portal vein are the site of increased vascular resistance. It seemed to us that the subtle changes in the portal venules of our patients indicate a primary lesion at this site. Boyer suggests that this type of portal hypertension is a sequela of previous unrecognized pylephlebitis. Those who espouse the "forward" theory of portal hypertension can argue that increased flow into the splanchnic bed is responsible for the portal hypertension; Tisdale, Klatskin and Glenn suggested this in 1959.[147]

We have previously been reluctant to consider the latter explanation because of the normal or decreased hepatic blood flow documented in the Nagoya patients, a few of our own, and those in Calcutta. We reasoned that portal hypertension due to a high splanchnic inflow would result in a very high blood flow through an undiseased liver. This reasoning is faulty, however, since the liver might respond to a high inflow with a functional increase in portal vein resistance that would keep total hepatic blood flow within normal limits. Eventually, structural changes in the portal vasculature, similar to those we have described, might develop as a secondary phenomenon. As mentioned, one of our patients with portal hypertension due to a traumatic hepatic artery–portal vein fistula has been found to have a nearly normal hepatic blood flow (1.650 ml./min. indocyanine green) and wedge pressure (9 mm. Hg above inferior vena cava pressure), together with histologic findings typical of "hepatoportal sclerosis."

Possibly a number of different diseases in different parts of the world are included under idiopathic portal hypertension.

EXTRAHEPATIC PORTAL HYPERTENSION

In this condition, the portal or splenic veins or both are occluded or have been changed into a fibrous cord or a collection of collateral channels sometimes called "cavernous transformation." The spleen is invariably enlarged and there are esophageal or gastric varices or both. Liver biopsy is normal or nearly normal and hepatic function tests are usually normal. Wedged hepatic vein pressure is normal and hepatic blood flow is mildly or moderately reduced. Splenoportography fails to opacify the obstructed segment of the portal circulation and shows numerous collateral channels. Intrasplenic pressure is raised. The clinical manifestations of extrahepatic portal hypertension consist of episodes of hematemesis, often appearing early in childhood or young adulthood, and recurring irregularly, sometimes at widely spaced intervals. The hematologic manifestations of hypersplenism are often present to a moderate degree but seldom produce symptoms.

The cause of extrahepatic portal block is usually unknown.[79, 143] A few patients give a history compatible with neonatal omphalitis but the association is so infrequent that we question its significance.[79] Localized splenic vein thrombosis adjacent to the pancreas is sometimes related to an episode of acute pancreatitis. In an occasional patient, the portal clot can be blamed on an associated Budd-Chiari syndrome, polycythemia vera or paroxysmal nocturnal hemoglobinuria. Portal vein thrombosis also may complicate cirrhosis of the liver, presumably as a consequence of stasis in the portal bed, or it may develop from invasion by hepatoma.

The cause of portal hypertension with portal block may seem obvious. Nevertheless, some facts are disconcerting. It is difficult to produce anything that resembles hypersplenism or permanent portal hypertension by ligating any branch of the portal system in animals.[23] Ravenna has pointed out that many examples of portal or splenic vein thrombosis in man are not accompanied by splenomegaly or esophageal varices.[109] Though ascites is typically not present in extrahepatic portal block and should not be, because of its presumed hepatic origin, a surprising number of patients with extrahepatic block do have ascites at some time during their illness.[4, 80, 144] Though hepatic tests are usually normal early in extrahepatic portal hypertension, they tend to become abnormal through the years, which suggests an intrahepatic lesion.[144] In our experience,

the minor pathologic changes in the portal areas that we have seen in idiopathic portal hypertension (i.e., hepatoportal sclerosis) are often seen in extrahepatic portal block.

In a recent publication my colleagues and I suggest that there may be no basic difference, with the exception of the portal vein occlusion, between idiopathic portal hypertension and extrahepatic portal obstruction.[80] Patients with "extrahepatic portal block" simply would be those in whom a superimposed portal thrombosis has developed. Many arguments can be marshalled against this suggestion, however. It seems unlikely that portal thrombosis would complicate idiopathic portal hypertension more often than it complicates the portal hypertension of cirrhosis of the liver. According to the concept we advanced, portal hypertension should be persistent on the hepatic side of the obstruction in the portal vein. Umbilical vein collateral circulation in the falciform ligament would be anticipated in an occasional patient, though it is generally agreed that a Cruveilhier-Baumgarten murmur is not heard in extrahepatic portal block. It will be interesting to attempt to measure portal pressure by the umbilical vein approach in patients with extrahepatic portal block.

CONSEQUENCES OF PORTAL HYPERTENSION

COLLATERAL CIRCULATION

A natural consequence of stasis and increased pressure in any venous bed is the development of connections to neighboring low pressure veins. The collateral circulation in long-standing portal hypertension is well developed though the size and location of the major collaterals varies considerably from patient to patient. It has been proposed that a well developed collateral flow can relieve portal hypertension, and patients have been described with large collaterals and relatively normal intrasplenic pressures.[149] However, since the stimulus for the development of collateral vessels is portal hypertension, it seems unlikely that the latter can ever be completely relieved by the collateral flow

The natural sites for the development of portal collateral vessels are areas where veins draining into the portal stream are in juxtaposition to veins draining into the caval system. The major locations for this are:

Submucosa of the Esophagus. Anastomoses form between the tributaries of the coronary vein (portal drainage) and azygos vein (superior vena cava drainage). This results in submucosal varices of the lower esophagus and upper stomach (Fig. 9–4). Collaterals from the spleen to the stomach contribute to this anastomotic plexus.

Submucosa of the Rectum. The lower

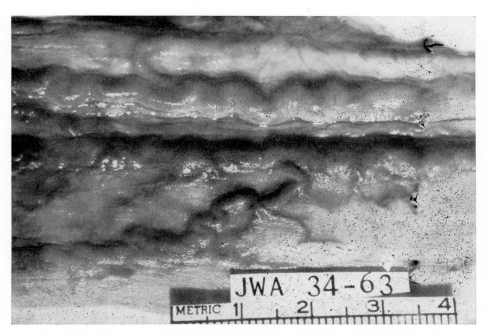

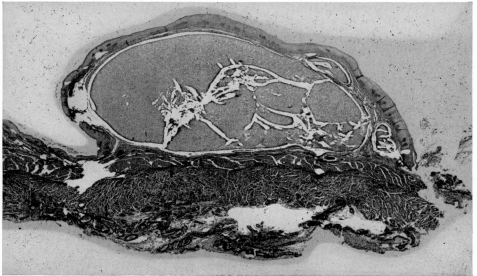

FIG. 9–4. *Top,* Varices in the lower esophagus at autopsy in a patient with alcoholic liver disease. The veins have been injected with a blood-agar mixture. *Bottom,* cross section through an injected varix.

portion of the rectum normally drains into the inferior vena cava via the inferior hemorrhoidal veins while the upper portion of the rectum drains into the portal system via the middle and superior hemorrhoidal veins. Anastomoses between these venous systems result in hemorrhoids.

Anterior Abdominal Wall. The umbilical vein remnant of the fetal circulation in the falciform ligament normally carries little or no blood but remains probe-patent. In portal hypertension it can serve as an anastomosis between the main left portal vein and the normotensive epigastric veins of the anterior abdominal wall that drain ultimately into the superior and inferior cavae.

Parietal Peritoneum. Connections between the portal and caval systems form in the posterior abdominal wall (veins of Retzius) and between the capsule of the liver and diaphragm (veins of Sappey).

Left Renal Vein. Large connections sometimes form between the splenic vein or other neighboring portal tributaries and the left renal vein. On rare occasions these are nearly as large as a surgical splenorenal shunt.

Increased Lymphatic Flow

The normal flow of hepatic lymph is toward the hilum and from there lymphatics traverse the hepatoduodenal and hepatogastric ligaments to join the cisterna chyli and thoracic duct. In portal hypertension of intrahepatic cause the flow of hepatic lymph is greatly increased. On postmortem studies, hilar lymphatics can be shown to be enlarged.[3] In life, the thoracic duct is dilated, lymph flow is markedly increased and lymphatic pressure is raised.[38] In our own experience we have seen thoracic duct lymph flow as great as 15 ml./min. and pressures that rise as high as 30 mm. Hg after 30 to 40 seconds of duct occlusion. It is presumed that most of this lymph flow is from the liver, though, in ascites, some of the increase may come from the peritoneum or omentum. The thoracic duct lymph is often blood-tinged in portal hypertension; the highest hematocrit we have observed is 19 mm. per cent. There is no good explanation for the sanguineous lymph, though it has been suggested that it results from peripheral veno-lymphatic connections rather than from leakage at the hepatic sinusoid.[37]

Since a natural response to the obstruction of venous return from any area of the body is an increase in lymph flow, the increased thoracic duct lymph flow in portal hypertension could be regarded as a manifestation of congestion of the liver. Since the major vascular obstruction in intrahepatic portal hypertension seems to be in the sinusoids or hepatic venules, the sinusoidal area can be considered "congested" and capable of forming more than the usual amount of hepatic lymph.

It would be interesting to know the thoracic duct pressure and lymph flow in extrahepatic portal hypertension; to my knowledge this has not been measured.

Ascites

Portal hypertension is a major factor in ascites formation. The leading current theory, which has much experimental backing, is that ascites forms as a consequence of sinusoidal hypertension and hepatic lymph formation in excess of what can be carried away by the hepatic lymphatics. Portacaval shunting usually relieves ascites and, in our experience, when it does not do so the residual hepatic sinusoidal pressure remains relatively high, as assessed by wedged hepatic vein pressure. Nevertheless, another factor or factors are operative in the production of ascites since at no fixed level of portal hypertension does ascites regularly appear. Whether this factor is the serum albumin level or something much more complex is unknown.

Increased Plasma Volume

This is a regular finding in chronic liver disease with portal hypertension and has been documented by many investigators.[41, 66, 85, 100] In our opinion, this is not a measurement artefact since we found the same degree of plasma volume increase in patients with or without ascites and no evidence of any significant loss of iodinated albumin into either the ascitic fluid or the thoracic duct lymph space during the 20 minutes required for equilibration.[66] Portal hypertension seems to provide a logical explanation for hypervolemia since it is invariably accompanied by dilatation of the entire portal venous bed and adjacent collateral veins.

We found the greatest increases in plasma volume in patients with esophageal varices and previous hemorrhage. We also found a reasonably good correlation between the plasma volume and the level of portal hypertension as assessed by wedged hepatic vein pressure. However, portal hypertension may not be the only reason for increased plasma volume in chronic liver disease. In our experience, some degree of hypervolemia persists after portacaval shunting, even after the side-to-side variety.[66] Also the degree of hypervolemia is apparently less in extrahepatic portal hypertension than in intrahepatic. Murray et al. found normal values for plasma volume in extrahepatic block,[85] whereas we found moderate increases. Unfortunately, Bradley's method for measuring splanchnic blood volume is not readily applicable to patients with extensive portal collateral circulation and it has proved technically difficult to measure the volume of the splanchnic venous bed at autopsy. If the volume of the dilated portal venous bed were great enough to account for the observed increase in plasma volume in portal hypertension then it would be unnecessary to seek another explanation of hypervolemia.

CLINICAL ASSESSMENT OF PORTAL HYPERTENSION

PHYSICAL FINDINGS

Most of the physical findings of chronic liver disease have some bearing on the presence of portal hypertension. Those with specific importance include:

Splenomegaly. Portal hypertension is not the only reason for splenic enlargement in chronic liver disease since the size of the spleen does not correlate well with the level of portal pressure. Palpable enlargement of the spleen is noted, however, in a great majority of patients with significant portal hypertension. Palpability of the spleen is enhanced for most examiners by using light pressure in the left upper quadrant while the patient lies on his right side and inhales deeply.

Ascites. Ascites is suggestive of portal hypertension unless explained by carcinoma, heart failure or inflammatory disease of the peritoneum. Shifting dullness is the best indicator of a moderate amount of ascites. The "fluid wave" is a relatively useless physical finding in my opinion, since I have never been able to elicit it except in obvious tense ascites. Careful insertion of a needle into either flank in the lower quadrant may be justifiable to document the presence of ascites when physical findings are uncertain and when its presence or absence is important.

Dilated Abdominal Veins. Many patients with portal hypertension have dilated veins in the flanks as a result of portal venous–parietal peritoneum connections or on the anterior abdominal wall as a result of umbilical vein–epigastric vein connections. Minor degrees of increased abdominal wall collateral circulation may be indistinguishable from normal veins made more prominent by stretching and thinning of the overlying skin in the patient without portal hypertension whose abdomen is distended. Abdominal collaterals are often seen more easily in infrared photographs (Fig. 9–5) or through the red goggles used by radiologists. Occasionally an extremely dilated and tortuous vein creates a lump on the abdominal wall that is best seen in lateral profile (Fig. 9–6). On one of our patients such a vein was mistaken for an umbilical hernia. Rarely the collateral veins take the shape of a "caput medusae" around the umbilicus.

When the veins are large, one can often hear the characteristic Cruveilhier-Baumgarten murmur. This is a continuous bruit, varying from low to high pitch, and most often heard somewhere between the umbilicus and the lower portion of the sternum. It is pathognomonic of intrahepatic portal hypertension with a large collateral vein in the falciform ligament. In some patients the bruit comes and goes, resulting in disputes between examiners as to its presence. It is often enhanced by having the patient raise his head from the pillow and it usually disappears completely when pressure is applied immediately above the umbilicus. There is often a palpable thrill over the area where the murmur is loudest.

Portal collateral veins must be differen-

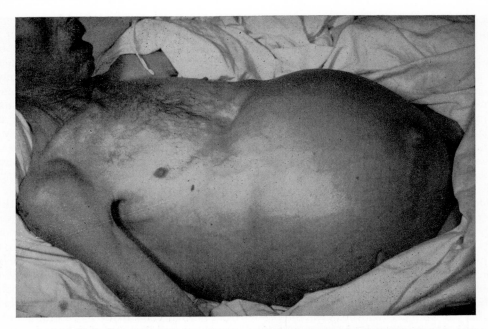

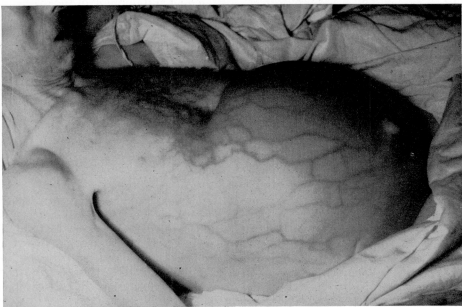

Fig. 9–5. Collateral abdominal veins on the anterior abdominal wall in a patient with alcoholic liver disease as recorded by black and white photography (*top*) and infrared photography (*bottom*).

tiated from collateral vessels that form after obstruction of the inferior vena cava. Vena caval collaterals tend to be more prominent in the flanks and less so in the central areas of the abdomen (Fig. 9–7). There are often dilated vessels over the back which are never seen with portal obstruction. In vessels below the umbilicus, the direction of flow is upward in vena caval collaterals and downward in portal collaterals. However, the

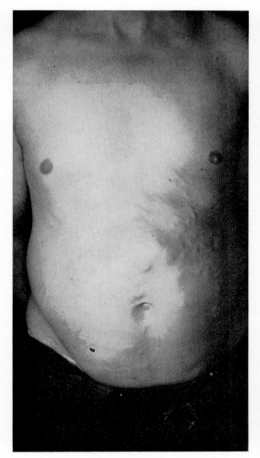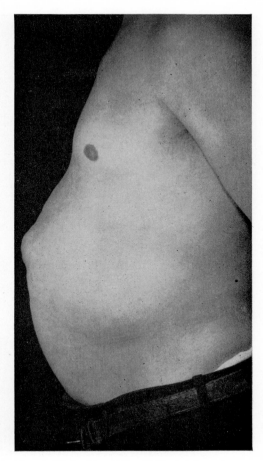

FIG. 9–6. Large abdominal collateral veins as seen anteriorly (*left*) and in profile (*right*). A Cruveilhier-Baumgarten murmur was heard over this vein.

valves in dilated veins may become ineffective and one cannot always ascertain the direction of the blood flow in a vessel by the usual technic of stripping it between 2 fingers. In vena caval obstruction, bruits are not heard over the dilated vessels and the femoral vein pressure should be elevated.

The sugar test has been reliable in our experience. During absorption of glucose from the gastrointestinal tract, sugar concentration should be higher in the portal vein and any of its collaterals than in the remainder of the circulatory system. Thirty minutes after ingestion of 50 Gm. of glucose by a fasting patient, peripheral vein and abdominal vein glucose concentrations are compared. If the abdominal vessels are portal collaterals, the sugar concentration should be substantially higher (usually 20 to 50 mg.%). Both values should be above normal to indicate that glucose is actually being absorbed.

DEMONSTRATION OF ESOPHAGEAL VARICES

This is not pathognomonic of portal hypertension. "Downhill varices" can occur when the superior vena cava is obstructed below the azygos vein. Palmer has pointed out that dilated veins are sometimes seen in the lower esophagus in patients with hiatus hernia without portal hypertension.[92] A few patients have been reported with esophageal varices that are unexplained.[94, 126]

Because of its simplicity, barium swallow is ordinarily used first to look for varices. A negative study, even by the cine technic, has

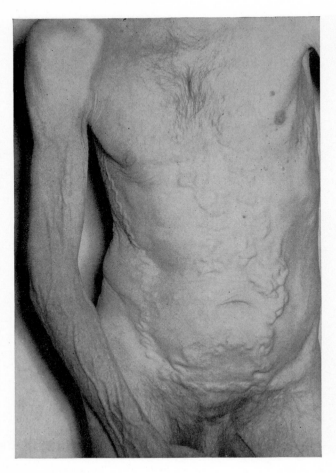

FIG. 9–7. Abdominal collateral veins resulting from long-standing inferior vena caval obstruction.

limited value because small or moderate sized varices are frequently missed on x-ray. Esophagoscopy is much more effective than barium swallow in demonstrating varices. Considerable endoscopic experience is required for optimum results, however, and it may be difficult to distinguish folds from varices.

SUPPLEMENTARY TECHNICS

In many patients, if definite esophageal varices are demonstrated by barium swallow or esophagoscopy and if the clinical picture is not complicated, further evaluation of the portal system is unnecessary. When more information is desired, the clinician has a wide choice of additional technics, as described in the first portion of this chapter. The most useful of these is probably splenic manometry followed by splenoportography. From this one gets information regarding the pressure in the portal system, the patency of the portal vein and the presence of collateral circulation. Esophageal varices are often seen directly or their presence inferred from the amount of contrast media seen in the coronary vein. In some centers splenoportography is considered routine in the investigation of patients with portal hypertension. In our clinic, we have had several examples of severe splenic bleeding requiring laparotomy. Though our experience is certainly not representative of what is reported in the literature, it has caused us to be rather selective in the application of splenoportography and to reserve it for patients who are likely to go to surgery.

Umbilical portography has not yet had widespread enough application to evaluate its clinical usefulness. It requires technical skill and may fail to opacify all of the portal vein and the collateral circulation. It is not likely to be as useful as splenoportography except in special circumstances such as the patient with previous splenectomy.

Hepatic vein catheterization is of limited usefulness. A major advantage, however, is the lack of any morbidity or significant discomfort to the patient. A definite elevation of wedged hepatic vein pressure is proof of portal hypertension though a normal wedge pressure does not eliminate the possibility of pre-sinusoidal or extrahepatic portal hypertension. The finding of portal hypertension, however, does not necessarily imply the presence of esophageal varices and one can not use the height of the wedge pressure to predict the likelihood of bleeding from esophageal varices. For us, the major clinical application of hepatic vein catheterization has been to follow the level of portal hypertension over a period of time. The procedure also has many research applications.

HEMORRHAGE FROM ESOPHAGEAL VARICES

CAUSE

Of the several theories for the cause of variceal hemorrhage, none is universally accepted and I think it is fair to say that we simply do not know why bleeding occurs. Liebowitz[67] and Orloff and Thomas[89] convincingly argued against a leading theory, that of acid peptic erosion of the varix wall. Two patients were recently reported with the combination of pernicious anemia, achlorhydria, cirrhosis and bleeding varices.[139]

It has always been our impression that larger varices are more likely to bleed, but we have no definite studies that prove this. Prolonged follow-up of patients after esophagoscopic demonstration of varices by Baker and colleagues[5] showed some correlation between size and bleeding tendency but not a marked one. Once varices are present, we have not been able to find any correlation between the level of wedge pressure and the likelihood of bleeding,[117] though the height of wedge pressure correlates well with the presence or absence of varices.

DIAGNOSIS

Bleeding esophageal varices have to be suspected in all patients with upper gastrointestinal hemorrhage. If alcoholic liver disease is confirmed, the differential diagnosis is narrowed to 4 major considerations: esophageal varices, alcoholic gastritis, peptic ulcer or the Mallory-Weiss syndrome. The first 2 are about equal in frequency in most series; peptic ulcer is somewhat less frequent and the Mallory-Weiss syndrome accounts for only 2 to 5 per cent of cases. In a patient with known, chronic, nonalcoholic liver disease, varices are about 4 times as likely a source for bleeding as peptic ulcer.

The type of bleeding is not very helpful in differential diagnosis except in the Mallory-Weiss syndrome when it sometimes follows repeated vomiting. Though there is usually hematemesis with varix bleeding, some patients have only melena. Bleeding from varices is not always voluminous and may be protracted, being evident only by strongly positive occult blood reactions in the feces.

The usual historical and physical evidences of chronic liver disease are searched for. Most important are jaundice, firmness of the liver edge, palpability of the spleen, ascites, auscultation of a C-B murmur, spider angiomata, hepatic fetor and asterixis. In the alcoholic, epigastric tenderness is more often due to hepatic necrosis than to peptic ulcer. Rarely in chronic liver disease, none of these findings is present, though more often than not this results from hurried or inadequate examination. In extrahepatic portal hypertension, enlargement of the spleen is usually the only abnormal physical finding and this can be missed as a consequence of splenic contraction from the hemorrhage.

In the laboratory, liver disease is detected and its severity assessed by hepatic tests. The most useful tests are serum proteins, bilirubin and prothrombin. It is important to draw blood for these before multiple transfusions are given. Values may be normal in extrahepatic portal hypertension and in occasional patients with well compensated cirrhosis. When the diagnosis of liver disease is in doubt and jaundice is not present, the

BSP test is useful. In patients without liver disease who are critically ill and hypovolemic, BSP retention may be moderately abnormal (up to 25 per cent retention at 30 minutes in our experience), but in patients with cirrhosis, retention is usually much greater than this during acute bleeding. Unquestionably, borderline values are not decisive. The blood ammonium level is useful in detecting liver disease. High values are informative and strongly suggest liver disease but normal values are of less help in diagnosis since they have been recorded in patients with definite cirrhosis and bleeding.[12] Emergency gastrointestinal x-ray is useful, though varices of significant size can be missed. Demonstration of a peptic ulcer is one of the most useful features of the emergency barium meal, though if cirrhosis is present, the ulcer is not necessarily the source of the bleeding.

Emergency esophagoscopy and gastroscopy can be extremely useful in experienced hands. These procedures are often difficult to arrange on an emergency basis, however, and for the inexperienced operator interpretation is considerably more difficult than when it is done electively. Not only may varices be difficult to identify, but it may be impossible to tell whether blood in the esophagus is coming from the stomach or from a varix. Nevertheless, in clinics where much endoscopy is performed, a great deal of confidence is placed in the results of emergency esophagoscopy and gastroscopy.[31, 35, 93] Mallory-Weiss lesions can be detected in this fashion, and sometimes emergency surgery is required for optimum therapy.

In the vast majority of patients, after careful and adequate examination, one can detect or rule out varices. However, short of a convincing esophagoscopic demonstration, there is no way to be certain that the varices are the source of the bleeding. Patients with alcoholic liver disease may be bleeding from gastritis or peptic ulcer. Differential diagnosis of the site of bleeding is particularly difficult if both peptic ulcer and esophageal varices are demonstrated. Response to balloon tamponade therapy is of some differential diagnostic value since prompt cessation of active bleeding strongly suggests varices. However, one is not always certain that bleeding is active when the tamponade tube is passed. Old blood in the stomach must be removed by lavage and continued fresh bleeding demonstrated before any confidence can be placed in the results of inflation of the balloon.

On occasion, one or more of the supplementary tests useful in the assessment of portal hypertension are required in a patient with hematemesis before an accurate diagnosis can be made. All of them indicate the presence and degree of portal hypertension but none allows a definite conclusion as to whether or not varices are bleeding.

PROGNOSIS

In alcoholic liver disease, mortality following hemorrhage from esophageal varices is very high. An average mortality of 73 per cent was calculated by Orloff and colleagues from a total of 8 reports in the literature that included slightly over 1,000 patients.[88] Much less data is available in the literature concerning nonalcoholic cirrhosis. Sherlock reports a 33 per cent mortality within 1 year of hemorrhage from varices in 120 patients, 75 per cent of whom were nonalcoholic.[136] In extrahepatic portal block, mortality from variceal hemorrhage is low.

Death following variceal hemorrhage is seldom directly due to exsanguination or shock. Hepatic failure is the usual cause of death, and is frequently complicated by aspiration pneumonia, sepsis or renal failure. Many patients bleed terminally as a manifestation of hepatic failure whereas in others bleeding seems to precipitate lethal hepatic coma even when bleeding has been controlled successfully.

There is a serious need for information regarding the natural history of esophageal varices after recovery from an episode of bleeding. It has been the custom in recent years to do interval portacaval shunt surgery in this type of patient so there has been little opportunity to develop actuarial data on patients treated conservatively. Such information should be forthcoming eventually from controlled trials of portacaval shunting that are now in progress in at least 2 areas.

Also follow-up information on patients with esophageal varices that have not bled will be available soon from 2 controlled trials of prophylactic portacaval shunt that are under way. Spontaneous reduction in portal hypertension and improvement in esophageal varices may occur in acute alcoholic liver disease,[65, 113] but this seems unlikely in any significant number of patients who have hemorrhaged from esophageal varices.

Medical Management

After initial evaluation of the patient with suspected bleeding varices, it is our custom to pass a soft rubber or plastic tube into the stomach through the nose for gastric aspiration and ice water lavage. (Nothing about our experience or that of others we have talked to suggests that this procedure ever precipitates hemorrhage by traumatizing varices.) After cleaning out the stomach, we leave the tube in place to monitor gastric content and to give medications in patients unable to swallow. It is removed if barium meal or esophagoscopy is performed.

After initial blood tests which include hemoglobin, hematocrit, bilirubin, serum proteins, prothrombin and sometimes BSP retention, we pass a long plastic tube from a peripheral vein into the central venous reservoir to monitor venous pressure and administer blood and fluids. Blood transfusions are given if there are clinical signs of hypovolemia or if the visible blood loss is large. Because hypervolemia is characteristic of chronic liver disease and there is a great possibility that excessive intravenous infusion may initiate variceal hemorrhage, we prefer not to give blood if the hemorrhage appears to be minor and if there are no clinical signs of hypovolemia. Also, one must take into account that serum hepatitis is a distressingly frequent complication after recovery from variceal hemorrhage in hospitals that use blood from commercial sources. Because of its hemostatic properties, fresh blood is preferable. When many units of blood are required, an occasional unit of fresh blood is even more desirable because the cirrhotic liver cannot rapidly manufacture the coagulation factors missing from stored blood.

It is important to remove as much of the shed blood from the GI tract as possible because of its contribution to hepatic encephalopathy. We clean the stomach out as well as possible and give an enema if the stool contains blood. A dose of magnesium sulfate is given through the stomach tube at the end of the lavage and is repeated in 8 hours.

Neomycin is given to reduce bacterial activity in the intestines. It can be given in tablet form orally, through the stomach tube after grinding up the tablets, or in solution as an enema. Most Eastern centers use doses of 8 to 12 Gm. daily; we use 2 to 4 Gm. daily. We know of no data showing which dose is best.

If active bleeding is evident after the first gastric lavage, one should consider a trial of vasopressin therapy. Vasopressin causes a decrease in splanchnic blood flow and a reduction in portal vein pressure that can be documented by hepatic vein catheterization.[114, 129, 132] A dose of 20 to 40 international units in 100 to 200 ml. of 5 per cent glucose in water is administered by intravenous drip over a 20 to 40 minute period. This causes blanching of the skin and intestinal cramps. Reputedly it can cause angina, though we have never seen this complication. Our impression and that of those who have published on its results is that it may stop variceal bleeding, though often only temporarily.[57, 77, 129, 133] The infusion can be repeated once or twice if bleeding recurs. There is concern that prolonged use of vasopressin might adversely reduce hepatic oxygen supply since it reduces hepatic blood flow; however, in catheterization studies, splanchnic oxygen consumption seems to remain constant in spite of reduced hepatic blood flow.[114] Results of repeated infusions might be different, however. Octapressin has some theoretical advantages over vasopressin because of lack of antidiuretic effect and appears to have the same action on the splanchnic bed.[148]

Balloon tamponade is used in most centers after vasopressin has failed or in place of or in conjunction with it. Two standard tubes available are the Sengstaken-Blakemore and the Linton tubes. We prefer the latter since it is somewhat simpler to handle and there is no danger of tracheal occlusion from the esophageal balloon should the tube slip partially out of the esophagus. Both seem to stop variceal bleeding effectively.

The gastric balloon of the Linton tube directly compresses varices in the lower esophagus, and blood flow into the upper vessels is probably markedly reduced by the pressure on the cardiac end of the stomach. When we use a Linton tube, we remove the monitoring tube and pass the deflated balloon tube through the lubricated nostril into the stomach. Some physicians prefer to pass it through the mouth, having applied topical anesthesia to lessen the gag reflex. The gastric balloon is inflated before passage to test for leaks. It is inflated again after the tube is well into the stomach, following which the tube is withdrawn until the balloon presses tightly against the cardia.

Pressure is maintained by attaching the tube to a face mask of some sort (Fig. 9–8) or to a 1 to 2 pound weight by means of a pulley system slung from the top of the bed (Fig. 9–9). If traction on the tube causes great distress in the patient it is best to start with a 1 pound weight and add more later. If bleeding is controlled, we maintain pressure for 18 to 24 hours and then discontinue traction and remove the air from the gastric balloon, leaving the tube in place. If bleeding recurs, the balloon is reinflated and tension is again applied. If tamponade fails to stop the bleeding, it may be helpful to add 100 ml. of air to the gastric balloon and increase the tension on the tube. If bleeding continues after this, we consider the possibility that the bleeding is from gastric varices outside the area covered by the balloon or from some other lesion such as peptic ulcer, gastritis or the Mallory-Weiss syndrome. We have seen instances, however, in which balloon tamponade was ineffective and yet no lesion other than esophageal varices was found at autopsy.

Both types of tamponade tubes can cause a wide range of complications including pneumonitis, aspiration, esophageal ulceration or rupture, and asphyxia.[28] Complications are more frequent with inexperience, inadequate nursing care and prolonged use of the tube. As with all indwelling gastric tubes, frequent irrigation is required to keep the gastric lumen free of clots.

In summarizing the results reported in the literature in the use of balloon tamponade in 311 patients, Orloff and colleagues point out that, though bleeding was controlled in a high percentage of patients, the overall mortality was 74 per cent.[88] It seems clear that hemorrhage from varices often sets in

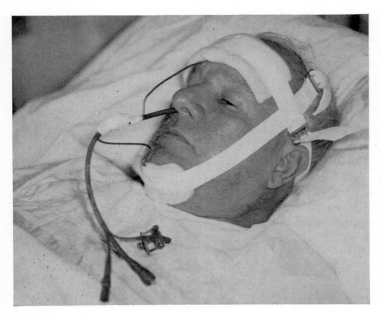

FIG. 9–8. Face mask for maintaining tension on esophageal tamponade tube. The tube is taped to the mask after it has been withdrawn far enough to achieve the desired tension on the gastric cardia.

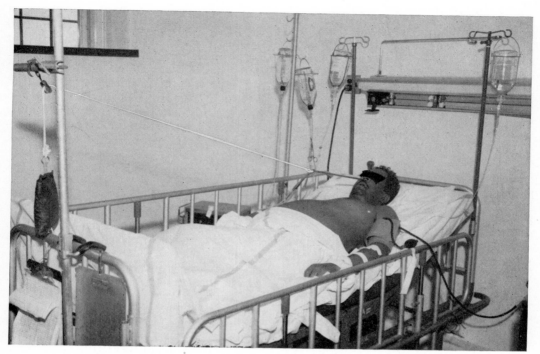

Fig. 9–9. Maintenance of traction on an esophageal tamponade tube with a 2-pound weight slung over a pulley attached to the bed.

motion a chain of events that culminates in fatal hepatic failure whether or not the bleeding is controlled.

Gastric hypothermia, with the same device that has been used for the treatment of bleeding peptic ulcer, has been tried in patients with hemorrhage from esophageal varices. Initial experience at our institution has been disappointing in that, though bleeding seemed to be reasonably well controlled, a high proportion of patients die from hepatic failure. Results are similar in the limited published experience.[157, 158]

General supportive care for patients with bleeding varices is limited. A moderate amount of parenteral glucose is presumably helpful, avoiding too great a surplus of water because of the potential development of hyponatremia from the reduced free water clearance characteristic of the ascitic cirrhotic. Potassium may be deficient in the alcoholic patient but, since renal failure is a common complication of variceal bleeding, replacement has to be monitored carefully. Moderate doses of water-soluble vitamins and folic acid can be added to the paren-

teral glucose given to the alcoholic patient and a single injection of vitamin K is probably wise for all cirrhotic subjects. The use of sedatives poses a problem because of the frequent development of hepatic coma in bleeding patients. Discomfort from the tamponade tube, irritable and irrational behavior at the onset of encephalopathy and incipient delirium tremens are all frequent events that require consideration of sedation in patients with bleeding varices. Phenobarbital, chloral hydrate, chlordiazepoxide and small doses of phenothiazines are among the safest drugs to use in these circumstances.

SURGICAL MANAGEMENT

Two surgical approaches have had considerable trial for the emergency treatment of bleeding varices: transesophageal varix ligation and emergency portacaval shunt.

Varix ligation can be performed abdominally[163] but ordinarily a chest incision is used. Relief of bleeding is immediate but temporary. The philosophy of its proponents is that it carries the patient through the acute episode of bleeding and provides an opportunity for elective portacaval shunt later. The major disadvantage is the addition of surgery and anesthesia for a patient in whom early hepatic failure from the bleeding episode may be developing already. Varix ligation has been used extensively by Linton and colleagues in patients in whom bleeding does not respond to therapy in the first 12 to 24 hours of hospitalization.[68] Orloff reported a comparison of nonoperative treatment and transesophageal ligation in a small series of patients with alcoholic liver disease and bleeding varices. Operative mortality was 46 per cent, whereas 86 per cent of the nonsurgical patients died.[88]

With admittedly limited experience with varix ligation, we have held the opinion that if any emergency surgery is performed it should be a portacaval shunt. Operative and anesthetic time is not significantly greater in experienced hands. Portacaval shunt provides satisfactory control of bleeding and a subsequent operation is avoided. We have reserved varix ligation for the occasion when a surgeon without portacaval shunt experience discovers unexpected variceal bleeding during laparotomy for presumed bleeding ulcer.

Our enthusiasm for emergency portacaval shunt has waxed and waned through the past 5 years. Enthusiasm is high when a patient with repeated bleeding episodes, who seems to be slipping into irreversible hepatic coma, survives after an emergency shunt. Enthusiasm ebbs when 2 or 3 consecutive patients expire postoperatively in hepatic coma. If emergency shunt is performed on "all comers" the surgical mortality will be discouragingly high. Orloff recently reported a mortality of 46 per cent in such a series.[88] He points out, however, that this is an improvement over the mortality of 84 per cent in a previously reported group from the same hospital treated medically. Mortality in series of selected patients is also high: Wantz and Payne, 41 per cent[159]; Rousselot, Gilbertson and Panke, 36 per cent[120]; Mikkelsen, 35 per cent[78]; and Preston and Trippel, 36 per cent.[105] We were impressed that Mikkelsen's patients could be divided retrospectively, on the basis of ascites, encephalopathy, serum albumin and serum bilirubin, into those considered as good risks

(18 patients, no postoperative deaths) and those who were poor risks (19 patients, 13 operative deaths). Good risk patients had no more than one of the following: ascites, encephalopathy, serum albumin less than 3 Gm./100 ml., serum bilirubin greater than 4 mg./100 ml. In general, they had had fewer transfusions and a shorter time elapsed between the onset of bleeding and the performance of surgery than the poor risk patients.

Our philosophy is as follows: with variceal bleeding a certain proportion of patients with chronic liver disease die from hepatic failure whether or not bleeding is controlled or whether or not surgery is performed. Many of these patients are relatively easy to recognize since they have jaundice, ascites, encephalopathy and poor hepatic tests. To us, emergency surgery seems useless. At the other extreme are patients with relatively good hepatic function who have an excellent chance of survival if bleeding is controlled and does not recur repeatedly. We prefer to treat such patients medically, using vasopressin and balloon tamponade. If bleeding stops promptly, we continue conservative treatment in the hope that they can undergo prolonged convalescence and we can consider elective portacaval shunt under optimum conditions. If bleeding does not stop within the first 24 hours or if it recurs, and the patient's status remains favorable, we attempt emergency portacaval shunt as promptly as possible. A certain number of patients do not fit easily into either of the above groups, and a decision for or against emergency portacaval shunt is difficult. An alternative approach is to perform emergency surgery in all such patients as soon as the bleeding varices are diagnosed.

Thoracic duct drainage has been used for the treatment of bleeding varices on the basis of the report by Dumont and Mulholland that variceal bleeding stopped in 2 patients during this procedure and that intrasplenic pressure fell in a third.[38] Denney et al. reported that bleeding from varices ceased during prolonged thoracic duct drainage in 6 patients.[37] Though no anatomical obstruction has been demonstrated in the thoracic duct of cirrhotic patients, the distention and increase in pressure suggest physiological obstruction in the sense that

Fig. 9–10. Wedged hepatic vein pressure before and after 30 minutes of thoracic duct drainage in 7 patients with alcoholic liver disease and portal hypertension.

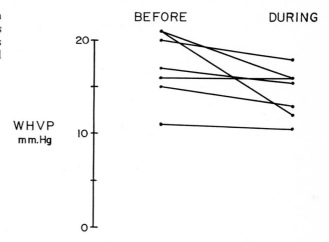

more lymph is produced than can drain easily into the subclavian vein. Venting the duct through a cannula decreases distention and presumably increases flow, probably by a siphon effect. It is conceivable that venting the duct lowers intrahepatic vascular resistance, and thus portal pressure, by decreasing lymphatic congestion in the liver. Our results have been disappointing, however. Thirty minutes of thoracic duct drainage failed to lower wedged hepatic vein pressure substantially (Fig. 9–10). Hepatic blood flow did not change in 4 patients.[166] Prolonged drainage of lymph without replacement can be dangerous because hypovolemia and shock could develop. We therefore advise against this form of therapy for bleeding varices, at least until more experimental work is available.

Patients with ascites often tolerate prolonged lymph drainage, much as they can tolerate paracentesis. None of our ascitic patients has had any natriuresis during lymphatic drainage, however, even when all of the lymph was replaced intravenously. We are not convinced, therefore, that it offers any advantage over paracentesis in the treatment of ascites.

ELECTIVE SURGERY FOR PORTAL HYPERTENSION

PORTAL-SYSTEMIC SHUNT

History

A number of European surgeons performed portacaval shunts in isolated patients in the early decades of the 20th century. In the United States the operation was first accomplished by Blakemore and Whipple in 1945.[11] During the subsequent 10 years a number of surgeons including Rousselot, Linton, Child, Welch, Pattison, Hallenbeck, Hunt, Walker and Eckman contributed to experience with portacaval shunting. Many surgeons are now skilled in the operation and it is performed in most medical centers. Technical improvements have led to a change from the thoraco-abdominal to an abdominal incision, to a shorter operative time and to a decrease in transfusion requirements. Under favorable circumstances, the operation is accomplished in one and a half hours.

General Effects

Morbidity and mortality from the operation is substantial, in part related to the technical competence of the operator and the anesthesia time required, but to a large degree due to the poor condition of the patient with chronic liver disease. Reported mortality figures vary from 7 to 20 per cent; in a review of 20 reports involving 1,244 patients, Grace, Muench and Chalmers calculated an average figure of 15.5 per cent.[48]

The incidence of variceal bleeding is markedly reduced after successful portalsystemic shunt. The most complete protection is provided by shunts that give the greatest portal bed decompression and that show the least tendency to thrombose. Shunt thrombosis is rare except when vein grafts

A. PORTAL HYPERTENSION
    BEFORE SURGERY

B. AFTER E-S PORTA-
    CAVAL SHUNT

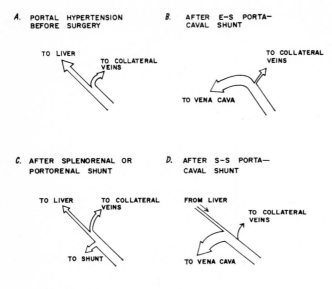

TO LIVER

TO COLLATERAL
VEINS

TO COLLATERAL
VEINS

TO VENA CAVA

FIG. 9–11. Diagrammatic representation of the portal circulatory changes accompanying portal hypertension and portal-systemic shunting.

C. AFTER SPLENORENAL OR
    PORTORENAL SHUNT

D. AFTER S-S PORTA-
    CAVAL SHUNT

TO LIVER   TO COLLATERAL
                VEINS

TO SHUNT

FROM LIVER

TO COLLATERAL
VEINS

TO VENA CAVA

E   PORTAL HYPERTENSION WITH UNUSUALLY HIGH HEPATIC
    VASCULAR RESISTANCE

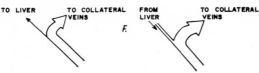

TO LIVER   TO COLLATERAL
                VEINS
                            F.

FROM
LIVER

TO COLLATERAL
VEINS

are used, when the connecting veins are angulated or when the shunt lumen is narrow, as it often is with the splenorenal connection. Esophageal varices do not disappear immediately after shunt; they tend to diminish gradually over a 3 to 12 month period and often remain indefinitely, even if hemorrhage does not recur.

Hepatic blood flow falls after portal-systemic shunt since portal blood is either entirely removed from the liver or less perfuses the organ because of a decreased pressure head. The amount of reduction in hepatic blood flow depends to a large extent on how much portal blood flow had already been reduced as a result of the liver disease. With end-to-side portacaval shunt all portal blood is removed from the liver, and in the remaining procedures portal flow is reduced in proportion to the degree to which the shunt lowers portal pressure (Fig. 9–11). If the shunt is large enough to offer very low resistance and if the portal vein is left open, hepatic arterial blood may flow

in a reverse direction in the portal vein, further lowering hepatic venous blood flow.

Theoretically hepatic arterial inflow could increase to compensate for reduction in portal flow following a shunt. To what extent this occurs is unknown, but in the patients we have studied by hepatic vein catheterization it has been insufficient to prevent a drop in hepatic venous flow. Prior to surgery, in patients with a high degree of hepatic venous outflow block, portal vein flow into the liver may be low or conceivably even reversed if some hepatic arterial blood leaves the liver by this route (Fig. 9–11). In such a patient an end-to-side portacaval shunt theoretically would not affect or would actually elevate hepatic venous flow. With other shunting procedures hepatic venous flow should still decrease because of increased ease of portal backflow. Occasionally this is the situation in cirrhosis since cross-clamping of the portal vein at surgery sometimes fails to raise the pressure on the intestinal side of the clamp.

Warren and Muller's data suggests that this is a reasonably frequent finding[161]; in our own patients, pressure dynamics of this type were seen in only 7 of 61.[81] Recent flow-meter studies of the portal vein by Moreno and co-workers[83] disclosed stagnant but forward flow in 7 of 85 patients with cirrhosis. They found no instances of retrograde flow.

Shaldon and co-workers proposed that the reduction in hepatic blood flow after porta-caval anastomosis was due to the closing of functionless intrahepatic shunts between the smaller branches of the portal vein and hepatic vein.[131] Their conclusions were derived from a single, thoroughly studied patient and should be tested in additional patients because of their potential importance. Oxygen consumption did not decrease in 10 patients that we studied before and after end-to-side portacaval shunt, even though hepatic blood flow fell 46 per cent.[110] Hepatic venous oxygen content fell, indicating an increased degree of extraction of oxygen from a smaller volume of blood. After side-to-side shunt, in our studies, splanchnic oxygen consumption appeared to decrease.[116] However, because of an uncertain amount of oxygen extracted from hepatic arterial blood flowing backward in the portal vein in these patients, little reliance can be placed on these results. Though in normal man hepatic vein oxygen content can fall to extremely low levels while hepatic oxygen consumption is maintained,[121] it is of some concern when oxygen delivery is decreased to the diseased liver with a distorted circulatory system.

Hepatic function, as assessed by standard tests, is regularly impaired immediately after portal-systemic shunt. This is presumed to be due to the trauma of surgery and anesthesia since there is usually a gradual improvement to preoperative levels thereafter.[42] BSP retention remains unusually high after shunt, however, in our experience. Whether this is entirely due to the decrease in hepatic blood flow or whether it indicates decreased hepatic functional reserve not easily assessed by the other biochemical tests is unknown. Of concern in present studies of prophylactic shunt is the apparent greater incidence of subsequent death from hepatic failure in the shunted patients.

Temporary ascites may appear postoperatively after any type of shunt. Whether it results simply from decreased hepatic function and lowered serum albumin or from cutting open the hilar lymphatics during the dissection is unknown. After the initial postoperative period the tendency to ascites formation is decreased by portal-systemic shunting, presumably as a consequence of decreased portal flow and decreased intrahepatic congestion. However, after end-to-side portacaval shunt, a moderate number of patients (approximately 5 per cent in our experience) fail to lose the tendency to ascites formation. A few even develop refractory ascites for the first time. Wedged hepatic vein pressure has been higher postoperatively in this group of patients than in those who do not develop ascites. This suggests that preoperative portal inflow was lower in such patients and that removal of portal blood by the shunt surgery has caused a smaller reduction in total hepatic blood flow, leaving the liver somewhat congested. Ascites usually responds favorably to side-to-side or double-barreled shunts, where hepatic blood flow is decreased most and where postoperative hepatic congestion, as assessed by wedge pressure, is least.

One of the most serious consequences of portal-systemic shunting is encephalopathy. In some patients these encephalopathic manifestations are mild and infrequent and present no major problem. Occasional patients have only one or 2 widely spaced episodes of severe hepatic coma with otherwise normal behavior. In many of the patients, however, the episodes are severe, recurrent and crippling. A few patients develop chronic neurologic syndromes with various combinations of myelopathy, chorea-athetosis, dysarthria and dementia.[155] The frequency of encephalopathy reported after shunt varies from 3 to 30 per cent. Grace and co-workers calculated an average figure of 19 per cent from a review of 13 reports comprising 733 patients.[48] Encephalopathy is more often severe in older patients.[135] We assume that it is more frequent with the largest shunts.

The frequency of peptic ulcer is thought to increase after portal-systemic shunt

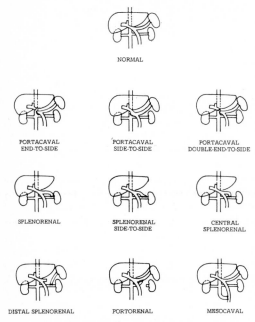

FIG. 9–12. Diagrammatic representation of 9 different types of portal-systemic shunts.

though there is a wide range in reported incidence from 3 to 15 per cent. Marked increase in gastric acid secretion can be consistently demonstrated in dogs after shunt and it has been postulated that an intestinally produced secretagogue, normally inactivated in the liver, is involved.[24] Studies of acid output in humans, however, show varying results. Ostrow, Timmerman and Gray found a considerable increase after shunt but only to levels within the general normal range; acid output in nonshunted cirrhotic patients was low.[91]

In a few patients marked iron storage has appeared after portacaval shunt.[125, 146, 150] This is a rare finding in our experience. It is unknown whether gastrointestinal iron absorption is increased by a shunt or whether this simply is an extreme example of the well-known tendency to iron storage exhibited by the cirrhotic, the shunt being a coincidence.

Types of Shunts (Fig. 9–12)

Portacaval, End-to-Side. This is the most commonly employed shunt and is technically the simplest. Thrombosis is rare if it is properly performed. It provides excellent

decompression of the portal system with a very low incidence of subsequent bleeding from varices. All portal blood flow is removed from the liver, which in a series of 10 patients studied by us, resulted in a 46 per cent decrease in hepatic blood flow. Splanchnic oxygen consumption did not fall in spite of this drop in blood flow.[110] There is usually some decrease in splenomegaly but leukopenia and platelet deficiency characteristic of "hypersplenism" do not always return to normal. This type of shunt does not completely protect against development of ascites.

Portacaval, Side-to-Side. Longmire and associates were the first to demonstrate the feasibility of side-to-side shunt in a sizeable group of patients.[70] Most surgeons consider this to be more difficult than the end-to-side shunt, particularly in patients in whom the 2 veins are separated anatomically by a large caudate lobe. In theory, the side-to-side shunt leaves a pathway for some portal blood to continue to flow into the liver and an opportunity for this flow to increase in case the hepatic vascular resistance decreases. In fact, however, little or no portal blood seems to flow into the liver. Several studies indicate that in 65 to 80 per cent of patients there is a reversed flow of blood from the liver toward the shunt orifice in the hepatic limb of the portal vein.[18, 83, 111] In the remainder, flow is static or toward the liver in small volume. Hepatic venous flow falls more after side-to-side shunt,[116] presumably because some hepatic arterial blood is diverted into the vena cava via the portal vein. Warren and co-workers suggest that backflowing hepatic arterial blood actually increases the total vascular irrigation of the liver and should be beneficial.[161] This depends, of course, on whether the hepatic arterial blood in question actually makes suitable contact with hepatocytes or whether it passes through functionless anastomoses. In our experience, in sampling the retrograde flowing blood via a catheter passed through the shunt orifice, extraction of oxygen and Bromsulphalein was always considerably less than their extraction in hepatic venous blood.[111] The volume of backflowing blood has been difficult to measure; the most accurate assessments appear to be those recently made by Moreno and colleagues with the electromagnetic flowmeter[83] where, in 13 patients, values ranged from 0.8 to 12.5 ml./kg. per minute. A large volume of hepatic arterial blood flowing to the portal vein admittedly might contribute as much to hepatic function as a smaller volume passing to the hepatic vein.

Side-to-side shunt results in lower wedge pressures, lower sinusoidal pressures and greater hepatic decompression, consonant with the greater fall in hepatic blood flow. This provides greater protection against ascites which is rare after successful side-to-side shunt.

We believe that side-to-side shunt disturbs hepatic physiology somewhat more than end-to-side shunt because of the greater fall in hepatic venous blood flow. In a follow-up of 2 groups of comparable patients given side-to-side and end-to-side shunt we have noted a greater incidence of encephalopathy after the side-to-side operation. The groups did not differ significantly in other respects. Encephalopathy was severe in 28 per cent of the side-to-side shunt patients compared to 8 per cent of the end-to-side patients.[115] Zuidema and Kirsh report almost identical findings.[169]

Portacaval, Double End-to-Side. McDermott introduced the "double-barreled" shunt for the treatment of ascites in 1958.[73] It should allow maximum decompression of the liver and should reduce hepatic venous blood flow even more than a side-to-side shunt. This is either an advantage or a disadvantage, depending on one's point of view. It is technically difficult but may be easier than side-to-side shunt in the patient whose portal vein does not lie close to the vena cava.

Splenorenal. Linton and colleagues and Hallenbeck have been the major proponents of the splenorenal shunt. It eliminates hypersplenism by removal of the spleen. Since the anastomosis is small, there is less fall in portal pressure and, presumably, some portal inflow into the liver continues. Hepatic blood flow probably falls less than after portacaval shunt. Bradley and co-workers found an average drop of 22 per cent in 5 patients.[15] Both Hallenbeck[51] and Linton[69] found a lesser incidence of encephalopathy after splenorenal than after portacaval shunt.

The major disadvantage of splenorenal shunt is the rather high tendency to throm-

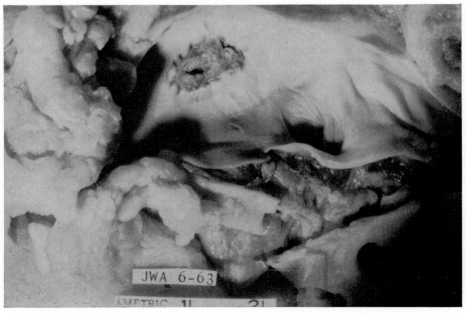

Fig. 9–13. Laminated thrombus in the orifice of a splenorenal shunt, viewed from the lumen of the renal vein. The size of the splenic vein at its anastomosis to the renal vein is 0.9×0.5 cm.

bosis (Fig. 9–13) which leads to a substantial incidence of recurrent variceal bleeding in all reported series. It is possible that the reported lower incidence of encephalopathy is due to the frequent thrombosis of this shunt. A splenorenal shunt is technically more difficult because of the smaller vein size, thinner walls and difficulty in making the connection without angulation of the splenic vein.

Splenorenal, Other Varieties. Mason advocates anastomosing the 2 veins side-to-side in order to obtain greater portal decompression and to obviate thrombosis of the anastomosis.[72] Clatworthy and Boles have used the central portion of the splenic vein, as close as possible to its junction with the superior mesenteric, for a "central splenorenal" shunt.[25] The splenic vein is larger and easier to work with at this site, particularly if the inferior mesenteric vein joins the superior mesenteric, as it often does.

Warren recently described a distal splenorenal shunt which he combines with division of the left gastric and splenic arteries and the coronary vein.[162] This operation is designed to decompress the area containing gastroesophageal varices without excessively reducing portal flow.

More experience is needed with all of these newer types of splenorenal shunt.

Portorenal. This type of shunt was recently described by Erlik, Barzilai and Shramek.[43] It may be technically easier than end-to-side or side-to-side portacaval shunt when the portal vein and vena cava are further apart than usual or when the caudate lobe is enlarged. The lumen is usually larger than that of a splenorenal shunt. There are enough collateral vessels to maintain the function of the left kidney. This is a theoretically promising type of shunt with which additional experience will undoubtedly be available soon.

Mesocaval. Marion[71] and Clatworthy[26] independently originated this shunt in 1953, for patients with extrahepatic block in whom both portal and splenic veins are unavailable. The end of the transected vena cava is swung anteriorly and cephalad below the pancreas to anastomose with the side of the superior mesenteric vein or with any identifiable large portal collateral in that area.

Voorhees and Blakemore[156] have described a reasonably extensive and satisfactory experience with this type of anastomosis in 34 patients. A low lying duodenal loop may make the shunt technically impossible unless the vena cava is brought through an aperture between the head of the pancreas and the third portion of the duodenum.[22]

Umbilical-Saphenous. Piccone and LeVeen[101] found that, in many patients, large volume flows (140 to 450 ml./min.) could be obtained through a catheter inserted into the dilated umbilical vein as far as the portal vein. In one patient, they were able to anastomose the umbilical channel to the saphenous vein tunneled under the skin of the abdomen and this connection stayed open for the 10 months that the patient lived. It seems doubtful that a shunt of this sort offers low enough resistance to effectively decompress the portal bed.

Selection of Patients for Portal-Systemic Shunt

In chronic liver disease, portal-systemic shunt should be elective only when liver function is stable or improving; otherwise mortality is unacceptably high. Under the most optimum circumstances, it ranges from 8 to 15 per cent. In alcoholic liver disease, a shunt should never be done electively during the early phases of decompensation when liver function may be worsening spontaneously. After a hemorrhage from varices, several weeks of convalescence are desirable except in the unusual patient who has good hepatic function that has not been adversely affected by the hemorrhage. Clearly there is a risk of a second hemorrhage during the delay; in our experience this has been less than the risk from early surgery. In alcoholic liver disease, the gradual tendency to improvement that is characteristically seen when drinking is stopped argues for the most prolonged delay possible. This is not necessarily true, of course, in nonalcoholic cirrhosis.

Results are best in patients who do not have ascites, jaundice or encephalopathy and in whom serum bilirubin is less than 1.8 mg.%, serum albumin greater than 3 gm.%, prothrombin time above 50 per cent, and BSP retention less than 30 per cent at

30 minutes. Test abnormalities greater than these do not contraindicate surgery, of course. Patients with a small liver do not fare as well after portal-systemic shunt but it could be argued that they need the greater protection against bleeding afforded by the operation. Whether or not preoperative hepatic blood flow measurements could be used to predict shunt mortality or results has not been investigated adequately.

Age appears to be a factor in predicting postoperative encephalopathy. The incidence is clearly increased in patients over 60 and may be somewhat increased in those between 50 and 60. No preoperative test consistently predicts postoperative encephalopathy. For several years we gave 6 Gm. of ammonium chloride daily for 3 days to all shunt candidates, looking for clinical encephalopathy. Several patients with negative tests did develop postoperative episodic stupor so we have concluded that this test is useless.

The most important factor in the ultimate outcome of alcoholic liver disease is whether or not the patient resumes drinking. We have been unable to predict which patients will return to drinking, so this is not a factor in our choice of shunt candidates. About half of our patients abstain for 2 years after surgery; we do not have precise figures for the "5 year cure" rate but it is disappointingly low.

In extrahepatic portal hypertension, mortality from variceal hemorrhage is low and portal-systemic shunt need not be done as an emergency. There is a high incidence of failure of shunts performed on infants, either because of thrombosis or because the vessel used for shunt is not large enough to decompress the portal bed. To have the largest possible blood vessels to work with, shunt surgery is postponed preferably until after the age of 10 years. The type of shunt used is dictated largely by the vessels available; preoperative or intraoperative portography is essential. Splenorenal or mesocaval shunts are most often used. When no vein is suitable for a shunt, it is difficult to decide whether such procedures as distal esophageal resection or transplantation of the spleen into the chest is indicated.

Prophylactic Portal-Systemic Shunt

Early enthusiasm for portal-systemic shunt surgery together with the known high mortality of the initial hemorrhage from varices led to the idea that a shunt operation should be performed as soon as varices are demonstrated. On the other hand, information from the study of Baker, Smith and Lieberman[5] suggested that only about 10 per cent of patients with esophageal varices bleed and die from the first hemorrhage within 2 to 3 years. Fortunately, 2 controlled trials of prophylactic shunt were begun in 1958 and 1959, and have been continued. Results of the study by the Boston Inter-Hospital Liver Group, published in 1965,[20] showed a somewhat better survival in the control patients. The study of Conn and Lindenmuth has shown similar results thus far and is continuing.[33] In the 2 studies, the results of which are remarkably similar, operative mortality has been low and protection against variceal bleeding excellent in the surgical group. Nevertheless, mortality has been slightly higher in the surgical group, apparently due to a greater incidence of hepatic failure. Routine application of prophylactic shunt does not seem warranted from this data.

Is Portal-Systemic Shunt Ever Indicated in Chronic Liver Disease?

Though shunts have been performed for over 20 years and are standard therapy in most medical centers, there is a surprising lack of controlled studies proving their efficacy. Shunts control variceal bleeding well but there is no proof that they affect overall survival. It is perhaps natural that no controlled studies were undertaken in the early days of portacaval shunting, since surgery seemed to offer the only solution to the serious problem of variceal hemorrhage. Many follow-up studies of shunts show a 5-year survival of approximately 40 per cent,[48] compared to the 15 to 35 per cent usually quoted for 1-year survival after the onset of variceal bleeding in nonoperated patients.[47, 108] Some investigators have reservations about the value of shunt surgery, however.[27, 87, 138] The mortality of shunted patients must be compared with that of the patients who survive hemorrhage and are in suitable condition for elective shunt. When all such patients are operated upon, it is impossible to compile statistics.

There have been efforts to compare the clinical course of shunted and nonshunted patients who have bled from varices. Cohn and Blaisdell estimated that survivors of variceal hemorrhage at San Francisco County Hospital who were judged to be in good enough condition for shunt surgery had a 30 per cent chance of 5-year survival on medical therapy alone.[27] Palmer and Jahnke developed a "control" group of 48 patients who had refused recommended portacaval shunt.[95] A brief 1-year follow-up of this group and a group of 44 patients who received end-to-side shunts suggested that the mortality in the surgical group was somewhat lower than that of the control group. However, many of the patients in both operated and control groups had not bled from varices. Satterfield, Mulligan and Butcher made a retrospective comparison of the course of 87 patients who had undergone portacaval shunt with that of 46 patients who had survived a hemorrhage from varices but had not undergone surgery.[124] The per cent survival at 5 years was about the same, with the operative group having fewer deaths from bleeding but more deaths from hepatic failure. The many limitations of a retrospective study of this type were recognized by the authors.

Edmunds and West published a 5-year comparison of 2 groups of 21 patients each, one of which received surgical and one medical therapy for bleeding varices.[40] Eight survived in the surgical group and 2 in the medical group. Encephalopathy was not assessed. In this study each group is probably too small for a definite conclusion.

Jackson and co-workers have reported the preliminary results of a Veterans Administration Hospital cooperative study on portacaval shunts.[55] This study involves a complex protocol that includes both prophylactic and therapeutic portacaval shunts with transfer of many patients from medical to surgical groups following hemorrhage, and loss of a number of surgical candidates through refusal of surgery. At the end of 3 years, in 156 cases, no appreciable difference in survival was detectable between medical and surgical groups. The final results are not yet in the literature.

Many investigators believe that, though portal-systemic shunt has many undesirable effects, it is the best solution to a serious problem. One reason for the lack of controlled studies has been the general feeling that it would be unfair to the patients not offered surgery. However, data developing from controlled trials of prophylactic portacaval shunt seem to make a comparable controlled study of therapeutic shunt mandatory. Though shunted patients have a low operative mortality and excellent protection from variceal hemorrhage, overall mortality is somewhat higher than that of control patients, largely because of an increased incidence of hepatic failure. This leads to the conclusion that the shunt favors hepatic failure. At least 2 additional controlled trials of portacaval shunt in patients with prior variceal hemorrhage have been started recently (Boston Inter-Hospital Liver Group and ourselves) and the Veterans Administration Hospital cooperative study is continuing. Nonalcoholic liver disease probably has to be studied separately, irrespective of the outcome of these investigations. Many individuals do very well after portacaval shunt so even if the controlled trials show overall better survival without surgery, there remains the problem of whether the operation can benefit specific groups of patients who are identifiable in advance. Shunt surgery may have to be evaluated for many more years.

OTHER SURGERY FOR PORTAL HYPERTENSION

Omentopexy has been used in an effort to increase collateral vessels between the portal and the systemic venous circuit. *Hepatic arterial ligation* was used on the theory that arterial-venous connections in the hepatic arterial bed are important in the genesis of portal hypertension. *The upper stomach* has been *transected and resutured* in an effort to interrupt the collateral vessels in which flow is toward the esophagus. All of these operations have been abandoned because of lack of demonstrable effect.

Segmental esophagogastrectomy with or without enteric interposition is used occasionally in patients with repeated variceal bleeding in whom no veno-venous shunt is possible. This is an extensive operative procedure with considerable risk. Nutritional problems postoperatively are significant. Varices may recur by growth of veins through the interposed segment of bowel. However, in selected patients with extrahepatic portal block, the benefit may be sufficient to justify this approach.

Splenectomy alone can not cure portal hypertension unless it is due to a localized splenic vein block. To the extent that it reduces splanchnic inflow it may be helpful, though it may create a situation favoring thrombosis in the main portal trunk, making any type of subsequent portacaval anastomosis impossible.

Transplantation of the spleen into the left chest is an attempt to stimulate portal–superior vena caval collateral flow. This operation is usually reserved for patients with extrahepatic portal block who have no suitable veins available for a veno-venous shunt. Its effectiveness is unknown since it has been performed in a limited number of patients.

Several surgeons have attempted to *arterialize the portal vein stump* after end-to-side portacaval shunt. Such an operation theoretically eliminates the reduced hepatic blood flow that follows portacaval anastomoses. There are technical difficulties in anastomosing arteries to veins, however, and animal work suggests that high arterial pressure and inflow may be injurious to the venous channels. Attempts to perfect this surgical approach seem to be worthwhile, however.

Portacaval transposition has been successful in a child with glycogen storage disease.[118] This operation is well tolerated in normal dogs and in dogs with cirrhosis of the liver. Theoretically it completely relieves portal hypertension while hepatic blood flow is well maintained. Potential drawbacks are the effects of vena caval hypertension on the kidneys and the shunting of all portal blood around the liver.

FUTURE RESEARCH IN PORTAL HYPERTENSION

Prevention of portal hypertension by control of chronic liver disease, seems to be an unattainable goal until the hepatitis virus is isolated and our cultural attitude toward alcohol is changed.

Since in idiopathic portal hypertension definite vascular lesions are not found, we must re-evaluate the standard concept that portal hypertension is primarily obstructive in origin. The possible importance of increased splanchnic inflow has to be considered and somehow evaluated.

From the standpoint of treatment of portal hypertension, the most pressing problem is to reach a decision, through controlled studies, regarding the wisdom of portal-systemic shunting. New technics for shunt operations are not likely to be particularly helpful unless they allow preservations of hepatic blood flow. Portacaval transposition seems to offer the greatest potential in this regard.

REFERENCES

1. Adler, D. C., Haverback, B. J., and Meyers, H. I.: Cineradiography of esophageal varices, J.A.M.A. *189*:77, 1964.
2. Aufses, A. H., Jr., Schaffner, F., Rosenthal, W. S.. and Herman, B. E.: Portal venous pressure in "pipestem fibrosis" of the liver due to schistosomiasis, Am. J. Med. *27*:807, 1959.
3. Baggenstoss, A. H., and Cain, J. C.: The hepatic hilar lymphatics of man: their relation to ascites, New Engl. J. Med. *256*:531, 1957.
4. Baggenstoss, A. H., and Wollaeger, E. E.: Portal hypertension due to chronic occlusion of the extrahepatic portion of the portal veins; its relation to ascites, Am. J. Med. *21*:16, 1956.
5. Baker, L. A., Smith, C., and Lieberman, G.: The natural history of esophageal varices, Am. J. Med. *26*:228, 1959.
6. Bayly, J. H., and Carbalhaes, O. G.: The umbilical vein in the adult: diagnosis, treatment and research, Am. Surg. *30*:56, 1964.
7. Beckett, A. G., Livingstone, A. V., and

Hill, K. R.; Acute alcoholic hepatitis, Brit. Med. J. 2:1113, 1961.

8. Benhamou, J. P., Girond, C., Guillemot, R., Nicollo, F., Tricot, R., Leger, L., and Fauvert, R.: Etudes sur l'hémodynamique portohépatique, Rev. franç. Étud. clin. biol. 7:524, 1962.

9. ———: Etudes sur l'hémodynamique portohépatique. VIII. La pression intra-hépatique, Rev. franç. Étud. clin. biol. 7: 1091, 1962.

10. Benhamou, J. P., Guillemot, R., Tricot, R., Leger, L., and Fauvert, R.: Hypertension portale essentielle, Presse méd. 70:2397, 1962.

11. Blakemore, A. H.: Portacaval shunt in surgical treatment of portal hypertension, Ann. Surg. 128:825, 1948.

12. Bordin, E. H.: Blood ammonia determinations as a diagnostic tool in the differentiation of upper gastrointestinal bleeding, Gastroenterology 37:457, 1959.

13. Boyer, J. L., Sen Gupta, K. P., Biswas, S. K., Pal, N. C., Basu Mallick, K. C., Iber, F. L., and Basu, A. K.: Idiopathic portal hypertension, Ann. Int. Med. 66: 41, 1967.

14. Bradley, S. E., Ingelfinger, F. J., Bradley, G. P., and Curry, J. J.: The estimation of hepatic blood flow in man, J. Clin. Invest. 24:890, 1945.

15. Bradley, S. E., Smythe, C. M., Fitzpatrick, H. F., and Blakemore, A. H.: The effect of a portacaval shunt on estimated hepatic blood flow and oxygen uptake in cirrhosis, J. Clin. Invest. 32: 526, 1953.

16. Bras, G., Berry, D. M., and Gyorgy, P.: Plants as aetiological factor in veno-occlusive disease of the liver, Lancet 1:960, 1957.

17. Bras, G., Brooks, S. E. H., and Watler, D. C.: Cirrhosis of the liver in Jamaica, J. Path. Bact. 82:503, 1961.

18. Britton, R. C., and Shirey, E. K.: Cine-portography in dynamics of portal flow following shunt procedures, Arch. Surg. 84:25, 1962.

19. Caesar, J., Barber, K. M., Baraona, E., and Sherlock, S.: The estimation of portal-systemic collateral flow in man using intrasplenic injection of radioactive indicator, Clin. Sci. 23:77, 1962.

20. Callow, A. D., Lloyd, J. B., Ishihara, A., Ponsdomeneeh, E., O'Hara, E. T., Chalmers, T. C., and Garceau, A. J.: Interim experience with a controlled study of prophylactic portacaval shunt, Surgery 57:123, 1965.

21. Campbell, G. S., Bick, H. D., Paulsen, E. P., Lober, P. H., Watson, C. J., and Varco, R. L.: Bleeding esophageal varices with polycystic liver: report of three cases, New Engl. J. Med. 259:904, 1958.

22. Cardillo, P. J., and Douglass, F. M.: Alternate anatomical approach to caval-mesenteric shunting, Surgery 60:317, 1966.

23. Child, C. G.: The Hepatic Circulation and Portal Hypertension, Philadelphia, Saunders, 1954.

24. Clarke, J. S.: Influence of the liver upon gastric secretion, Am. J. Med. 29:740, 1960.

25. Clatworthy, H. W., Jr., and Boles, E. T., Jr.: Extrahepatic portal bed block in children: pathogenesis and treatment, Ann. Surg. 150:371, 1959.

26. Clatworthy, H. W., Jr., Wall, T., and Watman, R. N.: A new type of portal-to-systemic venous shunt for portal hypertension, Arch. Surg. 71:588, 1955.

27. Cohn, R., and Blaisdell, F. W.: The natural history of the patient with cirrhosis of the liver with esophageal varices following the first massive hemorrhage, Surg. Gynec. Obstet. 106:699, 1958.

28. Conn, H. O.: Hazards attending the use of esophageal tamponade, New Engl. J. Med. 259:701, 1958.

29. ———: Ammonia tolerance as an index of portal-systemic collateral circulation in cirrhosis, Gastroenterology 41:97, 1961.

30. Conn, H. O., Binder, H., and Brodoff, M.: Fiberoptic and conventional esophagoscopy in the diagnosis of esophageal varices, Gastroenterology 52:810, 1967.

31. Conn, H. O., and Brodoff, M.: Emergency esophagoscopy in the diagnosis of upper gastrointestinal hemorrhage, Gastroenterology 47:505, 1964.

32. Conn, H. O., Greenspan, R. H., Clemett, A. R., Mitchell, J. R., and Brodoff, M.: Balloon tamponade in the radiological diagnosis of esophageal varices, Gastroenterology 50:29, 1966.

33. Conn, H. O., and Lindenmuth, W. W.: Prophylactic portacaval anastomosis in cirrhotic patients with esophageal varices, New Engl. J. Med. 272:1255, 1965.

34. Conn, H. O., Smith, H. W., and Brodoff, M.: Observer variation in the endoscopic

diagnosis of esophageal varices, New Engl. J. Med. *272*:830, 1965.

35. Dagradi, A. E., Stempien, S. J., and Owens, L. K.: Bleeding esophagogastric varices, Arch. Surg. *92*:944, 1966.

36. Dal Palu, C., Ruol, A., and Belloni, G.: Postsinusoidal portal hypertension in a patient with chronic lymphatic leukemia, Am. J. Dig. Dis. *8*:845, 1963.

37. Denney, M. K., Lucas, C. E., and Read, R. C.: Significance of hematochylia in Laennec's cirrhosis, Arch. Surg. *92*:657, 1966.

38. Dumont, A. E., and Mulholland, J. H.: Alterations in thoracic duct lymph flow in hepatic cirrhosis: significance in portal hypertension, Ann. Surg. *156*:668, 1962.

39. Edmondson, H. A., Peters, R. L., Reynolds, T. B., and Kuzma, O. T.: Sclerosing hyaline necrosis of the liver in the chronic alcoholic, Ann. Int. Med. *59*:646, 1963.

40. Edmunds, R., and West, J. P.: Treatment of bleeding esophageal varices: five-year comparison of medical and surgical procedures, J.A.M.A. *189*:854, 1964.

41. Eisenberg, S.: Blood volume in patients with Laennec's cirrhosis of the liver as determined by radioactive chromium-tagged red cells, Am. J. Med. *20*:189, 1956.

42. Ellis, D. S., Linton, R. R., and Jones, C. M.: Effect of venous shunt surgery on liver function in patients with portal hypertension, New Engl. J. Med. *254*:931, 1956.

43. Erlik, D., Barzilai, A., and Shramek, A.: Porto-renal shunt, a new technic for porto-systemic anastomosis in portal hypertension, Ann. Surg. *159*:72, 1964.

44. Fauvert, R., Benhamou, J. P., and Meyer, P., Fibrose hépatique congénitale, Rev. int. Hépat. *14*:395, 1964.

45. Fisher, B., Russ, C., Fedor, E., Wilde, R., Engstrom, P., and Fisher, E. R.: Further experimental observations on animals with arterialized livers, Surgery *38*:181, 1955.

46. Friedman, E. W., and Weiner, R. S.: Estimation of hepatic sinusoid pressure by means of venous catheters and estimation of portal pressure by hepatic vein catheterization, Am. J. Physiol. *165*:527, 1951.

47. Garceau, A. J., Chalmers, T. C., and The Boston Inter-Hospital Liver Group: The natural history of cirrhosis. I. Survival with esophageal varices, New Engl. J. Med. *268*:469, 1963.

48. Grace, N. D., Muench, H., and Chalmers, T. C.: The present status of shunts for portal hypertension in cirrhosis, Gastroenterology *50*:684, 1966.

49. Hales, M. R., Allan, J. S., and Hall, E. M.: Injection-corrosion studies of normal and cirrhotic livers, Am. J. Path. *35*:909, 1959.

50. Hallenbeck, G. A., and Adson, M. A.: Esophagogastric varices without hepatic cirrhosis, Arch. Surg. *83*:370, 1961.

51. Hallenbeck, G. A., Wollaeger, E. E., Adson, M. A., and Gage, R. P.: Results after portal-systemic shunts in 120 patients with cirrhosis of the liver, Surg. Gynec. Obstet. *116*:435, 1963.

52. Herrick, F. C.: Experimental study into cause of increased portal pressure in portal cirrhosis, J. Exp. Med. *9*:93, 1907.

53. Hunt, A. H.: A Contribution to the Study of Portal Hypertension, Edinburgh, Livingstone, 1958.

54. Imanaga, H., Yamamoto, S., and Kuroyanagi, Y.: Surgical treatment of portal hypertension according to state of intrahepatic circulation, Ann. Surg. *155*:42, 1962.

55. Jackson, F. C., Perrin, E. B., Jr., Dagradi, A. E., Smith, A. G., and Lee, L. E.: Clinical investigation of the portacaval shunt, Arch. Surg. *91*:43, 1965.

56. Jelliffe, D. B., Bras, G., and Mukherjee, K. L.: Veno-occlusive disease of the liver and Indian childhood cirrhosis, Arch. Dis. Childh. *32*:369, 1957.

57. Kehne, J. H., Hughes, F. A., and Gompertz, M. L.: Use of surgical pituitrin in the control of esophageal varix bleeding, Surgery *39*:917, 1956.

58. Kelty, R. H., Baggenstoss, A. H., and Butt, H. R.: The relation of the regenerated hepatic nodule to the vascular bed in cirrhosis, Proc. Mayo Clin. *25*:17, 1950.

59. Kerr, D. N. S., Harrison, C. V., Sherlock, S., and Walker, R. M.: Congenital hepatic fibrosis, Quart. J. Med. *30*:91, 1961.

60. Kimura, C., Shirotani, H., Hirooka, M., Terada, M., Iwahashi, K., and Maetani, S.: Membranous obliteration of the inferior vena cava in the hepatic portion, J. Cardiovasc. Surg. *4*:87, 1963.

61. Krook, H.: Estimation of portal venous pressure by occlusive hepatic vein cathe-

terization, Scand, J. Clin. Lab. Invest. 5: 285, 1953.

62. Lacroix, E., and Leusen, I.: La circulation hépatique et splanchnique, J. Physiol. (Paris) 57:115, 1965.

63. Lavoie, P., Jacob, M., Leduc, J., Legare, A., and Viallet, A.: The umbilicoportal approach for the study of splanchnic circulation: technical, radiological and hemodynamic considerations, Canad. J. Surg. 9:338, 1966.

64. Leevy, C. M., Zinke, M., Baber, J., and Chey, W. Y.: Observations on influence of medical therapy on portal hypertension in hepatic cirrhosis, Ann. Int. Med. 49:837, 1958.

65. Lemaire, A., and Housset, E.: La mesure de la pression portale par ponction du foie, Presse méd. 63:1063, 1955.

66. Lieberman, F. L., and Reynolds, T. B.: Plasma volume in cirrhosis of the liver: its relation to portal hypertension, ascites and renal failure, J. Clin. Invest. 46: 1297, 1967.

67. Liebowitz, H. R.: Pathogenesis of esophageal varix rupture, J.A.M.A. 175:874, 1961.

68. Linton, R. R., and Ellis, D. S.: Emergency and definitive treatment of bleeding esophageal varices, J.A.M.A. 160: 1017, 1956.

69. Linton, R. R., Ellis, D. S., and Geary, J. E.: Critical comparative analysis of early and late results of splenorenal and direct portacaval shunts performed in 169 patients with portal cirrhosis, Ann. Surg. 154:446, 1961.

70. Longmire, W. P., Jr., Mulder, D. G., Mahoney, P. S., and Mellinkoff, S. W.: Side-to-side portacaval anastomosis for portal hypertension, Ann. Surg. 147:881, 1958.

71. Marion, P.: Les obstructions portales, Sem. Hôp. Paris 29:2781, 1953.

72. Mason, E. E.: Splenectomy and side-to-side splenorenal shunt for portal hypertension, Surgery 60:536, 1966.

73. McDermott, W. V.: The treatment of cirrhotic ascites by combined hepatic and portal decompression, New Engl. J. Med. 259:897, 1958.

74. McIndoe, A. H.: Vascular lesions of portal cirrhosis, Arch. Path. 5:23, 1928.

75. McLean, E., Bras, G., and Gyorgy, P.: Veno-occlusive lesions in livers of rats fed Crotalaria fulva, Brit. J. Exp. Path. 40:242, 1964.

76. McMichael, J.: The portal circulation, J. Physiol. 75:241, 1932.

77. Merigan, T. C., Jr., Plotkin, G. R., and Davidson, C. S.: Effect of intravenously administered posterior pituitary extract on hemorrhage from bleeding esophageal varices, New Engl. J. Med. 266:134, 1962.

78. Mikkelsen, W. P.: Emergency portacaval shunt, Rev. Surg. 19:141, 1962.

79. ———: Extrahepatic portal hypertension in children, Am. J. Surg. 111:333, 1966.

80. Mikkelsen, W. P., Edmondson, H. A., Peters, R. L., Redeker, A. G., and Reynolds, T. B.: Extra- and intrahepatic portal hypertension without cirrhosis (hepatoportal sclerosis), Ann. Surg. 162: 602, 1965.

81. Mikkelsen, W. P., Turrill, F. L., and Pattison, A. C.: Portacaval shunt in cirrhosis of the liver; clinical and hemodynamic aspects, Am. J. Surg. 104:204, 1962.

82. Mino, R. A., Murphy, A. I., Jr., and Livingstone, R. G.: Sarcoidosis producing portal hypertension: treatment by splenectomy and splenorenal shunt, Ann. Surg. 130:951, 1949.

83. Moreno, A. H., Burchell, A. R., Rousselot, L. M., Panke, W. F., Slafsky, S. F., and Burke, J. H.: Portal blood flow in cirrhosis of the liver, J. Clin. Invest. 46: 436, 1967.

84. Mousa, A. H., and El-Garen, A.: The haemodynamic study of Egyptian hepatosplenic bilharziasis, J. Egypt. Med. Ass. 42:444, 1959.

85. Murray, J. F., Dawson, A. M., and Sherlock, S.: Circulatory changes in chronic liver disease, Am. J. Med. 24:358, 1958.

86. Myers, J. D., and Taylor, W. J.: An estimation of portal venous pressure by occlusive catheterization of an hepatic venule, J. Clin. Invest. 30:662, 1951.

87. Nachlas, M. M.: A critical evaluation of venous shunts for the treatment of cirrhotic patients with esophageal varices, Ann. Surg. 148:169, 1958.

88. Orloff, M. J., Halasz, N. A., Lipman, C., Schwabe, A. D., Thompson, J. C., and Weidner, W. A.: The complications of cirrhosis of the liver, Ann. Int. Med. 66: 165, 1967.

89. Orloff, M. J., and Thomas, H. S.: Pathogenesis of esophageal varix rupture, Arch. Surg. 87:301, 1963.

90. Orrego-Matté, H., Amenabar, E., Lara, G., Baraona, E., Palma, R., and Massad, F.: Measurement of intrahepatic pressure as index of portal pressure, Am. J. Med. Sci. 247:278, 1964.

91. Ostrow, J. D., Timmerman, R. J., and Gray, S. J.: Gastric secretion in human hepatic cirrhosis, Gastroenterology 38: 303, 1960.

92. Palmer, E. D.: Esophageal varices associated with hiatus hernia in the absence of portal hypertension, Am. J. Med. Sci. 235:677, 1958.

93. ———: Diagnosis of Upper Gastrointestinal Hemorrhage, Springfield, Ill., Thomas, 1961.

94. Palmer, E. D., and Brick, I. B.: Varices of the distal esophagus in the apparent absence of portal and of superior caval hypertension, Am. J. Med. Sci. 230:515, 1955.

95. Palmer, E. D., Jahnke, E. J., Jr., and Hughes, C. W.: Evaluation of clinical results of portal decompression in cirrhosis, J.A.M.A. 164:746. 1957.

96. Parker, R. G. F.: Occlusion of the hepatic veins in man, Medicine 38:369, 1959.

97. Parof, A., Chalut, J., Caroli, J., and Porcher, A.: Manometric splénique et splénoportographique dans les affections du système hemopoietique, les pyelophlebites, les cirrhoses du foie, Rev. int. Hepat. 5:617, 1955.

98. Paton, A., Reynolds, T. B., and Sherlock, S.: Assessment of portal venous hypertension by catheterization of hepatic vein, Lancet 1:918, 1953.

99. Patrassi, G., Dal Palu, C., Ruol, A., and Valdoni, P.: Pletora portale, Policlinico Sez. (prat.) 68:1920, 1961.

100. Perera, G. A.: The plasma volume in Laennec's cirrhohis of the liver, Ann. Int. Med. 24:643, 1946.

101. Piccone, V. A., Jr., and LeVeen, H. H.: Transumbilical portal decompression, Surg. Forum 17:372, 1966.

102. Polish, E., Christie, J., Cohen, A., and Sullivan, B., Jr.: Idiopathic presinusoidal portal hypertension (Banti's syndrome), Ann. Int. Med. 56:624, 1962.

103. Popper, H., Elias, H., and Petty, D. E.: Vascular pattern of cirrhotic liver, Am. J. Clin. Path. 22:717, 1952.

104. Popper, H., Szanto, P. B., and Parthasarathy, M.: Florid cirrhosis, a review of 35 cases, Am. J. Clin. Path. 25:889, 1955.

105. Preston, F. W., and Trippel, O. H.: Emergency portacaval shunt, Arch. Surg. 90:770, 1965.

106. Ramos, O. L., Saad, F., and Leser, W. P.: Portal hemodynamics and liver cell function in hepatic schistosomiasis, Gastroenterology 47:241, 1964.

107. Rather, L. J., and Cohn, R.: Some effects on the liver of the complete arterialization of its blood supply: III. Acute vascular necrosis, Surgery 34:207, 1953.

108. Ratnoff, O. D., and Patek, A. J., Jr.: Natural history of Laennec's cirrhosis of the liver: analysis of 386 cases, Medicine 21:207, 1942.

109. Ravenna, P.: Splenoportal venous obstruction without splenomegaly, Arch. Int. Med. 72:786, 1943.

110. Redeker, A. G., Geller, H. M., and Reynolds, T. B.: Hepatic wedge pressure, blood flow, vascular resistance and oxygen consumption in cirrhosis before and after end-to-side portacaval shunt, J. Clin. Invest. 37:606, 1958.

111. Redeker, A. G., Kunelis, C. T., Yamamoto, S., and Reynolds, T. B.: Assessment of portal and hepatic hemodynamics after side-to-side portacaval shunt in patients with cirrhosis, J. Clin. Invest. 43: 1464, 1964.

112. Reynolds, T. B., Balfour, D. C., Jr., Levinson, D. C., Mikkelsen, W. P., and Pattison, A. C.: Comparison of wedged hepatic vein pressure with portal vein pressure in human subjects with cirrhosis, J. Clin. Invest. 34:213, 1955.

113. Reynolds, T. B., Geller, H. M., Kuzma, O. T., and Redeker, A. G.: Spontaneous decrease in portal pressure with clinical improvement in cirrhosis, New Engl. J. Med. 263:734, 1960.

114. Reynolds, T. B., Geller, H. M., and Redeker, A. G.: The effect of vasopressin on hepatic hemodynamics in patients with portal hypertension, J. Clin. Invest. 39:1021, 1960.

115. Reynolds, T. B., Hudson, N., Mikkelsen, W. P., Turrill, F. L., and Redeker, A. G.: Clinical comparison of end-to-side and side-to-side portacaval shunt, New Engl. J. Med. 274:706, 1966.

116. Reynolds, T. B., Mikkelsen, W. P., Redeker, A. G., and Yamahiro, H. S.: The effect of side-to-side portacaval shunt on hepatic hemodynamics in cirrhosis, J. Clin. Invest. 41:1242, 1962.

117. Reynolds, T. B., Redeker, A. G., and Geller, H. M.: Wedged hepatic venous pressure: a clinical evaluation, Am. J. Med. 22:341, 1957.

118. Riddell, A. G., Davies, R. P., and Clark, A. D.: Portacaval transposition in the treatment of glycogen storage disease, Lancet 2:1146, 1966.

119. Rosenbaum, D. L., Murphy, G. W., and Swisher, S. N.: Hemodynamic studies of the portal circulation in myeloid metaplasia, Am. J. Med. 41:360, 1966.

120. Rousselot, L. M., Gilbertson, F. E., and Panke, W. F.: Severe hemorrhage from esophagogastric varices: its emergency management with particular reference to portacaval anastomosis, New Engl. J. Med. 262:269, 1960.

121. Rowell, L. B., Blackmon, J. R., and Bruce, R. A.: Indocyanine green clearance and estimated hepatic blood flow during mild to moderate exercise in upright man, J. Clin. Invest. 43:1677, 1964.

122. Ruprecht, A. L., and Kinney, T. D.: Esophageal varices caused by metastasis of carcinoma to the liver, Am. J. Dig. Dis. 1:145, 1956.

123. Safouh, M., Shehata, A., and Elwi, A.: Hepatic vein occlusion disease in Egyptian children, Arch. Path. 79:505, 1965.

124. Satterfield, J. V., Mulligan, L. V., and Butcher, H. R., Jr.: Bleeding esophageal varices: comparison of operative and nonoperative treatment, Arch. Surg. 90:667, 1965.

125. Schaefer, J. W., Amick, C. J., Oikawa, Y., and Schiff, L.: The development of hemochromatosis following portacaval anastomosis, Gastroenterology 42:181, 1962.

126. Schaefer, J. W., Bramschreiber, J., Mistilis, S., and Schiff, L.: Gastroesophageal variceal bleeding in the absence of hepatic cirrhosis or portal hypertension, Gastroenterology 46:583, 1965.

127. Schenk, W. G., Jr., McDonald, J. C., McDonald, K., and Drapanas, T.: Direct measurement of hepatic blood flow in surgical patients, Ann. Surg. 156:463, 1962.

128. Schlant, R. C., Galambos, J. T., Shuford, W. H., Rawls, W. J., Winter, T. S., III, and Edwards, F. K.: The clinical usefulness of wedge hepatic venography, Am. J. Med. 35:343, 1963.

129. Schwartz, S. I., Bales, H. W., Emerson, G. L., and Mahoney, E. B.: The use of intravenous Pituitrin in treatment of bleeding esophageal varices, Surgery 45:72, 1959.

130. Schwartz, S. I., and Greenlaw, R. H.: Evaluation of portal circulation by percutaneous splenic isotope injection, Surgery 50:833, 1961.

131. Shaldon, S., Chiandussi, L., Guevara, L., Caesar, J., and Sherlock, S.: The estimation of hepatic blood flow and intrahepatic shunted blood flow by colloidal heat-denatured human serum albumin labelled with I^{131}, J. Clin. Invest. 40:1346, 1961.

132. Shaldon, S., Dolle, W., Guevara, L., Iber, F. L., and Sherlock, S.: Effect of Pitressin on the splanchnic circulation in man, Circulation 24:797, 1961.

133. Shaldon, S., and Sherlock, S.: The use of vasopressin (Pitressin) in the control of bleeding from esophageal varices, Lancet 2:222, 1960.

134. ————: Portal hypertension in the myeloproliferative syndrome and the reticuloses, Am. J. Med. 32:758, 1962.

135. Sherlock, S.: Diseases of the Liver and Biliary System, ed. 3, Oxford, Blackwell, 1963.

136. ————: Hematemesis in portal hypertension, Brit. J. Surg. 51:746, 1964.

137. Sherlock, S., Feldman, C. A., Moran, B., and Scheuer, P. J.: Partial nodular transformation of the liver with portal hypertension, Am. J. Med. 40:195, 1966.

138. Siderys, H., Judd, D., Herendeen, T. L., Kilman, J. W., and Waldhausen, J. A.: The experimental production of elevated portal pressure by increasing portal flow, Surg. Gynec. Obstet. 120:514, 1965.

139. Smith, G. W., and Edwards, O. E.: Hemorrhage from varices in patients with achlorhydria, Gastroenterology 51:1054, 1966.

140. Stone, H. H., Jordan, W. D., Acker, J. J., and Martin, J. D.: Portal arteriovenous fistulas: review and case report, Am. J. Surg. 109:191, 1965.

141. Strauch, G. O.: Second thoughts on cirrhosis and portosystemic shunts, Surgery 58:773, 1965.

142. Taylor, W. J., Jackson, F. C., and Jensen, W. N.: Wilson's disease, portal hypertension and intrahepatic vascular ob-

struction, New Engl. J. Med. *260*:1160, 1959.

143. Thompson, E. N., and Sherlock, S.: The aetiology of portal vein thrombosis, with particular reference to role of infection in exchange transfusion, Quart J. Med. *33*:465, 1964.

144. Thompson, E. N., Williams, R., and Sherlock, S.: Liver function in extrahepatic portal hypertension, Lancet *2*: 1352, 1964.

145. Thompson, W. P., Caughey, J. L., Whipple, A. O., and Rousselot, L. M.: Splenic vein pressures in congestive splenomegaly (Banti's syndrome), J. Clin. Invest. *16*:571, 1937.

146. Tisdale, W. A.: Parenchymal siderosis in patients with cirrhosis after portasystemic shunt surgery, New Engl. J. Med. *265*: 928, 1961.

147. Tisdale, W. A., Klatskin, G., and Glenn, W. W. L.: Portal hypertension and bleeding esophageal varices: their occurrence in the absence of both intrahepatic and extrahepatic obstruction of the portal vein, New Engl. J. Med. *261*:209, 1959.

148. Tsakiris, A., Haemmerli, U. P., and Bühlmann, A.: Reduction of portal venous pressure in cirrhotic patients with bleeding from oesophageal varices by administration of a vasopressin derivative, phenylalanine-lysine-vasopressin, Am. J. Med. *36*:825, 1964.

149. Turner, M. D., Sherlock, S., and Steiner, R. E.: Splenic venography and intrasplenic pressure measurement in the clinical investigation of the portal venous system, Am. J. Med. *23*:846, 1957.

150. Tuttle, S. G., Figueroa, W. G., and Grossman, M. I.: Development of hemochromatosis in patient with Laennec's cirrhosis, Am. J. Med. *26*:655, 1959.

151. Tygstrup, N., Winkler, K., Mellemgaard, K., and Andreassen, M.: Determination of the hepatic arterial blood flow and oxygen supply in man by clamping the hepatic artery during surgery, J. Clin. Invest. *41*:447, 1962.

152. Ueda, H., Unuma, T., Iio, M., and Kameda, H.: Measurement of hepatic arterial and portal blood flow and circulation time via hepatic artery and portal vein with radioisotope, Jap. Heart J. *3*: 154, 1962.

153. Vennes, J. A.: Intrahepatic pressure: an

accurate reflection of portal pressure, Medicine *45*:445, 1966.

154. Viallet, A., Lavoie, P., Légaré, A., Bernier, J., Montgrain, P., and Joly, J. G.: Comparison of free portal pressure and wedged suprahepatic pressure in nine cases of cirrhosis, Un. méd. Canada *95*: 519, 1966.

155. Victor, M., Adams, R. D., and Cole, M.: The acquired (non-Wilsonian) type of chronic hepatocerebral degeneration, Medicine *44*:345, 1965.

156. Voorhees, A. B., Jr., and Blakemore, A. H.: Clinical experience with the superior mesenteric vein-inferior vena cava shunt in the treatment of portal hypertension, Surgery *51*:35, 1962.

157. Walker, G., Williams, R., Condon, R. E., Thompson, E. N., and Sherlock, S.: Gastric cooling in the treatment of bleeding from esophageal varices, Lancet *2*:328, 1964.

158. Wangensteen, S. L., and Smith, R. B., III: Intragastric cooling for upper gastrointestinal bleeding, Ann. N. Y. Acad. Sci. *115*:328, 1964.

159. Wantz, G. E., and Payne, M. A.: The emergency portacaval shunt, Surg. Gynec. Obstet. *109*:549, 1959.

160. Warren, J. V., and Brannon, E. S.: A method of obtaining blood samples directly from the hepatic vein in man, Proc. Soc. Exp. Biol. Med. *55*:144, 1944.

161. Warren, W. D., and Muller, W. H., Jr.: A clarification of some hemodynamic changes in cirrhosis and their surgical significance, Ann. Surg. *150*:413, 1959.

162. Warren, W. D., Zeppa, R., and Fomon, J. J.: Selective trans-splenic decompression of gastroesophageal varices by distal splenorenal shunt, Ann. Surg. *166*:437, 1967.

163. Welch, C. S.: Ligation of esophageal varices by the transabdominal route, New Engl. J. Med. *255*:677, 1956.

164. Whipple, A. O.: The problem of portal hypertension in relation to the hepatosplenopathies, Ann. Surg. *122*:449, 1945.

165. White. L. P., Phear, E. A., Summerskill, W. H. J., and Sherlock, S.: Ammonium tolerance in liver disease: observations based on catheterization of the hepatic vein, J. Clin. Invest. *34*:158, 1955.

166. Yamamoto, S., Redeker, A. G., and Reynolds, T. B.: The effect of thoracic duct drainage on hepatic hemodynamics

in cirrhosis, Gastroenterology *46*:305, 1964.

167. Yamamoto, S., and Reynolds, T. B.: Portal venography and pressure measurement at peritoneoscopy, Gastroenterology *47*:602, 1964.

168. Yamamoto, S., Yokoyama, Y., Takeshige, K., and Iwatsuki, S.: Budd-Chiari syndrome with obstruction of the inferior vena cava, Gastroenterology *54*:1070, 1968.

169. Zuidema, G. D., and Kirsh, M. M.: Hepatic encephalopathy following portal decompression: evaluation of end-to-side and side-to-side anastomosis, Am. Surg. *31*:567, 1965.

10

Portal Venography and Manometry

LOUIS M. ROUSSELOT, M.D., M.S., MED. SCI. D.,
AND *ALBERT R. BURCHELL*, M.D.

The diagnostic accuracy, clinical importance and dimensions of angiography have advanced greatly in the past few decades, especially in recent years. The pioneering work of dos Santos[27] who introduced the technic of translumbar aortography in 1929 was followed in the 1940's by technics of surgical exposure of peripheral arteries with retrograde passage of a catheter into the aorta.[15, 30, 33, 58] By this technic, Bierman's group in 1951 first catheterized selective visceral branches of the aorta.[10] In 1953 Seldinger revolutionized the technic with percutaneous nonoperative catheterization of the aorta,[70] a method which Odman utilized in selective study of branches of the aorta.[53] However, only in the past few years has this method included the demonstration and investigation of the previously inaccessible splanchnic arterial and portal venous systems.[12, 16, 37, 57]

Paralleling in history this arterial catheterization approach, other groups attempted to study the portal venous system more directly and met with earlier success. In 1936 and 1937 Thompson, Caughey, Whipple and Rousselot[61, 74] were the first to cannulate the splenic vein and to clinically record elevated splenic venous pressure in congestive splenomegaly. In 1945 Blakemore and Lord utilized laparotomy to study the portal venous system radiographically by a direct portal tributary injection.[11] In 1951 Abeatici and Campi,[1] Boulvin et al.,[14] and Leger[39] independently by a splenic pulp injection visualized the portal venous system and ob-

tained manometric studies successively in dogs, in patients at laparotomy, and finally percutaneously. The percutaneous approach was begun by Rousselot in the United States in 1952,[65] and is now the standard technic for study of the portal venous system. Numerous reports of large series, comprehensive reviews, monographs and textbook chapters attest to the diagnostic accuracy, safety and usefulness of the procedure.[6, 13, 31, 40, 41, 62, 66, 67, 78]

Both these major approaches to the demonstration and investigation of the splanchnic arterial and portal venous systems are being improved by unparalleled advances in radiographic technic. Hand operated cassette changers have given way to progressively better automatic cassette changers, which in turn are being replaced by cineradiography. In this technic image reproduction and the size of the field are constantly being improved. Image amplification has replaced simple fluoroscopy. Films are now developed automatically. Improved contrast media intensify opacification and diminish side effects. These advances have furthered technical facility and success in obtaining these special studies which in turn has engendered greater clinical and investigative interest in portal venography.

TERMINOLOGY AND HEMODYNAMIC CONSIDERATIONS

Portal venography is the radiologic visualization with a contrast medium of all or part of the portal venous system. The forms of portal venography currently employed in clinical medicine are classified according to the route by which radiopaque medium is introduced into the portal system.

Portal Portography

In portal portography the contrast medium is injected directly into the portal venous system, usually via a mesenteric branch cannulated at laparotomy. The directness of the injection usually results in excellent opacification of the portal vein, but also maximally disturbs the hemodynamic situation. Only in rare cases is any information obtained about the splenic vein.

Retrograde Portography

Retrograde portography involves a series of technics in which contrast medium is introduced intravascularly under sufficient injection pressure to produce unphysiologic retrograde filling of the portal system. This can be accomplished by inserting a needle percutaneously through the substance of the liver into an intrahepatic branch of the portal vein, or by retrograde catheterization of a hepatic vein with the injection of contrast medium when the catheter is in a wedged position. In cases of portal hypertension with diminution of portal venous inflow this retrograde opacification of the portal vein is facilitated, although it is feasible even in the normal subject.[50] Under circumstances of diminished portal venous inflow even the intrahepatic parenchymal deposition of contrast substance can result in such retrograde opacification of the portal venous system.[19, 49] By any of these technics only rarely is the splenic vein visualized by the pressure of injection. At present all these procedures are primarily investigative technics which allow for blood sampling, pressure recordings and a variety of research studies.

In transumbilical portal venography the umbilical vein is exposed surgically and dilated, and a large bore catheter is introduced retrogradely into the left main portal vein. From this vantage point and with a large bore catheter in place it is possible to achieve remarkably dense opacification but again by a retrograde injection technic which disrupts the hemodynamic situation.

Only rarely is the splenic vein visualized, but this can be accomplished by further retrograde passage of the catheter into the area of the spleen.[38]

Transcapillary Portography

Transcapillary portography involves the cannulation of the aorta, or in recent years selective aortic branches, such as the celiac, splenic and superior and inferior mesenteric arteries. The contrast medium injected into these arterial branches then transverses the splanchnic capillary bed, ultimately opacifying the portal and/or splenic veins. Since the high pressure of injection is dissipated as the contrast medium passes through the capillary bed, this technic does result in a functional physiologic study.

Splenic Portography

Splenic portography is the most commonly employed form of portal venography. By this method, the contrast medium is deposited into the splenic pulp, either percutaneously or under direct vision at laparotomy. As a practical consideration, it usually yields all the information clinically necessary for rational diagnosis and planning of therapy in suspected cases of portal hypertension. Most importantly, splenic portography obviates the introduction of the artefacts of direct intravascular injections, which are innately involved in portal and retrograde portography. In these intravascular technics, the force of the injection is directly into the portal system, producing a direct transmission of pressure which disturbs the physiologic situation under study. This may result in forceful retrograde filling of collateral vessels and give a false impression of the hemodynamic problem. In splenic portography the splenic pulp absorbs and cushions the pressure of injection, avoiding any direct transmission of pressure into the portal venous system, and thus allowing for functional hemodynamic visualization of the portal venous circulation.[62]

PERCUTANEOUS SPLENIC PORTOGRAPHY AND MANOMETRY

After more than 15 years of experimental and clinical evaluation, splenic portography and splenic pulp manometry have been almost universally accepted as the most informative means of diagnostically assessing anatomic variants and hemodynamic derangements in portal hypertension.

The use of this procedure has provided anatomic and pathophysiologic criteria for confirming or negating a presumed diagnosis of alterations in the portal venous system and, indeed, for diagnosing portal hypertension itself.

Splenic portography graphically depicts an important part of the pathophysiology of portal hypertension. This clinical syndrome reflects mechanical interference with the transhepatic flow of blood, either within the substance of the liver or external to it. This impediment to normal splanchnic flow toward the liver may result in a chronic pressure elevation in all, or part, of the splenoportal axis, depending on the site of obstruction. This elevated pressure in the portal venous system favors a retrograde flow of blood via preformed and newly developed portasystemic communication. Arteriovenous shunts, both intrahepatic and splanchnic, may play a role in cirrhotic portal hypertension but usually are secondary to portal bed block in the genesis of this condition. Thus by depositing contrast medium into the splenic pulp, one can opacify the flow of blood from the spleen along the splenoportal venous axis, and, in the majority of cases, visualize whether or not there is intra- or extrahepatic obstruction with hepatofugal flow, that is, retograde flow of blood away from the liver over collateral vessels. This is the hallmark of portal hypertension. By splenic portography one can detect portal hypertension by a graphic depiction of the fundamental hemodynamics and the pathophysiology. It can reveal the extent of collateralization and, of major importance to the surgeon, the size and patency of major vessels. The splenic portogram is a preoperative aid in surgical planning, for it establishes the availability of major vessels for shunting procedures and may detect inoperable situations.

The inherent dangers of any diagnostic procedure can be obviated largely by familiarity and proper attention to several details of technic. The following suggestions have evolved from our favorable experience with the technic in 1,070 splenic portograms per-formed in 901 patients on the surgical and medical services of St. Vincent's Hospital and Medical Center, New York City, 1952 to 1967.

INDICATIONS

Diagnosis. Splenic portography is primarily useful in confirming or negating a presumed diagnosis of portal hypertension, and in establishing the presence or absence of gastroesophageal varices.

Surgical Planning. Splenic portography is most useful as a preoperative aid in surgical planning, for it can delineate the level of splenoportal obstruction, establish the patency of major vessels for anastomosis, determine the presence or absence of varices and define avoidable inoperable situations. It is usually performed electively a few days prior to the proposed surgical procedure. Emergency splenic portography is obtained immediately before emergency surgery, if such becomes necessary.

Upper Abdominal Masses. Upper abdominal masses, hepatomegaly or splenomegaly not diagnosed by routine procedures, and, rarely, abdominal pain or ascites of undetermined origin may be clarified in certain situations by splenic portography. This has proved most useful in pancreatitis with or without pseudocyst and in neoplasms of the biliary tract, stomach, duodenum and body or tail of the pancreas. Local chronic occlusion of the splenic vein may occur with development of segmental splenic hypertension. Splenic portography has not proved very useful for clarifying small neoplasms of the upper abdomen.[67, 69]

Post Shunt Anastomotic Patency. This is readily determined by splenic portography and the degree of sustained pressure reduction documented by manometry.

CONTRAINDICATIONS

Contraindications to splenic portography include (1) severe abnormalities of the coagulation mechanism, especially a platelet count below 100,000/cu.mm. or a one-stage prothrombin time exceeding the control by 50 per cent, (2) a history of sensitivity to contrast medium, (3) a known tumor or abscess of the spleen, (4) renal insufficiency, (5) regional disease (e.g., pleurisy with or without effusion), (6) severe anemia, (7) a condition predisposing to rupture of the spleen (e.g., malaria, infectious mononucleosis, and (8) inability of the patient to cooperate. This last one is perhaps the most commonly encountered and must be respected. It frequently is observed in the agitated precomatose patient with irregularly spasmodic exaggerated respiratory excursions or other muscular contractions.

An impalpable spleen, massive ascites, deep coma, active hemorrhage and the presence of balloon tamponade or gastric hypothermia do not absolutely contraindicate the procedure, but require particular expertise on the part of the radiologist. An impalpable spleen requires careful fluoroscopic control and perhaps modification of the technic (see Technic). Massive ascites introduces at least a theoretical additional hazard, in that it results in a "floating spleen" negating the tamponade effect of the diaphragm and lateral chest wall upon the splenic puncture site which occurs in the average case without ascites.[67] Cases of deep coma or active hemorrhage with or without balloon tamponade challenge the most experienced clinician in deciding as to advisability, timing and performance of this procedure for the given patient.

PREPARATION

The patient is hospitalized and written permission is obtained. Routine coagulation studies include prothrombin time, platelet count and bleeding and clotting times. The subject is allowed nothing by mouth from midnight of the evening before the examination.

Premedication includes a barbiturate, meperidine hydrochloride (Demerol) and atropine in dosages appropriate to the size, age and general condition of the patient. Oversedating a patient with advanced liver disease with the barbiturate or narcotic may result in much blunting of the psyche and inability to cooperate with the safe conduct of the study. Diphenhydramine hydrochloride (Benadryl) is also given to minimize the possibility of allergic reaction to the contrast medium. Local 1 per cent procaine solution is the anesthesia of preference in adults; in children, a general anesthetic is the rule.

Sterile equipment consists of 4 towels, 3 cups for solutions, two 20-cc. syringes, a 50-cc. Luer-Lok syringe, two 3-way stopcocks, two 25-gauge hypodermic needles, a 6-inch length of rubber or plastic connecting tubing, a 10-inch length of B-D special flexible plastic connecting tube with Luer-Lok connection, 2 × 2 inch gauze pads, sponge forceps, water manometer, 1 per cent procaine solution, tincture of thimerosal (Merthiolate) (1:1,000), isotonic sodium chloride solution, and 50 cc. of a 75 per cent solution of diatrizoate sodium (Hypaque Sodium) (Fig. 10–1). A resuscitation tray containing sympathomimetic and antihistaminic drugs should always be on hand.

The day before the procedure, the patient is instructed in voluntary control of respiration, and again prior to the examination. The patient should practice voluntary midexcursion apnea, on command, several times, lest he misunderstand and take a deep inspiration or a sighing expiration during the procedure. The patient is advised of the importance of controlled gentle respiratory motions subsequently throughout the procedure. He is warned that transitory left upper-quadrant, transabdominal, or left shoulder pain, burning sensation or pressure may occur, as might a generalized sensation of warmth and facial flushing, with or without a metallic taste in the mouth. He must be cautioned not to move under such circumstances. This meticulous attention to enlist the fullest cooperation of the patient in completely controlling his respiratory motions is one of the 2 factors that contribute most to preventing technical errors and accidents.

TECHNIC

The patient is examined in the x-ray department on an x-ray table with a movable top and a rapid serial film changer. From 1952 to 1962 we used a standard x-ray table with a Bucky grid, 14 × 17 inch films, and a manually operated cassette changer. This technic resulted in superb films but required precision drilled team work. This is of proved merit and we advocate its use in hospitals not equipped with automatic units. Since 1962 we have used a Schonander automatic cassette changer. Although the quality

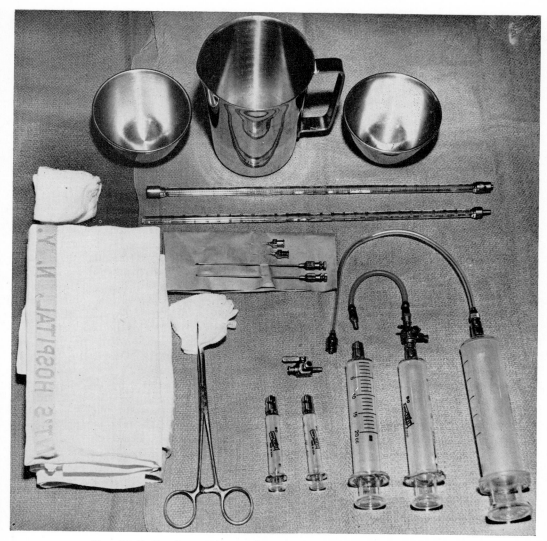

Fig. 10–1. Sterile equipment for percutaneous splenic portography.

of the films is not as good and the size of the field encompassed somewhat smaller (14 × 14), this has not affected the diagnostic accuracy of the procedure. It has greatly affected the photographic reproduction of the films, and forced us to repeat many of our previously used x-rays. However, the facility of using the Schonander technic has resulted in the more widespread use of the procedure and avoids exposing highly trained personnel to irradiation.

The use of 16 mm. or 35 mm. cinespleno-portography has proved to be most interest-ing in our experience. Phasic variations in portal venous flow, and occasionally most dramatic demonstrations of unusual hemo-dynamic variants have been observed. The small field encompassed by the cine technic, however, makes this method difficult to em-ploy and limits its usefulness. It necessitates scanning from the splenic bolus of contrast medium through the splenic vein, then at-tempting to move cephalad to follow coro-nary and varical flow, then shifting rapidly to the opposite side in time to observe portal flow and the intrahepatic transit. The use of an 11 inch screen would help to increase the size of the field but only at the loss of clarity of detail. The cine technic is not a clinical necessity but primarily an investigative tool.

The radiographic factors are MA 300, KVP 80, exposure time 0.1 sec., FFD 100 cm., film Eastman Kodak Royal Blue, filter 2 mm. aluminum, screen 35 × 35 cm. Radelin high speed Type TF Schonander. Exposures are obtained at 2, 4, 6, 8, 12, 16, 24 and 32 seconds from the start of the injection.

The patient is placed supine on the x-ray table with the left arm over the head and the right arm by the side. Vital signs are recorded. The table top and patient are then positioned over the film changer at an exactly reproducible location.

A scout film, centered at 2 fingerbreadths below the xyphoid process, is used to check the position of the patient and the exposure factors. It also serves as a plain film to identify the size and position of the spleen and to aid in the subsequent interpretation of the portogram.

The table top and patient are then moved back into position for anteroposterior projection fluoroscopy. Under image amplification the position of the hilum of the spleen in midexpiration is marked on the skin of the thorax or abdominal wall. The level of this anterior mark is usually in the same transverse plane as the lateral point of intersection of the left 9th intercostal space (determined by palpation) and the posterior axillary line. This spot is then marked and would be the usual site for puncture of a normal or small-sized spleen. The error in selecting the point of puncture tends to be in inserting the needle too far anteriorly. Rarely does one err by puncturing too far posteriorly. If the spleen is enlarged, then the point of puncture is marked at the mid-axillary line and the 9th intercostal space.

The operator then puts on a cap, mask and sterile gloves. A wide area of the skin of the left side is prepared with tincture of thimerosal. This area is then draped in a triangular fashion with 3 towels, so as to include the lower intercostal spaces, the xyphoid and the mark of the splenic hilum in the visible sterile field. A folded heavy

sheet is used to cover the x-ray table and thus protect the equipment in the field from being contaminated by the diffusion of bacteria through saturated drapes.

At the previously marked site for puncture, local infiltration anesthesia of the skin and the intercostal muscles is accomplished with 1 per cent procaine solution in adults. In children, the general anesthetic is begun.

A water manometer (with a 3-way stopcock and a 20-cc. syringe with saline solution), pressure transducer, or strain gauge is tested and connected to the 6-inch length of soft rubber tubing. This unit is set aside temporarily.

The patient is again cautioned about side effects and the necessity to control respirations. A 10-cm., 18-gauge spinal needle with stylet is chosen and inspected for burrs or other defects. Then it is inserted through the skin at the previously selected and anesthetized site of puncture. The patient is asked to hold his breath in the midpoint of a respiratory excursion, and the needle is advanced in one stroke toward the hilum of the spleen.

There are 2 methods for determining the exact direction of this single stroke of advancement of the needle. The first method is empiric but reliable. It involves lining up the point of puncture and the mark of the splenic hilum and introducing the needle in this direction but with about a 15° cephalad slant and a slight dorsal tilt for an average sized spleen. In cases of splenomegaly, the needle is directed somewhat more caudad and slightly anteriorly. In the other method, which is more direct, a target is selected under image amplification (such as the tip of a rib) that lines up the needle with the splenic hilum, and then the needle is advanced under continuous fluoroscopic control.[67] This could be further facilitated by the use of a television monitor. This latter technic need make no use of the skin marking of the splenic hilum, or it could be used as a double check. We have used this latter combination most often in recent years.

Once the splenic pulp is entered, no further resistance is encountered. The needle is advanced another 1 to 2 cm. in a normal-sized spleen, and 2 to 3 cm. in splenomegaly. Upon withdrawal of the stylet, the

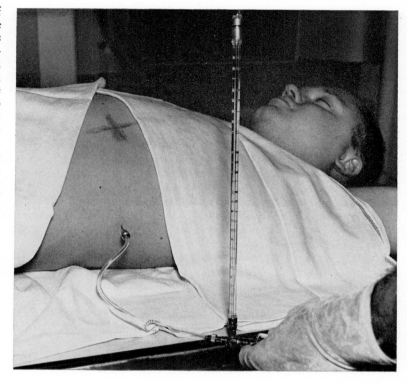

FIG. 10–2. Technic of percutaneous splenic pulp manometry. In this instance, the examination was performed in the x-ray department in conjunction with splenic portography. The zero point of the manometer has been placed at the level of the table (sterile drape removed for purposes of demonstration), and serial readings of splenic pulp pressure are being obtained.

operator releases his hold on the needle hub, and again the patient is instructed to resume gentle breathing. Failure to instruct the patient to resume breathing will prolong apnea beyond the few seconds necessary to insert the needle, and may result in a sudden involuntary deep inspiration. Subsequently during the course of the procedure whenever the needle is touched, the patient is instructed to stop breathing momentarily. If general anesthesia is being used, the anesthesiologist must produce controlled apnea when the needle is inserted, manipulated or removed. Complete control of the patient's respiratory motions and strict avoidance of touching the needle when the patient is breathing are the 2 key factors to safety in performing this study.

An immediate regular drop-by-drop return flow of blood from the freely swinging needle usually occurs, and indicates that the tip of the needle is within the splenic pulp. Rarely, a splenic pulp thrombus obstructs the lumen of the needle and prevents such initial backflow. In such an event, apnea is obtained again for a few seconds, and the needle is rotated along its long axis 180°. This usually results in a free backflow. Care is taken to prevent accumulation of such return flow of blood on the drapes.

Again the patient is instructed to hold his breath for the few seconds required to connect the previously assembled water manometer and tubing. The patient again breathes gently. The needle is cleared of any possible thrombus with an injection of 1 cc. of saline, and the zero point of the manometer is placed at table level (Fig. 10–2). Three sequential manometric determinations with intervening injections of 1 cc. of saline are then obtained. The meniscus is permitted to stabilize by free-fall from the 600-mm. level in the manometer but also is double-checked with a free-rise recording from a low level. The average of these readings is taken and corrected by subtracting 12 cm. This is the average distance from the table to the level of the anterior bodies of the 1st and 2nd lumbar vertebrae as measured in a series of 52 cadavers.[54] The 3 readings rarely vary by more than 2 cm. A normal range of splenic pulp pressure by this technic is 150 to 290 mm. saline. Some workers accept 250 mm. saline as the upper limit of normal.

Fifty cc. of 75 per cent Hypaque (warmed to body temperature) or 30 cc. of 50 per cent Hypaque for children is drawn into a 50-cc. Luer-Lok syringe. Caution is taken not to touch the plunger of the syringe to prevent the deposition of contrast medium or starch from the gloves. (Such a deposit could cause the plunger of the injecting syringe to "freeze.") The spring clip, normally employed to secure the plunger of the syringe, is removed to facilitate the rapid injecting technic. Then the syringe is attached to the special Becton-Dickinson flexible plastic tubing. (The use of the flexible tubing avoids a rigid unit, and thus prevents laceration of the splenic capsule as the needle subsequently swings with respiratory excursion. The Luer-Lok connections prevent "blowouts" during injection.) The plastic tubing is then filled with dye from the syringe. During a phase of voluntary apnea, the manometer and the tubing are disconnected from the needle, and the contrast-filled syringe and the flexible plastic tubing are connected quickly by the Luer-Lok. The patient resumes normal respiration.

Again, under image amplification 5 to 10 cc. of contrast medium is injected to test for good venous pickup of the contrast medium from the splenic pulp and the lack of significant extravasation, either pericapsular or back along the needle tract.

If these conditions are satisfied the procedure is then performed. If not, apnea is obtained again, and the needle is removed. Earlier maneuvers are repeated, and the needle is reinserted at a point 1 to 2 cm. from the previous puncture to minimize leakage from the first puncture site. This repeat test injection must confirm a satisfactory situation. For reasons of safety, no more than 3 punctures should be tried. Repeat puncture is indicated in about 1 of 20 examinations and is about 50 per cent successful.

Once a test injection is satisfactory under image amplification, the table top with the patient is moved back to the predetermined position over the Schonander rapid film changer. Forty or 45 cc. of 75 per cent

Hypaque is injected rapidly (10 to 15 seconds) by hand, and serial exposures are obtained. The needle is quickly removed while the patient holds his breath, and then he is allowed to resume normal breathing. Vital signs are checked. The films are developed and reviewed immediately. If extravasation is significant an additional film is then taken. In cases of failure, the study is never repeated the same day and at least a 48 hour interval is desirable.

The patient is returned to his room, kept at bed rest, and allowed only oral fluids until the next morning. Vital signs and serial hematocrit determinations are recorded at frequent, regular intervals.

Possible Modifications of this Technic

Of the many suggested modifications of the above technic, the following few merit special comment. (1) The use of a plastic hubbed needle,[2, 43, 71] that is, a needle within a plastic catheter, offers some definite advantages. Although its advocates stress the theoretical advantages of catheter flexibility in minimizing splenic laceration and bleeding, it seems to us that this flexibility obviates the far more common problem of pericapsular extravasation and retrograde injection of contrast medium back along the needle tract. By introducing a relatively soft flexible catheter through a splenic capsular puncture hole of smaller diameter than the outer diameter of the catheter, a "tight fit" should be created and maintained at the capsular level and a "tract" would be much less likely to develop than with a rigid metal needle. The use of such a plastic hubbed catheter holds promise and indeed we have recently adopted its use on a trial basis.

(2) The various technics for improving radiographic definition of vascular structures and for lessening post-portography splenic oozing, or both, such as an infusion of vasopressin[29] or the application of tourniquets to both thighs,[16] pose different problems. Both technics should improve the radiographic image but only at the price of completely disturbing the fundamental pathophysiology under study and thus compromising the fullest clinical usefulness of a then purely anatomic study. A splenic portogram obtained during pharmacologically

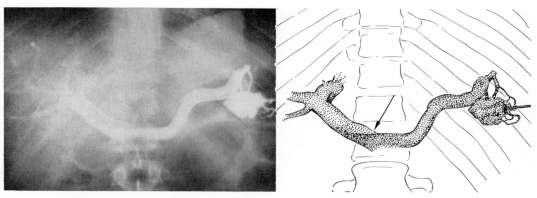

FIG. 10–4. Streamline phenomenon. This normal splenoportogram with accompanying diagrammatic interpretation demonstrates a radiolucent, linear streak (*arrow*) within an otherwise well-opacified and clearly defined portal vein. This hydraulic phenomenon is the result of nonmixing of the opacified blood from the splenic pulp and the nonopacified blood from the mesenteric veins. This is to be distinguished from partial thrombosis of the portal vein.

tortuosity, to become confluent with the portal vein. The angle of confluence is usually 90° to 150°; occasionally it is much more acute.[24, 25] Occasionally, the normal splenic vein is sigmoidal and dilated if during injection of the dye the injecting needle within the impaled spleen is pushed medially several centimeters, resulting in buckling of this vessel. This may occur naturally due to massive splenomegaly with resulting displacement of the vessel.

The portal vein is normally the largest vein of the portal system. It is generally straight in its course, either tubular or tapering slightly as it courses to its hepatoproximal termination and bifurcation. The walls of the normal vessel are sharply defined. Radiolucent linear streaks within an otherwise well-opacified and clearly defined portal vein represent the streaming phenomenon[55, 68] (Fig. 10–4). This physical, hydraulic phenomenon occurs because the density of the contrast-medium opacifying blood from the splenic pulp differs greatly from that of the nonopacified blood from the mesenteric vessels, preventing rapid mixing and allowing for layering. This initially appears as streaks of unmixed dye and blood. This may be mistaken for partial thrombosis of the portal vein, a condition that results in scalloped or notched irregularities, with radiolucencies along the wall of the vein

and occasionally within its lumen as well.

Not to be confused further with such irregularities of the wall of the portal vein are the radiolucent cupped defects occasionally identifiable as the site of entrance of the major mesenteric tributaries of the splenoportal axis. These occur especially at the entrance of the superior mesenteric and inferior mesenteric veins into the portal vein and actually represent simply another expression of the streamlining or nonmixing phenomenon.

As described, these major tributaries of the splenic and the portal veins normally are not opacified, except for an occasional slight transient reflux of contrast medium 1 to 2 cm. into either the inferior or the superior mesenteric vein visualized on one or two of the series of films. This normal variant is thought to be due to mild or transient elevations of portal pressure, possibly secondary to straining during the procedure and in no way is thought to represent hepatofugal flow of blood.

Both right and left branches of the portal vein and, rarely, the caudate branch may be visualized. Most frequently, the right branch is completely opacified. Indeed, frequently, the left lobe is not visualized at all. This appears to be merely a gravitational phenomenon, related to the patient's supine position, in which the right hepatic lobe is more dorsal than the left. Since the contrast medium has a high specific gravity, it flows preferentially to the right lobe.[7] Conversely, in the prone position, the left lobe is visualized more selectively.[8]

In the presinusoidal phase, the intrahepatic portal radicles are seen as a symmetrical, orderly, regular arborization of vessels in diminishing order of caliber. During sinusoidal transit of the contrast medium, the liver silhouette is diffusely opacified with little or no vessel structure apparent.

Splenic Portogram in Intrahepatic Obstruction

Probably the earliest portographic sign of intrahepatic obstruction is the distorted and uneven vasculogram and hepatogram phase observed in cases of portal cirrhosis that are as yet uncomplicated by frank portal hypertension.[62, 67] In such instances, the total obstructive element due to disruption of intrahepatic architecture has not progressed to the stage at which portal pressure is elevated and hepatofugal flow develops. Frequently, before the advent of portal hypertension, a sparse, irregular and patchy distortion of the vascular pattern within the liver (Fig. 10–5) and a mottled hepatogram phase pattern are seen (Fig. 10–6). No consistent presinusoidal or sinusoidal phase pattern has emerged from such studies to delineate the type of pathologic lesion (Laennec's cirrhosis, postnecrotic cirrhosis, biliary cirrhosis, schistosomal cirrhosis, etc.).

In more advanced cirrhosis, severe intrahepatic obstruction to the portal flow may result in portal hypertension (25 to 30 per cent) and a favoring of retrograde flow of splanchnic blood via preformed or newly developed portasystemic communications. As a result of this hepatofugal or reversed flow the contrast medium may opacify any or all of the tributaries of the splenoportal axis or a countless variety of newly evolved collaterals.

Despite this common pathophysiologic

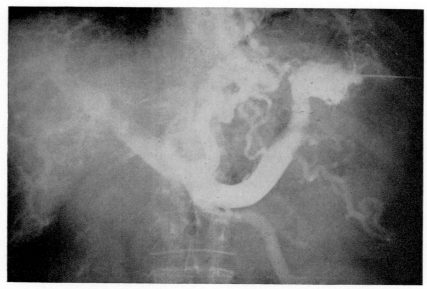

Fig. 10–5. Obstructive pattern in cirrhosis with portal hypertension. I. M. (Chart No. 132129). This 68-year-old woman was admitted following her second episode of upper gastrointestinal hemorrhage. Splenic pulp pressure was 350 mm. saline. Splenoportography reveals gastroesophageal varices and an inferior mesenteric collateral. Of special interest is the intrahepatic vasculogram phase which demonstrates considerable vascular distortion with marked deformity of the larger vessels and a paucity of smaller branches with an interlacing effect.

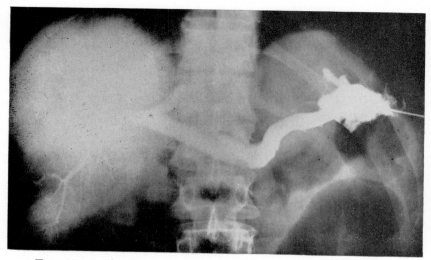

Fig. 10–6. Obstructive pattern in cirrhosis without portal hypertension. The distorted, patchy, mottled and uneven hepatogram sinusoidal phase of the portogram is seen in this patient with documented cirrhosis uncomplicated by portal hypertension with collateralization.

TABLE 10–1. DISTRIBUTION OF COLLATERAL SYSTEMS

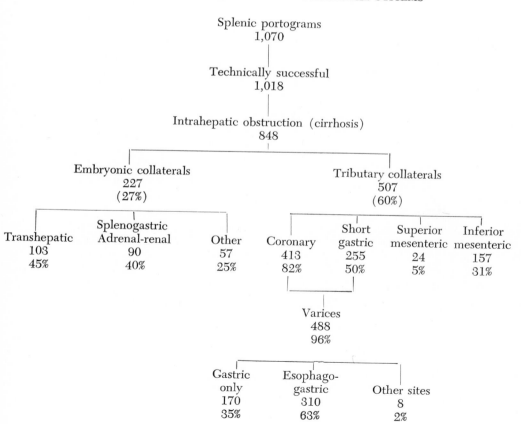

Splenic portograms
1,070

Technically successful
1,018

Intrahepatic obstruction (cirrhosis)
848

Embryonic collaterals   Tributary collaterals
227   507
(27%)   (60%)

Transhepatic   Splenogastric   Other   Coronary   Short   Superior   Inferior
103   Adrenal-renal   57   413   gastric   mesenteric   mesenteric
45%   90   25%   82%   255   24   157
               40%   50%   5%   31%

Varices
488
96%

Gastric   Esophago-
only   gastric   Other sites
170   310   8
35%   63%   2%

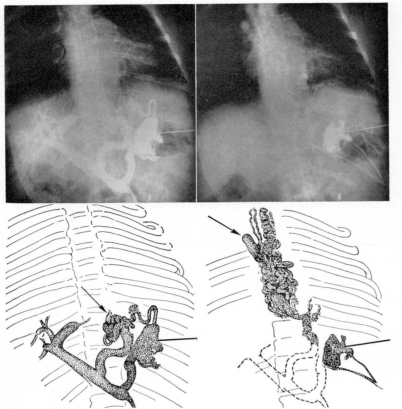

FIG. 10–7. The Coronary - gastroesophageal-azygos portasystemic collateral channel, M. I. (Chart No. 069145). This 76-year-old woman was admitted because of ascites and peripheral edema. She had never bled and was not anemic. Needle biopsy of the liver revealed postnecrotic cirrhosis. Splenic pulp pressure was 390 mm. saline. Splenic portography reveals a large coronary vein, filling massive gastroesophageal varices (*left*) which are seen to drain into the azygos vein (*right*). No surgical prophylactic intervention was advised; with resolution of ascites on a medical regimen, she was discharged to follow-up at our clinic.

basis, splenic portography in intrahepatic obstruction with portal hypertension reveals a wide range of patterns of diversion of portal blood away from the liver to the systemic circulation. A representative group of variants are statistically tabulated in Table 10–1 and are described and illustrated below.

Tributary Collateral Systems. The clinically most important and statistically most frequent of such portal-systemic collateral channels is the coronary-gastroesophageal-azygos system (Fig. 10–7). The clinical importance of this form of portal bypass of the liver, is, of course, the dreaded rupture of a gastroesophageal varix or varices, with massive hemorrhage. In our experience, gastric varices are more commonly demonstrated by portography than esophageal varices, occurring in more than 90 per cent of patients with a coronary-gastroesophageal-azygos collateral system. Gastric varices alone are present in 35 per cent of cases,

Esophageal varices have been visualized in only 65 per cent of patients in whom such portal-systemic collateralization has been documented by portography. A possible explanation of this phenomenon is that the contrast medium has become diluted before reaching the esophageal plexus, or that blood from gastric varices can be shunted directly to retroperitoneal veins, bypassing the esophageal plexus as suggested from our postmortem venographic studies.

The short gastric-gastroesophageal-azygos collateral venous system is only a variant of the coronary system, with blood being shunted away from the liver from the splenoportal axis via perisplenic vessels to the short gastric vessels and then on to the submucosal plexus of the stomach (Fig. 10–8). Frequently, the coronary and short gastric vessels simultaneously drain into gastroesophageal varices, which reach the systemic circulation by way of the azygos vein.

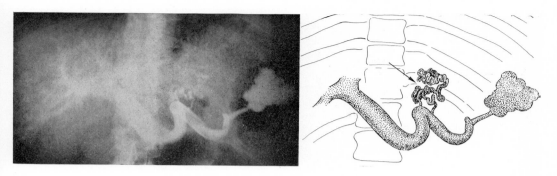

FIG. 10–8. The short gastric-gastroesophageal azygos portasystemic collateral channel. F. M. (Chart No. 114889). This 43-year-old nonalcoholic man was first admitted April 25, 1960, with ascites and peripheral edema with no history or evidence of bleeding. Needle biopsy of the liver revealed portal cirrhosis. Splenic pulp pressure was 380 mm. saline. The splenic portogram demonstrates a moderate-sized collection of gastric varices arising from short gastric vessels (arrow). There is no visualization of a coronary vein. Following diuresis, the patient was discharged, only to return subsequently with massive fatal hemorrhage.

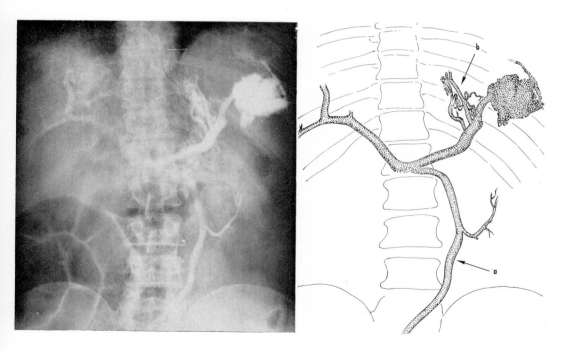

FIG. 10–9. Inferior mesenteric collateral system. J. C. (Chart No. 74760). This 53-year-old male was admitted with first episode of hematemesis and melena. Hepatomegaly, icterus and ascites were present on admission. Splenic pulp pressure was 396 mm. saline. Splenoportography demonstrates an extensive collateral channel via the inferior mesenteric venous system (a) extending into the pelvis. Gastric varices are seen to fill via the short gastric network of veins (b). The hemorrhage was managed successfully with tamponade and blood replacement, but the patient's general condition deteriorated, and he lapsed into coma and died.

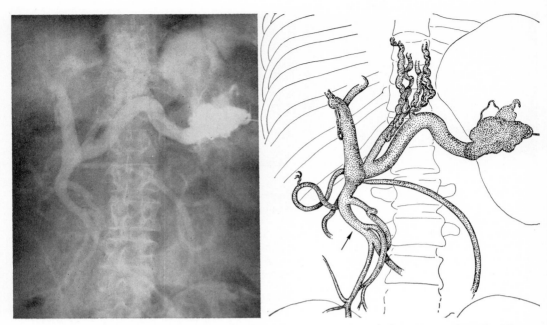

Fig. 10–10. Superior mesenteric collateral system. M. B. (Chart No. 050137). This 65-year-old nonalcoholic woman was admitted because of upper gastrointestinal hemorrhage. There was no evidence of stigmata of hepatic disease. Gastrointestinal series was uninformative. Splenic pulp pressure was 440 mm. saline. The portogram reveals the rather rare large superior mesenteric collateral (*arrow*), in addition to the extensive gastroesophageal varices that are filled by both the coronary and the short gastric vessels. The patient underwent an end-to-side portacaval shunt with a postshunt portal pressure of 280 mm. saline. This decompression of the portal bed has protected her from repeat hemorrhage in the 7½ year period of follow-up to date. At age 72, she is leading a normally active life.

The venous channels visualized in the gastroesophageal area are usually the submucosal varicosities and are of grave clinical importance. In addition to the submucosal esophageal varices, peri-esophageal vessels are frequently visualized.

For a classic analysis of varices, refer to Ruzicka's detailed evaluation of visualization of varices, diagnostic accuracy of splenoportography, radiographic characteristics of submucosal, perigastric, and peri-esophageal varices, and the rarer sites of varical complexes.[66]

The next most common collateral system noted is over the inferior mesenteric vein (Fig. 10–9). This most usually is visualized concomitant with some other form of collateralization, especially the gastroesophageal varices channel. Retrograde flow into the superior mesenteric, gastroepiploic, omental and pancreatic veins is visualized less frequently (Fig. 10–10).

Most of such backflow of blood from mesenteric, gastroepiploic, omental and pancreatic branches is assumed to eventually enter the systemic circulation through the usually functional communications at the level of the normal small portal-systemic venous communications, hemorrhoidal plexus and retroperitoneal areas in continuity with intra-abdominal viscera. Such communications are rarely visualized by splenoportography, because of their low flow rate involving a small volume of contrast medium which is further diluted by the tortuous length of these collaterals.

Embryonic Collateral Pathways. In addition to such diversion of portal blood by reversed flow into these normally patent venous tributaries of the portal system, splanchnic blood may bypass the liver in a hepatofugal fashion by opening closed, or partially closed, embryonic channels. This occurred in 227 (27 per cent) of our cir-

FIG. 10–11. The transhepatic collateral system. M. K. (Chart No. 189528). This 58-year-old alcoholic woman was admitted with a varical hemorrhage. Splenic pulp pressure was 310 mm. saline. The portogram demonstrates not only varices (better on earlier films of this study) but also a prominent transhepatic collateral (*arrow*), arising from the left portal and passing toward the umbilical area. There was no periumbilical hum or thrill. An end-to-side shunt was performed and she has done very well for the 3½ years of follow-up.

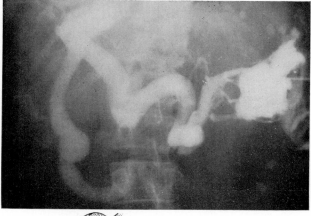

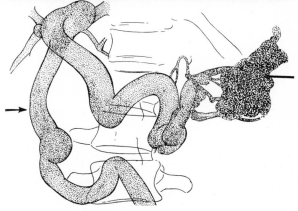

rhotic patients and were of 3 main types. In 45 per cent of such cases, the left intrahepatic branch of the portal vein communicates via the para-umbilical and the deep epigastric veins with the iliac veins and the vena cava (Cruveilhier-Baumgarten syndrome). The absolute incidence of this collateral may well be greater than our experience documents since routine portography in the supine position results in gravitational selective visualization of the right intrahepatic portal branch. If studies are done in the prone position,[49a] with more selective filling of the left intrahepatic portal branch, a higher incidence of visualization of the umbilical vein should be anticipated. We have designated this as the transhepatic collateral system (Fig. 10–11). In approximately 40 per cent of embryonic channels (Fig. 10–12) there is a splenic diversion into the left renal vein, frequently via the left adrenal vein. In the remaining 25 per cent of these embryonic collaterals, the final site of portal-systemic communications cannot be determined (Fig. 10–13).

Despite the frequent extreme size of these so-called natural shunts, they do not decompress a hypertensive portal venous system and do not prevent gastroesophageal varices or severe varical hemorrhage. The average portal pressure for a subgroup of these 227 patients previously reported was 390 mm.; the incidence of varices, 85 per cent; and the incidence of varical hemorrhage, 70 per cent. These vessels appear to shunt a sizeable volume of blood but via dilated and tortuous pathways, at low rates of flow, with considerable eddying. In short, they cannot alleviate portal hypertension.[63]

Splenic Portogram in Extrahepatic Obstruction

The hallmark of simple extrahepatic obstruction is the development of bridging

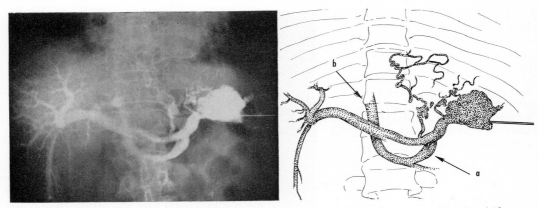

Fig. 10–12. Splenic–left adrenal–renal embryonic collateral system. C. R. (Chart No. 098962). This 72-year-old man was admitted with hepatomegaly, nausea and vomiting. He had never bled. Liver biopsy revealed portal cirrhosis. Splenic pulp pressure was 260 mm. saline. The splenic portogram reveals a natural shunt via an embryonic pathway via the left adrenal-renal vein (a) to the inferior vena cava (b). There is evidence of varices arising from the short gastric vessels. The patient subsequently died apparently from a heart attack without ever bleeding.

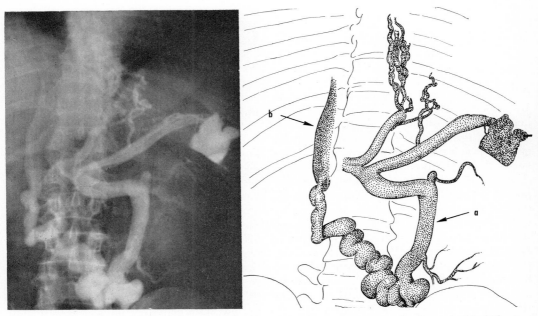

Fig. 10–13. Unidentifiable site of embryonic portasystemic communications. A. M. (Chart No. 114311). This 67-year-old alcoholic was admitted because of progressive ascites without bleeding. Needle biopsy of the liver revealed portal cirrhosis. Splenic pulp pressure was 430 mm. saline. Splenic portography demonstrates a large natural shunt (a) extending into the left pelvis with tortuous communications with the inferior vena cava (b). The portal vein is not visualized. As indicated in the text, this does not confirm complete thrombosis of the portal vein but rather may simply represent a hemodynamic variant.

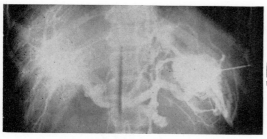
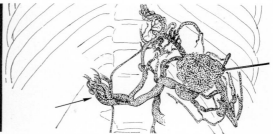

FIG. 10–14. Cavernomatous transformation of the portal vein. S. K. (Chart No. 126669). This 11-year-old child was referred for admission because of bright-red hematemesis. Physical examination and gastrointestinal series were unremarkable. Liver chemistries were normal. Splenic pulp pressure was 340 mm. saline. Splenoportography demonstrates extensive gastroesophageal varices with cavernomatous transformation of the portal vein with a convoluted agglomeration of venous structures (*arrow*) replacing the normal single portal vein. Gastroesophageal varices are demonstrated. At operation, a Marion procedure (caval mesenteric shunt) was accomplished.

collaterals. These collateral vessels initially exhibit retrograde flow but only proximal to the site of obstruction. The flow pattern then reverts to an essentially hepatopetal type. Accordingly the splenoportographic pattern of extrahepatic obstructive portal hypertension varies according to the degree and the anatomic site of obstruction. The intricate and frequently bizarre collateral network that develops proximal to the site of obstruction depends on whether the block is proximal or distal to normally occurring tributaries of the splenoportal axis, or potentially available embryonic pathways of collateralization.

Of course, the transhepatic collateral is never visualized in cases of extrahepatic obstruction, since this portal-systemic communication originates from the left branch of the portal vein (intrahepatic). The degree of obstruction is reflected in greatly delayed, minimal or even absent opacification of the intrahepatic portal radicles, which are filled only via bridging collaterals, along the gastrohepatic omentum to the liver capsule. However, failure of the contrast medium to visualize the portal vein or to opacify the liver is not absolute evidence of an extrahepatic block, as is discussed subsequently.

Occasionally, intrahepatic and extrahepatic obstruction coexist, as in cirrhosis (intrahepatic obstruction) with acquired portal vein thrombosis (extrahepatic obstruction).

Extrahepatic obstructive patterns are frequently identifiable as specific pathologic entities and may be either congenital or acquired, such as portal vein thrombosis, cavernomatous transformation of the portal vein, agenesis or stenosis of the portal vein, splenic vein thrombosis or, rarely, bifid veins or veins with endovenous septa.

Congenital Lesions. These are usually manifest in infancy and childhood.

Cavernomatous transformation of the portal vein results in a pattern of mottled opacification of a convoluted agglomeration of racemose venous structures that have replaced the normal single portal (or rarely splenic) vein (Fig. 10–14). The contrast-ladened blood from the spleen is seen to flow toward the cavernoma, frequently with only a small aliquot passing through it to the liver, but a large portion of the splanchnic flow is diverted away from the site of obstruction via collateral vessels, usually the coronary-gastroesophageal-azygos system. This is a pathologic as well as a roentgen entity.[35]

In stenosis, aplasia or agenesis of the portal vein the portal vein is not visualized as such but clearly defined, large, linear and tortuous bridging collaterals develop along the right border of the gastrohepatic ligament, around the common bile duct and in the retroperitoneal area, between the liver and the duodenum (Fig. 10–15). Again, in this form of extrahepatic portal obstruction, a large portion of the splanchnic flow is de-

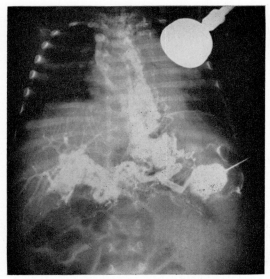
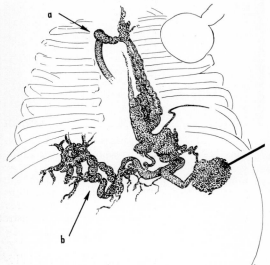

Fig. 10–15. Portal vein stenosis or agenesis. M. M. (Chart No. 125824). This 16-month-old child was referred for splenic portography. At time of premature birth at another hospital, he was noted to have ascites and hepatosplenomegaly. There was no umbilical infection. At age 10 months, the patient was severely anemic and ascitic with evidence of hypersplenism. Liver chemistries were normal. Barium swallow revealed varices. The child had massive gastroesophageal varices and the azygos was visualized (*a*). Large bridging collaterals replaced the stenosed portal vein (*b*).

flected away from the liver via the coronary-gastroesophageal-azygos system.

Other rare anomalies of the portal vein include aneurysm, a location anterior to the duodenum and pancreas, double portal vein, bifid vein, endovenous septa and direct drainage into the inferior vena cava.

Acquired Lesions. The primary acquired condition is thrombosis, which may be complete or incomplete and either localized or involving any or all segments of the spleno-portal axis. Most commonly it is a complication of cirrhosis, with a 5 to 10 per cent incidence of at least partial portal vein bland thrombosis. It is commonly found in cirrhosis complicated by hepatoma. We have been fortunate in studying, via 3 splenic portograms, over an 11-month period, the evolution of an incomplete thrombus (Fig. 10–16). Acquired obstructions may also occur secondary to pylephlebitis, pancreatitis, pancreatic cyst, trauma or tumor.

Portal Vein Thrombosis. Complete thrombosis of the portal vein generally results in a pattern of collateral vessels similar to that seen in agenesis of the portal vein. The entire vessel may be obliterated with bridging collaterals developing either between

Fig. 10–16. Evolution of portal vein thrombosis. M. C. (Chart No. 12951). This 76-year-old woman was admitted because of repeated episodes of upper gastrointestinal hemorrhage and intractable ascites. Splenic pulp pressure was 480 mm. saline. Splenic portography November, 1956 (A) revealed short gastric vessels leading to a small collection of varices. The portal vein was normal. Because of the patient's advanced age and general condition, she was denied surgery. She was readmitted April, 1957, with recurrent hemorrhage. Splenic portography (B) now revealed extensive varices and an indentation or mural thrombus on the lateral wall (*arrow*) of the portal vein. In October, 1957, the patient bled again, and splenic portography (C) now revealed typical notching and irregularity of intraluminal thrombosis of the portal vein (*arrow*).

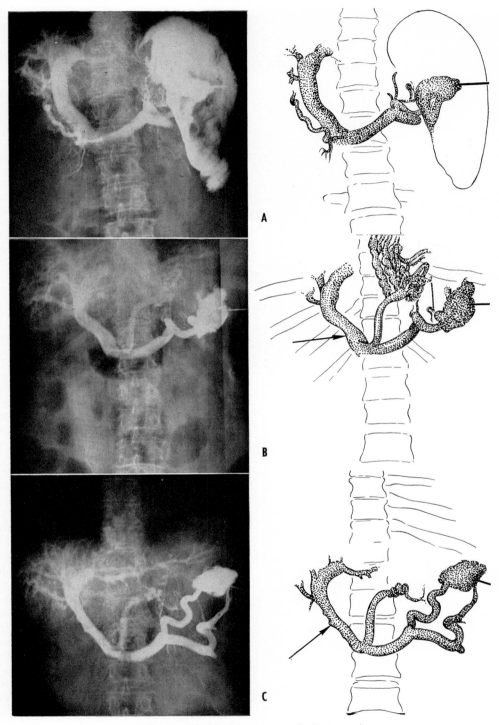

FIGURE 10–16. (*Caption on facing page*)

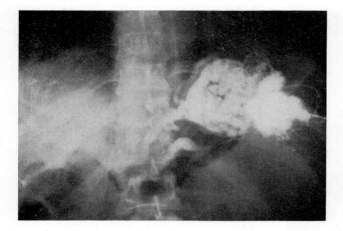

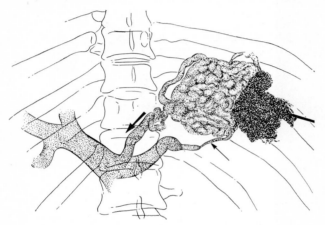

FIG. 10–17. Splenic vein occlusion. M. L. (Chart No. 156476). This 51-year-old male alcoholic was admitted with a varical hemorrhage. There was splenomegaly but no other stigmata of liver disease. Liver chemistries were near normal values. The splenic pulp pressure was 500 mm. saline. The portogram illustrates splenic vein obstruction (*small arrow*) with channeling of splenic venous flow in a retrograde fashion through the short gastric veins into a massive conglomeration of gastric varices. This varical complex is drained via the coronary vein (*large arrow* indicating direction of flow determined by serial films) into the portal vein and then on to the liver.

As developed in the text, this indicates that there is no portal vein or intrahepatic obstruction and that the only site of obstruction is in the splenic vein. In this case it was secondary to pancreatitis with cyst formation in the tail of the pancreas. The patient was treated by splenectomy which cured the hemodynamic problem and by caudad pancreatico-cystectomy which cured the underlying local problem. He has not bled again in the more than 5 years of follow-up.

the splenic vein and liver, superior mesenteric vein and liver, or, rarely, coronary vein and liver. Since these attempts to span the obstruction and carry blood to the liver are functionally inadequate, hepatofugal patterns of collateralization are typically visualized also, arising from any previously described embryonal or tributary pathway.

Incomplete portal vein thrombosis results in scalloped or notched irregularities and radiolucencies along the wall margins of the vein and occasionally within its lumen. Frequently the splenic vein is dilated and the diameter of the portal vein decreases. Occasionally calcification of the vein wall and recanalization are detected. May we reiterate that partial thrombosis of the portal vein should not be confused with the streamlined phenomenon, or the concave defects seen at the site of entrance of the tributaries of the portal vein.

Simple nonvisualization of the portal vein is not evidence of thrombotic occlusion. Indeed in more than 85 per cent of all such cases the portal vein is anatomically patent. A functional variation in local hemodynamics may result in nonvisualization, a point of great clinical significance since a direct portacaval anastomosis is feasible. This problem is discussed at greater length under Limitations of Splenic Portography.

Splenic Vein Thrombosis. Again bridging collaterals are characteristic, although in this situation they span the obstruction between the splenic and portal veins. Typically, bypass is via tributary and not embryonal collaterals: (a) from the splenic pulp deposit to short gastric and gastric varices then via the coronary vein to the portal vein or (b) from the splenic pulp deposit to the gastroepiploic to superior mesenteric vein to portal vein. Again these attempts at bridg-

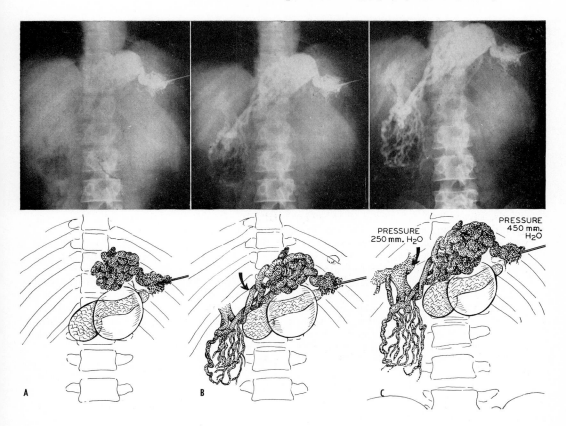

FIG. 10–18. Portal normotension with segmental splenic hypertension. P. T. (Chart No. 125322). This 41-year-old man had undergone exploratory laparotomy at another hospital for intermittent tarry stools. Exploration was normal except for splenomegaly. The liver was unremarkable. The patient continued to bleed postoperatively and was referred for further evaluation. Liver chemistries were normal. Splenic pulp pressure was 450 mm. saline. The splenic portogram reveals (A) a deposit of dye in the splenic pulp with rapid filling of massive gastric varices. However, subsequent exposures (B) and (C) demonstrate that the direction of flow in these varices is normal, i.e., to the liver. Contrast medium is seen to reach the portal vein (*arrow*) via bridging collaterals with opacification of the liver. Thus the portographic criteria of portal hypertension are not met, since there is normal hepatopetal flow of splanchnic blood.

A preoperative diagnosis of splenic vein obstruction with segmental splenic hypertension and portal venous system normotension was made. At operation the portal pressure was found to be normal (250 mm.) and the splenic vein was compressed and occluded by a pancreatic cyst, as shown in the diagrammatic representation. A cyst-jejunostomy was performed. The segmental splenic hypertension was cured by splenectomy. This case illustrates the importance of careful application of the hemodynamic principles of diagnosis previously discussed. It also poses a problem of the occasional patient whose elevated splenic pulp pressure determination gives a false impression of portal hypertension and requires portographic examination for definitive diagnosis.

ing the site of obstruction are usually functionally inadequate and hepatofugal collateralization occurs, arising proximal to the obstruction (Figs. 10–17 and 10–18).

Segmental Splenic Hypertension. Isolated splenic vein obstruction, at a point splenoproximal to the coronary and/or the superior mesenteric vein, can result in the interesting and clinically important situation of segmental splenic hypertension. Under

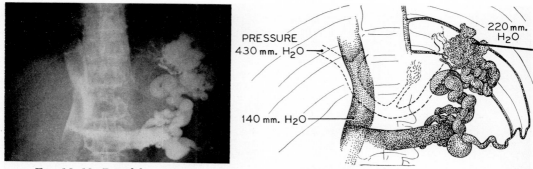

Fig. 10–19. Portal hypertension with segmental splenic normotension. M. McM. (Chart No. 140364). This 57-year-old alcoholic male was admitted with a 2-day history of hematemesis. Liver chemistries were grossly abnormal. There were multiple stigmata of chronic liver dysfunction. GI series with esophagram was noninformative. Splenic pulp pressure was 220 mm. saline. Splenoportography demonstrated a large tortuous splenorenal collateral which drained both into intercostal vessels to the hemiazygos system, and more importantly into the left renal vein to the inferior vena cava.

At exploratory laparotomy the liver was grossly cirrhotic. The portal pressure was found to be 430 mm. Portal portography revealed a small but normal patent portal vein with a coronary vein and varices (diagrammatically represented by the superimposed dotted line outline). This situation was interpreted to represent intrahepatic block with portal hypertension. In contrast with the previous case (Fig. 10–18), portal hypertension was present in the face of segmental decompression of the spleen or part of the spleen by the splenorenal venous communication. However, this splenorenal natural shunt was ineffectual in decompressing the portal system and preventing varical hemorrhage. An end-to-side portacaval shunt was effected as treatment for the portal hypertension.

these conditions, the pressure in the splanchnic venous system splenoproximal to the point of obstruction is elevated, while splenodistal to the obstruction (in the portal vein), it is normal. Varices and a coronary vein may well be visualized by portography, but serial films or cineradiography indicate that the flow in the coronary vein is in the normal direction toward the portal vein and liver. Thus the coronary vein must be beyond the site of obstruction, that is, the splenic vein. Clinically, this is a most important distinction, since obviously a portacaval shunt under such circumstances would aggravate the condition and facilitate still greater flow through the varical complex. The indicated treatment is twofold: (1) splenectomy which removes the only venous structures splenoproximal to the obstruction that can drain into the varical system, and (2) treatment of the underlying process that resulted in the venous obstruction (e.g., caudal pancreatectomy, excision of splenic artery aneurysm, drainage of pancreatic cyst).

The opposite situation of *segmental splenic normotension* with portal hypertension is fortunately rare. This occurs if a large, naturally occurring shunt decompresses the splenic area so that the pulp pressure reading is normal. Radiographically the large splenic natural shunt is always visualized and the remainder of the splenoportal system usually is not. The situation can be clarified by documenting portal hypertension by other radiographic technics such as the venous phase of superior mesenteric arteriography or by direct determination of the portal venous pressure at laparotomy. If the portal venous system is visualized it will indicate hepatofugal collateralization generally via the coronary varical system. Although effective in segmentally lowering splenic venous pressure, such a situation has consistently (7 cases) proved ineffectual in decompressing the portal system and preventing varical hemorrhage (Fig. 10–19).

Extrinsic Obstructive Factors. Extravascular compression by tumor or direct vessel invasion by carcinoma of biliary or pancreatic origin occasionally completely obstructs either the splenic or the portal veins.

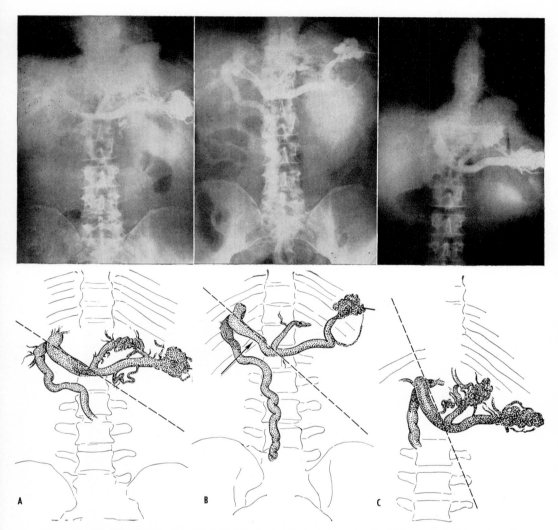

Fig. 10–20. Displacement of portal vein by hepatoma. A. F. (Chart No. 77368). This 49-year-old alcoholic male was first seen because of ascites in April, 1958. Liver chemistries were grossly abnormal. Needle biopsy of the liver revealed Laennec's cirrhosis. Gastrointestinal series was unremarkable. Splenic pulp pressure was 310 mm. saline, and splenoportogram (A) showed gastroesophageal varices, a large transhepatic collateral and a normal portal vein.

The patient was readmitted February, 1959, free of ascites for elective inguinal herniorrhaphy. Follow-up splenic pulp pressure was 322 mm. Splenoportogram (B) revealed indentation of lateral wall of portal vein, suggestive of extrinsic pressure or intraluminal filling defect. There was also minimal change in the angulation of the portal vein's long axis.

The patient was readmitted October, 1960, because of right upper-quadrant abdominal pain. The alkaline phosphatase was 20.2 B.U. Splenic pulp pressure was 320 mm. Splenoportography (C) now revealed severe shift of the portal vein axis to a more vertical direction, suggesting extrinsic pressure or displacement of the portal vein.

In November, 1960, the patient hemorrhaged for the first time and died. At postmortem examination, hepatoma of the right lobe of the liver was found to be displacing the portal vein.

The splenoportal axis may be displaced, constricted or distorted, with incomplete obstruction, as a sequel to expanding tumors in these same sites (Fig. 10–20).

Combined Intra- and Extrahepatic Obstruction. Alcoholic patients are occasionally encountered with both cirrhosis (intrahepatic block) and pancreatitis or pancreatic cysts with splenic vein obstruction (extrahepatic block). Then both splenic segmental hypertension and generalized portal hypertension are evident. We have seen only 2 such cases. Neither splenectomy alone (for the splenic component) nor portacaval shunt alone (for the generalized portal component) is adequate treatment of the condition; both must be performed as well as possible surgical correction of the local obstructing lesion.

Of course, in the much more common situation of cirrhosis (intrahepatic block) and bland portal vein thrombosis (extrahepatic block), the splenic portographic pattern represents no diagnostic problem. Therapy need not be directed at 2 components since the extrahepatic obstruction has not resulted in segmentation of the splenoportal axis.

The Splenic Portogram for Other Conditions

Neoplasia

Primary and metastatic neoplasms of the liver are demonstrated sometimes by splenoportography.[67, 69] The sinusoidal or hepatogram phase might reveal radiolucent filling

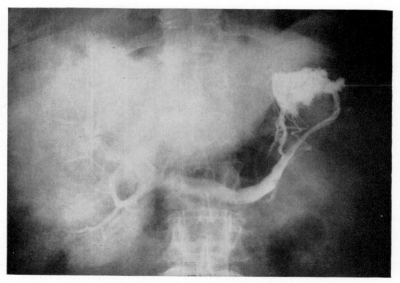

Fig. 10–21. Metastatic carcinoma of the liver. T. H. (Chart No. 96846). This 65-year-old man was admitted with a 2-month history of watery diarrhea and weight loss. Examination revealed stenosing rectal carcinoma at 5 cm. from the anal verge. Alkaline phosphatase was 10.2 B.U. Splenic portography was performed in search of probable hepatic metastasis. Splenic pulp pressure was 283 mm. saline. Splenoportography included a vasculogram phase that showed definitely abnormal bowing and compression effect on several individual branches of the inferior portion of the right lobe. In the hepatogram phase (*above*), the right lateral margin of the liver is poorly defined, with irregular filling defects. The left lobe appears grossly normal. At laparotomy, the right lobe of the liver was riddled with metastases, especially in the inferior and lateral portions. The left lobe was uninvolved.

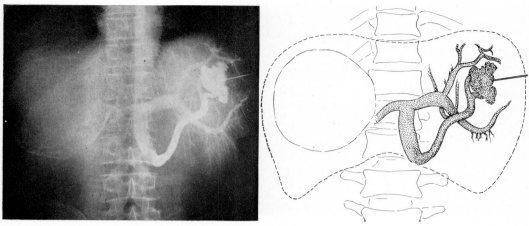

FIG. 10–22. Hydatid cyst of liver. The right lobe of the liver has been virtually completely replaced by the cyst, with nonvisualization of the intraparenchymal branching of the right portal vein. Accordingly, the left portal vein is visualized unusually well. The portal vein is displaced into a position more vertical than usual.

defects in an otherwise diffusely opacified liver (Fig. 10–21). The intrahepatic portal branches, or even the portal vein itself, may be displaced (Fig. 10–20).

Ruzicka discusses this problem at length.[67] He considers the sinusoidal phase to be most useful for the detection of neoplasms in the liver. Generally the lesion must be greater than 1.5 cm. in diameter, unless several smaller lesions have coalesced. He also states that this technic is limited in that usually the left lobe of the liver cannot be visualized. Hepatoscintigraphy, hepatic arteriography, retrograde hepatic venography and trans-

umbilical portography all seem to be superior technics for evaluating hepatic neoplasia.

Splenoportography is useful in occasional cases of hydatid cyst, portal vein aneurysm, hemangioma or amebic abscess of the liver (Fig. 10–22).[18, 42, 62, 73]

Shunt Patency

By splenoportography one can confirm closure or patency of a portacaval anastomotic shunt in the postshunt bleeder. If the shunt is patent and functioning, splenoportography outlines clearly the splenic vein,

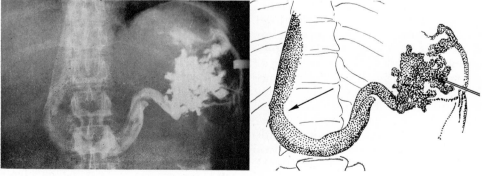

FIG. 10–23. Postshunt percutaneous splenic portogram. R. O. (Chart No. 113615). This 55-year-old woman was referred from another hospital for evaluation of post portacaval shunt bleeding. Splenic pulp pressure was 176 mm. saline. Splenoportography shows rapid flow through a widely open shunt (arrow) with good visualization of the inferior vena cava. Subsequent diagnostic studies revealed a peptic duodenal ulcer to be the site of bleeding.

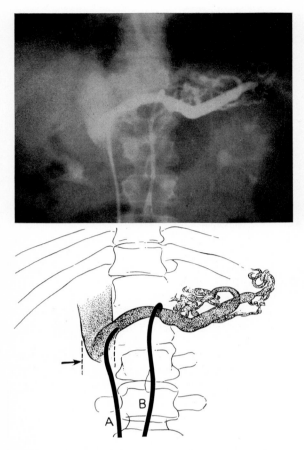

Fig. 10–24. Postshunt catheterization of the anastomosis. A. M. (Chart No. 137778). This 50-year-old man was readmitted for post portacaval shunt hemorrhage. Since he had undergone a previous splenectomy for hypersplenism, splenic portography was not possible. Catheter B was introduced into a femoral artery and threaded up the aorta into the superior mesenteric artery. The transcapillary venous phase of this study proved inadequate for evaluation of shunt patency so that the alternate venous study was performed. Catheter A was introduced percutaneously through a femoral vein and threaded up to and through the anastomosis. The force of retrograde injection had resulted in opacification of minute caudad peripancreatic vessels, but with the end of the pressure injection these vessels were seen to drain toward the widely patent anastomosis and vena cava (*arrow*). The pressure in the portal vein was normal.

the portal trunk, the site of anastomosis and the proximal inferior vena cava, without evidence of hepatofugal flow via collaterals (Fig. 10–23). If the shunt is closed or inadequate, persistent collateralization with retrograde flow over a collateral network is present, and the shunt is not visualized. Splenic pulp pressure determinations obtained as part of the portography study offer additional confirmation or negation of the patency of the shunt and the presence or absence of portal hypertension. Shunt patency can also be demonstrated by the transcapillary venous phase of selective splanchnic arteriography or by direct catheterization of the anastomosis via the femoral vein and inferior vena cava (Fig. 10–24).

LIMITATIONS OF SPLENIC PORTOGRAPHY

Sometimes splenic portography fails to render the desired information such as major vein patency and the presence and extent of portal collateralization. These situations may be enumerated as follows: (1) nonvisualization of portal vein or of both portal and splenic veins; (2) inconsistent findings in repeat examinations; (3) normal portographic pattern in spite of the presence of varices; (4) technical failure.

Nonvisualized Major Vein

The most common and clinically most significant limitation of splenic portography is the occasional failure of a technically satisfactory study to visualize the portal vein (Fig. 10–25) or even the entire splenoportal axis (Fig. 10–26).[19, 62] In this situation, there are no definite signs of thrombosis such as scalloped vessel margins, recanalization or especially bridging collateralization. There simply is no radiographic information available about the portal vein or portal and splenic veins. In the past nonvisualization was frequently assumed to

Fig. 10–25. The non-visualized but patent portal vein. C. K. (Chart No. 213189). This 54-year-old male had a long history of resistant ascites secondary to alcoholic cirrhosis. His splenic pulp pressure was 350 mm. saline. The portogram depicts (1) nonvisualization of the portal vein, (2) massive varices filling from a large coronary system, and (3) a varical—left adrenorenal natural shunt. Since the coronary vein was the collateral that resulted in such massive runoff, the splenic vein remained well visualized although the portal vein was not opacified. At the time of the side-to-side shunt, the portal vein proved patent, with a small flow toward the liver recorded by the electromagnetic flowmeter. He has remained free of ascites for the 2½ years of follow-up.

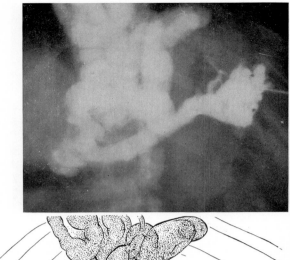

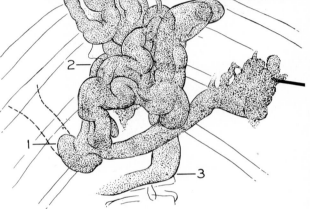

represent complete occlusion. On this basis, patients were denied even attempts at portacaval anastomosis. Subsequent surgical explorations or postmortem findings frequently demonstrated the complete patency and normalcy of the portal vein and portal and splenic veins. This experience prompted us to review this problem in 1965[19] about which we now have additional information and can interpret more clearly.

Statistical Data. In the current series of 1,018 technically successful splenic portograms, the portal vein was not visualized in 64 patients (6.3 per cent). In 53 of these 64 patients in whom anatomic patency of the vessel could be verified either at operation or at autopsy, the portal vein was proved to be patent in 44 cases (83 per cent). Of 265 patients whose condition both allowed and required portacaval shunt, in 36 cases (13.6 per cent) the portal vein was not visualized.

In these 36 patients requiring a decision regarding surgical intervention, the portal vein was found to be patent, despite radiographic nonvisualization, in 33 instances (92 per cent). (See schematic summary, Table 10–2.)

Further analysis indicates that for 13 of the 64 patients (22 per cent) with a nonvisualized portal vein, the splenic vein is also not visualized. Of particular importance is that 11 of these 13 patients (85 per cent) have a prominent spleno-adreno-renal shunt or an unidentifiable natural shunt arising from the splenic area.

In all the remaining 51 cases of isolated portal venous nonvisualization, the coronary-azygos system was prominent. A spleno-adreno-renal natural shunt was present in only 2 instances (4 per cent).

Theoretical Explanation. The several suggested explanations of this phenomenon

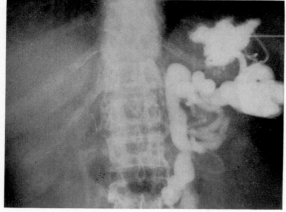

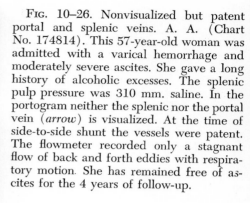

Fig. 10–26. Nonvisualized but patent portal and splenic veins. A. A. (Chart No. 174814). This 57-year-old woman was admitted with a varical hemorrhage and moderately severe ascites. She gave a long history of alcoholic excesses. The splenic pulp pressure was 310 mm. saline. In the portogram neither the splenic nor the portal vein (*arrow*) is visualized. At the time of side-to-side shunt the vessels were patent. The flowmeter recorded only a stagnant flow of back and forth eddies with respiratory motion. She has remained free of ascites for the 4 years of follow-up.

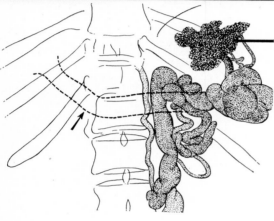

can be categorized into 3 theories. (1) Non-visualization is the simple result of the presence of a large collateral system through which contrast medium bypasses the splenic pulp. The point at which this collateral interposes along the course of the splenoportal axis determines the extent of nonvisualization. If it arises splenoproximal to the splenic vein, no part of the splenorenal axis is visualized. If it arises at the junction of the splenic and portal veins, the splenic vein is visualized but the portal is not. It would be further assumed that mesenteric "unstained" blood continues to flow primarily to the liver.

(2) This explanation concurs in part with the first but postulates further that the mesenteric "unstained" blood is primarily diverted away from the liver. With this assumption, if the dominant collateral arises splenoproximal to the splenic vein, some mesenteric blood might flow through a co-existing varical system and/or segmentally reverse its natural direction of flow and course back along the splenic vein to the splenic natural shunt. If the dominant collateral system vessel arises at the coronary level, mesenteric flow would be primarily over this route. In either collateral situation, the flow in the portal vein would be greatly diminished but toward the liver, and the flow in the splenic vein might even be segmentally reversed.

(3) It has been proposed that the contrast medium deposited in the spleen could not enter and opacify the portal vein or portal and splenic veins because of the stronger opposition of true reverse portal flow of hepatic arterial blood either perfusing the sinusoids or bypassing them via arteriovenous intrahepatic shunts and then coursing back down the portal vein.

From studies in cirrhotic patients including direct electromagnetic portal flow deter-

TABLE 10–2. DISTRIBUTION OF PATIENTS WITH NONVISUALIZATION
PHENOMENON

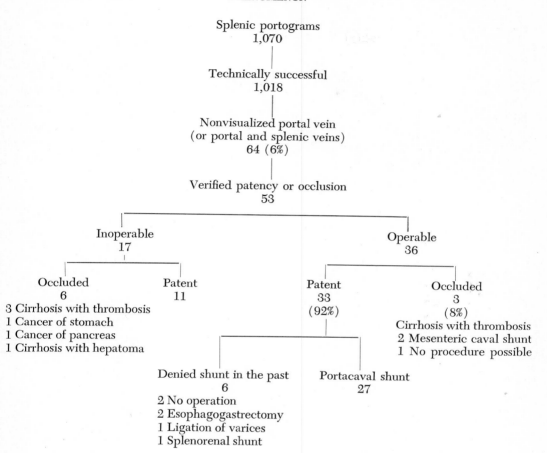

Splenic portograms
1,070

Technically successful
1,018

Nonvisualized portal vein
(or portal and splenic veins)
64 (6%)

Verified patency or occlusion
53

Inoperable
17

Operable
36

Occluded
6
3 Cirrhosis with thrombosis
1 Cancer of stomach
1 Cancer of pancreas
1 Cirrhosis with hepatoma

Patent
11

Patent
33
(92%)

Occluded
3
(8%)
Cirrhosis with thrombosis
2 Mesenteric caval shunt
1 No procedure possible

Denied shunt in the past
6
2 No operation
2 Esophagogastrectomy
1 Ligation of varices
1 Splenorenal shunt

Portacaval shunt
27

minations and special radiographic technics (hepatic intraparenchymal deposition of contrast and the venous phase of selective mesenteric arteriography), there has been accumulating evidence that this phenomenon of nonvisualization is best explained by the second of the above theories. The contrast-stained blood from the splenic deposit is diverted away from the liver by a strategically placed collateral interposed along the course of the splenoportal axis, and determining the extent of nonvisualization. However—and this is the key to the management of the problem—much of the mesenteric venous return is also diverted away from the liver, so that the flow of even "unstained" mesenteric blood through the

portal vein is greatly reduced or even ceases completely (Fig. 10–27, A and B).

This interpretation is supported by an earlier report of 92 direct electromagnetic flowmeter determinations of direction and volume of portal venous flow[45] and our current series of 128 such studies (Fig. 10–28). In no cases did we record a true reverse flow in the portal vein itself prior to anastomosis. These data do not support the third theory. In patients with a nonvisualized portal vein, portal flow was greatly reduced, slightly more than half the value of those shunted with a normally visualized portal vein. Those patients with both portal and splenic nonvisualization had still greater reduction in portal flow, less than half of

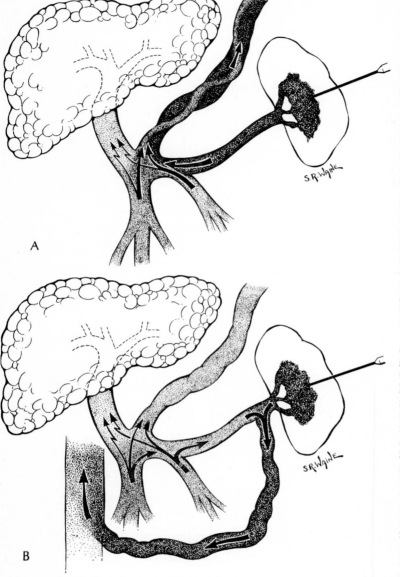

FIG. 10–27. Hemodynamic mechanism explaining the nonvisualization phenomenon. As explained in the text, accumulating evidence from different sources indicates the validity of the following explanation. (A) Nonvisualization of the portal vein but visualization of the splenic vein occurs when a particularly large coronary vein diverts from the liver nearly all the dye-stained blood after it has opacified the splenic vein. In addition, most of the mesenteric venous flow is likewise diverted although some small aliquot (*broken arrrows*) may continue towards the liver (cf. Fig. 10–25).
(B) Nonvisualization of both the portal and splenic veins occurs when a particularly large spleno-adreno-renal or other perisplenic natural shunt diverts from the liver the dye-stained blood at a point immediately beyond the splenic bolus. In addition, most of the mesenteric flow is likewise diverted from the liver, either through a coronary system and/or in a segmentally reversed manner along the splenic vein to the natural shunt. A small aliquot of mesenteric flow (*broken arrows*) may continue toward the liver (Cf. Fig. 10–26).

those with isolated portal nonvisualization, suggesting still further diversion of mesenteric flow away from the liver, and perhaps in a segmentally reverse flow back to the splenic natural shunt.

Our experience with more than 150 intrahepatic depositions of contrast medium supports the observation that spontaneous reverse flow in the portal vein does not occur or is extremely rare in cirrhosis even under circumstances of portal vein nonvisualization.[19, 46, 47, 49] This interpretation is confirmed by the fact that in the many hundreds of reported selective celiac or hepatic arteriograms there has never been a pre-shunt demonstration of reverse flow in the portal vein itself in cirrhosis, unless complicated by hepatic vein thrombosis (Budd-Chiari syndrome). The technic of intrahepatic deposition of contrast, also revealed that with peak pressures of injection reflux of contrast medium back down the portal vein could be made to occur regularly in cases of nonvisualization. With the completion of the disruptive injecting pressure, forward flow would be evident. This was interpreted to be indirect suggestive evidence of a severe reduction in portal venous inflow in the situation of portal nonvisualization confirming the theorized diversion of mesenteric flow.[19]

Portal portography has also demonstrated diversion of mesenteric flow away from the liver. In one of our cases the operative x-ray showed only the superior mesenteric vein and the coronary-varical system without any visualization of what subsequently proved to be a normal portal vein. In another case operative portal portography failed to visualize a patent portal vein and also showed segmental reverse flow of the mesenteric injection back along the splenic vein to a large spleno-adreno-renal natural shunt. This interpretation could be criticized legitimately since in portal portography vascular injection disrupts the underlying hemodynamic situation.

Yet this interpretation has been confirmed most emphatically by the venous phase of selective superior mesenteric arteriography. This technic is nondisruptive and does allow for a physiologic interpretation of the venous phase since the pressure of injection is dissipated with passage of the contrast medium through the intestinal capillary bed. Bron et al.[17] and Boijsen and Ekman[12] have each reported a case of splenoportographic nonvisualization of the entire splenoportal axis in which the venous phase of superior mesenteric arteriography revealed slight forward visualization of the portal vein and, most significantly, segmentally reversed flow of mesenteric blood back along the course of the splenic vein. We have experienced 3 similar cases, further documenting that mesenteric flow is largely diverted away from the liver in the situation of nonvisualization of major vessels.

Clinical Approach to this Problem. We

have entered into the above lengthy discussion of the hemodynamic situation in the nonvisualized major veins, and have particularly stressed the direction of mesenteric blood flow, because an understanding of these pathophysiologic data is necessary for a rational clinical approach to this seemingly difficult problem. If splenoportography, the usually reliable standard of diagnostics in portal hypertension, fails to provide information concerning patency of major veins and availability for a shunting procedure, the clinician has several alternate pathways of pursuing the problem. Traditionally it has been assumed that this phenomenon represents vessel occlusion and that a shunt is not feasible. However, in 92 per cent of such operable situations the portal vein is available for shunting. The clinician may decide to attempt further radiographic diagnostic studies. The usual approach in this respect has been operative portal portography. In our experience this has proved reliable in only 67 per cent of cases, and misleading in the remaining 33 per cent. Although this represents a total of only 6 cases, in 2 of them the operative portal portogram revealed only collateral runoff without visualization of a subsequently proved normal patent portal vein. In retrospect this is not surprising since hemodynamic data have established that mesenteric flow in this condition is primarily away from the liver. With continuing accumulation of information we have lost our enthusiasm for operative portal portography, because it prolongs anesthetic and operative time while providing a low rate of diagnostic accuracy. It might be argued that this technic would be universally successful if the injecting catheter were advanced all the way into the portal vein. Unfortunately the technical and operative conditions of the procedure frequently preclude this. If attempted, the catheter's position is usually not confirmed until the x-ray film is developed. If further catheter manipulation and film exposure is required, the procedure becomes unwieldy, prolonged and possibly hazardous to the patient. Thus we have generally abandoned this procedure for the problem of nonvisualization.

The clinician might decide to obtain a

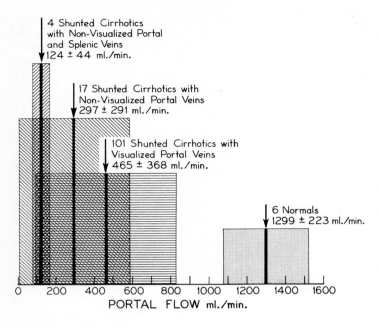

4 Shunted Cirrhotics
with Non-Visualized Portal
and Splenic Veins
124 ± 44 ml./min.

17 Shunted Cirrhotics with
Non-Visualized Portal Veins
297 ± 291 ml./min.

101 Shunted Cirrhotics with
Visualized Portal Veins
465 ± 368 ml./min.

6 Normals
1299 ± 223 ml./min.

PORTAL FLOW ml./min.

FIG. 10–28. Correlation of nonvisualization phenomenon and volumes of portal vein flow. A square-wave electromagnetic flowmeter with noncannulating probes was used to measure portal venous flow in 6 normal patients and in 122 cirrhotics prior to a portacaval shunt. Of the cirrhotics, in 101 the portal vein was visualized and in 17 it was not; in 4 neither the portal nor the splenic vein was visualized. The mean value of portal vein flow and standard deviation is expressed in ml./min. for each group. Although for all the cirrhotic patients portal flow was greatly below normal, the most exaggerated reduction was noted in cases of nonvisualization. When nonvisualization involved both major veins there was a most extensive diversion of splanchnic flow with an extreme reduction in portal flow. We did not record any instances of reversed portal vein flow.

selective splanchnic arteriogram preoperatively. In this situation, a celiac or a splenic selective catheterization study would yield no further diagnostic information since hemodynamically it is no different than a splenic portogram. Accordingly, a selective superior mesenteric arteriogram is preferred. Here again the basic pathophysiology and pathohemodynamics compromise a favorably high diagnostic rate, since mesenteric flow is primarily away from the liver. In the cases reported to date it has been only 60 per cent reliable. This represents only 5 cases, however; one of Bron, Jackson, et al.[17] and one of Boijsen, Ekman, et al.,[12] each of which was successfully resolved by arteriography, and 3 of our own of which only one was diagnostic. Hopefully, further advances in this approach will increase its clinical usefulness, although the basic pathohemodynamics of mesenteric venous flow theoretically preclude an exceedingly high rate of positive diagnoses.

Another radiographic diagnostic approach to this problem would be the use of transumbilical portal venography. In theory, this study affords a near perfect rate of depicting the anatomic state of the portal vein. Despite recent reports of fairly sizable series,[20, 34, 56] there unfortunately has not been recorded to date a case of the use of this technic in splenoportographic major vessel nonvisualization.

The direct transhepatic portal injection technic of Bierman,[9] the intrahepatic deposition technic of Moreno,[49] and the retrograde hepatic venous wedged catheter technic[59, 75] are essentially investigative and none seems to offer clinical application to the solution of nonvisualization.

Another approach to the clinical management of a patient with a nonvisualized portal vein would involve no further attempts at preoperative diagnostic radiographic studies. Inasmuch as none of these supplementary studies approximates the 92 per cent diagnostic accuracy rate of exploratory laparotomy, the surgeon may well resolve this dilemma by a limited subcostal incision and immediate palpation and visualization of the portal vein. If the vein is patent, the incision may be extended, and the dissection and shunt completed. If the vein is occluded an alternate anastomosis (mesenterico-caval) could be established. We have successfully followed this policy for the past several years. As part of continuing studies in this field we are evaluating the preoperative use of the venous phase of selective splanchnic arteriography and transumbilical portal venography in hopes of defining criteria that will increase their diagnostic accuracy in those cases in which splenic portography proves indecisive.

Other Possible Limitations

Inconsistent Findings. We have seen one case in which the initial splenic portogram revealed almost complete diversion of contrast medium around the liver via a large splenorenal communication. However, a second examination resulted in prompt visualization of the splenoportal axis with demonstration of gastroesophageal varices. Whether this difference in portographic findings was a result of local variations in hemodynamics or a reflection of the point of splenic puncture remains obscure. The compartmentalized structure of the splenic pulp with its segmented open-end drainage[28] may account for this phenomenon, especially in patients with portal hypertension. More specifically, injection into one portion of the spleen may result in preferentially greater visualization of the local collateral system (e.g., vasa brevia superiorly) as compared with another form of preferential opacification of collaterals if a different segment of the spleen were injected (e.g., splenorenal collateral inferiorly). Fortunately, this problem has occurred in less than 1 per cent (9 instances). Its solution remains unclear.

Bleeding Varices but a Normal Portogram. This is reported rarely and may be related to the above described phenomenon.[26] A more probable explanation, based on posterior gravitational layering of the contrast with an anterior origin of the coronary vein, has been proposed recently.[49a] The presence of varices could then be documented by prone portography.

Failure Rate. The splenic portogram was unsatisfactory because of technical factors in less than 5 per cent of our cases (1,018 of

1,070 examinations were successful). Such a rate can be maintained consistently and perhaps even lowered by never-ending attention to the smallest detail of technic and by an alertness for that "spontaneous degeneration" that tends to afflict all successful clinical procedures that gradually come to be regarded as "routine."

PORTAL PORTOGRAPHY AND MANOMETRY

This direct intravascular injection introduces innate artefacts and cannot be considered a physiologic assessment of splenoportal hemodynamics. However, it does depict with great clarity the anatomic pattern of a moiety of the extrahepatic portal venous system, especially the superior mesenteric vein and the portal vein. The coronary vein and gastric varices may be seen, but the splenic vein rarely fills.

As mentioned, the indications and usefulness of portal portography are steadily diminishing. In the past, it was used routinely in cases in which the splenic portogram suggested portal vein thrombosis. We have concluded that this is rarely necessary. The question of portal vein thrombosis is most readily and definitively settled by an experienced surgeon's immediate, direct, operative visualization and palpation of the vessel. The same holds true for the problem of a nonvisualized portal vein, a situation in which portal portography has even proved misleading. In the situation of dense, frozen adhesions encasing the hepatoduodenal ligament, the surgeon might wisely not even further consider a time-consuming and hazardous dissection, but immediately abandon all attempts at a portacaval shunt, and proceed with an alternate anastomosis (mesenterico-caval).

The patient who has had a splenectomy or in whom a splenic portogram would be uniquely hazardous, or had proved technically unobtainable has traditionally been considered a candidate for operative portal portography. An increasing number of these problem cases are currently being resolved by preoperative evaluation of the transcapillary venous phase of selective splanchnic arteriography, which avoids the prolongation of anesthetic and operative time involved in portal portography.

The necessary equipment is prepared. A pressure-recording unit, consisting of a 20-cc. Luer-Lok syringe, a 3-way stopcock, Luer-Lok plastic connecting tubing, a short-bevel 18-gauge polyethylene catheter and a water manometer, is filled with saline. Likewise, a 50-cc. syringe with a Luer-Lok plastic tubing connector is filled with 50 cc. of 50 to 75 per cent Hypaque in preparation for the injection of contrast medium. A sterile centimeter rule is included.

Celiotomy is performed with the patient supine. The film cassette is centered at the xyphoid. A loop of jejunum is selected approximately 30 to 40 cm. from the ligament of Treitz. The bowel is elevated, the mesentery drawn taut, and its mesenteric vascular pattern is inspected carefully by transillumination. A large vein connecting the middle and outer arcade is chosen for cannulation. In this process, gentle handling of tissues is of paramount importance, since vasospasm can be triggered readily by rough manipulation. A 3-cm. incision is made through the peritoneum of the mesentery to one side of the selected vessel. A 3-cm. segment of vein without tributaries is mobilized from its adjacent artery, and a 3-0 silk ligature is passed around the proximal end (i.e., toward the root of the mesentery), placing a half tie, but not drawing it taut. With gentle traction on the latter suture, a V-shaped incision is made through the anterior wall of the vein, and a 15- or 18-gauge polyethylene catheter (depending on vein diameter) is introduced rapidly into the lumen and advanced for a distance of about 6 cm. The proximal ligature is "snugged" up, securing the catheter in place.

If an explosive anesthetic agent is employed, the anesthetist is advised to shift temporarily to a nonexplosive technic about 20 minutes before anticipated exposure of the film. The catheter is attached to the previously prepared manometer unit filled with normal saline. Three free-fall determinations of portal pressure are recorded. An additional correction is made for the measured vertical distance between the portal vein and the zero point of the manometer. The cannula is flushed with normal saline, and the pressure recording unit is replaced by the injection unit, while the anesthetist maintains controlled apnea. Fifty cc. of 50 to 75 per cent Hypaque (30 cc. 50 per cent Hypaque in children) is injected rapidly in 5 to 7 seconds. Film is exposed toward the end of the injection. A 200-MA portable x-ray unit is employed, permitting an exposure time of less than 1 second. Respirations are resumed. Again, the vein is cleared with normal saline, the catheter removed, the initial tie in the proximal ligature drawn taut, and a square knot completed. The peritoneal edges are reapproximated over the vein with one or 2 interrupted 4-0 silk sutures.

Performed in this manner, portal portography is extremely safe and informative. Thrombosis of the injected vein is reported rarely; we never encountered this.

EVALUATION OF THE PORTAL SYSTEM UNDER EMERGENCY CONDITIONS

The prompt diagnosis of the nature and site of acute upper gastrointestinal hemorrhage and the determination of therapy is often of lifesaving importance. Portal hypertension and gastroesophageal varices should be tested for early, since the clinical course and medical and surgical management and prognosis of varical bleeding differs greatly from that of hemorrhage from other causes (peptic ulcer, neoplasm, erosive gastritis, esophagitis, etc.). The mortality rate with the first varical hemorrhage is 30 to 50 per cent.[41] The usual associated cirrhosis of the liver further compromises the patient's ability to withstand hemorrhage, and, unless bleeding is controlled early, hepatic damage may be irreversible.

The establishment of the presence or absence of gastroesophageal varices may be elusive in the phase of severe active bleeding. For example, the history and physical findings may suggest cirrhosis when bleeding is from a site other than varices. Physical findings consistent with a diagnosis of cirrhosis do not establish the coexistence of portal hypertension with bleeding varices.

Indeed, only 20 to 30 per cent of cirrhotics have portal hypertension.[41] Furthermore, peptic ulcer is present in 15 to 20 per cent of cirrhotic patients; the incidence in the general population is 10 per cent.[41] A less common factor limiting differential diagnosis of upper gastrointestinal hemorrhage is that some patients who bleed from varices may present nothing in the history nor exhibit any physical finding suggestive of cirhosis or an extrahepatic obstruction as the genesis of portal hypertension and varices.

Emergency Splenic Pulp Manometry

The conventional methods of differential diagnosis (barium contrast roentgenography, esophagoscopy, trial balloon tamponade and liver function tests) have limitations. Splenic pulp manometry is a direct, determinative, practical and safe emergency method of differentiating varices from other sites of upper gastrointestinal hemorrhage.

The rationale of the use of splenic pulp manometry is based on the following factors. Our group has shown that there is linear correlation between splenic pulp pressure, direct portal pressure and the degree of portal collateralization as demonstrated by combined percutaneous splenic pulp manometry and portography.[48] Indeed, the highest levels of portal tension are recorded in patients who bled from gastroesophageal varices. Furthermore, splenic pulp pressure is a reliable index of actual portal vein pressure.[3, 23, 48, 72, 76] These factors suggest that emergency percutaneous splenic pulp manometry alone might yield valuable diagnostic information concerning the presence or the absence of varices in patients with acute and severe bleeding from the upper gastrointestinal tract.

The technic of the procedure is identical with that described for the manometric phase of percutaneous splenoportography. However, there is no need for special facilities or personnel as might be necessary for emergencies requiring splenic portography or liver function studies, endoscopy or transcapillary arteriography. It spares many patients the risks and discomfort of an unnecessary trial diagnostic balloon tamponade.[21] Also one can rapidly and accurately establish a diagnosis in the acutely ill patient who

cannot be transported to the x-ray department for conventional roentgenograms, serial splenoportography or selective arteriography. The patient can be examined on the emergency room stretcher or in bed with a board for support of the patient and establishment of an accurate baseline.

On our surgical and medical services, splenic manometry as a primary diagnostic test in a series of over 200 patients who had recently bled or were actively bleeding from the upper gastrointestinal tract has been 90 per cent accurate in detecting or negating gastrointestinal varices.[64] Splenic pulp pressure in patients subsequently proved to be bleeding from varices was consistently higher (mean, above 425 mm. saline) than that of patients bleeding from other sites (mean, 175 mm.). All patients whose pressure was less than 250 mm. bled from a source other than varices. The small zone of fallibility, 250 to 290 mm., included less than 10 per cent of the total group. In these patients, subsequent serial splenoportography was required in determining the presence or absence of varices (Fig. 10–29).

Demonstration of an elevated portal pressure in a patient bleeding from the upper gastrointestinal tract does not, of course, rule out bleeding from a site other than gastroesophageal varices. However, experience at our clinic indicates that in portal hypertension by far the most probable site of bleeding is varices. A normal portal pressure, with rare exceptions, rules out varical hemorrhage.

The presence of hemorrhagic shock does not invalidate the accuracy of splenic pulp manometry in detecting portal hypertension and varices as the cause of hemorrhage. Wigger's physiological studies have shown that in the dog the portal pressure, after a temporary decline, tends to return toward control values during a period of hemorrhagic shock.[77] Our observation of markedly elevated portal pressures in 15 patients bleeding massively from varices and with low systolic arterial pressures tend clinically to confirm this important aspect of the reliability of the technic.

The frequency of the need for this procedure cannot be judged from the large size of our series. Since our data include

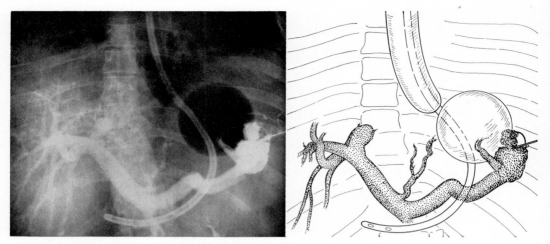

FIG. 10–29. Emergency splenic pulp manometry and portography. This film shows the possible value of splenic portography in demonstrating gastroesophageal varices under emergency conditions. The examination can be performed even with the Sengstaken-Blakemore tube in place, either with the balloon inflated (as above) or momentarily deflated.

the investigative evaluation of the diagnostic accuracy of the technic, many cases included in the initial phases of the study did not involve ambiguity of diagnosis. Their inclusion as controls, however, served to establish the reliability of the technic. In more recent years, we have been restricting the use of the procedure and seeking criteria for its rational use. Currently we employ emergency splenic pulp manometry only in those cases of upper gastrointestinal hemorrhage in which the diagnosis is in doubt and in which the clinical situation demands serious therapeutic measures. Accordingly, before deciding upon emergency surgical intervention, and before employing balloon tamponade or gastric hypothermia, we seek to distinguish between a varical or nonvarical site of hemorrhage by the quickest, easiest and most reliable technic, namely, emergency splenic pulp manometry. In cases in which the site of bleeding is known or in cases in which hemorrhage is subsiding, we no longer routinely perform immediate emergency splenic pulp manometry. Of course, many of these patients require subsequent elective splenic portography and manometry.

In summary, our extended and continuing clinical experience over the years confirms that emergency splenic pulp manometry can determine the presence or absence of gas-troesophageal varices, and result in more effective management of these difficult problems.

EMERGENCY SELECTIVE ARTERIOGRAPHY

In recent years, the emergency use of arteriography has been successful in localizing the site of active intestinal hemorrhage.[4, 5, 36, 51, 52] The most attractive feature of this approach is the direct nature of the study. When successful, it results in striking visualization of extravasation of blood and contrast medium from a vascular structure into the lumen of the intestinal tract. This can be obtained for either an arterial or venous bleeding point since both phases of the splanchnic circulation are visualized. It has proved more helpful in problems of arterial bleeding, probably because the contrast medium is less diluted in the arterial phase, resulting in superior opacification.

Of course, the patient must be actively bleeding at the time of the examination. The rate of hemorrhage sufficient to produce a satisfactory study in the experimental animal is reportedly 0.5 to 6 ml./min., depending on the site of selective catheterization.[32, 51, 52] The success of the technic is mostly independent of the size of the lesion or the presence of blood clots within the lumen of the intestinal tract.

The disadvantages of the emergency use

of this procedure are primarily 2 interrelated aspects of the study. First, a patient with severe active hemorrhage must be transported to the x-ray department. This must involve some compromise in nursing care and observation. In borderline hypovolemia and hypotension, such movement may result in frank shock. Secondly, highly specialized facilities must be available and specially trained personnel are needed.

Finally, the diagnostic failure rate especially with regard to the more difficult venous evaluation remains unknown. Our own impression, based on limited experience, is that it is considerably higher than with emergency splenic pulp manometry. Emergency arteriography appears to be approximately 60 per cent accurate, whereas emergency splenic pulp manometry has been 90 per cent accurate. The latter continues to be our primary emergency diagnostic study although we are continuing to investigate the usefulness of emergency selective arteriography.

RETROGRADE PORTOGRAPHY

As discussed, most retrograde portography technics are primarily investigative and have no immediate clinical application. The exception is transumbilical portal venography which has recently enkindled renewed interest.[20, 34, 56]

The primary attraction of transumbilical venography is its capacity to opacify densely the intrahepatic and usually part of the extrahepatic portal venous system. That this might prove to be of comparable or greater merit than hepatic scintography or arteriography for the delineation of hepatic metastasis remains to be established.

It has also been suggested but curiously never confirmed that transumbilical venography is diagnostic in cases of splenic portographic nonvisualization of the portal vein or portal and splenic veins. It is even more curious that this technic has never been reported to have portrayed portal venous congenital or acquired extrahepatic obstruction. Both situations might possibly be clarified by this technic which further experience may prove to be a major advance in this field of diagnosis.

Some words of caution, however, and discussion of the limitations of this technic are appropriate. (1) The method involves a direct, intravascular, retrograde injection, which affords maximal opacification of vessels but negates any physiologic interpretation by its disruptive pressure of injection. Further investigation may prove, however, that at the completion of the injection, the pre-existing hemodynamic state is re-established and can be depicted radiographically, probably best by the cine technic. (2) This procedure might well prove unreliable if not misleading in elucidating cases of segmental splenic hypertension or combined intra- or extrahepatic obstruction. (3) Theoretical objections such as placing a surgical wound on the abdomen prior to a proposed shunt with the potentiality of wound infection and the possibility that the massive direct portal injection of contrast medium might initiate a late chemical phlebitis with portal vein or anastomotic inflammatory thrombosis await further evaluation. (4) The currently reported technical failure rate of 12 to 20 per cent[34, 56] far exceeds that of 4 to 5 per cent for splenic portography.

Perhaps umbilical venography will prove most useful as a complement to splenic portography and/or the venous phase of selective splanchnic arteriography in selected problem situations such as the nonvisualized major vein; or as an independently valuable study in cases of hepatic neoplasm.

TRANSCAPILLARY PORTOGRAPHY

Perhaps the most significant development in portal venography during the past few years is the reintroduction and refinement of the historic technic of transcapillary portography. The transition from Rigler's original aortic injection[60] to selective celiac, mesenteric or splenic arterial catheterization[10, 12, 16, 37, 53, 57] has resulted in a much higher rate of successful venous visualization and vastly improved venous concentration of contrast medium.

Discussion of the hemodynamics of this technic, of its role in the problem cases of splenic portography major vessel nonvisualization and its usefulness in the emergency setting of acute hemorrhage are integrated

SITE OF CATHETER	NUMBER OF CASES	NUMBER WITH DIAGNOSTIC SPLENOPORTAL VENOUS PHASE	PER-CENTAGE
Aortic	10	1	10
Celiac	119	67	56
Splenic	9	6	67
Mesenteric	59	32	55
Combined celiac and mesenteric	48	28	58

into preceding sections of this chapter. Further discussion of the incidence of failure and of factors determining a successful study is now in order.

Although the technic is reportedly universally successful in visualizing the venous system,[16] our experience with approximately 200 such studies for a variety of indications has not resulted in such a success rate. Table 10–3 records our success rate of venous visualization at the different sites of selective catheterization and injection. All sites have approximately a 60 per cent success rate with the exception of the aortic injections which of course represent failures of selective catheterization attempts. This 40 per cent rate of venous nonvisualization far exceeds the 6 per cent rate of such failure for percutaneous splenic portography and represents the major disadvantage and limitation of the transcapillary technic.

Recognizing the inherent merits of this approach, however, many groups including our own continue to search for factors that govern this failure rate. So far this has not resulted in any well codified method of operation or in a striking increase in successful studies.

Studies of optimal quality are generally obtained by catheterizing a large splenic artery. Indeed, when accompanied by a large splenic vein with presumably high flow rates the technical quality of the transcapillary study may even exceed that of a high quality percutaneous splenic portogram (Fig. 10–30). In other seemingly similar instances, this does not occur and the large spleen seems to act like a sponge, absorbing the arterial injection rapidly but releasing the contrast medium into the venous system so slowly visualization is poor or impossible. If the splenic artery is injected in cases of splenic portographic major venous nonvisualization, the identical pattern is reproduced.

A celiac catheterization study is slightly less selective and usually results in varying degrees of lesser opacification than a splenic injection. If the splenic artery is the dominant branch of the celiac trunk, the diversion of contrast medium over the other branches may be minimal and result in an excellent study. If the splenic artery is small and especially if the hepatic artery is quite large and sequestrates much of the contrast medium, visualization of the splenoportal axis will be poor or impossible. In such instances, the supplemental use of superior mesenteric catheterization for a simultaneous double catheter injection may prove useful.

Superior mesenteric catheterization alone may give definite information concerning the superior mesenteric and portal veins themselves but only rarely affords any visualization of the splenic vein (Fig. 10–31). Accordingly this study alone might result in missing the diagnosis especially of splenic vein obstruction.

Many factors that determine the success of this technic in cases of portal hypertension will become known only during the course of the study. Accordingly, the transcapillary approach requires a knowledgeable, resourceful, persistent and flexible radiologist, who can modify and extend his technic to particular anatomic and hemodynamic situations.

CONCLUSION

Percutaneous splenic portography and manometry are invaluable as an elective diagnostic technic in safely and accurately assessing the anatomic and hemodynamic situation in suspected portal hypertension. It is of further diagnostic value in extrahepatic obstruction, where the site of block may be clearly defined. In selected cases, the com-

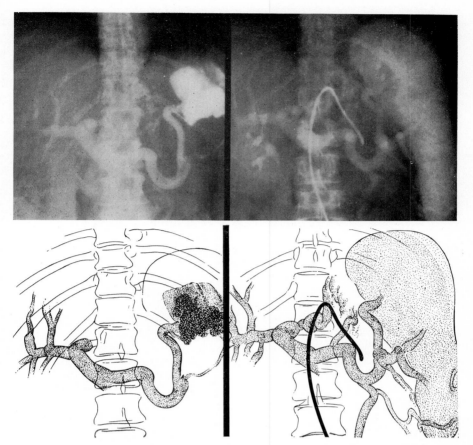

Fig. 10–30. Venous phase of splenic arteriography. A. H. (Chart No. 226813). This 58-year-old cirrhotic patient had endured several admissions and many years of outpatient treatment for medically refractory ascites. She had never experienced a varical hemorrhage. Splenic pulp manometry indicated a pressure of 420 mm. saline. The splenic portogram (*left*) revealed a technically good study allowing for a diagnosis of portal hypertension on the basis of hepatofugal collateral flow over varices, and patency of the splenic and portal veins. The venous phase of selective splenic arteriography (*right*) resulted in an even more striking demonstration of the same information. Unfortunately, such findings are not consistently observed, due to a variety of factors discussed in the text. This patient underwent a side-to-side shunt with a good drop in portal pressure, a reversal of flow in the hepatic limb of the portal vein, and relief of previously intractable ascites.

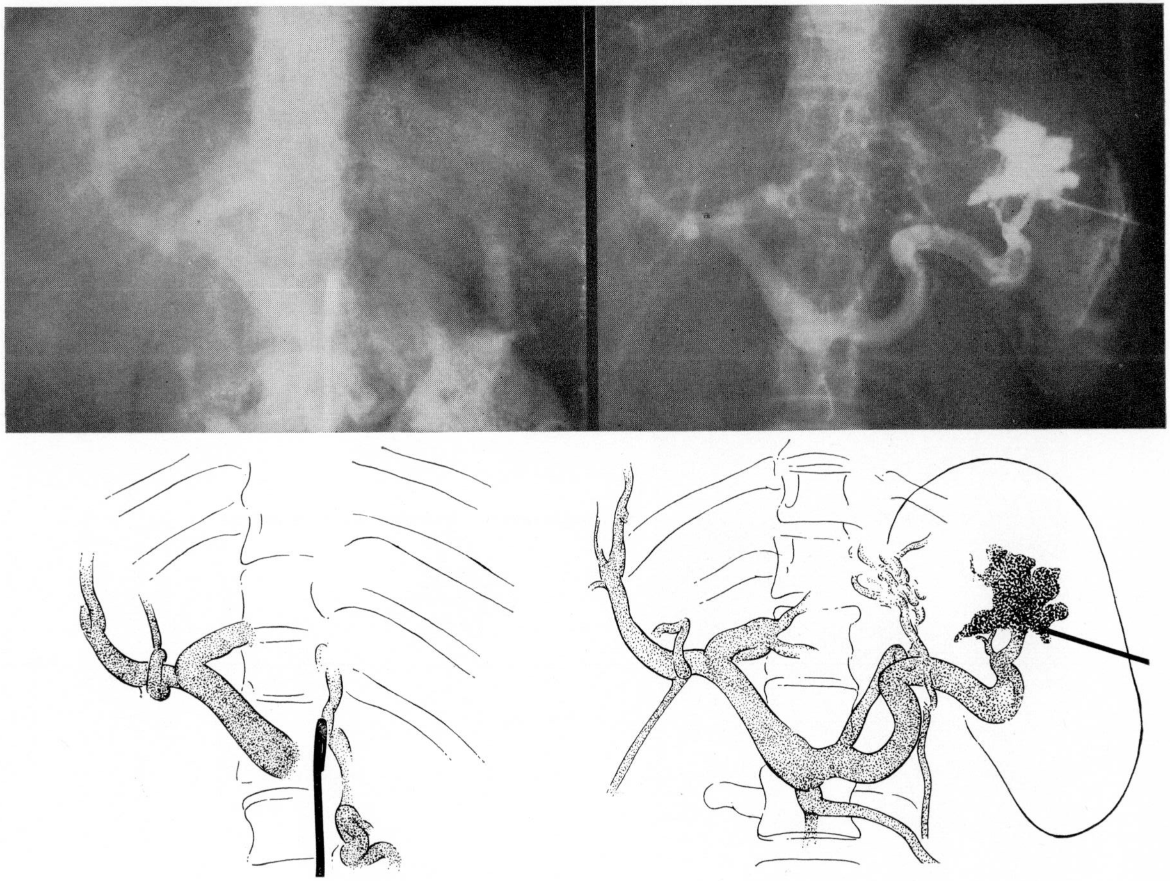

Fig. 10–31. Venous phase of superior mesenteric arteriography. L. B. (Chart No. 230288). This 52-year-old woman experienced a varical hemorrhage in 1965 at which time she was explored elsewhere without preoperative splenic portography. On the basis of this exploration, an experienced surgeon was convinced that her portal vein was thrombosed and that no surgical procedure was technically feasible. Following a recurrent hemorrhage she was referred to St. Vincent's for further evaluation. The superior mesenteric arteriogram (*left*) demonstrated a perfectly normal vein, obviously patent and without thrombosis. The splenic vein was not visualized, however. The splenic portogram (*right*) provided the complete information depicting hepatofugal flow, indicating portal hypertension and also documenting both splenic and portal vein patency. An end-to-side portacaval shunt was effected without difficulty and without subsequent hemorrhage.

These studies illustrate 2 independent points: (1) a mesenteric arterial injection by itself does not routinely give information concerning the patency of the splenic vein and so cannot rule out independent or coexisting extrahepatic obstruction; (2) the treatment of patients with suspected portal hypertension demands the use of appropriate radiographic studies such as splenic portography to confirm or negate the diagnosis and to establish the patency of major veins for portal anastomosis.

plementary value of portal portography has been demonstrated. Finally, splenic pulp manometry has proved to be a singularly accurate, safe and discriminatory emergency test in the differential diagnosis of variceal versus nonvariceal upper gastrointestinal hemorrhage. Newer complementary diagnostic technics including the transcapillary venous phase of selective visceral arteriography and retrograde transumbilical portal venography are being developed. A plea is made that splenic portography with 16 years of proved usefulness be utilized as the standard for comparing and evaluating the future role of these promising new approaches to the further understanding of the portal venous system.

REFERENCES

1. Abeatici, S., and Campi, L.: Sur les possibilités de l'angiographie hépatique: la visualisation du système portal, Acta radiol. *36*:383, 1951.
2. Amplatz, K.: The catheter needle *in* Schobinger, R. A., and Ruzicka, F. F., Jr. (eds.): Vascular Roentgenology, p. 89, New York, Macmillan, 1964.
3. Atkinson, M., and Sherlock, S.: Intrasplenic pressure as index of portal venous pressure, Lancet *1*:1325, 1954.
4. Baum, S., Nusbaum, M., Blakemore, W. S., and Finkelstein, A. K.: The preoperative radiographic demonstration of intra-abdominal bleeding from undetermined sites by percutaneous selective celiac and superior mesenteric arteriography, Surgery *58*:797, 1965.
5. Baum, S., Roy, R., Finkelstein, A. K., and Blakemore, W. S.: Clinical application of selective celiac and superior mesenteric arteriography, Radiology *84*:279, 1965.
6. Bergstrand, I.: Splenoportography, *in* Abrams, H. L. (ed.): Angiography, Boston, Little, Brown, 1961.
7. Bergstrand, I., and Ekman, C. A.: Percutaneous lieno-portal venography, Acta radiol. *43*:377, 1955.
8. ———: Portal circulation in portal hypertension, Acta radiol. *47*:1, 1957.
9. Bierman, H. R., Kelly, K. H., Coblents, A., White, L. P., and Fisher, A.: Transhepatic venous catheterization and venography, J.A.M.A. *158*:1331, 1955.
10. Bierman, H. R., Miller, E. R., Byron, R. L., Jr., Dod, K. S., Kelly, K. H., and Black, D. H.: Intra-arterial catheterization of viscera in man, Am. J. Roentgenol. *66*:555, 1951.
11. Blakemore, A. H., and Lord, J. W., Jr.: Technic of using Vitallium tubes in establishing portacaval shunts for portal hypertension, Ann. Surg. *122*:476, 1945.
12. Boijsen, E., Ekman, C. A., and Olin, T.: Coeliac and superior mesenteric angiography in portal hypertension, Acta chir. scand. *126*:315, 1963.
13. Bookstein, J. J., and Whitehouse, W. M.: Splenoportography, Radiol. Clin. N. Amer. *2*:447, 1964.
14. Boulvin, R., Chevalier, M., Gallus, P., and Nagel, M.: Le portagraphie per voie splénique transpariétale, Acta chir. belg. *50*:534, 1951.
15. Broden, B., Hanson, H. E., and Kornell, J.: Thoracic aortography, Acta radiol. *29*:181, 1948.
16. Bron, K. M., and Fisher, B.: Arterial portography: indications and technique, Surgery *61*:137, 1967.
17. Bron, K. M., Jackson, F. C., Haller, J., Perez-Stable, E., Eisen, H. B., and Poller, S.: The value of selective arteriography in demonstrating portal and splenic vein patency following nonvisualization by splenoportography, Radiology *85*:448, 1965.
18. Bunnag, T. S., Koaparisuthi, V., Arthachinta, S., Chienpradit, K., and Binbakaya, L.: Percutaneous splenic portography in amebic liver abscess, Am. J. Roentgenol. *80*:324, 1958.
19. Burchell, A. R., Moreno, A. H., Panke, W. F., and Rousselot, L. M.: Some limitations of splenic portography. I. Incidence, hemodynamics and surgical implications of the nonvisualized portal vein, Ann. Surg. *162*:981, 1965.
20. Chiandussi, L., Juliani, G., Greco, F., Cravero, D., Sardi, G., and Toscano, G.: Hepatic portography by direct catheterization of the portal vein through the round ligament of the liver (ligamentum teres), Am. J. Roentgenol. *99*:625, 1967.
21. Conn, H. O.: Hazards attending use of esophageal tamponade, New Engl. J. Med. *259*:701, 1958.
22. Coomaraswamy, R. P., Del Guercio, L. R. M., Miller, H., State, D., and Elkin, M.: Splenoportography and portal vein throm-

bosis in patients with cirrhosis of the liver, Surg. Gynec. Obstet. *118*:560, 1964.

23. Davis, W. D., Jr., Batson, H. M., Jr., and Schindel, W.: Studies on portal pressure. I. Relation of intrasplenic pulp pressure to portal venous pressure, and use of splenic explant in the study of portal venous pressure, J. Lab. Clin. Med. *44*:786, 1954.

24. Doehner, G. A., Ruzicka, F. F., Hoffman, G., and Rousselot, L. M.: The portal venous system: its roentgen anatomy, Radiology *64*:675, 1955.

25. Doehner, G. A., Ruzicka, F. F., Jr., Rousselot, L. M., and Hoffman, G.: The portal venous system: on its pathological roentgen anatomy, Radiology *66*:206, 1956.

26. Doppman, J. L., and Shapiro, R.: Bleeding esophageal varices in the presence of normal splenoportogram; a case report, Am. J. Roentgenol. *86*:1103, 1961.

27. dos Santos, R., Lamas, A., and Pereira Caldas, J.: Arteriografia da aorta e dos vasos abdominais, Med. contemp. *47*:93, 1929.

28. Dreyer, B.: The segmental nature of the spleen, Blood *18*:468, 1961.

29. Edlich, R. F., Ferlic, R. M., and Bernstein, E. F.: Vasopressin as an adjunct to splenoportography, Arch. Surg. *92*:802, 1966.

30. Fariñas, P. L.: A new technique for the arteriographic examination of the abdominal aorta and its branches, Am. J. Roentgenol. *46*:641, 1941.

31. Ferguson, D. J., and Ranniger, K.: Portography in portal hypertension, Surg. Clin. N. Amer. *44*:45, 1964.

32. Jaffe, B. F., Youker, J. E., and Margulis, A. R.: Aortographic localization of controlled gastrointestinal hemorrhage in dogs, Surgery *58*:984, 1965.

33. Jonsson, G.: Visualization of coronary arteries, Acta radiol. *29*:536, 1948.

34. Kessler, R. E., and Zimmon, D. S.: Umbilical vein catheterization in man, Surg. Gynec. Obstet. *124*:594, 1967.

35. Klemperer, P.: Cavernomatous transformation of the portal vein, its relation to Banti's disease, Arch. Path. *6*:353, 1928.

36. Koehler, P. R., and Salmon, R. B.: Angiographic localization of unknown acute gastrointestinal bleeding sites, Radiology *89*:244, 1967.

37. Kreel, L., and Williams, R.: Arteriovenography of the portal system, Brit. Med. J. *2*:1500, 1964.

38. Legare, A.: Personal communication to F.

F. Ruzicka, Jr. as quoted in Splenoportography *in* Margulis, A. R., and Burhenne, J. (eds.): Alimentary Tract Roentgenology, St. Louis, Mosby, 1967.

39. Leger, L. H.: Phlebographie portale par injection splénique intraparenchymateuse, Mém. Acad. chir. *77*:586, 1951.

40. ———: Splenoportography: Diagnostic Phlebography of the Portal Venous System, Springfield, Ill., Thomas, 1966.

41. Liebowitz, H. R., and Rousselot, L. M.: Bleeding Esophageal Varices—Portal Hypertension, Springfield, Ill., Thomas, 1959.

42. ———: Saccular aneurysm of portal vein with agnogenic myeloid metaplasia, N. Y. State J. Med. *67*:1443, 1967.

43. Maxwell, J. W., Jr., and Jackson, F. C.: Splenoportography using a plastic hubbed catheter, Surg. Gynec. Obstet. *124*:362, 1967.

44. Miller, H., Coomaraswamy, R. P., Del Guercio, L. R. M., Elkin, M., and State, D.: Value of biplane splenoportography, Radiology *81*:953, 1963.

45. Moreno, A. H., Burchell, A. R., Rousselot, L. M., Panke, W. F., Slafsky, S. F., and Burke, J. H.: Portal blood flow in cirrhosis of the liver, J. Clin. Invest *46*:436, 1967.

46. Moreno, A. H., Burchell, A. R., Van der Wonde, R., and Burke, J. H.: Respiratory regulation of splanchnic and systemic venous return, Am. J. Physiol. *213*:455, 1967.

47. Moreno, A. H., Rousselot, L. M., Burchell, A. R., Bono, R. F., and Burke, J. H.: Studies on the outflow tracts of the liver. 1. On a method for the functional demonstration of the outflow tracts of the liver and its application to the study of hepatic hemodynamics in normal and cirrhotic rats, Ann. Surg. *155*:412, 1962.

48. Moreno, A. H., Rousselot, L. M., and Panke, W. F.: Studies on portal hypertension. II. Correlation between severity of pathologic involvement of the portal system and variations in tension, Surg. Clin. N. Amer. *38*:421, 1958.

49. Moreno, A. H., Ruzicka, F. F., Rousselot, L. M., Burchell, A. R., Bono, R. F., Slafsky, S. F., and Burke, J. H.: Functional hepatography. A study of the hemodynamics of the outflow tracts of the human liver by intraparenchymal deposition of contrast medium, with attempts at functional evaluation of the outflow block

concept of cirrhotic ascites and the accessory outflow role of the portal vein, Radiology *81*:65, 1963.

49a. Moskowitz, H., Chait, A., Margulies, M., and Mellins, H. Z.: Prone splenoportography, Radiology *90*:1132, 1968.

50. Ney, H. R.: Rontgenologischer Nachweis portovenoser und intervenoser Nebenschlusse in der Leber, Acta radiol. *49*: 227, 1958.

51. Nusbaum, M., and Baum, S.: Radiographic demonstration of unknown sites of gastrointestinal bleeding, Surg., Forum *14*:374, 1963.

52. Nusbaum, M., Baum, S., Blakemore, W. S., and Finkelstein, A. K.: Demonstration of intra-abdominal bleeding by selective arteriography. Visualization of celiac and superior mesenteric arteries, J.A.M.A. *191*: 389, 1965.

53. Odman, P.: Percutaneous selective angiography of the coeliac artery, Acta. radiol. Suppl. *159*, 1958.

54. Panke, W. F., Bradley, E. G., Moreno, A. H., Ruzicka, F. F., Jr., and Rousselot, L. M.: Technique, hazards, and usefulness of percutaneous splenic portography, J.A.M.A. *169*:1032, 1959.

55. Panke, W. F., Moreno, A. H., and Rousselot, L. M.: The diagnostic study of the portal venous system, Med. Clin. N. Amer. *44*:727, 1960.

56. Piccone, V. A., Le Veen, H. H., White, J. J., Skinner, G. B., and MacLean, L. D.: Transumbilical portal hepatography; a significant adjunct in the investigation of liver disease, Surgery *61*:333, 1967.

57. Pollard, J. J., and Nebesar, R. A.: Catheterization of splenic artery for portal venography, New Engl. J. Med. *271*:234, 1964.

58. Radner, S.: Thoracal aortography by catheterization from the radial artery, Acta radiol. *29*:178, 1948.

59. Rappaport, A. M.: Hepatic venography, Acta radiol. *36*:165, 1951.

60. Rigler, L. G., Olfelt, P. C., and Krumbach, R. W.: Roentgen hepatography by injection of a contrast medium into the aorta, Radiology *60*:363, 1953.

61. Rousselot, L. M.: Role of congestion (portal hypertension) in so-called Banti's syndrome; clinical and pathologic study of thirty-one cases with late results following splenectomy, J.A.M.A. *107*:1788, 1936.

62. Rousselot, L. M., and Burchell, A. R.: Portal venography and manometry, *in* Schiff, L. (ed.); Diseases of the Liver, ed. 2, Philadelphia, Lippincott, 1963.

63. Rousselot, L. M., Moreno, A. H., and Panke, W. F.: Studies on portal hypertension. IV. The clinical and physiopathologic significance of self-established (nonsurgical) portal systemic venous shunts, Ann. Surg. *150*:384, 1959.

64. Rousselot, L. M., Panke, W. F., and Moreno, A. H.: Further evaluation of splenic pulp manometry as a differential diagnostic test of acute upper gastrointestinal bleeding, Am. J. Gastroent. *35*:474, 1961.

65. Rousselot, L. M., Ruzicka, F. F., and Doehner, G. A.: Portal venography via the portal and percutaneous splenic routes, Surgery *34*:557, 1953.

66. Ruzicka, F. F., Jr.: Technique (percutaneous splenoportography), *in* Schobinger, R., and Ruzicka, F. F., Jr. (eds.): Vascular Roentgenology, New York, Macmillan, 1964, p. 588.

67. ————: Splenoportography *in* Margulis, A. R., and Burhenne, J. (eds.): Alimentary Tract Roentgenology, St. Louis, Mosby, 1967.

68. Ruzicka, F. F., Jr., Doehner, G. A., and Rousselot, L. M.: Portal venography: anatomic and physiologic consideration in interpretation, Am. J. Dig. Dis. *1*:3, 1956.

69. Ruzicka, F. F., Jr., Gould, H. R., Bradley, E. G., and Rousselot, L. M.: Value of splenic portography in the diagnosis of intrahepatic and extrahepatic neoplasm, Am. J. Med. *29*:434, 1960.

70. Seldinger, S. I.: Catheter replacement of the needle in percutaneous arteriography, Acta radiol. *39*:368, 1953.

71. ————: A simple method of catheterization of the spleen and liver, Acta radiol. *48*:93, 1957.

72. Taylor, F. W., and Egbert, H. L.: Portal tension, Surg. Gynec. Obstet. *92*:64, 1951.

73. Thomas, T. V.: Aneurysm of the portal vein: report of two cases, one resulting in thrombosis and spontaneous rupture, Surgery *61*:550, 1967.

74. Thompson, W. P., Caughey, J. L., Whipple, A. O., and Rousselot, L. M.: Splenic vein pressure in congestive splenomegaly (Banti's syndrome), J. Clin. Invest. *16*: 571, 1937.

75. Tori, G.: Hepatic venography in man, Acta radiol. *39*:89, 1953.

76. Turner, M. D., Sherlock, S., and Steiner, R. E.: Splenic venography and intrasplenic pressure measurement in the clinical investigation of the portal venous system, Am. J. Med. *23*:846, 1957.

77. Wiggers, C. J., Opdyke, D. F., and Johnson, J. R.: Portal pressure gradients under experimental conditions, including hemorrhagic shock, Am. J. Physiol. *146*:192, 1946.

78. Zeid, S. S., Felson, B., and Schiff, L.: Percutaneous splenoportal venography, with additional comments on transhepatic venography, Ann. Int. Med. *52*:782, 1960.

11

Ascites: The Kidney in Liver Disease

W. H. J. SUMMERSKILL, D.M. (*Oxon.*), F.R.C.P. (*Lond.*), F.A.C.P.

Ascites refers to accumulation of free fluid within the peritoneal cavity (Gr. *askitēs*, from *askos* bag). Although liable to occur in any liver disease, ascites is the commonest major complication of cirrhosis and implies a poor prognosis.[107, 121]

Ascites is mentioned in some of the earliest medical literature.[32] Hippocrates recognized an association between liver disease and dropsy; Celsus described in detail the methods of paracentesis most likely to succeed; and Erasistratus of Alexandria attributed ascites more specifically to the stonelike hardness of the liver, commenting that "the blood is prevented from going forward into the liver owing to the narrowness of the passages." Galenic theories were upheld for a long time, until physicians of the seventeenth century contributed original ideas to the pathogenesis and treatment of ascites. Lower[83] initiated the investigative approach, producing ascites in dogs by ligating the vena cava above the liver, the prototype of many experimental preparations; Sydenham deduced that "the terrible habit of swilling spiritous liquors" predisposed to the condition[136]; and Brown anticipated subsequent controversy by reviving Graeco-Roman reservations regarding paracentesis as definitive therapy.[17] Flint is usually credited with having first documented (in 1863) functional renal failure as a complication of ascites.[44]

PHYSICAL FINDINGS

By the nineteenth century, clinicians had established most of the diagnostic criteria still commonly employed in differentiating ascites from other conditions, including abdominal cysts, pregnancy, distention of the bladder and obesity. Murchison listed progressive enlargement of the abdomen, eversion or hernia of the umbilicus, exertional dyspnea and thoracic breathing.[95] He drew attention to the importance of percussing for dullness over the flanks with the patient in the supine position and of evoking the shift of dullness in response to gravity as the patient assumed the lateral or knee-elbow position. The method of eliciting a fluid thrill also was described, together with the tendency of the umbilicus to approximate more closely the pubic synthesis than the sternum, in contrast to upward displacement of the umbilicus by ovarian cysts.

At present the maneuvers of choice depend particularly on personal experience, and volumes of fluid exceeding 1.5 liters can usually be detected. Lately it has been claimed that as little as 120 ml. of fluid can be identified by use of the "puddle" sign,[74] and, where doubt exists, roentgenograms occasionally show evidence of haziness or obliteration of normal structures. Rarely, but especially in obese patients, aspiration of the abdomen is considered necessary for diagnosis.

Additional findings in patients with ascites include incisional, inguinal or femoral herniae, the development of pale abdominal striae, and scrotal edema. Large volumes of fluid, which may exceed 30 liters, render the abdominal organs inaccessible to palpation, although they may be ballotable; the recti

355

muscles may divaricate, together with elevation of the diaphragm. The latter change rotates the heart, thus displacing the apex beat, and, by raising intrapleural pressure, leads to a compensatory rise in right cardiac filling pressure with engorgement of the neck veins.[120] Gaseous distention of the abdomen and other functional gastrointestinal disorders, presumably of mechanical origin, are frequent. Predisposition to hiatal hernia and gastroesophageal reflux, which may cause erosions and hemorrhage from varices, have been postulated on the same basis.[115] Prominent venous channels developing on the anterior abdominal wall are derived either from the portal vein, due to portal hypertension, or from the inferior vena cava. Caval collateral vessels are attributed to compression of the inferior vena cava by the increased intra-abdominal pressure, and this mechanism, together with hypoalbuminemia, is thought to be responsible for the frequent coexistence of dependent edema.

Pleural effusion, occurring on the right side in the majority of instances, is present in approximately 10 per cent of patients with cirrhosis and ascites.[62] Sometimes this is symptomatic, and occasionally the fluid may have a serosanguineous or chylous appearance. Studies of the movement of ^{131}I, albumin, carbon particles or air between the abdominal and thoracic cavities have failed to specify a single mechanism for such effusions.[62, 77] Johnston and Loo interpreted their data as indicating upward movement of fluid through diaphragmatic lymphatics, whereas Lieberman and associates state that acquired diaphragmatic defects (which are occasionally induced by transthoracic hepatic biopsy) are responsible and often can be demonstrated at thoracoscopy or autopsy. Another possibility is that fluid transudes into the pleural cavity as a result of portal hypertension affecting the azygous and hemiazygous venous systems.

DIFFERENTIAL DIAGNOSIS

Since Cabot[20] reviewed the causes of ascites comprehensively, hepatic, neoplastic and cardiac diseases continue to account for most cases, and the preponderance of patients with cirrhosis[20, 121] has been reaffirmed in a recent series studied by Berner and associates.[11] Less commonly, renal, metabolic, nutritional, inflammatory, vascular or collagen disorders lead to accumulation of abdominal fluid; extravasations of urine, bile or blood occasionally are responsible. The primary disease leading to ascites can be determined by routine methods in most instances and thus lies beyond the scope of this chapter.

When the etiology is obscure, inspection of the ascitic fluid, followed by standard histologic, chemical and bacteriologic procedures is sometimes helpful. If trauma and rare congenital defects are excluded, bloody or chylous ascites almost invariably indicates a neoplasm. True chylous ascites results from lymphatic obstruction and has a fat content that is usually twice that of the plasma and exceeds 400 mg./100 ml.[97] Pseudochylous ascites may be associated with cirrhosis; the fluid appears milky because of excessive amounts of neutral fat, but the lipid content does not exceed that of the plasma.[149]

Peritonitis, usually due to enteric organisms, can develop insidiously in patients with cirrhosis and ascites. There is often concomitant fever and leucocytosis, but the fluid may appear clear, especially with pneumococcal infections.[42a]

Cytologic findings in ascitic fluid are becoming more reliable now that false results due to morphologic variations, including bizarre forms of mesothelial cells undergoing metaplasia, are being eliminated. However, confirmation of malignant disease remains difficult until the process is far advanced[67]; furthermore, hepatoma is seldom confirmed by this method.[61] Chemical studies also may distinguish the cause of ascites,[64] especially when the findings in blood and ascitic fluid are compared.[111] Higher ratios between ascitic fluid and blood for concentrations of enzymes, proteins and fats are characteristic of malignant ascites, whereas an ammonia content exceeding 3 times that of blood is consistent with acute lesions of the gastrointestinal tract requiring surgical treatment.[87]

FIG. 11–1. Intra-abdominal factors that affect the movement of fluid across the peritoneum.

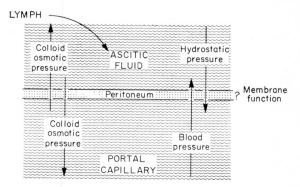

PATHOGENESIS

Circumstances primarily responsible for accumulation of ascites are speculative, despite identification of several relevant disorders of hydrostatic and osmotic equilibrium associated with hepatic disease. These changes are considered in relation first to their influence on fluid accumulating locally within the abdomen and second to the general retention of sodium and water within the body.

Intra-abdominal Factors. Transport of fluid between the peritoneal cavity and portal circulation is explicable mainly by Starling's equilibrium.[124] This equilibrium normally is maintained by the plasma colloid osmotic pressure minus the ascitic fluid colloid osmotic pressure balancing the portal-capillary pressure minus the intra-abdominal hydrostatic pressure (Fig. 11–1).

Changes associated with liver disease alter this equilibrium so that fluid transudes from the capillaries into the peritoneal cavity. In the normal person, a portal-capillary pressure of approximately 30 mm. Hg on the arterial side allows protein-free fluid to filtrate into the pericapillary space; reabsorption occurs in the venous limb, where the pressure drops below the colloid osmotic pressure of the plasma proteins. Since the portal-venous pressure in hepatic disease is often greatly elevated above the normal (mean, 7 mm. Hg) because of portal hypertension, fluid is not reabsorbed effectively into the venous end of the capillaries. That portal hypertension contributes to the formation of ascites is evident from the fact that ascites usually disappears after portal-

systemic shunt procedures.[93, 151] However, portal hypertension due to extrahepatic obstruction of the portal vein rarely causes ascites in patients or experimental animals in the absence of liver disease,[7, 147] and experimental ascites can be induced without elevation of portal pressure.[147]

Additional factors, particularly those related to hepatic function, are, therefore, pertinent. Of these, the most relevant to Starling's concept is hypoalbuminemia associated with impaired hepatic synthesis of protein, since the plasma colloid osmotic pressure depends mainly on the serum albumin concentration. By measuring both portal pressure and serum albumin concentrations, some authors believe the threshold for formation of ascites can be predicted.[4, 112] For example, Atkinson and Losowsky[4] postulated the following critical equation:

$$\frac{10 \times \text{serum albumin (Gm./100 ml.)} + 4}{\text{intrasplenic pressure (cm. } H_2O)} = 1.$$

They found that ascites formed at values below unity. Their data allowed effective separation of patients with and without ascites (Fig. 11–2), although others, including Cherrick and associates,[26] found such measurements less reliable, even when including calculation of net fluid transfer pressure across the peritoneum.

In ascites, Starling's equilibrium is further deranged by protein in ascitic fluid, the concentration of albumin being roughly proportional to that in serum.[4] The concentration of albumin in ascitic fluid often exceeds the amount that would be anticipated in a transudate, and as much as a third of the total body exchangeable albumin may be contained in the ascitic fluid, thus raising

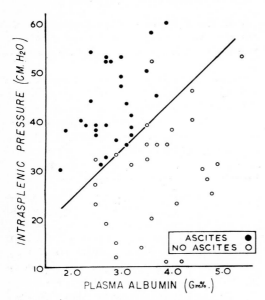

FIG. 11–2. Plasma-albumin concentration and portal vein pressure in relation to formation of ascites. (Courtesy of M. Atkinson and M. S. Losowsky.)

the colloid osmotic pressure of ascitic fluid (Fig. 11–1). These facts, together with the surprisingly swift equilibration of albumin between ascitic fluid and blood,[12, 114] may reflect increased hepatic formation of lymph in some patients, with permeation of protein directly from the hepatic and hilar lymphatics to the peritoneal cavity. Excellent reviews of the several mechanisms believed to be responsible are available.[35, 157]

While the contribution of lymph to formation of ascites has been demonstrated vividly by Mallet-Guy and co-workers[86] in experimental acute hepatic congestion, chronic liver disease is less conducive to such gross evidence of the phenomenon and its relevance under such circumstances has been questioned.[82] However, the lymphatic channels at the hepatic hilus increase in cirrhosis and ascites,[6] and surgeons have visualized lymph leaking from clusters of such vessels as well as from subcapsular hepatic lymphatics in patients with cirrhosis[35]; hepatic lymph flow increases also with experimental cirrhosis.[98] Since the extensive hepatic sinusoidal bed is permeable to plasma protein and normally

contains blood at low pressure, it is postulated that postsinusoidal venous outflow obstruction increases the filtration pressure, thereby forcing fluid into the interstitial space, from whence it drains into the lymphatics. The increased resistance to sinusoidal drainage in hepatic diseases may be attributable to regenerating nodules, fibrosis, swollen liver cells, venous thrombosis or even to changes in pressure effected by the development of hepatic arterial-sinusoidal communications.[35]

As much as 80 per cent of hepatic lymph is diverted through the diaphragmatic lymphatics, which communicate with the thoracic duct; large molecules, such as protein, are returned to the general circulation preferentially by this route. Some indication of the capacity of the lymphatic drainage system of the abdomen is exemplified in the rat by clearance of whole blood introduced into the peritoneum at a rate of 20 mg./kg./ 24 hours.[157] Dumont and Mulholland[35] cannulated the thoracic duct in patients with cirrhosis, portal hypertension and ascites, and found large channels, sometimes approximating the caliber of the subclavian vein, in which hemorrhagic lymph flowed at a rate up to 12 times the normal rate (1 ml. or less per minute). Pressures ranged from the upper limit of normal (15 cm. saline) to 70 cm., and venting the duct sometimes caused a "small geyser of lymph" to erupt. Since draining lymph externally occasionally led to reduction in size of the liver, diminution of ascites, a fall in portal (splenic pulp) pressure and cessation of bleeding from varices, an adverse disproportion between drainage capacity and excess production of lymph in cirrhosis has been implicated in the pathogenesis of portal hypertension as well as of ascites.[35]

Ascitic fluid has the characteristics of an ultrafiltrate of plasma augmented by varied amounts of protein, and thus represents an expansion of the extracellular space. Far from resembling a stagnant pool, its constituents are in dynamic equilibrium with the remainder of the body. Movement of material between the abdominal cavity and the general circulation is mediated by the peritoneum as well as by the lymphatic system. Isotope studies indicate that 40 to 80 per cent of the water is exchanged with that in the blood each hour.[106] Thus, active transport mechanisms, especially those affecting movement of sodium and water across the peritoneal membrane, theoretically oppose or encourage formation of ascites, and it has been postulated that integrity of the membrane is prejudiced and that cell permeability varies in patients with impaired hepatic function.[114] Relatively few studies have been made of transport kinetics of the peritoneum, but Shear and colleagues, who cited earlier work, have demonstrated that sodium transport in experimental preparations can be modified by both physical and pharmacologic agents.[118]

Retention of Sodium and Water. Retention of fluid within the body, characteristic of ascites, is associated not only with derangements of hydrostatic equilibrium within the abdomen, as described, but also with physiologic and biochemical changes involving endocrine metabolism and renal function. The sequence whereby these mechanisms are initiated and thereafter interact to maintain or intensify the ascitic state cannot be defined; important contributory factors have been delineated, but essential information is lacking. Why accumulation of fluid within the abdomen should evoke hormonal and hemodynamic adjustments that apparently aggravate the situation rather than compensate for it is not explainable.

In ascitic patients, total body water and total body exchangeable sodium are greatly increased[13, 28, 138]; plasma volume also is increased.[36, 92] Regardless of sodium intake, it is not rare for patients with ascites to excrete as little as 1 mEq. of sodium per 24 hours. Except under complicated circumstances (p. 369), water is retained secondarily to sodium through readjustment of the renal osmoregulatory mechanisms that maintain isotonicity. The major factors believed to govern excretion of sodium are (1) changes in glomerular filtration rate and (2) mineralocorticoid hormone activity; a "third factor"[16, 34] has recently been invoked to explain maintenance of the normal interplay between plasma (or effective extra-

cellular fluid) volume and sodium and water balance. Alterations in each of these mechanisms have been demonstrated in cirrhosis and ascites.

Glomerular filtration rate is often, but not invariably, reduced in ascites, thus limiting the quantity of solute available for excretion.[9, 10, 102, 117] The abnormality is more prominent when ascites is relatively difficult to treat and is attributed primarily to a reduction in estimated renal plasma flow, although in some patients with ascites clearances of inulin and para-aminohippuric acid are normal (Fig. 11–3). Of greater importance in sodium retention is secondary hyperaldosteronism, a prominent feature in the majority of patients with ascites.[84, 154] Large amounts of aldosterone are found in the urine, and decreased plasma disappearance curves, together with the increased amounts of unconjugated hormone excreted, suggest that failure of the diseased liver to inactivate aldosterone contributes partially to its activity.[30] In addition, concentrations of plasma renin, angiotensin and angiotensinase are elevated[14, 18, 48] and pathologic changes consistent with hyperaldosteronism have been described, including increases in the juxtaglomerular indices and width of the zona glomerulosa of the adrenal cortices.[55] Diminished renal perfusion is implicated most commonly as the stimulus to secondary hyperaldosteronism[72]; surprisingly, although renal blood flow is reduced in many patients with ascites (Fig. 11–3), this fails to correlate directly with increased tubular absorption of sodium.[9, 117]

More general relationships between adrenal function and formation of ascites may be inferred from the diuresis which follows bilateral adrenalectomy or the use of drugs which suppress adrenal function.[57, 58, 88, 131] However, since such responses are somewhat nonspecific or incomplete, attention has been directed toward additional mechanisms. These comprise the effects of mineralocorticoid hormones, unidentified as yet but capable of stimulating reabsorption of sodium in the proximal renal tubule, and of certain extra-adrenal endocrine mechanisms, including the possibilities that fluid retention is due, in part, to estrogens[105] that are detoxicated by the liver or that vasopressin participates, especially when relative overhydration and hyponatremia develop (see p. 369).

It is convenient to postulate impairment of "third factor" activity[16] to explain the discrepancies in current knowledge of formation of ascites, thereby implicating failure of the proximal renal tubule to reduce reabsorption of sodium in response to expansion of plasma or effective extracellular fluid volume. As evidence partially consistent with this view, McCloy and co-workers[92] demonstrated increased plasma volume in patients with cirrhosis, including those with ascites or impaired renal plasma flow, and found that further augmenting plasma volume by raising serum colloid osmotic pressure with albumin or by raising plasma osmolality with hypertonic saline resulted in subnormal and temporary responses in renal tubular and circulatory function.[91]

The nature of a "third factor" is speculative, but experimental evidence suggests that it is a humoral substance that affects active transport of sodium by the renal tubule and is activated by changes in the effective extracellular fluid volume. Impairment of "third factor" in cirrhosis could be related to abnormalities of hepatic function or of portal circulation, since evidence from animal experimentation suggests that extracellular fluid volume is partially regulated by osmoreceptors within the liver or by a diuretic factor released from it that is sensitive to changes in the composition of portal blood.[54, 94, 155] Such mechanisms may be impaired in cirrhosis and portal hyper-

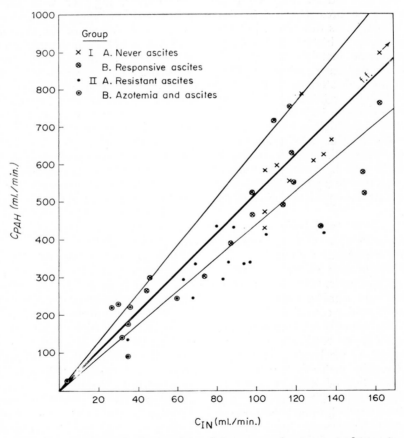

Fig. 11–3. Renal plasma flow (clearance of para-aminohippuric acid, C_{PAH}), glomerular filtration rate (clearance of inulin, C_{IN}), and filtration fraction (f.f.) in cirrhosis.

tension. The high plasma volume in cirrhosis appears to be linked more closely with the presence and degree of portal hypertension[79] than with other factors, although it is not necessarily affected by reduction of portal pressure through portal-systemic shunt operations. The possibility that sodium and water are absorbed abnormally from the gastrointestinal tract in cirrhosis is not supported by preliminary studies.[123, 137]

TREATMENT

General Principles. Metabolic studies have proved the efficacy of many methods of choice for removing excess water and sodium from patients with ascites. However, the degree to which these measures prolong survival rather than introduce new complications is less scientifically documented, as is the extent to which ascites represents a necessary physiologic adjustment by the body to altered circumstances, rather than a damaging, pathologic state. Therapy, therefore, is restricted to the minimum necessary and effective for the individual, and specific measures are adjuvant to those employed for the associated liver disease which causes retention of fluid.

Ascites may accumulate suddenly as a sequel to sudden deterioration in liver function associated with alcoholism, gastrointestinal hemorrhage, surgical procedures or intercurrent illness. In such instances, it may suffice to treat the precipitating factor and temporarily restrict sodium intake. Rarely is recovery spontaneous.[103] In some instances, mild ascites persists relatively unchanged for several months and requires only alert supervision and a nutritious diet, including a modest reduction of sodium.

More frequently, ascites develops insidiously and progresses to the point of discomfort. Sodium is then restricted more rigorously; and diuretic agents are used to procure a steady weight loss of up to 7 kg. weekly. Since newer drugs are very potent, detectable fluid is retained within the abdomen as a precaution against volume and sodium depletion. If the patient is treated in a hospital, upon dismissal he should be well educated in the details of therapy, which should have been modified to conditions pertaining at home. Ascites commonly becomes increasingly refractory to medical management. Progression of the hepatic disease is usually responsible, but the possibility of hepatoma is sometimes pertinent. Additional palliative or more radical procedures are then considered.

Diet and Nutrition. The importance of restricting the dietary intake of sodium is dictated by the avid sodium retention of patients with ascites and confirmed by wide experience,[31] despite the theoretic drawback of aggravating hyperaldosteronism. Fluid intake is reduced only in specific instances (see p. 370). Restriction of sodium usually prevents further accumulation of fluid and may initiate diuresis, especially when liver function improves concomitantly. Although a diet that contains less than 10 mEq. of sodium may be ideal in the hospital, technical difficulties and the lack of palatability make it impractical for most patients under domestic conditions. Diets that contain at least 20 mEq. usually are preferred for maintenance, and can be made more attractive by the use of salt substitutes and special sodium-depleted foods. Failure of treatment usually reflects deviation from the dietary regimen, and frequent consultations are advisable to review and, if indicated, to arrange analysis of the sodium content of the diet, drinking water or drugs taken incidentally. Protein, calorie and vitamin intake must be emphasized, especially for alcoholic and other undernourished patients, for this may improve liver function with coincident disappearance of ascites, together with abstention from alcohol, although it sometimes takes several months.[31, 132]

Proteins depleted of sodium can be prescribed when high protein and low sodium requirements of the diet conflict. Starch hydrolysates may be used to increase caloric intake in anorectic patients, and vitamins can be given as supplements. The protein requirement depends on age, sex, physique and the type of liver disease or its complications. Intakes of more than 100 Gm. seldom increase retention of nitrogen, even in previously malnourished patients, whereas those with cryptogenic cirrhosis may require less[45, 132]; in contrast, high protein diets can precipitate hepatic coma.[133]

TABLE 11–1. EFFECTS OF THERAPY IN PATIENTS WITH ASCITES REQUIRING DIURETICS*

DIURETIC AGENT	SUPPLEMENTAL THERAPY	PER CENT OF PATIENTS		
		SATIS-FACTORY DIURESIS	HYPO-KALEMIA	ALKALOSIS
Thiazide	None	25	90	10
	Potassium	25	30	5
Spironolactone or triamterene	None	15	...	...
Thiazide plus spironolactone or triamterene	None	75	20	60
	Potassium	75	...	40
	Potassium and lysine monohydrochloride	75	...	...
Ethacrynic acid or furosemide	None	100	100	90
	Potassium	100	50	70
	Potassium and lysine monohydrochloride	100	40	10
Ethacrynic acid or furosemide plus spironolactone or triamterene	None	100	30	80
	Potassium	100	10	60
	Potassium and lysine monohydrochloride	100	...	...

* Lieberman, F. L., and Reynolds, T. B.: Unpublished data (personal communication).

Additional factors designed to improve or maintain protein metabolism include the administration of albumin, ascitic fluid or protein hydrolysates by vein and the use of anabolic agents. Acute or repeated infusions of albumin or ascitic fluid have been abandoned in all but exceptional circumstances because of the side effects, expense and lack of sustained action.[27, 91, 121, 145] Trials of anabolic agents[43, 152] have yielded conflicting results, and the drugs may be hepatotoxic.[104]

Diuretic Therapy. Comprehensive reviews of the actions and efficacy of various diuretic agents have been published recently by Earley[37] and by Laragh.[71] Lieberman and Reynolds[78] have reported on the use of newer diuretics in cirrhosis and ascites; and the yield from their more recent and extensive experiences is summarized in Table 11–1. All diuretics currently used diminish reabsorption of sodium ions by the renal tubule, thus promoting isotonic losses of sodium and water in the urine. However, they differ in modes and sites of action, side effects and therapeutic indications.

Organomercurials, such as Thiomerin, impede reabsorption of sodium beyond the proximal tubule and simultaneously inhibit secretion of potassium; these effects are enhanced by acidifying agents. Unfortunately, repeated parenteral administration is required and these agents are being replaced by more potent drugs which can be given by mouth. Thiazide derivatives reduce reabsorption of sodium and chloride mainly in the distal part of the loop of Henle and proximal portion of the distal tubule. Their action at this location also compromises generation of dilute fluid by the tubule. In addition, thiazides inhibit carbonic anhydrase activity, thereby limiting tubular secretion of hydrogen ion and increasing loss of bicarbonate and potassium. The site of action and effects of furosemide are similar to those of the thiazides; since a relatively high rate of excretion of chloride is promoted, hypochloremic alkalosis may develop. Since both act proximal to the sodium-potassium exchange site, excretion of potassium also is increased.

Ethacrynic acid exerts its main effects more proximally in the loop of Henle and also may precipitate both potassium depletion and hypochloremic alkalosis, probably by discrete mechanisms.[78] The aldosterone antagonist spironolactone and the pteridine derivative triamterene exert their major effects distally at the site of sodium-potassium exchange. Loss of potassium is therefore diminished and the diuretic effect depends on sufficient sodium reaching the distal site. Prednisone and similar steroid medications were once useful in conjunction with earlier diuretic agents; their actions probably include some suppression of endogenous mineralocorticoid production, an increase in glomerular filtration rate and promotion of free water clearance by the kidney, but the newer, more potent compounds usually render steroids superfluous as diuretic agents.

Ideally diuretic therapy brings about a slow and uncomplicated diuresis, during which excess body sodium and water are excreted while essential substances are retained, and thereafter a steady balance between sodium intake and sodium excretion is maintained by the judicious control of diet and medications. The smallest and least frequent dose of the safest effective drug is chosen. Diuretics are usually taken in the morning, so that sleep is undisturbed by diuresis, and some believe the response is better if the patient can be kept supine. Usually, treatment is initiated with thiazides. Potassium depletion is a possibility (Table 11–1), since body-exchangeable potassium is often low in liver disease (Fig.

11–4), because of dietary deficiency, secondary hyperaldosteronism, the prior use of diuretics, or severe impairment of hepatic function.[23, 24] The simultaneous administration of spironolactone or triamterene with a thiazide reduces loss of potassium and is advisable during diuresis, whereas supplementation of dietary potassium (up to 100 mEq./day) is usually preferable for subsequent maintenance. When spironolactone or triamterene is administered alone, the increase in excretion of sodium is often limited.

If patients are resistant to such treatment, the more potent but dangerous drugs, ethacrynic acid or furosemide, are almost invariably effective (Fig. 11–5). There is insufficient evidence to indicate which is preferable. With either, triamterene or spironolactone should be prescribed to conserve potassium and, when starting therapy, oral potassium chloride supplements also are advisable. Since the magnitude of the response may not be predictable, lysine monohydrochloride (up to 100 mEq./day) is given as a precaution against unexpectedly large diuresis leading to hypochloremic alkalosis and hypovolemia.

Of the complications of diuretic therapy (Fig. 11–5), potassium depletion is the most frequent and is guarded against by appropriate combinations of diuretic agents, with

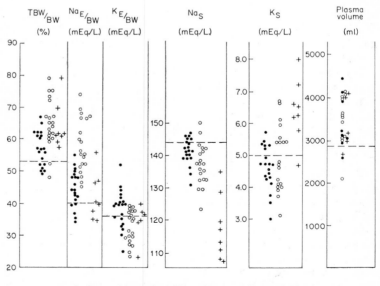

Fig. 11–4. Total body water (TBW), exchangeable sodium (Na_E), and exchangeable potassium (K_E) in relation to body weight (BW); serum concentrations of sodium (Na_S) and of potassium (K_S); and corrected plasma volume in patients with cirrhosis.

○ Ascites   + Azotemia   ● No ascites   — — Mean normal value

oral supplements of potassium when necessary. Less commonly, spironolactone or triamterene causes potassium retention and hyperkalemia. Cessation of therapy, perhaps with additional measures (see p. 370), is then indicated, since the situation is potentially hazardous.[8] When excess sodium and chloride is excreted, hypochloremic alkalosis develops. Lysine monohydrochloride is the treatment of choice since the acidifying agents usually recommended (ammonium chloride or acetazolamide) can precipitate the hepatic coma syndrome. Excessive doses of the stronger diuretics may even cause true depletion of volume and sodium. For these reasons, during treatment detectable fluid should be retained within the abdomen of all patients with ascites. Even if diuresis is not massive, dilutional hyponatremia may develop in association with impairment of renal circulatory function in ascites patients who are receiving diuretic agents.[8, 9, 78] For the management of these complications, see p. 370.

Hepatic coma is not infrequently pre-cipitated by diuretic agents, especially thiazides, ethacrynic acid and furosemide (Table 11–1). The causes are complex and uncertainly interrelated, but may reflect hypokalemia, depletion of potassium, an increased contribution of ammonia from the kidney to the systemic circulation and changes in extracellular and intracellular pH, which could facilitate transport of ammonia into the cells of the central nervous system. In most instances, cessation of diuretic therapy and temporary reduction of dietary intake of protein suffice for treatment; sometimes additional measures, including enemas and the administration of broad-spectrum antibiotics, are necessary.

Less frequent complications of diuretic therapy include hyperuricemia, decreased glucose tolerance and, rarely, nephrotoxicity, vasculitis or pancreatitis.[37, 71]

Surgical Measures. Paracentesis abdominis has been practiced and condemned regularly for nearly 2,000 years. Hazards include infection, hemorrhage, perforation of an abdominal viscus and precipitation or

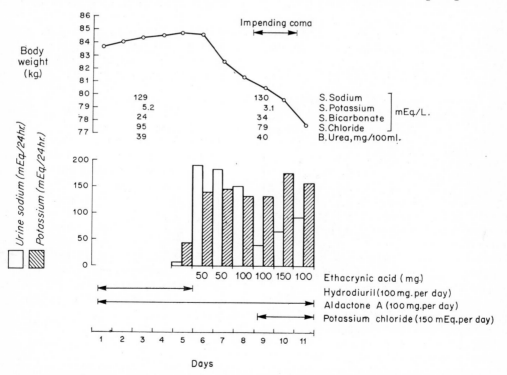

Fig. 11–5. Effects and complications of diuretic therapy in cirrhosis with ascites. *B.*, blood; *S.*, serum.

aggravation of disorders of water and electrolyte metabolism or renal function, with possible peripheral vascular collapse or hepatic coma (see p. 370). Gabuzda and associates documented the metabolic consequences of removing large amounts of fluid, electrolytes and protein by paracentesis and later considered the management of complications.[46] Hemodynamic changes resulting from paracentesis include increases in cardiac output and stroke volume, probably related to augmentation of the venous return, with concomitant reductions in portal and inferior vena cava pressure.[66] Complications are minimized by careful procedure, including slow withdrawal of fluid at a rate not exceeding 2 liters in 24 hours.

Other than for diagnostic purposes, serious distress due to the volume of ascites constitutes the major indication for paracentesis; it is prudent to remove only sufficient fluid to alleviate discomfort, as a prelude to standard treatment. The withdrawal of small volumes of fluid at frequent intervals advocated by Caroli[22] is most clearly indicated when ascites accumulates massively in patients with oliguria and azotemia during terminal hepatic failure.

Infrequently, ascites is difficult to manage despite apparently adequate hepatic function, the latter being judged more by general nutrition, the absence of jaundice or previous coma, and satisfactory blood coagulation mechanisms than by chemical tests. In such patients, definitive surgical treatment of ascites occasionally is considered, with the reservation that such operations do not improve the underlying liver disease. Portal-systemic shunts usually relieve ascites; the discouraging operative mortality exceeding 40 per cent in patients resistant to medical treatment reported by Blakemore[15] may have been reduced by subsequent changes in technic.[93, 151] As an alternative, bilateral adrenalectomy[57, 88] is rarely successful; postoperative management is intricate, and the procedure has been abandoned. Portacaval anastomosis may be relevant when gastroesophageal varices are demonstrated and massive hemorrhage has occurred. In alcoholics, simultaneous but slow improvements in both liver function[31]

and degree of portal hypertension[110] indicate deferment of major surgical treatment until the response to medical therapy and the sincerity of abstention from alcohol can be assessed. Recovery from ascites may be related to abstinence rather than to surgical treatment, whereas major procedures are seldom warranted when continued alcoholism leads inevitably to hepatic failure.

Prognosis and Complications. The prognosis in ascites is poor; only 50 per cent of the patients reported by Ratnoff and Patek survived for 6 months.[107] Despite progress in therapy, there is little evidence that the outlook has improved, especially when the onset of ascites is insidious and when increasing resistance to treatment develops.[25, 27, 121]

The majority of patients die from hepatic coma, gastrointestinal hemorrhage or other complications more directly attributable to the associated hepatic disease than to retention of fluid.[130] However, renal circulatory failure with the ultimate development of oliguria and azotemia is a frequent accompaniment[8, 56, 102] and has been reviewed recently.[127] Chalmers expressed the opinion that almost every patient with progressive cirrhosis had terminal oliguria and uremia,[25] while more than half of the patients dying from cirrhosis reviewed by Shear and associates had evidence of renal failure.[119] It has been concluded that advances in therapy are responsible,[140] because newer diuretics cause a fall in plasma volume and hence renal circulatory failure, but no increase in the incidence of the complication was discerned from 1958 to 1962 in more than 100 patients who died from cirrhosis at the Cleveland Metropolitan General Hospital.[119]

Prognosis, since it is largely determined by liver function, is most favorable when ascites develops in response to hepatic diseases or precipitating factors for which specific measures of treatment are available, and is more hopeful in the alcoholic who can abstain than in nonalcoholic patients with cirrhosis.[132]

THE KIDNEY IN LIVER DISEASE

Liver-Kidney Interrelationships. Before considering precipitating factors and mechanisms for the renal failure to which patients with cirrhosis and ascites are curiously prone, it is necessary to be aware of the numerous associations known or postulated between diseases or disordered function of the liver and kidney and, simultaneously, to reject indiscriminate use of the term "hepatorenal syndrome" until specific interrelationships between the 2 organs are confirmed by experimental and clinical data.[8, 89, 119, 127] Primary diseases of both the liver and kidney, which may occur with more than coincidental frequency,[42] or systemic disorders involving both organs are most readily classified. An association is recognized also between renal tumors and abnormal tests of hepatic function, [76, 125, 134] which may be corrected by surgical removal of the tumor.

By contrast, azotemia that develops during hepatic failure usually is not attributable to any characteristic change in renal pathology, although certain circumstances incidental to and often inseparable from hepatic disease may predispose to kidney lesions.[25, 122, 126, 130, 140] Thus, therapeutic measures or complications of hepatic disease may lead to renal circulatory failure, tubular necrosis or nephropathy, and these are often assumed to be sequelae to decreases in plasma volume or arterial blood pressure. Depletion of potassium or sodium secondary to dietetic or diuretic therapy, the nephrotoxicity of neomycin and other drugs, paracentesis abdominis or other surgical procedures, and, especially, hemorrhage from gastroesophageal varices have been thought to be responsible in these regards.[8, 9, 42, 68, 89, 116, 119, 129, 140, 144] The specificity of the effect on the kidney of jaundice, caused by parenchymal disease of the liver or obstruction of the extrahepatic biliary system, can be defined less confidently. Azotemia appears to occur with undue frequency after operations on the biliary tract, and it is postulated that bilirubinemia predisposes the kidney to tubular necrosis in the presence of hypovolemia and arterial hypotension.[33, 148, 153] Bile salts have recently been reported to be nephrotoxic in animals.

Although arterial blood pressure is not consistently decreased in azotemia,[8] and despite high or normal plasma volume in cirrhosis,[36, 91] azotemia has often been accepted as occurring invariably on a prerenal basis, as a sequel to reduction of the theoretically effective extracellular fluid volume. However, applications of newer technics, together with more careful assessment of the role of possible precipitating mechanisms, indicate that renal failure frequently develops spontaneously as an intrinsic part of hepatic failure.[28, 129, 130] Such a relationship is now accepted,[8, 119, 143] although in individual cases it frequently is difficult to appraise the contribution of exogenous factors; and differentiation between tubular necrosis and spontaneous development of renal failure is less precise[8, 116, 119] than ideally depicted (Table 11–2). For example, scrutiny of 76 cases of cirrhosis and azotemia did not reveal any cause for renal failure other than its association with advanced hepatic disease in a third of the patients[8]; in the remainder, exogenous factors, of which gastrointestinal hemorrhage was the most frequent, could not be exonerated. Others have not found a plausible explanation for azotemia except its association with hepatic failure in comparable proportions of cases.[116, 119] Indeed, the extrarenal factors once accorded prime etiologic importance often may be agonal or only reflect a previously prejudiced state of renal function.[8, 9] Hence, glomerular filtration rate and estimated renal plasma flow may be reduced in cirrhosis prior to clinically evident deterioration[9, 119, 142] and may be of such degree (Fig. 11–3) that the term "preazotemia" has been applied.[8]

Renal Circulatory Failure. The salient features of renal circulatory failure in cirrhosis or, much less commonly, in other hepatic diseases[127] are well defined.[8, 42, 56, 89, 101, 102, 119] Ascites is almost invariable and is usually refractory to treatment; other complications, including hepatic coma and portal hypertension, are frequent. Jaundice may or may not be present, but hepatic function is severely impaired by most clinical and biochemical criteria.

Initially, fatigue and anorexia are associated with hyponatremia, hypokalemia, hypochloremia and elevated concentrations of blood urea and serum creatinine. Patients may later experience nausea, vomiting and thirst; simultaneously the biochemical abnormalities become more pronounced. Less

TABLE 11–2. DIFFERENTIATION BETWEEN SPONTANEOUS RENAL FAILURE AND RENAL
TUBULAR NECROSIS IN HEPATIC DISEASE

	SPONTANEOUS RENAL FAILURE	RENAL TUBULAR NECROSIS
Jaundice	Possible	Often
Ascites	Usually	Possible
Hepatic function	Poor	Variable
Precipitating factors	Possible	Yes
Course	Variable	Rapid
Arterial hypotension	Late	Early
Oliguria	Late	Early
Specific gravity of urine	>1.010	±1.010
Protein, casts and blood cells in urine	No	Yes
Tubular reabsorption of sodium	Increased	Decreased
Tubular reabsorption of potassium	<sodium	>sodium
Osmolality of urine	High (maybe >plasma)	Low (<plasma)
Glomerular filtration rate and estimated renal plasma flow	Low	Low
Filtration fraction	Often high	Often low
Extraction ratio for PAH	Normal	Low
Specific renal histologic change	No	Sometimes

often, hyperkalemia[89, 129, 130] or, rarely, hypernatremia[141] is found; the pH of whole blood is variable but often abnormal[8, 129] and, occasionally, unexplained anemia is reported.[8, 130]

With further deterioration, the neuropsychiatric disorder, electroencephalographic changes and elevated blood ammonia concentrations, consistent with and indistinguishable from hepatic coma, appear. Hyperammonemia is presumably sustained by hydrolysis of the increased amounts of urea excreted into the gut,[2, 150] although the contrasting possibility that a metabolic abnormality associated with hepatic coma adversely affects renal function has been proposed.[119] During this late phase, oliguria and arterial hypotension are evident and deepening coma with an unfavorable outcome is the rule.[8, 89, 119] Features of hepatic failure still predominate and death not infrequently results from massive gastrointestinal hemorrhage.[8, 119] It has been emphasized that oliguria and arterial hypotension often appear only in the final stage of the spontaneous syndrome,[8] thus contrasting with earlier concepts that azotemia invariably had a prerenal basis.

Renal Function. Urinalysis, tests of renal function and histologic examination of the kidney, when interpreted in relation to the clinical findings, assist in establishing the diagnosis and may differentiate renal tubular necrosis from spontaneous renal circulatory failure (Table 11–2). Equivocal results are not uncommon[8, 42, 119] and may reflect that more than one factor operates in the development of azotemia. The wide variety of gross or histologic changes in the kidneys in hepatic disease include several of dubious relevance; even the presence of tubular necrosis is seldom obvious on histologic examination.[89] Significantly greater numbers of renal glomerular lesions are found at autopsy in patients who have had hepatic disease; splitting, fraying or thickening of the basement membrane was observed in 28 per cent of one series.[63]

More recently Salomon and colleagues[113] identified glomerular changes in renal biopsy tissue from all of 24 patients with hepatic disease. Studies by electron microscopy revealed deposits in the capillary wall and mesangium, thickening of the basement membranes and an increased mesangial matrix. However, these glomerular changes, like other morphologic findings, have not been correlated with abnormalities of renal function or with the type, duration or severity of the hepatic disease.[63, 113] Recently a cadaveric kidney transplanted from a patient with cirrhosis and renal circulatory failure functioned promptly in the recipient.

Conventional tests of renal function often show reduced clearances of inulin, PAH, creatinine and urea in ascites[9, 10, 53, 70, 117, 143]; additional features may be expected when azotemia is on an extrarenal basis and attributable to tubular necrosis (Table 11–2). Progressive deterioration in clearance values has been correlated with the severity of the clinical condition (Fig. 11–3), as indicated by the presence of ascites, its resistance to treatment, and the presence of azotemia.[9] A disorder of renal hemodynamic function[9, 70, 117, 143] is assumed from the absence of diagnostic features on urinalysis, the apparent adequacy of the functioning renal mass when examined histologically, and the frequently high filtration fraction.[9] Total renal plasma flow[10] and the renal fraction of cardiac output are reduced,[10, 69] although cardiac output and indices,[10, 69, 117] mean arterial blood pressure,[10] and systemic vascular resistance[10] are usually within the normal range. However, an increased blood flow to the splanchnic or other regions cannot be excluded as leading to the low renal component of cardiac output.

The cause of the progressive decrease in renal perfusion cannot yet be specified. The concept that osmoreceptors, sensitive to reductions in the theoretical effective extracellular fluid volume caused by loss of water and electrolytes into the peritoneum, initiate the reduction in renal blood flow is attractive but currently it is not susceptible to proof or to refutation. Hyponatremia and hypoalbuminemia undoubtedly may affect circulatory and tubular function of the normal kidney.[38, 39, 49, 65, 109] However, in cirrhosis plasma volume is high,[36, 92] and raising serum osmolality or plasma colloid osmotic pressure has not produced impressive or sustained effects on either renal hemodynamics or sodium and water reabsorption in cirrhosis.[27, 91, 146, 156] Renal hemodynamic function also is unlikely to be impaired greatly as a result of compression of the renal venous outflow by the hydrostatic effects of ascites, for renal vein pressures are neither consistently nor sufficiently above the normal range.[10] Moreover, glomerular filtration rate (GFR) and estimated renal plasma flow (ERPF) are little influenced by disappearance of ascites,[9] although some aspects of renal function may improve.[51]

Baldus and colleagues,[10] finding total renal vascular resistance significantly elevated in patients with severe impairment of renal hemodynamic function, believed that an increase in resistance offered by the renal vasculature could be responsible. The site of increased resistance is unknown and the abnormality cannot be designated as compensatory or causal. Vasoactive material liberated from, or inadequately inactivated by, the failing liver demands consideration. An alternative theory might implicate an interrelationship between the renal and hepatic circulations mediated through the autonomic nervous system. Thus, occlusion of the portal vein or ligation of the hepatic artery strikingly reduces renal blood flow in the dog and the effect is abolished by sympathectomy and splanchnicectomy.[99, 100] Subsequently, hepatic periarterial nerve crush alone has been shown to be as effective as hepatic anoxia in evoking renal vasoconstriction.[59]

Shear and associates,[117] who found low extraction ratios in 3 patients and frequently subnormal filtration fractions and who cited evidence adduced by others from the impairment of renal concentrating ability in cirrhosis,[60] suggested that increased medullary blood flow and shunting of blood around the glomerular capillaries account for renal circulatory failure. This suggestion contrasts with the normal extraction ratios of PAH and differences in arterial and renal vein oxygen found by Baldus and associates,[10] findings that make it less likely that arteriovenous communication within the kidneys, comparable to that occurring in other organs in cirrhosis, is a cause of the renal circulatory disorder.

Abnormalities of renal tubular function are fundamental in the formation of ascites (see p. 359), but it is not certain that they are related to impaired renal circulation. Overly tenacious retention of sodium, with relatively greater amounts of potassium in the urine, persists despite progressive reductions in GFR and ERPF.[9] Osmolar

The Kidney in Liver Disease 369

clearance is low[9, 117] and tubular reabsorption of urea may be increased in oliguric patients.[9] Martini has expressed the view that excessive tubular reabsorption of sodium and water by the kidneys is "basic" to the development of azotemia,[89] but it is also relevant that diuretic therapy or adrenalectomy affects water and electrolyte excretion without consistently affecting other aspects of renal function. Current concepts implicate diminished renal perfusion as a stimulus to secondary hyperaldosteronism, but no data correlate this with sodium retention, perhaps because tubular reabsorption of sodium also occurs proximally, being controlled by an unknown mechanism such as "third factor." Similarly, the curious natriuresis and lack of pressor response which follow administration of angiotensin in patients with cirrhosis and ascites, while coinciding with renal vasoconstriction and a fall in ERPF without a change in GFR,[1, 73] sequester no evident clue to the interrelationships of impaired renal functions.

The defective renal tubular excretion of water in cirrhosis, characterized by reductions in maximal urine flow and free water clearance, bears a highly significant relationship to the reduction in GFR rather than to the rate of sodium excretion.[9, 117] This pattern of abnormal excretion of water in cirrhosis is consonant with excess vasopressin activity[42, 75] and probably accounts for the hyponatremia and relative overhydration that precede or are associated with the development of azotemia. Under such circumstances, the osmolality of the urine may approximate or exceed that of the plasma. Moreover, often in cirrhosis the urine is not highly concentrated, an abnormality evidently not related to changes in GFR, excretion of sodium or free water clearance, but consistent with the increase in medullary blood flow.

Water and Electrolyte Metabolism. The gross abnormalities of water and electrolyte metabolism with cirrhosis and ascites (Fig. 11–4) are central to the condition, and awareness of their characteristics is essential to management. Total body water and exchangeable sodium are increased[13, 28] and hyponatremia is the rule in azotemia, with serum sodium concentrations (Na_S) usually

falling below 130 mEq./liter.[8, 28, 56, 89, 119, 128, 130] Hyponatremia is of the dilutional variety and has therefore been termed "paradoxical"; overhydration may be aggravated by thirst, and the osmolality of plasma sometimes is less than that of the urine.[9] Overhydration and hyponatremia cause inconstant and nonspecific complaints[75]; in animals, hyponatremia may augment tissue catabolism,[81] thereby increasing the concentration of urea in the blood.

Total body exchangeable potassium (K_E) is difficult to refer to conventional parameters in the presence of ascites,[24] but values appear low[23, 24, 96] and the deficit often approximates 500 mEq.[24] Dietary inadequacies, diuretic therapy or secondary hyperaldosteronism may lead to potassium depletion, but a greater correlation with the degree of impairment of hepatic function has also been claimed[24] and supplemental potassium may not replete body stores in such patients.[24, 96] Potassium deficiency must be evaluated as a causal factor for several abnormalities of azotemic patients, including extracellular alkalosis,[23] hyperammonemia,[5] hepatic coma[108] and renal tubular dysfunction, but its contribution to symptomatology and the frequency of therapeutic response to potassium therapy in hepatic failure may have been overstated.[23, 128] As with Na_S, serum concentrations of potassium (K_S) are unreliable as indicators of body stores in cirrhosis (Fig. 11–4).[24] Serum concentration of potassium is usually low and is abnormal in approximately half the patients[23, 24]; hyperkalemia may develop with azotemia and lead to cardiac conduction defects or even death.[9, 128–130, 140] Hypochloremia also is common,[9] but chloride deficiency is seldom demonstrated convincingly; the likelihood must be considered in patients receiving diuretics, especially ethacrynic acid,[78] and when extracellular alkalosis is present.[3] Respiratory alkalosis of uncertain cause is frequent, but variable disorders of acid-base equilibrium occur in hepatic failure and none is characteristic of ascites or azotemia.[9, 23, 40]

Despite greater hyponatremia and hyperkalemia, Na_E is usually increased and K_E is often decreased in azotemia. Values for Na_E and K_E do not necessarily differ from those associated with ascites in patients without azotemia, but relatively less water and more sodium may be excreted during diuretic therapy when renal circulatory function is impaired.[28, 128-130] There is also a slight indication that changes in K_S and Na_S partially reflect transpositions of sodium and potassium between the intracellular and extracellular fluid compartments.[28]

Prognosis and Treatment of Renal Circulatory Failure. Azotemia that develops spontaneously during hepatic failure has been described variously as "an almost certain portent of death,"[90] "lethal"[119] and "terminal."[122] Improvement has occasioned case reports[29, 47, 50] since the syndrome is irreversible without exception in some series.[52, 119] However, in others azotemia has not been uniformly fatal.[9, 128, 129] The outlook is considered less bleak if a well-defined precipitating factor is identified and treated, as in some cases with tubular necrosis.[116] The duration of azotemia varies from a few days to more than 6 weeks[9, 117] and death is attributable primarily to hepatic failure, the prognosis being related most clearly to the degree of reversibility of the hepatic disease and the prospect of comparable improvement in renal function.[9, 10] Blood pressure, output of urine, duration of azotemia or height of blood urea concentrations apparently discriminate less effectively between survivors and nonsurvivors.[9]

The development of dilutional hyponatremia is "ominous" in ascites[75] and the prospect is particularly grave when values drop below 125 mEq./liter.[9, 89, 128] Although recovery of 9 of 15 patients with hyponatremia of this degree was reported in one series, mortality was greatly increased in the presence of azotemia.[126] Under such circumstances, the serum sodium concentration is one of the less unreliable tests of "liver function" when used as an index of the severity and prognosis of the hepatic disease. Since hyponatremia is due to overhydration and since the latter is related to impairment of GFR, it is not surprising that defective excretion of a water load also implies a poor prognosis.

The grave outlook may reflect also the inadequacy of current treatment. Standard conservative measures[9, 119, 127, 128] are de-

signed to permit maximal time for the recovery of hepatic function on which the outcome appears to depend. As a precaution, paracentesis or other procedures considered likely to precipitate the syndrome are avoided in vulnerable patients, and vigorous treatment is instituted for complications such as gastrointestinal hemorrhage, which also may lead to azotemia. Other developments incident to hepatic failure, including hepatic coma, call for prompt management by standard procedures; recently, new approaches to the control of hyperammonemia by reducing urease activity with diets,[85] using enzyme inhibitors[135] or inducing immunity to urease[139] have been proposed. The effect of diuretics on renal function is unknown and variable, but since it may provoke decreases in GFR and plasma volume, albeit usually reversible,[78, 144] such therapy is prudently withheld in azotemia. Continued restriction of dietary sodium is advisable for patients with ascites in most instances.

Restriction of fluid intake is mandatory for overhydration and oliguria; it is considered for any patient whose serum sodium concentration falls below 130 mEq./liter or whenever the output of urine is less than 500 ml. in 24 hours, regardless of the blood urea concentration. Attempts to increase plasma colloid osmotic pressure and serum osmolality by infusions of albumin, albumin and saline or ascitic fluid have variable effects on volume of urine, GFR and excretion of sodium,[29, 144, 146, 156] but the duration and magnitude of these changes are seldom of practical significance in patients with the greatest impairment of renal function.[27, 47, 91, 145] Administration of saline to patients with ascites is hazardous; it is permissible only if a well-defined sodium deficit is demonstrated[119] and when accompanied by restricted intake of fluids. Potassium is supplemented if deficiency is evident, and is given cautiously, lest hyperkalemia develop.[9, 28] This complication may require the administration of ion exchange resins, glucose and insulin.

The disappointing results of standard procedures should not deter an empirical attitude toward therapy. Norepinephrine, aminophylline, mannitol, metaraminol and prednisone influence various aspects of renal circulatory or tubular function in health and in some disease states, but their effects have appeared inconsistent in cirrhosis and discouraging in impaired renal function[9, 21, 70, 90, 119, 130, 144]; trials of other compounds and use of newer pressor agents are justifiable. Hemodialysis, when not precluded by problems related to blood coagulation, or peritoneal dialysis should control several metabolic disorders, including those pertaining to water, electrolytes, ammonia and urea. Although information is limited and disappointing,[116, 119, 121] greater experience should be gained in selected cases. The more experimental approaches, including use of the porcine liver, cross-circulation procedures and hepatic transplantation in hepatic and renal failure,[19, 41, 80] should be limited to specialized centers, but represent important potential sources of original contributions which may be translated in the future to better management of azotemia in hepatic failure.

REFERENCES

1. Ames, R. P., Borkowski, A. J., Sicinski, A. M., and Laragh, J. H.: Prolonged infusions of angiotension II and norepinephrine and blood pressure, electrolyte balance, and aldosterone and cortisol secretion in normal man and in cirrhosis with ascites, J. Clin. Invest. 44:1171, 1965.

2. Aoyagi, T., Engstrom, G. W., Evans, W. B., and Summerskill, W. H. J.: Gastrointestinal urease in man. Part I. Activity of mucosal urease; Part II. Urea hydrolysis and ammonia absorption in upper and lower gut lumen and the effect of neomycin, Gut 7:631; 635, 1966.

3. Atkins, E. L., and Schwartz, W. B.: Factors governing correction of the alkalosis associated with potassium deficiency; the critical role of chloride in the recovery process, J. Clin. Invest. 41:218, 1962.

4. Atkinson, M., and Losowsky, M. S.: The mechanism of ascites formation in chronic liver disease, Quart. J. Med. 30: 153, 1961.

5. Baertl, J. M., Sancetta, S. M., and Gabuzda, G. J.: Relation of acute potassium depletion to renal ammonium metabolism in patients with cirrhosis, J. Clin. Invest. 42:696, 1963.

6. Baggenstoss, A. H., and Cain, J. C.: The hepatic hilar lymphatics of man: their relation to ascites, New Engl. J. Med. 256:531, 1957.

7. Baggenstoss, A. H., and Wollaeger, E. E.: Portal hypertension due to chronic occlusion of the extrahepatic portion of the portal vein: its relation to ascites, Am. J. Med. 21:16, 1956.

8. Baldus, W. P., Feichter, R. N., and Summerskill, W. H. J.: The kidney in cirrhosis. I. Clinical and biochemical features of azotemia in hepatic failure, Ann. Int. Med. 60:353, 1964.

9. Baldus, W. P., Feichter, R. N., Summerskill, W. H. J., Hunt, J. C., and Wakim, K. G.: The kidney in cirrhosis. II. Disorders of renal function, Ann. Int. Med. 60:366, 1964.

10. Baldus, W. P., Summerskill, W. H. J., Hunt, J. C., and Maher, F. T.: Renal circulation in cirrhosis: observations based on catheterization of the renal vein, J. Clin. Invest. 43:1090, 1964.

11. Berner, C., Fred, H. L., Riggs, S., and Davis, J. S.: Diagnostic probabilities in patients with conspicuous ascites, Arch. Int. Med. 113:687, 1964.

12. Berson, S. A., and Yalow, R. S.: The distribution of I^{131} labeled human serum albumin introduced into ascitic fluid: analysis of the kinetics of a three compartment catenary transfer system in man and speculations on possible sites of degradation, J. Clin. Invest. 33:377, 1954.

13. Birkenfeld, L. W., Leibman, J., O'Meara, M. P., and Edelman, I. S.: Total exchangeable sodium, total exchangeable potassium, and total body water in edematous patients with cirrhosis of the liver and congestive heart failure, J. Clin. Invest. 37:687, 1958.

14. Biron, P., Baldus, W. P., and Summerskill, W. H. J.: Plasma angiotensinase activity in cirrhosis, Proc. Soc. Exp. Biol. Med. 116:1074, 1964.

15. Blakemore, A. H.: Portacaval shunting for portal hypertension, Surg. Gynec. Obstet. 94:443, 1952.

16. Bricker, N. S.: The control of sodium excretion with normal and reduced nephron populations: the pre-eminence of third factor (Editorial), Am. J. Med. 43:313, 1967.

17. Brown, J.: Cirrhosis of the liver *in* Major, R. H. (ed.): Classic Description of Disease, ed. 2, pp. 691-693, Springfield, Ill., Thomas, 1939.
18. Brown, J. J., Davies, D. L., Lever, A. F., and Robertson, J. I. S.: Variations in plasma renin concentration in several physiological and pathological states, Canad. Med. Ass. J. 90:201, 1964.
19. Burnell, J. M., Thomas, E. D., Ansell, J. S., Cross, H. E., Dillard, D. H., Epstein, R. B., Eschbach, J. W., Jr., Hogan, R., Hutchings, R. H., Motulsky, A., Ormsby, J. W., Poffenbarger, P., Scribner, B. H., and Volwiler, W.: Observations on cross circulation in man, Am. J. Med. 38:832, 1965.
20. Cabot, R. C.: The causes of ascites: a study of five thousand cases, Am. J. Med. Sci. 143:1, 1912.
21. Carbone, J. V., and Matthews, H. B.: The use of prednisone to initiate or potentiate diuresis in chronic hepatic disease with ascites, Gastroenterology 38:52, 1960.
22. Caroli, J.: Le traitement des ascites cirrhotiques par les ponctions fractionnées et très rapprochées, Rev. méd. Suisse rom. 71:345, 1951.
23. Casey, T. H., Summerskill, W. H. J., Bickford, R. G., and Rosevear, J. W.: Body and serum potassium in liver disease. II. Relationships to arterial ammonia, blood pH, and hepatic coma, Gastroenterology 48:208, 1965.
24. Casey, T. H., Summerskill, W. H. J., and Orvis, A. L.: Body and serum potassium in liver disease. I. Relationship to hepatic function and associated factors, Gastroenterology 48:198, 1965.
25. Chalmers, T. C.: Pathogenesis and treatment of hepatic failure, New Engl. J. Med. 263:23; 77, 1960.
26. Cherrick, G. R., Kerr, D. N., Read, A. E., and Sherlock, S.: Colloid osmotic pressure and hydrostatic pressure relationships in the formation of ascites in hepatic cirrhosis, Clin. Sci. 19:361, 1960.
27. Clermont, R. J., Vlahcevic, Z. R., Chalmers, T. C., Adham, N. F., Curtis, G. W., and Morrison, R. S.: Intravenous therapy of massive ascites in patients with cirrhosis. II. Long term effects on survival and frequency of renal failure, Gastroenterology 53:220, 1967.
28. Clowdus, B. F., II, Summerskill, W. H. J., Casey, T. H., Higgins, J. A., and Orvis, A. L.: Isotope studies of the development of water and electrolyte disorders and azotemia during the treatment of ascites, Gastroenterology 41:360, 1961.
29. Cohn, J. N.: Hepatorenal failure following portacaval shunt: hemodynamic considerations and the application of ascitic fluid infusion, Med. Ann. D.C. 33:567; 594, 1964.
30. Coppage, W. S., Jr., Island, D. P., Cooner, A. E., and Liddle, G. W.: The metabolism of aldosterone in normal subjects and in patients with hepatic cirrhosis, J. Clin. Invest. 41:1672, 1962.
31. Davidson, C. S.: Diet in the treatment of liver disease, Am. J. Med. 25:690, 1958.
32. Dawson, A. D.: Historical notes on ascites (editorial), Gastroenterology 39:790, 1960.
33. Dawson, J. L.: Post-operative renal function in obstructive jaundice: effect of a mannitol diuresis, Brit. Med. J. 1:82, 1965.
34. de Wardener, H. E., Mills, I. H., Clapham, W. F., and Hayter, C. J.: Studies on the efferent mechanism of the sodium diuresis which follows the administration of intravenous saline in the dog, Clin. Sci. 21:249, 1961.
35. Dumont, A. E., and Mulholland, J. H.: Hepatic lymph in cirrhosis *in* Popper, H., and Schaffner, F. (eds.): Progress in Liver Diseases, vol. II, pp. 427–441, New York, Grune & Stratton, 1965.
36. Dykes, P. W.: A study of the effects of albumin infusions in patients with cirrhosis of the liver, Quart. J. Med. 30:297, 1961.
37. Earley, L. E.: Diuretics, New Engl. J. Med. 276:966; 1023, 1967.
38. Earley, L. E., and Friedler, R. M.: Changes in renal blood flow and possibly the intrarenal distribution of blood during the natriuresis accompanying saline loading in the dog, J. Clin. Invest. 44:929, 1965.
39. ———: Studies on the mechanism of natriuresis accompanying increased renal blood flow and its role in the renal response to extracellular volume expansion, J. Clin. Invest. 44:1857, 1965.
40. Eichenholz, A.: Respiratory alkalosis, Arch. Int. Med. 116:699, 1965.
41. Eiseman, B., Liem, D. S., and Raffucci, F.: Heterologous liver perfusion in treat-

ment of hepatic failure, Ann. Surg. *162*: 329, 1965.

42. Eisner, G. M., and Levitt, M. F.: The cirrhotic nephropathy *in* Popper, H., and Schaffner, F. (eds.): Progress in Liver Diseases, vol. I, pp. 119–133, New York, Grune & Stratton, 1961.

42a. Epstein, M., Calia, F. M., and Gabuzda, G. J.:Pneumococcal peritonitis in patients with postnecrotic cirrhosis, New Engl. J. Med. *278*:69, 1968.

43. Fenster, L. F.: The nonefficacy of short-term anabolic steroid therapy in alcoholic liver disease, Ann. Int. Med. *65*:738, 1966.

44. Flint, A.: Clinical report on hydro-peritoneum, based on an analysis of 46 cases, Am. J. Med. Sci. *45*:306, 1863.

45. Gabuzda, G. J., Jr., and Davidson, C. S.: Protein metabolism in patients with cirrhosis of the liver, Ann. N. Y. Acad. Sci. *57*:776, 1954.

46. Gabuzda, G. J., Jr., Traeger, H. S., and Davidson, C. S.: Hepatic cirrhosis: effects of sodium chloride administration and restriction and of abdominal paracentesis on electrolyte and water balance, J. Clin. Invest. *33*:780, 1954.

47. Galambos, J. T., and Wilkinson, H. A., III: Reversible hyponatremia and azotemia in a patient with cirrhosis and ascites, Am. J. Dig. Dis. *7*:642, 1962.

48. Genest, J., de Champlain, J., Veyrat, R., Boucher, R., Tremblay, G. Y., Strong, C. G., Koiw, E., and Marc-Aurèle, J.: Role of the renin-angiotensin system in various physiological and pathological states *in* Hypertension: Proc. of the Council for High Blood Pressure Research, Cleveland, O., Nov. 1964; Am. Heart Assoc., vol. 13, p. 97, 1965.

49. Goldsmith, C., Rector, F. C., Jr., and Seldin, D. W.: Evidence for a direct effect of serum sodium concentration on sodium reabsorption, J. Clin. Invest. *41*: 850, 1962.

50. Goldstein, H., and Boyle, J. D.: Spontaneous recovery from the hepatorenal syndrome; report of four cases, New Engl. J. Med. *272*:895, 1965.

51. Gordon, M. E.: The acute effects of abdominal paracentesis in Laennec's cirrhosis upon exchanges of electrolytes and water, renal function, and hemodynamics, Am. J. Gastroent. *33*:15, 1960.

52. Goresky, C. A., and Kumar, G.: Renal failure in cirrhosis of the liver, Canad. Med. Ass. J. *90*:353, 1964.

53. Gornel, D. L., Lancestremere, R. G., Papper, S., and Lowenstein, L. M.: Acute changes in renal excretion of water and solute in patients with Laennec's cirrhosis, induced by the administration of the pressor amine, metaraminol, J. Clin. Invest. *41*:594, 1962.

54. Haberich, F. J., Aziz, O., and Nowacki, P. E.: Über einen osmoreceptorisch tätigen Mechanismus in der Leber, Pflügers Arch. ges. Physiol. *285*:73, 1965.

55. Hartroft, W. S., and Hartroft, P. M.: New approaches in the study of cardiovascular disease: aldosterone, renin, hypertension and juxtaglomerular cells, Fed. Proc. *20*:845, 1961.

56. Hecker, R., and Sherlock, S.: Electrolyte and circulatory changes in terminal liver failure, Lancet *2*:1121, 1956.

57. Henley, K. S., Streeten, D. H. P., and Pollard, H. M.: Hyperaldosteronism in liver disease: the treatment of refractory ascites by adrenalectomy and by the administration of spirolactones, Gastroenterology *38*:681, 1960.

58. Holub, D. A., and Jailer, J. W.: Sodium and water diuresis in cirrhotic patients with intractable ascites following chemical inhibition of aldosterone synthesis, Ann. Int. Med. *53*:425, 1960.

59. Hori, M., Austen, W. G., and McDermott, W. V., Jr.: Role of hepatic arterial blood flow and hepatic nerves on renal circulation and function: I. Acute studies in the dog. II. Chronic studies in the dog, Ann. Surg. *162*:849; 949, 1965.

60. Jick, H., Kamm, D. E., Snyder, J. G., Morrison, R. S., and Chalmers, T. C.: On the concentrating defect in cirrhosis of the liver, J. Clin. Invest. *43*:258, 1964.

61. Johnson, W. D.: The cytological diagnosis of cancer in serous effusions, Acta Cytol. (Balt.) *10*:161, 1966.

62. Johnston, R. F., and Loo, R. V.: Hepatic hydrothorax: studies to determine the the source of the fluid and report of thirteen cases, Ann. Int. Med. *61*:385, 1964.

63. Jones, W. A., Rao, D. R. G., and Braunstein, H.: The renal glomerulus in cirrhosis of the liver, Am. J. Path. *39*:393, 1961.

64. Kay, H. E. M.: The value of paper electrophoresis of serum proteins in diagnosis of ascites, Brit. Med. J. *2*:1025, 1954.

65. Kessler, E., Nelson, W. P., III, and

Rosano, C. L.: Urinary electrolytes at low rates of urine flow after expansion of extracellular volume, J. Lab. Clin. Med. 65:804, 1965.

66. Knauer, C. M., and Lowe, H. M.: Hemodynamics in the cirrhotic patient during paracentesis, New Engl. J. Med. 276: 491, 1967.

67. Konikov, N., Bleisch, V., and Piskie, V.: Prognostic significance of cytologic diagnoses of effusions, Acta Cytol. (Balt.) 10:335, 1966.

68. Kunin, C. M., Chalmers, T. C., Leevy, C. M., Sebastyen, S. C., Lieber, C. S., and Finland, M.: Absorption of orally administered neomycin and kanamycin, with special reference to patients with severe hepatic and renal disease, New Engl. J. Med. 262:380, 1960.

69. Lancestremere, R. G., Davidson, P. L., Earley, L. E., O'Brien, F. J., and Papper, S.: Renal failure in Laennec's cirrhosis. II. Simultaneous determination of cardiac output and renal hemodynamics, J. Clin. Invest. 41:1922, 1962.

70. Lancestremere, R. G., Klingler, E. L., Jr., Frisch, E., and Papper, S.: Simultaneous determination of cardiac output and renal function in patients with Laennec's cirrhosis during the administration of the pressor amine, metaraminol, J. Lab. Clin. Med. 61:820, 1963.

71. Laragh, J. H.: The proper use of newer diuretics, Ann. Int. Med. 67:606, 1967.

72. Laragh, J. H., Cannon, P. J., and Ames, R. P.: Interaction between aldosterone secretion, sodium and potassium balance, and angiotensin activity in man: studies in hypertension and cirrhosis, Canad. Med. Ass. J. 90:248, 1964.

73. Laragh, J. H., Cannon, P. J., Bentzel, C. J., Sicinski, A. M., and Meltzer, J. I.: Angiotensin II, norepinephrine, and renal transport of electrolytes and water in normal man and in cirrhosis with ascites, J. Clin. Invest. 42:1179, 1963.

74. Lawson, J. D., and Weissbein, A. S.: The puddle sign: an aid in the diagnosis of minimal ascites, New Engl. J. Med. 260: 652, 1959.

75. Leaf, A.: The clinical and physiologic significance of the serum sodium concentration, New Engl. J. Med. 267:24; 77, 1962.

76. Lemmon, W. T., Jr., Holland, P. V., and Holland, J. M.: The hepatopathy of

hypernephroma, Am. J. Surg. 110:487, 1965.

77. Lieberman, F. L., Hidemura, R., Peters, R. L., and Reynolds, T. B.: Pathogenesis and treatment of hydrothorax complicating cirrhosis with ascites, Ann. Int. Med. 64:341, 1966.

78. Lieberman, F. L., and Reynolds, T. B.: The use of ethacrynic acid in patients with cirrhosis and ascites, Gastroenterology 49:531, 1965.

79. ———: Plasma volume in cirrhosis of the liver: its relations to portal hypertension, ascites, and renal failure, J. Clin. Invest. 46:1297, 1967.

80. Liem, D. S., Waltuch, T. L., and Eiseman, B.: Function of ex-vivo pig liver perfused with human blood, Surg. Forum 15:90, 1964.

81. Linhart, J. W., and Welt, L. G.: The effect of hyponatremia and cellular dilution on tissue catabolism in the rat, Trans. Ass. Am. Phycns 76:184, 1963.

82. Losowsky, M. S., and Davidson, C. S.: The source of ascitic fluid in cirrhosis of the liver (Editorial), Arch. Int. Med. 110:279, 1962.

83. Lower, R.: Traité du coeur (French translation from the Latin), p. 121, Paris, E. Michallet, 1679.

84. Luetscher, J. A., Jr., and Johnson, B. B.: Observations on the sodium-retaining corticoid (aldosterone) in the urine of children and adults in relation to sodium balance and edema, J. Clin. Invest. 33: 1441, 1954.

85. Macbeth, W. A. A. G., Kass, E. H., and McDermott, W. V., Jr.: Treatment of hepatic encephalopathy by alteration of intestinal flora with Lactobacillus acidophilus, Lancet 1:399, 1965.

86. Mallet-Guy, P., Devic, G., Feroldi, J., and Desjacques, P.: Étude expérimentale des ascites: sténoses veineuses posthépatiques et transposition due foie dans le thorax, Lyon chir. 49:153, 1954.

87. Mansberger, A. R., Jr.: Value of peritoneal fluid ammonia levels in the differential diagnosis of the acute abdomen, Ann. Surg. 155:998, 1962.

88. Marson, F. G. W.: Total adrenalectomy in hepatic cirrhosis with ascites, Lancet 2:847, 1954.

89. Martini, G. A.: Gibt es ein hepatorenales Syndrom? Dtsch. med. Wschr. 87:2408, 1962.

90. Mashford, M. L., Mahon, W. A., and

Chalmers, T. C.: Studies of the cardiovascular system in the hypotension of liver failure, New Engl. J. Med. 267: 1071, 1962.

91. McCloy, R. M., Baldus, W. P., Maher, F. T., and Summerskill, W. H. J.: Effects of changing plasma volume, serum albumin concentration, and plasma osmolality on renal function in cirrhosis, Gastroenterology 53:229, 1967.

92. McCloy, R. M., Baldus, W. P., Tauxe, W. N., and Summerskill, W. H. J.: Plasma volume and renal circulatory function in cirrhosis, Ann. Int. Med. 66: 307, 1967.

93. McDermott, W. V., Jr.: The double portacaval shunt in the treatment of cirrhotic ascites, Surg. Gynec. Obstet. 110: 457, 1960.

94. Milies, E.: A new diuretic factor of hepatic origin, Acta physiol. lat.-amer. 10: 178, 1960.

95. Murchison, C.: Clinical Lectures on Diseases of the Liver, ed. 3, London, Longmans, Green, 1885, 702 pp.

96. Nagant De Deuxchaisnes, C., Collet, R. A., Busset, R., and Mach, R. S.: Exchangeable potassium in wasting, amyotrophy, heart-disease, and cirrhosis of the liver, Lancet 1:681, 1961.

97. Nix, J. T., Albert, M., Dugas, J. E., and Wendt, D. L.: Chylothorax and chylous ascites: a study of 302 selected cases, Am. J. Gastroent. 28:40, 1957.

98. Nix, J. T., Mann, F. C., Bollman, J. L., Grindlay, J. H., and Flock, E. V.: Alterations of protein constituents of lymph by specific injury to the liver, Am. J. Physiol. 164:119, 1951.

99. Onnis, M., Shumacker, H. B., Jr., and Bounous, G.: Response to occlusion of the portal vein: blood pressure and renal blood flow, Arch. Surg. 85:897, 1962.

100. ———: Blood pressure and renal blood flow response to occlusion of visceral arteries, Ann. Surg. 157:56, 1963.

101. Papper, S.: The role of the kidney in Laennec's cirrhosis of the liver, Medicine 37:299, 1958.

102. Papper, S., Belsky, J. L., and Bleifer, K. H.: Renal failure in Laennec's cirrhosis of the liver. I. Description of clinical and laboratory features, Ann. Int. Med. 51: 759, 1959.

103. Pecikyan, R., Kanzaki, G., and Berger, E. Y.: Electrolyte excretion during the spontaneous recovery from the ascitic phase of cirrhosis of the liver, Am. J. Med. 42:359, 1967.

104. Popper, H., and Schaffner, F.: Drug-induced hepatic injury, Ann. Int. Med. 51:1230, 1959.

105. Preedy, J. R. K., and Aitken, E. H.: The effect of estrogen on water and electrolyte metabolism. II. Hepatic disease, J. Clin. Invest. 35:430, 1956.

106. Prentice, T. C., Sri, W., and Joiner, E. E.: Quantitative studies of ascitic fluid circulation with tritium-labeled water, Am. J. Med. 13:668, 1952.

107. Ratnoff, O. D., and Patek, A. J., Jr.: The natural history of Laennec's cirrhosis of the liver: an analysis of 386 cases, Medicine 21:207, 1942.

108. Read, A. E., Laidlaw, J., Haslam, R. M., and Sherlock, S.: Neuropsychiatric complications following chlorothiazide therapy in patients with hepatic cirrhosis: possible relation to hypokalaemia, Clin. Sci. 18:409, 1959.

109. Rector, F. C., Jr., Van Giesen, G., Kiil, F., and Seldin, D. W.: Influence of expansion of extracellular volume on tubular reabsorption of sodium independent of changes in glomerular filtration rate and aldosterone activity, J. Clin. Invest. 43:341, 1964.

110. Reynolds, T. B., Geller, H. M., Kuzma, O. T., and Redeker, A. G.: Spontaneous decrease in portal pressure with clinical improvement in cirrhosis, New Engl. J. Med. 263:734, 1960.

111. Rovelstad, R. A., Bartholomew, L. G., and Cain, J. C.: Helpful laboratory procedures in the differential diagnosis of ascites, Proc. Mayo Clin. 34:565, 1959.

112. Ruol, A., Dal Palu, C., Curri, G., Zerbini, E., and Casson, F.: Validita della legge di Starling per la interpretazione patogenetica della ascite, Inst. Patologica Medica Dell'Universita di Padova, 1960.

113. Salomon, M. I., Sakaguchi, H., Churg, J., Dachs, S., Grishman, E., Mautner, W., Paronetto F., and Rosenthal, W. S.: Renal lesions in hepatic disease: A study based on kidney biopsy, Arch. Int. Med. 115:704, 1965.

114. Schoenberger, J. A., Kroll, G., Sakamoto, A., and Kark, R. M.: Investigation of permeability factor in ascites and edema using albumin tagged with I131, Gastroenterology 22:607, 1952.

115. Scobie, B. A., Schlegel, J. F., Code, C. F., and Summerskill, W. H. J.: Pressure

376   Ascites: The Kidney in Liver Disease

changes of the esophagus and gastroesophageal junction with cirrhosis and
varices, Gastroenterology 49:67, 1965.

116. Shaldon, S., and Walker, G.: Jaundice
and acute renal failure *in* Martini, G. A.
(ed.): Aktuelle Probleme der Hepato-
logie; Ultrastruktur Steroidstoffwechsel,
Durchblutung, Leber, und Niere, pp.
118–123, Stuttgart, Thieme, 1962.

117. Shear, L., Hall, P. W., III, and Gabuzda,
G. J.: Renal failure in patients with cirrhosis of the liver. II. Factors influencing
maximal urinary flow rate, Am. J. Med.
39:199, 1965.

118. Shear, L., Harvey, J. D., and Barry, K.
G.: Peritoneal sodium transport: enhancement by pharmacologic and physical agents, J. Lab. Clin. Med. 67:181,
1966.

119. Shear, L., Kleinerman. J., and Gabuzda,
G. J.: Renal failure in patients with cirrhosis of the liver. I. Clinical and pathologic characteristics, Am. J. Med. 39:184,
1965.

120. Sherlock, S.: Circulatory studies on pa-
tients with ascites *in* Ciba Foundation
Symposium: Liver Disease, pp. 182–184,
London, Churchill, 1951.

121. ———: Diseases of the Liver and
Biliary System, ed. 3, Oxford, Blackwell
Scientific Publications, 1963, 714 pp.

122. Sherlock, S., and Shaldon, S.: The aetiology and management of ascites in patients with hepatic cirrhosis: a review,
Gut 4:95, 1963.

123. Spät, A., Saliga, M., Sturcz, J., and
Sólyom, J.: Effect of aldosterone on intestinal transport of sodium and potassium, Lancet 2:96, 1963.

124. Starling, E. H.: On the absorption of
fluids from the connective tissue spaces,
J. Physiol. (London) 19:312, 1896.

125. Stauffer, M. H.: Nephrogenic hepatosplenomegaly (Abstract), Gastroenterology 40:694, 1961.

126. Summerskill, W. H. J.: Pathogenesis and
treatment of disorders of water and electrolyte metabolism in hepatic disease,
Proc. Mayo Clin. 35:89, 1960.

127. ———: Hepatic failure and the kidney,
Gastroenterology 51:94, 1966.

128. Summerskill, W. H. J., Baldus, W. P.,
and Feichter, R. N.: Renal function in
cirrhosis with ascites: clinical, biochemical and physiologic changes *in* Martini,
G. A. (ed.): Aktuelle Probleme der Hep-
atologie: Ultrastruktur Steroidstoffwech-

sel, Durchblutung, Leber, und Niere,
pp. 90–98, Stuttgart, Thieme, 1962.

129. Summerskill, W. H. J., Clowdus, B. F.,
and Casey, T. H.: Clinical and metabolic
changes during the development of azotemia in hepatic failure with ascites,
Proc. Mayo Clin. 35:783, 1960.

130. Summerskill, W. H. J., Clowdus, B. F.,
II, and Rosevear, J. W.: Long-term medical management and complications of
"resistant" ascites, Gut 2:285, 1961.

131. Summerskill, W. H. J., and Crabbe, J.:
Effects of amphenone therapy on urinary
excretion of aldosterone and sodium in
hepatic cirrhosis with ascites, Lancet 2:
1091, 1957.

132. Summerskill, W. H. J., Davidson, C. S.,
Dible, J. H., Mallory, G. K., Sherlock, S.,
Turner, M. D., and Wolfe, S. J.: Cirrhosis of the liver: a study of alcoholic and
nonalcoholic patients in Boston and London, New Engl. J. Med. 262:1, 1960.

133. Summerskill, W. H. J., Davidson, E. A.,
Sherlock, S., and Steiner, R. E.: The neuropsychiatric syndrome associated with
hepatic cirrhosis and an extensive portal
collateral circulation, Quart, J. Med. 25:
245, 1956.

134. Summerskill, W. H. J., and Shorter, R.
G.: Progressive hepatic failure: Its asso-
ciation with undifferentiated renal tumor,
Arch. Int. Med. 120:81, 1967.

135. Summerskill, W. H. J., Thorsell, F.,
Feinberg, J. H., and Aldrete, J. S.: Effects of urease inhibition in hyperammonemia: clinical and experimental
studies with acetohydroxamic acid, Gastroenterology 54:20, 1968.

136. Sydenham, T.: The Works of Thomas
Sydenham, M.D. (Translated by R. G.
Latham), vol. 2, p. 164, London, The
Sydenham Society, 1850.

137. Talley, R. B., Schedl, H. P., and Clifton,
J. A.: Small intestinal glucose, electro-
lyte, and water absorption in cirrhosis,
Gastroenterology 47:382, 1964.

138. Talso, P. J., Spafford, N., Ferenzi, G.,
and Jackson, H. O.: Paradoxical hyponatremia associated with congestive heart
failure and with cirrhosis of the liver,
Metabolism 5:58, 1956.

139. Thomson, A., and Visek, W. J.: Some
effects of induction of urease immunity
in patients with hepatic insufficiency,
Am. J. Med. 35:804, 1963.

140. Vesin, P., Giboudeau, M., Renault, H.,
and Cattan, R.: Le syndrome "élévation

de la kaliémie-azotémie-oligurie" dans les cirrhoses ascitiques: mécanisme et conséquences thérapeutiques (échec des spirolactones), Bull. Soc. méd. hôp. Paris 76:1013, 1960.

141. Vesin, P., Roberti, A., Kac, J., and Viguié, R.: Coma avec azotémie, hypernatrémie et hyperchlorémie chez un cirrhotique, Sem. Hôp. Paris 41:1220, 1965.

142. Vesin, P., Traverso, H., Combrisson, A., Besson, P., Hirsch-Marie, H., and Cattan, R.: Le rein du cirrhotique étude de la filtration glomérulaire, Sem. Hôp. Paris 38:3595, 1962.

143. Vesin, P., Traverso, H., Hirsch-Marie, H., and Cattan, R.: L'insuffisance rénale circulatoire spontanée du cirrhotique: son évolution, Sem. Hôp. Paris 38:3598, 1962.

144. Vesin, P., Traverso, H., and Roberti, A.: Action des glucocorticoïdes et des salidiurétiques sur la filtration glomérulaire et le volume plasmatique dans la cirrhose ascitique, Schweiz. med. Wschr. 95:1157, 1965.

145. Vlahcevic, Z. R., Adham, N. F., Chalmers, T. C., Clermont, R. J., Moore, E. W., Jick, H., Curtis, G. W., and Morrison, R. S.: Intravenous therapy of massive ascites in patients with cirrhosis. I. Short term comparison with diuretic treatment, Gastroenterology 53:211, 1967.

146. Vlahcevic, Z. R., Adham, N. F., Jick, H., Moore, E. W., and Chalmers, T. C.: Renal effects of acute expansion of plasma volume in cirrhosis, New Engl. J. Med. 272:387, 1965.

147. Volwiler, W., Grindlay, J. H., and Bollman, J. L.: The relation of portal vein pressure to the formation of ascites—an experimental study, Gastroenterology 14:40, 1950.

148. Walker, J. G.: Renal failure in jaundice, Proc. Roy. Soc. Med. 55:570, 1962.

149. Waterhouse, C., Jaenike, J. R., and Marinetti, G.: Studies on the nature and origin of pseudochylous ascites, Trans. Ass. Am. Phycns 71:312, 1958.

150. Webster, L. T., Jr., and Gabuzda, G. J.: Relation of azotemia to blood "ammonium" in patients with hepatic cirrhosis, Arch. Int. Med. 103:15, 1959.

151. Welch, C. S., Welch, H. F., and Carter, J. H.: The treatment of ascites by side to side portacaval shunt, Ann. Surg. 150:428, 1959.

152. Wells, R.: Prednisolone and testosterone propionate in cirrhosis of the liver: a controlled trial, Lancet 2:1416, 1960.

153. Williams, R. D., Elliott, D. W., and Zollinger, R. M.: The effect of hypotension in obstructive jaundice, Arch. Surg. 81:334, 1960.

154. Wolff, H. P., Koczorek, K. R., and Buchborn, E.: Aldosterone and antidiuretic hormone (adiuretin) in liver disease, Acta endocr. (Kbh.) 27:45, 1958.

155. Wolfman, E. F., Jr., Zuidema, G. D., Oneal, R. M., Turcotte, J., Kowalczyk, R., and Child, C. G., III: Sodium excretion after intrasplenic and systemic injections of sodium chloride in normal dogs and after portacaval shunt, Surgery 50:231, 1961.

156. Yamahiro, H. S., and Reynolds, T. B.: Effects of ascitic fluid infusion on sodium excretion, blood volume, and creatinine clearance in cirrhosis, Gastroenterology 40:497, 1961.

157. Yoffey, J. M., and Courtice, F. C.: Lymphatics, Lymph and Lymphoid Tissue, ed. 2, Cambridge, Mass., Harvard Press, 1956, 510 pp.

12

Hepatic Coma

CHARLES S. DAVIDSON, M.D., AND *GEORGE J. GABUZDA*, M.D.

DEFINITION

In severe acute or chronic liver disease, whatever the etiology, characteristic neuropsychiatric findings and peculiar changes in state of consciousness often herald the onset of coma. The coma may continue for a few days to several weeks, and frequently terminates in death. "Hepatic coma" refers to this serious complication of advanced liver disease. The early stages of the condition are called "impending hepatic coma" or "precoma." "Hepatic encephalopathy" and "portal-systemic encephalopathy" have been employed frequently in recent years to refer to this and closely related syndromes.

Other terms have been used to describe this condition. In 1866 Leyden proposed the term "cholemia" for the comatose state.[77] He attributed the coma to retention of bile acids in the blood and pointed out its clinical resemblance to uremia. There is no evidence that retention of bile acids is implicated in the pathogenesis of hepatic coma; therefore, the term "cholemia" is meaningless from the point of view of etiology. The term "liver failure" implies conditions such as jaundice, hemorrhagic diathesis or massive liver cell necrosis which need not accompany hepatic coma, as will become evident in subsequent discussion. "Hepatargy" is a term that did not become generally accepted.[56]

Though not all patients are or even become comatose, "hepatic coma" is most widely accepted as embracing all the clinical manifestations of this syndrome. Accordingly, "hepatic coma" is used here collectively to refer to all stages that occur in advanced liver disease during the sequence: prodrome, impending coma, stupor, coma (Table 12–1).

Hepatic coma is one of the most frequent terminal episodes of primary liver disease. Patek and Ratnoff found that 36 per cent of their patients with cirrhosis died in hepatic coma.[99] It is the usual terminal event when viral hepatitis ends fatally, and it is observed in Wilson's disease (hepatolenticular degeneration), biliary cirrhosis and hemochromatosis. The series of 60 patients studied by Adams and Foley at the Boston City Hospital consisted of 48 with cirrhosis, of whom all but 7 were chronic alcoholics, 3 with hemochromatosis, 4 with infectious hepatitis, 1 with biliary cirrhosis, 1 with toxic hepatitis, and 3 with acute or subacute atrophy of the liver.[1] The preponderance of alcoholics probably reflects the population of the hospital where the study was made. Because of its frequency the hepatic coma appearing in alcoholic cirrhosis has been best described and qualified and is the prototype of the remainder.

CLINICAL MANIFESTATIONS

ONSET AND DEVELOPMENT

Recognition of early stages of hepatic coma is essential for successful therapy and preventive measures. Table 12–1 is a partial classification of the stages of this condition.

Prodrome. The onset of hepatic coma is usually gradual and may be almost imperceptible. Murphy et al. noted loss of affect

378

TABLE 12–1. STAGES IN ONSET AND DEVELOPMENT OF HEPATIC COMA

	MENTAL STATE	TREMOR	E. E. G. CHANGES
Prodrome (often only in retrospect)	Euphoria, occasionally depression Confusion, absent or difficult to detect Slight slowing of mentation Untidiness	Often present but slight	Usually absent
Impending coma	Confusion Usually euphoria Drowsiness Inappropriate behavior	Usually present and easily elicitable	Almost always present
Stupor	Sleeps most of time but arousable Confusion, marked	Usually present if patient can cooperate	Almost always present
Semicoma or coma	Unconsciousness May respond to noxious stimuli or, when deep, may not respond	Usually absent (no muscle tone)	Often present

and a defect in judgment in the early stages.[90] Euphoria (sometimes marked) is frequent, although the patients may be depressed and apathetic. Patients are often untidy and behave inappropriately. Sometimes sleep is upset, the patient being drowsy or even sleeping through long periods of the day but being wakeful, noisy and confused during the night. Often many of these abnormalities are absent or difficult to detect. In acute forms of liver disease, particularly acute atrophy, seizures, mania, sometimes with hallucinations, may be observed before the onset of coma.[1]

Impending Hepatic Coma. This stage is more specific. Mental confusion is evident and is characterized in its early stages merely by slowness of response but soon progresses to confusion with regard to time, place or person. The detailed and accurate clinical observations of Adams and Foley have helped immeasurably to clarify and characterize the early stages of hepatic coma.[1]

A characteristic tremor is almost invariably observed. Although irregular involuntary movements had been noted by a number of authors for many years, Adams and Foley first clearly described the tremor.[1] Their description follows:

Concomitant with the change in the state of consciousness there appeared in the majority of cases a characteristic type of involuntary movement. This was most consistently and most effectively demonstrated by having the patient hold his arms and hands outstretched with the fingers spread apart. Depending upon the severity of the process, as this posture was maintained there appeared at irregular intervals of a fraction of a second to seven seconds, a series of movements consisting usually of lateral deviations of the fingers, flexion-extension of the fingers at the metacarpophalangeal joint, and flexion-extension of the wrist. The movements are rapid and arrhythmic—at one phase, for example, flexion, when the arms were outstretched in a pronated position, was always more rapid than the other. They tended to occur in bursts, at a rate of one or two per second. There were, however, intervals during which none of these movements were seen. In the more severe cases, as the arms were outstretched, there was the flexion-extension movement at the elbow and at the shoulder.

They observed these same rhythmic movements in the legs when the recumbent patient was asked to dorsiflex his foot, in the face upon strong closure of the eyelids as well as upon retraction of the corners of the mouth, pursing the lips, or protruding the tongue.

Although frequent, the "flapping tremor" ("asterixis") is not observed in every patient with impending coma. When deep coma ensues, the tremor usually disappears because the patient is unable to sustain a posture to bring out the tremor. With recovery, the tremor usually disappears but may continue for days or occasionally even months. The tremor is not specific, for an identical or similar tremor has been seen by Adams and Foley in uremia, polycythemia with heart failure and mental confusion, and in hypokalemic stupors.[1] Similar observations have been made by us and others.[27, 34, 128, 131, 134] Nevertheless, it is so characteristic of impending hepatic coma that its presence in severe liver disease must be heeded.

The third characteristic of impending hepatic coma is an abnormality in the electroencephalogram first described by Foley, Watson and Adams[47] and consisting of "paroxysms of bilaterally synchronous, symmetrical, high voltage, slow waves in the delta range of 1½ to 3 per second . . . interspersed with or . . . superimposed on relatively normal (alpha) waves."[1] In the early stages these "slow rollers" often occur in bursts and appear first in the frontal regions; later they spread laterally and posteriorly until the entire record is of slow activity. In some patients these changes are not evident during any stage of hepatic coma. However, Adams and Foley found that of 25 patients 22 had typical waves at some phase.[1] These electroencephalographic abnormalities are seen occasionally in other neurologic disturbances, particularly those of a metabolic nature.

Although mental confusion, the flapping tremor, and the electroencephalographic changes may not all be present and are not individually necessarily specific for hepatic coma, the combination of the 3 in a patient with severe liver disease makes the diagnosis of impending hepatic coma almost inevitable, and if any one or 2 occur in such a patient the physician suspects impending hepatic coma and modifies treatment accordingly.

If impending hepatic coma is untreated, it may last for from a few hours to days, weeks or longer with minor or major fluctuations in the state of consciousness. Modern treatment has strikingly shortened the duration of impending coma, which may be completely reversible or controllable to a significant extent (see Treatment).

Coma. Characteristically, as time goes on the confusion deepens, the patient sleeps for longer periods of time, and becomes difficult and then impossible to arouse. Coma may vary from a state in which reflexes are present, and the patient responds to painful stimuli with movements or a cry or moan, to deep coma with areflexia, absent corneal reflexes and failure to respond to any stimulus. During this stage of coma most patients appear to the casual observer as though sleeping peacefully. Temperature, pulse and respirations may not be abnormal. At times, particularly when complicating infections ensue, fever may occur together with tachycardia and tachypnea. Hyperventilation and respiratory alkalosis are observed in some patients.[63, 149]

Rigidity of the limbs is seen frequently and varies considerably in the patient from time to time. When deep coma ensues, little or no rigidity is evident. During the earlier stages passive movements of the limbs may be resisted, but only occasionally is true cogwheel rigidity present. Convulsions may be seen. Adams and Foley report that about a third of their patients at one time or another had convulsions, usually near the terminal stage of the coma.[1] Others report a much lower incidence. The deep tendon reflexes also vary considerably. Sometimes hyperreflexia is present. At other times reflexes are absent, sometimes on one side and sometimes bilaterally. Ankle clonus occurred in about 20 per cent and extensor plantar responses in 75 per cent of Adams and Foley's patients. Walshe found ankle clonus in most patients, often before the plantar response became abnormal.[152] Indeed, if these patients are watched carefully, most show some reflex changes and plantar extension, sometimes unilateral and at other times bilateral. Grasping and sucking reflexes are sometimes elicited.

Occasionally patients in hepatic coma die with no apparent precipitating cause other than prolonged coma. Most patients have a terminal episode of bronchopneumonia or bacteremia, and some of massive gastrointestinal bleeding.

Chronic Neuropsychiatric Syndromes. Patients suffering intermittently for long periods of time from precoma, either related to portal systemic shunts consequent to liver disease or to portal vascular surgery, may exhibit unusual, atypical syndromes including relatively irreversible neurologic disorders.[97, 110, 150, 168] Acute psychoses and paraplegia may occur. The patients may demonstrate dementia, dysarthria, grimacing, ataxia of gait, intention tremor, choreoathetosis, mild pyramidal tract signs and diffuse electroencephalographic abnormalities. Muscular rigidity, grasp reflexes, nystagmus and persisting asterixis are signs seen less commonly. Rarely, combined systemic disease of the spinal cord and permanent myelopathy are found.

In some cases the signs and symptoms are adequately controlled with treatment by dietary protein restriction and oral neomycin, but in others relief from these measures is only partial. Some patients are permanently disabled by these neuropsychiatric complications, presumably from irreparable neurological damage.

Read et al. warn that any neuropsychiatric syndrome that develops in liver disease should be considered related to the liver disease and portal systemic shunting until proved otherwise.[110] Occasionally the onset of a neuropsychiatric disorder is the first indication of disease of the liver or the portal circulation.

COURSE AND PROGNOSIS

Characteristically hepatic coma tends to fluctuate, particularly in the early stages. Thus, a patient may be alert and have a barely detectable flapping tremor in the morning hours only to be confused and even stuporous with a severe tremor in the evening or night. Even deep coma usually fluctuates in depth from time to time. A patient who has been in deep coma for a few hours or even a few days wakes if treated, and all signs of hepatic coma usually disappear. Generally speaking, the deeper and longer the coma the less likely is a favorable response. Hence, the longer the coma, the poorer the prognosis. The fluctuations in depth of coma and the spontaneous remissions make the study of the disease and especially assessment of the efficacy of therapy extremely difficult and cast doubt on some of the therapeutic measures that have been proposed (see Treatment).

TABLE 12–2. HEPATIC COMA: PRECIPITATING FACTORS

1. Nitrogen Overload
   A. Exogenous
      a. Dietary protein excess
      b. Gastrointestinal bleeding
      c. Ammonium salts, urea
   B. Endogenous
      a. Increased enterohepatic circulation urea (azotemia)
      b. Increased renal vein ammonium output:
         Potassium deficiency
         Alkalinization of urine
2. Fluid and Electrolyte Abnormalities
   A. Hypovolemia, dehydration
   B. Hyponatremia
   C. Potassium deficiency
   D. Alkalosis-acidosis
   E. Following paracentesis
   F. Following induced diuresis
3. Narcotics (including paregoric), hypnotics, sedatives, analgesics
4. Acute Infections
   A. Viral
   B. Bacterial: pneumonia, urinary tract, enteritis, meningeal, coliform septicemia
5. Surgical Operations
6. Diuretic Agents: Mercurials, acetazolamide, thiazides, aldosterone antagonists, ethacrynic acid, furosemide
7. Intra-abdominal Disease
   A. Perforated viscus
   B. Peritonitis
      a. Coliform
      b. No demonstrable cause
   C. Acute pancreatitis
   D. Hepatoma

PRECIPITATING FACTORS

Murphy et al., in the study of 40 patients with hepatic coma at the Boston City Hospital, found that in about half of them the coma appeared spontaneously; that is, no precipitating factor was found.[90] The coma in the other 20 patients was described as "complicated," which indicates that it was precipitated by factors such as severe infection, massive upper gastrointestinal bleeding or major operation. These and other precipitating factors are listed in Table 12–2. For the possible mechanisms by which these factors induce coma, see Pathogenesis.

Usually the onset and course of hepatic coma in complicated cases are more rapid than in that arising apparently spontaneously. However, the prognosis is considerably better in the former, presumably because many of the complicating factors are amenable to therapy. The use of antibiotics in the treatment of infection, correction of abnormalities of electrolyte and water balance, and transfusions and other measures in acute gastrointestinal bleeding favorably influence the prognosis in the complicated cases. Sedatives, as mentioned, appear to play a part in inducing hepatic coma or may prolong the course and make more likely a fatal termination.

LABORATORY FINDINGS

The usual laboratory tests are of little help, either in diagnosis of hepatic coma or in prognosis except in establishing the presence and severity of the liver disease and in assessing the status of precipitating factors and complications such as pneumonia or gastrointestinal bleeding. Anemia is common in liver disease, but apparently is not specifically related to the onset of coma except when acute gastrointestinal bleeding is a precipitating factor. That is, the chronic macrocytic anemia of liver disease is as common in patients with hepatic coma as in those without.

In a similar manner the white blood cell count is specifically related to the comatose state only as an evidence of infection (for example, bronchopneumonia) or of the particularly active form of cirrhosis of alcoholics emphasized by Phillips and Davidson[103] in which leukocytosis, jaundice and terminal coma are the rule. Murphy et al. found that the white count tends to rise in many of the patients with hepatic coma they studied.[90] White counts of 20,000 were not unusual in their series, leukocytosis being usually a sign of terminal infection.

The blood nonprotein nitrogen concentration may remain normal throughout a period of hepatic coma even when it ends fatally, although usually a gradual rise is noted which is more abrupt terminally. Several mechanisms may account for this. First, oliguria, as is discussed later, commonly accompanies hepatic coma. Second, acute gastrointestinal hemorrhage may be a factor. Third, if caloric intake is insufficient, protein may be burned for energy. Mild acidosis is a common accompaniment of terminal hepatic coma, although patients may be carried for days in deep coma without a significant reduction in the carbon dioxide combining power or blood pH. Hypoglycemia is not characteristic of hepatic coma, nor is hyperglycemia seen more often than it is in liver disease with a normal mental state. Respiratory alkalosis reportedly accompanies precoma and coma in some patients.[63, 149]

Severe hypoglycemia with hypoglycemic coma is seen occasionally in patients with severe liver disease, usually those with fibrosis of the pancreas as well (especially hemochromatosis). This is an unusual occurrence, and the comatose state is not true hepatic coma but responds rapidly to administration of glucose solutions.

In general, liver function tests in hepatic coma, although greatly disturbed and indicating the severity of the liver disease, appear to be unrelated to the onset, course or prognosis of the comatose state.

Jaundice and bilirubinemia usually roughly parallel the activity of the liver disease but do not bear any particular relation to hepatic coma except that in active liver disease irreversible coma is more likely to develop than in the chronic, more stable variety. Hepatic coma often supervenes in chronic cirrhosis without jaundice or bilirubinemia, although in previously nonjaundiced patients bilirubin concentration may increase slightly or occasionally moderately during the coma.

The commonly used liver function tests, such as serum enzyme levels, blood prothrombin activity, thymol turbidity, cephalin flocculation and Bromsulphalein retention likewise parallel the activity or severity of the liver disease and are related to hepatic coma only in this sense. Urine urobilinogen is extremely variable. In a few cases reported by Kelly et al. the nonurobilinogen Ehrlich-reacting substances in the urine were increased to exceptionally high values.[68] The blood alpha amino nitrogen concentration is usually normal or slightly increased in hepatic coma, except in patients with acute atrophy of the liver in which excessively high values are found frequently. Except in this latter instance, the total blood alpha-amino-nitrogen is not directly related to the onset, course or prognosis. Free phenolic compounds in the blood as measured by Murphy et al.[90] were either normal or somewhat elevated but did not differ significantly from the values obtained in the same patients before the onset of coma. The normal or slightly elevated blood phenol values contrast with the high concentrations found in uremia by Murphy et al.[90] and Nesbitt[94] and colleagues.

In routine examination, the urine is usually normal except for the changes in urine urobilinogen noted above and the presence of bilirubin. Small quantities of albumin and occasionally casts and other formed elements may be seen but are not observed with sufficient regularity or consistency to relate them to the comatose state. In general, then, the results of routine examinations of blood and urine as well as the standard liver function tests are related to the coma only insofar as they give evidence of severity and activity of the underlying liver disease.

Most patients with hepatic coma present with varied patterns of alterations in blood electrolytes, but some have patterns that are normal in every respect.[110] Abnormalities may reflect manifestations of the liver disease (or of alcoholism) such as poor intake, nausea, vomiting, diarrhea. Others may result from therapy with diuretic agents, parenteral fluids or abdominal taps, or from metabolic defects secondary to the liver disease itself, such as organic acidosis. Significance of alterations from the normal must be judged in light of these interrelations. As coma becomes protracted and management more complex, abnormalities are likely to become more numerous and profound. As in other laboratory tests, no special pattern of alterations in blood electrolytes relates specifically or clearly to hepatic coma. Hyponatremia, hypokalemia, metabolic acidosis or respiratory alkalosis are the most common accompaniments of severe liver disease with coma. The clinical significance of these and their management are discussed more fully under Treatment.

PATHOLOGY

Liver. Hepatic coma may arise as a complication and frequently as a terminal episode in almost any severe primary liver disease. The pathologic and histologic changes in the liver are those of the specific liver disease. No known specific changes in the liver are attributable to or otherwise related to the state of consciousness. In Laennec's cirrhosis, for example, hepatic coma may arise and end fatally in the chronic, static form of liver disease in which extensive fibrosis is present, but relatively healthy-appearing liver cells are interspersed in islands between the extensive fibrous tissue. Perhaps more commonly the coma is a terminal event in the more active form with jaundice and leukocytosis[82, 103] and in acute atrophy of the liver from poisoning or in pregnancy or with massive hepatic necrosis from viral hepatitis. Since hepatic coma may arise in apparently static liver disease as well as in acute liver disease, the term "liver failure" is not synonymous with hepatic coma, and should be used only when there is clinical or other evidence of progressive disease.[29]

Brain. Adams and Foley have studied extensively the pathology of the brain and other nervous tissues.[1] They found little of diagnostic importance upon gross examination of the brain. In some jaundiced patients the dura seemed to have a pale greenish hue. Various adventitious lesions, such as infarct and evidences of old trauma to the cerebral cortex, were observed. Wernicke's encephalopathy was found in 2 instances. Microscopically, an increase in number and size of the protoplasmic astrocytes were seen in all parts of the cerebral cortex, the putamen, globus pallidus, caudate nucleus, amygdaloid and sublenticular nuclei, thalamic and subthalamic nuclei, red nucleus, substantia nigra, tectum of the midbrain, pontine nuclei, dentate and roof nuclei of the cerebellum, the Purkinje layer of the cerebellum in some cases, the nuclei of Goll and Burdach, and the inferior olivary nuclei. The hypothalamic nuclei, interlaminar nuclei of the thalamus, and the somatic nuclei of brain stem and spinal cord were not involved to any significant degree.

The fibrous astrocytes in the white matter

usually retained their natural appearance. The number of protoplasmic astrocytes was nearly doubled in the hepatic coma cases as compared with the non-coma cases of liver disease and the controls without liver disease, and they averaged 35 per cent larger in size. Degeneration of nerve cells in the cerebral cortex, thalami and lenticular, red and dentate nuclei were observed in all of the more severe and protracted cases of hepatic coma. In some areas this was associated occasionally with a focus of protoplasmic astrocytes. In the less severe or prolonged cases nerve cell loss or degeneration was not as clearcut. Myelin stains failed to disclose important abnormalities. Specific changes in the oligodendroglia were those only of slight swelling. No specific changes in the blood vessels were related to hepatic coma. Swollen astrocytes were not found in the brains from patients who had had severe cerebral anoxia, uremia, diabetic acidosis, porphyria, delirium tremens, Korsakoff's psychosis, vitamin B deficiency or Wernicke's disease, hypoglycemia, fatal head injury, arsenical poisoning, bacterial meningitis or status epilepticus. They felt that "the brain lesion is then highly characteristic of advanced liver disease, but is not specific." Attempts to elucidate the cause of the swollen astrocytes were not productive of an answer but pointed to a metabolic defect affecting the nervous system in severe liver disease.

Kidney. Renal function abnormalities can often be demonstrated in advanced liver disease with or without hepatic coma.[8, 98, 120] Renal failure sometimes precipitates hepatic coma and is often associated with its progressive development, but azotemia is not an inevitable accompaniment of hepatic coma. Patients dying with hepatic coma show no specific gross or microscopic pathologic changes in the kidney that relate to the hepatic coma. Renal function sometimes deteriorates without apparent cause. In these patients often the kidneys have either no histologic abnormalities or minor alterations insufficient to account for the functional abnormalities. Some patients with severe liver disease with or without coma have nonspecific glomerular basement membrane thickening. Others show histologic evidence

of tubular injury. The latter most probably is a consequence of shock, dehydration, electrolyte imbalance, etc., rather than of the coma. Patients with intense jaundice at time of death may show so-called "bile nephrosis." This is considered a finding not specifically related to the hepatic coma or to the renal failure.

Other Tissues. Specific changes in other tissues either are not present or have not been found, other than as they relate to severe liver disease. Thus, bile staining of tissues is found in jaundiced patients. Endocrine changes, as observed in liver disease, are found at autopsy, but as yet no specific pathologic findings in tissues other than the brain appear to be related to hepatic coma itself.

DIFFERENTIAL DIAGNOSIS

Impending hepatic coma should be diagnosed when a patient with liver disease develops mental confusion, the characteristic flapping tremor, and (if possible to record) the electroencephalographic changes described under Clinical Manifestations. When the patient is in deep coma at the first examination or when these characteristic signs are absent, differentiation from other cerebral lesions must be made carefully. Any common condition leading to coma—for example, a cerebrovascular accident, diabetic coma, insulin shock, oversedation—may occur in severe liver disease and be confused with hepatic coma, occasionally even after careful study.

Chronic alcoholics with liver disease require special consideration in making the diagnosis of hepatic coma. This group of patients is, of course, susceptible to delirium tremens, acute alcoholic hallucinosis, alcohol induced hypoglycemia, Wernicke's syndrome and Korsakoff's psychosis. The mental confusion in Wernicke's encephalopathy may resemble that of hepatic coma, but the characteristic ophthalmoplegia, nystagmus and ataxia that are almost always present in this condition when it is full blown make the differentiation from hepatic coma relatively simple. The ophthalmoplegia of Wernicke usually responds within minutes or hours to intravenous administration of thiamine. The other manifestations improve more gradually with alcohol abstinence and the provision of an adequate diet. The manifestations of delirium tremens are well enough known not to require detailed consideration in the differentiation from hepatic coma. The tremor of delirium tremens is much more rapid and is accompanied by a degree of agitation and motor activity uncommonly seen in hepatic coma. Hallucinations and delusions so regularly seen in acute alcohol withdrawal are rare in hepatic coma. The memory defect and confabulation that are characteristic of Korsakoff's psychosis are not components of hepatic coma. Any alcoholic may have peripheral neuritis with or without severe liver disease. When hepatic coma accompanies one or several of the conditions mentioned, exact diagnosis is especially difficult.

Cerebral trauma in a patient with manifest liver disease may be confused easily with hepatic coma. It is particularly important to recognize this because many alcoholics develop severe liver disease and also are often subjected to head trauma. Moreover, the lowered prothrombin concentration, reduced platelet count and other hemostatic abnormalities so commonly found in liver disease may cause severe or progressive bleeding following even minor trauma. If previous trauma is possible, and if progressive disturbances in consciousness lead to coma, a skull fracture with either brain contusion or laceration is suspected, and prompt measures taken to make the diagnosis.

The cerebrospinal fluid as examined by the usual tests is usually normal in hepatic coma. Adams and Foley examined the spinal fluid in more than 25 cases and found the pressure to be normal, no cells and the protein content within normal limits. Xanthochromia was present in a few patients with intense jaundice. Walshe has found an abnormal content of amino acids in hepatic coma.[154]

Perhaps the most important traumatic cerebral lesion confused with hepatic coma is subdural hematoma. In this case the traumatic history may be insignificant or so long in the past as to be forgotten. The mental confusion associated with a subdural hemorrhage is sometimes indistinguishable from that of impending coma. A penetrating history taken from the relatives of the patient may lead to the history of trauma, and careful and repeated physical examinations must be made in an effort to find localizing signs. However, even a history of trauma, together with localizing signs, may be a concomitant of hepatic coma as noted above (Clinical Manifestations), so that even conscientious and painstaking clinical examination may not serve to differentiate these two—indeed, the two coexist occasionally. Finding erythrocytes, especially if crenated, in the spinal fluid may support the diagnosis of subdural hemorrhage. If subdural hematoma is reasonably suspected, burr holes should be made with a careful search for a clot.

The tremor of Wilson's disease resembles somewhat that seen in impending hepatic coma. In the former, however, the tremor is usually greatly exaggerated and has other characteristics that may serve to differentiate it from the latter. Moreover, the tremor is of long duration, and mental confusion is not a part of Wilson's disease at least until the terminal stages. This differential should not be difficult to make.

PATHOGENESIS

Most current hypotheses incriminate *abnormalities in ammonia metabolism* in the pathogenesis of hepatic coma. In numerous clinical and laboratory studies in recent years the significance of ammonia as an etiologic factor has been evaluated.[50] Stimulus for this intensive effort came from observations that a reversible syndrome indistinguishable clinically from impending hepatic coma resulted from administration of nitrogenous substances (ammonium cycle resins, ammonium chloride, diammonium citrate, urea, dietary protein) to patients with hepatic cirrhosis.[54, 104, 117] Subsequently blood ammonium levels in liver disease were found to be elevated, especially in hepatic coma in which the level usually correlated with the state of consciousness.[116, 118, 144] Also, increased blood ammonium levels correlated closely with episodes of stupor in a patient with surgically constructed Eck fistula, which added considerable support to this hypothesis.[85]

In retrospect, the role of the liver in ammonia metabolism had been studied by biochemists for many years.[114, 140] Portal vein blood of dogs was found to contain much more ammonia than the hepatic vein.[64] Moreover, ammonia in the blood increased in dogs after an Eck fistula was constructed.[48, 93] These observations supported the concept that an important function of the liver is removal of ammonia, a potentially toxic substance that originates in the gastrointestinal tract. Later other workers demonstrated that this function involved conversion of ammonia to urea in liver.[73]

In a series of brilliant studies of the completely hepatectomized dog, Bollman, Mann, Magath and collaborators clearly demonstrated the role of the liver in deamination of amino acids and urea formation from ammonia.[14, 15, 16, 83] They found a high ammonia content in the blood of these dogs which they believed arose largely from the gastrointestinal tract. The decrease in blood urea concentration after hepatectomy in dogs was found to be abolished following bilateral nephrectomy.[15] In this circumstance the concentration of blood urea remained unchanged, which indicates that this substance was not formed after the liver had been removed. Finally, the demonstration by Krebs and Henseleit[73] that liver tissue alone can form urea from ammonium salts established the liver as the site of urea formation as originally suggested by von Schroder.[151]

The development of anorexia, emesis and lethargy after Eck fistula or hepatectomy in dogs that had been fed protein, introduced the concept of "protein intoxication." It was considered that protein breakdown products in the gastrointestinal tract were absorbed and not removed in these animals. Because of its toxicity ammonia was considered as one of the possible causes of this phenomenon.

Rowntree, in his discussion of terminal hepatic disease, notes that Frerichs in 1851 observed twitching and convulsions in dogs given intravenous ammonium carbonate.[113] Monguio and Krause studied the significance of the blood ammonia content as a method of evaluating liver function.[88] They studied dogs—normal, with liver injury and after an Eck fistula. High blood ammonia concentrations were found after chronic meat feeding, and the term "meat poisoning" arose. The authors note:

> In the event that our opinion that a meat diet produces ammonia poisoning in dogs whose livers have been injured should be verified by experiments, then it will become urgently imperative that all patients suffering from functional disturbances of the liver, especially cases of severe injuries to the parenchyma and cirrhosis, should have protein food reduced to small portions.

The *toxicity of ammonia* is well established. Ammonium salts given intravenously to animals produce convulsions and death. Moreover, intravenous administration of urease which rapidly converts blood urea to ammonia and produces a rise in blood ammonia concentrations is also fatal after convulsions.[23, 139] The effect of urease can be prevented by the prior immunization of the animal with small but gradually increasing doses of crystalline urease which incites the formation of an antiurease.[71]

A simplified summary of the metabolism of ammonia and its relation to hepatic coma may be helpful at this point. Ammonia arising from ingested ammonium salts or produced by bacteria in the gastrointestinal tract is absorbed into the portal circulation and is presented at once to the liver. Most of the ammonia is removed from the portal blood by the liver so that little if any escapes into the general circulation. Ammonia presented to the systemic circulation is sometimes formed by other tissues; for example, by muscle after exercise, normal kidney, or kidney in the presence of metabolic acidosis or potassium deficiency. This is also removed from the blood by the liver.

By far the largest amount of ammonia is converted to urea. Urea is formed through the "orinthine cycle." Urea synthesis requires energy and utilizes ATP. Ammonia and carbon dioxide first combine with glutamic acid. The carbamyl group is transferred to ornithine, which adds another ammonia to form arginine. The enzyme arginase, present in considerable amounts in the liver, splits off urea from arginine, and ornithine is reconstituted.

In parenchymal liver disease increased quantities of ammonium in the systemic circulation reach peripheral tissues, e.g., brain, muscle, kidney, as consequences of portosystemic shunting and failure of the liver to metabolize adequately ammonia delivered to it from the gut or other sources. The excessive amounts of ammonia delivered to the brain induce untoward alterations in cerebral metabolism by some undefined mechanism. In "susceptible" patients with liver disease, these alterations cause the neurologic symptoms, signs and electroencephalographic changes characteristic of hepatic coma.

Elevated blood ammonia concentrations in diseases of the liver have been reported by a number of observers.[49, 70, 72, 147] Patients with severe Laennec's cirrhosis after oral ingestion of ammonium chloride or urea may develop drowsiness, confusion and clonic muscular jerkings.[104, 146, 148] These symptoms usually were associated with elevation of the blood ammonia concentration. That the effect of ammonium is not due to acidosis is shown by the observations of Phillips et al.[104] and of Schwartz et al.[116] The rise in blood ammonia concentration found by van Caulaert et al.[146] after the ingestion of ammonium chloride by patients with atrophic cirrhosis and by Kirk and Sumner[71] in studies of ammonium tolerance in cirrhosis was attributed to shunting of blood through collateral channels to the general circulation.

Studies in patients with severe cirrhosis[54, 104, 117] and in a patient with an Eck fistula[85] have shown clearly that the syndrome of impending hepatic coma and even deep coma may be induced by the administration of ammonium chloride, diammonium citrate or urea and after increases in dietary protein. Following the administration of these nitrogenous substances, blood ammonia concentrations rose in most of these patients. Likewise in spontaneous hepatic coma the blood ammonia concentration is usually elevated—in many instances, above that observed in severe liver disease without cerebral manifestations.[144] The state of consciousness correlates with blood ammonium content better than with any other biochemical measurement made to date.[104, 116, 144] A relation of ammonium level to clinical state is more evident if blood ammonium is determined serially. The degree of elevation associated with neuropsychiatric symptoms may vary from patient to patient, and in a given patient from time to time. The reasons for these variations are not known. Perhaps they are related to the rate at which the blood ammonium content is elevated, duration of elevation, factors influencing diffusion of ammonium into cells, failure of blood levels to reflect accurately intracellular concentrations, cerebral susceptibility to ammonium, or the patient's adaptation to the abnormality.

Potentially toxic substances other than ammonium are also considered in the pathogenesis of hepatic coma, but their importance is not nearly as well documented. For example, methionine administration induces coma in susceptible patients and the coma may be prevented by antibiotic administration.[101] This effect of methionine may be due to ammonia release in the gastrointestinal tract, but small molecular weight sulfur compounds, such as dimethylsulfide and methylmercaptan may be implicated. These compounds were postulated by Challenger and Walshe to relate to fetor hepaticus.[24]

Investigators have suggested for many years that compounds derived from tryptophan metabolism in the bowel, such as indole and indolyl derivatives, are toxic. Walshe and colleagues found that some of these compounds depressed the respiration of rat brain slices *in vitro* far more than ammonium.[155] The similarity of the tremor of hepatic coma to that seen in Wilson's hepatolenticular degeneration suggests a common etiology, but there is no evidence for this. The abnormalities in copper metabolism observed in Wilson's disease do not occur in severe cirrhosis. In fact, since hepatic coma can accompany any severe liver disease, this eliminates metabolic abnormalities related to but one form of liver disease. Thus, marked amino-acidemia is characteristic of acute necrosis of the liver but is not always seen in the coma of cirrhosis.[90] However, using paper chromatography, Walshe has observed distinct abnormalities in the blood content of individual amino acids, but no specific abnormality related to the coma.[154]

Hypoglycemia with coma is an occasional finding in alcoholics and in hemochromatosis but is rarely seen in the usual patient with cirrhosis. Treatment of hepatic coma with glucose solutions alters the state of consciousness only in the rare instances in which hypoglycemia does occur.[90] As noted, the term cholemia has been applied to hepatic coma, suggesting the flooding of the blood with material such as bilirubin and bile salts which are usually excreted by the liver into the gastrointestinal tract. However, hepatic coma frequently occurs in the absence of bilirubinemia, so that failure to excrete these substances cannot be implicated as an important etiologic factor.

The usual liver function tests (e.g., Bromsulphalein, cephalin flocculation, thymol turbidity and flocculation, enzyme levels and prothrombin concentration) do little more, as a rule, than demonstrate that severe liver disease is present. They offer no help in deciding whether or not hepatic coma will occur. Moreover, no specific change in the already deranged liver function tests occurs when coma supervenes, except as they become more abnormal in cases of progressive liver disease, such as acute atrophy or necrosis. In the ordinary patient with cirrhosis there is little if any change in these tests when they are compared before and in deep coma. A slight or occasionally moderate rise in serum bilirubin concentration may be observed, but commonly there is no change at all. The lack of aid from these tests in understanding hepatic coma is due to their nonspecificity.

A number of *metabolic abnormalities* in severe liver disease has been studied, and some may be particularly deranged in hepatic coma. The relation of these, if any, to hepatic coma is unclear. Elevations of blood pyruvate and lactate were observed in hepatic coma by Snell and Butt,[132] and of pyruvate and alpha-keto-glutarate by Smith,[130] Summerskill,[138] and Dawson[31] and their colleagues.

In three patients with hepatic coma studied by Amatuzio et al. blood pyruvate rose progressively and markedly after glucose administration; this did not occur in conscious patients with severe liver disease.[2] A deficiency of thiamine, which as cocarboxylase (diphosphothiamine) is necessary for the metabolism of pyruvate, seems to be unlikely to account for this, because almost invariably large amounts of thiamine are administered to these patients. The possibility that thiamine is poorly converted into cocarboxylase in hepatic coma has not been investigated, although a partial defect in thiamine phosphorylation has been demonstrated in chronic cirrhosis.[165] Lipoic acid, a component that combines with thiamine in the sequential disposition of ketoacids, does not correct the abnormality of pyruvate and lactate metabolism that occurs after giving a glucose load.[21]

It is clear that ammonium salts and certain other nitrogenous substances, including protein taken by mouth, may produce untoward effects in patients with severe liver disease, especially those with spontaneous or surgically made portacaval anastomosis.[54, 85, 104, 117] Not all patients with severe liver disease to whom these substances are administered develop hepatic coma. The exact incidence of this complication in various types of liver disease is not established. In fact, the susceptible population may well be small. Although this reaction does not occur regularly and its exact mechanism remains obscure, it is reproducible and well documented. It is not surprising, therefore, that ammonia metabolism in severe liver disease has been studied extensively.

Ordinarily the nitrogen contained in foods is the ultimate source of ammonium that must be metabolized. Ammonium salts taken by mouth are absorbed as such, probably high in the gastrointestinal tract. Urea and protein ingested are changed to ammonia by the effects of bacterial enzymes on urea and on amino and amide nitrogen groups. The gastrointestinal tract is a major source of blood ammonium, the ammonium content of portal blood being higher than that of any other vascular site. Furthermore, the ammonium content of portal blood draining the lower intestinal tract is higher than that draining the upper intestinal tract.

Gastric juice contains significant amounts of ammonium at levels that are considerably higher than those in arterial blood.[45, 79, 89, 107, 137] The ammonium in gastric juice is related to the level of urea in blood. It originates in part from circulating urea as a result of bacterial and possibly nonbacterial urease activity in mucosal cells, and possibly also in part from circulating ammonia. When gastric juice passes into the duodenum and jejunum, the ammonium it contains becomes available for absorption.

Circulating urea diffuses readily into the gastrointestinal lumen where it is hydrolyzed to ammonium and carbon dioxide. In man about 25 per cent of urea synthesized undergoes enterohepatic circulation: it is hydrolyzed in the gut and the resultant ammonium is reabsorbed and delivered to the liver via the portal circulation to be resynthesized to urea. Thus, in azotemia, a considerable quantity of ammonium may become available from this source.[78, 162] Renal failure may precipitate clinical manifestations of hepatic coma, or if these manifestations pre-exist, they may be aggravated. As might be expected, blood ammonia levels in cirrhosis and azotemia are high. Neuropsychiatric signs and symptoms are sometimes reversible, if azotemia is correctable. These mechanisms are also exemplified by patients with liver disease who have ureteroenterostomies and develop ammonium intoxication.[84, 129] This results from ammonium overload originating from hydrolysis of urea delivered to the colon by the diversion of urine.

Certain features of ammonium metabolism by the *kidney* also pertain to hepatic coma. In the normal person, the kidney is an important source of blood ammonium since renal vein blood contains more ammonium than arterial blood. This is related to ammonium production from glutamine and to a lesser extent from other amino acids, a normal function of the kidney. Normally ammonium is a buffer for excretion of hydrogen ion. Excretion of ammonium is closely related to the pH gradient between tubular cells and tubular fluid; in urine with a low pH the ammonium content is high and vice versa. Internal ammonium

overloading might result from diversion of ammonium from urine to renal venous outflow, or from increased renal ammonium production or availability to renal venous blood. Diversion of ammonium from urine to renal venous outflow is illustrated by the pharmacologic effects of acetazolamide. This induces bicarbonate diuresis and alkalinization of the urine. Urinary ammonium output decreases and ammonium content of renal vein blood promptly increases. This sequence may well explain the induction of hepatic coma in susceptible patients given this agent.[160]

Potassium deficiency also is related indirectly to hepatic coma because this cation affects renal ammonium metabolism.[7, 53] In potassium deficiency resulting from drug-induced diuresis,[7] renal potassium wasting[53] or enteric potassium losses,[5] renal production of ammonium or availability of ammonium to tubular fluid and to renal venous outflow is increased. This relation betwen potassium and ammonium is reflected by decreased blood potassium and elevated blood ammonium levels that are reciprocally related. In these circumstances the kidney is a significant internal source of ammonium which may induce the hepatic coma syndrome. The altered biochemical changes and the untoward clinical phenomenon are reversed readily if potassium salts are administered in adequate doses.

Potassium deficiency also illustrates the possible effects of alterations in *acid-base status* on ammonium toxicity.[156] In potassium deficiency, extracellular fluid is relatively alkaline and intracellular fluid relatively acid. The pH gradient favors diffusion and trapping of ammonia in cells from extracellular fluid. Thus, a given level of ammonium in blood may be rendered more toxic by potassium deficiency. This situation is readily reversed as extracellular alkalosis and potassium deficiency are corrected.

In hepatic coma other abnormalities in acid-base balance may occur. Patients frequently have metabolic alkalosis associated with hyperventilation.[63, 149] The etiology and significance of this are not known. Respiratory alkalosis should not be corrected by CO_2 inhalation since this has a deleterious effect in patients with hepatic precoma.

Increased quantities of organic acids resulting from abnormal metabolism of substrates by liver or from progressive renal failure with azotemia may cause metabolic acidosis. Acidosis is usually corrected as the hepatic disease or renal complications improve.

The clinical significance of all changes in acid-base balance on intracellular ammonium metabolism have not been established definitively. The physician must evaluate the etiology and estimate whether or not a given alteration is serious enough to warrant correction.

Kidney function is often abnormal in hepatic insufficiency.[8, 98, 120] In some patients it can be attributed to pre-existing primary kidney disease or to extrarenal factors. Others demonstrate evidences of acute tubular necrosis following episodes of precoma, bleeding, shock, dehydration, electrolyte imbalance, etc. In still others renal function deteriorates progressively without apparent cause. Renal function for this third group is characterized by decreased renal plasma flow and glomerular filtration rate, low urinary sodium concentration, relatively high urinary specific gravity, and diminished excretion of a water load. The cause of this water intolerance, oliguria and azotemia in hepatic coma is not known.

Oliguria and moderate azotemia are common although not universal concomitants of hepatic coma. In fact, during its development or at some time before termination many patients become oliguric with rising blood nonprotein nitrogen and creatinine concentrations. The rise in nonprotein nitrogen is due almost entirely to a rise in blood urea concentration. Since oliguria usually persists in spite of an adequate water intake and restriction of sodium intake, it is not due to dehydration or to fluid accumulation associated with sodium retention. When more fluids are administered than the kidneys will excrete, fluid accumulates progressively. When fluid intake is high and oliguria marked, and severe sodium restriction is adhered to, extracellular water increases and consequently extracelluar electrolytes are less concentrated. Hyponatremia and occasionally hypokalemia may be seen in this circumstance. As is noted under Treatment,

beneficial effects may follow the correction of these electrolyte disturbances.

The production of a *vasodepressor substance* VDM by the anoxic liver has been demonstrated by Shorr and colleagues.[127] This substance is also a powerful antidiuretic. Whether its activity increases in severe liver disease, especially in hepatic coma, is not known. Nevertheless, increased production of VDM may be a factor that accounts for the oliguria. That it is not the only factor seems reasonable, since the hypotension that is observed with increased VDM activity is not the rule with hepatic coma, although blood pressure may be reduced during the genesis of hepatic coma.

In some patients who have *spontaneous hepatic coma*—i.e., in whom no precipitating cause is found—a normal urinary output is maintained, nonprotein nitrogen concentration does not rise and electrolyte balance is normal. In fact, no physiologic or biochemical abnormalities are observed except for the development of deep coma which may be fatal. Careful observations of such patients leads one to believe that, although the factors outlined above must be given important consideration in the management of hepatic coma, they are not primarily involved in pathogenesis.

Renal failure may have other deleterious actions in relation to liver disease, specifically, in relation to hepatic coma.[162] Potassium retention, although unusual in hepatic disease, may occur during oliguria, if the potassium intake is high. Renal failure likewise leads to greatly enhanced secretions of urea into the stomach where it is acted upon by gastric urease liberating ammonia which may then be absorbed rapidly. As noted by Lieber and Davidson, "Uremia, even of a moderate degree, thus appears as a potential danger for patients with liver disease, and prevention of this complication seems indicated."[78]

Hepatic coma is an affliction of the central nervous system that occurs in some patients with severe liver disease. Accordingly, interrelationships of the brain and liver must be considered with special reference to how *cerebral metabolism* is disrupted. The significant pathologic lesions found consistently in the brain are an increase in number and size of protoplasmic astrocytes, and, less regularly, disappearance of nerve cells.[1, 150] The possible relation of these changes to alterations in cerebral metabolism is not known. Cerebral oxygen uptake is decreased in hepatic coma without strict relation to blood ammonium levels or arteriovenous ammonium differences across the brain.[41] The brain takes up ammonium at increasing arterial concentrations.[11, 161] This capacity to extract ammonium is less efficient in "spontaneous coma" than in coma precipitated by increasing nitrogen load, e.g., protein feeding, gastrointestinal bleeding.[161] An understanding of ammonium metabolism in brain, especially under conditions of ammonium excess, is of obvious pertinence.

In hepatic coma glutamic acid is highly concentrated in brain tissue. Although glucose is the usual source of energy for brain, Weil-Malherbe has shown that glutamic acid sustains respiration of brain slices and is metabolized to a considerable extent in certain circumstances.[163] Glutamic acid in brain has another important function, the disposition of ammonium. The main route for ammonium disposal involves conversion of alpha-keto-glutarate to glutamic acid and then to glutamine. Several co-enzymes and co-factors are necessary for the enzymatic reactions involved in ammonium removal and metabolism. Many of the removal reactions require energy, specifically high energy phosphate.

The hypothesis has been proposed that the alterations in cerebral metabolism causing hepatic coma result from depletion of the citric acid cycle by way of conversion of alpha-keto-glutarate to glutamic acid and glutamine.[11] Much work has been directed at evaluating this hypothesis. Flock and colleagues found a very high glutamine content in the brains of dogs that died after hepatectomy.[46] Walshe, using paper chromatography, found a marked increase of glutamine in the blood and particularly in the spinal fluid in hepatic coma.[154] However, Seegmiller and colleagues were unable to show any correlation between the blood glutamine content and state of consciousness.[118] In fact, blood glutamine seemed much less likely to parallel the clinical manifestations of hepatic coma than did the blood ammonia concentration. Increased amounts of glutamine are also found in the spinal fluid of patients with hepatic coma, but levels of alpha-keto-glutarate are also elevated.[134, 154]

Thus, measurements of the amounts of ammonium, glutamine, alpha-keto-glutarate and other keto-acids and amino acids in blood and spinal fluid demonstrate abnormalities, but the patterns of change are not consistent. This limitation is possibly related to failure of blood and spinal fluid levels to reflect intracellular cerebral concentrations. Several investigators have utilized *in vivo* systems in an attempt to overcome this limitation. Eiseman and co-workers infused ammonium salts into the carotid arteries of dogs.[26, 35] Cerebral alpha-keto-glutarate decreased and pyruvate and glutamine increased. Glutamate concentration did not change, nor did blood alpha-keto-glutarate or glutamine. Schenker and associates induced ammonium intoxication in rats and mice and measured various chemical substances in different regions of the brain after stupor developed.[115, 126] Adenosine triphosphate (ATP) and phosphocreatine were altered in base areas of brain as compared to cortical areas, whereas glucose and glycogen concentrations in cortex and base were comparable. Ammonium failed to depress cortical or brain stem alpha-keto-glutarate, and decreased ATP only in the brain stem. ATP depletion was not related to cortical or basilar alpha-keto-glutarate concentrations. These findings provide evidence that toxic doses of ammonium affect cerebral energy metabolism *in vivo*, and, furthermore, that the effect is preferentially localized at the base of the brain. The findings do not support the idea that cerebral alpha-keto-glutarate depletion resulting in decreased ATP synthesis accounts for ammonium toxicity.

Goetcheus and Webster considered an alternate mechanism for the effect of ammonium on cerebral metabolism.[60] They postulated that excess ammonium causes an increased cerebral concentration of gamma-aminobutyrate, a compound present almost exclusively in brain and possessing neuroinhibitory properties. The serum gamma-aminobutyrate levels were not elevated in hepatic coma. Rats in whom cirrhosis was induced by carbon tetrachloride also demonstrated normal concentrations of this metabolite in their brains. Other hypotheses include impaired acetylcholine synthesis[20]; abnormal metabolism of 5-hydroxytryptophan, the precursor of 5-hydroxytryptamine (serotonin)[19]; and impaired decarboxylation of alpha-keto-glutarate.[87] Geiger demonstrated that maintenance of function and survival of perfused cat brain depends on substances elaborated by liver, possibly cytidine and uridine.[57, 58] These findings suggest that in severe liver disease the brain may be deprived of an essential metabolite.

In summary, there is substantial evidence that ammonium alters cerebral metabolism in hepatic coma. This is manifest clinically as alterations in behavior and mental status, various neurologic findings including a coarse flapping tremor, and a characteristic electroencephalographic change. There are theoretical mechanisms whereby ammonium excess affects cerebral metabolism adversely. Information derived from clinical studies and from experiments using *in vivo* and *in vitro* systems is not sufficiently definitive to permit acceptance of any of the hypotheses. The exact mechanism(s) by which ammonium excess affects cerebral metabolism is unknown.

TREATMENT

Preventive

Many patients with severe liver disease appear to develop coma spontaneously. However, as discussed under Pathogenesis, a host of factors may predispose toward, hasten the development of or actually induce this frequently terminal complication. The relation of these factors to the genesis of hepatic coma will become clearer as more is known of the condition. Even at present for the majority of patients a predisposing event or factor may be etiologically important and might have been correctable or avoided. Therefore, it behooves the physician to become familiar with all of the possible predisposing agents and mechanisms so

that they can be avoided as far as possible. This is not practical in all circumstances because some of them, such as paracentesis, are necessary for the treatment of other manifestations of chronic liver disease; and others, for example, massive upper gastrointestinal hemorrhage, are not yet classifiable as preventable conditions.

The Use of Hypnotics, Analgesics, Sedatives and Anesthetic Agents in Liver Disease. All of the common hypnotics, sedatives and analgesics may be tolerated poorly and even contribute to the induction of hepatic coma in susceptible patients.[90] Often these agents are needed by the patients who should not receive them. The excitement, the noisy, irrational and inappropriate behavior so often observed especially at night in the early stages of hepatic coma urgently require that a sedative be given in order that the patient, his neighbors or the doctors and nurses may find relief. Frequently, it is in this circumstance after the administration of the sedative that stupor and then deep coma appear and may become irreversible and fatal. (Whether the sedative induces hepatic coma or merely accelerates progression into deep coma is unknown.)

The same chain of events may occur less commonly in patients with severe liver disease who have no evidence of impending hepatic coma. Therefore, the physician must exercise extreme care in administering sedatives, analgesics or hypnotics. Under certain circumstances sedation is necessary, and one should know which agent to choose and what dose to administer. The pharmacology of these drugs with particular reference to their metabolism by the liver is discussed briefly here.

Morphine and some of its close derivatives are probably the worst offenders in the genesis of hepatic coma.[23, 36, 67] Morphine is conjugated in the liver before it is excreted.[10, 95, 96] Gross found that conjugation of morphine in animals greatly decreased after liver damage.[61] In man the action of morphine is prolonged in severe liver disease. Not uncommonly, a patient given as little as ⅛ grain of morphine sleeps for a day or two.

Methadone is probably in a class with morphine in liver disease, for it appears to be metabolized by the liver also.[18] In contrast with morphine and presumably methadone, meperidine (Demerol) does not appear to require the liver for excretion; or, if it does, the requirement is quantitatively much smaller than for morphine.[157] It seems possible to give comparatively larger doses of meperidine in severe liver disease without inducing prolonged sleep.

In addition to its prolonged action morphine has a second contraindication—its antidiuretic action.[59] Whether the oliguria so commonly seen in hepatic coma is a cause or effect is not clear. Nevertheless, accentuation of oliguria by morphine administration would seem to be poor clinical practice. The use of the antidote for morphine poisoning, N-allylnormorphine[3] has not been documented in the treatment of morphine poisoning in severe liver disease; but, considering its effect in other instances of morphine poisoning, a fair trial should be given.

There is good evidence for the generalization that the long-acting, short-chain barbiturates are excreted largely by the kidney, while those with a more rapid onset and shorter action and larger molecules tend to be handled by the liver.[22, 106, 112] The thiobarbiturates (for example, Pentothal Sodium) are also detoxified by the liver.[124] Therefore, if barbiturates must be used, one should choose those with the greatest renal excretion, such as barbital and phenobarbital. Pentothal and pentobarbital presumably would be among those less easily excreted in severe liver disease. Whether there is, in fact, any delay in handling the various barbiturates in patients with severe liver disease as compared with normal individuals seems to be doubtful from the work of Sessions et al.[118a] Nevertheless, patients who have been given either frequent small doses or a relatively large dose of a barbiturate have developed hepatic coma; whether coma was induced by the barbiturate or accelerated by it is not known. Of course, for a great many patients with liver disease who have been given barbiturates hepatic coma does not develop. Moreover, in many circumstances the need for hypnotics justifies administration of barbiturates irrespective of the possible development of hepatic coma. The physician who recognizes the possibility

of coma guards the dosage and frequency of administration carefully. Similar precautions apply to glutethimide. Paraldehyde is also a bad offender, because it presumably is metabolized to a considerable extent by the liver and is used so often as a sedative in alcoholics who may have severe liver disease.[76] In many instances hepatic coma appears to have been induced or accelerated by paraldehyde. When paraldehyde has been used, often the characteristic odor can be detected on the breath for several days, which indicates that it is eliminated slowly from the body.

Chloral hydrate is a chlorinated hydrocarbon. Although the small doses used for sedation are not likely to have a direct heptatotoxic effect, it is metabolized by conjugation in the liver. This limits its use in patients with liver disease.

In general, the dosage for most hypnotic sedatives and analgesics should be considerably less for patients with severe liver disease than for normals, both in quantity and frequency of administration. For example, 50 or even 25 mg. of meperidine may give a satisfactory analgesic effect. The barbiturates do not appear to be as effective in smaller than usual doses, but their frequency of administration must be controlled carefully. Prolonged sleep has followed continued administration over several days of only a half grain of phenobarbital 3 times daily.

Many psychomimetric, antiemetic and antihistaminic drugs have become available in recent years. They are readily absorbed from the gut lumen, and the liver is a main site for their metabolism. About 60 per cent of phenothiazine taken orally is removed from the portal circulation by liver. Phenothiazines also undergo an enterohepatic circulation. They are demethylated and conjugated with glucuronic acid. Meprobamate and antihistamines are metabolized in liver by hydroxylation and also conjugated as glucuronides. Tolerance of patients with liver disease for the newer agents, e.g., phenothiazines, meprobamate, benzodiazepines, dibenzazepines, antihistamines, is not evaluated adequately. Amine oxidase inhibitors are known to have propensity to cause untoward effects and should be avoided.

Some of the agents mentioned may control the agitation due to alcohol withdrawal or the gastrointestinal symptoms that seriously limit oral intake of food and fluid. Agents that are least likely to induce hepatic injury are given preference. However, precautions that apply to use of hypnotics and sedatives also apply here: sufficient indication for use, careful adjustment of dose and close observation of the patient's response. Drugs of the types mentioned are strictly avoided in patients with neuropsychiatric findings of hepatic coma or precoma.

In conclusion, the use of analgesics, hypnotics, sedatives and psychomimetric drugs in severe liver disease may be hazardous and should be avoided, if at all possible. When their use is clearly indicated, care is given to the dosage and frequency of administration, and prior to this the patient should be examined carefully for evidence of impending hepatic coma.

Patients with liver disease tolerate surgical operations poorly. This may be due in part to the prior administration of hypnotics and analgesics. Only under rare circumstances should morphine be used, particularly as meperidine seems to be a safe substitute. Again, dosage of these agents should be reduced, particularly with regard to frequency of administration.

The effect of anesthetic agents on the liver has not been studied extensively. Chloroform particularly, as well as some other inhalation anesthetics, produce liver damage. Fairlie and colleagues found abnormalities in Bromsulphalein excretion after surgical operation and with ether, cyclopropane and spinal anesthesia.[37] Bromsulphalein excretion can be decreased in febrile states, shock and a number of other circumstances, particularly when the circulation to the liver is altered, as well as after liver damage itself. The Bromsulphalein test may not be a valid criterion of the effect of the anesthetic agent. Certainly, chloroform is never used in patients with liver disease, if it is advised under any circumstances. Whether ether is less harmful to the liver than the other commonly used inhalation anesthetics is debated. Some clinicians consider cyclopropane less harmful than ether.[13]

Halothane is a commonly used anesthetic agent. In an extensive retrospective survey halothane and other anesthetic agents were compared with regard to incidence of fatal massive hepatic necrosis and overall death rate.[136] Massive hepatic necrosis due to any cause was rare. In most cases this was associated with prolonged traumatic surgery, profound hypotension, liberal use of pressor substances, congestive heart failure, anoxia or some combination of these. Massive liver necrosis in the others could not be attributed to these causes. A few cases might have resulted from coincidental viral hepatitis, in others halothane was suspected. Rarely does halothane induce fatal liver necrosis; however, if necrosis occurs it is likely to be severe and massive. The patients exhibit a fulminant course with hepatic coma as one of the terminal events. Independent clinical observations show that halothane probably does produce liver damage at a low level of incidence. Until the relative propensities of halothane and other agents to induce hepatic injury are better established caution about the use of this agent is warranted, especially in considering a second exposure. If unexplained fever and jaundice or other evidences of hepatic dysfunction develop after halothane is used, it should probably not be given again.[30] (See Chap. 14.)

Anesthetic agents are used judiciously and with caution and respect. Adequate oxygenation must be maintained, hypotension prevented and blood loss replaced adequately during surgical procedures.

Acute infection is an important precipitating factor of hepatic coma. All acute infections in liver disease are handled expeditiously, and appropriate antibiotics are used in the usual therapeutic amounts. Every effort is made to keep the urinary output satisfactory during a febrile episode, although overloading with fluid is avoided when oliguria not associated with dehydration is present.

Nitrogenous Substances. As discussed under Pathogenesis concerning the relation of ammonia metabolism to hepatic coma, great care is exercised in administering ammonium salts or urea to patients with liver disease. Only a small number of patients develop hepatic coma when ammonium salts are administered, but there is no way to judge susceptibility of individual patients. Ammonium chloride is commonly used to induce metabolic acidosis in order to potentiate the diuretic effects of organic mercurials. In patients with liver disease oral administration of a solution of calcium chloride (containing 1 or 2 mEq. of chloride per ml.) is preferred for this purpose, since it does not induce hepatic coma.

Evidences of mental confusion and of the characteristic tremor are searched for at frequent intervals if nitrogenous substances are given. Under no circumstance are they given to severely ill patients or particularly to those with signs of impending hepatic coma. The problem of dietary protein is discussed below under General Therapeutic Measures.

Acute gastrointestinal bleeding is an important predisposing factor to hepatic coma. The bleeding may be from ruptured esophageal varices, from peptic ulcer, which is more common in patients with liver disease than in those without, from gastritis (particularly in alcoholics), or less commonly from other sites. Patients with severe liver disease may bleed extensively and recover after transfusions and other therapeutic measures, only to lapse into coma 24 to 48 hours later. The etiology of the coma in this circumstance probably is related to factors of blood loss and attendant shock and oliguria, to other metabolic aberrations and to the large amount of protein deposited in the gastrointestinal tract which may release ammonia. Treatment is aimed at therapy for shock with blood transfusions and other measures, stopping the bleeding, and, when practical, removal of the blood from the colon by enema.

It is extremely difficult to decide upon emergency surgery when severe liver disease is accompanied by upper gastrointestinal tract bleeding. The decision must be made on a highly individual basis after careful consultation between surgeon and internist, and then only when the patient's condition has improved and there is some hope that a relatively brief operation will prevent a recurrence of bleeding.

Paracentesis. Hepatic coma follows all too frequently within 24 to 48 hours after paracentesis in patients with severe liver disease. Reduction in plasma volume and oliguria are usual after large quantities of ascitic fluid are removed from the peritoneal cavity,[55, 92] presumably because ascitic fluid accumulates again rapidly at the expense of the plasma after paracentesis. Hyponatremia, particularly when sodium intake is restricted, may follow the ingestion of water during this period of oliguria. These factors may play an important part in producing impending coma or even coma following this procedure.

The physician is cautious before undertaking paracentesis; if it can relieve dyspnea or severe anorexia it probably should be done. If the patient is in the early stages of hepatic coma, the decision is extremely difficult and an individual one. In this circumstance the removal of small quantities of fluid from time to time may accomplish the same result more slowly but with less likelihood of upsetting the metabolic balance. Often adequate relief of symptoms follows removal of only 1 or 2 liters of ascitic fluid. This may suffice for the time in the severely ill or precomatose patient who may be seriously jeopardized by vigorous therapy with paracentesis or diuretic agents.

Diuretics. Diuretics are often used for treating ascites and edema accumulation in cirrhosis. However, in some susceptible patients many of these agents induce precoma or, occasionally, deep coma. If an episode of impending hepatic coma is related to administration of a diuretic agent, or occurs for some other reason while the agent is being given, it is discontinued and any electrolyte disturbances promptly corrected. These agents are not used if impending hepatic coma is evident, even if ascites and edema are significant. Fluid accumulation is controlled in most cases by strict attention to sodium and fluid intakes.[28, 55, 120] These conservative measures entail the least risk when precoma or coma exist.

Neuropsychiatric manifestations have followed the use of chlorothiazides,[54, 108] carbonic anhydrase inhibitors,[105, 160] mercurial diuretics,[7] spironolactone, ethacrynic acid and furosemide.[122] There is little information available in regard to the relative propensity of each agent to induce untoward effects and to the incidence of adverse effects in the population treated.[122] The exact mechanism(s) by which diuretic drugs precipitate impending hepatic coma is not known. Some information about this aspect is available for certain of the drugs. Induction of potassium deficits by chlorothiazides and organic mercurials is reciprocally related to elevated blood ammonium levels and clinical symptoms of hepatic coma.[7, 109] These are readily reversed by administration of potassium salts in adequate amounts. [7, 53, 108] In these instances ammonium overload results from the increased production of ammonium by kidney that occurs with potassium deficiency.[7, 53] Other drugs that induce renal potassium wasting, such as ethacrynic acid and furosemide, may well induce untoward effects by the same mechanism, although these agents have not been specifically investigated. Not all patients who develop hypokalemia exhibit signs of hepatic coma, but there is no way to distinguish those who will from those who will not.

Oral potassium supplements are given simultaneously when agents that induce renal potassium wasting are prescribed. If blood potassium levels decline in spite of supplementation with potassium salts the agent is temporarily discontinued and the supplement continued until depletion is corrected. One report indicates that broad-spectrum antibiotics diminish or even prevent a rise in blood ammonium and onset of precoma in many patients given chlorothiazide.[81] The reason for this effect is unclear. In our experience fewer untoward effects occur when potassium wasting drugs such as thiazides, ethacrynic acid or furosemide are given in conjunction with potassium-saving agents such as spironolactone or triamterene, but even here the patient must be carefully observed clinically and blood electrolytes monitored. Bicarbonate diuresis, increased urine pH, metabolic acidosis, and a diversion of ammonium from urine to renal venous outflow results from use of carbonic anhydrase inhibitors. This diversion may yield an endogenous systemic ammonium overload. There is also evidence that metabolism of ammonium by peripheral tissues, including brain, is affected by thiazides and acetazolamide.[105, 108, 109, 160]

Diuretic agents have certain potential hazards in common. Induction of a brisk and persistent diuresis may lead to plasma volume depletion, compromise of renal perfusion, oliguria, azotemia and sodium depletion which may precipitate or aggravate the manifestations of hepatic coma. These drugs are discontinued immediately if any of these changes is detected.

Potassium Deficiency. The relation of potassium deficiency to the hepatic coma syndrome and to ammonium metabolism is discussed under Pathogenesis and Diuretics. Potassium deficiency resulting from causes other than use of diuretic agents may also be associated with impending hepatic coma, presumably because it affects ammonium metabolism. Body stores of potassium are limited in cirrhotic patients. These patients, whose food (and potassium) intakes are often inadequate, may also have nausea, vomiting and diarrhea which favor the development of potassium deficits. These are especially likely to occur in liver disease associated with excessive intake of alcoholic beverages.

GENERAL THERAPEUTIC MEASURES

Exacting nursing care is a *sine qua non*, particularly when deep coma is present. Not only general measures are important, such as keeping the patient clean, preventing decubitus, etc., but also measurements of body weight, intake, output and the vital signs are of the utmost value. Only with these measures can the physician make the essential calculations necessary to understand the patient's condition. Hepatic coma is treated best on a metabolic ward with trained personnel and complete laboratory aid, but these facilities are seldom available. However, good nursing, the usual laboratory facilities and an attentive physician should be satisfactory.

The first principle in the treatment of hepatic coma is meticulousness by all personnel concerned: care for the patient's general condition, care that all that happens to the patient is known and recorded, and care to observe, record and treat all complications. A flow sheet for recording clinical and laboratory data, including intake of fluid, electrolytes and nutrients and the volume of urine and quantity of feces is essential. All observations are made at frequent intervals, beginning at the earliest stage of the disease—during impending coma or earlier, if possible.] The following observations are among those considered important:

Clinical Observations. These are made once daily; if the clinical state is changing rapidly, more frequent, even hourly, examinations are made. The extent and magnitude of the characteristic tremor is recorded, and the state of consciousness classified approximately according to Table 12–1. When the patient no longer responds, the deep tendon reflexes, the sucking, grasping, plantar and corneal reflexes are examined.

Minor mental confusion is difficult to evaluate. Simple mathematical problems, such as subtracting sevens from 100, sometimes brings out a mild confusional state in a patient who can answer correctly questions as to time, place and person. Sometimes, even though the patient answers the usual questions satisfactorily, a slight clouding of consciousness is apparent by the relative slowness with which the answers are given. A certain untidiness about the person himself and his belongings is sometimes observed. Inappropriate behavior may be a clue to early hepatic coma, and often a curious staring, glassy-eyed appearance is evident—the so-called "faraway" look.

Intake and Output. The intake and the output of all fluids, electrolytes and nutrients are listed so that fluid and electrolyte balance can be judged and caloric and protein requirements satisfied. Daily urine volume is recorded, and the volumes tallied at regular intervals. Urine specific gravity is noted, and urinary sediment examined frequently. Insensible loss of fluid is estimated, and the amount of fluid contributed by the oxidation of food is calculated. In this way an intake and output balance sheet can be maintained, and one will not err on the side of dehydration or of fluid intoxication. If the patient is incontinent of urine, or if there is other reason to doubt that collections will be complete, an indwelling catheter with constant drainage is used in spite of the possibility of bladder or renal infection. Daily irrigations with a 1:1,000 dilution of Zephiran solution often prevent infection.

Laboratory Observations. Daily determinations should be made of the blood hematocrit, blood nonprotein nitrogen and creatinine concentrations, blood carbon dioxide content, and, when possible, body weight. The hematocrit serves as another index of possible hemoconcentration or hemodilution, and the nonprotein nitrogen and the blood carbon dioxide combining power are helpful in estimating kidney clearance of end products of nitrogen metabolism and regulation of the acid-base balance of the body. Serum sodium, potassium and chloride concentrations are determined frequently. As noted, hyponatremia is common in hepatic disease, especially when ascites is present. In hepatic coma hyponatremia is sometimes severe, particularly following paracentesis or after large quantities of fluids are given. Hypokalemia may result from continuing fluid losses from the upper or lower gastrointestinal tract.

Blood sugar is measured occasionally, particularly early in the course to eliminate the rare hypoglycemia as a causative factor. Every stool is examined, if possible, for the presence of blood. It is sometimes useful to know the total daily sodium excretion; for most patients with ascites and edema this can be assumed to be only a minute quantity, but in other situations it is relatively normal and occasionally is excessive, especially when acute renal tubular necrosis is also present.

Intake of Electrolytes, Water and Nutrients. If the patient is in semicoma or deep coma and cannot eat or be fed satisfactorily, a stomach tube may be used. Appropriate quantities of food and medications such as neomycin and potassium chloride solution can then be given orally. Antacids can also be instilled in patients with gastrointestinal bleeding. The presence of varices—as revealed by roentgenograms or suggested by portal hypertension or the severity of the liver disease—need not contraindicate intubation. If the tube is well lubricated, pliable and gently handled there is relatively little danger from intubation.

Intravenous feedings may be used when desired or necessary. Because adequate supplies of a suitable fat emulsion for parenteral use are not available, sufficient calories cannot be supplied intravenously. Glucose, saline solution and protein hydrolysates may be given, care being taken to judge the required fluid and electrolyte intake as well as that of the other nutrients, especially protein. When solutions are administered by tube or intravenously the rate must be relatively slow so that the liver and other tissues are not flooded at times with large quantities of nutrients.

Water. Many patients with chronic liver disease have a decreased tolerance to water. This tends to be more marked in hepatic coma. In order to avoid water intoxication and hyponatremia, fluids administered to patients with impending or deep hepatic coma must be restricted somewhat. Most patients tolerate approximately 1,500 ml./day. If the urine volume is low, one should suspect dehydration, a marked decrease in water tolerance or severe hyponatremia and sodium depletion. In this complicated circumstance accurate records of fluid intake and output and fluid balance are invaluable. If relatively large quantities of fluid have been given and if the blood hematocrit has been falling, one can suspect overhydration and hyponatremia. A very low serum sodium concentration corroborates this hypothesis and one may decide to administer hypertonic saline in an effort to bring about an electrolyte concentration closer to normal. This treatment of hyponatremia strikingly improves the state of consciousness of occasional patients with hepatic coma.[92] If the urine volume is low, and if fluid intake has been restricted severely, one can suspect dehydration, and an increase of fluid intake can be given a trial for 24 hours; but if this does not lead to a concomitant and proportional increase in urine output, it is evident that water tolerance is greatly reduced. In this circumstance continuing the high fluid intake would lead inevitably to fluid retention, hemodilution and hyponatremia.

Sodium. If ascites and edema are present, sodium intake is restricted to approximately 250 mg./day or less. One must then follow body weight, fluid intake and output, blood hematocrit and, if possible, daily sodium excretion, to prevent hyponatremia and sodium depletion.

If ascites and edema are not present, moderate quantities of sodium can be administered. If this leads to diminished urine volume and gain in weight, it may be assumed that fluid is being retained and that ascites and edema will result. In this circumstance sodium is restricted to prevent these clinical manifestations.

Potassium. Potassium is supplemented if potassium deficiency is established by clinical findings, decreased blood potassium level and appropriate electrocardiographic changes. Potassium salts given in adequate amounts readily reverse the untoward biochemical and clinical manifestations of the deficiency *per se*, and often also those of hepatic coma or precoma when this coexists. Oral supplements are preferable to intravenous supplements, but potassium chloride solution is given intravenously, if necessary, providing the rate of infusion is slow. When oliguria or hyponatremia are present, potassium is given only if evidence of deficiency is convincing, and even then caution is used until the urine flow rate is adequate.

The total body potassium deficit cannot yet be determined accurately in clinical situations. A total body deficit of several hundred milliequivalents is not unusual in liver disease complicated by poor intake and excessive enteric losses. Potassium deficits may also be incurred from increased urinary excretion secondary to metabolic alkalosis or to use of certain diuretic drugs. About 150 to 300 mEq. of potassium given in divided doses over a period of 2 to 3 days usually relieves jeopardy from this cause providing losses do not continue. The dosage can be decreased progressively as clinical and laboratory responses become evident. Reversal of impending coma symptoms is likely to be evident over a period of 3 to 5 days as potassium is repleted.

Alkalosis commonly, but not inevitably, accompanies potassium deficiency. In these instances the potassium deficit may not be remedied completely until alkalosis is corrected. Use of the citrate, bicarbonate or gluconate salts of potassium tends to foster alkalosis. Potassium chloride is the supplement of choice when alkalosis coexists, because chloride affects the excretion of bicarbonate in the urine.

Calories. The caloric requirements for

TABLE 12–3. VITAMINS FOR PATIENTS WITH HEPATIC COMA

Oral		Parenteral	
Thiamine HCl	2 mg.	Thiamine HCl	5 mg.
Riboflavin	2 mg.	Riboflavin	5 mg.
Niacinamide	20 mg.	Niacinamide	100 mg.
Ascorbic acid	50 mg.	Calcium pantothenate	20 mg.
Calcium pantothenate	5 mg.	Pyridoxine	2 mg.
Pyridoxine HCl	0.5 mg.	Ascorbic acid	300 mg.
Folic acid	0.25 mg.	Folic acid	1.5 mg.
Vitamin B_{12}	2 mcg.	Vitamin B_{12}	1 mcg.
Vitamin A	5,000 units		
Vitamin D	400 units		
Vitamin K	2 mg.		

From Committee on Therapeutic Nutrition: Publication 234, Washington, D.C., Food and Nutrition Board, National Research Council.

done in conjunction with intubation used to establish the site of bleeding or with esophageal tamponade used to control bleeding. Cathartics and enemas should usually be used early in the management of patients with hepatic coma. They should not, however, be continued repeatedly or beyond a day or so lest significant losses of fluid and electrolytes from the gastrointestinal tract cause further metabolic complications. These measures should probably be avoided in patients with active gastrointestinal bleeding or suspected of having peritonitis, situations in which it is inadvisable to enhance intestinal motility.

Vitamin Administration. This is seldom a problem, for most of these patients receive large or even massive doses of vitamins as a routine. At least adequate amounts of the commonly administered vitamins should be supplied, either orally or parenterally, particularly if the patient has come to the hospital after a heavy drinking spree or with an unknown dietary history or one of poor food intake. Massive doses need not be given. For quantities recommended by the Committee on Therapeutic Nutrition,[141] see Table 12–3.

OTHER THERAPEUTIC MEASURES

Glucose. It has been the custom for many years to give fairly large amounts of glucose parenterally to patients with severe liver disease, particularly those with hepatic coma. Many physicians, especially Jones,[66] have recommended it. At least occasional patients with hepatic coma may benefit from the intravenous administration of glucose. Possibly coincidental restriction of dietary protein intake and the influence of glucose in decreasing tissue protein breakdown account for this. Also glucose reportedly stimulates the combination of ammonia with glutamic acid to form glutamine,[163] the latter presumably acting as a storehouse for ammonia and removing it from the blood where it may be toxic. If the ammonia concentration is high and is contributing to the comatose state, glucose administration might aid in its removal.

Adrenocorticotropic Hormone (ACTH) and Cortisone. It is difficult to evaluate the efficacy of these hormones in the treatment of hepatic coma.[100, 133, 158] Ducci reported patients with viral hepatitis and coma who responded to large doses of cortisone (600 mg./day).[33] Several other patients have responded to similar amounts. Whether smaller doses are effective is not known. Most patients who have been given either hormone in any dosage have shown no clinical change. Occasionally patients with liver disease may even have been made worse.[17] It may be that these hormones are most effective in viral hepatitis and less so in coma associated with cirrhosis in chronic alcoholics. Further trial is indicated.

Albumin. In ascites and edema normal human serum albumin occasionally induces diuresis, but the dangers are thought by some to outweigh the advantages, the chief danger being massive upper gastrointestinal hemorrhage, usually from varices.[38] In hepatic coma albumin has been tried, generally without success, but occasional patients who have fallen into coma following bleeding episodes or following paracentesis have improved considerably following the administration of 25 or 50 Gm. of normal human serum albumin intravenously. Why albumin is effective is unclear. Perhaps it relieves the oliguria resulting from lowered plasma volume after bleeding or paracentesis.

Glutamic Acid. Walshe reported beneficial results in hepatic coma following the intravenous administration of 20 Gm. of glutamic acid (as sodium glutamate) and suggested that it be given further therapeutic trial.[153] Were ammonia the toxic agent, glutamic acid might act by combining with it to form glutamine. In fact, glutamate lowers high blood ammonia content. However, a number of further observations do not give encouragement so far as the effectiveness of glutamic acid in the treatment of hepatic coma in chronic alcoholics is concerned.[159] So far no clearcut or lasting benefit attributable to glutamic acid is substantiated.

Arginine. Arginine is an intermediate in the urea synthesis cycle. The use of this amino acid is based on the potential it has for enhancing urea formation from ammonia. Najarian and Harper, following some experimental studies of their own and of others, reported a clinical study of the effect of arginine on the blood ammonia and hepatic coma.[91] They reported good results. Others have substantiated this, but some have found no demonstrable effect either on blood ammonia or on coma in liver disease.[12, 111, 166, 167] The best controlled clinical studies indicate that use of arginine does not convincingly alter response to treatment or outcome. Formation of urea from arginine depends upon hepatic arginase activity. Availability of this enzyme may well be limited in severe liver disease.

The use of arginine or glutamic acid is not likely to make a critical difference in patients who do not respond to reduction in protein intake, administration of antibiotic, bowel cleansing, blood replacement and measures to correct and control fluid and electrolyte balance.

Hemodialysis. Hemodialysis has been tried as a means for decreasing blood ammonia levels and treating hepatic coma.[25, 69] Although ammonia level may be lowered temporarily with dialysis, clinical responses have not been consistent enough to encourage general acceptance of this method. Actually, patients with severe liver disease are prone to complications from the dialysis procedure, such as hemorrhagic diathesis. When oliguria and azotemia complicate hepatic coma, dialysis may be considered as a means of managing the renal failure. In these instances also results are not generally encouraging.

Exchange Transfusions. The treatment of fulminating liver failure with exchange transfusions has received attention recently and is being investigated.[9, 145] Some patients with fulminant hepatitis awaken following exchange transfusions. It may be that life has been saved by maintaining the patient until massive necrosis subsides and liver cell regeneration becomes established.

To date, a majority of patients who have had exchange transfusions have not survived. Until additional data is accumulated on the use of exchange transfusions no conclusions can be made about indications for the use of this method or its efficacy. However, a distinction between liver failure and hepatic coma should be kept in mind. Fulminant liver failure due to massive necrosis, for example, may have as one of its preterminal manifestations hepatic coma, but the latter occurs much more frequently as an episodic complication of acute or reversible liver disease. Unusual measures are inadvisable for the treatment of hepatic coma, except when other manifestations of fulminant hepatic failure occur and the more conservative measures discussed above have been given a trial.

Colon Surgery. Since most of the ammonia (and other possibly toxic substances from bacterial action) arise from the colon, Atkinson and Goligher and others have done colectomy or colon bypass procedures on patients who are disabled with recurrent attacks of hepatic stupor and coma following portacaval anastomosis.[6, 86, 121] Prior to the operation sufficient protein could not be given to maintain nutrition, but after surgery protein balance increased considerably and nutrition improved. In general, however, reduction of protein intake together with use of an oral broad-spectrum antibiotic is the treatment of choice; this controls most chronic neuropsychiatric symptoms. Colon surgery is considered only for the occasional desperate case.

Other Measures. Several additional approaches to decreasing availability of ammonia from the gastrointestinal tract have been described recently. Immunity to urease has been induced with graded doses of jackbean meal urease in patients with hepatic disease.[142] Acetohydroxamate has been suggested for use since it inhibits bacterial urease.[4, 42] Others propose decreasing the organisms with urease activity by altering the bacterial flora of the gut by feeding *Lactobacillus acidophilus*.[80] These approaches need much more extensive clinical evaluation to determine whether they can be recommended as beneficial adjuncts in the management of patients with liver disease complicated by acute or recurrent episodes of coma.

REFERENCES

1. Adams, R. D., and Foley, J. M.: The neurological disorder associated with liver disease, *in* Metabolic and Toxic Diseases of the Nervous System, vol. 32, Proc. Assoc. Res. Nerv. & Ment. Dis., Baltimore, Williams & Wilkins, 1953.
2. Amatuzio, D. S., Shrifter, N., Stutzman, F. L., and Nesbitt, S.: Blood pyruvic acid response to intravenous glucose or insulin in the normal and in patients with liver disease and with diabetes mellitus, J. Clin. Invest. 31:751, 1952.
3. American Medical Association Council on Drugs: Nalorphine hydrochloride, *in* New and Nonofficial Drugs, Philadelphia, Lippincott, 1962.
4. Aoyagi, T., and Summerskill W. H. J.: Inhibition by acetohydroxamic acid of human mucosal and faecal urease-specific activity, Lancet 1:296, 1966.
5. Artz, S. A., Paes, I. C., and Faloon, W.

W.: Hypokalemia-induced hepatic coma in cirrhosis, Gastroenterology 51:1046, 1966.
6. Atkinson, M., and Goligher, J. C.: Recurrent hepatic coma treated by colectomy and ileorectal anastomosis, Lancet 1:461, 1960.
7. Baertl, J. M., Sancetta, S. M.. and Gabuzda, G. J.: Relation of acute potassium depletion to renal ammonium metabolism in patients with cirrhosis, J. Clin. Invest. 42:696, 1963.
8. Baldus, W. P., Feichter, R. N., and Summerskill, W. H. J.: The kidney in cirrhosis. I. Clinical and biochemical features of azotemia in hepatic failure, Ann. Int. Med. 60:353, 1964.
9. Berger, R. L., Liversage, R. M., Jr., Chalmers, T. C., Graham, J. H., McGoldrick, D. M., and Stohlman, F., Jr.: Exchange transfusion in the treatment of fulminating hepatitis, New Engl. J. Med. 274:497, 1966.
10. Bernheim, F., and Bernheim, M. L. C.: Note on the in vitro inactivation of morphine by liver, J. Pharmacol. Exp. Ther. 83:85, 1945.
11. Bessman, S. P., and Bessman, A. N.: The cerebral and peripheral uptake of ammonia in liver disease with an hypothesis for the mechanism of hepatic coma, J. Clin. Invest. 34:622, 1955.
12. Bessman, S. P., Shear, S., and Fitzgerald, J.: Effect of arginine and glutamate on the removal of ammonia from the blood in normal and cirrhotic patients, New Engl. J. Med. 256:941, 1957.
13. Blakemore, A. H.: Discussion *in* Tr. 7th Liver Injury Conf., New York, Macy, 1948.
14. Bollman, J. L., and Mann, F. C.: Studies on the physiology of the liver. XVIII. The effect of removal of the liver on the formation of ammonia, Am. J. Physiol. 92:92, 1930.
15. Bollman, J. L., Mann, F. C., and Magath, T. B.: Studies on the physiology of liver. Effect of total removal of liver on formation of urea, Am. J. Physiol. 69:371, 1924.
16. ———: Studies on the physiology of the liver. XV. The effect of total removal of the liver on deaminization, Am. J. Physiol. 78:258, 1926.
17. Bongiovanni, A. M., Blondheim, S. H., Eisenmenger, W. J., and Kunkel, H. G.;

Effects of ACTH in patients with liver disease, J. Clin. Invest. 29:798, 1950.

18. Bonnycastle, D. D., and Delia, C. W.: Effect of hepatectomy upon the analgetic action of l-methadone, Proc. Soc. Exp. Biol. Med. 74:589, 1950.

19. Borges, F. J., Merlis, J. K., and Bessman, S. P.: Serotonin metabolism in liver disease, J. Clin. Invest. 38:715, 1959.

20. Braganca, B. M., Faulkner, J., and Quastel, J. H.: Effects of inhibitors of glutamine synthesis on inhibition of acetylcholine synthesis in brain slices by ammonium ions, Biochim. Biophys. Acta 10:83, 1953.

21. Bravo, M., Orrego-Matte, H., and Walshe, J. M.: Carbohydrate intermediates in hepatic cirrhosis: Role of lipoic acid, J. Lab. Clin. Med. 57:213, 1961.

22. Cameron, G. R., and DeSaram, G. S. W.: The effect of liver damage on the action of some barbiturates, J. Path. Bact. 48: 49, 1939.

23. Carnot, P., Gerard, P., and Moissonnier, S.: Action de l'urease du soja sur l'organisme animal, Ann. Inst. Pasteur 35:37, 1921.

24. Challenger, F., and Walshe, J. M.: Foeter hepaticus, Lancet 1:1239, 1955.

25. Ching, N. P., Nealon, T. F., Jr., and Gibbon, J. H., Jr.: An extracorporeal device for hepatic coma, J.A.M.A. 183:350, 1963.

26. Clark, G. M., and Eiseman, B.: Studies in ammonia metabolism. IV. Biochemical changes in brain tissue of dogs during ammonia-induced coma, New Engl. J. Med. 259:178, 1958.

27. Conn, H. O.: Asterixis in non-hepatic disorders, Am. J. Med. 29:647, 1960.

28. Davidson, C. S.: Cirrhosis of the liver treated with prolonged sodium restrictions, J.A.M.A. 159:1257, 1955.

29. ———: Hepatic coma: thoughts on terminology, A.M.A. Arch. Int. Med. 104: 515, 1959.

30. Davidson, C. S., Babior, B., and Popper, H.: Concerning halothane hepatotoxicity, New Engl. J. Med. 275:1497, 1966.

31. Dawson, A. M., De Groote, J., Rosenthal, W. S., and Sherlock, S.: Blood pyruvic acid and alpha-ketoglutaric acid levels in liver disease and hepatic coma, Lancet 1:392, 1957.

32. Dawson, A. M., McLaren, J., and Sherlock, S.: Neomycin in the treatment of hepatic coma, Lancet 2:1262, 1957.

33. Ducci, H.: Cortisone in hepatitis; recovery in five comatose cases, Merck Rep. 62:21, 1953.

34. Dutton, R., Jr., Nicholas, W., Fisher, C. J., and Renzetti, A. D., Jr.: Blood ammonia in chronic pulmonary emphysema, New Engl. J. Med. 261:1369, 1959.

35. Eiseman, B., Osofsky, H., Roberts, E., and Jelinek, B.: Cerebral free amino acids in dogs following infusion of ammonia, J. Appl. Physiol. 14:251, 1959.

36. Fagin, I. D., and Thompson, F. M.: Cirrhosis of the liver; an analysis of 71 cases, Ann. Int. Med. 21:285, 1944.

37. Fairlie, C. W., Barss, T. P., French, A. B., Jones, C. M., and Beecher, H. K.: Metabolic effects of anesthesia in man. IV. A comparison of the effects of certain anesthetic agents on the normal liver, New Engl. J. Med. 244:615, 1951.

38. Faloon, W. W., Eckhardt, R. D., Cooper, A. M., and Davidson, C. S.: The effect of human serum albumin, mercurial diuretics and a low sodium diet on sodium excretion in patients with cirrhosis of the liver, J. Clin. Invest. 28:595, 1949.

39. Farquhar, J. D., Stokes, J., Jr., Whitlock, C. M., Jr., Bluemle, L. W., Jr., and Gambescia, J. M.: Studies on the use of aureomycin in hepatic disease. III. A note on aureomycin therapy in hepatic coma, Am. J. Med. Sci. 220:166, 1950.

40. Fast, B. B., Wolfe, S. J., Stormont, J. M., and Davidson, C. S.: Antibiotic therapy in the management of hepatic coma, A.M.A. Arch. Int. Med. 101:467, 1958.

41. Fazekas, J. F., Ticktin, H. E., Ehrmentraut, W. R., and Alman, R. W.: Cerebral metabolism in hepatic insufficiency, Am. J. Med. 21:843, 1956.

42. Fishbein, W. N., Carbone, P. P., and Hochstein, H. D.: Acetohydroxamate: Bacterial urease inhibitor with therapeutic potential in hyperammonaemic states, Nature 208:46, 1965.

43. Fisher, C. J., and Faloon, W. W.: Control of blood ammonia in cirrhosis by oral neomycin, Clin. Res. Proc. 4:147, 1956.

44. ———: Episodic stupor following portacaval shunt: observations on etiology and therapy, New Engl. J. Med. 255:589, 1956.

45. Fleshler, B., and Gabuzda, G. J.: Effect of ammonium chloride and urea infusions on ammonium levels and acidity of gastric juice, Gut 6:349, 1965.

46. Flock, E. V., Block, M. A., Mann, F. C.,

Grindlay, J. H., and Bollman, J. S.: The effect of glucose on the amino acids of plasma after total hepatectomy, J. Biol. Chem. 198:427, 1952.

47. Foley, J. M., Watson, C. W., and Adams, R. D.: Significance of electroencephalographic changes in hepatic coma, Tr. Am. Neurol. Assoc. 75:161, 1950.

48. Folin, O., and Denis, W.: Protein metabolism from the standpoint of blood and tissue analysis. The origin and significance of the ammonia in the portal blood, J. Biol. Chem. 11:161, 1912.

49. Fuld, H.: Über die diagnostische Verwertbarkeit von Ammoniakbestimmungen im Blut, Klin. Wschr. 12:1364, 1933.

50. Gabuzda, G. J.: Hepatic coma: clinical considerations, pathogenesis and management, in Dock, W., and Snapper, I. (Eds.): Advances in Internal Medicine, p. 11, Chicago, Year Book, 1962.

51. Gabuzda, G. J., Jr., and Davidson, C. S.: Protein metabolism in patients with cirrhosis of the liver, Ann. N. Y. Acad. Sci. 57:776, 1954.

52. Gabuzda, G. J., Gocke, T. M., Jackson, G. G., Grigsby, M. E., Del Love, B., Jr., and Finland, M.: Some effects of antibiotics on nutrition in man, A.M.A. Arch. Int. Med. 101:476, 1958.

53. Gabuzda, G. J., and Hall, P. W., III: Relation of potassium depletion to renal ammonium metabolism and hepatic coma, Medicine 45:481, 1966.

54. Gabuzda, G. J., Jr., Phillips, G. B., and Davidson, C. S.: Reversible toxic manifestations in patients with cirrhosis of the liver given cation-exchange resins, New Engl. J. Med. 246:124, 1952.

55. Gabuzda, G. J., Jr., Traeger, H. S., and Davidson, C. S.: Hepatic cirrhosis: effects of sodium chloride administration and restriction and of abdominal paracentesis on electrolyte and water balance, J. Clin. Invest. 33:780, 1954.

56. Gaustad, V.: Transient hepatargy, Acta med. scand. 135:354, 1949.

57. Geiger, A., Magnes, J., Taylor, R. M., and Veralli, M.: Effect of blood constituents on uptake of glucose and on metabolic rate of the brain in perfusion experiments, Am. J. Physiol. 177:138, 1954.

58. Geiger, A., and Yamasaki, S.: Cytidine and uridine requirement of the brain, J. Neurochem. 1:93, 1956.

59. Giarman, N. J., Mattie, L. R., and Stephenson, W. F.: Studies on the anti-diuretic action of morphine, Science 117:225, 1953.

60. Goetcheus, J. S., and Webster, L. T., Jr.: γ-Aminobutyrate and hepatic coma, J. Lab. Clin. Med. 65:257, 1965.

61. Gross, E. G.: Effect of liver damage on urinary morphine excretion, Proc. Soc. Exp. Biol. Med. 51:61, 1942.

62. Hegsted, D. M., Tsongas, A. G., Abbott, D. B., and Stare, F. J.: Protein requirements of adults, J. Lab. Clin. Med. 31:261, 1946.

63. Heinemann, H. O.. Emirgil, C., and Mijnssen, J. P.: Hyperventilation and arterial hypoxemia in cirrhosis of the liver, Am. J. Med. 28:239, 1960.

64. Horodynski, W., Salaskin, S., and Zaleski, J.: Über die Verteilung des Ammoniaks im Blut und den Organen normaler und hungernder Hunde, Z. Physiol. Chem. 35:246, 1902.

65. Jacobson, E. D., Chodas, R. B., and Faloon, W. W.: An experimental malabsorption syndrome induced by neomycin, Am. J. Med. 28:524, 1960.

66. Jones, C. M.: The treatment of acute hepatic insufficiency and its relation to prognosis, Am. J. Dig. Dis. 3:624, 1936–37.

67. ———: Liver intoxication, New Engl. J. Med. 230:766, 1944.

68. Kelly, W. D., Lewis, J. H., and Davidson, C. S.: The determination of urine urobilinogen, J. Lab. Clin. Med. 31:1045, 1946.

69. Kiley, J. E., Pender, J. C., Welch, H. F., and Welch, C. S.: Ammonia intoxication treated by hemodialysis, New Engl. J. Med. 259:1156, 1958.

70. Kirk, E.: Amino acid and ammonia metabolism in liver diseases, Acta med. scand., Suppl. 77, 1936.

71. Kirk, J. S., and Sumner, J. B.: Antiurease, J. Biol. Chem. 94:21, 1931.

72. Koyama, T.: Über den Wert der Bestimmung des Ammoniakstickstoffgehaltes des Blutes für die Beurteilung der Leberfunktionen und ihre Bedeutung für die Leberkrankheiten, Tohoku J. Exp. Med. 29:343, 1936.

73. Krebs, H. A., and Henseleit, K.: Untersuchungen über die Harnstoffbildung im Tierkörper, Z. Physiol. Chem. 210:33, 1932.

74. Kunin, C. M., Chalmers, T. C., Leevy, C. M., Sebastyen, S. C., Lieber, C. S., and Finland, M.: Absorption of orally ad-

ministered neomycin and kanamycin with special reference to patients with severe hepatic and renal disease, New Engl. J. Med. 262:380, 1960.

75. Last, P. M., and Sherlock, S.: Systemic absorption of orally administered neomycin in liver disease, New Engl. J. Med. 262:385, 1960.

76. Levine, H., Gilbert, A. J., and Bodansky, M.: The pulmonary and urinary excretion of paraldehyde in normal dogs and in dogs with liver damage, J. Pharmacol. Exp. Ther. 69:316, 1940.

77. Leyden, E.: Beiträge zur Pathologie des Icterus, Berlin, A. Hirschwald, 1866.

78. Lieber, C. S., and Davidson, C. S.: Complications resulting from renal failure in patients with liver disease, A.M.A. Arch. Int. Med. 106:749, 1960.

79. Lieber, C. S., and Lefèvre, A.: Ammonia as a source of gastric hypoacidity in patients with uremia, J. Clin. Invest. 38: 1271, 1959.

80. Macbeth, W. A. A. G., Kass, E. H., and McDermott, W. V., Jr.: Treatment of hepatic encephalopathy by alteration of intestinal flora with lactobacillus acidophilus, Lancet, 1:399, 1965.

81. Mackie, J. E., Stormont, J. M., Hollister, R. M., and Davidson, C. S.: Production of impending hepatic coma by chlorothiazide and its prevention by antibiotics, New Engl. J. Med. 259:1151, 1958.

82. Mallory, F. B.: Cirrhosis of the liver. Five different types of lesions from which it may arise, Bull. Johns Hopkins Hosp. 22: 1, 1911.

83. Mann, F. C.: Studies in the physiology of the liver. I. Technic and general effects of removal, Am. J. Physiol. 55:285, 1921.

84. McDermott, W. V., Jr.: Diversion of urine to the intestines as a factor in ammoniagenic coma, New Engl. J. Med. 256:460, 1957.

85 McDermott, W. V., Jr., and Adams, R. D.: Episodic stupor associated with an Eck fistula in the human with particular reference to the metabolism of ammonia, J. Clin. Invest. 33:1, 1954.

86. McDermott, W. V., Jr., Victor, M., and Point, W. W.: Exclusion of the colon in the treatment of hepatic encephalopathy, New Engl. J. Med. 267:850, 1962.

87. McKhann, G. M., and Tower, D. B.: Ammonia toxicity and cerebral oxidative metabolism, Am. J. Physiol. 200:420, 1961.

88. Monguio, J., and Krause, F.: Über die Bedeutung des NH₃-Gehaltes des Blutes für die Beurteilung der Leberfunktion, Klin. Wschr. 13:1142, 1934.

89. Mossberg, S. M., Thayer, W. R., Jr., and Spiro, H. M.: Azotemia and gastric acidity: the effect of intravenous urea on gastric acid and gastric ammonium production in man, J. Lab. Clin. Med. 61: 469, 1963.

90. Murphy, T. L., Chalmers, T. C., Eckhardt, R. D., and Davidson, C. S.: Hepatic coma: clinical and laboratory observations on forty patients, New Engl. J. Med. 239:605, 1948.

91. Najarian, J. S., and Harper, H. A.: A clinical study of the effect of arginine on blood ammonia, Am. J. Med. 21:832, 1956.

92. Nelson, W. P., III, Rosenbaum, J. D., and Strauss, M. B.: Hyponatremia in hepatic cirrhosis following paracentesis, J. Clin. Invest. 30:738, 1951.

93. Nencki, M., Pawlow, J. P., and Zaleski, J.: Über den Ammoniakgehalt des Blutes und der Organe und die Harnstoffbildung bei den Säugetieren, Arch. exp. Path. Pharmak. 37:26, 1896.

94. Nesbitt, S.: Excretion of coproporphyrin in hepatic disease: urinary excretion in liver insufficiency with neurological manifestations, Arch. Int. Med. 71:62, 1943.

95. Oberst, F. W.: Free and bound morphine, J. Pharmacol. Exp. Ther. 73:401, 1941.

96. ————: Fate of morphine, J. Pharmacol. Exp. Ther. 74:37, 1942.

97. Pant, S. S., Bhargava, A. N., Singh, M. M., and Dhanda, P. C.: Myelopathy in hepatic cirrhosis, Brit. Med. J. 1:1064, 1963.

98. Papper, S., Belsky, J. L., and Bleifer, K. H.: Renal failure in Laennec's cirrhosis of the liver. I. Description of clinical and laboratory features, Ann. Int. Med. 51: 759, 1959.

99. Patek, A. J., Jr., and Ratnoff, O. D.: The natural history of Laennec's cirrhosis of the liver, Medicine 21:207, 1942.

100. Pessar, T., and Hessing, J. W.: Massive doses of cortisone in hepatic coma, Ann. Int. Med. 48:1254, 1958.

101. Phear, E. A., Ruebner, B., Sherlock, S., and Summerskill, W. H. J.: Methionine toxicity in liver disease and its prevention by chlortetracycline, Clin. Sci. 15:93, 1956.

102. Phear, E. A., Sherlock, S., and Summerskill, W. H. J.: Blood-ammonium levels in liver disease and "hepatic coma," Lancet 1:836, 1955.

103. Phillips, G. B., and Davidson, C. S.: Nutritional aspects of cirrhosis in alcoholism. Effect of a purified diet supplemented with choline, Ann. N. Y. Acad. Med. 57: 812, 1954.

104. Phillips, G. B., Schwartz, R., Gabuzda, G. J., Jr., and Davidson, C. S.: The syndrome of impending hepatic coma in patients with cirrhosis of the liver given nitrogen substances, New Engl. J. Med. 247:239, 1952.

105. Posner, J. B., and Plum, F.: The toxic effects of carbon dioxide and acetazolamide in hepatic encephalopathy, J. Clin. Invest. 39:1246, 1960.

106. Pratt, T. W.: A comparison of the action of pentobarbital (Nembutal) and sodium barbital in rabbits as related to the detoxicating power of the liver, J. Pharmacol. Exp. Ther. 48:285, 1933.

107. Rappoport, W. J., and Kern, F., Jr.: Gastric urease activity in normal subjects and in subjects with cirrhosis, J. Lab. Clin. Med. 61:550, 1963.

108. Read, A. E., Haslam, R. M., Laidlaw, J., and Sherlock, S.: Chlorothiazide in control of ascites in hepatic cirrhosis, Brit. Med. J. 1:963, 1958.

109. Read, A. E., Laidlaw, J., Haslam, R. M., and Sherlock, S.: Neuropsychiatric complications following chlorothiazide therapy in patients with hepatic cirrhosis: possible relation to hypokalaemia, Clin. Sci. 18:409, 1959.

110. Read, A. E., Sherlock, S., Laidlaw, J., and Walker, J. G.: The neuropsychiatric syndromes associated with chronic liver disease and an extensive portal-systemic collateral circulation, Quart. J. Med. 36: 135, 1967.

111. Reynolds. T. B., Redeker, A. G., and Davis, P.: A controlled study of the effects of L-arginine on hepatic encephalopathy, Am. J. Med. 25:359, 1958.

112. Richards, R. K., and Appel, M.: The barbiturates and the liver, Curr. Res. Anesth. Analg. 20:64, 1941.

113. Rowntree, L. G.: Certain clinical and terminal pictures in hepatic disease, Med. Clin. N. Amer. 13:1399, 1929–30.

114. Salaskin, S.: Über das Ammoniak in physiologischer and pathologischer Hinsicht und die Rolle der Leber im Stoffwechsel stickstoffhaltiger Substanzen, Z. Physiol. Chem. 25:449, 1898.

115. Schenker, S., McCandless, D. W., Brophy, E., and Lewis, M. S.: Studies on the intracerebral toxicity of ammonia, J. Clin. Invest. 46:838, 1967.

116. Schwartz, R., Phillips, G. B., Gabuzda, G. J., Jr., and Davidson, C. S.: Blood ammonia and electrolytes in hepatic coma, J. Lab. Clin. Med. 42:499, 1953.

117. Schwartz, R., Phillips, G. B., Seegmiller, J. E., Gabuzda, G. J., Jr., and Davidson, C. S.: Dietary protein in the genesis of hepatic coma, New Engl. J. Med. 251: 685, 1954.

118. Seegmiller, J. E., Schwartz, R., and Davidson, C. S.: The plasma ammonia and glutamine content in patients with hepatic coma, J. Clin. Invest. 33:984, 1954.

118a. Sessions, J. T., Minkel, H. P., Bullard, J. C., and Ingelfinger, F. J.: The effect of barbiturates in patients with liver disease, J. Clin. Invest. 33:1116, 1954.

119. Shaffer, J. M., Bluemle, L. W., Jr., Sborov, V. M., and Neefe, J. R.: Studies on the use of Aureomycin in hepatic disease. IV. Aureomycin therapy in chronic liver disease, Am. J. Med. Sci. 220:173, 1950.

120. Shear, L., Kleinerman, J., and Gabuzda, G. J.: Renal failure in patients with cirrhosis of the liver. I. Clinical and pathologic characteristics, Am. J. Med. 39: 184, 1965.

121. Sher, M. H., Serlin, O., and Sensenig, D. M.: Exclusion of the colon for chronic hepatic encephalopathy, Am. J. Surg. 112: 83, 1966.

122. Sherlock, S., Senewiratne, B., Scott, A., and Walker, J. G.: Complications of diuretic therapy in hepatic cirrhosis, Lancet 1:1049, 1966.

123. Sherlock, S., Summerskill, W. H. J., White, L. P., and Phear, E. A.: Portal-systemic encephalopathy. Neurological complications of liver disease, Lancet 2: 453, 1954.

124. Shideman, F. E., Kelly, A. R., and Adams, B. J.: The role of the liver in the detoxication of thiopental (Pentothal) and two other thiobarbiturates, J. Pharmacol. Exp. Ther. 91:331, 1947.

125. Shils, M. E.: Renal disease and the metabolic effects of tetracycline, Ann. Int. Med. 58:389, 1963.

126. Shorey, J., McCandless, D. W., and

Schenker, S.: Cerebral α-ketoglutarate in ammonia intoxication, Gastroenterology 53:706, 1967.

127. Shorr, E., Zweifach, B. W., Furchgott, R. F., and Baez, S.: Hepatorenal factors in circulatory homeostasis. IV. Tissue origins of vasotropic principles, VEM and VDM, which appear during evolution of hemorrhagic and tourniquet shock, Circulation 3:42, 1951.

128. Sievers, M. L., and Vander, J. B.: Toxic effects of ammonium chloride in cardiac, renal and hepatic disease, J.A.M.A. 161: 410, 1956.

129. Silberman, R.: Ammonia intoxication following ureterosigmoidostomy in a patient with liver disease, Lancet 2:937, 1958.

130. Smith, L. H., Ettinger, R. H., and Seligson, D.: A comparison of the metabolism of fructose and glucose in hepatic disease and diabetes mellitus, J. Clin. Invest. 32: 273, 1953.

131. Smythe, C. McC., and Baroody, N. B.: Hepatic-type "flapping tremor" occurring in patients without hepatic disease, J.A.M.A. 165:31, 1957.

132. Snell, A. M., and Butt, H. R.: Hepatic coma: Observations bearing on its nature and treatment, Trans. Ass. Am. Phycns 56:321, 1941.

133. Spellberg, M. A.: Observations on the treatment of hepatic coma: the favorable effect of corticotropin and corticoids and the responsiveness of adrenal cortex to corticotropin during hepatic coma, Gastroenterology 32:600, 1957.

134. Stauffer, J. C., and Scribner, B. H.: Ammonia intoxication during treatment of alkalosis in a patient with normal liver function, Am. J. Med. 23:990, 1957.

135. Stormont, J. M., Mackie, J. E., and Davidson, C. S.: Observations on antibiotics in the treatment of hepatic coma and on factors contributing to prognosis, New Engl. J. Med. 259:1145, 1958.

136. Subcommittee on the National Halothane Study of the Committee on Anesthesia, National Academy of Sciences—National Research Council: Summary of the national halothane study; possible association between halothane anesthesia and postoperative hepatic necrosis, J.A.M.A. 197:775, 1966.

137. Summerskill, W. H. J., Aoyagi, T., and Evans, W. B.: Ammonia in the upper gastrointestinal tract of man: quantitations and relationships, Gut 7:497, 1966.

138. Summerskill, W. H. J., Wolfe, S. J., and Davidson, C. S.: The metabolism of ammonia and alpha-keto-acids in liver disease and hepatic coma, J. Clin. Invest. 36:361, 1957.

139. Tauber, H., and Kleiner, I. S.: Toxicity of crystalline urease, J. Biol. Chem. 92: 177, 1931.

140. Thannhauser, S. J.: Die chemischen Leistungen der normalen Leber für die Vorgänge des intermediaren Stoffwechsels, Klin. Wschr. 12:49, 1933.

141. Therapeutic Nutrition, Committee on: Publication 234, Washington, D.C., Food and Nutrition Board, National Research Council, 1952.

142. Thomson, A., and Visek, W. J.: Some effects of induction of urease immunity in patients with hepatic insufficiency, Am. J. Med. 35:804, 1963.

143. Tisdale, W. A., Fenster, L. F., and Klatskin, G.: Acute staphylococcal enterocolitis complicating oral neomycin therapy in cirrhosis, New Engl. J. Med. 263:1014, 1960.

144. Traeger, H. S., Gabuzda, G. J., Jr., Ballou, A. N., and Davidson, C. S.: Blood "ammonia" concentration in liver disease and liver coma, Metabolism 3:99, 1954.

145. Trey, C., Burns, D. G., and Saunders, S. J.: Treatment of hepatic coma by exchange blood transfusion, New Engl. J. Med. 274:473, 1966.

146. van Caulaert, C., and Deviller, C.: Ammoniémie expérimentale après ingestion de chlorure d'ammonium chez l'homme à l'état normal et pathologique, C. R. Soc. Biol. 111:50, 1932.

147. van Caulaert, C., Deviller, C., and Halff, M.: Le taux de l'ammoniémie dans certaines affections hépatiques, C. R. Soc. Biol. 111:735, 1932.

148. ————: Troubles provoqués par l'ingestion de sels ammoniacaux chez l'homme atteint de cirrhose de Laennec, C. R. Soc. Biol. 111:739, 1932.

149. Vanamee, P., Poppell, J. W., Glicksman, A. S., Randall, H. T., and Roberts, K. E.: Respiratory alkalosis in hepatic coma, A.M.A. Arch. Int. Med. 97:762, 1956.

150. Victor, M., Adams, R. D., and Cole, M.: The acquired (non-Wilsonian) type of

chronic hepato-cerebral degeneration, Medicine *44*:345, 1965.

151. von Schroder, W.: Über die Bildungs-stätte des Harnstoffs, Arch. exp. Path. Pharmak. *15*:364, 1882.
152. Walshe, J. M.: Observations on the symptomatology and pathogenesis of hepatic coma, Quart. J. Med. *20*:421, 1951.
153. ———: The effect of glutamic acid on the coma of hepatic failure, Lancet *1*: 1075, 1953.
154. ———: Disturbances of amino acid metabolism following liver injury, Quart. J. Med. *22*:483, 1953.
155. Walshe, J. M., De Carli, L., and Davidson, C. S.: Some factors influencing cerebral oxidation in relation to hepatic coma, Clin. Sci. *17*:11, 1958.
156. Warren, K. S.: Ammonia toxicity and pH, Nature *195*:47, 1962.
157. Way, E. L., Gimble, A. I., McKelway, W. P.. Ross, H., Sung, C., and Ellsworth, H.: The absorption, distribution and excretion of Demerol, J. Pharmacol. Exp. Ther. *96*:477, 1949.
158. Webster, L. T., Jr., and Davidson, C. S.: The effect of cortisone and hydrocortisone on hepatic coma, Gastroenterology *33*: 225, 1957.
159. ———: The effect of sodium glutamate on hepatic coma, J. Clin. Invest. *35*:191, 1956.
160. ———: Production of impending hepatic coma by a carbonic anhydrase in-hibitor, Diamox, Proc. Soc. Exp. Biol. Med. *91*:27, 1956.
161. Webster, L. T., Jr., and Gabuzda, G. J.: Ammonium uptake by the extremities and brain in hepatic coma, J. Clin. Invest. *37*:414, 1958.
162. ———: Relation of azotemia to blood "ammonium" in patients with hepatic cirrhosis, A.M.A. Arch. Int. Med. *103*:15, 1959.
163. Weil-Malherbe, H.: Significance of glutamic acid for the metabolism of nervous tissue, Physiol. Rev. *30*:549, 1950.
164. White, L. P., Phear, E. A., Summerskill, W. H. J., and Sherlock, S.: Ammonium tolerance in liver disease: observations based on catheterization of the hepatic veins, J. Clin. Invest. *34*:158, 1955.
165. Williams, R. H., and Bissell, G. W.: Thiamine metabolism, Arch. Int. Med. *73*:203, 1944.
166. Wolfe, S. J., Fast, B. B., Stormont, J. M., and Davidson, C. S.: Treatment of hepatic coma; use of Krebs' urea cycle intermediates (*l*-arginine, *dl*-ornithine), J. Lab. Clin. Med. *51*:672, 1958.
167. Zieve, L., Mendelson, D. F., and Goepfert, M.: Shunt encephalomyelopathy. I. Recurrent protein encephalopathy with response to arginine, Ann. Int. Med. *53*:33, 1960.
168. ———: Shunt encephalomyelopathy. II. Occurrence of permanent myelopathy, Ann. Int. Med. *53*:53, 1960.

13

Viral Hepatitis

JAMES W. MOSLEY, M.D., AND *JOHN T. GALAMBOS*, M.D.

Viral hepatitis may be clinically defined as an acute infectious illness in which hepatic cell necrosis is responsible for the most frequent, prominent and characteristic symptoms. It is caused by at least two virus-like (filterable) agents which produce homologous but not heterologous immunity and which also differ in epidemiologic characteristics. When distinguishable, the etiologically separate forms are most commonly designated as "infectious hepatitis" and "serum hepatitis." The hepatitides produced by other viruses and virus-like agents are not discussed in this chapter.

HISTORY

INFECTIOUS HEPATITIS

It is frequently said that infectious hepatitis was described in the Hippocratic writings. Only one writer, however, has cited any possibly relevant passage as a basis for such a statement. Cockayne[59] in 1912 pointed to the description of a benign form of epidemic jaundice in *De internis affectionibus.*

This type of jaundice is called epidemic because it occurs in all seasons. It is caused above all else by over-indulgence, excesses of wine, and after a chill. From the first moment the body changes color and becomes yellow; the eyes become markedly jaundiced; the disease appears under the hair and under the nails. There are chills and low-grade fever. The patient is weak. The head aches; the urine is yellow and thick. This form of jaundice is less dangerous than the preceding and is cured if quickly treated. (Translated from the Littré Edition.)

It is difficult to apply contemporary diag-

noses to historical epidemics, as Rath has emphasized.[319] The symptoms mentioned in this instance are scarcely diagnostic of infectious hepatitis, and others more common or characteristic were not listed. The Greek writer makes a particular point of the fact that jaundice was present "from the first moment," whereas a preicteric phase lasting 3 to 7 days is usual in infectious hepatitis. Even the description as "epidemic" is not necessarily helpful. Shrewsbury* has pointed out: "There is little doubt that the term 'epidemic' in Hippocratic Greek was not identical in its meaning with our use of it. In that day, it bore a much closer relation to season and climate, and a much slighter relation to numerical incidence." Therefore, a description of infectious hepatitis as early as Hippocratic times must be considered as no more than possible.

Caution must also be used in attempting to identify more recent episodes, although other causes of epidemic jaundice, such as yellow fever, leptospirosis or louse-borne relapsing fever, usually have case fatality rates that are distinctively higher. In the *Handbook of Geographical and Historical Pathology*, published in the 1880's, Hirsch listed 34 epidemics of jaundice, the earliest of which occurred on Minorca during the summer of 1745.[171] Hirsch pointed out that in some of these outbreaks "the malady ran the course of a simple catarrhal icterus; or it showed the marked signs of gastrointestinal catarrh complicated with jaundice."

An extensive compilation of epidemics of jaundice is found in the *World-Atlas of Epidemic Diseases* by Bachmann.[17] His list includes two epidemics from the seven-

* Shrewsbury, J. F. D.: Personal communication.

410

teenth century, 25 from the eighteenth century, and 53 from 1802 to 1874. Although some of these were probably due to other agents (including that of serum hepatitis), it seems likely that most represented infectious hepatitis.

The earliest recorded epidemic of benign jaundice in the United States appears to be that cited by Faulkner as having occurred in Norfolk, Virginia, in 1812.[100] There are brief descriptions or references to 10 other epidemics prior to 1861, although one can infer from descriptions by American physicians that epidemics were not common. There were, however, more than 70,000 cases in the Union Army during the Civil War.[363] During the first year of the War, morbidity due to jaundice was as high as 8 per cent in some contingents.[417]

Benign jaundice in sporadic form was also recognized in the nineteenth century. The misconception that such cases were due to swelling of the ostium of the common bile duct was originated by Bamberger in 1855 and perpetuated by Virchow in 1865.[394] Virchow autopsied 4 cases and found mucus plugs in the bile duct in all instances; he did not describe the liver in any of these cases.

The views of Bamberger and Virchow did not go unchallenged in the nineteenth and early part of the twentieth centuries. Various writers recognized the common identity of epidemic and sporadic jaundice, placed the seat of one or both diseases in the liver, and suggested that they were caused by an infectious agent. Those whose views were particularly perceptive included Botkin, Heitler and Flindt. As a result of Botkin's contributions to the concept of infectious hepatitis, the disease is known in Russia as Botkin's disease. Cockayne distinguished sporadic and epidemic catarrhal jaundice from Weil's disease, and appreciated a relationship of the former to acute yellow atrophy.[59]

A hepatogenous basis of both epidemic and benign sporadic jaundice was, in fact, recognized so frequently in the late nineteenth and early twentieth centuries that it is surprising that the concept of catarrhal jaundice persisted for so long. Apparently the name "catarrhal jaundice" was perpetu-

ated by textbooks, and was too widely used to be displaced easily.[353] This was certainly true in the English-speaking world.

In the first edition of his *Principles and Practice of Medicine* in 1892, Osler included catarrhal jaundice among "Diseases of the Bile-Passages." Here he stated that the disease is "due to swelling and obstruction of the terminal portion of the common duct." He concluded that it was almost always an extension of gastroduodenal catarrh, and indicated that it occurred most frequently in young persons and could occur in epidemics.

Osler's concepts and wording remained essentially unchanged until after his death. McCrae, as editor of the tenth edition in 1925, modified the definition of catarrhal jaundice as follows: "Jaundice due to hepatitis and cholangitis, possibly sometimes associated with obstruction of the terminal portion of the common duct." "Epidemic Catarrhal Jaundice" appeared separately in the eighth edition in 1916 among "Diseases of Doubtful Etiology," and was described as being due to common source transmission. Nevertheless, catarrhal jaundice still was listed in the semicentennial edition in 1942 as a disease of the biliary passages, and duodenal installation of magnesium sulfate was recommended as being of "great value" to relax the sphincter. That semicentennial edition coincided with the redefinition of epidemic jaundice, catarrhal jaundice and acute yellow atrophy into presently used terms and concepts.

SERUM HEPATITIS

The history of serum hepatitis can be traced with certainty no earlier than 1883, when Luerman described an epidemic in Bremen among factory workers inoculated with a smallpox vaccine containing human serum.[238] Another epidemic of postvaccinal jaundice occurred in Merzig the same year.[187] Such a relatively late emergence would fit with the common idea that serum hepatitis with its dependence on parenteral transmission could not have maintained itself earlier. Venesection, however, had been practiced by barber surgeons for several centuries prior to this time. Nor would the earlier opportunities for parenteral transmission have been confined to Western countries, for scarification and tattooing for ritual purposes or beautification are of considerable antiquity and widespread distribution.

In retrospect, it is easy to trace serum hepatitis in western Europe in the early twentieth century. Soon after the introduction in 1909 of arsphenamine for the treatment of syphilis, the occurrence of jaundice in proximity to therapy was noted.[174] Early and late forms of postarsenical jaundice were then recognized.[326] Some instances of the former were probably drug-induced, particularly when jaundice followed the initiation of treatment by only a few days (Milian's syndrome). Most cases of post-arsphenamine jaundice, however, seem likely to have been viral in etiology. Infectious, as well as serum hepatitis was probably transmitted by the technics used in clinics: Stokes et al.[372] and Ruge[339] pointed to correlations with the level of epidemic jaundice in the community. Probably, however, the agent of serum hepatitis was responsible for the larger number of cases. In some instances both infectious and serum hepatitis may have been transmitted simultaneously, as has been subsequently demonstrated.[412] Icterus also complicated other forms of parenteral treatment for venereal diseases. Jaundice was reported after use of acriflavine,[274] bismuth[219] and penicillin.[180] By the time penicillin came into use, however, the transmission of viral hepatitis was sufficiently well understood that corrective measures could be instituted within a relatively short period of time.

Artificially transmitted malaria as a treatment for neurosyphilis, introduced in 1917, was also accompanied by jaundice in a far higher proportion of cases than would be anticipated from experience with naturally acquired disease. Icterus was particularly frequent in service personnel in whom malaria was induced during World War II. Chalmers in 1947 demonstrated a distribution of intervals from inoculation similar to that anticipated for serum hepatitis.[49]

From the 1920's through the late 1940's, jaundice was noted as a complication of diabetes mellitus among hospitalized and clinic patients.[92, 391] For example, in 1938 Graham observed 28 cases at his diabetic clinic in London.[133] He pointed to the absence of this illness among diabetics in his private practice, and suspected that the cause was persistence of a small amount of disinfectant in the syringes used for administering insulin. Changing the procedure to storage in industrial alcohol and flushing with ether failed to halt transmission, and Graham concluded that personal contact was most probably responsible, even though patients with jaundice did not necessarily attend the clinic on the same day. As early as 1923, however, Flaum, Malmros and Persson stopped the occurrence of cases in their clinic by revising the procedure for sterilizing needles used to obtain capillary blood for glucose determinations.[105]

Therapy of rheumatoid arthritis with intravenous gold was also complicated by jaundice in the 1930's and early 1940's.[146] Of historic interest are the reports of Hench[167] and others that icterus had a beneficial effect on rheumatoid arthritis. As a result, patients with this disease were among the first volunteers used in British experiments to establish the nature of the etiologic agent.[241]

After new vaccines were introduced in the 1930's, postvaccinal jaundice reappeared. With live, attenuated strains of yellow fever virus, human serum was used as a stabilizer in some instances, and pooled convalescent serum was administered separately to modify the severity of infection. Icterus after vaccination was first seen in 1934 by Findlay and associates, but was dismissed as fortuitous until cases became so numerous in 1936 and 1937 that coincidence could no longer be invoked.[102] The same occurrence was observed in Brazil during the late 1930's.[109, 367] The culmination of epidemiologic experience with this entity was the use of pooled serum in vaccine produced by the United States Army in 1941, from which at least 28,585 icteric cases resulted.[186] The actual total was probably larger.[303] Postvaccinal jaundice also appeared at this time in Russia where a method for immunization against sand-fly fever had been developed. Separate injections of virus-containing blood obtained in the acute stage of the illness, and pooled convalescent serum were given. Sergiev, Tareev and co-workers reported 109 cases of jaundice among vaccinated persons in 1940.[354] As a consequence serum hepatitis is known in Eastern Europe as Sergiev-Tareev disease.

Convalescent serum used to treat or prevent infectious diseases came into relatively wide use in the 1930's and 1940's. Pooling insured greater uniformity of antibody titers and produced larger supplies. Two separate epidemics of postserum jaundice were reported in Great Britain. Forty-four cases and 10 deaths were clearly associated with prior administration of pooled measles convalescent serum.[243, 314] Pooled serum continued to be used, however, and another striking epidemic occurred 4 years later when two lots of pooled mumps convalescent serum were given to troop units threatened with incapacity by a mumps epidemic.[25] The attack rate of icteric disease among soldiers who received the material was 44.7 per cent.

Finally, the practice of pooling plasma for field treatment of battle casualties was given impetus by World War II, as the need for cross-matching was obviated. Early in the War, the only preparation available was small-pool (10 to 25 donors) liquid plasma, for which some refrigeration was required. Later when lyophilization made possible much wider use, large quantities were prepared and pools became much bigger (hundreds of donors). As a result, post-transfusion jaundice became widely prevalent among battle casualties. In June 1945, 23 per cent of all cases of viral hepatitis in Army hospitals were plasma-associated.[344]

Thus, epidemic jaundice, postarsenical jaundice, postvaccinal jaundice and homologous serum (nonhemolytic) jaundice presented themselves as a group of epidemiologic entities. Because of World War II, these problems became exaggerated in magnitude and led to studies which defined the etiologic basis.

ETIOLOGY

During the early part of the twentieth century, efforts to discover the cause of epidemic jaundice were focused upon bacterial agents. Although various species, especially several of the *Salmonella* group, were sometimes isolated from more than one patient in any given outbreak,[343] no serotype could be consistently related to the disease. It seems likely that in many instances infections by such enteric bacteria were acquired simultaneously with the agent of infectious hepatitis, as is now known to have been the case in one epidemic of water-borne disease.[112]

Failure to identify a bacterial agent led several investigators during the 1920's and 1930's to suggest that a virus was responsible for epidemic jaundice. Isolation attempts employed laboratory animals and the embryonated hen's egg; tissue culture technics were not feasible except on a limited scale until antibiotics became available. Successful transmission to pigs was claimed by Andersen[9] in 1937, but efforts at substantiation in other laboratories were unrewarding.

An infectious etiology was suggested by the occurrence of the disease in epidemic form. Transmission of the disease to a laboratory worker who worked with serum from a known case was reported in 1931.[101] Yunet and Yunet observed apparent transmission by a blood transfusion in 1938.[419] Nevertheless, alternate hypotheses were widely entertained. Although Eppinger was largely responsible for whatever recognition was accorded in the 1920's and 1930's to hepatic rather than biliary origin for epidemic jaundice, he and his group believed that it was caused by intoxication. Lainer's[222] failure to transmit the disease to volunteers by administration of blood and duodenal fluid taken from patients 3 to 10 days after the onset of jaundice supported Eppinger's concept of a noninfectious etiology. No reason for the lack of success can be suggested from Lainer's report.

The first experimental transmission may have been achieved by Japanese workers in 1940. Yoshibumi and Shigemoto administered filtered samples of blood, urine or pharyngeal secretions to a total of 20 children.[418] Three of 10 subjects inoculated with blood developed jaundice 8, 11 and 23 days later. The unusually short incubation periods in 2 of the 3 cases, as well as mention of epidemic jaundice being prevalent in the area, create uncertainty about the validity of this work.

The first successful transmission is usually credited to Voegt.[395] In 1941 he administered to 4 volunteers 5 ml. of unfiltered duodenal fluid taken from a patient 24 to 30 days after onset of symptoms. Symptoms developed in two of the recipients 25 to 28 days after ingesting the material, and all four had transient, mild abnormalities of liver function tests. He also administered blood or plasma from 2 patients to four volunteers on two separate occasions. Hepatitis may have been transmitted to one volunteer who had mild conjunctival icterus on the 19th day after the first inoculation. The other 3 volunteers had abnormal flocculation tests.

Both sets of experiments in Japan and Germany were limited in scope and neither approached the problem of postarsphenamine or homologous serum jaundice. Comprehensive work to characterize adequately the etiology of epidemic and other forms of jaundice was carried out by British and American teams of investigators. Their work is the basis of present concepts, to which relatively few significant additions have been made. Out of the British and American work during World War II emerged the definition of two distinct virus-like agents. The characteristics defined in these experiments were sufficient to explain almost all of the epidemiologic observations to that time, and most of those since.

Table 13–1 shows the basis for the distinction between the two agents. One of the most fundamental is the lack of sufficient antigenic similarity to provide cross-protection on challenge. (On this basis alone, one distinguishes three types of polioviruses, even though they do not differ in their clinical manifestations, incubation periods or modes of transmission.) In three groups of experiments, 26 volunteers re-challenged with infectious hepatitis materials remained well, while 3 of 6 who had recovered from infectious hepatitis showed disease when given the agent of serum hepatitis.[153, 240, 282] Conversely, 29 volunteers re-challenged with serum hepatitis materials in three experiments were immune,[153, 240, 282] but 7 of

8 who had recovered from serum hepatitis became ill when challenged in two experiments[148, 282] with the infectious hepatitis agent.

In experiments during World War II infectious and serum hepatitis viruses were also clearly distinguished on the basis of infectivity when ingested. In numerous volunteer experiments oral administration of fecal suspensions transmitted infectious hepatitis. On the other hand, no illnesses occurred when feces from 10 cases of serum hepatitis were administered to 40 volunteers by mouth in three separate sets of experiments.[152, 239, 286] Further, serum of known infectivity (27 definite cases among 43 volunteers when administered by the parenteral route) failed to produce jaundice among 23 volunteers in three experiments[152, 282, 304] when given by mouth.

Finally, a characteristic difference in incubation period was observed. In eight experiments orally and parenterally administered materials from patients with infectious hepatitis resulted in symptoms in 59 volunteers 15 to 37 days later.[148, 150, 152, 153, 162] On the other hand, when serum from patients or volunteers with serum hepatitis was administered parenterally to 76 volunteers symptoms occurred 28 to 160 days later.[152, 162, 239, 240, 282, 298] It was initially thought that the route of inoculation explained this difference. Serum from cases of epidemic jaundice, however, resulted in disease 20 to 34 days later when given parenterally and 21 to 34 days when given by mouth.[147]

On the basis of these results, the existence of two etiologic entities differing in their epidemiologic as well as immunologic characteristics was postulated.[149, 282] The term most commonly applied to the form transmitted by the fecal-oral route with its shorter incubation period is "infectious hepatitis" (IH). The form that is transmitted exclusively by the parenteral route and that has the longer incubation period was initially called "homologous serum hepatitis," to distinguish it from hemolytic jaundice produced by heterologous serum. More recently it has been more simply designated as "serum hepatitis" (SH). These terms are the most commonly used.

TABLE 13–1. BASIS FOR DIFFERENTIATION OF INFECTIOUS HEPATITIS AND SERUM HEPATITIS

CHARACTERISTICS	INFECTIOUS HEPATITIS (VIRUS A DISEASE)	SERUM HEPATITIS (VIRUS B DISEASE)	COMMENTS BASED ON RECENT OBSERVATIONS
Classic distinctions based on volunteer experiments in World War II			
Subsequent immunity to: infectious hepatitis serum hepatitis	Yes No	No Yes	A few persons have had three apparently distinct episodes of jaundice.[155, 227, 334] One to 5 per cent of patients give a past history of jaundice that suggests two episodes of infectious hepatitis.
Agent infectious by oral route	Yes	No	Occasional instances[103, 113, 261, 314] of apparent person-to-person transmission of serum hepatitis have been observed. Recent data by Krugman et al.[214] indicates excretion in stool and oral infectivity of agent having 41 to 125 day incubation period.
Agent excreted in feces	Yes	No	
Incubation period	15–37 days	28–160 days	Twenty to 45 days more common for IH in subsequent experience. Distribution of cases of transfusion-associated disease does not fit that expected on basis of classic experiments.[266]
Subsequently defined distinctions			
Case fatality rate	Very low; 0.1 to 0.2 percent in general population.	Variable, but high in most instances; 0.3 to 37 percent, usually 10 to 12 percent in transfusion-associated disease.[52]	Debility may contribute to high rate in transfusion-associated disease, but does not explain all instances.
Protection by immune serum globulin	Unequivocally demonstrated. Doses as small as 0.005 ml./lb. body weight effective.[85, 108]	Probably not effective. If any effect, large and repeated doses required.	Effectiveness against serum hepatitis doubtful; immune serum globulin administration for prophylaxis of transfusion-associated disease not advised.[322]
Disease in newborn due to transplacental transmission	Exceedingly rare	Occasionally occurs.	Difference probably due to frequency with which infection becomes overt disease.

During the 1950's the terms "virus A hepatitis" and "virus B hepatitis" were introduced for infectious and serum hepatitis, respectively. These designations were intended to avoid the implication that serum hepatitis was the only form transmissible by the parenteral route. If the designations *infectious hepatitis* and *serum hepatitis* are used, it is important to remember that both types are transmissible by inoculation.

Since World War II several additional distinctions between infectious and serum hepatitis have been observed. The *case fatality rate* in infectious hepatitis is very low, probably being no higher than 1 to 2 per 1,000 cases. The only exception is in certain groups of pregnant women.[424] The case fatality rate for serum hepatitis is usually significantly higher than that for infectious hepatitis.[52] In part this has been attributed to debility of patients when the disease is transfusion-associated.[28] Even the rate of 3 per 1,000 among healthy soldiers in World War II given yellow fever vaccine[345] was only slightly higher than that for infectious hepatitis. A similarly low rate has recently been observed in Swedish athletes who acquired serum hepatitis through wound infections.[129] Debility cannot, however, account for all instances in which the case fatality rate has been high. In one epidemic of iatrogenic disease in psychiatric patients, 37 per cent of those who became clinically ill died.[81] For children given icterogenic pooled serum, the case fatality rate was 19 per cent in one outbreak,[243] and soldiers had a rate of 17 per cent in another unrelated episode.[25]

Infectious and serum hepatitis also differ in their potential prevention by *immune serum globulin (ISG)*. Icteric infectious hepatitis is easily prevented by doses as small as 0.005 ml./lb. of body weight given in the incubation period.[85, 108] Prevention of serum hepatitis, on the other hand, has never been unequivocally demonstrated.[269] In general, the more carefully controlled studies have been negative.[84, 175, 374] If ISG is protective, it is so only in large, repeated doses.

Finally, infectious hepatitis may differ from serum hepatitis in likelihood of disease transmitted from mother to fetus. Even when infectious hepatitis occurs late in pregnancy, definite transmission is reported only rarely.[295, 388] More frequently, follow-up fails to uncover evidence of disease in the neonatal period. Fifteen infants that were stillborn of an icteric mother or died within 1 week after delivery were examined during the Delhi epidemic.[246] None showed histopathologic evidence of hepatitis.

A number of cases of neonatal hepatitis, especially of the giant-cell type, that have been attributed to serum hepatitis in the past are now recognized to have other etiologies. There remain a number of instances, however, in which serum hepatitis seems a possible cause. This supposition is strengthened by the experimental demonstration[373] of viremia in the asymptomatic mother and viremia in the child who became jaundiced at 1 month of age. The occurrence of neonatal hepatitis in siblings suggests that the carrier state may result in disease among successive infants born to mothers with this condition.

Many common viruses cross the placental barrier.[200] Probably both the IH and SH agents infect the fetus transplacentally. Present information still suggests a distinction in their likelihood of producing *disease* in the infant.

The concepts derived from volunteer studies during World War II may have to be modified according to recent evidence of Krugman and associates.[214] An immunologically distinct agent that produces hepatitis after intervals of 41 to 125 days (to onset of transaminase abnormality) has been transmitted by oral administration of fecal filtrates. This finding in two separate trials lends experimental support to several epidemiologic observations previously discounted. Propert in 1938 observed apparent transmission of jaundice induced by convalescent measles serum to 2 uninoculated children in the same institution after an interval of 2 months.[314] Freeman found hepatitis in the wives of 4 servicemen who received icterogenic yellow fever vaccine.[113] One of the vaccinated men from whom transmission presumably occurred was not jaundiced. Mirick and Shank reported

TABLE 13–2. CHARACTERISTICS OF INFECTIOUS AND SERUM HEPATITIS AGENTS

CHARACTERISTIC	INFECTIOUS HEPATITIS AGENT (VIRUS A)	SERUM HEPATITIS AGENT (VIRUS B)
Filterability		
Seitz EK filter	Passed[162, 284]	Passed[102]
Berkefeld M	Not done	Passed[298]
Chamberland No. 2	Passed[149]	Not done
Gradocol membrane with pore size of 52 mμ	Not done	Passed[255]
Ether 10%, 24 hours at 4°C.	Survived[242] (Infectivity may have been diminished)	Not done
Triple ether extraction of serum	Not done	Survived[242]
Acid stability	Presumptive survival pH 4 overnight[91]	Not done
Temperature stability		
Autoclaving, 15 psi, 30 min.	Inactivated	Inactivated
Dry heat, 160°C., 60 min.	Inactivated[340]	Inactivated[340]
Boiling, 20 min.	Inactivated[412]	Inactivated[412]
Boiling, 5 min.	Unknown	Presumably survived[94]
60°C., 10 hours	Not done	Inactivated[124]
60°C., 4 hours	Not done	Survived[275]
56°C., 1 hour	Not done	Survived[240, 345]
56°C., 30 min.	Survived[149]	Survived
Chlorination		
Water with high organic content breakpoint chlorination	Inactivated[280]	Not done
1 ppm. total residual, 30 min.	Survived[280]	Not done
With low organic content 1.1 ppm. total residual, 30 min.	Inactivated[280]	Not done
Storage of plasma at 31.6°C., 6 months	Not done	Survived[323]
Ultraviolet irradiation of plasma	Not done	Survived[277]
Beta-propiolactone	Not done	Inactivated[234]
Tricresol 0.2 %	Not done	Survived[102]
Thimerosal 1:2,000	Not done	Survived[25]
Nitrogen mustard, 500 mg./l.	Not done	Survived[83]

person-to-person transmission of hepatitis induced by pooled plasma.[261] In addition to these instances are occasional reports of person-to-person transmission of transfusion-associated hepatitis after intervals more appropriate for serum hepatitis than infectious hepatitis.

The discrepancy between the clearcut results of experiments during World War II[282, 286, 304] on the communicability of serum hepatitis and the more recent ones at Willowbrook State School is unexplained. Nevertheless, it appears that serum hepatitis, even if transferable by the fecal-oral route, is far less often *transmitted from person-to-person* than infectious hepatitis.[41, 137, 240] A quantitative difference, therefore, still remains, and possibly there is a qualitative distinction not yet defined.

ETIOLOGIC AGENTS

Attempts at Laboratory Isolation. The agents of viral hepatitis have been the object of a persisting and unrewarding series of efforts at laboratory isolation.[267] Almost every virology laboratory in the world has attempted, usually repeatedly, to demonstrate replication of the agents in either laboratory animals or tissue culture systems, or both. Thus far, none of the claimed successes has received independent confirmation. All of the organisms isolated appear to have been adventitious agents in patients from whom specimens were collected or contaminants of laboratory systems used by the investigators. Although both Drake et al.[84] and McLean and associates[33, 383] utilized experiments with human volunteers to support their claims, other laboratories could not verify their methods. The reported successes have led to statements in the literature that the agents have been isolated, but all thus far must be discounted.

The only report of possible success in isolation attempts that has not been withdrawn or lacked reproducibility in other laboratories is that of Deinhardt and associates.[74] By means of serum transaminase assays and biopsies, a transmissible hepatitis has been established in marmosets. Although presumably derived from human materials, the relationship of the agent in marmosets to the human disease has not yet been determined. It may represent a latent agent of the marmoset.[259]

Characteristics of the Agents. In the nineteenth century the word "virus" was used to designate any microbial agent that produced disease. It was then found that some agents passed bacteria-tight filters, and these were appropriately called "filterable viruses." In recent years, the designation has been reserved for those filterable microbes that are so dependent upon host systems that they contain only one type of nucleic acid. The volunteer experiments indicate that the agents of infectious and serum hepatitis are filterable.[149, 255, 298] They are, therefore, known to be viruses in at least the earlier sense of the term. Whether they are true viruses in the more recent and restricted sense is not known, although probable.

IH and SH viruses were among the first to be recognized as heartier than other microbial agents with which laboratory work was commonly carried out in the 1930's and early 1940's. As a result, their resistance to physical and chemical inactivation is sometimes exaggerated. Viruses described in recent years, such as SV_{40} appear to be much more resistant than either hepatitis agent.

Knowledge of the hepatitis agents is limited, because experiments require human volunteers and circumstances must be fortuitous to establish their characteristics. The available information is summarized in Table 13–2. It has usually been assumed that the IH agent resembles or is classifiable as an enterovirus. Its excretion in feces and infectivity by the oral route are compatible with this concept. Suggestive also is the evidence for ether stability,[242] although MacCallum and co-workers thought that the procedure may have reduced titer. Overnight stability at pH 4 (the pH of orange juice) may be inferred from epidemiologic evidence.[91]

EPIDEMIOLOGY

ROUTES AND PERIOD OF INFECTIVITY

Information concerning the period of infectivity for infectious and serum hepatitis is limited. In most instances, it is derived from volunteer studies, and represents experiments in which materials from patients were pooled. This limitation must be kept in mind when interpreting statements concerning duration of virus excretion and viremia.

Infectious Hepatitis. *Excretion of Virus in Feces.* Excretion of virus in the feces during the incubation period has been examined by Krugman, Ward and associates.[217] Three volunteers developed jaundice 39, 41 and 46 days, respectively, after experimental infection. Stools from the three had been collected on the 11th and 25th days after oral administration of virus.

The pool of feces collected on the 11th day produced no abnormalities in 8 new volunteers. Stools from the 25th day given to 13 subjects caused icteric disease in one and anicteric (or inapparent) infection in three. Thus, the virus was not excreted as early as 28 to 35 days prior to onset of icterus, but was present in feces 14 to 21 days before jaundice. In the preicteric and early icteric phases of infectious hepatitis, excretion of virus has been demonstrated many times.[150, 151, 282] Stools collected on the first and third days of jaundice,[303] and from the first through eighth days of jaundice[217] were infectious for volunteers. Thus, the virus is excreted in the feces at least as late as the onset of icterus, and may continue for several days thereafter. In addition, a specimen taken 8 days after jaundice may have contained virus.[303] It was administered together with a larger pool, however, so that the result cannot be unequivocally interpreted as positive, even though the other material administered alone in a second experiment was negative.

Tests have not been carried out with fecal specimens collected during the interval between the early illness and convalescence. Fecal pools from the recovery phase of infectious hepatitis, however, have been uniformly negative. Such studies in volunteers have included tests of feces collected from: One patient 25 and 26 days after onset of symptoms (19 and 20 days after onset of jaundice)[151]; five patients 26 through 29 days after onset of symptoms[151]; three patients 19 through 33 days after jaundice appeared[216]; one patient 32 days after jaundice and at a time when the pyruvic transaminase was 750 Karmen units[216]; and two patients 33 and 43 days after jaundice.[286] Thus, stools from 12 patients 3 or more weeks after onset of symptoms were not found to contain demonstrable virus.

Chronic fecal excretion has been experimentally demonstrated only in 2 young children with laboratory evidence of "chronic" hepatitis.[373] This finding was supported by epidemiologic evidence of transmission to other children in the same orphanage.[27] An additional instance of probable excretion (as evidenced by transmission to contacts) by a child with chronic hepatitis has been observed by one of the authors. On the other hand, studies by Neefe and associates of 3 volunteers with persistent symptoms, abnormal flocculation tests and mild abnormalities on liver biopsy, showed no evidence for chronic excretion of the virus.[285] A filtrate of 23 fecal specimens collected from the 3 men 92 to 342 days after onset failed to produce definite evidence of hepatic damage in 5 volunteers.

Viremia in the incubation period of infectious hepatitis has been most extensively explored in the studies at Willowbrook State School. A specimen taken 25 days before onset of jaundice produced hepatitis in 1 of 6 subjects.[128] A pool of serum taken from 3 children 21 to 28 days before jaundice was negative in 8 volunteers, but a second pool from the same subjects 14 to 21 days prior to jaundice was positive.[216] Havens failed to demonstrate viremia in one volunteer 17 days prior to onset of jaundice (11 days prior to symptoms).[151] This result is not necessarily in conflict with the findings of Krugman and co-workers, as the time at which viremia begins probably varies from patient to patient. Specimens have also been positive in volunteer studies when obtained 3 days prior to onset of symptoms, [111] and 3 to 7 days prior to onset of jaundice.[216] Inadvertent transmission through blood donations has indicated viremia 11 days[145] and 2 days[111] prior to onset of symptoms.

Viremia has been repeatedly demonstrated in the preicteric and early icteric phase. A pool of serum from 3 patients collected 1 through 8 days after onset of symptoms produced jaundice in all of 3 volunteers.[151] Krugman et al. found hepatitis in 1 of 10 subjects given serum taken on the third day after jaundice appeared.[217] Neefe and Stokes produced jaundice in 2 of 6 volunteers given a pool of 39 serum specimens collected "before and after" onset of hepatitis, but failed to find evidence of hepatitis in three volunteers given single specimens from patients during the "first or second week" of illness.[284] A convalescent specimen taken from one patient 31 days after onset of symptoms (25 days after jaundice) was negative in 3 volunteers.[151]

Chronic viremia with an agent having all

the characteristics of IH virus has not been unequivocally demonstrated. Serum specimens taken 66 to 141 days after onset were negative in one set of studies.[298] Creutzfeldt and co-workers found one donor with postnecrotic cirrhosis and chronic viremia, as evidenced by hepatitis in 8 of 54 recipients of his blood.[66] The man had had a clinical attack of hepatitis some 17 years before, which may or may not have been infectious hepatitis and may or may not have been related to his carrier state. Incubation periods in recipients ranged from 24 to 64 days, and provide evidence, therefore, which is difficult to interpret. Such carriers, if their viremia is related to infectious hepatitis, must be infrequent in the population. In a number of countries blood donors with a history of infectious hepatitis are accepted if this disease occurred more than 1 year prior to donation. This practice does not appear to have been associated with a higher rate of transfusion-associated hepatitis. In the United States, however, such persons are usually excluded as donors.

Viruria occurs commonly in the course of many viral infections, and would not be unexpected in infectious hepatitis. Findlay and Willcox reported transmission with urine to 3 of 6 volunteers.[104] Other investigators during World War II in three sets of experiments involving 29 volunteers were unable to reproduce this result.[151, 241, 284] More recently, Giles and co-workers infected 1 of 12 volunteers with urine collected on the day when jaundice developed.[128] Urine appears to be, therefore, poorly infective. Viruria has been thought to have epidemiologic importance only in one episode in which unconventional contamination of potato salad was suspected.[192]

Nasopharyngeal washings from cases of infectious hepatitis reportedly produced anicteric or inapparent hepatitis in 2 of 7 volunteers studied by MacCallum and Bradley.[241] They found no evidence of transmission, however, in two other experiments involving 15 additional subjects. Havens had negative results in one experiment involving 3 volunteers,[151] and Neefe and Stokes found no evidence of transmission in two sets of experiments using a total of 8 subjects.[284] One of the two pools of washings tested by the latter investigators included specimens taken late in the incubation period, as well as the preiteric and icteric phase of illness.

This failure to demonstrate infectivity of nasopharyngeal secretions has been the most important evidence against earlier opinions that the disease is spread by the respiratory route.

Serum Hepatitis. This disease with its longer incubation period is associated with a longer period of viremia. It was transmitted in one instance[287] with blood taken 87 days prior to onset of symptoms, and with specimens collected 60 and 16 days prior to onset in two other experiments.[152, 304] In two instances, natural transmission by blood donations occurred 1 to 2 years prior to onset of what appeared to be the initial clinical episode of hepatitis.[283]

Chronic viremia for periods of over 5 years has been documented in some blood donors.[165, 373] In most instances, there is no history of a past illness suggestive of acute or chronic hepatitis. Many carriers of serum hepatitis virus do have abnormalities of liver function tests, which can persist for at least 4 years. Unfortunately, other carriers have no abnormalities and cannot be so identified.

INCUBATION PERIOD

Definition. The incubation period in viral hepatitis has been defined variably as the interval from infection (1) to onset of first *symptoms*, (2) to onset of *jaundice* or (3) to the first detected *abnormality in one or more laboratory tests*. One must consider these differences in definition when comparing various findings, for the incubation period would vary from study to study on this basis alone. For one volunteer observed by Stokes and co-workers, the interval from inoculation to onset of first symptoms was 33 days[373]; jaundice did not appear, however, until the 68th day. Although 35 days between appearance of symptoms and jaundice is unusually long, this case illustrates the potential discrepancy.

We prefer to define the incubation period as the interval to onset of symptoms, for such a definition (1) conforms to that applied to other infectious diseases, (2) has been used in the literature with sufficient frequency to permit broad comparisons, (3) obviates any need to define incubation period of anicteric cases on a basis different from that of icteric cases, and (4) poses no problem when one is dealing with the occasional anicteric case in which there is icteric relapse.

The interval to onset of jaundice is preferred by some investigators. They feel that jaundice is a dramatic alteration likely to be remembered by the patient, and is easily dated because it is often the immediate reason for consulting a physician. This is undoubtedly true in many instances; in others, however, the onset of jaundice is insidious. Jaundice may not be noticed by the patient until it is marked or is called to his attention by someone else. Although no data are available, it is our impression that the majority of patients can date the onset of ill health with reasonable accuracy, but detect jaundice in themselves only after the serum bilirubin is considerably elevated.

The detection of a laboratory abnormality has the advantage of being based on an objectively assessable event. This advantage is more than offset, however, by the fact that the interval defined in this way is dependent upon the frequency with which testing is carried out. If specimens are collected only once a week, the "incubation period" is overestimated by as much as 6 days in some instances. Furthermore, the time at which one test usually becomes abnormal can differ markedly from the time at which another shows deviation. The serum transaminases, for example, may be elevated up to 10 days prior to illness, but bilirubinuria does not usually occur until several days after symptoms.

Laboratory tests are utilized more commonly to define the latent period in cases of subclinical or inapparent infection. In such instances, the particular abnormality used as an index should be related to the development of the comparable abnormality in clinically apparent cases, rather than to incubation period defined in terms of either onset of symptoms or onset of jaundice.

Incubation Period of Infectious Hepatitis. Several early estimates of the incuba-

tion period in infectious hepatitis were in substantial agreement with recent definitions. Lindstedt in 1919 found that cases resulting from limited exposure during a Norwegian epidemic had onset of symptoms 14 to 28 days later.[230] Similarly, Pickles, during the early 1930's, found that illness in a rural area of England resulted 26 to 35 days after contact.[307] In the common vehicle epidemic in Canada reported by Fraser in 1931, the interval from onset of simultaneously acquired gastroenteritis to onset of jaundice was 18 to 35 days, with an average of 25 to 27 days.[112]

In the volunteer studies during World War II, the incubation period of infectious hepatitis was 15 days (onset of symptoms) to 47 days (onset of jaundice).[242] In most instances the incubation period was 20 to 33 days.[151, 282]

Some exceptions to these observations concerning incubation period of experimentally induced infectious hepatitis have been recorded. Of 4 volunteers to whom a pool of serum from 2 patients with presumed infectious hepatitis was given parenterally, 3 developed jaundice 64, 75 and 92 days later.[241] No details concerning donors of the specimens are given. Two of 4 volunteers given serum from a mentally defective child had onset 63 to 69 days later.[242] The child was found to have hyperbilirubinemia 4 days later and was presumably infected as part of an institutional outbreak. Finally, Oliphant produced illness 85 to 106 days after parenteral administration of a serum specimen collected during the epidemic of infectious hepatitis among Allied military personnel in Italy.[297] The apparent discrepancy between these results and those cited previously has several possible explanations. As the infectious material in all instances was serum administered parenterally, the illness of the donor may have been mistakenly diagnosed as infectious hepatitis. It is also possible that the donors were carriers of serum hepatitis in whom infectious hepatitis supervened. Thirdly, they may represent instances of contact transmission of an agent that has the incubation period of serum hepatitis.[214]

In naturally-transmitted disease, the period to onset of symptoms usually ranges from 20 to 45 days, with a mode of approximately 28 days. The incubation period is most easily assessed when there has been a common-vehicle epidemic, with exposure limited to 1 or 2 days.[18, 91, 320, 389, 402]

Incubation Period of Serum Hepatitis. Serum hepatitis was observed to have an incubation period of 2 to 6 months in the postvaccinal epidemics of 1883.[187, 238] A similar lag to onset was observed in volunteer studies in the 1940's and early 1950's. In a group of six experiments, the onsets in 77 volunteers infected during World War II ranged from 28 days[298] to 160 days[297]; in the majority the interval was 60 to 110 days.[152, 162, 239, 240 282] Other volunteer experiments[83, 277] using materials containing the SH agent gave generally similar results, although there were some exceptions[276] as is discussed below. The intervals observed in epidemics such as those which followed use of contaminated yellow fever vaccine were similar.[109, 345]

Recent observations of incubation periods in transfusion-associated viral hepatitis reveal a distribution in which the relative contributions of the IH and SH agents cannot be easily defined. On the basis of most of the volunteer studies cited above, a bimodal curve would be anticipated, with the first peak after an interval of approximately 28 days and a second peak some 70 to 90 days after transfusion. Instead, one sees a unimodal distribution with skew to the right, and single peak 45 to 49 days after transfusion (Figure 13–1). Retrospectively, it is apparent that similarly "short" incubation periods were characteristic of cases induced by blood from carriers identified by Neefe and associates.[283] Of 6 original blood recipients, 4 developed hepatitis less than 50 days after transfusion. Of 21 volunteers who developed icteric or anicteric hepatitis after inoculation of serum from the same carriers, 10 had onset within 50 days.[276]

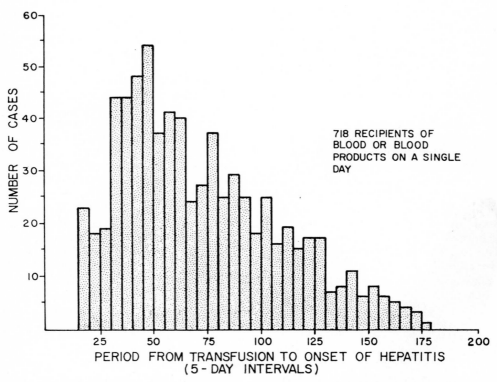

FIG. 13–1. Incubation periods of transfusion-associated viral hepatitis among 718 recipients of blood or blood products on a single day.[266]

Analysis of the large number of cases made available through the national surveillance system in the United States has indicated a difference in incubation periods associated with whole blood or unpooled derivatives, and those associated with pooled plasma and its derivatives (Fig. 13–2).[266] The average interval from transfusion to onset was 69 days in those receiving blood only, and 102 days in those receiving pooled derivatives only. Patients who received both blood and pooled derivatives had an average incubation period of 84 days. Approximately 37 per cent of recipients of blood or unpooled products had onset of disease less than 50 days after transfusion, in contrast to less than 10 per cent of those given pooled derivatives only. The other epidemiologic characteristics of cases with short incubation periods do not necessarily permit the assumption that they represent infections with the IH agent. No adequately supported explanation can be offered at present for the distribution of incubation periods in blood-associated hepatitis.

Factors That Affect the Incubation Period. Experimental and epidemiologic observations indicate that the incubation periods of other infectious agents are affected by: (1) the amount of virus in the inoculum, (2) the route of inoculation and (3) the strain of virus. It seems likely that these factors also modify, at least to some extent, the incubation periods of infectious and se-

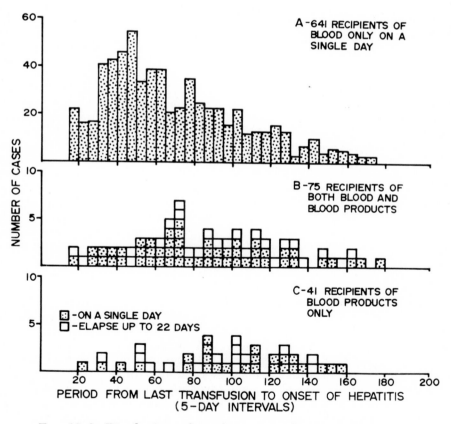

FIG. 13–2. Distributions of incubation periods in recipients of (A) whole blood or unpooled derivatives only; (B) whole blood *and* potentially icterogenic blood products; and (C) potentially icterogenic blood products (pooled irradiated plasma or fibrinogen) only.[266]

TABLE 13–3. TITRATIONS OF THE INFECTIOUS HEPATITIS AGENT. INFLUENCE OF DOSE ON INCUBATION PERIOD (ADAPTED FROM WARD AND KRUGMAN[405])

STRAIN	MATERIAL	INVESTIGATORS	DOSE	No. OF SUBJECTS	INCUBATION PERIODS (IN DAYS) ICTERIC PATIENTS	ANICTERIC PATIENTS
BE	Serum	Havens[153]	0.5 ml.	2	30*	—
			0.1 ml.	2	21*	—
			0.01 ml.	2	26*	—
Akiba	Serum	Gordon et al.[131]	0.02 ml.	4	33, 37	—
			0.002 ml.	5	35	—
			0.0002 ml.	4	—	—
WBRK	Serum	Krugman et al.*	0.25 ml.	9	38, 42, 43	31, 38, 38
			0.025 ml.	10	45, 49, 49, 49, 55, 55	—
			0.0025 ml.	11	—	43
WBRK	Feces	Ward et al.[406]	4.0 Gm.	13	42, 42, 44, 46, 47 54, 54, 54, 58, 58	—
			2.0 Gm.	5	39, 39, 46	—
			1.0 Gm.	11	39, 39, 43, 49	—
			0.1 Gm.	8	39	—
			0.001 Gm.	8	—	—
			0.00001 Gm.	8	—	—

* Cited by Ward and Krugman.[405]

rum hepatitis. The few systematic observations that have been made, however, do not suggest a great influence.

Because titrations of infectious material require large numbers of human volunteers, relatively few have been carried out. These are summarized in Table 13–3. Variations of as much as 100-fold did not affect infectivity of the IH agent in two of the three experiments with this agent. Some influence of dose on the length of incubation period is suggested in the Willowbrook study (WBRK strain), but its effect, as judged by the composite experience, does not appear to be as marked as would be expected by analogy with other agents.

In the only titration[83] of the SH agent, no effect of dilution by as much as 10^{-6} was seen. The number of volunteers, however, was small. Murray and co-workers believed that a reduction in virus titer by ultraviolet irradiation of pooled plasma resulted in lengthening of the modal incubation period in volunteers from 70–79 to 100–109 days.[277]

The influence of dose of SH agent upon incubation period is of greatest importance in relation to the frequency of "short" incubation periods following transfusion of whole blood. It has been suggested that the interval may be less in some cases because of the much larger inoculum presumably contained in a whole unit. Such an effect would explain the incubation periods of 35 to 43 days in volunteers given 1.0 ml. of a 1:4 dilution of serum from a patient whose illness began 10 days after transfusion of an entire unit of whole blood.[111] On the other hand, the volunteers infected by Murray and co-workers[276] did not necessarily have shorter incubation periods following administration of 1 ml. of serum than did patients whose hepatitis was produced by an entire unit from the same chronic carriers. No conclusion is possible at present.

The effect of route of infection on incubation period was examined during volunteer studies in the 1940's because of the suggestion that the difference between infectious and serum hepatitis could be due to the difference in route of infection. A serum pool that produced hepatitis in 2 of 3 volunteers after 26 and 33 days when given orally, resulted in disease after 28,

28, 35 and 37 days in 10 volunteers who received the same dose parenterally.[282] In a separate experiment,[148] orally administered serum produced disease after 23, 24, 29 and 34 days, and parenterally after 20, 20, 21, 24, 25 and 31 days. These results indicate that route of infection could not account for the difference in incubation period between the IH and SH agents, and also does not affect the incubation period of infectious hepatitis.

Strain differences may affect the incubation period. Krugman and co-workers have observed the IH virus in their institution to have a relatively long incubation period at Willowbrook State School.[217] Part of this difference may be explained by the use of onset of jaundice rather than onset of symptoms in mentally-retarded children. Even so, the Willowbrook agent appears to have a longer incubation period, which is possibly attributable to strain variation.

Modes of Transmission

Contact-Associated Hepatitis. As discussed, the agent of infectious hepatitis has been demonstrated in the feces, and is infective when ingested. There is experimental support, therefore, for the concept that fecal-oral transmission has a major role in the transmission of this disease. This suggests that its epidemiologic pattern resembles that of typhoid fever, the classic model for fecal-oral transmission, and also poliomyelitis. In view of the fact that our environment is generally much more fecally contaminated than we wish to admit, this mechanism possibly accounts for all person-to-person transmission.

Person-to-person transmission of infectious hepatitis is limited in most instances to close contacts. These include household members, persons living in the same dormitory or other communal quarters, and play contacts of children. Such restricted spread is characteristic of diseases transmitted by the fecal-oral route. Explosive outbreaks due to respiratory transmission, such as those that occur with measles, are seldom seen with infectious hepatitis. Spread due to classroom contact is not frequent, although school-centered epidemics do occur. Disease attributable to office exposure is

unusual. Since transmission is limited to close contacts and the incubation period is relatively long, infectious hepatitis spreads leisurely through the community. Several months are usually required to reach the peak of the outbreak, and a comparable period of time for the wave to recede.

Spread to household contacts is also relatively leisurely. Figure 13–3 shows the distribution of subsequent cases in households in relation to the index case. This example is taken from an epidemic in Missouri in 1951[208]; other epidemics in the United States and abroad have had similar patterns.[366, 376] Other cases in the family occur as a large wave of secondary illnesses and a smaller group of tertiary infections. Household members in whom the onset is less than 15 days after that of the index case are usually regarded as having co-primary rather than secondary infections. Recent evidence for early fecal excretion[217] suggests that some such infections are secondary, and are acquired 2 to 3 weeks before the first person in the family becomes ill. However, most household cases occur one full incubation period or more after the index case. This finding suggests that the patient is most infectious for close contacts about the time of onset of symptoms.

Spontaneous transmission 1 to 2 weeks prior to onset has been documented only in instances in which exposure was to mentally-retarded children.[22, 216] The extent of fecal soiling of the environment by this group is a possible explanation of the greater ease with which they seem to transmit the disease relatively early in the incubation period.

It has been postulated from time to time that respiratory transmission may occur. This was the conclusion of Pickles, whose epidemiologic observations in rural England suggested that casual contact was sufficient.[307] Failure to demonstrate transmission by nasopharyngeal secretions administered to volunteers has led most observers to dismiss this possibility. Ipsen, Donovan and James observed two instances in which very casual contact resulted in transmission.[184] Aach and co-workers more recently observed an explosive epidemic in which airborne transmission seemed the most likely mechanism.[1] Conclusions concerning this route must await further study.

Primate-Associated Hepatitis. This epidemiologic entity became established in 1961 with the description of 11 cases among persons having contact with newly-imported chimpanzees.[168] Other episodes were recognized retrospectively as early as 1953,[166] and many cases have been documented since.[71, 271, 338] The total number of persons known to have been infected by primates exceeds 140. Most cases have been in professional animal handlers, veterinarians and scientists working with the animals. Chimpanzees have been most frequently implicated, but Colombian woolly monkeys, Celebes apes, and the gorilla have also been involved in outbreaks.

The illness acquired by contact with non-human primates is clinically indistinguishable from infectious hepatitis, and is believed to be due to the IH agent. Although an extrahuman reservoir of the human virus is possible, a more likely explanation is transmission from man to primate and then back to man. Chimpanzees are presumably involved most frequently because of the mode of their capture, as well as the extent of their contact in captivity with humans. In most instances, the animals implicated show no evidence of illness interpretable as hepatitis. Since the disease can be transmitted to man, they may have inapparent infection. This supposition is supported by the paucity of significant abnormalities in newly-captured chimpanzees when given material of known infectivity.[73] Relatively minor abnormalities of various laboratory tests are seen with some frequency,[14, 169] but their specificity is doubtful.

Water-Borne Infectious Hepatitis. The first adequately described epidemic of water-borne hepatitis was observed in 1916[10]; other episodes have been repeatedly reported since that time.[268] This mode of transmission results from both contamination of the usual supplies of drinking water and ingestion of contaminated water not intended for consumption. In the United States most cases of water-borne disease are produced by private supplies,[328, 389] but municipal systems have been involved in at least two instances.[272, 309] It is, in fact, surprising that water-borne hepatitis does not occur more frequently. There are many instances of salmonellosis and "viral" gastroenteritis produced by sewage contamination of supplies without subsequent hepatitis.[268]

Shellfish-Associated Hepatitis. This epidemiologic entity was first described in Sweden in 1956, when some 600 cases followed ingestion of sewage-contaminated oysters.[120, 332] No further episodes were recognized until 1961, when an oyster-associated epidemic of 81 cases[252] and a clam-associated epidemic of over 300 cases occurred simultaneously in the United States.[81] Subsequently, there have been two other clam-associated epidemics of major proportions in the United States.

In addition to the problem of epidemic hepatitis, the occurrence of endemic shellfish-associated disease in the United States is also documented. Low level contamination appears to result in cases widely scattered both in time and place of onset. The association of such cases with prior ingestion of clams or oysters can be established only by epidemiologic analyses of surveillance data. The epidemiologic history of shellfish ingestion during the 6 weeks prior to onset, however, should suggest the possibility to the clinician and to the local health department.

Both epidemic and endemic shellfish-associated hepatitis have more frequently been due to *raw* clams than *raw* oysters. Since clams burrow, they concentrate in estuarial waters near sewage outfalls. Harvesting of clams from public waters by part-time workers opens greater possibilities for illegal operations. Oysters, in contrast, attach themselves to rock, and beds in the northeastern United States are generally restricted to privately-owned or privately-leased waters.

An association of *steamed* clams with infectious hepatitis was suspected by Rindge and co-workers,[327] and subsequently documented by Koff and associates.[210] Koff and Sears have demonstrated that the temperature of the body of the animal at the time of "gaping" is below that which could be expected to inactivate virus.[211] The more thorough the cooking, the safer (but less palatable) the product.

Shellfish-associated hepatitis has not been reported outside the United States since the Swedish epidemic in 1956, but is suggested by the frequency with which Americans who acquire the infection abroad give a history of shellfish ingestion during an interval compatible with the incubation period.

Mechanical Transmission by Insects. This mode of transmission has been suggested in some instances. Whitehead and Crouch observed 47 cases in native men in Port Sudan, and noted that none occurred in native women or Europeans.[413] They commented that these latter groups did not eat in the market place where many *flies* were present. Kirk described the epidemic among New Zealand troops at El Alamein in 1942.[201] The area occupied by these troops was strewn with corpses and feces from the German troops previously encamped there. The Germans had had a high incidence of infectious hepatitis, and flies were extremely prevalent. Hepatitis was not a problem in other portions of the line where flies were equally numerous but there were no human bodies or feces scattered over the ground. On the other hand, during a summer camp epidemic Neefe and Stokes could not demonstrate the virus in flies collected from a trap adjacent to the camp kitchen.[284] The flies were homogenized and their filtrate administered orally to five volunteers, of whom none developed clinical or laboratory evidence of hepatitis.

The evidence from work with poliomyelitis suggests that flies play no significant role in transmission of enteric viruses. Paffenbarger and Watt found no effect of intensive control measures on the expected course of a poliomyelitis epidemic.[301] Earlier, diarrheal disease due to shigellosis had been reduced significantly through such a program.[407]

Tarshis believed that *cockroaches* had a role in transmitting infectious hepatitis in a Los Angeles housing project.[382] The disease decreased following control measures directed against this insect. Koff and co-workers, however, found no evidence for such

TABLE 13–4. CLASSIFICATION OF HUMAN BLOOD AND BLOOD DERIVATIVES ACCORDING TO THEIR RISK OF TRANSMITTING VIRAL HEPATITIS

"AVERAGE RISK" MATERIALS (NOT POOLED OR TREATED)

1. Whole blood (fresh or stored)
2. Packed red blood cells
3. Single donor plasma
4. Platelet-rich plasma
5. Fresh frozen plasma

"HIGH RISK" DERIVATIVES (POOLED, INADEQUATELY TREATED)

1. Irradiated pooled plasma
2. Pooled plasma stored at "room" temperature for 6 months
3. Pooled plasma stored at 31.6° C. for 6 months
4. Fibrinogen
5. Antihemophilic globulin

"SAFE" DERIVATIVES (POOLED, ADEQUATELY TREATED)

1. Serum albumin*
2. Plasma protein fraction*
3. Thrombin*
4. Profibrinolysin and fibrinolysin*
5. Immune globulin†
6. Hyperimmune globulin (mumps, tetanus, vaccinia, etc.)†

* Sterilized by heating for 10 hours at 60° C.
† Cohn-fractionated (cold ethanol).

association.[210] The frequency of cockroach infestation in households in which infectious hepatitis occurred was the same as that among interviewed controls.

Possibly under some circumstances mechanical transmission by insects contributes to spread. Such situations, if they do occur, appear to be unusual.

Transfusion-Associated Hepatitis. Human blood and blood derivatives in present use may be classed according to their risk of transmitting viral hepatitis (see Table 13–4).

"Average risk" materials are whole blood itself and derivatives that are prepared without pooling of individual units. Estimates of the risk in the United States have been derived from a series of separate investigations at university hospitals or large medical centers, a number of which are sum-

TABLE 13-5. RISK OF VIRAL HEPATITIS FROM TRANSFUSION OF WHOLE BLOOD—
REPRESENTATIVE STUDIES IN THE UNITED STATES

PERIOD OF STUDY	INVESTIGATOR	CITY	COMPLETENESS OF FOLLOW-UP	TYPE OF DONOR POPULATION	AVERAGE NUMBER OF UNITS PER PATIENT	No. OF TRANSFUSED PATIENTS IN STUDY	No. OF CASES OF ICTERIC HEPATITIS	ATTACK RATE PER 100 PERSONS	ATTACK RATE PER 1,000 UNITS GIVEN
1946–1956	Allen and Sayman[5]	Chicago	97.7%	Mixed	3.1	1,894	47	2.5	8.2
1952–1954	Strumia et al.[377]	Philadelphia	60.4%	Not stated	2.6	1,237	11	0.9	3.3
1953–1956	Hoxworth et al.[177]	Cincinnati	93.2%	Unpaid	2.2	3,349	19	0.6	2.6
1954–1956	Jennings et al.[188]	Detroit	Not stated	Not stated	3.1	796	10	1.3	4.0
1955	Maxwell[253]	Milwaukee	70.7%	Unpaid	5.4	1,171	13	1.1	2.4
1955–1960	Mirick[262]	Baltimore	Prospective	Mixed	4.8	587	22	3.7	7.9
1956	Bang et al.[19]	New York	68.7%	Mixed	2.8	1,371	39	2.8	8.7
1957–1961	Adashek and Adashek[2]	Los Angeles	52.4%	Unpaid	18.0	644	12	1.9	1.0
1959–1960	Ward[262]	Los Angeles	Prospective	Mixed	4.0	146	9	6.2	15.3
1959–1960	McCollum[262]	New Haven	Prospective	Mixed	3.2	83	2	2.4	7.5
1963–1965	Holland et al.[175]	Bethesda	Prospective	Mixed	23.3	83	6	7.2	3.2

marized in Table 13–5. The overall attack rate of viral hepatitis varies from 0.6 to 13.6 per 100 persons transfused, or, 1.0 to 15.3 cases per 1,000 units administered. To some extent, these differences are attributable to method of study and depend upon: the method of follow-up, the definition of a case and the range of incubation periods accepted. On the other hand, methodologic differences can by no means account for all of the variation observed. Recognized factors that affect rates, at least in some studies, include: (1) the frequency of alcoholics, drug addicts and prisoners in the donor population and (2) the total number of transfusions given to the patient.

In several studies, the use by commercial blood banks of "skid row" individuals as paid donors has resulted in appreciably higher rates of viral hepatitis.[60, 220] Blood from prisoners in some penal institutions used as a donor source by community or volunteer blood banks may carry a comparably high risk,[4, 347] so the problem of high risk donors is not necessarily limited to blood banks that pay for donations. The collection agency's interest in the quality of its blood and its vigor in following up suspected carriers are the best guarantees of as low an incidence as can be obtained.

Logically the more units administered, the greater the risk; this association was not demonstrated until the study of Allen and Sayman.[5] Their attack rates by number of units given are shown in Table 13–6. The only deviation from the expected increase

was in those receiving more than 5 units of blood. A relationship of attack rate to units administered was also observed by Mirick, Ward and McCollum,[262] whose results are also shown in Table 13–6. These data emphasize that in general the more blood administered, the greater is the risk.

"High risk" derivatives are produced when plasma from individual units is separated and pooled. Under these circumstances, a single unit containing the virus of human hepatitis could contaminate the entire batch. The frequency with which units from such pools are contaminated is much higher than that of an equivalent number of nonpooled units; the frequency increases with the size of the pool.

High risk products in current use are pooled plasma, fibrinogen and antihemophilic globulin concentrates. The repeated attempts to find processes for inactivating the viruses of hepatitis in pooled plasma have been unavailing. Initially ultraviolet irradiation appeared to be effective as judged by the results of human volunteer experiments.[299] Subsequent experience with additional volunteer studies and follow-up of icterogenic lots has demonstrated that plasma so treated, at least under conditions of commercial production, still has a higher than average risk. Similarly, initial work with storage for 6 months at "room" temperature, or under more carefully controlled conditions at 31.6° C. (90° F.), suggested that such material was safe,[4, 177] but a carefully controlled, prospective investi-

TABLE 13–6. RISK OF VIRAL HEPATITIS IN RELATION TO NUMBER OF UNITS OF BLOOD TRANSFUSED

UNITS ADMINIS-TERED	ALLEN AND SAYMAN[5]			MIRICK, WARD, McCOLLUM[262]		
	Number of Patients Transfused	Cases of Icteric Hepatitis	Attack Rate per 100 Persons	Number of Patients Transfused	Cases of Icteric Hepatitis	Attack Rate per 100 Persons
1	880	12	1.4			
2	572	15	2.7			
3	218	7	3.2	785	15	2.5
4	323	8	2.5			
5	135	9	6.7			
6–9	253	16	5.1	263*	8*	3.0*
10 or more	166	10	6.0	57	4	7.0

* 6 to 10 units in data presented by Mirick, Ward and McCollum.

gation showed that this process was also ineffective.[324] Irradiated pooled plasma treated with beta-propiolactone is reportedly safe,[234] but the study has not been confirmed and the material is commercially unavailable. No effective method for sterilizing fibrinogen or antihemophilic globulin preparations is available.

Whole blood and its unpooled derivatives are usually used in the same geographic area in which they are collected. Pooled plasma and fibrinogen, on the other hand, are usually prepared from widely collected donations and distributed routinely to all parts of the country. In contrast to the wide variation from hospital to hospital in the incidence of viral hepatitis following transfusion of whole blood, attack rates from high risk products could be expected to be more uniform. Data from published studies of plasma and fibrinogen generally bear this out.

Dialysis-Associated Hepatitis. A high rate of viral hepatitis has been widely reported in patients with kidney disease who undergo repeated dialyses. The incidence of this complication appears to be approximately proportional to the extent to which blood is used.[306] There is also a high risk of hepatitis for hospital personnel working in dialysis units,[191] presumably through abrasions, punctures and lacerations.

Transplantation-Associated Hepatitis. A case of serum hepatitis in an untransfused patient receiving a bone graft has been reported.[360] The increasing use of organ transplants suggests that transplantation-associated hepatitis should be sought in other instances, although it is difficult to document because of the frequency with which recipients are transfused with blood and icterogenic blood products.

Instrument-Associated Hepatitis. Any instrument that breaks the skin of one person and then breaks the skin of another without being sterilized has the potential for transmitting both the IH and SH agents. The variety of instruments implicated in transmission is wide, and will undoubtedly be extended if epidemiologic alertness to the possibility is maintained.

A history of an injection or dental procedure during the 6 months prior to onset is not of itself adequate to suggest that this was the source of infection. A frequency greater than that in a comparable population without hepatitis must be demonstrated also. Nevertheless, a detailed epidemiologic history is worth obtaining from each patient regarding visits to physicians, dentists, clinics and hospitals. If several cases occur among patients of any given physician or facility, it is worthwhile to investigate.

Syringe-Associated Hepatitis. As described above, the wide prevalence of jaundice in venereal disease clinics in World War II led to early recognition of this epidemiologic form of viral hepatitis. For example, Howells and Kerr in England reported in 1946 that 47 of 120 patients with hepatitis had a history of a penicillin injection in the preceding 6 months.[176] The interval from inoculation to symptoms was 62 to 157 days. Most of the patients had been treated at the same venereal disease clinic, where an individual needle was used for each injection but the same syringe for about 5 patients. An epidemic in the late 1940's among Army personnel was caused by a 10-dose-per-syringe technic for giving tetanus toxoid.[47] Incubation periods were characteristic of infectious rather than serum hepatitis. Sherwood described in 1948 an outbreak of 4 cases among diabetic patients who received insulin by a multiple-dose-per-syringe technic.[358]

The mechanism by which hepatitis is transmitted by syringe was investigated by Hughes, who demonstrated aspiration of needle contents into the syringe while the needle is removed.[180] Red cells were found in the syringe contents following 17 of 39 intramuscular injections, although no blood was grossly visible and aspiration was not attempted. Hughes also found that red cells migrated spontaneously from the tip of the needle into the syringe in as little as 45 seconds. In view of transmission of icteric serum hepatitis to 5 of 10 volunteers by only 0.00004 ml. of whole blood,[83] the frequency of syringe-associated hepatitis is not surprising.

With widespread adoption of adequate technics for sterilization and use of disposable equipment for injections, syringe-associated hepatitis appears to be relatively infrequent in the United States. Koff and co-workers found no indication of physician- or hospital-associated disease among patients in the Boston area.[210] The national surveillance data, although uncontrolled, similarly do not indicate persistence of a general problem. Nevertheless, parenteral transmission does occur whenever good technic is ignored. An outbreak in 1959 involved patients of a physician in Maine.[89] A major epidemic was produced by a psychiatrist who had 41 cases among 329 patients in his practice, with 15 deaths.[81]

Syringe-associated hepatitis is frequent in some areas outside the United States. Zuckerman reported a greater than expected frequency of injections in Royal Air Force personnel with hepatitis.[425] Use of the multiple-dose-per-syringe technic was common in RAF clinics and hospitals, and undoubtedly accounts for this excess of cases in those exposed by a parenteral procedure. Nicolau and co-workers reported a high incidence of parenterally transmitted hepatitis in Rumania.[292] Part of the high incidence of viral hepatitis among Americans in residence abroad[56, 110] may be due to serum hepatitis associated with medical or diagnostic procedures.

Hepatitis Associated with Dental Treatment. This form of transmission has been reported intermittently.[106, 384] Sultz found a greater than expected frequency of dental visits in patients with hepatitis in Buffalo,[378] but dental visits could not be implicated in Boston.[210]

Tattoo-Associated Hepatitis. The frequency with which contaminated tattoo needles and vials of dye transmit hepatitis is probably greater than can be documented. In addition to cases related to professional parlors,[330, 365] amateur efforts with improvised equipment may be responsible.[347]

Addiction-Associated Hepatitis. Viral hepatitis among drug addicts was recognized in the 1950's, primarily among illicit users of narcotics in New York City.[7, 11, 227] To an increasing extent this epidemiologic entity has been described from other parts of the United States[334, 347, 368] and abroad.[29]

The problem of transmission by unsterilized, often improvised, equipment is widely associated with non-narcotic drugs used parenterally at gatherings of devotees. Surveillance data indicate that 10 to 15 per cent of all patients with reported hepatitis in New York City, New Jersey and the Los Angeles area are *easily* identified as addicts; the total problem is undoubtedly even larger.

The relative extents to which the IH and SH viruses contribute to total cases among addicts is unknown. In most instances drugs are used daily, so that the time of probable exposure cannot usually be determined. In one prison the epidemiologic pattern suggested that most cases were due to serum hepatitis.[347] In the open community and among younger addicts both types of hepatitis undoubtedly occur; some persons experience two or even three attacks.[155, 227, 334] A high frequency of abnormal liver function tests between attacks in addicts suggests that some second or third episodes may be recurrences rather than new infections. No method for resolving the question of reinfection or recurrence is available.

Track-Finder's Hepatitis. Since 1962, there have been several reports of an unusual frequency of viral hepatitis among participants in the Scandinavian sport of track-finding (*orienteering*).[116, 329, 392] The competitors run a course of their own devising over rugged terrain, past a number of checkpoints located 1 to 2 kilometers apart. Clothing usually consists of short socks, shorts and a short-sleeved shirt. Most meets are held in wooded areas; over 90 per cent of the participants indicated frequent or occasional scratches and cuts. When facilities were limited, the track-finders washed in small pools of stagnant water, and used a small number of basins.

An association began to be recognized late in 1957, and by 1963 an estimated 568 cases had occurred. The pattern of illnesses had the epidemiologic characteristics of serum rather than infectious hepatitis. By preventive measures this epidemiologic entity was virtually abolished, although relaxation of these rules permitted a new epidemic of 41 cases in 1965–1966.[329]

Biting Insects. Theoretically biting insects have a role in transmitting both infectious and serum hepatitis, and this possibility has been suggested, particularly as a medium

TABLE 13–7. AGE-SPECIFIC ATTACK RATES PER 100 PERSONS. COMMON VEHICLE EPIDEMICS OF INFECTIOUS AND SERUM HEPATITIS. ICTERIC CASES

Age Group	INFECTIOUS HEPATITIS			SERUM HEPATITIS		
	Sweden[141] 1941	USA[273] 1946	India[361] 1955–56	Virgin Islands[298] 1942	Brazil[109] (Vaccine Lot 489) 1940	Brazil[109] (Vaccine Lot 494) 1940
0– 4	10.5	1.1	1.6*	7.0	2.2	0.8
5– 9	27.3	6.3		8.4		
10–14	41.5	9.5		11.8	5.6	1.2
15–19	43.4	16.0	2.8*	18.8	12.2	2.5
20–29	39.0	8.3		21.1	12.5	2.2
30–39	24.7	4.7		22.8	13.0	2.5
40–49	14.3	0.6	1.8*	22.8		
50–59	0.0	0.4		21.4		
60 and over		0.0		12.2	16.7	1.9

* Rates for Region I, Delhi, calculated from investigator's data.

for survival of the SH agent. The only experimental attempt at parenteral transmission used bed bugs, and was negative.[44] Therapeutic malaria transferred by syringe and needle resulted in transmission of jaundice, but transmission of malaria by mosquitoes under controlled conditions did not.[49] Since an interval of several weeks would have been allowed for development of the protozoal parasite in the mosquito, this result does not exclude mechanical transfer when two or more persons are bitten during a brief period. However, it is unlikely that biting insects have any significant role in transmission of infectious or serum hepatitis.

EPIDEMIOLOGIC PATTERNS

Age. Age is a well-known factor in the incidence of the icteric form of viral hepatitis. The extent can be estimated when relatively uniform exposure of all age groups is assumed. This situation has been most closely approximated in epidemics of water-borne infectious hepatitis and vaccine-associated serum hepatitis. Table 13–7 presents the data from six studies which included sufficiently large numbers of cases for the results to be meaningful. In all of these, the incidence of icteric hepatitis in children was significantly less than that in young adults.

Table 13–7 indicates that attack rates in those less than 5 years of age have ranged from approximately a third to one-forty-seventh of the maximum rate in older children or adults. Stated conversely, for every case of icteric disease among 100 children of preschool age at risk in common-vehicle epidemics, there were 3 to 47 cases among 100 adults. Attack rates for school-age children were also generally lower than the maximal rates in adults, but less dramatically so. The relative frequency of inapparent and anicteric infections, therefore, diminishes with increasing age. The wide variations in these examples of ratios of inapparent infection to overt disease, point out the inaccuracy of applying the finding in one epidemic to other situations.

A second factor that affects age distribution is acquired immunity. Table 13–7 shows a diminishing attack rate of infectious hepatitis in older adults, which suggests a decreasing proportion of susceptible persons in older groups. In fact, given equal exposure, the rates of icteric hepatitis in young adults would probably be even higher in relation to those in children in a totally susceptible population. A similar diminution with increasing age in attack rate was not seen in the epidemic of serum hepatitis, against which any substantial amount of immunity in older adults would not be anticipated.

Waning immunity has been suggested as

an explanation for higher attack rate among adults than children in water-borne epidemics in India.[78, 361] This argument is based on the assumption that infectious hepatitis is highly endemic in such an area and that experience with it is essentially universal by an early age. Such an assumption derives from the presumed analogy with poliomyelitis under similar environmental circumstances.[305] This type of age distribution in water-borne epidemics, however, is not peculiar to India; a similar distribution was found in Sweden[141] and in the United States.[273] Further, if waning of immunity were a significant factor in age-specific attack rates during common-vehicle epidemics, one would expect the highest incidence in the oldest age group. Instead, incidence decreases progressively with age beyond early adulthood in all such occurrences. Additional evidence against a waning of acquired immunity to infectious hepatitis has been provided by an epidemic at Fort Yukon, Alaska. Maynard found a much lower attack rate among persons 17 years of age and over.[254] The last epidemic of infectious hepatitis had been approximately 16 years previously.

The third factor that influences age-specific attack rates is the opportunity for exposure. In most communities of the United States and also of Europe, the predominance of cases is among school-age children. This is probably due to not only the greater availability of susceptible persons in this age group, but also to more frequent opportunities to acquire infection.

Age-specific attack rates in the community-wide epidemic during 1944 and 1945 in Tama, Iowa,[72] are given in Table 13–8. Age distribution of primary cases may be used as an index of those groups in which transmission is occurring in the community. From the table it is evident that *inter*familial spread was in this instance confined almost entirely to those 5 through 14 years of age. *Intra*familial spread involved a much broader age group. This pattern is probably typical of most community outbreaks in the United States, when unmodified by administration of immune serum globulin to household contact.

Secondary attack rates in Table 13–8

TABLE 13–8. AGE-SPECIFIC ATTACK RATES IN A COMMUNITY-WIDE EPIDEMIC TAMA, IOWA, 1944–45*

AGE GROUP	ATTACK RATE PER 100 PERSONS		
	Entire Community	Primary † Cases	Household Contacts
0– 4	5.9	1.3	20.8
5– 9	23.5	14.9	37.7
10–14	20.0	4.9	49.2
15–19	3.3	—	21.0
20–29	2.0		
30–39	4.8	0.5	15.9
40–49	2.4		
50 and over	1.2		

* From Davis and Hanlon.[72]
† Calculated from investigator's data.

among preschool children and adults are lower than among school-age children. This may be explained on the basis of a higher inapparent infection-overt disease ratio among the former, and greater frequency of acquired immunity among the latter. An additional factor that influences this pattern, however, is lack of equal exposure for all family members. Ipsen has demonstrated that the secondary household attack rate from a disease as contagious as measles varies inversely with the difference in age between siblings.[183] Schneider and Mosley found a low rate of inapparent as well as clinically diagnosable hepatitis among preschool household contacts.[352] "Social distance" appears to be a factor even within a household.

Although school-age children are important in interfamilial spread of the disease, transmission does not necessarily occur frequently in the classroom itself. School-ground and neighborhood play contact appear to be much more important. Dana and Mosley, in unpublished studies, found that the likelihood of a second case in a classroom within 2 months of an index case was only 1 per cent, even without excluding other types of contact responsible for some of the infections. When subsequent cases do occur in schools and classrooms, distribution, as shown in Figure 13–4, fails to show the type of clustering seen in household contacts (see Fig. 13–3).

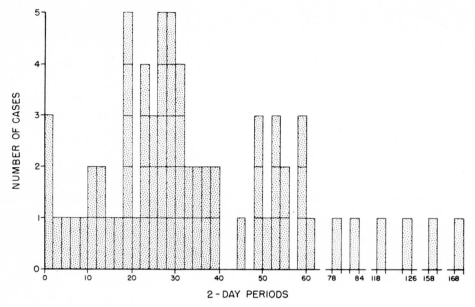

Fig. 13–3. Intervals between onset of symptoms in index and subsequent cases of infectious hepatitis in 37 families in Cooper County, Missouri, 1951. (From Knight et al.[208]).

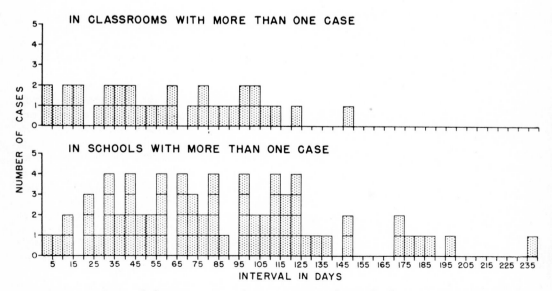

Fig. 13–4. Intervals between onset of symptoms in index and subsequent cases in schools and classrooms having more than one case, Kenton County, Kentucky, 1956–57. (Unpublished data, Hepatitis Unit, NCDC.)

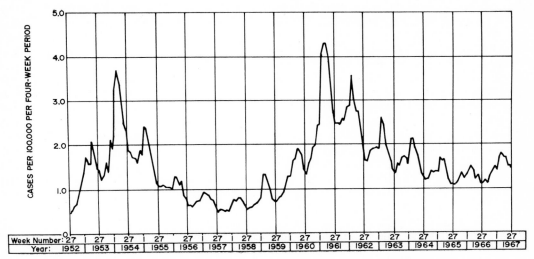

Fig. 13–5. Case rate of reported cases of viral hepatitis in the United States by 4-week periods from July 1952 through June 1967 (*Morbidity and Mortality Weekly Report*, NCDC).

This suggests that transmission does not usually occur in classrooms as readily as it does in households.

In most common-vehicle epidemics, cases are confined to relatively narrow age groups due to the circumstances under which contaminated food and water are ingested. Raw shellfish are usually not consumed by children. As a result, the five shellfish-associated epidemics recognized thus far have involved mostly adults. A sudden change in the age-distribution pattern of infectious hepatitis may, in fact, provide a clue that common-source transmission has occurred, as is illustrated in the report by Mason and McLean.[252]

Presumably serum hepatitis is much more frequent in adults than in children because adults have greater opportunities to acquire the disease. Transfusions and the use of injections in medical therapy are far more frequent among adults. Dental care is more frequently required. Tattooing and illicit use of narcotics or other agents parenterally are almost exclusively adolescent and adult practices.

Secular Trends. Viral hepatitis has been a nationally reportable disease in the United States only since 1952. Figure 13–5 shows the pattern of the morbidity trend from July of that year through June, 1967. Because the seasonal increase begins in the autumn months and reaches a peak in January, the data are more reliably analyzed on the basis of an epidemiologic year extending from July of one calendar year through June of the following calendar year. Figure 13–5, therefore, presents data for the United States in terms of epidemiologic rather than calendar years.

There have been two epidemic cycles in the United States, the first with a peak in epidemiologic year 1953–54 and the second in 1960–61. The 1966–67 reversal of the downtrend in the second cycle suggests the beginning of a third cycle. Whether such regularity existed in the past or will continue is unknown. Seven- to 8-year cycles, however, are not necessarily the usual patterns in other countries. Scandinavia appears to have much longer cycles, with peaks occurring 10 to 30 years apart. Israel, on the other hand, has alternate high and low years, a pattern similar to that of measles. More data over a longer period are necessary both to define and to understand these variations.

PATHOGENESIS

If the agent of infectious hepatitis behaves like polioviruses when entering the body through the alimentary tract, initial multiplication probably occurs in the lymphatic tissue of the intestine as well as the mesenteric nodes.[32, 411] It has not been established whether polioviruses and other enteroviruses multiply in epithelial cells of the intestine.

Intradermal and hypodermal introduction of viruses usually result in initial multiplication in the regional lymphatics. Viremia occurs subsequently and affords the agent access to all tissues. During viremia the agent may be in plasma or in the leukocytes, or both. Multiplication of measles virus in leukocytes has been demonstrated *in vitro*,[135] and may explain the chromosome breaks observed in 30 to 70 per cent of white cells taken on the third to fifth day of rash.[291] Breaks have similarly been reported in leukocytes from patients with infectious hepatitis.[358]

In yellow fever, Tigertt and co-workers found the virus in reticuloendothelial cells of lymph nodes, spleen and liver.[385] Initial multiplication in the liver was confined to the Kupffer cells, and only later was the virus said to have been demonstrable in the parenchymal cells. On the other hand, the virus of Rift Valley fever, which is hepatotropic in lambs and mice, appears early in the liver and is never demonstrable in the Kupffer cells.[256]

In human viral hepatitis, it has been presumed that the basic derangement is in the parenchymal cell. Morphologic evidence that the viruses multiply in the liver, however, has been lacking. Although the Councilman-like eosinophilic bodies have been thought to represent inclusion bodies,[26] electron microscopy fails to reveal viral particles and suggests a different explanation for this structure (see below).[30, 206] No true cytoplasmic or intranuclear inclusions have been demonstrated. Although several claims have been advanced that viral particles can be found in the liver in infectious and serum hepatitis,[16] further study has indicated that the material involved is probably glycogen.

Because it is difficult to identify virus particles, it has been suggested that the agents of viral hepatitis may not multiply in the liver. Such a hypothesis assumes that a toxin results from extrahepatic multiplication, with the changes in the liver being secondary to its release. No method for testing this hypothesis is available. Mere failure to demonstrate virus particles by electron microscopy, however, is not sufficient basis for assuming that this hypothesis is valid. The virus of yellow fever has not yet been unequivocally demonstrated in hepatocytes by electron microscopy.[257] The number of particles in a cell, the size and morphology of the virus, and its tendency to form structured aggregates are all important determinants of whether intracellular virus can be identified.

Although viruses are obligate intracellular parasites that divert processes of the host cell to their own replication, infection is not synonymous with damage. A true virus contains only one type of nucleic acid surrounded by a protein coat. Following entry into the cell, which is often by a process that resembles pinocytosis, the protein coat is removed by enzymes of the host. The nucleic acid then induces replication of itself as well as the protein components. Experimental evidence suggests that these materials are synthesized from the soluble nucleotide and amino acid pools of the cell, without degradation of components of the host cell being necessary. The virus also relies upon energy processes of the host for synthesis. The nucleic acid and protein coat may be assembled in either the nucleus or the cytoplasm, depending on the particular virus in question.

For some viruses maturation is followed by lysis of the cell. In other instances viral particles are released over a period of time through the cell membrane. Finally, some viruses replicate extensively within cell systems without causing any change in the cell's appearance by light microscopy. No special significance, therefore, can be attached to the failure thus far to observe inclusions or virus-like particles in the liver in viral hepatitis.

PATHOLOGY OF VIRAL HEPATITIS

Until World War II lack of general recognition that liver damage causes the jaundice in viral hepatitis stemmed, at least in part, from the infrequency with which catarrhal and epidemic jaundice could be studied at autopsy. If the discrepancy between the concept embodied in the term "catarrhal jaundice" and the findings on postmortem examination had been noticed more frequently by pathologist and clinician, the delay in accepting a hepatic origin would undoubtedly have been less.

Various circumstances in World War II resulted in large numbers of cases of both infectious and serum hepatitis, so that even a low case fatality rate resulted in accumulation of a considerable amount of necropsy material. Thus, Lucké based his 1944 study on specimens from 125 fatal cases in which the disease had been acquired from contaminated yellow fever vaccine.[236] Although the range of materials available to other investigators was not so extensive, it was sufficient to permit a number of workers to

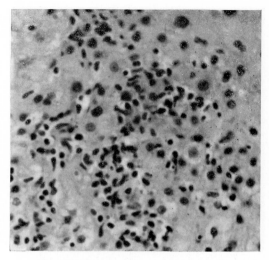

FIG. 13–7. *Spotty necrosis.* Predominantly mononuclear inflammatory exudate accumulated in "spotty areas" in the liver cell plates replacing hepatocytes which have disappeared without telltale marks. These inflammatory cells also infiltrate between hepatocytes in adjacent liver cell plates. (Hematoxylin and eosin. Original magnification × 200.)

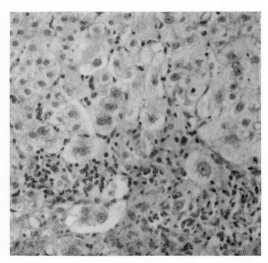

FIG. 13–6. *Typical virus hepatitis.* In the hepatic lobules there are scattered areas of spotty accumulation of predominantly mononuclear inflammatory cells. The lack of zonal distribution of necrosis is typical, but not diagnostic, of viral hepatitis. The lobular orientation of the liver cell plates is somewhat disturbed, but not distorted. This biopsy is from a 31-year-old woman with acute infectious hepatitis. (Hematoxylin and eosin. Original magnification × 100.)

characterize the usual changes in the fatal form of the disease.

An additional and broader basis for study of histopathologic alterations in viral hepatitis was laid in 1939 by Iversen and Roholm when they developed liver biopsy into a clinically applicable technic.[185] These investigators, as well as Dible, McMichael and Sherlock,[79] obtained extensive information by examining needle aspiration specimens from nonfatal cases. This supplementation of the material available from autopsies permitted thorough delineation of the histopathologic changes in viral hepatitis by the late 1940's. Relatively little has been added since that time to what can be learned by light microscopy. Electron microscopy has contributed nothing to the specificity of diagnosis in viral hepatitis.

Histopathologic examination holds a far more important position with regard to diagnosis of viral hepatitis than to that in other infectious diseases. The reasons for this are not difficult to define: (1) Because of continued failure to isolate the viruses,

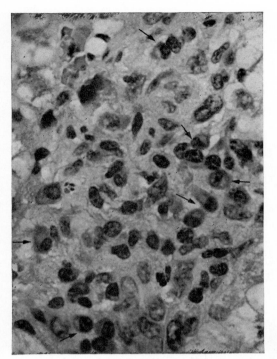

FIG. 13–8. *Mononuclear inflammatory exudate.* At high magnification many plasma cells can be seen among other mononuclear cells. The biopsy is from a 28-year-old male with acute infectious hepatitis. (Hematoxylin and eosin. Original magnification × 450.)

conveniently discussed in terms of four categories.

TYPICAL VIRAL HEPATITIS

In this discussion "typical viral hepatitis" refers to the group of findings most commonly seen. The characteristic morphologic abnormality is single cell degeneration and "spotty" necrosis. Inflammatory cells accumulate in areas where groups of hepatocytes have vanished from the liver cell plates (Fig. 13–6). Such changes are distributed randomly throughout the lobule. The inflammatory exudate in the lobule is almost always predominantly mononuclear (Fig. 13–7). Among the mononuclear cells are varying proportions of lymphocytes, macrophages and plasma cells (Fig. 13–8), but polymorphonuclear (PMN) leukocytes and eosinophils are also present. This intra-

laboratory technics for identification of the etiologic agents or specific serologic tests are not available. (2) Although the clinical picture of viral hepatitis is relatively characteristic, at times there is enough uncertainty to cause diagnostic difficulties, especially when sporadic disease occurs in an adult. (3) The histopathologic picture is sufficiently characteristic to permit a definite diagnosis from a biopsy specimen in most instances. (4) The development of easier technics have made this procedure widely available.

Although the diagnosis of viral hepatitis is best established at present by liver biopsy, no single type of histopathologic lesion is characteristic of the disease. The diagnosis is based on the co-existence of various morphologic abnormalities, and also upon their distribution. The patterns of morphologic lesions in viral hepatitis may be

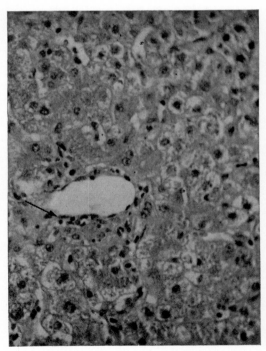

FIG. 13–9. *Minimal central phlebitis.* Several mononuclear cells and an occasional PMN leukocyte accumulated under the endothelial lining of an efferent vein (*arrow*) in a 52-year-old patient with serum hepatitis. (Hematoxylin and eosin. Original magnification × 200.)

lobular inflammatory exudate is not confined to the liver cell plates, but is also seen in the space of Disse and in the sinusoids. Rarely, isolated areas of necrosis are seen where PMN leukocytes may be the predominant type of inflammatory cell. Although eosinophils are commonly seen, their accumulation is not associated with eosinophilia in peripheral blood.

Central phlebitis is a characteristic lesion of viral hepatitis. When seen, it is an aid in diagnosis. The endothelium of the efferent vein is unaffected, but an inflammatory exudate accumulates between the liver cell plate and the vein (Fig. 13–9). This reaction will appear to be more severe when it coincides with necrosis of smaller or larger groups of hepatocytes adjacent to the efferent vein. Under these conditions, the inflammatory exudate evoked by parenchymal necrosis and central phlebitis merge (Fig. 13–10).

The differences of staining qualities of

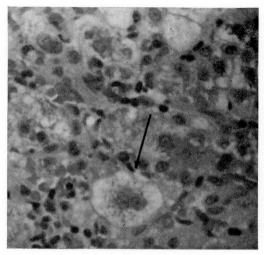

FIG. 13–11. *Balloon cell.* Adjacent to small areas of necrosis a large, pale, double-nucleated cell is seen (*arrow*). Thin strands of eosinophilic cytoplasm are widely separated by fine vacuolization. The biopsy is from a 28-year-old male during the acute icteric phase of infectious hepatitis. (Hematoxylin and eosin. Original magnification × 200.)

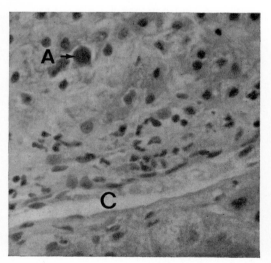

FIG. 13–10. *Central phlebitis and single cell degeneration.* A longitudinally cut efferent vein is in the center of the field (*C*). PMN leukocytes and mononuclear cells have accumulated under the endothelial lining cells and extend into the adjacent parenchyma. They have replaced hepatocytes in the liver cell plates. Extruded from the liver cell plate is an acidophilic body (*A*). (Hematoxylin and eosin. Original magnification × 200.)

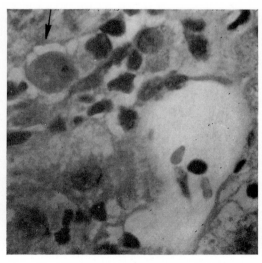

FIG. 13–12. An *acidophilic (Councilman) body* (*arrow*) is seen adjacent to a slightly dilated sinusoid. Liver cell necrosis is evident by the accumulation of mononuclear cells and PMN leukocytes. These cells surround an eosinophilic body which also contains a nuclear fragment and a vacuole. (Hematoxylin and eosin. Original magnification × 450.)

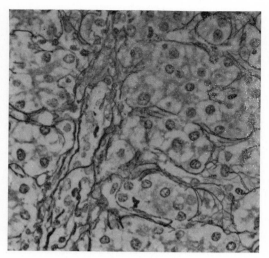

FIG. 13–13. *Reticulum collapse.* The absence of hepatocytes from the liver cell plates is marked by the "collapse" of the reticulum fibers. These fibers normally lie between the liver cell plates and sinusoidal lining cells in close association with the latter and appear as single thin lines along both sides of the hepatocytes on light microscopy. When hepatocytes have disappeared, these reticulum fibers approach each other or "collapse." This biopsy is from a 26-year-old man during the acute phase of infectious hepatitis. (Weigert's silver impregnation. Original magnification × 200.)

adjacent liver cells may be marked. Some hepatocytes enlarge; this varies in extent from cell to cell. When extreme, such enlarged cells contain small fragments or thin strands of eosinophilic cytoplasm, and are called "balloon cells." Some balloon cells have two nuclei and may contain pigment granules (Fig. 13–11). The enlargement of these cells is not due to the accumulation of fat or glycogen, but is the result of: (1) vacuolization and disruption of the endoplasmic reticulum, (2) an apparent decrease in the number of ribosomes, (3) decreased density of the mitochondria and (4) wide separation of cytoplasmic organelles.[189]

As single liver cells degenerate, the cytoplasmic basophilia disappears, making the cytoplasm dark red in hematoxylin-eosin stained sections. The nucleus of these cells is usually either pyknotic or fragmented. In some instances, the nuclear material is completely extruded. Occasionally, vacuolization is seen in the dense cytoplasm (Fig. 13–12). These hyalinized cells are called "acidophilic bodies" or Councilman bodies because they resemble the acidophilic bodies found in the mid-zone of the lobule in yellow fever. These acidophilic bodies are commonly seen in viral hepatitis, but are not specific for it. They are also seen in other viral, bacterial and parasitic infections[53] and in alcoholic hepatitis. Electron microscopy of acidophilic bodies shows changes interpreted as due to cytoplasmic dehydration.[206]

More frequently, hepatocytes vanish from liver cell plates without a trace and their absence is manifested by the collapse of the reticulum fibers and by accumulation of inflammatory cells. In some instances, however, few or no inflammatory cells accompany the reticulum collapse (Fig. 13–13).

Regeneration proceeds together with necrosis of the liver parenchyma. Groups of young or multinucleated hepatocytes are frequently seen adjacent to areas of necrosis and inflammation. Vigorous regenerative activity may be evidenced by the increased frequency of karyokinesis without cytokinesis, and hyperkaryokinesis. The former is manifested by increased numbers of multinucleated and even giant cells (Fig. 13–14), and the latter by more frequently occurring polyploid cells. Increased rate of mitosis is seen and multipolar mitoses are evident.[247]

Necrosis, degeneration, regeneration and inflammation in close proximity distort the normal architectural pattern and result in a lobular disarray. In scattered areas of the lobules the liver cells arrange themselves in an acinus-like pattern (Figs. 13–15 and 13–16). The pseudoacinus formation may be pronounced in some and absent in other cases of viral hepatitis. It is not limited to certain epidemics.

Under the electron microscope the early lesions of viral hepatitis are characterized by peculiar clumping of the endoplasmic reticulum. Cystic dilatation and fragmentation of the endoplasmic reticulum in surviving cells suggests an anatomic basis for impairment of several specific functions such as protein and steroid synthesis, glucuronide conjugation, and detoxification.[348]

The portal areas are enlarged and edematous and have an accumulation of inflammatory cells which often extends into the periphery of the lobule. In some cases ductular proliferation can be seen and an inflammatory exudate accumulates around the basement membrane of small ductules (Fig. 13–17). The significance of this pericholangitis during the acute stage of the illness is not clear; it may well be part of a generalized portal inflammation.

Kupffer cells are enlarged and protrude into the sinusoidal lumen. Many of these cells contain PAS-positive material which is not glycogen. After several weeks of viral hepatitis, some Kupffer cells contain a "dirty brown" pigment on hematoxylin-eosin stained sections. This pigment has also been called "wear and tear pigment" and is thought to be lipofuscin.[236, 364] This type of pigment in the Kupffer cells is not found in viral hepatitis alone. Its presence indicates previous parenchymal necrosis from various causes. Nevertheless, it is often helpful in the differential diagnosis of jaundice during the later stages of viral hepatitis.

During the later stages the same lesions are seen as during the acute phase of viral hepatitis. The extent and severity of the lesions, however, is much milder. The usual findings are: lipofuscin in the Kupffer cells; scattered areas of "spotty" necrosis containing mononuclear cells; slight enlargement of portal tracts with many plasma cells and histiocytes; and, irregularity of the liver cell

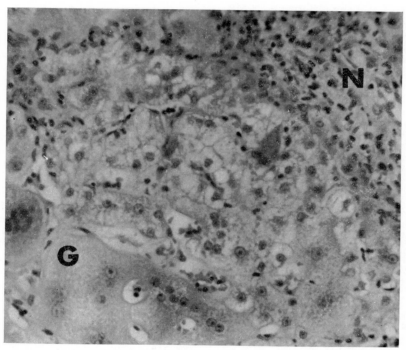

Fig. 13–14. *Degeneration and regeneration.* In the upper right (*N*), hepatocytes are not detectable and this area of necrosis is filled with mononuclear cells, PMN leukocytes and a few plasma cells. In the center of the illustration morphologically normal, well-glycogenated hepatocytes are seen in the liver cell plates. In the lower left of the illustration (*G*), there are large cells with indistinct cell walls and multinucleated giant cells. The biopsy is from a 33-year-old woman with infectious hepatitis. (Hematoxylin and eosin. Original magnification × 200.)

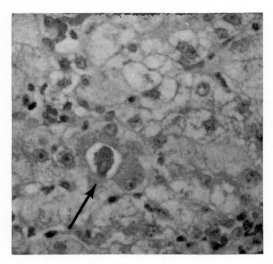

FIG. 13–15. *Pseudoacinus and microcalculus.* Adjacent to an area of spotty necrosis a pseudoacinus is seen (*arrow*). In the center of the pseudoacinus is an irregular, elliptical "microcalculus" with irregular edges. The biopsy was obtained during the cholestatic phase of serum hepatitis in a 64-year-old man. (Hematoxylin and eosin. Original magnification × 200.)

plates with an increased number of multinucleated regenerating cells. These changes may be associated with elevated serum transaminases in patients who remain asymptomatic. Such changes in hepatic histology can be seen months and even years after the acute episode of viral hepatitis. These lesions do not progress to the life-threatening, debilitating complications of viral hepatitis such as chronic hepatitis or postnecrotic cirrhosis.

Some patients with only moderate hepatocellular necrosis are very ill; others with extensive inflammatory reactions and "spotty" parenchymal necrosis feel well and have good appetites. Despite these exceptions, the density and intensity of spotty accumulation of inflammatory cells in the lobule usually correlates reasonably well with the clinical picture of the patient.

More frequently, there is discrepancy between the severity of morphologic lesions and the degree of abnormality of "liver function" tests, especially the transaminases. Such discrepancy may be due to sampling error. It is also possible that the clinical manifestations of the disease and

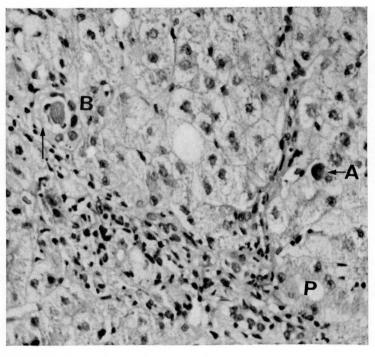

FIG. 13–16. *Pseudoacinus and cholangitis.* The illness began 2 weeks after transfusions and had a severe course. Impending coma and ascites developed. Other areas of the specimen show submassive necrosis. Note an acidophilic body (*A*) and a pseudoacinus (*P*). The portal tract contains a predominantly PMN leukocytic inflammatory exudate. A perilobular bile ductule (*B*) contains a large "microcalculus." A part of the ductular epithelium shows necrosis (*vertical arrow*) and is infiltrated with PMN leukocytes. This biopsy was obtained 7 weeks after the onset of transfusion-associated viral hepatitis in a 52-year-old man. (Hematoxylin and eosin. Original magnification × 200.)

the abnormalities in the usual liver function tests may be dependent not only on the extent and severity of the "spotty" parenchymal necrosis, but also on the functional capacity of the apparently intact, surviving hepatocytes.

The morphologic changes in anicteric hepatitis or in the prodromal stage before the onset of jaundice are the same type, but usually less severe than described above. Cholestasis is not seen in these specimens.

CHOLESTATIC HEPATITIS

Cholestasis is a term applied to the presence of "bile thrombi" or "microcalculi" in dilated bile canaliculi. This appearance is produced by mechanical obstruction of one of the major bile ducts (extrahepatic cholestasis). The picture can also be seen in the absence of mechanical interference with bile flow (intrahepatic cholestasis). Therefore, this histologic finding, by itself, cannot differentiate extrahepatic mechanical obstruction from primary intrahepatic cholestasis.

"Microcalculi" consist of bilirubin-containing coagulum which fills the dilated canaliculus. The microvilli are flattened or completely absent in these canaliculi. "Microcalculi" are usually most frequent near the central vein. In some cases a large microcalculus is surrounded by several hepatocytes arranged in a gland-like pattern (Fig. 13–15). This appearance gives rise to the descriptive term "pseudo-acinus." In addition to this intracanalicular bile stasis, golden yellow bilirubin containing pigment can be seen in the hepatocytes and in the Kupffer cells.

Occasionally, cholestasis in viral hepatitis is manifested by "microcalculi" in bile ductules. In rare cases, such cholestasis is associated with necrosis and inflammation (cholangitis) of the ductular epithelium (Fig. 13–16).

Cholestasis in viral hepatitis is commonly associated with the characteristic morphologic complex described above under Typical Viral Hepatitis. In some cases lesions other than cholestasis are difficult to find, although long and meticulous search may reveal parenchymal cell necrosis. The portal areas contain many PMN leukocytes

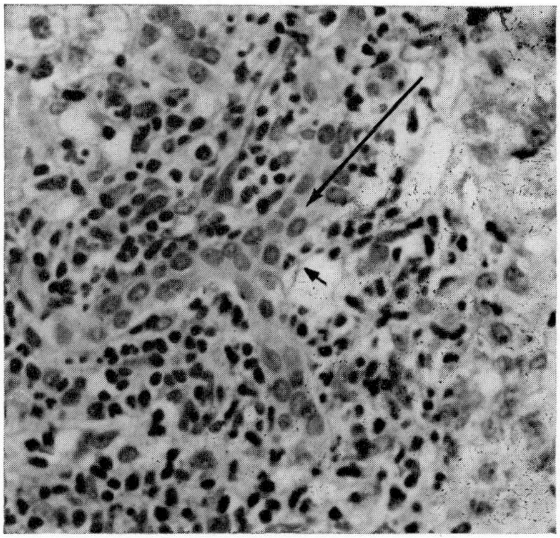

FIG. 13–17. *Portal inflammation.* Numerous PMN leukocytes and mononuclear cells are scattered throughout the portal tract. Several PMN leukocytes are adjacent to the basement membrane of a bifurcating, tangentially-cut bile ductule (*long arrow*), giving the appearance of pericholangitis (*short arrow*). The limiting plate, the sharp demarcation of the portal tract from the liver cell plates, is obscured by the extension of the portal inflammatory exudate into the hepatic lobule. This biopsy is from a 26-year-old man with acute infectious hepatitis. (Hematoxylin and eosin. Original magnification × 200.)

which frequently aggregate around bile ductules. The differentiation of the cholestatic form of viral hepatitis from drug-induced cholestasis is very difficult in such cases.[336]

The mechanism of intrahepatic cholestasis in viral hepatitis has not been defined. It may be related to primary damage of the microvilli of the bile canaliculi or may be secondary to dysfunction of the bile secretory apparatus of the hepatocyte itself. The latter is manifested by a change of the physicochemical composition of freshly secreted bile which precipitates in the canaliculi.

SUBMASSIVE AND MASSIVE HEPATIC NECROSIS

The pathology of histologically devastating forms of viral hepatitis can be divided

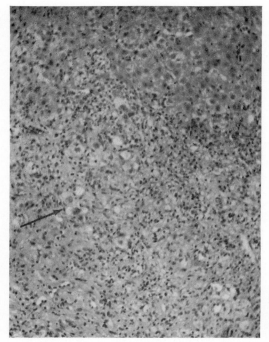

FIG. 13–18. *Submassive hepatic necrosis.* Necrosis of all or parts of several adjacent lobules can be seen next to liver parenchyma, which shows only scattered areas of "spotty" necrosis. In the area of massive confluent necrosis small islands of hepatocytes survived. Some of these cells show "ballooning" (*arrow*). A prominent mononuclear inflammatory exudate is seen throughout the area of necrosis. The ground substance in this area contained a high concentration of glycosaminoglycans. (Hematoxylin and eosin. Original magnification × 100.)

into submassive and massive hepatic necrosis.

Submassive Hepatic Necrosis. In this form of the disease, some lobules may show "spotty necrosis" and changes described under Typical Viral Hepatitis. In many areas complete lobules, parts of lobules or several adjacent lobules are destroyed by the disease.[117, 387] The demarcation may be sharp between the areas of confluent multilobular necrosis and "spotty necrosis" (Fig. 13–18). In the former only the collapsed framework of reticulum remains to indicate the site of absent hepatocytes. Broad strands

of collapsed reticulum extend between adjacent portal areas and between portal tracts and central veins. Such "bridging" must not be confused with normal portal connective tissue when the portal tract is cut tangentially.

In submassive hepatic necrosis the response of the hepatic mesenchyma is different from that seen in the typical viral hepatitis. A characteristic abnormality is the change of the biochemical composition of the ground substance both in the areas of submassive injury and in the edematous portal tract.[118] The pathognomonic feature of this type of response is the accumulation of large amounts of glycosaminoglycans (probably proteoglycans as proteinpolysac-

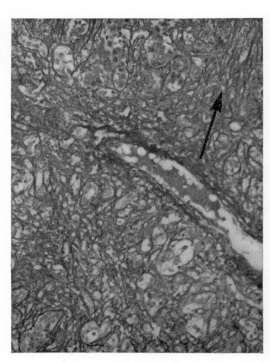

FIG. 13–19. *Submassive hepatic necrosis.* Reticulum collapse is prominent in this area of multilobular necrosis. Small islands of surviving hepatocytes are engulfed in a disorganized framework of reticulum. In other areas the original parallel lobular orientation of the reticulum fibers is still discernible (*arrow*). (Weigert's silver impregnation. Original magnification × 100.)

charide macromolecules). Glycosaminoglycans are not seen in "spotty necrosis" nor are they demonstrable in every area of reticulum collapse in submassive necrosis.[117] This type of connective tissue response is characteristic of the early stages of scar formation. It is not clear whether the preexisting reticulum fibers are converted to collagen bundles, or newly synthesized collagen polymerizes into highly crosslinked bundles. As fibroblasts appear, the lesion progresses into a fibrous septum; in some instances, however, the lesion may resolve completely.[118, 386]

In the early phase of submassive necrosis the collapsed reticulum fibers surround small groups of surviving liver cells (Fig. 13–19). The area in which this reticulum collapse occurs seems to be the periphery of the hepatic acinus of Rappaport.[317] In this stage the van Gieson reaction, which is reasonably specific for collagen,[315] does not stain fibers within the glycosaminoglycan-rich ground substance. This lesion is reversible and must not be confused with frank nodule and collagenous septum formation, which is irreversible.[118] In older lesions, however, collagen is readily demonstrable by this method.

Both the areas of "spotty" and submassive necrosis contain numerous lymphocytes and variable numbers of plasma cells, macrophages, eosinophilic and PMN leukocytes (Fig. 13–18). A similar inflammatory exudate is seen in the enlarged and edematous portal areas. The prominent cellular exudate is not uniformly distributed in all areas of necrosis and collapse. In some areas the mononuclear cells tend to form follicle-like aggregates. They accumulate along blood vessels or interlobular bile ductules.

Duplications of small interlobular ductules are common. Cholestasis is frequently seen and may be prominent. "Microcalculi" may be seen not only in dilated canaliculi, but also in intralobular or sublobular ductules (Fig. 13–16).

Massive Hepatic Necrosis. This variant was first described by Rokitansky in 1842, who named it "acute yellow atrophy."[331] This term is inaccurate because at autopsy the liver does not look yellow, but brownish, and is not atrophic, but necrotic. The most detailed study of this form of viral hepatitis was that of Lucké and Mallory.[237] At autopsy the liver capsule is usually finely wrinkled. As the liver is removed and placed on the table, it does not hold its shape because of a flabby consistency. Histologic examination shows that almost all the hepatocytes have disappeared, and a reticulum framework is the only remnant of the hepatic lobule. The portal triads are preserved and the hepatic arteries, portal veins and bile ducts in them show little change. The spaces between the sinusoids are filled with scavenger cells and necrotic debris. The sinusoids in some regions are congested with red blood cells. The massive necrosis of the liver parenchyma is unexpectedly accompanied by little inflammatory reaction. Neither the vigorous PMN leukocytic response nor the biochemical alterations of the hepatic mesenchyma seen in submassive necrosis can be identified. In widely scattered areas, single or small groups of lymphocytes may be seen. Here and there, small groups of surviving hepatocytes can be found; these usually are close to portal tracts. Occasionally the remaining parenchymal cells show evidence of regenerative activity (Fig. 13–20). On morphologic grounds massive hepatic necrosis of viral hepatitis cannot be differentiated from that which follows the administration of drugs or anesthetic agents.

Massive hepatic necrosis applies to the pathologic findings in patients who die in hepatic failure. It is reasonable to suspect that the same morphologic picture would be found in those with fulminant hepatic failure who survive. This suspicion cannot be documented, however, because the prolonged prothrombin time which accompanies hepatic failure precludes liver biopsy. One of us treated a patient who recovered from fulminant hepatitis (rapidly developing, severe jaundice; deep coma lasting over 5 days; SGOT > 5000 K.U.; oliguria; creatinine > 12 mg./100 ml.). Three weeks after coma was alleviated by exchange transfusion, the liver biopsy showed almost normal hepatic architecture. There were only widely scattered areas of focal necrosis, portal inflammation and cholestasis; the vast majority of hepatocytes

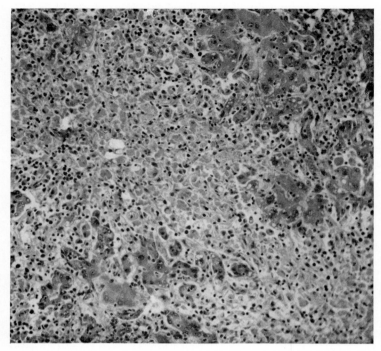

Fig. 13–20. *Massive hepatic necrosis.* This illustration shows one of the few small groups of surviving hepatocytes. Some are vacuolated; others have two to four hyperchromatic nuclei, which suggests regenerative activity. This liver elsewhere contained only portal structures and necrotic parenchyma. Here, poorly stained cytoplasmic remnants, necrotic hepatocytes with pyknotic nuclei and proteinaceous coagulum are filling the space between the surviving hepatocytes. "Scavenger" cells are seen in the necrotic debris where liver cell plates used to be. No significant inflammatory exudate can be seen, although, in widely scattered areas, small groups of lymphocytes accumulate. Glycosaminoglycans are not detectable in the ground substance. This morphologic picture is not characteristic of the etiology of massive hepatic necrosis. (Hematoxylin and eosin. Original magnification × 100.)

were normal in appearance. At that time in convalescence there was no evidence of either massive or submassive necrosis. Clinical and biochemical recovery were complete. Complete regeneration has been described by others,[193, 195] but similarly without documentation.

The absence of the usual mesenchymal changes in massive necrosis which precede the development of fibrosis and cirrhosis argues in favor of complete recovery if survival occurs. If death can be delayed, the liver cell plates can regenerate along pre-existing collapsed reticulum fibers. Patients who survived for up to 140 days after fulminant hepatic failure did not show the development of cirrhosis.[64] Only minimal fibrosis was detectable.

Possibly in patients who survive fulminant hepatic failure but develop postnecrotic cirrhosis, the histopathologic changes were those of submassive hepatic necrosis and were accompanied by its typical active mesenchymal response. Here, hepatocellular regeneration and scar formation proceed

simultaneously, resulting in nodular regeneration and septum formation. The evidence to date, therefore, does not permit a quantitative estimate of the incidence of cirrhosis following massive hepatic necrosis. Indeed, there is no convincing evidence yet that cirrhosis follows such a lesion.

CLINICAL ASPECTS

Infection by the agents of viral hepatitis produces a spectrum of clinical and laboratory manifestations. These range in severity from asymptomatic infection to fulminant disease leading to death in a few days. For convenience, the clinical aspects of the disease are discussed under the following headings:

Typical Viral Hepatitis
  Inapparent Hepatitis
    Not detectable by currently available methods
    Detectable by available laboratory tests

Symptomatic Hepatitis
    Anicteric (not clinically jaundiced)
    Icteric
Atypical Viral Hepatitis
    Benign Variants
        Cholestatic Hepatitis
        Prolonged Hepatitis
        Relapsing Hepatitis
        Unresolved Viral Hepatitis
        Posthepatitis Hyperbilirubinemia
        Prolonged Hypertransaminasemia
        Prolonged or Recurrent Symptoms
           without Laboratory Abnormalities
    Life-Threatening Variants
        Fulminant Viral Hepatitis
        Submassive Hepatic Necrosis
        Chronic Hepatitis
        Postnecrotic Cirrhosis

TYPICAL VIRAL HEPATITIS

This term denotes the most frequent form in which the infection occurs in the community, as well as the most frequent form in which the disease presents itself to the clinician. Cases of typical viral hepatitis can be divided conveniently into the groups indicated above, which roughly correspond to the severity of infection. Such a classification should not be interpreted rigidly, for the category to which any patient may be assigned depends not only upon the severity of the disease, but also upon the frequency of examinations and astuteness of the examiner.

Inapparent Hepatitis. This term refers to an infection that produces no symptoms. It can be recognized only by detecting one or more abnormalities in liver function tests in patients who have been exposed to the disease. The term "anicteric" hepatitis has often been used to describe "inapparent" hepatitis. It seems useful, however, to distinguish those persons with sufficient involvement to produce illness from those with no symptoms; in this discussion "anicteric" hepatitis is restricted to the former group.

Inapparent infections were documented by abnormalities in liver function tests and histopathologic examination of biopsy specimens in volunteer experiments during World War II. In addition, liver function tests have been used to study institutional[77, 85, 130, 218, 244] and familial outbreaks,[352] and recipients of blood and blood products.[65, 143, 359]

Such investigations have been considerably assisted by the availability of a convenient assay for serum transaminase activity since 1956. Its superior sensitivity over serum bilirubin and flocculation procedures was demonstrated by Krugman and associates in an asymptomatic child with documented viremia.[217] It may be no more sensitive than measurement of sulfobromophthalein (BSP) retention, and is probably less specific for hepatic injury except in the presence of fever. Serum transaminase assay is much more convenient than other procedures, for a fasting specimen is not needed and serum activity diminishes relatively slowly during storage even at room temperature.

The frequency of inapparent hepatitis detectable by transaminase abnormality in relation to symptomatic anicteric or icteric hepatitis has varied widely in published reports. Some investigators have found fewer than one inapparent infection for every clinically apparent case.[352] Others have found 10 to 30 persons with transaminase elevation alone for every icteric patient.[77, 143, 359] As discussed previously in relation to Table 13–7, it seems probable that the ratio of inapparent to symptomatic infections varies from epidemic to epidemic.

Remember, however, that transaminase elevations, particularly milder and transient elevations, occur in a variety of infections. Transaminase abnormalities, therefore, must be viewed with caution unless the observations are well controlled. This is particularly true when large numbers of "anicteric cases" are found in the presence of only a few icteric cases, especially among adults.

The agents of viral hepatitis may also produce infection so mild that it is not detectable either clinically or by any laboratory tests for hepatic dysfunction. Such infections will be defined only when procedures for virus isolation or demonstration of antibody response become available.

Symptomatic Viral Hepatitis. When infection with the agents of hepatitis produces

TABLE 13–9. SYMPTOMS REPORTED BY 415 ICTERIC AND 35 ANICTERIC PATIENTS. EPIDEMICS OF TYPICAL INFECTIOUS HEPATITIS. HEPATITIS UNIT, NCDC, 1955–1963

	ICTERIC PATIENTS			ANICTERIC PATIENTS		
SYMPTOM	Number Questioned	Number Experiencing Symptom	Per cent Experiencing Symptom	Number Questioned	Number Experiencing Symptom	Per cent Experiencing Symptom
Brown urine	415	389	94	35	27	77
Lassitude	415	378	91	35	32	91
Loss of appetite	415	372	90	35	28	80
Nausea	415	360	87	35	21	60
Weakness	257	198	77	—	—	—
Fever	415	316	76	35	21	60
Vomiting	415	295	71	35	19	54
Headache	415	294	70	35	19	54
Chilliness	381	250	66	31	10	32
Abdom. discomfort	415	271	65	35	29	83
Abdom. pain	257	168	65	—	—	—
Whitish stools	415	217	52	31	8	26
Myalgia	158	82	52	35	13	37
Drowsiness	67	33	49	17	11	65
Irritability	92	40	43	22	9	41
Itching	395	164	42	31	8	26
Constipation	383	110	29	—	—	—
Diarrhea	101	25	25	—	—	—
Arthralgia	34	7	21	—	—	—
Sore throat	138	27	20	—	—	—
Nasal discharge	138	20	14	31	4	13
Cough	106	8	7	—	—	—

symptoms, the illness may be anicteric or icteric. The latter term does not imply hyperbilirubinemia alone; it should be restricted to patients with clinically detectable jaundice of conjunctivae, mucous membranes or skin.

The relative frequency of various symptoms in some 450 patients with icteric and anicteric illnesses in an epidemic setting was determined by the Hepatitis Unit, NCDC. The results are shown in Table 13–9.

Anicteric Viral Hepatitis. The symptoms of anicteric viral hepatitis are essentially the same as those of the icteric disease. The clinical course is qualitatively similar, but of lesser duration in most instances. The high percentage of bilirubinuria (Table 13–9) in the patients recognized as having anicteric hepatitis during NCDC investigations is undoubtedly an exaggeration of

its "true" frequency. In surveys by which this group of anicteric cases was defined, bilirubinuria itself was an important criterion leading to the diagnosis of what otherwise was an "undifferentiated" acute illness. In the Boston study of hospitalized adults, a history of contact with a sick, non-jaundiced child was significantly more frequent among adults with icteric hepatitis than among controls.[210] This finding suggests that anicteric hepatitis in children is often not recognized as such.

Icteric Viral Hepatitis. Most persons with icteric viral hepatitis have symptoms, although jaundice is occasionally observed in an asymptomatic individual. The level of hyperbilirubinemia necessary to result in clinically detectable jaundice varies with the alertness of the examiner, the conditions of the examination and the natural pigmentation of the patient. In general, conjunctival jaundice becomes detectable at serum bilirubin concentration of 2.0 to 4.0 mg./100 ml.[142]

ONSET. The symptoms of infectious hepatitis and serum hepatitis are similar. One noteworthy exception may be in the mode of onset. When questioned, the patient with infectious hepatitis is sometimes able to recall having tired more easily during the several days prior to onset. It is not common, however, for this premonitory fatigability to have been sufficiently severe for him to have relinquished any of his usual activities. The transition from health to acute illness takes place within a period of 24 hours in about 60 per cent of patients. Level of physical activity presumably does not affect the mode of onset, for the frequency of abrupt appearance of symptoms was the same in prison volunteers[279] as in the general population.[132, 422]

The onset of symptoms is usually more insidious in serum hepatitis than in infectious hepatitis. This was the case in one study of transfusion-associated disease whether the incubation period was longer or shorter than 60 days.[132] The mode of onset, however, cannot be used to differentiate between infectious and serum hepatitis in the individual patient.[381]

In experimentally-induced serum hepatitis, a transient illness with mild symptoms was sometimes observed early in the incubation period. Neefe et al. found headache, loss of appetite, nausea and occasionally vomiting in 8 of 9 volunteers within 50 days after inoculation.[287] In 7 of 9 volunteers the mild symptoms developed after 12 to 35 days. These complaints lasted 1 to several days, and were accompanied by mild abnormalities of liver function tests. In at least one instance, viremia was present during such a minor illness 23 days after inoculation and 87 days before the major illness. After the minor illness, the patients either remained well or had one or more brief recurrences until the onset of the major phase of the illness 73 to 110 days after inoculation. The occurrence of minor illness is reminiscent of the premonitory symptoms and transient rash observed in measles which is thought to be related to the initial viremia. The minor illness in serum hepatitis is rarely observed clinically, presumably because patients are not under such careful scrutiny.

ACUTE PHASE OF ILLNESS. Symptoms in infectious hepatitis usually last 2 to 7 days before the onset of jaundice. In one series in which children predominated, the median duration of the preicteric phase was 5 days.[264] The interval from first symptoms to jaundice exceeded 10 days, however, in 14 per cent of cases (Fig. 13–21). In a group of British servicemen it exceeded 8 days in about 12 per cent of patients.[426]

The main features of the clinical disease are well known. Careful attention to less frequent details has been lacking in recent years, and studies of pathophysiologic mechanisms have been almost nonexistent. The relative frequencies of complaints among icteric patients represented in Table 13–9 are similar to those reported by others.[229] Considering the varying circumstances under which such data have been collected, uniformity is remarkable.

Flu-like symptoms predominate in the early phase of the acute illness. Fever or feverishness occurs in two-thirds to three-fourths of patients with infectious hepatitis, and is more prominent in the first few days of illness. The temperature is usually 37.5° to 38.5° C. (99.5° to 101.3° F.), but occasionally is 39° to 40° C. (102° to 104° F.). Chilliness accompanies the early phases in about half of those patients with fever, but shaking chills are uncommon. Headache is frequent, but usually not severe.

Nasal discharge, sore throat or cough is seen during the prodromata of 10 to 20 per cent of patients, and have been said to occur more among children.[157] These symptoms are mild, and are not usually mentioned spontaneously by the patient. Bronchitis and pneumonitis attributable to the hepatitis agents have not been described.

Loss of appetite is one of the most frequent of all symptoms, as is true in other forms of parenchymal cell injury. Possibly anorexia is induced by a "toxin" produced by the impaired liver or by the failure of the hepatocyte to "detoxify" an abnormal product. The patient not only lacks appe-

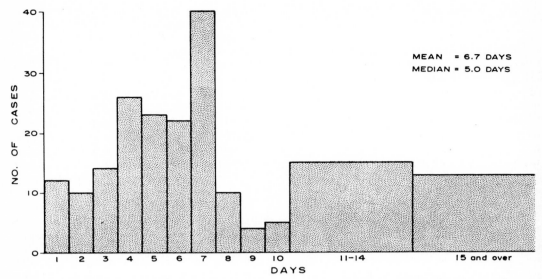

FIG. 13–21. Number of days between onset of symptoms and appearance of overt jaundice among 194 patients with infectious hepatitis, Detroit, 1937–38. (From data presented by Molner and Meyer[264].)

tite, but finds food repugnant when presented to him. Merely the smell of food often induces nausea. Greasy or "heavy" foods are tolerated poorly by most patients. Anorexia is usually more marked later in the day, so that it is common for a patient to eat well at breakfast but poorly at other meals. In addition to aversion to food, patients are also offended by cigarette smoke and other strong odors.

Vomiting in typical viral hepatitis is neither severe nor protracted. When vomiting becomes progressively more severe for several days, it may indicate a more serious, atypical form of viral hepatitis. The mechanism of nausea and vomiting cannot be fully defined, but one contributing factor may be gastritis and duodenitis. Acute superficial gastritis was found by gastroscopy during the preicteric and acute phase of the illness in seven of nine patients[209] and in three of six volunteers with experimentally-induced infectious hepatitis.[158] The gastric mucosa was normal in the latter group by gastroscopy before infection. Cytologic studies and histologic examinations of suction biopsies show changes in mucosal cells and inflammation.[13, 63] Roentgenologic examination suggests antral gastritis and duodenitis.[158, 308]

Abdominal discomfort or *pain*, particularly in the upper right quadrant, is common. Such discomfort may be increased by or noticed only upon motions which produce jarring or "jogging" of the liver. Change of bowel habits, either to constipation or diarrhea, is seen in about one-fourth of patients. These are of short duration; diarrhea, if it occurs, is rarely severe.

The *urine* becomes sufficiently brownish ("dark") for the change in color to be noticed in 94 per cent of patients with clinically detectable jaundice. This often occurs one to several days before jaundice of eyes or skin is noted. In 29 of 398 cases bilirubinuria preceded jaundice by 7 to 14 days.[163] Similar observations were made in 1846 when Budd described the "colouring matter of bile" in the urine before "the skin becomes yellow."[42] Bilirubin concentration in the urine is initially too low to be detected by casual observation, but laboratory tests can correctly demonstrate its presence.

Patients are usually found to have become aware of their jaundice by having noticed that their "*eyes turned yellow.*" This is due to icterus of their conjunctivae, and not to "scleral" icterus. Jaundice can be detected in the mucous membrane before the skin becomes noticeably icteric. In some patients

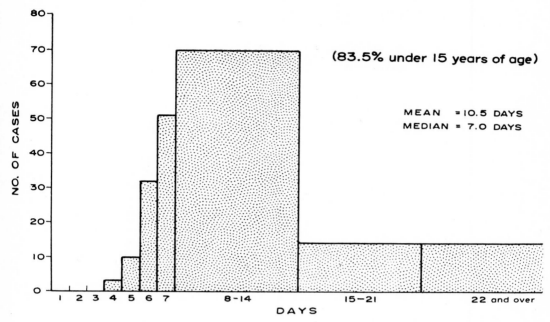

FIG. 13–22. Duration in days of overt jaundice among 194 cases of infectious hepatitis, Detroit, 1937–38. Most of the patients (83.5 per cent) were under 15 years of age. (From data presented by Molner and Meyer.[264])

jaundice can be detected first by observing the tympanic membranes.

The *onset of jaundice* may be associated with progression, persistence or rapid disappearance of all distressing symptoms. Those patients who become asymptomatic with the onset of jaundice and whose diagnosis was not made until they became jaundiced find it curious that they were ambulatory when they felt "terrible" but confined to bed when they feel well. When symptoms persist or progress, usually the malaise and gastrointestinal complaints are those which remain.

The duration of jaundice in infectious hepatitis in the majority of patients is exaggerated by reports in the literature. Most studies have been based largely on hospitalized cases, which ordinarily represent the more severe forms of the disease. In addition, concern with sequelae of hepatitis often prolongs hospitalization. Most children recover within 2 weeks and most adults within 4 to 6 weeks. This is illustrated in Figure 13–22 by data from the study of Molner and Meyer.[264]

Grey or *yellow stools* are observed during the first week of jaundice by 20 to 40 per cent of persons with clinical jaundice. The return of normal fecal color is one sign of recovery. In most patients this occurs during the second or third week of the illness.

Itching results in almost half the patients[229]; it is usually transient and mild. A few patients, however, are severely distressed by pruritus and may have excoriations. Itching commonly occurs as jaundice begins to appear, or as it begins to recede. Some patients also develop transient skin rashes. The most common one is a macular erythema; however, a papular rash is sometimes seen. Urticarial eruptions are uncommon; these usually develop during the preicteric phase.[107, 163] A single case of erythema nodosa has been described.[163]

Irritability and *drowsiness* may be early symptoms of impending hepatic coma; however, these symptoms are often seen early in typical viral hepatitis and do not necessarily denote the potentially serious form of the disease. Asterixis, however, is seen only in severe disease. Apathy may last into the icteric stage.

Depression is common. Any mature adult

would be concerned if faced with the prospect of an illness lasting several weeks; in some patients, however, fear and depression are greatly exaggerated beyond the expected. Such symptoms are self-limited and require no specific treatment, although depression may persist for weeks and extend into convalescence. Depression was profound in 2.8 per cent of cases in one large series.[103] Frank delirium and psychosis are rare, but have been described.[107, 224]

Symptoms suggestive of *meningitis* occasionally develop.[351] Meningismus was described once among 1,365 cases.[224] The spinal fluid is usually normal, but may be icteric and contain lymphocytes.[43, 107, 333, 410] Encephalitis is rare, but has been observed.[39, 43, 44, 103, 410] Peripheral neuritis is likewise uncommon, but has been described.[39, 43, 226, 371]

Sudden increase of jaundice in acute viral hepatitis may be the result of *hemolysis* rather than increasing severity of the hepatic component of the disease. Such hemolysis is most frequently associated with glucose-6-phosphatase dehydrogenase (G-6-PD) deficiency of the erythrocytes.[144, 316, 341] Following severe hemolysis, G-6-PD abnormalities may not be detectable in the anemic patient due to destruction of most of the deficient red cells.

A sudden increase of jaundice may be due to agglutination of erythrocytes in hepatic sinusoids, in patients with SS or SC hemoglobin, rather than worsening of the viral hepatitis. A precipitous rise of serum bilirubin concentration to over 40 mg./100 ml. was observed by one of the authors in an 18-year-old Negro male with SS hemoglobinopathy during the acute icteric phase. Rapid and progressive improvement occurred without corticosteroid treatment.

Rarely, thrombocytopenia,[6] pancytopenia [75, 202] or aplastic anemia[228] develops during viral hepatitis.

Upper gastrointestinal bleeding is unusual. Occult gastrointestinal blood loss could not be detected by ^{51}Cr-labeled erythrocytes in 5 patients.[48] Melena was observed only once in 432 patients of Findlay et al.,[103] and one of 838 of Fox et al.[109] In an outbreak of serum hepatitis among 398 soldiers, one patient with gastrointestinal

hemorrhage and another with a bleeding nose required transfusions.[163] In patients with a history of recent ulcer activity, some caution is warranted in the authors' experience. Three patients with hepatitis following transfusions for bleeding peptic ulcers have been observed who died from uncontrollable upper gastrointestinal hemorrhage during the acute illness.

Electrocardiographic changes during the acute phase of hepatitis consisting of bradycardia, P-R prolongation or T wave depression, have been described.[173, 235] These changes returned to normal during convalescence. In fatal cases myocarditis has been described.[342] There is no evidence for significant cardiac involvement, however, in typical hepatitis.

Changes of *carbohydrate metabolism* have been observed during viral hepatitis. During the postabsorptive state, hyperglycemia is more common than hypoglycemia.[423] A "diabetic" glucose tolerance curve during viral hepatitis must be interpreted with caution. This abnormality is likely to be due to the poor carbohydrate intake rather than to diabetes mellitus. The insulin requirement may increase in a diabetic during acute hepatitis, but returns to the previous level as the patient improves. Diabetic ketoacidosis was not described in diabetic patients.[139] Although it has been claimed that hepatitis runs a more stormy clinical course among diabetics,[194] this finding may have been due to a greater frequency of serum hepatitis among diabetics at the time of the study. The outcome of the disease in diabetics does not appear to be different from nondiabetic patients of similar age and state of general health.

PHYSICAL EXAMINATION. Almost all patients with acute viral hepatitis have tenderness over the liver. It may be elicited by palpation of the right upper quadrant of the abdomen or by fist percussion over the right hypochondrium. This tenderness often poses a problem in attempts to palpate the edge of the liver, for the patient is reluctant to breathe with his diaphragm. Even a cooperative patient will spontaneously use his thoracic muscles to "take a deep breath" if the physician's hand is pressing below his right rib-cage. The greater the descent of the diaphragm, the more severe the discomfort. Unless the patient is explicitly shown how to breathe with his diaphragm and reassured about the discomfort that such inspiration may cause, the examiner may not be able to palpate the enlarged liver.

In the average adult the liver is commonly enlarged to 12 to 14 cm. in vertical length by percussion of the upper edge in the mid-clavicular line and by palpation of the lower edge of the liver 2 to 4 cm. below the costal margin. The liver edge may be sharp or rounded, but never irregular. Although the liver usually feels firmer than normal, it does not have the firm, rubbery consistency that it has in cirrhosis. While hepatomegaly is common, it is rarely massive in viral hepatitis. Before the diagnosis of viral hepatitis is accepted in such cases, it should be confirmed by biopsy.

In some patients it is said that the liver is not palpable because it is "too soft." As a rule, inflammation and edema in the liver are sufficiently acute to make the capsule tense. These changes produce tenderness and an increase in firmness of the liver. Only massive necrosis leads to a small and soft liver.

The spleen is palpable in 5 to 15 per cent of the patients and the posterior cervical lymph nodes may be mildly enlarged. Generalized or marked lymphadenopathy is not a feature of viral hepatitis.

Spider angiomata often develop in patients during acute hepatitis; the frequency is generally underestimated because these lesions are not specifically sought. These lesions disappear in convalescence[163] and do not indicate chronic liver disease. Palmar and malar erythema also occur without relation to severity. Transient gynecomastia in convalescence has been described in two patients with serum hepatitis.[205]

A physical finding suggestive of the diagnosis of viral hepatitis in drug addicts is the occurrence of hematomas, ecchymoses or scars along the course of veins. Most such lesions occur on the left forearm of a right-handed person. Occasional addicts, especially prisoners who would suffer punitive measures if their practice were discovered, use femoral or neck veins.

ABNORMALITIES IN LABORATORY TESTS. Several investigators have observed shortened survival of ^{51}Cr-labeled *erythrocytes* in a high percentage of patients with typical viral hepatitis.[48, 63, 198] The hematocrit and hemoglobin concentrations, however, are usually within normal limits[147, 173]; only in one study, 19 of 25 American soldiers in Korea had decreases below 40 per cent associated with reticulocytosis during the second or third week of illness.[63]

Although a total *white cell count* within normal limits is usual in viral hepatitis, leukopenia was documented as early as 1923.[190] A decrease in leukocytes, although not necessarily to leukopenic levels, was found to develop with onset of fever in experimentally induced viral hepatitis.[159] The count returned to its usual level by the end of the first week of jaundice. The fall in white cell levels in the early stages of viral hepatitis is due to granulocytopenia, so that relative lymphocytosis results. Many of the lymphocytes appear large and atypical ("virucytes").[232] The relative lymphocytosis and atypical lymphocytes are characteristic of viral hepatitis, but occur in other viral diseases as well.

Typical viral hepatitis should be diagnosed with caution when leukocytosis is present. The white cell count is slightly elevated occasionally in typical viral hepatitis, but higher levels most often denote a more severe, atypical form of hepatitis or an entirely different etiology of the illness.

Examination of the urine occasionally shows a few red cells or mild proteinuria. The frequency of hematuria and proteinuria in the study[63] of American soldiers in Korea is not typical of the usual urinary findings during viral hepatitis in this country.

Most patients have an increased urinary excretion of urobilinogen before and at the time of the onset of jaundice. Later, urobilinogen disappears from the urine as the stools become acholic in the obstructive phase.[369]

Bilirubinuria is often seen during the preicteric phase of viral hepatitis. Bilirubinuria during the early phase of hepatitis has been described at direct and total serum bilirubin concentrations much lower than those found later when bilirubin is no longer in the urine.[125] Several explanations have been offered for this disparity between serum and urine bilirubin levels.

Bilirubinuria early in the disease may be due to a lowered renal threshold for bilirubin as a result of direct renal involvement by the disease. Support for the hypothesis of renal damage during acute hepatitis has come from recent studies using percutaneous renal biopsy, which show histopathologic changes in the kidney during infectious hepatitis.[63] However, changes in renal histology have not yet been correlated with bilirubin excretion.

An alternative explanation for the disparate urine and serum bilirubin levels is based on a qualitative difference in the bilirubin metabolites presented to the kidneys during the early phase of viral hepatitis, compared with those present later in the disease.[99] Although it has subsequently been demonstrated[346] that bilirubin diglucuronide has a higher renal clearance than the monoglucuronide, serial determinations of these components have demonstrated no change in their relative proportions with convalescence.[31] Because bilirubin monoglucuronide seems to be a chemical artifact, this reasoning fails to clarify the problem.[134] On the other hand, in 15 patients with hepatitis the urinary excretion of bilirubin was directly and linearly related to the estimated filtered load; that is to say, it was proportional to the plasma direct bilirubin concentration multiplied by glomerular filtration rate.[401]

The mechanism of bilirubinuria during the early phase of hepatitis may be due to a rise of plasma concentration of bile salts, which increases the dialysability of direct bilirubin.[114] The dialysable serum bilirubin increased when its renal excretion was prevented by ureteral ligation.[115] If the plasma bile salts were increased during the early cholestatic phase of hepatitis, but not during convalescence, it would explain bilirubinuria with low direct bilirubin plasma levels during the early phase and the absence of bilirubinuria during convalescence when plasma direct bilirubin levels are higher.

Steatorrhea is transient. Poor fat absorption may explain in part the intolerance to fatty foods during the early phase of the illness.[61]

The *serum bilirubin* determination is one of the most frequently utilized laboratory tests. It is also one of the most difficult to carry out reproducibly at levels within or near the normal range. In addition, bilirubin deteriorates quickly on storage, so that the procedure should be performed using freshly obtained serum. For these reasons, results should be interpreted with more than usual caution.

An increase is sometimes seen in the direct reacting component of serum bilirubin when the total concentration is within normal limits. This abnormality may be found in some patients with anicteric hepatitis, and in others during the preicteric phase of an icteric illness. With onset of the icteric phase, the serum concentration usually rises for 10 to 14 days in the average adult. The rate of decline from the peak level is more gradual, and often requires 2 to 4 weeks. In most patients the maximum concentration of bilirubin is less than 10 mg./100 ml.[381] It is unusual for the serum level to reach a high value or to remain constant for a prolonged period of time. If the serum bilirubin concentration reaches a plateau, the possibility of an atypical form of hepatitis should be considered. Particularly in older women, however, typical viral hepatitis may be associated with high levels of serum bilirubin which show little change for weeks. Liver biopsy reveals only the typical spotty necrosis of viral hepatitis, and liver function becomes subsequently normal.

Studies using prolonged *infusions of sulfobromophthalein* (BSP) have been helpful in understanding pathophysiology of viral hepatitis. Hepatic storage (S) of the dye and the excretory function (Tm) are impaired early. Changes of both S and Tm correlated with the serum bilirubin concentration, but Tm alone correlated with alkaline phosphatase activity. During convalescence, the storage function returned to normal before excretory function did. This could be interpreted to indicate a more rapid restoration of cellular function and vascular perfusion than biliary drainage.

The usual test for BSP retention can be helpful in evaluating an illness thought to be anicteric hepatitis. BSP retention is a sensitive index of liver function and can be of great value in the clinical appraisal of the patient. This test is occasionally useful to determine the rate of recovery of hepatic excretory function during the convalescent phase when serum bilirubin approaches normal. The determination of BSP retention has no particular value in the average clinically jaundiced patient with typical viral hepatitis. However, the BSP retention was normal in 39 per cent of 956 patients whose total bilirubin was between 1.5 and 3.0 mg./100 ml., and in 44 per cent of those whose direct bilirubin concentrations were between 1.0 and 1.7 mg./100 ml.[160]

The gallbladder usually can be visualized during viral hepatitis if BSP retention is less than 20 per cent.[248] The stage of the disease seems to be more important in permitting opacification of the gallbladder or bile ducts than the height itself of the serum bilirubin concentration. For example, radiographic examination of the biliary system during hepatitis was thought to be futile if the serum bilirubin concentration is over 3 mg./100 ml.[93]; yet, 13 of 17 cholecystograms showed good visualization in patients whose serum bilirubin concentrations were 5 to 10.9 mg./100 ml.[321]

The most popular laboratory test to detect parenchymal injury of the liver is assay of the *serum transaminase* activities.[55] This popularity is generally well founded upon the experience accumulated thus far, although the claim[355] that they represent the most sensitive index cannot truly be substantiated on the basis of controlled studies. The assays are sufficiently sensitive, are as specific an index as is generally needed, and are within the technical capability of every hospital laboratory.

Hypertransaminasemia may precede the onset of symptoms of infectious hepatitis by 7 to 10 days.[130, 244, 352] The peak level is usually reached in the first week after symptoms begin. The height of the activity may have some statistical correlation with severity of disease as judged by the presence or absence of clinical illness. There is, however, no necessary correlation, as is evident

from finding levels as high as 3,000 KU in household contacts of infectious hepatitis who were asymptomatic.[352] The height of transaminase activity should not, therefore, be regarded as prognostic, nor as an indication for corticosteroid therapy.

As the acute illness subsides, the serum transaminase activity usually returns to and remains within normal limits. The decrease in level may be more rapid than that of the serum bilirubin concentrations.[244] However, in one-fourth to a half of patients, after an initial fall, a secondary rise of the serum transaminase has been observed,[245, 270, 325] and varies markedly in duration. The persistence of the serum transaminase elevation during the convalescent and postconvalescent phase is nevertheless compatible with complete clinical recovery.

The *serum alkaline phosphatase* activity may be normal in typical viral hepatitis, but in the majority of patients it is slightly elevated.[122] Usually, it does not exceed twice the upper limit of normal for any of the usual assay procedures.[356, 426] Transient elevations are often seen concurrently with a transient decrease of bile pigment content of the stool when looked for during the early cholestatic phase of the typical disease. In association with intrahepatic cholestasis, marked elevations of serum alkaline phosphatase activities are observed. Specific alkaline phosphatase activities, such as ATP-ase or 5-nucleotidase, or the test of stability of alkaline phosphatase activity at 60° C., contribute in only a selected group of patients when bone alkaline phosphatase activity in the serum is increased. Although alkaline phosphatase elevations are the rule during the early acute phase of hepatitis, none of 625 soldiers studied had hypercholesterolemia.[122]

The electrophoretic separation of *serum proteins* shows no marked changes in most patients. In some cases of typical viral hepatitis, and in prolonged or more severe hepatitis, decreased albumin and increased gamma-globulin levels are seen. The gamma globulin concentration may reach twice the normal limit without indicating a change to a persistent chronic disease. Gamma globulins over 3.5 Gm./100 ml. with albumin below 2.5 Gm./100 ml., however, indicate a disease other than typical viral hepatitis. The underlying disease should be confirmed by biopsy under such conditions.

The *turbidity and flocculation procedures*, widely used in the 1940's and 1950's, are now much less extensively employed. Their poor reproducibility is one factor contributing to their eclipse. More important is the fact that the same or better information is now provided by the serum transaminase assays and serum protein electrophoresis.

A wide variety of *agglutination* technics have been proposed as adjuncts in the diagnosis of viral hepatitis. In some instances these have been considered specific due to adsorption of virus on the particles on erythrocytes. One of the most widely evaluated such procedures was the rhesus cell agglutination test of Hoyt and Morrison.[178] Recently introduced is the HIM test of Bolin and co-workers,[35] based on agglutination of latex particles by antibodies to one of the "candidate" viruses.[34] None of these various technics is specific, and none appears to provide more help in diagnosis than the more familiar flocculation and turbidity tests.

Atypical Viral Hepatitis

Atypical viral hepatitis can be divided into two major groups: (a) prolongations of a self-limited, benign disease and (b) the development of a serious, life-threatening, acute or chronic illness.

Benign Variants of Viral Hepatitis. *Cholestatic Viral Hepatitis*. The term "cholestatic hepatitis" is commonly used in two ways: (1) to refer to a clinical picture in which the course of the disease and the laboratory findings simulate those associated with mechanical obstruction of a major bile duct; and (2) to describe a characteristic set of histopathologic findings in the liver. The latter findings are frequently *but not necessarily* associated with a clinical and laboratory picture suggestive of mechanical obstruction. It was initially assumed that the clinical picture and pathologic changes in the liver went *pari passu*, as liver biopsy was carried out only in clinically atypical cases. Biopsy on a more routine basis in two epidemics, however, revealed that the histopathologic findings of cholestasis could be associated with clinically typical viral hepatitis.[86, 87] The present discussion refers to the clinically atypical variant.

In cholestatic viral hepatitis the clinical course is prolonged, with more marked and persistent jaundice. Itching is often prominent and may be persistent. The serum bilirubin concentration is usually 10 to 15 mg./100 ml., and may be higher; it rarely exceeds 25 mg./100 ml. The serum lipoprotein and cholesterol levels are usually elevated. The serum alkaline phosphatase activity is almost always elevated, and at times the increase is marked. The serum gamma-globulin concentration may be elevated and increased levels of the alpha and beta globulins are also common.

Difficulties in diagnosis are most pronounced in sporadic cases, especially those in which right upper quadrant pain or discomfort is prominent. Fortunately, cholestatic hepatitis sometimes does occur in patients with an epidemiologic history suggestive of viral hepatitis, or after a typical acute onset with gastrointestinal and flu-like symptoms. The liver is often palpable and tender; when the liver is not palpable, tenderness can usually be elicited. Jaundice in cholestatic hepatitis is not associated with progressive enlargement of the liver.

Prolonged Viral Hepatitis. The term "prolonged hepatitis" refers to cases that are atypically lengthy; laboratory abnormalities persist and symptoms and physical findings continue. The point in the clinical course at which "typical" becomes "prolonged" is, however, difficult to define. The duration of acute hepatitis is known to vary with age; the acute illness and convalescence lasts longer in adults than in children. The duration of illness probably also varies with the strain of virus, although this opinion is difficult to document. Therefore, we have arbitrarily used 4 months as the time at which adults would be considered as having a prolonged course.

In prolonged viral hepatitis, disease may be evident for 12 months or longer. The symptoms are those seen in the latter part of typical viral hepatitis. Appetite is adequate; malaise is variable, but usually mild or absent. Lassitude and fatigability may be pronounced. Jaundice is usually not deep. The liver may remain palpable, but usually it diminishes in size after the first weeks of illness. The laboratory abnormalities may show some fluctuation, but the trend in general is toward slow improvement. Rises of serum bilirubin and serum transaminase levels often follow undue physical exertion on the part of the impatient patient. Liver biopsy shows scattered areas of mononuclear cell infiltrate, spotty necrosis and increased cellularity of portal areas. Some of the Kupffer cells are enlarged and many contain greyish-yellow pigment having the characteristics of lipofuscin.

Prolonged hepatitis represents only a lengthening of the acute illness, and does not constitute a separate entity. This attitude can be justified not only by clinical experience, but also by available data. The length of illness in the large group of patients studied by Barker and associates[20] conforms not to a bimodal curve but rather a skewed unimodal distribution. Mathematical analysis suggests that an illness that lasts 4 months or longer would be expected in 3 to 5 per cent of cases.[117]

This self-limited, although prolonged, variant of viral hepatitis must be differentiated from progressive, destructive disease which frequently runs a chronic, irreversible course. The term "chronic hepatitis" should be reserved for the latter, although it is unfortunately sometimes used in referring to the former. The optimistic outlook which accompanies the management of a self-limited illness, with its excellent long-term prognosis, should not be clouded by the grim uncertainties of a chronic, active, irreversible disease. In chronic hepatitis one may accept the risk of toxicity of pharmacologic agents with questionable therapeutic benefits, but such risk is unjustified in prolonged hepatitis. Eventual recovery within 1 year is the rule in this form of the illness, although in a few cases it extends even longer.

Relapsing Hepatitis. This term refers to illness in which the patient who has apparently recovered completely following an acute episode of viral hepatitis manifests a recurrence of the original symptoms and findings on one or more occasions. Recurrences are, however, usually milder than the original attack. The rises of bilirubin and serum transaminase levels usually do not exceed the values found during the first episode. The relapse does not denote a different type of disease, but probably means incomplete recovery from the original illness, despite an asymptomatic interval. In some patients a second and rarely a third relapse occurs in the succeeding weeks or months.

Relapses sometimes are precipitated by too early ambulation or excessive physical activity. At times they have been blamed on consumption of alcoholic beverages. An increased frequency of relapse has been also described in patients whose acute illness was treated with corticosteroids.[96, 97, 98]

The incidence of relapses has varied in different groups of patients. Depending on the frequency of observations, the methods of examination and the criteria used to estimate the relapse, the incidence was 1.5 to 18 per cent.[154, 157, 173] In general, clinical relapse occurs only in a small proportion of cases. In selected groups the relapse rate may be high. For example, in one group of 350 patients with a mean duration of illness of 56 days, the relapse rate was 13.4 per cent.[221] These patients, like the ones with prolonged viral hepatitis, recover completely.

Relapsing viral hepatitis should be differentiated from a second attack due to another agent. Patients can acquire at once, or within a short period, infections both with infectious and with serum hepatitis viruses.[412] This is particularly true of addiction-associated disease. Due to the long incubation period of serum hepatitis, one may misinterpret the illness as a relapse of the first illness (*i.e.*, of infectious hepatitis). The longer the interval between the two icteric illnesses, the more likely that the second illness is not a relapse but a separate infection.

Unresolved Viral Hepatitis (Prolonged or Recurrent Abnormal Laboratory Tests with or without Symptoms). Unresolved hepatitis is a term recently introduced by Redeker to describe mild, nonprogressive biochemical relapses, which are accompanied by symptoms in some instances and histopathologic abnormalities.[323] Retrospectively, this term probably could be applied to 40 patients with "delayed recovery" described by Mallory.[247] He found changes in liver biopsies consistent with mild viral hepatitis 100 to 500 days after the onset of the disease. The findings included periportal and spotty intralobular inflammation, and focal hyaline necrosis. Redeker's group of patients with incomplete recovery were largely discovered through serial liver function tests as part of a routine follow-up. Liver biopsies at the time of biochemical abnormalities showed changes diagnostic of mild viral hepatitis. Such episodes have been found to recur over several years without any evidence of progression into chronic active hepatitis or postnecrotic cirrhosis. These biochemical and morphologic recurrences have been associated with symptoms in some patients; others, however, remained asymptomatic. There is no information whether patients with unresolved hepatitis have transient or persistent viremia, virurrhea or viruria.

Posthepatitis Hyperbilirubinemia. Some patients who have apparently recovered from acute viral hepatitis and who no longer have any symptomatic or biochemical abnormalities related to the disease have recurrent indirect hyperbilirubinemia for months or years.[24, 181, 196, 397] At times, exertion appears to precipitate jaundice. Other than mild icterus, the findings on physical examination are within normal limits. The liver is not enlarged or tender during these episodes. Laboratory tests demonstrate indirect hyperbilirubinemia, usually less than 4 to 5 mg./100 ml. The hematocrit is normal, patients do not have reticulocytosis and the fecal urobilinogen excretion is within normal limits. The bilirubin infusion tests show a characteristic depression of the rate of bilirubin disappearance from the circulation. After months or years, this abnormality may subside. The patient can live a perfectly normal life.

Prolonged Hypertransaminasemia. In years past when the serum turbidity and flocculation procedures were widely used, prolonged or recurrent abnormalities of these laboratory tests were comomn after recovery from viral hepatitis. Initially, significance was attached to elevated values; experience, however, indicated that these abnormalities of themselves had no clinical significance.

With the increasing usefulness and popularity of serum transaminases, a new entity consisting of unexplained elevations of the serum transaminase activities could perhaps have been anticipated. For patients who recover from acute viral hepatitis secondary increases of the serum transaminase may be prolonged.[245, 270, 325, 352] These elevations can persist for weeks or months without any clinical evidence of disease. Abnormal BSP retention did not accompany the delayed return of serum transaminase to normal in the American studies,[270, 325] but did so in some patients in a French investigation.[245]

Such isolated abnormalities are often viewed with concern by the physician, who may restrict activity or even enforce bed rest for a person who feels well. The caution which has been exercised concerning serum transaminase abnormalities is understandable in view of initial emphasis upon necrosis as the major or only mechanism for elevation of serum activity. The mechanism of late elevations remains to be elucidated, as does the relationship of the entity to unresolved hepatitis. Possibly, hypertransaminasemia and unresolved hepatitis represent the same type of abnormality. In neither case is restriction of activity warranted, for the course is benign.

Prolonged or Recurrent Symptoms Without Documented Liver Disease (Prolonged Convalescence, Posthepatitis Syndrome). By definition, patients in this category have symptoms, but *no* biochemical or morphologic evidence of liver disease. The incidence of isolated abnormalities of one of the so-called liver function tests is no more frequent than in asymptomatic patients who recovered from viral hepatitis.[356] In terms of frequency, this syndrome was thought to be the most important sequel of viral hepatitis, and was compared to the "effort syndrome" among the soldiers of World War I.[157] After the second World War, the term "posthepatitis syndrome" was suggested.[357]

Some patients apparently recover from

the acute illness and all the laboratory features of the disease return to normal limits, but they have chronic complaints. Their symptoms include: depression; mild anorexia; failure to regain their initial weight, or even further weight loss; lack of return of libido; and fatty food intolerance (for foods such as bacon or pork chops, although they tolerate well rich desserts and ice cream). Occasionally, the liver edge is palpable, but hepatomegaly cannot usually be demonstrated. The liver is normal in shape and consistency. Liver biopsy shows no abnormalities of note which cannot be seen in other patients who recovered from viral hepatitis and are asymptomatic.

Some investigators, including one of us (J.W.M.), feel that this prolonged convalescence is an intrinsic feature of viral hepatitis. They point to the infrequency of similar emotional disturbances following recovery from other illnesses of comparable severity, and the occurrence of depression in persons previously and subsequently free from this complaint. Other investigators, including the second author (J.T.G.), feel that it is more likely that the illness provides the neurotic patient with an acceptable excuse for disability, and point to the frequency of prolonged convalescence following industrial accidents. In either case the proper approach is to reassure the patient that the symptoms will disappear with time, as in fact they do in most instances.

Life-Threatening Variants of Viral Hepatitis. *Fulminant Viral Hepatitis.* This term is applied to the clinical picture in which the disease runs a rapidly downhill course and is fatal, usually within 3 weeks. Occasionally, alterations of consciousness dominate and death occurs before jaundice becomes detectable. Among the 196 cases reported by Lucké and Mallory during World War II, over half the deaths occurred within 10 days of onset of symptoms, and three-quarters of the patients died within 3 weeks.[237] The symptoms of fulminant hepatitis may be present from the beginning, or develop during the course of what appeared to be typical viral hepatitis.

The illness may begin with mild malaise and anorexia, but progresses within a few days to somnolence, stupor and coma. The danger signals which may indicate the development of fulminant hepatitis are: insomnia (sedation may precipitate deep coma), severe vomiting, excessive irritability, confusion, asterixis, drowsiness, and convulsions (most often seen in children). One of the most ominous signs heralding massive hepatic necrosis is the rapid decrease in size of a previously enlarged, tender liver.

Fever develops in most patients with fulminant hepatitis. Leukocytosis with neutrophilia is a usual finding. This finding contrasts with the normal or low level of leukocytes, with relative lymphocytosis, in typical viral hepatitis.

Gastrointestinal bleeding may develop in association with a marked decrease of serum fibrinogen concentrations as a result of diffuse intravascular coagulation. Occasionally the one-stage prothrombin time remains within 60 per cent of normal until just before death. More commonly, the prothrombin time is prolonged because of the deficiency of clotting factors II, V and VII. Verstraete et al. have pointed out that the coagulation factors depressed in liver disease are those consumed in formation of fibrin.[393] They have also found that the half-life of fibrinogen is shortened in liver disease.

Hyperventilation with low serum bicarbonate concentration may be the result of respiratory alkalosis of hepatic coma, but in some patients it is due to lactic acidosis. To distinguish between these two conditions, one must measure the pH of arterial blood. Lactic acidosis is suspected if: (1) the serum bicarbonate falls rapidly, (2) the concentrations are below 12 mEq/L., (3) there is an unexplained anion gap, and (4) the urine pH is low. Lactic acidosis progresses rapidly and is fatal unless promptly corrected with infusion of sodium bicarbonate. Ringer's lactate is ineffective in the treatment of lactic acidosis. When oliguria and azotemia are associated with this disease, edema and ascites may accumulate because of salt and water overload. Hyponatremia may develop because of the infusion of large volumes of glucose in water.

Submassive Hepatic Necrosis (Subacute Hepatitis). Patients in this category must be defined on the basis of histopathologic diagnosis, for the course is so variable that a clinically accurate term that aptly characterizes it is lacking. "Subacute hepatitis" is the closest approximation to an appropriate clinical designation, but fails to convey to the contemporary physician a sense of the seriousness of this variant.

For many patients with subsequent evidence of submassive hepatic necrosis, the onset is characteristic of typical viral hepatitis. In others, nonspecific symptoms of anicteric hepatitis, such as anorexia, malaise and lassitude, may last for weeks or months. During this prolonged preicteric phase the illness becomes progressively more debilitating. Occasionally the first clinical manifestation of the disease is unexplained ascites.

Later phases of the disease may simulate typical viral hepatitis, but with a more protracted, stormy course. In contrast with typical hepatitis, fever lasts longer than a few days; anorexia, nausea and vomiting are more persistent, and enlargement of the spleen is thought to be more frequent.

The serum transaminase levels fluctuate during the course of the disease. The alkaline phosphatase may be normal or markedly elevated. Extremely high serum levels of alkaline phosphatase were seen by one of us in association with clubbing and "pulmonary" osteoarthropathy. The serum albumin concentration is usually lowered, and gamma-globulin levels are high. Some of these patients have positive tests for LE factor, rheumatoid factor or Wassermann antibody.

There is no unequivocal clinical or laboratory feature, nor is there a sufficiently typical combination of these abnormalities which would confirm the diagnosis of submassive hepatic necrosis. The only definite diagnostic tests is a liver biopsy.

The necrosis is not confined, as in typical viral hepatitis, to small "spotty" areas scattered throughout the liver cell plates, but involves large confluent areas of the liver parenchyma. Despite the variability of the clinical course, submassive necrosis apparently develops early in the course of the disease. The variant develops more frequently in women than in men, and usu-

ally in women who are over 40 years of age.[386] The disease runs a subacute course in about one-third of patients, and terminates in death within a few months.

Chronic Hepatitis and Postnecrotic Cirrhosis (Chronic Active Hepatitis). These are diseases or the spectrum of a disease likely due to several etiologic agents or factors. The IH and SH viruses are among the probable causes; it seems unlikely, however, that they account for all or even a majority of cases unless inapparent infection leads to this result far more frequently than episodes clinically diagnosable as viral hepatitis.[204] The latter possibility has been suggested, but cannot be substantiated from present data. The proportion of cases of chronic hepatitis and postnecrotic ("posthepatitic") cirrhosis due to *recognized* viral hepatitis is small; the proportion of cases of viral hepatitis that progress to chronic active hepatitis must be very small.

The onset of illness may be acute and indistinguishable from that seen in typical viral hepatitis. However, the onset may be prolonged and vague, with a protracted preicteric period like that described above in submassive hepatic necrosis. Some patients, particularly children, are diagnosed after the incidental discovery of asymptomatic hepatosplenomegaly.

The incidence of the disease is unknown and the age distribution is not clear. The disease has been seen in prepubertal children, among teenagers, as well as in adult males and females. Chronic active hepatitis was described as occurring predominantly in girls.[23, 400] Later, the same disease was described in both boys and girls following viral hepatitis.[414] Many of the patients remain relatively asymptomatic for various periods of time. The liver and spleen are moderately or markedly enlarged. Early in the course of the disease patients usually do not have ascites, spider angiomata or encephalopathy.

There is no irrefutable evidence from serial biopsies in individual patients or epidemiologic studies of large groups that *typical infectious hepatitis* progresses to chronic active hepatitis or postnecrotic cirrhosis. If this sequence does take place, it occurs in numbers so small that statistical analysis of epidemics of infectious hepatitis have not demonstrated this progression.[8, 54, 69, 281, 288, 421]

On the other hand, it is well recognized that chronic active hepatitis or postnecrotic cirrhosis develops following the serious variants of viral hepatitis, i.e., submassive hepatic necrosis and chronic hepatitis. It seems likely that events that lead to postnecrotic cirrhosis are determined early in the course of the hepatitis. Both submassive hepatic necrosis and chronic hepatitis are thought to represent an atypical response of the host to viral hepatitis. Two suggested hypotheses are: (1) an abnormal immune response (as discussed in Chapter 16) and (2) an altered hepatic mesenchymal response.

The second of these hypotheses postulates an excessive mesenchymal reaction relative to the parenchymal injury.[117, 118] This atypical mesenchymal response can be detected with histochemical technics as early as 6 to 7 days after hepatocellular damage. The mesenchymal response of submassive necrosis and chronic hepatitis is not observed in typical viral hepatitis, whether the biopsy is taken early or late in the course of the clinical disease. This hepatic mesenchymal reaction is characterized by the accumulation in the perisinusoidal space of highly negatively charged macromolecules (glycosaminoglycans) which surround not only injured but also morphologically intact hepatocytes. Because of the density of their electronegative charges, such a layer of macromolecules could act comparably to ion-exchange resins. Consequently, these moieties may have a significant effect on parenchymal metabolism.

The role of glycosaminoglycans as surface blocking and triggering agents for cell division has been documented.[231] This explanation is supported by Tisdale's observation[386] of low mitotic counts in livers with submassive hepatic necrosis, in contrast to those with acute viral hepatitis. The observation that glycosaminoglycans stimulate the fibrous organization and regulate fiber formation and fiber size would also support this theory.[118, 136, 140, 416]

A cycle of mesenchymal response–parenchymal injury would explain the progressive nature and the persistent activity of chronic hepatitis. It is not clear whether the abnormal mesenchymal response is due to humoral or immunologic factors or some other genetically determined cause. Nevertheless, the mechanism for the chronic progressive nature of submassive hepatic necrosis and chronic hepatitis seems to lie in the hepatic mesenchyma.

MANAGEMENT OF VIRAL HEPATITIS

Therapy is not specific. Management is based on: (1) analogies with other forms of liver disease in man or in the experimental animal, (2) clinical impressions gained during the management of individual patients with viral hepatitis, and (3) clinical studies. The most reliable data are, of course, derived from clinical studies, but few are adequately controlled. In addition, almost all the conclusions based on well-controlled studies are limited in application because they have dealt with the disease in otherwise healthy young men. One must use caution in applying the conclusions gained from such studies, despite their scale, to patients whose illness is caused by a different strain of virus and whose age, sex and general health vary from those of the study subjects.

In general, ordinary viral hepatitis is managed by rest, food and drugs. Therapy consists of: (1) What one must do and (2) what one must not do.

TYPICAL VIRAL HEPATITIS

General Measures. Rest is one of the most time-honored features in the management of human disease. Indeed, perhaps the best evidence for the occurrence of infectious hepatitis in Hippocratic times is the controversy over bed rest. The Coan school generally maintained that patients should be allowed ambulation *ad libitum*, whereas the Cnidian school insisted on strict bed rest.

It is usually not necessary to insist that a person acutely ill with viral hepatitis remain in bed, for he feels too ill to stir about. Personal pressures due to business or family affairs, however, sometimes prevent the patient from obtaining adequate bed rest at this stage of the illness. The patient should be in bed as long as he feels he needs to be in bed. Hospitalization is sometimes the only way to provide adequate rest, especially for mothers of young children.

As the patient begins to feel better, he may also desire to have bathroom privileges, to sit up for meals or to move about for an increasing number of other reasons. Whether rigidly enforced bed rest during these periods is superior to ambulation is a moot question.

In general, there are three points of view concerning bed rest: (1) That bed rest be rigidly enforced even though the patient feels well enough to ambulate, (2) that the patient be forced out of bed and made to ambulate even though he feels too ill or fatigued to do so and (3) that ambulation proceed according to the patient's sense of well-being and his rate of improvement.

Bed rest until liver function tests return to normal or stabilize at levels near normal was first suggested out of experience in the Mediterranean Theater in World War II.[20, 21, 45] Hepatitis patients among troops who had been debilitated by the severe physical demands of war were permitted early ambulation, which seemed to increase the frequency of relapse and other sequelae. This concept was reinforced by the theoretical consideration that the erect position decreases hepatic blood flow by 40 per cent[38, 68] and more recently by evidence that exercise decreases the flow by 80 to 85 per cent.[335, 399] Assuming that any decrease in hepatic blood flow lengthens the course of hepatitis, it follows that the upright position and physical exercise prolong hepatic debility.

The average duration of hospital bed rest for soldiers with viral hepatitis rose from 30 days in 1943–44, to 50 days in the Mediterranean Theater in 1943–45, to 60 days in Europe in 1947–49, to 89 days in the Orient in 1950–51.[154] Since the early 1950's,[50] however, the emphasis on strict bed rest and prolonged confinement has been increasingly challenged. For patients who walked about the ward as they wished,

regardless of the severity of jaundice, the course of the illness was not affected as long as they rested in bed after each meal.[50, 288] Indeed, it has been claimed that hard physical exercise during acute viral hepatitis has no deleterious effect.[289] Nevertheless, Swift et al. found some worsening when patients with high serum bilirubin concentrations exercised, but no such untoward effect was detectable if the serum bilirubin concentration was less than 3 mg./100 ml.[381]

The conflicting studies have resulted in a wide range of opinions and formulae concerning the time of ambulation. Some authorities have specific yardsticks regarding the duration of bed rest during acute illness and the duration of convalescence. Others have used specific levels of serum bilirubin, BSP retention and/or transaminase activity. Such conventions are poorly supported by available evidence and seem excessively rigid. Any of the laboratory indices mentioned may remain elevated for prolonged periods without any necessary relationship to evidence of clinically significant disease.

The studies in military personnel may not be uncritically transposed to an older civilian population. To date, however, no evidence is available that increase of hepatic blood flow during recumbency accelerates the rate of healing of viral hepatitis. Furthermore, the prolonged bed rest by itself results not only in physical debility, but is emotionally disturbing to some patients and may also lead to economic hardship.

One must not condone prolonged bed rest in viral hepatitis beyond the overt clinical illness. Patients with good appetite and a sense of well-being, regardless of the depth of jaundice, may ambulate in their rooms within the limits of physical fatigue. Such limited activity has not been shown to be deleterious. Even during the acute illness, if the patient's physical strength permits, he can use the bathroom or a bedside commode. When the patient's sense of well being returns and laboratory abnormalities improve, one should determine whether ambulation alters the rate of improvement. After performing an out-of-bed task, the patient should rest in bed before proceeding to the next activity. Gradual ambulation can hasten rather than slow recovery.

Generally, certain laboratory tests are helpful. Most useful are the serum transaminases and the serum bilirubin. In some patients, however, the serum transaminases show a secondary rise after 2 or 3 weeks of illness; this does not necessarily indicate any deterioration of the patient's general condition. Indeed, elevations may occur during continued clinical improvement. The test for BSP retention helps in evaluating such patients, but it cannot be repeated frequently because the danger of anaphylaxis increases with each injection.

Results of physical examination of the liver and laboratory procedures permit progressive ambulation of the improving patient. When in doubt, one should reduce ambulation in an attempt to increase the rate of improvement. If increased bed rest does not prove superior to ambulation, the patient may resume activities that will permit the rate of improvement obtainable with bed rest. These considerations are particularly important in prolonged hepatitis, which may last for months.

Return to bed rest with only bathroom privileges is advisable in hepatitis relapses, but increasing ambulation is permitted again when the patient and his laboratory tests improve, provided improvement continues during progressive ambulation.

Weakness and easy fatigability are common after viral hepatitis, particularly for patients who have been kept in bed for long periods of time. They result more often from prolonged bed rest than from the ravages of a self-limited disease.

Diet. Acutely ill patients with viral hepatitis should receive over 16 carbohydrate calories (4 Gm. of glucose) per kg. of body weight. Early in the disease, anorexia, nausea and vomiting may cause problems in achieving this goal. Although the patient is nauseated, he usually can take some food by mouth. Hard candy, carbonated drinks and fruit juices are often retained when other foods are not. If food is not retained, intravenous glucose is used to supplement the oral calories and also to provide hydra-

tion, and 10 per cent glucose in water is given as a source of water and energy. Potassium and sodium chloride should be added to the glucose solution to replace losses by vomiting.

Because some patients with severe viral hepatitis cannot excrete a normal water load, the administration of large amounts of hypotonic glucose in water may induce water intoxication. For this reason, 10 per cent rather than 5 per cent glucose should be used. Rarely is urine output reduced to a point at which administration of 10 per cent glucose in water is contraindicated. Excessive hydration is indicated by (1) an unexplained rise in body weight and (2) a decline of serum sodium concentration and hematocrit. Concentrated glucose infusion is required only in submassive or massive hepatic necrosis.

As vomiting subsides and appetite returns, the diet recommended is 1 Gm. protein/kg. body weight and 30 to 35 calories/kg. body weight. This amount of food divided into five or six small feedings, rather than three large meals, is more likely to be consumed.

In the civilian population, a high calorie intake, particularly of proteins, is of questionable value. A forced high protein (150 Gm.) and high calorie (3,000) diet had a slight effect on the rate of convalescence of soldiers with infectious hepatitis.[50] On the other hand, a similar diet did not compare favorably with an *ad libitum* diet in 67 volunteers with serum hepatitis.[225] The duration of illness of the high calorie diet group was either longer than or similar to controls in these experiments. The disadvantage of possible weight gain during inactivity outweighs the possible advantages of such culinary largesse. The strain of virus has a greater effect on the duration of illness than the food intake.

Regulation of fat in the diet is based on an analogy with management of gallbladder disease and on the fact that experimental liver disease among rodents does not improve on a high fat–low protein diet.[420] It is doubtful that this is an adequate basis on which to treat hepatitis patients on a low fat–high protein diet. An ill patient with poor appetite would much rather avoid "heavy" or "greasy" food. Under these conditions, the low fat diet has its basis in common sense rather than scientific observations. For a group of patients with viral hepatitis who consumed a high fat diet, BSP clearance did not improve any more slowly and probably did so more rapidly than the controls.[172]

One of the traditionally important "do not's" in the dietary management of viral hepatitis is consumption of alcoholic beverages. Havens[154] has pointed out that others have emphasized the harmful effects of ethanol without adequate evidence. A single intravenous infusion of 80 mg. of ethanol per kg. body weight (equivalent to two martinis) in acute viral hepatitis had no demonstrable effect on the activities of two serum transaminases and two dehydrogenases.[119] Nevertheless, larger amounts of ethanol are deleterious to hepatic metabolism and morphology in human subjects regardless of dietary intake.[337]

After a patient recovers completely from viral hepatitis, alcohol ingestion has not been demonstrated to be more harmful than for the general population. The practice of forbidding alcoholic beverages for 1 year or more after full recovery from viral hepatitis is not based on acceptable clinical studies. Gardner et al. did not find a relationship between the drinking habits of 114 soldiers and the appearance of residuals 6 to 12 months after recovery from viral hepatitis.[121] However, excessive alcoholic intake soon after jaundice subsides has been followed by relapse of the hepatitis in a few cases.[70]

There is no evidence that vitamin supplements contribute to the therapy of viral hepatitis. The customary administration of water-soluble vitamins by mouth is harmless in well-nourished individuals and may help patients with previously poor dietary habits.

Vitamin K is usually administered in viral hepatitis whenever the prothrombin time is depressed. A single injection of 10 mg. of menadione intramuscularly or the same amount of phytonadione (vitamin K_1) intravenously is justified because of the evidence for impaired absorption of fat during acute hepatitis.[61] If marked improvement in prothrombin time follows, the basis for the diagnosis should be reconsidered, for such a result is unlikely to occur in hepatocellular damage. Repeated injections in an attempt to force the prothrombin time to respond are not only useless but may be harmful. For some patients with hepatocellular disease the prothrombin time is further prolonged for 24 to 48 hours after vitamin K is administered.[390] In premature infants menadione competes with bilirubin for glucuronide conjugation, and sometimes causes an increase in hyperbilirubinemia.

Drugs. *Corticosteroids.* Corticosteroid administration in the typical form of viral hepatitis may result in a more rapid decrease of the transaminase activity and bilirubin concentration in the serum.

Following ACTH or corticosteroid therapy, serum bilirubin strikingly decreased in half to two-thirds of patients with viral hepatitis.[51, 415] When a rapid decrease was observed, it began within 1 to 2 days and lasted 1 to 3 days. The average decline was 32 per cent per day, compared with 22 per cent per day in the hyperbilirubinemia due to other causes. The initial, rapid decrease was followed by a second phase characterized by a much slower decline averaging 7.4 per cent per day. Corticosteroids did not affect the slow phase of bilirubin decrease, the biliary or urinary excretion of bilirubin or erythrocyte breakdown.[415] A statistically significant difference in rate of decline of bilirubin, transaminases and aldolase could not be demonstrated by De Ritis and co-workers,[76] although the mean was slightly faster in all indices among patients receiving prednisone.

No reliable evidence is available that corticosteroids either slow the rate of liver cell necrosis in typical viral hepatitis or increase the rate of liver cell regeneration. The incidence of relapse of viral hepatitis increased when the original illness was treated with corticosteroids.[96, 97]

Corticosteroid therapy is not indicated in typical acute viral hepatitis.[350] It does not shorten the illness sufficiently to risk the complications of these agents. Corticosteroids apparently are beneficial when the disease is unusually severe, the jaundice continues to deepen after 3 weeks, and anorexia and vomiting are not controlled by conservative management. These considerations become even more important indications if the patient is over 45 years of age. Once started, for whatever reason, corticosteroid therapy should be continued for 3 to 4 weeks with gradually decreasing doses. If therapy is suddenly stopped, the probability of relapse increases.

Estrogens. The administration of estrogens to women with chronic active liver disease resulted in an increase of serum bilirubin concentrations.[23] For many normal women BSP retention becomes abnormal following the institution of anti-ovulatory drugs, and some may become jaundiced due to liver cell necrosis. The American Medical Association has accordingly advised against the use of oral contraceptives in "hepatic disease."[62] On the other hand, anti-ovulatory drugs used to prevent pregnancy in a group of young women with chronic liver disease in Switzerland did not significantly alter liver function tests.[250] An Expert Committee of the World Health Organization also expressed an opinion that estrogens do not aggravate the course of viral hepatitis.[58]

On the basis of these conflicting data, it seems advisable not to administer "birth control pills" during the acute phase of viral hepatitis. Evidence is not sufficient to exclude the toxic effect of estrogens on an already diseased liver.[294] Furthermore, there is little likelihood that this type of prophylaxis would be needed under the circumstances. After recovery from viral hepatitis, anti-ovulatory drugs may be instituted for the first time, or can be re-instituted. The serum bilirubin and one of the transaminase activities should be followed. If the bilirubin and transaminase levels continue to rise, however, the anti-ovulatory drugs should be discontinued. Abnormal BSP retention is common during administration of these drugs even in women who have not had hepatitis, and is not necessarily a contraindication to their continued use.

Antiemetics. Nausea and vomiting in typical viral hepatitis usually subsides within a few days. Antihistamines have

proved useful in ameliorating these symptoms. If avoidance of oral intake and antihistamines do not provide sufficient relief, phenothiazines may help.

Antibiotics. Broad-spectrum antibiotics were administered in several viral diseases, including viral hepatitis, as soon as they became available in the late 1940's. No evidence has emerged from these studies to justify their use in viral hepatitis.

Fresh Blood. In severe viral hepatitis prothrombin time may be prolonged due to deficiencies in clotting factors II, V and VII, and, sometimes, fibrinogen. If bleeding occurs, it is important to transfuse patients with fresh blood, fresh frozen plasma or prothrombin concentrate. Blood collected under vacuum in a glass container rapidly loses its factor V content. Even in plastic containers in 24 hours the viability of platelets is seriously impaired and the activity of AHF is appreciably diminished.[263] The recommended hemostatic level of factor V is at least 5 to 10 per cent,[36] or 25 per cent of normal[408]; and of factor VII 10 to 20 per cent of normal.[233] The disappearance rate of infused factor V was T ½ = 16 hours; factor VII had a two-phase decay curve for the first T ½ = 4 hours, and the second T ½ = 39.5 hours.[37]

Immune Serum Globulin (ISG) in the Treatment of Active Illness. From experience with other viral diseases, it would be anticipated that immune serum globulin (ISG) is of no value in the treatment of viral hepatitis. This is, in fact, the finding in the large-scale studies of both acute[127] and chronic hepatitis.[396] As much as 45 ml. of ISG was of no demonstrable benefit. This experience was confirmed in a smaller series of patients also given corticosteroids at the United States Army Hepatitis Center in Germany.[95]

The report of a marked effect of convalescent serum on the outcome of canine hepatitis is unverified.[265] Even if the result is confirmed for the animal model, the experience cited above does not suggest that similar effect could be anticipated in human hepatitis.

ISG for Protection of Contacts. The attending physician should assume responsibility for seeing that ISG is administered to household contacts. The dosage is discussed in the last section of this chapter.

Reporting of Cases. Infectious and serum hepatitis are notifiable diseases in all States of the United States. Each case should be reported to the local health authority, on the postal card form used for acute communicable diseases. The physician in charge of care is responsible for making such reports. As discussed below, control measures in the community are dependent upon as complete a picture of hepatitis morbidity as can be obtained.

RELAPSING OR PROLONGED VIRAL HEPATITIS

The same measures used for acute hepatitis are applicable in relapsing or prolonged hepatitis. There is a tendency, however, to be less critical in evaluating the possible benefits of corticosteroids in the latter group. A sufficient number of patients has not been studied to persuade one that corticosteroid therapy shortens the course of an otherwise prolonged viral hepatitis. Remember that prolonged hepatitis is a self-limited, although protracted, disease.

Bed rest for months is debilitating by itself; its purpose is to accelerate recovery and prevent postnecrotic cirrhosis. If the clinical condition is not improved by bed rest, ambulation should be permitted. The extent of ambulation depends on the behavior of the clinical and laboratory manifestations of the disease.

CHOLESTATIC VIRAL HEPATITIS

Cholestasis due to viral hepatitis is primarily a problem in differential diagnosis. The only therapeutic maneuver that is uniquely helpful in cholestatic hepatitis is the use of cholestyramine when pruritus becomes clinically significant. Patients with transient steatorrhea are helped by reducing intake of the usual dietary fats. Steatorrhea is rarely severe enough to warrant supplementary administration of medium-chain fatty acids.

Corticosteroid therapy was associated with decrease of jaundice in some patients with this form of hepatitis,[300] but many others have not shown such gratifying responses. In a group of 5 patients with cholestatic hepatitis, one showed no decreased serum bilirubin concentration with either ACTH or corticosteroid treatment. In the remaining 4, the initial rapid decrease of serum bilirubin averaged 10 per cent per day and was followed by a slower rate of decrease. Neither corticosteroids nor ACTH has an apparent effect on the second phase of this response.[379, 415] Nevertheless, corticosteroids continue to be used in this form of hepatitis despite the absence of reliable data confirming their effectiveness.

FULMINANT VIRAL HEPATITIS

General Measures. The cornerstones of therapy are: (1) to maintain an adequate blood volume and urine flow; (2) to provide at least 16 carbohydrate calories (4 Gm. glucose) per kg. per day; (3) to avoid oral protein intake; and (4) to administer 8 to 10 Gm./day neomycin by mouth or by stomach tube. Neomycin enemas may alter the intestinal flora more rapidly and ameliorate hepatic encephalopathy. Peritoneal dialysis is of no value in inducing recovery in this fulminant disease.

Daily weight, daily hematocrit and frequent serum electrolyte measurements are obtained. Because renal failure is frequent, the creatinine and urine volume are determined daily. Patients should be watched for bleeding tendency which may be due to either a decrease of clotting factors II, V and VII or a rapid decrease of plasma fibrinogen concentration as a result of diffused intravascular clotting.

Lactic acidosis may appear and progress rapidly unless treated with large amounts of sodium bicarbonate intravenously.

Corticosteroids. Theoretically this therapy delays parenchymal necrosis, promotes regeneration and suppresses tissue injury due to immunologic or inflammatory insults. No evidence supports this. Although corticosteroids are generally used in fulminant hepatitis, their therapeutic value has not been established.

Ducci and Katz enthusiastically recommended the use of massive doses of corticosteroids in fulminant hepatic failure due to massive hepatic necrosis.[88] Katz et al. believed that the recovery of 7 of 19 patients with fulminant viral hepatitis was related to corticosteroid therapy.[199] Additional reports of survival from fulminant hepatic necrosis following corticosteroid therapy appear in the literature.[98] Unfortunately, others, including the authors, have not had similar success with moderate or massive doses of corticosteroids in treating fulminant hepatitis.

Growth Hormone. This hormone is administered in the hope that it may accelerate regeneration of the hepatic parenchyma. Growth hormone, indeed, accelerates regeneration of resected liver in hypophysectomized rats. To date, there is no evidence that growth hormone is deficient in fulminant hepatitis or that parenchymal regeneration is accelerated by growth hormone in humans with this disease.

Exchange Transfusions. Successful treatment of a patient in hepatic coma with exchange transfusion was first reported in January, 1958[223]; the procedure did not become popular, however, until 1966. The rationale for this approach is the removal of nondialyzable "toxic" compounds that may inhibit hepatic parenchymal regeneration or other essential metabolic functions, for example, in the nervous system. It is hoped that the removal of any deleterious factors will delay death sufficiently to allow hepatic regeneration and recovery. No specific "toxic material" removed by exchange transfusion has been identified to date. Whatever this material may be, it was not removed either by hemodialysis or by peritoneal dialysis, which have induced neither recovery of consciousness nor survival in comatose patients.

Following exchange transfusions, comatose patients with fulminant hepatic failure may regain consciousness for varying periods of time. Some who respond relapse into coma and die; others recover. Whether the case fatality rate is reduced by this form of drastic therapy remains to be seen. If the criteria for selection of patients for exchange transfusion are relaxed, patients who would otherwise survive will be exposed to the possible complications and dangers of exchange transfusions.

Extensive clinical experience must be accumulated to define the exact criteria for selection of patients. The currently recognized indication for exchange transfusion is progressive or fulminant hepatic failure associated with hepatic coma.

Technic of Exchange Transfusion. A Cournand needle or a catheter is put into an artery and a catheter is placed in a large central vein. If a renal dialysis team is available in the hospital, they may insert a silastic Teflon cannula to produce an arteriovenous arm shunt. Blood can be removed from the arterial side intermittently and fresh blood infused with the aid of a motor-driven pump in the venous side. This equipment speeds the exchange and reduces fatigue on the part of the physicians caring for the patient. The venous catheter can also be used to monitor central venous pressure.

For each exchange 75 to 100 ml./kg. of fresh, heparinized blood is used. Effort should be made to preserve platelets. The clotting time is controlled by repeated protamine injections. The exchange should proceed as rapidly as technical factors permit. Several exchanges have been performed on successive days before improvement became noticeable. Once exchange transfusion has been performed, it should be repeated on subsequent days, although no clearcut, immediate improvement takes place. Patients may respond only to a third or fourth exchange or, rarely, even later.

The venous and arterial catheters can be kept in place for weeks. When blood is not being administered or withdrawn, the catheters can be filled with heparinized saline and closed. The central venous catheter can also be used to administer hypertonic glucose solutions.

Recently, plasma exchange has been recommended. This procedure consists of the infusion of 300 ml. of fresh frozen plasma for each 500 ml. blood removed. The patient's plasma is discarded and packed red cells are infused. When fulminant hepatic failure is caused by viral hepatitis, plasma exchange is probably more hazardous for laboratory personnel than exchange of whole blood.

Complications of Exchange Transfusions. (1) The risks of exchange transfusions are few. Hematoma may develop at the puncture site, but this can be prevented by careful management. Arterial catheters can be kept in place for 4 weeks without untoward effect. Infection can be a serious problem, however, so that extreme care must be exercised to avoid infection at the puncture site. If infection develops or is strongly suspected, the catheter must be immediately removed.

Some patients develop hypoglycemia and will require the administration of glucose in high concentrations. This hypoglycemia may not be adequately controlled by the infusion of 5 per cent glucose alone. If serum albumin concentration begins to fall, an adequate concentration is maintained with the infusion of concentrated albumin solutions.

BLEEDING DIATHESIS. Following the infusion of fresh blood, the initially prolonged prothrombin time usually improves transiently. Following exchanges, thrombocytopenia develops in almost every patient. It may be related to agglutination of platelets by specific or nonspecific antibodies, to intravascular coagulation,[393] or to mechanical destruction in the transfusion procedure. The thrombocytopenia is usually transient, but if bleeding occurs, the infusion of platelet concentrates or blood collected within 6 hours is required.[263]

SUBMASSIVE HEPATIC NECROSIS

Treatment of submassive hepatic necrosis is generally that of severe typical viral hepatitis. The major difference is the apparent, although not yet conclusively documented, benefit attributed to corticosteroid therapy. Fifty to 60 mg. of prednisone is given per day and the therapy is continued with gradually decreasing doses for months. The duration of treatment should be gauged not only by clinical examination and biochemical analysis of liver function but also by liver biopsy. The progressive downhill course of the disease has been arrested or reversed in patients while they were given corticosteroid therapy.

In addition to the apparent beneficial effect of corticosteroids on the clinical illness, these hormones may effect the development of chronic sequelae of this severe hepatic lesion. Here again, lack of well-controlled studies makes it uncertain whether corticosteroids prevent the development of

cirrhosis. Despite such treatment, submassive hepatic necrosis usually progresses to postnecrotic cirrhosis. However, some patients with well-documented submassive hepatic necrosis recover normal hepatic function and morphology after receiving corticosteroids.[117, 386] For the therapy of late sequelae of this form of hepatitis, see Chapter 16.

PREVENTION

In an era of rapid advances in viral diseases, it is commonplace to think almost exclusively in terms of vaccination for prevention. For the foreseeable future, however, no vaccine is likely to be available against infectious or serum hepatitis. There has usually been a delay of 5 to 10 years between the growth of a virus in tissue culture and general availability of a vaccine derived from it. The polioviruses were first cultivated in tissue culture in 1948; a vaccine was not licensed until 1955. The virus of measles was isolated in 1954; a measles vaccine was licensed in 1963. The problem of assessing the safety of either an inactivated or a live, attenuated vaccine against infectious hepatitis will probably be even greater than usual because of the question of late sequelae from inapparent, smoldering infection. For serum hepatitis, active immunization of the general population may not be feasible even if a vaccine is developed, because of numerous practical problems.

There are many approaches to the prevention of viral infections other than active immunization. This is certainly true for serum hepatitis and to a lesser extent for infectious hepatitis. Instrument-associated hepatitis, for example, whether due to the SH or IH agent, is theoretically entirely preventable. Transfusion-associated hepatitis, at least in relation to whole blood and some blood products, cannot be eliminated; there are, however, ways to reduce its incidence. Water- and food-borne infectious hepatitis, although infrequent, represent epidemiologic forms of infectious hepatitis which can be controlled.

Each epidemiologic entity requires an approach suitable to the mode of transmission. For example, measures that prevent instrument-associated hepatitis have no relevance to water-borne hepatitis. The way in which infection is acquired in the individual case, therefore, has implications for the prevention of other potential cases from the same source. Preventive measures, if they are to be effectively directed, must be based on a continuing search for those modes of transmission contributing to viral hepatitis in the particular community.

Table 13–10 indicates the preventive measures applicable to each epidemiologic form of infectious and serum hepatitis. Certain aspects of these approaches deserve further comment. For details concerning use of immune serum globulin, see the last section of this chapter.

Personal and Environmental Hygiene

Good personal hygiene should reduce the incidence of infectious hepatitis, as it does of other diseases transmitted by the fecal-oral route. In contact-associated hepatitis, fecal particles are presumably transferred to the mouth from hands contaminated by direct contact with the infected person, or soiled indirectly through objects in the environment. Consistent with this concept are the high attack rates often observed among young children, among groups in lower socioeconomic levels, and in institutions housing persons intellectually or emotionally incapable of practicing good hygiene.

There seems no reason to doubt that poor hygienic habits on the part of either the infected person or his susceptible contacts contribute to an increased risk for the latter group. It is by no means clear, however, that *excessive* cleanliness greatly reduces the likelihood of infection after known exposure.

Most susceptible persons living in the same household as a patient with infectious hepatitis are infected by the time the diagnosis is made. Under any circumstance, all household members should receive immune serum globulin for prophylaxis. Rigid isolation, therefore, is not necessary. The patient's dishes and linen do not require separate handling, as long as soap and hot water are used routinely in the household.

Separate toilet facilities are not needed, although hand washing may be emphasized to reduce the intensity of exposure.

Supervised hand washing at schools in the face of an epidemic may help reinforce a habit desirable from the standpoint of preventing all enteric infections; epidemiologic evidence suggests that the practice does little to alter the course or extent of an outbreak of infectious hepatitis. "Disinfection" of desks, door knobs and other objects in the school room similarly contributes nothing.

Handling of Recently Imported Primates

Recently imported nonhuman primates, particularly chimpanzees, are a potential source of infectious hepatitis (as well as other diseases). For at least 60 days after their entry into the United States contacts should be restricted to the minimum required for care. Several victims of chimpanzee-associated hepatitis acquired their infection during coffee-breaks or lunch hours through unauthorized play with these animals.

If a person must handle a primate, he should wear protective clothing and wash his hands carefully after contact with the animal's paws, fur or cage. In this situation good personal hygiene and environmental sanitation do appear to be of value. Routine immune serum globulin (ISG) should be administered to handlers only when the volume of newly imported animals is high and cleanliness fails. The effect of ISG administration to chimpanzees is unknown.

Water and Food Sanitation

The same engineering practices that have contributed to safety of drinking water supplies from the standpoint of typhoid fever and gastroenteritis are applicable to prevention of infectious hepatitis transmitted by drinking water. Early recognition of a water-borne epidemic is of importance from two standpoints: (1) Because of the long incubation period of infectious hepatitis, contamination has often ended before cases begin to occur. In other instances, however, contamination is intermittent or

TABLE 13–10.   APPROACHES TO PREVENTION OF INFECTIOUS AND SERUM HEPATITIS
BASED ON MODE OF TRANSMISSION

EPIDEMIOLOGIC ENTITY (MODE OF TRANSMISSION)	ETIOLOGIC AGENT(S)	APPROACHES TO PREVENTION
Contact-associated hepatitis	IH virus	1. Administer ISG to household contacts.
Primate-associated hepatitis	IH virus	1. Restrict contacts of nonhuman primates for 60 days after importation. 2. House in animal quarters permitting good sanitation. 3. Limit physical contact of handlers to minimum for care; wear protective devices to prevent fecal soiling of clothing; wash hands carefully after contact. 4. Administer ISG to persons having continued exposure to newly-imported animals if above measures fail to achieve control.
Water-borne hepatitis	IH virus	1. Monitor public and private water supplies for evidences of fecal pollution. 2. Avoid uncertain or infrequently used supplies. 3. Observe reported cases for unexpected clustering or shift in age distribution. 4. Administer ISG to persons exposed to supply when epidemic wave is recognized.
Shellfish-associated hepatitis	IH virus	1. Vigorously police contaminated (closed) waters. 2. Avoid raw or partially cooked shellfish of uncertain quality, especially abroad. 3. Question patients for history of ingestion of raw or steamed clams or oysters within 50 days of onset. 4. Observe reported cases for clustering of cases with history of shellfish ingestion.
Food-borne hepatitis (other than shellfish-associated)	IH virus	1. Enforce good food sanitation practices. 2. Observe reported cases for unexpected clusterings or shift in age distribution. 3. Administer ISG to persons exposed to food when epidemic wave is recognized.
Blood-associated hepatitis	SH virus IH virus	1. Enforce high standards of donor quality. 2. Report all cases of blood-associated hepatitis (10 to 180 days) to bank supplying blood and health department. 3. Maintain donor registers, with exclusion of recognized carriers (similar to typhoid carrier register in relation to food handling). 4. Administer blood only when necessary. 5. Administer no more blood than necessary. 6. Monitor hemoglobin and hematocrit determinations for accuracy as index of need for transfusion.
Plasma-associated hepatitis	SH virus	1. Substitute heat-sterilized product (plasma protein solution or albumin).

TABLE 13–10 *Continued*

EPIDEMIOLOGIC ENTITY (MODE OF TRANSMISSION)	ETIOLOGIC AGENT(S)	APPROACHES TO PREVENTION
Fibrinogen-associated hepatitis AHG-associated hepatitis	SH virus	1. Administer only when hypofibrinogenemia is specific cause of bleeding. 2. Substitute single unit fresh frozen plasma if feasible. 3. Administer all units from one lot. 4. Record manufacturer and lot number of all recipients. 5. Observe contaminated (icterogenic) lots.

Syringe-associated hepatitis
Instrument-associated hepatitis
	SH virus
	IH virus
		1. Sterilize any instrument that breaks the skin or mucous membranes, or that is contaminated with blood or tissue fluids.
		  a. boil 30 minutes.
		  b. autoclave 15 psi for 30 minutes.
		  c. dry heat 160° C. for 60 minutes.
		2. Use disposable equipment *once*.
		3. Avoid multiple-dose-per-syringe technic.

Addiction-associated hepatitis	SH virus IH virus	1. Educate drug-addicts to danger of sharing unsterilized syringes.
Tattoo-associated hepatitis	SH virus IH virus	1. Supervise sterilization practices of tattoo parlors. 2. Educate drug-addicts to danger of sharing unsterilized equipment or dyes (often improvised).

persistent, so that detection of the fault can prevent further cases. (2) If an epidemic is recognized early, administration of ISG may prevent disease in some exposed persons.

In some instances, water-borne epidemics of infectious hepatitis are preceded by "herald waves" of gastroenteritis. Water-borne epidemics of gastroenteritis occur far more frequently than those of infectious hepatitis, and should not be considered of themselves an indication for ISG administration.

Food-borne epidemics of infectious hepatitis have been recognized with increasing frequency in recent years; they are, nevertheless, uncommon. They undoubtedly are decreased in frequency by: (1) good personal hygiene on the part of food handlers; (2) minimizing the extent that food is actually handled; and (3) preventing sewage contamination of foods in storage, especially those served without cooking. In some food-borne epidemics, a food handler

has been recognized to have had overt disease; in the remainder, no source of contamination could be identified.

No information is available concerning the frequency with which infection is transmitted by an overtly ill food handler, but it appears to be rare. It seems advisable, therefore, to withhold ISG from persons eating food in the establishment unless it is clear that a person with poor hygienic habits has definitely handled food served without further cooking. Although a food handler who develops infectious hepatitis should be prohibited from handling food until fully recovered, there appears to be no benefit in exclusion beyond convalescence. To the extent that volunteer experiments are applicable, their results indicate that fecal excretion of virus ends not long after onset of jaundice.

Shellfish-associated hepatitis is more difficult to prevent. Although shellfish sanitation practices undoubtedly contributed to the decline of shellfish-borne typhoid fever, general sanitation improvements, with decrease in the frequency of the typhoid bacillus in sewage, must also have had a role. Application of quality standards to growing areas, patrol and inspection, all contribute to shellfish safety. The problems of preventing illegal harvesting are so numerous, however, that other solutions must be found. Several hundred cases of shellfish-associated hepatitis occur each year in the United States; consumption of raw shellfish abroad may also result in an increased risk of disease. The best guarantee is purchase of shellfish to be eaten raw or with minimal heating from a supplier of known reputation.

Transfusion-Associated Disease

In the absence of a specific virologic procedure for detection of carriers, many blood banks have adopted "liver function" tests as screening procedures. The studies of their value have yielded conflicting results. Strumia et al.,[377] and Jennings and co-workers[188] concluded from their investigations that the thymol turbidity tests could be helpful, and Bang et al.[19] found the serum aspartic transaminase of value. These tests have not appeared useful in identifying carriers, however, in the hands of other investigators[40, 197, 253] and their worth from a practical point of view is doubtful.

A number of other methods are presently available for lowering the incidence of post-transfusion viral hepatitis. They should be applied to the maximal extent.

Enforcement of Adequate Standards of Donor Quality. Although hospital blood banks would like to be able to meet their needs through replacement and volunteer donors, almost none can do so. They must rely on additional sources of blood, such as the Red Cross, community blood banks and commercial blood banks. It is the responsibility of the hospital blood bank and the physician to know the integrity, professional competence and financial practices of blood banks from which they obtain blood and blood derivatives.

Identification of Known or Suspected Carriers Through Central Registries. The carrier state of viral hepatitis may persist over a prolonged period of time. It is extremely important, therefore, that carriers of hepatitis virus be identified and excluded from future donations.

It is impractical for most hospitals to conduct follow-up studies of all persons who receive blood from their banks. It is possible, however, to question all cases of viral hepatitis concerning prior transfusion of blood or blood products. This is an ethical, and should be a legal obligation. Such cases should be reported as serum or transfusion-associated hepatitis to the local health department, and to the blood bank that supplies the units received.

Few hospitals notify the blood bank that supplies blood if the recipient develops transfusion-associated hepatitis. Even if the blood bank does exclude such a person by a notation on its own records, it seldom informs the donor himself that his blood is potentially hazardous. Nor are other blood banks notified of the donor's likelihood of being a carrier. Therefore, possible or even probable carriers are not being excluded effectively.

Carrier registries similar to those for food handlers who harbor the agent of typhoid fever are just beginning to be established. On a statewide basis they exist so far only in New Jersey and Rhode Island. However, cooperative arrangements do exist on a less extensive scale. Such programs are important in reducing the incidence of transfusion-associated viral hepatitis.

Use of Blood And Blood Derivatives Only When Necessary. Potentially icterogenic materials should be used only if clearly necessary. If whole blood or other "average risk" materials must be used, the minimal amount that will accomplish the purpose should be given.

In general, it is agreed that initiation of transfusion *with the intention* of administering only a single unit within the patient's immediately foreseeable course is a questionable practice. If, however, after transfusion is begun it becomes apparent that only 1 unit is required, then 1 unit is all that should be given. Administering a second unit approximately doubles the patient's risk of developing hepatitis (Table 13–6).

A "high risk" blood derivative (irradiated pooled plasma or fibrinogen) should not be used if a safer substitute (albumin, plasma protein fraction, or fresh frozen plasma) will accomplish the same purpose. If the immunoglobulin fraction is needed, ISG can be separately administered. If a "high risk" derivative must be used, all units administered should be from the same lot.

Accurate Laboratory Determination for Indicating the Need for Blood and Blood Derivatives. Many factors not immediately apparent affect the frequency of transfusion, which in turn, determines the total number of cases of transfusion-associated hepatitis. This is illustrated by the findings of Mann and co-workers concerning the relationship between reported values for hemoglobin from the hospital laboratory and the transfusion rate.[249] On two occasions during their study re-standardization raised the reported hemoglobin values. After each re-standardization the transfusion rate decreased up to 35 per cent. The investigators showed that a decrease of only 5 per cent in reported hemoglobin levels due to technical difficulty during a 48-hour period resulted in 2 patients in their hospital who received blood unnecessarily. A quality-control program obviated most of the inaccuracies and permitted rapid detection of deviations from accuracy in the procedure.

The necessity for constant supervision of the hemoglobin determination has been emphasized by Sundermann.[380] Standards sent out by the Proficiency Testing Service of the American Society of Clinical Pathologists have indicated a gradual increase in the frequency of errors in clinical hemoglobinometry. Sundermann attributes this to greater use of commercially prepared standard solutions by hospital laboratories. Obviously a quality-control program must include checks against both intra- and extramural standards.

Adequate Transfusion Records. The ability to identify the recipient of a given unit of blood, *and*, conversely, the unit number or numbers received by a given patient are both indispensable parts of defining the problem of transfusion-associated hepatitis.

Carriers can be identified only if blood can be traced from donor to recipient and from recipient back to donor. The work of a hospital transfusion committee[404] requires a list of recipients and the units of blood and blood derivatives administered to each. While all hospitals keep some records concerning whole blood, such records are frequently unsatisfactory. The card or ledger entry usually indicates cross-matching of a unit for a given patient, but often does not state definitely whether the blood was given to that patient. One may have to resort to the patient's chart to see whether blood was administered. Even in the chart, the doctor's orders or the nurse's notes may have to be scrutinized. Occasionally, the only adequate indication that a transfusion was given will be found in the accounting office.

When pooled plasma, fibrinogen and antihemophilic globulin are used, the name of the manufacturer and the lot number should be recorded. The lot of these "high risk" derivatives can then be identified if hepatitis develops subsequently. If the same lot is common to other cases, the unused units should be promptly withdrawn from the shelves. In many hospitals, however, these products are dispensed by the pharmacy instead of the blood bank, without adequate records being kept of recipients, the manufacturer or the lot number. As a consequence, it is usually extremely difficult to establish attack rates due to these products, or to incriminate specific lots so that the unused portion can be withdrawn. It is to be strongly urged, therefore, that plasma, fibrinogen and antihemophilic globulin be dispensed only through hospital blood banks, with maintenance of similar records as for whole blood. It should be possible to identify recipients of a particular lot, and to identify the lot and manufacturer for any given recipient.

STERILIZATION OF INSTRUMENTS AND EQUIPMENT

An instrument that breaks the skin of one person should be sterilized before being introduced under the skin of a second. The evidence concerning the adequacy of various procedures is derived from two major sources: (1) experimental studies in which bacterial spores have most frequently been used as the model and (2) epidemiologic observations of situations in which transmission of viral hepatitis was prevented by instituting or changing some practice. As usual, the evidence is not as ample as one would like in order to make many of the necessary practical decisions. The data are sufficient, however, to define acceptable standards in most instances.

Syringes, needles, instruments and other equipment should be disassembled and cleaned of gross blood. This permits better heat penetration and reduces the amount of protection afforded to viruses by organic material in their milieu. Such cleaning is potentially hazardous to persons carrying out the cleaning operation.[170] Gloves should be worn at all times in handling blood-contaminated equipment, for immersion of apparently unabraded hands in contaminated cleaning solutions may well be responsible for many infections of medical and paramedical personnel. In some hospitals equipment is autoclaved prior to cleaning.

There is evidence that disinfectant solutions are not adequate to inactivate the hepatitis agent. Phenol, tricresol and thimerosal were all found ineffective in early studies (Table 13–2). A recent investigation of the effect of polyethoxy-ethanol-iodine (Wescodyne) on enteroviruses showed that the presence of other organic matter caused rapid loss of virucidal potential.[403] Ineffectiveness probably results also from sequestration of some virus particles in protein precipitates, making them inaccessible to further inactivation by chemical agents. Viable virus persisted on glassware despite overnight immersion in a solution of prescribed strength.

Boiling for 20 to 30 minutes appeared to be effective in inactivating the hepatitis agents.[412] On the other hand, boiling for 5 minutes presumably was not effective in at least one instance.[94] Similarly, autoclaving at 15 psi for 30 minutes and dry heat at 160° for 60 minutes were effective measures in venereal disease clinics in the 1940's. Any of the three methods is acceptable.

Fragile equipment that would be damaged by heating is frequently sterilized with ethylene oxide. Of particular pertinence to the problem of viral hepatitis is its position as the most acceptable approach to sterilization of plastic parts in heart-lung machines. Because many factors such as concentration, temperature, pressure and humidity influence the effectiveness of ethylene oxide against bacterial spores, there are some reservations about its efficiency in average daily use.[362] Its ability to inactivate viruses has been studied very little. Vaccinia and Columbia SK viruses on a glass surface were inactivated by a 10 per cent concentration in 8 hours, but not in 6 hours.[203] Poliovirus suspended in albumin or fibrinogen showed linear rates of inactivation proportional to concentration of ethylene oxide at 20° C., but even the highest concentration (1 per cent) allowed survival of 5 to 1,000 $TCID_{50}$.[15] The possibility of ineffective "sterilization" should be considered, therefore, whenever the incidence of transfusion-associated hepatitis is higher than anticipated in patients undergoing heart surgery.

IMMUNE SERUM GLOBULIN

Satisfactory preparations of concentrated antibodies became available when technics for large-scale separation of plasma protein components were developed in the early 1940's. There was concern about using this material, however, because pooled convalescent serum for mumps and measles was known to cause viral hepatitis. In contrast to expectations, no cases of jaundice were observed. Attention was accordingly directed toward the possibility that contaminating virus was neutralized and that immune serum globulin (ISG) could be used to prevent viral hepatitis.

The first trial of ISG for prevention of infectious hepatitis was in 1944 during a common-vehicle epidemic at a summer camp in Pennsylvania.[284] Of 53 exposed persons who received the material, only 3 (5.7 per cent) subsequently experienced hepatitis with jaundice. In contrast, 45 per cent of the other 278 persons had icteric disease. These results were quickly confirmed in two other studies.[126, 161] Thus, the effectiveness of ISG was established by field trials within a short time of becoming available. No serious question of its value for the prevention of infectious hepatitis has subsequently been raised.

ISG in the United States is produced from both plasma donations and placental blood. The relative proportions from the two sources varies from lot to lot and from manufacturer to manufacturer. Regulations require that each production pool include plasma or blood from at least 1,000 donors, and most lots represent the immunologic experience of much larger populations. All manufacturers use modifications of the cold alcohol technic of Cohn for separation of plasma protein components. American preparations contain 16.5 ± 1.5 Gm. of protein per 100 ml., of which at least 90 per cent must have the electrophoretic characteristics of gamma globulin. Most of the immunoglobulins are of the IgG class, but low levels of IgA and IgM are found in most lots.[164] Relatively wide variations in the concentration of antibodies have been observed in the past.[260, 349] To minimize such discrepancies, minimum levels of antibody to diphtheria toxin, measles virus, and one poliovirus type are now required of each lot. Such antibodies, however, are not necessarily an index of potency against infectious hepatitis.

Although all lots of ISG are theoretically contaminated with SH virus, no instance of hepatitis definitely attributable to prior administration of Cohn-fractionated material has been reported. That the lots of ISG are safe was confirmed by experimental studies in which ISG was prepared from known icterogenic plasma pool.[278] Adverse reactions are generally limited to pain and tenderness at the injection site. Hematomas are seen occasionally, especially in patients who had received anticoagulants and were given large amounts of ISG at a single site. The few reported cases of anaphylactic shock may have been due to inadvertent intravenous injection.

The stimulation of antibodies to heterologous immunoglobulin types in the Gm system has been demonstrated.[3, 370] On this basis, the question of later adverse reactions to transfusion has been raised, although no definitely documented case has been reported. An even more likely consequence would be the shortening of passive immunity, although this has not yet been demonstrated either.

MECHANISM OF PROTECTION AFFORDED BY IMMUNE SERUM GLOBULIN

It is assumed that ISG is protective because it contains antibody to infectious hepatitis. This appears to be why ISG is effective against other infectious agents, and no precedent exists for postulating any other method by which it modifies or prevents infectious hepatitis. Passive immunity afforded by antibody is an assumption, and it is conceivable, even if unlikely, that a protein with properties other than those of neutralizing antibody could be responsible for protection.

If antibody is the means of protection, then infectious hepatitis and measles are the only two diseases in which ISG obtained from the general population is protective in relatively small doses. From this it is assumed that experience with infectious hepatitis is general and that immunity is long-lasting. It is also of interest that ISG from a population in one area of the world seems to protect adequately against infectious hepatitis that occurs in other, distant areas.[272]

Passive immunization protects by suppressing infection or the clinical manifestations. There is adequate evidence that in many cases of infection by the IH virus, ISG suppresses only the clinical illness. This was first documented by Drake and Ming during an institutional outbreak.[85] Using liver function tests to detect inapparent hepatitis, they demonstrated that attack rates in immunized persons were similar to those in unimmunized persons. Inapparent infections occurred during the first 8 weeks after globulin administration in persons who received a dose of 0.005 ml./lb. of body weight, but continued for 13 weeks in the group that received 0.01 ml./lb. The incidence of anicteric hepatitis (illness without clinical jaundice) during the first 4 weeks after administration of ISG was also lower in those who received the larger dose. These observations suggest that with a larger dose not only are clinical manifestations suppressed, but also infection. Possibly, however, the findings represent only more complete suppression of detectable abnormalities, of which the laboratory manifestations are one group.

By serum transaminase assay, inapparent infection in persons who received ISG has been confirmed extensively. Schneider and Mosley found that for household contacts who received ISG in a community-wide epidemic, the incidence of serum aspartic transaminase abnormality was equivalent to that for those to whom protection had not been given.[352] Almost all such abnormalities were observed within 36 days after onset of the index case, which indicates that most of these persons were in the incubation phase at the time ISG was given. Krugman and co-workers likewise found that at an institution for the mentally retarded transaminase and other laboratory abnormalities occurred at the same rate among those who received ISG on admission as inpatients who were not protected.[217] In this situation, infection followed passive immunization, which indicates that modification is also applicable to those not already effectively exposed to it. The fact that ISG permits asymptomatic infections does not exclude the possibility, however, that larger doses administered prior to infection or early in the incubation period may suppress infection entirely. Suppression of infection itself in some instances would be anticipated on the basis of experience with ISG prophylaxis of measles.

The person with inapparent infection due to ISG modification would be presumed to excrete virus to the same extent as an individual with naturally acquired infection. The infected individual who would be confined to bed if he became ill remains in contact with others at school, work and in social situations. It has, therefore, been suggested that use of ISG promotes the spread of infectious hepatitis.[293] Paktoris observed, however, that ISG administered to half of a school population lowered the incidence of infectious hepatitis not only

in the recipients but also in the uninoculated.[302] It must be postulated, therefore, that ISG alters the extent or duration of virus excretion.

Even before these demonstrations, inapparent infection was suspected on the basis of subsequent absence of icteric illness despite continued exposure. Stokes and associates suggested that partial passive immunity conferred by ISG was supplanted by active immunity as a result of "low-grade" infection ("passive-active" immunization).[375] They challenged part of an institutional population protected by ISG more than 1 year earlier, and found a significantly lower rate of induced infectious hepatitis than in a control group. Such protection could be explained only on the basis of active immunity due to inapparent infection.

Some investigators believe that passive-active immunity occurs in the absence of naturally acquired infection. They assume that ISG preparations behave as vaccines because of the presence of neutralized or partly neutralized IH virus in plasma pools.[67] Limited replication of the agent administered in ISG would presumably result in long-term immunization. The findings of Wehrle and Hammon, however, fail to substantiate long-term immunization in the absence of contact with infectious hepatitis in proximity to ISG administration.[409] They determined the incidence in later years of infectious hepatitis among large groups of children given ISG to prevent poliomyelitis. The rate was similar to that in the control group that received gelatin placebo. Passive-active immunization on a short-term basis due to virus in ISG has also been assumed.[207] Theoretically this is unlikely, and is contradicted by the evidence for long-term immunity in those receiving ISG who have natural exposure.[67]

Immune Serum Globulin Administered in the Incubation Period of Infectious Hepatitis (After infection has already occurred). ISG has been found effective in a number of studies on prophylaxis among household contacts. The effectiveness* has usually been 80 to 90 per cent; some varia-

* Percent Effectiveness $= \left(\dfrac{\text{Attack rate in untreated} - \text{Attack rate in treated}}{\text{Attack rate in untreated}} \right) \times 100$

tion is due to differences in the definition of "failures." Experience indicates that 0.005 to 0.01 ml./lb. of body weight protects as adequately as larger doses.[85, 108] Recommendations that doses of 0.02 ml./lb. be given to children and 0.06 ml./lb. to adults[215] were based on studies in which ISG was administered prior to exposure, and in which the globulin preparation used may have been substandard.[272] For practical purposes 0.5 ml. is given to children who weigh less than 50 lb., 1.0 ml. to older children who weigh less than 100 lb., and 2.0 ml. to all adults.

Since the incubation period is relatively long, ISG can be administered to many susceptibles prior to onset of symptoms. This is particularly true for household contacts. ISG can be given to persons exposed to a common source if it is recognized sufficiently early. The course of several epidemics due to a common vehicle has been truncated by administration of globulin to those known to have been exposed.[273, 318] The earlier in the incubation period ISG is given, the more likely it is to have a protective effect.[212] It is worthwhile, however, to administer ISG up to 6 weeks after known exposure (Fig. 13–3).

Immune Serum Globulin Administered Prior to Infection. ISG prevents disease when administered prior to exposure. Its use for this purpose, particularly among Americans abroad, has increased greatly in recent years.

The half-life of ISG is often used as a guide to the duration of protection and the time for administration of subsequent doses. The most frequently cited values are those obtained by Dixon and co-workers using [131]I: 20.3 days in children and 13.1 days in adults.[80] Results using ^{35}S labeling of autogenously synthesized gamma globulin indicate slower metabolism.[12, 398] Martin et al., measuring antibody by biologic assay, found various rates of degradation for antibodies with different antigenic affinities.[251] The mean half-life of antibodies ranged from 21.7 days for Coxsackie A10, to 44.9 days for adenovirus type 2.

There is no reason to assume that the half-life of antibody to infectious hepatitis deviates significantly from the values for other antibodies. The pertinence of these data, however, to the need for readministration of ISG cannot be evaluated without two other pieces of information not presently available: (1) the level of antibody obtained after administration of a given dose of a particular ISG preparation and (2) the minimum level of antibody that is protective. It is necessary to know *how many half-lives* must elapse after a given dose before there is significant risk of overt disease if exposure takes place.

The duration of ISG protection should ideally be determined in a group all of whom are continually and uniformly exposed to challenge. While such ideal conditions are not found, they seem to be most closely approximated by prolonged institutional epidemics. When ISG is administered to part of an institutional population during an epidemic, the time at which cases begin to occur at the *same* rate in the immunized group as in the control may be taken as the end of passive protection.

Studies of institutional epidemics indicate prolonged periods of protection with ISG. Stokes et al.[375] observed absence of cases for 7 to 12 months after 0.01 ml./lb. of body weight; Drake and Ming,[85] for 15 weeks after 0.005 and 0.01 ml./lb.; and Krugman, Ward and associates,[218] for 5 to 12 months after 0.06 ml./lb. More recently, Krugman has presented data showing that 0.02 and 0.06 ml./lb. both protected residents of Willowbrook State School for 5 months.[213] Employees of the School appeared to have a substantial reduction in incidence when given 5 ml. of ISG at 6-month intervals.

INDICATIONS FOR PROPHYLAXIS OF INFECTIOUS HEPATITIS

During the 1950's ISG was probably under-utilized in situations in which it would have been of value, especially with regard to prevention of disease in household contacts. During the 1960's the extent of its use has rapidly increased, so that even the *possibility* of exposure is now sometimes considered adequate justification for ISG administration. The public is widely aware of its availability, and because the material is innocuous the physician may yield to the patient's demand when he would not otherwise do so. The indications for use of ISG, therefore, need careful reconsideration.

Household Contacts. In the United States, secondary attack rate among household contacts is frequently high. Rates of icteric disease have been as great as 45 per cent among children. The incidence of secondary infections is lower in adults, but nonetheless 5 to 20 per cent. As a result the usual practice in the United States is to administer ISG to all persons living in households in which cases occur. Administration of ISG in a dose of approximately 0.01 ml./lb. to all household contacts as soon as the index case is diagnosed is easily justified. Indeed, protection of susceptible household contacts is an integral part of the care of the patient.

In some instances, it is considered unnecessary to administer ISG to adults because of the low attack rate in this group. Although the incidence is lower in persons 20 years of age and over, it is sufficiently high after household exposure to warrant protection. The illness in adults is more serious and of greater economic consequences for the family. Even grandparents or other older adults living in the household should receive ISG. Instances of severe or even fatal illnesses in older, unprotected persons have come to our attention.

It has also been argued that ISG should not be given to children in the household. It is felt that their illness is mild, and that they should acquire permanent immunity from active infection. Administration of ISG, however, does not prevent infection in either household or institutional contacts, and immunity appears to be comparable.

School Contacts. Although school-centered epidemics occur in the United States, epidemiologic evidence suggests that neighborhood play contact among children of school age is of more importance than classroom contact. For this reason, it does not appear justified to administer ISG on a school-wide or classroom-wide basis unless there is clear evidence that infections are being acquired at the school itself.

In contrast, in Czechoslovakia, Poland and Russia nursery and school contact is thought to spread infectious hepatitis more than household contact. As a result, school-wide administration of ISG has been widely practiced in Eastern European countries. The data suggest that the incidence of infectious hepatitis is reduced in this way.[302] As indicated, however, this practice apparently reduces the amount of circulating IH virus, as evidenced by a lower attack rate in groups that have not received this material, and over a prolonged period could result in a highly susceptible population.

Work Contacts. Infectious hepatitis is infrequently transmitted by casual contact such as that which occurs in an office. The few reported situations suggest respiratory rather than fecal-oral transmission.[123] Although use of common toilet facilities frequently causes concern to co-workers of the hepatitis patient, administration of ISG is not justified.

Institutions. Institutions are comparable to households in the intimacy of contact, and high attack rates similar to secondary rates in households sometimes occur. Explosive epidemics are particularly likely when hygiene is poor, as among the mentally retarded or regressed psychiatric patients, or when sanitation is substandard. When infectious hepatitis threatens to become rampant, use of ISG is justified.

In general, infectious hepatitis in institutions for retarded or psychiatric patients shows three patterns: (1) freedom from disease for long periods, followed by explosive epidemics; (2) sporadic cases with occasional epidemics of limited extent; and (3) continuous endemic hepatitis. The third pattern is usually seen only in large institutions with high rates of admission and discharge.

In institutions largely or entirely free of the disease, ISG is administered to cottage, dormitory or ward mates of patients with infectious hepatitis in the hope of restricting the disease to one building. Such attempts, however, are often unsuccessful. Retarded patients appear to be the most likely persons to transmit the disease in the incubation period, and it is spread commonly by patients who work or visit in other parts of the institution before jaundice is recognized. Institution-wide administration whenever hepatitis occurs in an inmate, however, is expensive. Delay, therefore, is justified until the infection is clearly propagating itself, for cases sometimes remain isolated or are limited to small clusters. Whether institution-wide administration of ISG in institutions with endemic infection can abolish the disease is unknown.

Common Source or Common-Vehicle Exposure. ISG is indicated for persons exposed to a recognized common source of infection such as a group of infected chimpanzees or a common-vehicle such as water or food. Illnesses in such situations have undoubtedly been prevented by this measure. Prevention of cases is one of the major reasons for continual alertness to the possible occurrence of common-vehicle epidemics.

Water- and food-borne outbreaks of infectious hepatitis have been preceded by a "herald" wave of gastroenteritis. In contrast, however, water- and food-borne gastroenteritis is rarely followed by infectious hepatitis. Similarly, a few food-borne epidemics of infectious hepatitis have followed disease in a food handler; more commonly, no overt case was recognizable, or was recognized only in retrospect. In many instances a food handler has developed hepatitis without transmitting it. In view of these facts, it seems justified from the public health point of view not to administer ISG to persons potentially exposed until the first case occurs in the group. Since the incubation period is relatively long, most cases can be prevented; the alternative is large-scale and repetitive overuse of the material.

Immune Serum Globulin Prophylaxis in Persons for Whom Exposure is Anticipated. To an ever greater extent, ISG is being given to persons or groups believed to have an increased risk of exposure. In some instances this anticipation of risk is well founded upon experience; in other situations, such use is probably not justified. Unfortunately, data are lacking to define the attack rate in many situations in which risk *may* be increased.

Travel or Residence Abroad. The systematic use of ISG to prevent infectious hepatitis among persons in high risk areas was begun by the Swedish. As early as 1956, a contingent of Swedish troops serving under United Nations' auspices in the Gaza Strip received this material, and it was used regularly after 1957.[207] The incidence of viral hepatitis was reduced from 4.0 per cent among unprotected Swedish soldiers to 0.1 per cent. Marked reductions were achieved in other Scandinavian contingents for which the practice was adopted.

Through the late 1950's, the frequent occurrence of viral hepatitis among some Americans abroad was often mentioned, but no reports appeared in the medical literature. Some use of ISG to protect individual travelers probably began during this time. By 1961, when the first groups of Peace Corps Volunteers went abroad, the possibility that infectious hepatitis could be a significant hazard was sufficiently well known that ISG was made available for individual units on an optional basis. Some unprotected contingents remained free of the disease; two unprotected groups in South America, however, had rates of 14 per cent. As a result, the measure became mandatory in 1962.

Data have recently been collected on the incidence of viral hepatitis in American missionaries, who have generally served abroad without having ISG prophylaxis. The overall risk for Protestant missionaries and their dependents was 1.6 per cent per year in one study.[56, 57] Rates were highest among younger adults, and varied with the area of residence as indicated in Figure 13–23. The incidence in per cent per year among adults ranged from 8.0 in North Africa and the Middle East to 0.5 in Japan. Frame found overall rates of 2.0 to 3.8 per cent among American missionaries in Ethiopia and the Sudan.[110]

It is difficult to generalize from these limited data to other groups in order to make recommendations. The risk varies from area to area and from time to time in any given area because of long-term secular trends and seasonal factors. The type of travel accommodations should also affect the risk. Table 13–11 is a guide to ISG prophylaxis abroad. It probably represents as adequate a set of recommendations as can be formulated from insufficient data.

For convenience, ISG immunization is usually given just prior to departure overseas. Ideally, however, it should be administered during the second month of travel or residence in view of the paucity of cases in the first 2 months abroad. If travel or

residence abroad is prolonged ISG should be administered again every 6 months. A single injection of ISG appears to protect for this length of time.

In no area of the world is infection sufficiently frequent to dependably provide immunization during the first 6 months. Continued administration of ISG is necessary

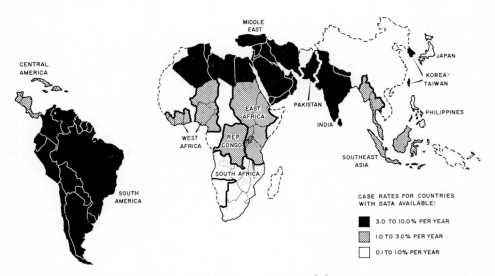

Fig. 13–23. Case rates of viral hepatitis among adult American missionaries in various geographic areas abroad, 1945–64. (From Cline et al.[56])

TABLE 13–11. GUIDELINES FOR ISG PROPHYLAXIS OF INFECTIOUS HEPATITIS FOR U.S. RESIDENTS TRAVELING OR LIVING IN FOREIGN COUNTRIES[322]
(See text for additional details)

INDIVIDUAL'S WEIGHT (lb.)	ISG DOSE (ml.) Short-term Travel (1–2 Months)	Extended Travel or Residence (3–6 Months)†	ROUTINE ISG PROPHYLAXIS* Indicated	Not Indicated
			AFRICA ASIA	EUROPE NORTH AMERICA Canada
Up to 50	0.5	1.0	NORTH AMERICA Central America Mexico (rural)	Caribbean Islands Mexico (urban)
50–100	1.0	2.5		
Over 100	2.0	5.0	PACIFIC REGION Philippine Islands South Pacific Islands SOUTH AMERICA	PACIFIC REGION Australia Japan New Zealand

* In all travel, care should be exercised in consuming uncooked foods and water of uncertain quality.
† Repeat every 6 months of travel or residence.

for protection during the entire period of residence and subsequent periods of sojourn abroad.

As little as 0.01 ml./lb. has protected in institutional outbreaks for 6 months or longer.[375] Similarly, Kluge observed good protection for up to 6 months with doses of approximately 0.007 to 0.02 ml./lb.[207] Thus, 0.02 to 0.03 ml./lb. every 6 months seems to be a reasonable recommendation. A convenient dose for adults is 5.0 ml. Larger doses (up to 0.06 ml./lb.) have been thought to protect for a longer period. Although this concept should be true *a priori*, the data do not substantiate the necessity for nor any advantage of higher doses.

Medical and Paramedical Personnel. In general, one should rely on measures other than administration of ISG for prevention of infectious hepatitis.[46] When fecal soiling of the environment is extensive, it may be necessary to administer ISG to lower the incidence of infectious hepatitis in exposed personnel. Apparently a dose of 5.0 ml. every 6 months is as adequate as larger or more frequent injections.

Chimpanzee Handlers. Routine administration of ISG to personnel who care for recently imported chimpanzees has been widely adopted. Good hygienic and sanitation practices in proper animal quarters probably provide adequate protection in most instances. When the disease cannot otherwise be controlled, 5.0 ml. of ISG every 6 months should be used.

ATTEMPTED PROPHYLAXIS OF SERUM HEPATITIS

The initial study of ISG for prevention of serum hepatitis was carried out among World War II battle casualties by Grossman, Stewart and Stokes soon after the material became available.[138] The results suggested that immune globulin helped to ameliorate or prevent subsequent serum hepatitis. Ten ml. of immune globulin was given to alternate patients at varying times after blood and/or plasma had been received, and again 1 month subsequently. The maximum period of follow-up was 175 days and the minimum was 85 days after admission.

A second study by Duncan and co-work-ers employing a single 10 ml. dose of immune globulin demonstrated no difference in the incidence of serum hepatitis among treated and untreated patients.[90] One 10 ml. dose was given alternately to newly admitted battle casualties who had been transfused. The minimum period of follow-up was 207 days. Of the 2,406 patients who received globulin, 1.2 per cent developed icteric hepatitis. Of 2,374 controls, 0.9 per cent became ill. Incubation periods, however, among those who received ISG appeared to be significantly more prolonged than among those not receiving globulin.

Because of the discrepant results among these studies, Stokes and co-workers carried out a number of well-controlled studies using human volunteers.[374] In none of these could it be shown that ISG was protective or altered incubation periods. Attack rates and incubation periods were similar in control and treated groups.

It was postulated that the failure to protect against the strain of serum hepatitis used in the preceding experiments was due to a lack of experience with this virus in the donor population from which the globulin was derived. Accordingly, studies were carried out with "hyperimmune" globulin prepared from plasma of volunteers infected with the same strain 4 months to 6 years earlier.[82] No protection was demonstrated even when 2 ml. of "hyperimmune" globulin was mixed in the same syringe with 0.04 ml. of infectious serum.

Because of these negative results, no further work was carried out until a cooperative study was initiated in Baltimore by Mirick, and continued by Ward in Los Angeles and McCollum in New Haven.[262] Ten ml. of globulin was administered to 623 patients at the time of transfusion and again 1 month later, while 622 patients served as a control group. The incidence of icteric hepatitis was 1.1 and 4.0 per cent, respectively. The incidence was similar for all forms of the disease (icteric, anicteric and inapparent hepatitis). Apparently ISG was protective.

The results of Mirick and co-workers prompted Holland et al. to re-study the problem, also using two doses of 10 ml. each approximately 1 month apart; no effect of ISG was demonstrated.[175]

These conflicting results pose a problem for the internist and the surgeon. In general, the more adequately controlled studies have failed to demonstrate protection even with two doses. Therefore, ISG should *not* be given for attempted prophylaxis of serum hepatitis. This position has also been taken by the Public Health Service Advisory Committee on Immunization Practices[322] and other responsible groups. Attempts to compromise by recommending use of ISG for some "high risk groups"[313] ignores the quality of the negative evidence. The likelihood of protection is not proportional to the need. In addition, many potential legal difficulties are associated with such a position.

REFERENCES

1. Aach, R. D., Evans, J., and Losee, J.: An epidemic of infectious hepatitis possibly due to airborne transmission, Am. J. Epidemiol. 87:99, 1968.
2. Adashek, E. P., and Adashek, W. H.: Blood transfusion hepatitis in openheart surgery, Arch. Surg. 87:792, 1963.
3. Allen, J. C., and Kunkel, H. G.: Antibodies to genetic types of gamma globulin after multiple transfusions, Science 139:418, 1963.
4. Allen, J. G., Enerson, D. M., Barron, E. S. G., and Sykes, C.: Pooled plasma with little or no risk of homologous serum jaundice, J.A.M.A. 154:103, 1954.
5. Allen, J. G., and Sayman, W. A.: Serum hepatitis from transfusions of blood, J.A.M.A. 180:1079, 1962.
6. Alt, H. L., and Swank, R. L.: Thrombocytopenic purpura associated with catarrhal jaundice: Report of a case, Ann. Int. Med. 10:1049, 1937.
7. Altschul, A., Roster, P. D., Paley, S. S., and Turner, L.: Incidence of hepatitis among narcotic addicts in the Harlem Hospital, New York, Arch. Int. Med. 89:24, 1952.
8. Andersen, J., and Vellar, O.: Viral hepatitis: A follow-up study of 373 notified cases in Oslo 1949–53, Acta med. scand. 182:691, 1967.
9. Andersen, T. T.: The etiology of *Hepa-titis epidemica*, Acta med. scand. 93:209, 1937.
10. Andersson, O.: Epidemic of jaundice, Nord. hyg. T. 2:252, 1921.
11. Appelbaum, E., and Kalkstein, M.: Artificial transmission of viral hepatitis among intravenous diacetylmorphine addicts, J.A.M.A. 147:222, 1951.
12. Armstrong, S. H., Jr., Kukral, J., Hershman, J., McLeod, K., and Wolter, J.: Comparison of the persistence in the blood of gamma globulins labeled with S[35] and I[131] in the same subjects, J. Lab. Clin. Med. 44:762, 1954.
13. Astaldi, G., Grandini, U., Poggi, C., and Strosselli, E.: Intestinal biopsy in acute hepatitis, Am. J. Dig. Dis. 9:237, 1964.
14. Atchley, F. O., and Kimbrough, R. D.: Experimental study of infectious hepatitis in chimpanzees, Lab. Invest. 15:1520, 1966.
15. Auerswald, W., and Doleschel, W.: On the sterilizing effect of ethylene oxide on virus suspended in protein solutions, Med. Exp. 6:193, 1962.
16. Babudieri, B., Fiaschi, E., Nacarato, R., and Scuro, L. A.: Presence of virus-like bodies in liver cells of patients with infectious hepatitis, J. Clin. Path. 19:577, 1966.
17. Bachmann, L.: Infectious hepatitis in Europe *in* Rodenwaldt, E. (ed.): World-Atlas of Epidemic Diseases, Part I, p. 67, Hamburg, Falk-Verlag, 1952.
18. Ballance, G. A.: Epidemic of infective hepatitis in an Oxford college, Brit. Med. J. 1:1071, 1954.
19. Bang, N. U., Ruegsegger, P., Ley, A. B., and LaDue, J. S.: Detection of hepatitis carriers by serum glutamic oxalacetic transaminase activity, J.A.M.A. 171:2303, 1955.
20. Barker, M. H., Capps, R. B., and Allen, F. W.: Acute infectious hepatitis in the Mediterranean Theater, J.A.M.A. 128:997, 1945.
21. ———: Chronic hepatitis in the Mediterranean Theater: A new clinical syndrome, J.A.M.A. 129:653, 1945.
22. Batten, P. J., Runte, V E., and Skinner, H. G.: Infectious hepatitis: Infectiousness during the presymptomatic phase of the disease, Am. J. Hyg. 77:129, 1963.
23. Bearn, A. G., Kunkel, H. G., and Slater, R. J.: The problem of chronic liver disease in young women, Am. J. Med. 21:3, 1956.

24. Beck, K., and Kuhn, H. A.: Beitrag zur Pathogenese der funktionellen Hyperbilirubinemie, Z. klin. Med. *155*:547, 1959.

25. Beeson, P. B., Chesney, G., and McFarlan, A. M.: Hepatitis following injection of mumps convalescent plasma, Lancet *1*:814, 1944.

26. Benda, L., Gerlach, F., Rissel, E., and Thaler, H.: Ueber Untersuchungen zur Frage der Virusaetiologie der Hepatitis epidemica, Arch. ges. Virusforsch. *4*:89, 1949.

27. Bennett, A. M., Capps, R. B., Drake, M. E., Ettinger, R. H., Mills, E. H., and Stokes, J., Jr.: Endemic infectious hepatitis in an infants' orphanage. II. Epidemiologic studies in infants and small children, Arch. Int. Med. *90*:37, 1952.

28. Berk, J. E.: Hepatitis following transfusion, Gastroenterology *8*:296, 1947.

29. Bewley, T. H., Ben-Arie, O., and Marks, V.: Morbidity and mortality from heroin dependence. 3: Relation of hepatitis to self-injection techniques, Brit. Med. J. *1*:730, 1968.

30. Biava, C., and Mukhlova-Montiel, M.: Electron microscopic observations on Councilman-like acidophilic bodies and other forms of acidophilic changes in human liver cells, Am. J. Path. *46*:775, 1965.

31. Blacklidge, V. Y.: The clinical significance of Eberlein's method of determining the three main fractions of serum bilirubin, J. Pediat. *62*:666, 1963.

32. Bodian, D.: Poliovirus in chimpanzee tissues after virus feeding, Am. J. Hyg. *64*:181, 1956.

33. Boggs, J. D., Capps, R. B., Weiss, C. F., and McLean, I. W., Jr.: Status report on tissue-cultivated hepatitis virus. II. Clinical trials, J.A.M.A. *177*:678. 1961.

34. Bolin, V. S., Alsever, J. B., Barger, J. B., and Jarvis, T. B.: Studies on serum and infectious hepatitis viruses of man. I. Preliminary report on the isolation of serum and infectious hepatitis viruses from man in tissue culture, Transfusion *1*:360, 1961.

35. Bolin, V. S., Chase, B. S., and Alsever, J. B.: A virus-latex agglutination test for detecting antibodies against isolates associated with viral hepatitis, Am. J. Clin. Path. *49*:635, 1968.

36. Borchgrevink, C. F., and Owren, P. A.: Surgery in a patient with factor V (proaccelerin) deficiency, Acta med. scand. *170*:743, 1961.

37. Bowie, E. J. W., Thompson, J. H., Jr., Didisheim, P., and Owen, C. A., Jr.: Disappearance rates of coagulation factors: Transfusion studies in factor-deficient patients, Transfusion *7*:174, 1967.

38. Bradley, S. E.: Effect of posture and exercise upon blood flow through the liver, p. 53, Seventh Liver Injury Conference, New York, Macy, 1948.

39. Brain, R.: Discussion on recent experiences of acute encephalomyelitis and allied conditions, Proc. Roy. Soc. Med. *36*:319, 1943.

40. Brandt, K.-H., Meulendijk, P. N., Poulie, N. J., Schalm, L., Schulte, M. J., Zanen, H. C., and Streefkerk, J.: Data on the determination of SGOT and SGPT activity in donor blood for the possible prevention of post-transfusion hepatitis, Acta med. scand. *177*:321, 1965.

41. Brightman, I. J., and Korns, R. F.: Homologous serum jaundice in recipients of pooled plasma, J.A.M.A. *135*:268, 1947.

42. Budd, G.: Diseases of the Liver, p. 368, Philadelphia, Lea & Blanchard, 1846.

43. Byrne, E. A. J., and Taylor, G. F.: An outbreak of jaundice with signs in the nervous system, Brit. Med. J. *1*:477, 1945.

44. Cameron, J. D. S.: Infective hepatitis, Quart. J. Med. *12*:139, 1943.

45. Capps, R. B., and Barker, M. H.: The management of infectious hepatitis, Ann. Int. Med. *26*:405, 1947.

46. Capps, R. B., Bennett, A. M., and Stokes, J., Jr.: Endemic infectious hepatitis in an infants' orphanage: I. Epidemiologic studies in student nurses, Arch. Int. Med. *89*:6, 1952.

47. Capps, R. B., Sborov, V., and Scheiffley, C. S.: A syringe-transmitted epidemic of infectious hepatitis, J.A.M.A. *136*:819, 1948.

48. Cawein, M. J., III, Hagedorn, A. B., and Owen, C. A., Jr.: Anemia of hepatic disease studied with radiochromium, Gastroenterology *38*:324, 1960.

49. Chalmers, T. C., Jr.: The occurrence of jaundice in therapeutic and natural malaria, J. Clin. Invest. *26*:1055, 1947.

50. Chalmers, T. C., Eckhardt, R. D., Reynolds, W. E., Cigarroa, J. G., Jr., Deane, N., Reifenstein, R. W., Smith, C. W., and Davidson, C. S.: The treatment of acute infectious hepatitis. Controlled studies of the effects of diet, rest, and physical reconditioning on the acute course of the disease and on the incidence of relapses

and residual abnormalities, J. Clin. Invest. *34*:1163, 1955.

51. Chalmers, T. C., Gill, R. J., Jernigan, T. P., Svec, F. A., Jordan, R. S., Waldstein, S. S., and Knowlton, M.: Evaluation of a four-day ACTH test in the differential diagnosis of jaundice, Gastroenterology *30*:894, 1956.

52. Chalmers, T. C., Koff, R. S., and Grady, G. F.: A note on fatality in serum hepatitis, Gastroenterology *49*:22, 1965.

53. Child, P. L., and Ruiz, A.: Acidophilic bodies, Arch. Path. *85*:45, 1968.

54. Chuttani, H. K., Sidhu, A. S., Wig, K. L., Gupta, D. N., and Ramalingaswami, V.: Follow-up study of cases from the Delhi epidemic of infectious hepatitis of 1955-6, Brit. Med. J. *2*:676, 1966.

55. Clermont, R. J., and Chalmers, T. C.: The transaminase tests in liver disease, Medicine *46*:197, 1967.

56. Cline, A. L., Mosley, J. W., Housworth, W. J., Weddingen, E. J., and Luby, J. P.: Viral hepatitis among American missionaries abroad: Attack rates by geographic area and year of residence, Paper presented at the 15th Annual Meeting, Am. Soc. Tropical Medicine and Hygiene, San Juan, Puerto Rico, Oct. 31–Nov. 4, 1966.

57. Cline, A. L., Mosley, J. W., and Scovel, F. G.: Viral hepatitis among American missionaries abroad: a preliminary study, J.A.M.A. *199*:551, 1967.

58. Clinical aspects of oral estrogens, World Health Organization, Tech. Rep. Series, No. 326, p. 12–13, 1966.

59. Cockayne, E. A.: Catarrhal jaundice, sporadic and epidemic and its relation to acute yellow atrophy of the liver, Quart. J. Med. *6*:1, 1912.

60. Cohen, S. N., and Dougherty, W. J.: Transfusion hepatitis arising from addict blood donors, J.A.M.A. *203*:427, 1968.

61. Colwell, A. R.: Fecal fat excretion in patients with jaundice due to viral hepatitis, Gastroenterology *33*:591, 1957.

62. Committee on Human Reproduction: Control of fertility, J.A.M.A. *194*:462, 1965.

63. Conrad, M. E., Schwartz, F. D., and Young, A. A.: Infectious hepatitis: A generalized disease, Am. J. Med. *37*:789, 1964.

64. Cook, G. C., and Sherlock, S.: Jaundice and its relation to therapeutic agents, Lancet *1*:175, 1965.

65. Creutzfeldt, W.: Die Transfusions Hepatitis und ihre Verhütung, Internist *7*:1, 1966.

66. Creutzfeldt, W., Schmitt, H., Richert, J., Kaiser, K., and Matthew, M.: Transmission of hepatitis over ten years by a blood donor with posthepatitis cirrhosis, German Med. Monthly *8*:30, 1963.

67. Csapo, J., Budai, J., Nyerges, G., Richter, R., and Toth, I.: Active immunization experiments against epidemic hepatitis: I. Mode of action of gamma globulin, Acad. Sci. Hungary *17*:45, 1961.

68. Culbertson, J. W., Wilkins, R. W., Ingelfinger, F. J., and Bradley, S. E.: The effect of the upright position upon the hepatic blood flow in normotensive and hypertensive subjects, J. Clin. Invest. *30*:305, 1951.

69. Cullinan, E. R., King, R. C., and Rivers, J. S.: The prognosis of infective hepatitis: preliminary account of a long-term follow-up, Brit. Med. J. *1*:1315, 1958.

70. Damodaran, K., and Hartfall, S. J.: Infective hepatitis in garrison of Malta, Brit. Med. J. *2*:587, 1944.

71. Davenport, F. M., Hennessy, A. V., Christopher, N., and Smith, C. K.: A common source multi-household outbreak of chimpanzee-associated hepatitis in humans, Am. J. Epidemiol. *83*:146, 1966.

72. Davis, D. J., and Hanlon, R. C.: Epidemic infectious hepatitis in a small Iowa community, Am. J. Hyg. *43*:314, 1946.

73. Deinhardt, F., Courtois, G., Dherte, P., Osterrieth, P., Ninane, G., Henle, G., and Henle, W.: Studies of liver function tests in chimpanzees after inoculation with human infectious hepatitis virus, Am. J. Hyg. *75*:311, 1962.

74. Deinhardt, F., Holmes, A. W., Capps, R. B., and Popper, H.: Studies on the transmission of human viral hepatitis to marmoset monkeys. I. Transmission of disease, serial passage, and description of liver lesions, J. Exp. Med. *125*:673, 1967.

75. Deller, J. J., Jr., Cirksena, W. J., and Marcarelli, J.: Fatal pancytopenia associated with viral hepatitis, New Engl. J. Med. *266*:297, 1962.

76. De Ritis, F., Giusti, G., Mallucci, L., and Piazza, M.: Negative results of prednisone therapy in viral hepatitis, Lancet *1*:533, 1964.

77. De Ritis, F., Mallucci, L., Coltorti, M., Gusti, G., and Caldera, M.: Anicteric virus hepatitis in a closed environment as

shown by serum transaminase activity, Bull. W. H. O. *20*:589, 1959.

78. Dhamdhere, M. R., and Nadkarni, M. G.: Infectious hepatitis at Aurangabad: Report of an outbreak, Indian J. Med. Sci. *16*:1006, 1962.

79. Dible, J. H., McMichael, J., and Sherlock, S.: Pathology of acute hepatitis: Aspiration biopsy studies of epidemic, arsenotherapy and serum jaundice, Lancet *2*: 402, 1943.

80. Dixon, F. J., Talmage, D. W., Maurer, P. H., and Deichmiller, M.: The half-life of homologous gamma globulin (antibody) in several species, J. Exp. Med. *96*:313, 1952.

81. Dougherty, W. J., and Altman, R.: Viral hepatitis in New Jersey 1960–61, Am. J. Med. *32*:704, 1962.

82. Drake, M. E., Barondess, J. A., Bashe, W. J., Jr., Henle, G., Henle, W., Stokes, J., Jr., and Pennell, R. B.: Failure of convalescent gamma globulin to protect against homologous serum hepatitis, J.A.M.A. *152*:690, 1953.

83. Drake, M. E., Hampil, B., Pennell, R. B., Spizizen, J., Henle, W., and Stokes, J., Jr.: Effect of nitrogen mustard on virus of serum hepatitis in whole blood, Proc. Soc. Exp. Biol. Med. *80*:310, 1952.

84. Drake, M. E., Kitts, A. W., Blanchard, M. C., Farquhar, J. D., Stokes, J., Jr., and Henle, W.: Studies on the agent of infectious hepatitis. II. The disease produced in human volunteers by the agent cultivated in tissue culture or embryonated hen's eggs, J. Exp. Med. *92*:283, 1950.

85. Drake, M. E., and Ming, C.: Gamma globulin in epidemic hepatitis: Comparative value of two dosage levels, apparently near the minimal effective level, J.A.M.A. *155*:1302, 1954.

86. Dubin, I. N.: Intrahepatic bile stasis in acute nonfatal viral hepatitis; its incidence, pathogenesis and correlation with jaundice, Gastroenterology *36*:645, 1959.

87. Dubin, I. N., Sullivan, B. H., LeGolvan, P. C., and Murphy, L. C.: The cholestatic form of viral hepatitis: Experiences with viral hepatitis at Brook Army Hospital during the years of 1951 to 1953, Am. J. Med. *29*:55, 1960.

88. Ducci, H., and Katz, R.: Cortisone, ACTH and antibiotics in fulminant hepatitis, Gastroenterology *21*:357, 1952.

89. Dull, H. B.: Syringe-transmitted hepatitis: A recent epidemic in historic perspective, J.A.M.A. *176*:413, 1961.

90. Duncan, G., Christian, H. A., Stokes, J., Jr., Rexer, W. F., Nicholson, J. T., and Edgar, A.: An evaluation of immune serum globulin as a prophylactic agent against homologous serum hepatitis, Am. J. Med. Sci. *213*:53, 1947.

91. Eisenstein, A. B., Aach, R. D., Jacobsohn, W., and Goldman, A.: An epidemic of hepatitis in a general hospital. Probable transmission by contaminated orange juice, J.A.M.A. *185*:171, 1963.

92. Eldh: cited by Selander, P., *in* Hepatitis epidemica, Kinderärztl. Prax. *8*:202, 1937.

93. Eltorm, H., Kjerulf-Jensen, K., and Tygstrup, N.: Cholecystography in patients suffering from acute epidemic hepatitis, Dan. Med. Bull. *2*: 8, 1955.

94. Epidemic of homologous serum hepatitis, Foreign Letters, J.A.M.A. *137*:209, 1948.

95. Evans, A. S., Nelson, R. S., Sprinz, H., and Cantrell, F. P.: Adrenal hormone therapy in viral hepatitis. IV. The effect of gamma globulin and oral cortisone in the acute disease, Am. J. Med. *19*:783, 1955.

96. Evans, A. S., Sprinz, H., and Nelson, R. S.: Adrenal hormone therapy in viral hepatitis. I. The effect of ACTH in the acute disease, Ann. Int. Med. *38*:1115, 1953.

97. ———: Adrenal hormone therapy in viral hepatitis. II. The effect of cortisone in the acute disease, Ann. Int. Med. *38*: 1134, 1953.

98. ———: Adrenal hormone therapy in viral hepatitis. III. The effect of ACTH and cortisone in severe and fulminant cases, Ann. Int. Med. *38*:1148, 1953.

99. Farquhar, J. D.: Renal studies in acute infectious (epidemic) hepatitis, Am. J. Med. Sci. *218*:291, 1949.

100. Faulkner, L.: On epidemic jaundice, Maryland & Virginia M. J. *15*:355, 1860.

101. Findlay, G. M., Dunlop, J. L., and Brown, H. C.: Observations on epidemic catarrhal jaundice, Trans. Roy. Soc. Trop. Med. Hyg. *25*:7, 1931.

102. Findlay, G. M., and MacCallum, F. O.: Note on acute hepatitis and yellow fever immunization, Trans. Roy. Soc. Trop. Med. Hyg. *31*:297, 1937.

103. Findlay, G. M., Martin, N. H., and Mitchell, J. B.: Hepatitis after yellow fever inoculation: relation to infective

hepatitis, Lancet 2:301, 340 and 365, 1944.

104. Findlay, G. M., and Willcox, R. R.: Transmission of infective hepatitis by faeces and urine, Lancet 1:212, 1945.

105. Flaum, A., Malmros, H., and Persson, E.: Eine nosocomiale Ikterus-Epidemie, Acta med. scand., Suppl. 16:544, 1926.

106. Foley, F. E., and Gutheim, R. N.: Serum hepatitis following dental procedures: a presentation of 15 cases, including three fatalities, Ann. Int. Med. 45:369, 1956.

107. Ford, J. C.: Infective hepatitis. 300 Cases in an outer London borough, Lancet 1:675, 1943.

108. Fowinkle, E. W., and Guthrie, N.: Comparison of two doses of gamma globulin in prevention of infectious hepatitis, Pub. Health Rep. 79:634, 1964.

109. Fox, J. P., Manso, C., Penna, H. A., and Para, M.: Observations on the occurrence of icterus in Brazil following vaccination against yellow fever, Am. J. Hyg. 36:68, 1942.

110. Frame, J. D.: Hepatitis among missionaries in Ethiopia and Sudan, J.A.M.A. 203:819, 1968.

111. Francis, T., Jr., Frisch, A. W., and Quilligan, J. J., Jr.: Demonstration of infectious hepatitis virus in presymptomatic period after transfer by transfusion, Proc. Soc. Exp. Biol. Med. 61:276, 1946.

112. Fraser, R.: A study of epidemic catarrhal jaundice, Canad. J. Pub. Health 22:396, 1931.

113. Freeman, G.: Epidemiology and incubation period of jaundice following yellow fever vaccination, Am. J. Trop. Med. 26:15, 1946.

114. Fulop, M., and Sandson, J.: The effect of bile salts on the binding of bilirubin by plasma proteins, Clin. Sci. 33:459, 1967.

115. Fulop, M., Sandson, J., and Brazeau, P.: Dialysability of conjugated bilirubin from plasma of jaundiced dogs and patients, Lancet 1:1017, 1964.

116. Gabinus, O., and Jonsson, T.: Serum hepatitis through wound infection, Lancet 1:43, 1962.

117. Galambos, J. T.: Chronic persisting hepatitis, Am. J. Dig. Dis. 9:817, 1964.

118. ————: Acid mucopolysaccharides and cirrhosis of the liver, Gastroenterology 51:65, 1966.

119. Galambos, J. T., Asada, M., and Shanks, J. Z.: The effect of intravenous ethanol on serum enzymes in patients with normal or diseased liver, Gastroenterology 44:267, 1963.

120. Gard, S.: Discussion in Hartman, F. W., et al. (eds.): Hepatitis Frontiers, Henry Ford Hosp. Int. Symposium, Boston, Little, Brown, 1957.

121. Gardner, H. T., Rovelstad, R. A., Moor, D. J., Streitfeld, F. A., and Knowlton, M.: Hepatitis among American occupation troops in Germany, Ann. Int. Med. 30:1009, 1949.

122. Gardner, H. T., Swift, W. E., Jr., Modica, M., Levintow, L., and Knowlton, M.: Serum cholesterol and cholesterol esters in viral hepatitis, Am. J. Med. 8:584, 1950.

123. Gauld, R. L.: Epidemiological field studies of infectious hepatitis in the Mediterranean Theater of operations, Am. J. Hyg. 43:248, 1946.

124. Gellis, S. S., Neefe, J. R., Stokes, J., Jr., Strong, L. E., Janeway, C. A., and Scatchard, G.: Chemical, clinical, and immunological studies on the products of human plasma fractionation. XXXVI. Inactivation of the virus of homologous serum hepatitis in solutions of normal human serum albumin by means of heat, J. Clin. Invest. 27:239, 1948.

125. Gellis, S. S., and Stokes, J., Jr.: Methylene blue test in infectious (epidemic) hepatitis, J.A.M.A. 128:782, 1945.

126 Gellis, S. S., Stokes, J., Jr., Brother, G. M., Hall, W. M., Gilmore, H. R., Beyer, E., and Morrissey, R. A.: The use of human immune serum globulin (gamma globulin) in infectious (epidemic) hepatitis in the Mediterranean Theater of operations. I. Studies in prophylaxis in two epidemics of infectious hepatitis, J.A.M.A. 128:1062, 1945.

127. Gellis, S. S., Stokes, J., Jr., Forster, H. W., Jr., Brother, G. M., and Hall, W. M.: The use of human immune serum globulin (gamma globulin) in infectious (epidemic) hepatitis in the Mediterranean Theater of operations. II. Studies on treatment in an epidemic of infectious hepatitis, J.A.M.A. 128:1158, 1945.

128. Giles, J. P., Liebhaber, H., Krugman, S., and Lattimer, C.: Early viremia and viruria in infectious hepatitis, Virology 24:107, 1964.

129. Gille, G., Ringertz, O., and Zetterberg, B.: Serum hepatitis among Swedish

track-finders. II. A clinical study, Acta med. scand. *182*:129, 1967.

130. Goldberg, D. M., and Campbell, D. R.: Biochemical investigation of outbreak of infectious hepatitis in a closed community, Brit. Med. J. *2*:1435, 1962.

131. Gordon, I., Patterson, R. P., Dorrance, W. R., Whitney, E., and Gauvreau, A. C.: Evaluation of the embryonated hen's egg as a host for the agent of infectious hepatitis, J. Lab. Clin. Med. *49*:597, 1947.

132. Grady, G. F., Chalmers, T. C., and the Boston Interhospital Liver Group: Viral hepatitis in a group of Boston hospitals. II. A prospective controlled epidemiologic study, New Engl. J. Med. *272*:662, 1965.

133. Graham, G.: Diabetes mellitus: a survey of changes in treatment during the last fifteen years, Lancet *2*:1, 1938.

134. Gregory, C. H.: Studies of conjugated bilirubin. III. Pigment I, a complex of conjugated and free bilirubin, J. Lab. Clin. Med. *61*:917, 1963.

135. Gresser, I., and Chany, C.: Isolation of measles virus from the washed leucocytic fraction of blood, Proc. Soc. Exp. Biol. Med. *113*:695, 1963.

136. Gross, J.: Discussion of: Metabolism of collagen in mammalian tissues by Robertson, W. V. B. *in* Connective Tissue: Intracellular Macromolecules, p. 114, Boston, Little, Brown, 1964.

137. Grossman, C. M., and Saward, E. W.: Homologous serum jaundice following the administration of commercial pooled plasma: A report of eight cases including one fatality, New Engl. J. Med. *234*:181, 1946.

138. Grossman, E. B., Stewart, S. G., and Stokes, J., Jr.: Post-transfusion hepatitis in battle casualties and study of its prophylaxis by means of human immune serum globulin, J.A.M.A. *129*:991, 1945.

139. Hahn, H., and Scherer, E.: Hepatitis bei diabetes mellitus, Z. Verdavvngskr. *11*:22, 1951.

140. Hall, D. A.: The Chemistry of Connective Tissue, Springfield, Ill., Thomas, 1961.

141. Hallgren, R.: Epidemic hepatitis in the county of Vasterbotten in Northern Sweden: an epidemiological and chemical study, Acta med. scand., Suppl. *140*:1, 1942.

142. ———: Epidemic hepatitis in the county

of Vasterbotten in Northern Sweden; II, Acta med. scand. *115*:21, 1943.

143. Hampers, C. L., Prager, D., and Senior, J. R.: Post transfusion anicteric hepatitis, New Engl. J. Med. *271*:747, 1964.

144. Hansbarger, E. A., and Hyun, B. H.: Acute hemolytic anemia in viral hepatitis, Virginia Med. Monthly *90*:134, 1963.

145. Harden, A. G., Barondess, J. A., and Parker, B.: Transmission of infectious hepatitis by transfusion of whole blood, New Engl. J. Med. *253*:923, 1955.

146. Hartfall, S. J., Garland, H. G., and Goldie, W.: Gold treatment of arthritis: a review of 900 cases, Lancet *2*:838, 1937.

147. Havens, W. P., Jr.: Infectious hepatitis in the Middle East: a clinical review of 200 cases seen in a military hospital, J.A.M.A. *126*:17, 1944.

148. ———: Experiment in cross immunity between infectious hepatitis and homologous serum jaundice, Proc. Soc. Exp. Biol. Med. *59*:148, 1945.

149. ———: Properties of the etiologic agent of infectious hepatitis, Proc. Soc. Exp. Biol. Med. *58*:203, 1945.

150. ———: Elimination in human feces of infectious hepatitis virus parenterally introduced, Proc. Soc. Exp. Biol. Med. *61*:210, 1946.

151. ———: Period of infectivity of patients with experimentally induced infectious hepatitis, J. Exp. Med. *83*:251, 1946.

152. ———: Period of infectivity of patients with homologous serum jaundice and routes of infection in this disease, J. Exp. Med. *83*:441, 1946.

153. ———: Immunity in experimentally induced infectious hepatitis, J. Exp. Med. *84*:403, 1946.

154. ———: Infectious hepatitis, Medicine *27*:279, 1948.

155. ———: Viral hepatitis: multiple attacks in a narcotic addict, Ann. Int. Med. *44*:199, 1956.

156. ———: Viral hepatitis, Yale J. Biol. Med. *34*:314, 1961.

157. ———: Viral hepatitis: clinical patterns and diagnosis, Am. J. Med. *32*:665, 1962.

158. Havens, W. P., Jr., Kushlan, S. D., and Green, M. R.: Experimentally induced infectious hepatitis: roentgenographic and gastroscopic observations, Arch. Int. Med. *79*:457, 1947.

159. Havens, W. P., Jr., and Marck, R. E.: The leukocytic response of patients with

experimentally induced infectious hepatitis, Am. J. Med. Sci. *212*:129, 1946.

160. Havens, W. P., Jr., Miller, W. N., Swift, W. E., Jr., Gardner, H. T., and Knowlton, M.: Factors influencing retention of bromsulfalein in the blood of patients with viral hepatitis, Am. J. Med. 8:591, 1950.

161. Havens, W. P., Jr., and Paul, J. R.: Prevention of infectious hepatitis with gamma globulin, J.A.M.A. *129*:270, 1945.

162. Havens, W. P., Jr., Ward, R., Drill, V. A., and Paul, J. R.: Experimental production of hepatitis by feeding icterogenic materials, Proc. Soc. Exp. Biol. Med. *57*: 206, 1944.

163. Hayman, J. M., and Read, W. A.: Some clinical observations on an outbreak of jaundice following yellow fever vaccination, Am. J. Med. Sci. *209*:281, 1945.

164. Heiner, D. C., and Evans, L.: Immunoglobulins and other proteins in commercial preparations of gamma globulin, J. Pediat. *70*:820, 1967.

165. Heisto, H., and Julsrud, A. C.: Silent carriers of hepatitis virus B, Acta med. scand. *164*:349, 1959.

166. Held, J. R.: The public health implications of nonhuman primates in the transmission of hepatitis to man, Scientific Proceedings 100th Annual Meeting Am. Veterinary Med. A., p. 183, 1963.

167. Hench, P. S.: Analgesia accompanying hepatitis and jaundice in cases of chronic arthritis, fibrositis, and sciatic pain, Proc. Staff Meetings Mayo Clin. 8:430, 1933.

168. Hillis, W. D.: An outbreak of infectious hepatitis among chimpanzee handlers at a United States Air Force Base, Am. J. Hyg. 73:316, 1961.

169. ————: Viral hepatitis associated with sub-human primates, Transfusion 3:445, 1963.

170. Hinton, W. A.: Acute infectious hepatitis, a hazard for workers in blood testing laboratories, The Pub. Health Lab. 5:2, 1947.

171. Hirsch, A.: Handbook of Geographical and Historical Pathology (Translated from the second German edition by Creighton, C.), vol. 3, p. 417, London, New Sydenham Society, 1886.

172. Hoagland, C. L., Labby, D. H., Kunkel, H. G., and Shank, R. E.: An analysis of the effect of fat in the diet on recovery

in infectious hepatitis, Am. J. Pub. Health *36*:1287, 1946.

173. Hoagland, C. L., and Shank, R. E.: Infectious hepatitis: a review of 200 cases, J.A.M.A. *130*:615, 1946.

174. Hofmann, A.: Icterus mit letalem Ausgung nach Salvarsan, Münch. med. Wschr. 58:1773, 1911.

175. Holland, P. V., Rubinson, R. M., Morrow, A. G., and Schmidt, P. J.: Gamma-globulin in the prophylaxis of post-transfusion hepatitis, J.A.M.A. *196*:471, 1966.

176. Howells, L., and Kerr, J. D. O.: Hepatitis after penicillin injections, Lancet *1*:51, 1946.

177. Hoxworth, P. I., Haesler, W. E., Jr., and Smith, H., Jr.: The risk of hepatitis from whole blood and stored plasma, Surg. Gynec. Obstet. *109*:38, 1959.

178. Hoyt, R. E., and Morrison, L. M.: Reaction of viral hepatitis sera with M. rhesus erythrocytes, Proc. Soc. Exp. Biol. Med. 93:547, 1956.

179. Hsia, D. Y. -Y., Taylor, R. G., and Gellis, S. S.: Long-term follow-up study on infectious hepatitis during pregnancy, J. Pediat. *41*:13, 1952.

180. Hughes, R. R.: Postpenicillin jaundice, Brit. Med. J. 2:685, 1946.

181. Hult, H.: Cholémie simple familiale (Gilbert) and posthepatic states without fibrosis of liver, Acta med. scand. *138* (Suppl. 244):1, 1950.

182. Iber, F. L., and Mendeloff, A. J.: Prevention and treatment of viral hepatitis, Arch. Int. Med. *109*:310, 1962.

183. Ipsen, J., Jr.: Social distance in epidemiology. Age of susceptible siblings as the determining factor in household infectivity of measles, Hum. Biol. *31*:162, 1959.

184. Ipsen, J., Donovan, W. R., and James, G.: Sociologic factors in the spread of epidemic hepatitis in a rural school district, J. Hyg. *50*:457, 1952.

185. Iverson, P., and Roholm, K.: On aspiration biopsy of the liver, with remarks on its diagnostic significance, Acta med. scand. *102*:1, 1939.

186. Jaundice following yellow fever vaccination, Editorial, J.A.M.A. *119*:1110, 1942.

187. Jehn: Eine Icterusepidemie in wahrscheinlichem Zusammenhang mit vorausgegangener Revaccination, Dtsch. med. Wschr. *11*:339, 354, 1885.

188. Jennings, E. R., Hindman, W. M., Zak, B., Reed, J., and Brines, O. A.: The thymol turbidity test in screening of blood donors, Am. J. Clin. Path. 27:489, 1957.

189. Jezequel, A. M., Albot, G., and Nezelof, C.: Les cellules clarifées dans l'hépatite parenchymateuse: étude comparée en microscopie optique et electronique, Presse méd. 68:567, 1960.

190. Jones, C. M., and Minot, G. R.: Infectious "catarrhal" jaundice: an attempt to establish a clinical entity, Boston Med. Surg. J. 189:531, 1923.

191. Jones, P. O., Goldsmith, H. J., Wright, F. K., Roberts, C., and Watson, D. C.: Viral hepatitis: a staff hazard in dialysis units, Lancet 1:835, 1967.

192. Joseph, P. R., Millar, J. D., and Henderson, D. A.: An outbreak of hepatitis traced to food contamination, New Engl. J. Med. 273:188, 1965.

193. Kalk, H.: Biopsy findings during and after hepatic coma and after acute necrosis of the liver, Gastroenterology 36:214, 1959.

194. ———: Die chronischen Verlaufsformen der Hepatitis Epidemica in Beziehung zu ihren anatomischen Grundlagen, Dtsch. med. Wschr. 72:308, 1947.

195. Kalk, H., and Wildhirt, H. E.: Beobachtungen zur Regenerationsfahigkeit der menschlichen leber, Gastroenterologia 85:250, 1956.

196. ———: Die posthepatitische hyperbilirubinamie, Z. klin. Med. 153:354, 1955/56.

197. Katz, R., Ducci, H., Bennett, H., and Rodriguez, J.: Incidence of hepatitis following transfusions of whole blood, Am. J. Clin. Path. 27:406, 1957.

198. Katz, R., Velasco, M., Guzman, C., and Alessandri, H.: Red cell survival estimated by radiochromium in hepatobiliary disease, Gastroenterology 46:399, 1964.

199. Katz, R., Velasco, M., Klinger, J., and Alessandri, H.: Corticosteroids in the treatment of acute hepatitis in coma, Gastroenterology 42:258, 1962.

200. Kibrick, S.: Viral infections in the fetus and newborn in Polland, M. (ed.): Perspectives in Virology, vol. II, p. 140, Minneapolis, Burgess, 1961.

201. Kirk, R.: Spread of infective hepatitis, Lancet 1:80, 1945.

202. Kivel, R. M.: Hematologic aspects of acute viral hepatitis, Am. J. Dig. Dis. 6:1017, 1961.

203. Klarenbeek, A., and van Tongeren, H. A. E.: Viricidal action of ethylene oxide gas, J. Hyg. 52:525, 1954.

204. Klatskin, G.: Subacute hepatic necrosis and postnecrotic cirrhosis due to anicteric infections with the hepatitis virus, Am. J. Med. 25:333, 1958.

205. Klatskin, G., and Rappaport, E. M.: Gynecomastia due to infectious hepatitis of the homologous serum type, Am. J. Med. Sci. 214:121, 1947.

206. Klion, F. M., and Schaffner, F.: The ultrastructure of acidophilic "Councilman-like" bodies in the liver, Am. J. Path. 48:755, 1966.

207. Kluge, T.: Gamma-globulin in the prevention of viral hepatitis. A study on the effect of medium-sized doses, Acta med. scand. 174:469, 1963.

208. Knight, V., Drake, M. E., Belden, E. A., Franklin, B. J., Romer, M., and Copple, L. O.: Characteristics of spread of infectious hepatitis in schools and households in an epidemic in a rural area, Am. J. Hyg. 59:1, 1954.

209. Knight, W. A., and Cogswell, R. C.: Preliminary observations of the gastric mucosa in patients with infectious hepatitis, J.A.M.A. 128:803, 1945.

210. Koff, R. S., Grady, G. F., Chalmers, T. C., Mosley, J. W., Swartz, B. L., and the Boston Interhospital Liver Group: Viral hepatitis in a group of Boston hospitals. III. Importance of exposure to shell fish in a non-epidemic period, New Engl. J. Med. 276:703, 1967.

211. Koff, R. S., and Sears, H. S.: Internal temperature of steamed clams, New Engl. J. Med. 276:737, 1967.

212. Krasna, V., and Radkovsky, J.: Evaluation of the effectiveness of gamma globulin in the prevention of infectious hepatitis in Prague in 1953–1956, J. Epid. Microbiol. Immunol. 6:295, 1957.

213. Krugman, S.: Discussion presented at Symposium on Hepatitis in the Tropics, Bull. N. Y. Acad. Med. (In press.)

214. Krugman, S., Giles, J. P., and Hammond, J.: Infectious hepatitis: evidence for two distinctive clinical, epidemiological and immunological types of infection, J.A.M.A. 200:365, 1967.

215. Krugman, S., and Ward, R.: Infectious hepatitis: current status of prevention

with gamma globulin, Yale J. Biol. Med. *34*:329, 1961/62.

216. Krugman, S., Ward, R., and Giles, J. P.: Natural history of infectious hepatitis, Am. J. Med. *32*:717, 1962.

217. Krugman, S., Ward, R., Giles, J. P., Bodansky, O., and Jacobs, A. M.: Infectious hepatitis: detection of virus during incubation period and in clinically inapparent infection, New Engl. J. Med. *261*:729, 1959.

218. Krugman, S., Ward, R., Giles, J. P., and Jacobs, A. M.: Infectious hepatitis. Studies on the effect of gamma globulin and on the incidence of inapparent infection, J.A.M.A. *174*:823, 1960.

219. Kulchar, G. V., and Reynolds, W. J.: Bismuth hepatitis, J.A.M.A. *120*:343, 1942.

220. Kunin, C. M.: Serum hepatitis from whole blood: incidence and relation to source of blood, Am. J. Med. Sci. *237*:293, 1959.

221. Kunkle, H. G., Labby, D. H., and Hoagland, C. L.: Chronic liver disease following infectious hepatitis. I. Abnormal convalescence from initial attack, Ann. Int. Med. *27*:202, 1947.

222. Lainer, F.: Zur Frage der Infektiosität des Ikterus, Wien. klin. Wschr. *53*:601, 1940.

223. Lee, C., and Tink, A.: Exchange transfusion in hepatic coma: report of a case, Med. J. Australia *1*:40, 1958.

224. Leibowitz, S., and Gorman, W. F.: Neuropsychiatric complications of viral hepatitis, New Engl. J. Med. *246*:932, 1952.

225. Leone, N. C., Ratner, F., Diefenbach, W. C., Eads, M. G., Lieberman, J. E., and Murray, R.: Clinical evaluation of a high-protein, high-carbohydrate, restricted fat diet in the treatment of viral hepatitis, Ann. N. Y. Acad. Sci. *57*:948, 1954.

226. Lescher, F. G. The nervous complications of infective hepatitis, Brit. Med. J. *1*:554, 1944.

227. Levine, R. A., and Payne, M. A.: Homologous serum hepatitis in youthful heroin users, Ann. Int. Med. *53*:164, 1960.

228. Levy, R. N., Sawitsky, A., Florman, A. L., and Rubin, E.: Fatal aplastic anemia after hepatitis, New Engl. J. Med. *273*:1118, 1965.

229. Lichtman, S. S.: Diseases of the Liver, Gallbladder and Bile Ducts, vol. 1, Table 29, p. 486, Philadelphia, Lea & Febiger, 1953.

230. Lindstedt, F.: Beitrag zur Kenntnis des Icterus Catarrhalis mit besonderer Rucksicht auf die Incubationszeit dessen epide-

231. Lippman, M.: A proposed role for mucopolysaccharides in the initiation and control of cell division, Trans. N. Y. Acad. Sci. *27*:342, 1965.

232. Litwins, J., and Leibowitz, S.: Abnormal lymphocytes ("virocytes") in virus diseases other than infectious mononucleosis, Acta haematol. 5:223, 1951.

233. Loeliger, E. A., Esch, B. v. d., Romeny-Wachter, C. Ch. t. H., and Booij, H. L.: Factor VII. Its turnover rate and its possible role in thrombogenesis, Thromb. Diath. Haemorrh. *4*:196, 1960.

234. LoGrippo, G. A.: Human plasma treated with ultraviolet and propiolactone, J.A.M.A. *187*:722, 1964.

235. Louis, V.: Elektrokardiographische Befunde bei der Hepatitis Epidemica, Schweiz. med. Wschr. *75*:986, 1945.

236. Lucké, B.: Pathology of fatal epidemic hepatitis, Am. J. Path. *20*:471, 1944.

237. Lucké, B., and Mallory, T.: The fulminant form of epidemic hepatitis, Am. J. Path. *22*:867, 1946.

238. Luerman: Eine Icterusepidemie, Berl. klin. Wschr. *22*:20, 1885.

239. MacCallum, F. O.: Transmission of arsenotherapy jaundice by blood: failure with faeces and nasopharyngeal washings, Lancet *1*:342, 1945.

240. MacCallum, F. O., and Bauer, D. J.: Homologous serum jaundice: transmission experiments with human volunteers, Lancet *1*:622, 1944.

241. MacCallum, F. O., and Bradley, W. H.: Transmission of infective hepatitis to human volunteers, Lancet *2*:228, 1944.

242. MacCallum, F. O., McFarlan, A. M., Miles, J. A. R., Pollock, M. R., and Wilson, C.: Infective hepatitis: studies in East Anglia during the period 1943-47, Medical Research Council Special Report Series, No. 273, H. M. S. Office, London, 1951.

243. MacNalty, A. S.: Acute infective jaundice and administration of measles serum, Ann. Rep. Chief Med. Offr. Min. Health, p. 38, H. M. Stationery Office, London, 1938.

244. Madsen, S., Bang, N. U., and Iversen, K.: Serum glutamic oxaloacetic transaminase in diseases of the liver and biliary tract, Brit. Med. J. *1*:543, 1958.

245. Maitre, A., Giraud, J., Colette, B., Quaglino, B., and Fort, V.: Infectious hepa-

titis. I. Study of variations of glutamic oxaloacetic transaminase (GOT) and glutamic pyruvic transaminase (GPT): 155 case studies, Sem. Hôp. Paris 38:2790, 1962.

246. Malkani, P. K., and Grewal, A. K.: Observations on infectious hepatitis in pregnancy, Indian J. Med. Res., Suppl. 45: 77, 1957.

247. Mallory, T. B.: The pathology of epidemic hepatitis, J.A.M.A. 134:655, 1947.

248. Mandel, W., Gaines, L. M., Jr., and Marilley, R. J., Jr.: Evaluation of oral cholecystography in liver disease, Arch. Int. Med. 97:335, 1956.

249. Mann, J. D., Woodson, G. S., Hoffman, R. G., and Martinek, R. G.: The relation between reported values for hemoglobin and the transfusion rate in a general hospital, Am. J. Clin. Path. 32:225, 1959.

250. Markoff, N.: Oral contraceptives in liver disease, Schweiz. med. Wschr. 97:1502, 1967.

251. Martin, C. M., Gordon, R. S., Felts, W. R., and McCullough, N. B.: Studies on gamma globulins. I. Distribution and metabolism of antibodies and gamma globulin in hypogammaglobulinemic patients, J. Lab. Clin. Med. 49:607, 1957.

252. Mason, J. O., and McLean, W. R.: Infectious hepatitis traced to the consumption of raw oysters, Am. J. Hyg. 75:90, 1962.

253. Maxwell, N. G.: Incidence of serum hepatitis in recipients of thymol turbidity-screened blood or aged liquid plasma, Am. J. Clin. Path. 34:518, 1960.

254. Maynard, J. E.: Infectious hepatitis at Fort Yukon, Alaska—report of an outbreak, 1960–1961, Am. J. Pub. Health 53:31, 1963.

255. McCollum, R. W.: The size of serum hepatitis virus, Proc. Soc. Exp. Biol. Med. 81:157, 1952.

256. McGavran, M. H., and Easterday, B. C.: Rift Valley fever virus hepatitis. Light and electron microscopic studies in the mouse, Am. J. Path. 42:587, 1963.

257. McGavran, M. H., and White, J. D.: Electron microscopic and immunofluorescent observations on monkey liver and tissue culture cells infected with the Asibi strain of yellow fever virus, Am. J. Path. 45:501, 1964.

258. Mella, B., and Lang, D. J.: Leukocyte mitosis: Suppression in vitro associated with acute infectious hepatitis, Science 155:80, 1967.

259. Melnick, J. L., and Park, W. P.: Hepatitis virus studies in marmosets, Paper presented at the Eighth International Congress on Tropical Medicine and Malaria, Teheran, September 7–15, 1968.

260. Meyer, H. M., Brooks, B. E., Douglas, R. D., and Rogers, N. G.: Measles serologic standards, Am. J. Dis. Child. 103:495, 1962.

261. Mirick, G. S., and Shank, R. E.: An epidemic of serum hepatitis studied under controlled conditions, Trans. Am. Clin. Climat. Assoc. 71:176, 1959.

262. Mirick, G. S., Ward, R., and McCollum, R. W.: Modification of post-transfusion hepatitis by gamma globulin, New Engl. J. Med. 273:59, 1965.

263. Mollison, P. L.: Blood Transfusion in Clinical Medicine, pp. 111–112, Philadelphia, Davis, 1967.

264. Molner, J. G., and Meyer, K. F.: Jaundice in Detroit, Am. J. Pub. Health 30:509, 1940.

265. Morris, T. Q., Gocke, D. J., and Sardi, G. F.: Exchange transfusion treatment of fulminating viral hepatitis in the dog, J. Clin. Invest. 46:1098, 1967.

266. Mosley, J. W.: New patterns of transfusion-associated hepatitis, Epatologia 12: 527, 1966.

267. ———: The search for human hepatitis viruses, Arch. ges. Virusforsch. 22:252, 1967.

268. ———: Transmission of viral diseases by drinking water in Berg, G. (ed.): Transmission of Viruses by the Water Route, p. 5, New York, Interscience, 1967.

269. Mosley, J. W., and Dull, H. B.: Transfusion-associated viral hepatitis, Anesthesiology 27:409, 1966.

270. Mosley, J. W., Dull, H. B., Doege, T. C., and Kuykendall, H. D.: Elevations of serum transaminase activities following infectious hepatitis, Gastroenterology 41:9, 1961.

271. Mosley, J. W., Reinhardt, H. P., and Hassler, F. R.: Chimpanzee-associated hepatitis: an outbreak in Oklahoma, J.A.M.A. 199:695, 1967.

272. Mosley, J. W., Reisler, D. J., Brachott, D., Roth, D., and Weiser J.: Comparison of two lots of immune serum globulin for prophylaxis of infectious hepatitis, Am. J. Epidemiol. 87:539, 1968.

273. Mosley, J. W., Schrack, W. D., Jr., Den-

sham, T. W., and Matter, L. D.: Infectious hepatitis in Clearfield County, Pennsylvania. I. A probable water-borne epidemic, Am. J. Med. *26*:555, 1959.

274. Murray, D. H.: Acriflavine: its use, by intravenous injection in the treatment of gonorrhea, J. Roy. Army Med. Cps. *54*:19, 1930.

275. Murray, R., and Diefenbach, W. C.: Effect of heat on the agent of homologous serum hepatitis, Proc. Soc. Exp. Biol. Med. *84*:230, 1953.

276. Murray, R., Diefenbach, W. C. L., Ratner, F., Leone, N. C., and Oliphant, J. W.: Carriers of hepatitis virus in the blood and viral hepatitis in whole blood recipients. 2. Confirmation of carrier state by transmission experiments in volunteers, J.A.M.A. *154*:1072, 1954.

277. Murray, R., Oliphant, J. W., Tripp, J. T., Hampil, B., Ratner, F., Diefenbach, W. C. L., and Geller, H.: Effect of ultraviolet radiation on the infectivity of icterogenic plasma, J.A.M.A. *157*:8, 1955.

278. Murray, R., and Ratner, F.: Safety of immune serum globulin with respect to homologous serum hepatitis, Proc. Soc. Exp. Biol. Med. *83*:554, 1953.

279. Neefe, J. R.: Viral hepatitis *in* Schiff, L. (ed.): Diseases of the Liver, 2nd ed., p. 425, Philadelphia, Lippincott, 1963.

280. Neefe, J. R., Baty, J. B., Reinhold, J. G., and Stokes, J., Jr.: Inactivation of the virus of infectious hepatitis in drinking water, Am. J. Pub. Health *37*:365, 1947.

281. Neefe, J. R., Gambescia, J. M., Kurtz, C. H., Smith, H. D., Beebe, G. W., Jablon, S., Reinhold, J. G., and Williams, S. C.: Prevalence and nature of hepatic disturbance following acute viral hepatitis with jaundice, Ann. Int. Med. *43*:1, 1955.

282. Neefe, J. R., Gellis, S. S., and Stokes, J., Jr.: Homologous serum hepatitis and infectious (epidemic) hepatitis: studies in volunteers bearing on immunological and other characteristics of the etiological agents, Am. J. Med. *1*:3, 1946.

283. Neefe, J. R., Norris, R. F., Reinhold, J. G., Mitchell, C. B., and Howell, D. S.: Carriers of hepatitis virus in blood and viral hepatitis in whole blood recipients. I. Studies on donors suspected as carriers of hepatitis virus and as sources of posttransfusion viral hepatitis, J.A.M.A. *154*: 1066, 1954.

284. Neefe, J. R., and Stokes, J., Jr.: An epidemic of infectious hepatitis apparently due to a water-borne agent, J.A.M.A. *128*:1063, 1945.

285. Neefe, J. R., Stokes, J., Jr., Garber, R. S., and Gellis, S. S.: Studies on the relationship of the hepatitis virus to persistent symptoms, disability, and hepatic disturbance ("chronic hepatitis syndrome") following acute infectious hepatitis, J. Clin. Invest. *26*:329, 1947.

286. Neefe, J. R., Stokes, J., Jr., and Reinhold, J. G.: Oral administration to volunteers of feces from patients with homologous serum hepatitis and infectious (epidemic) hepatitis, Am. J. Med. Sci. *210*:29, 1945.

287. Neefe, J. R., Stokes, J., Jr., Reinhold, J. G., and Lukens, F. D. W.: Hepatitis due to the injection of homologous blood products in human volunteers, J. Clin. Invest. *23*:836, 1944.

288. Nefzger, M. D., and Chalmers, T. C.: The treatment of acute infectious hepatitis: ten-year follow-up study of the effects of diet and rest, Am. J. Med. *35*:299, 1963.

289. Nelson, R. S., Sprinz, H., Colbert, J. W., Jr., Cantrell, F. P., Havens, W. P., Jr., and Knowlton, M.: Effect of physical activity on recovery from hepatitis, Am. J. Med. *16*:780, 1954.

290. Newman, J. L.: Infective hepatitis: the history of an outbreak in the Lavant valley, Brit. Med. J. *1*:61, 1942.

291. Nichols, W. S., Levan, A., Hall, B., and Ostergren, G.: Measles-associated chromosome breakage, Hereditas *48*:367, 1962.

292. Nicolau, S. S., Zavate, O., Constantinescu, N., Micu, I., Birzu, N., Rusu, F., and Ovanescu, A.: Investigations on infective hepatitis transmitted by the parenteral route, Stud. Cercet. Inframicrobiol. *12*: 421, 1961.

293. Noble, H. B., and Peterson, D. R.: Evaluation of immune serum globulin for control of infectious hepatitis, Pub. Health Rep. *80*:173, 1965.

294. Ockner, R. K., and Davidson, C. S.: Hepatic effects of oral contraceptives, New Engl. J. Med. *276*:331, 1967.

295. Olin, G.: Hepatitis epidemic presumably spread by water, Acta med. scand., Suppl. *196*:381, 1947.

296. Oliphant, J. W.: Infectious hepatitis: experimental study of immunity, Pub. Health Rep. *59*:1614, 1944.

297. Oliphant, J. W.: Jaundice following administration of human serum, Bull. N. Y. Acad. Med. 20:429, 1944.

298. Oliphant, J. W., Gilliam, A. G., and Larson, C. L.: Jaundice following administration of human serum, Pub. Health Rep. 58:1233, 1943.

299. Oliphant, J. W., and Hollaender, A.: Experimental inactivation of etiologic agent in serum by ultraviolet irradiation, Pub. Health Rep. 61:598, 1946.

300. Overholt, E. L., and Hardin, E. B.: Cholangiolitic hepatitis: Clinicopathologic studies and response to steroid therapy in four cases, Arch. Int. Med. 103: 859, 1959.

301. Paffenbarger, R. S., and Watt, J.: Poliomyelitis in Hidalgo County, Texas, 1948; epidemiologic observations, Am. J. Hyg. 58:269, 1953.

302. Paktoris, E. A.: Current problems in epidemiology and prevention of Botkin's disease, Vestn. Akad. med. Nauk. 18:55, 1963.

303. Paul, J. R., and Gardner, H. T.: Viral hepatitis in Coates, J. B., Jr. (ed.): Preventive Medicine in World War II, vol. V. Communicable Diseases Transmitted through Contact or by Unknown Means, p. 411, Washington, D.C., Office of the Surgeon Gen., Dept. of the Army, 1960.

304. Paul, J. R., Havens, W. P., Jr., Sabin, A. B., and Philip, C. B.: Transmission experiments in serum jaundice and infectious hepatitis, J.A.M.A. 128:911, 1945.

305. Paul, J. R., and Horstmann, D. M.: A survey of poliomyelitis virus antibodies in French Morocco, Am. J. Trop. Med. Hyg. 4:512, 1955.

306. Petersen, J. L., Grady, G. F., and Chalmers, T. C.: Hepatitis and chronic hemodialysis, Gastroenterology 54:163, 1968.

307. Pickles, W. N.: Epidemic catarrhal jaundice: An outbreak in Yorkshire, Brit. Med. J. 1:944, 1930.

308. Poschl, M.: Roentgenuntersuchungen des Magen-Daruckanals bei Icterus infectiosus, Röntgenpraxis 14:401, 1942.

309. Poskanzer, D. C., and Beadenkopf, W. G.: Waterborne infectious hepatitis epidemic from a chlorinated municipal supply, Pub. Health Rep. 76:745, 1961.

310. Potter, H. P., Jr., Cohen, N. N., and Norris, R. F.: Chronic hepatic dysfunction in heroin addicts. Possible relations to carrier state of viral hepatitis, J.A.M.A. 174:2049, 1960.

311. Preisig, R., Rankin, J. G., Sweeting, J., and Bradley, S. E.: Hepatic hemodynamics during viral hepatitis in man, Circulation 34:188, 1966.

312. Preisig, R., Williams, R., Sweeting, J., and Bradley, S. E.: Changes in sulfobromophthalein transport and storage by the liver during viral hepatitis in man, Am. J. Med. 40:170, 1966.

313. Prevention of high fatality rate in serum hepatitis, Editorial, J.A.M.A. 185:1037, 1963.

314. Propert, S. A.: Hepatitis after prophylactic serum, Brit. Med. J. 2:677, 1938.

315. Puchtler, H., and Sweat, F.: Histochemical specificity of staining methods for connective tissue fibres, resorcin-fuchsin and van Gieson's picrofuchsin, Histochemie 4: 24, 1959.

316. Raffensperger, E. C.: Acute acquired hemolytic anemia in association with acute viral hepatitis, Ann. Int. Med. 48:1243, 1958.

317. Rappaport, A. M.: Acinar units and the pathophysiology of the liver in Rouiller, C. (ed.): The Liver, vol. 1, Chap. 6, p. 266, New York, Academic, 1963.

318. Raska, K., Helcl, J., Jezek, J., Kubelka, Z., Litov, M., Novak, K., Radkousky, J., Sery, V., Zejdl, J., and Zikmund, V.: A milkborne infectious hepatitis epidemic, J. Hyg. Epidem. (Praha) 10:413, 1966.

319. Rath, G.: Moderne diagnosen historischer Seuchen, Dtsch. med. Wschr. 81:2065, 1956.

320. Read, M. R., Bancroft, H., Doull, J. A., and Parker, R. F.: Infectious hepatitis—presumably food-borne outbreak, Am. J. Pub. Health 36:367, 1946.

321. Readinger, H. M., Swift, W. E., Jr., Gardner, H. T., and Sheedy, J. A.: Oral cholecystography in patients with viral hepatitis, Am. J. Med. 8:611, 1950.

322. Recommendation of the Public Health Service Advisory Committee on Immunization Practices, Morb. Mort. Wkly. Rep. 17:290, 1968.

323. Redeker, A. G.: Unresolved viral hepatitis, Presented to the Western Association of Physicians, Jan. 31, 1968, Carmel, California.

324. Redeker, A. G., Hopkins, C. E., Jackson, B., and Peck, P.: A controlled study of the safety of pooled plasma stored in the

494 **Viral Hepatitis**

liquid state at 30–32°C for six months, Transfusion 8:60, 1968.

325. Reisler, D. M., Strong, W. B., and Mosley, J. W.: Transaminase levels in the post convalescent phase of infectious hepatitis, J.A.M.A. 202:37, 1967.

326. Rheder, H., and Beckmann, W.: Über spatikterus bei lues nach Salvarsan-Quecksilberkur, Z. klin. Med. 84:234, 1917.

327. Rindge, M. E., Clem, J. D., Linkner, R. E., and Sherman, L. K.: A case study on the transmission of infectious hepatitis by raw clams: Report from Greenwich, Connecticut, Public Health Service Publication, Washington, D.C., 1963.

328. Rindge, M. E., Mason, J. O., and Elsea, W. R.: Infectious hepatitis: report of an outbreak in a small Connecticut school, due to waterborne transmission, J.A.M.A. 180:33, 1962.

329. Ringertz, O., and Zetterberg, B.: Serum hepatitis among Swedish track-finders. I. An epidemiological study, New Engl. J. Med. 276:540, 1967.

330. Roberts, R. H., and Still, H.: Homologous serum jaundice transmitted by a tattooing needle, Canad. Med. Ass. J. 62:75, 1950.

331. Rokitansky, K.: Handbuch der speciellen pathologischen Anatomie, vol. 3, p. 313, Vienna, Braumuller and Seidel, 1842.

332. Roos, B.: Hepatitis epidemic conveyed by oysters, Svenska Lakar. 53:989, 1956.

333. Rosenberg, D. G., and Galambos, J. T.: Yellow spinal fluid: diagnostic significance of cerebrospinal fluid in jaundiced patients, Am. J. Dig. Dis. 5:32, 1960.

334. Rosenstein, B. J.: Viral hepatitis in narcotics users: an outbreak in Rhode Island, J.A.M.A. 199:698, 1967.

335. Rowell, L. B., Blackmon, J. R., and Bruce, R. A.: Indocyanine green clearance and estimated hepatic blood flow during mild to maximal exercise in upright man, J. Clin. Invest. 43:1677, 1964.

336. Rubin, E.: Interpretation of the liver biopsy: diagnostic criteria, Gastroenterology 45:400, 1963.

337. Rubin, E., and Lieber, C. S.: Alcohol-induced hepatic injury in nonalcoholic volunteers, New Engl. J. Med. 278:869, 1968.

338. Ruddy, S. J., Mosley, J. W., and Held, J. R.: Chimpanzee-associated viral hepatitis in 1963, Am. J. Epid. 86:634, 1963.

339. Ruge, H.: The connection between syphilis, Salvarsan and so-called catarrhal jaundice on the basis of 2,500 cases observed in the German Navy from 1919 to 1929, Urol. cutan. Rev. 36:355, 1932.

340. Salaman, M. H., Williams, D. I., King, A. J., and Nicol, C. S.: Prevention of jaundice resulting from antisyphilitic treatment, Lancet 2:7, 1944.

341. Salen, G., Goldstein, F., Haurani, F., and Wirts, W.: Acute hemolytic anemia complicating viral hepatitis in patients with glucose-6-phosphatase dehydrogenase deficiency, Ann. Int. Med. 65:1210, 1966.

342. Saphir, O., Amromin, G. D., and Yokoo, H.: Mycocarditis in viral (epidemic) hepatitis, Am. J. Med. Sci. 231:168, 1956.

343. Sarrailhé, A., and Clunet, J.: La "Jaunisse des camps" et l'épidémie de paratyphoiide des Dardanelles, Bull. Soc. Med. Par. 40:45, 1916.

344. Sartwell, P. E.: Infectious hepatitis in relation to blood transfusion, Bull. U. S. Army Med. Dept. 7:90, 1947.

345. Sawyer, W. A., Meyer, K. F., Eaton, M. D., Bauer, J. H., Putnam, P., and Schwentker, F. F.: Jaundice in the army personnel in the western region of the United States and its relation to vaccination against yellow fever, Am. J. Hyg. 39:337, 1944.

346. Schachter, D.: Estimation of bilirubin mono- and diglucuronide in the plasma and urine of patients with nonhemolytic jaundice, J. Lab. Clin. Med. 53:557, 1959.

347. Schafer, I. A., and Mosley, J. W.: A study of viral hepatitis in a penal institution, Ann. Int. Med. 49:1162, 1958.

348. Schaffner, F.: Intralobular changes in hepatocytes and the electron microscopic mesenchymal response in acute viral hepatitis, Medicine 45:547, 1966.

349. Schiff, G. M., Sever, J. L., and Huebner, R. J.: Rubella virus: neutralizing antibody in commercial gamma globulin, Science 142:58, 1963.

350. Schiff, L.: The use of steroids in liver disease, Medicine 45:565, 1966.

351. Schlenker, H.: Meningitis als Austakt. zu Hepatitis Epidemica und Poliomyelitis, Schweiz. Med. Wschr. 74:47, 1944.

352. Schneider, A. J., and Mosley, J. W.: Studies of variations of glutamic-oxalacetic transaminase in serum in infectious hepatitis, Pediatrics 24:367, 1959.

353. Selander, P.: Hepatitis epidemic, Kinderärztl. Prax. 8:202, 1937.

354. Sergiev, P. G., Tareev, E. M., Gontaeva,

A. A., Liushitz, I. M., Savinskii, G. N., Trofimovskii, A. I., and Tsimerman, A. I.: Epidemic hepatitis in relation to immunizations with human sera, Ter. Arkh. 18:595, 1940.

355. Serum enzymes in diagnosis, Editorial, J.A.M.A. 174:2146, 1960.

356. Sherlock, S.: Diseases of the Liver and Biliary System, 3rd ed., Philadelphia, Davis, 1963.

357. Sherlock, S., and Walshe, V.: The post-hepatitis syndrome, Lancet 2:482, 1946.

358. Sherwood, P. M.: An outbreak of syringe-transmitted hepatitis with jaundice in hospitalized diabetic patients, Ann. Int. Med. 33:380, 1950.

359. Shimizu, Y., and Kitamoto, O.: The incidence of viral hepatitis after blood transfusions, Gastroenterology 44:740, 1963.

360. Shutkin, N. M.: Homologous-serum hepatitis following the use of refrigerated bone-bank bone, J. Bone Joint Surg. 36A: 160, 1954.

361. Sidhu, A. S.: Sample survey on the incidence of infectious hepatitis in Delhi (1955–56), Indian J. Med. Res., Suppl. 45:31, 1957.

362. Skaliy, P.: Ethylene oxide as a hospital sterilizing agent, Hospital 41:100, 1967.

363. Smart, C.: The medical and surgical history of the war of the rebellion, Part III, vol. 1, pp. 874-879, Washington, D.C., Government Printing Office, 1888.

364. Smetena, H. F.: The histopathology of acute non-fatal hepatitis, Bull. N. Y. Acad. Med. 28:482, 1952.

365. Smith, B. F.: Occurrence of hepatitis in recently tattooed service personnel, J.A.M.A. 144:1074, 1950.

366. Snow, D. J. R.: Infective hepatitis: a discussion on its mode of spread in families, Med. J. Australia 2:139, 1953.

367. Soper, F. L., and Smith, H. H.: Yellow fever vaccination with cultivated virus and immune and hyperimmune serum, Am. J. Trop. Med. 18:111, 1938.

368. Steigmann, F., Hyman, S., and Goldbloom, R.: Infectious hepatitis (homologous serum type) in drug addicts, Gastroenterology 15:642, 1950.

369. Steigmann, F., and Popper, H.: Intrahepatic obstructive jaundice, Gastroenterology 1:645, 1943.

370. Stiehm, E. R., and Fudenberg, H. H.: Antibodies to gamma-globulin in infants and children exposed to isologous gamma-globulin, Pediatrics 35:229, 1965.

371. Stokes, J. F., Owen, J. R., and Holmes, E. G.: Neurological complications of infective hepatitis, Brit. Med. J. 2:642, 1945.

372. Stokes, J. H., Ruedemann, R., and Lemon, W. S.: Epidemic infectious jaundice and its relation to the therapy of syphilis, Arch. Int. Med. 26:522, 1920.

373. Stokes, J., Jr., Berk, J. E., Malamut. L. L., Drake, M. E., Barondess, J. A., Bashe, W. J., Wolman, I. J., Farquhar, J. D., Bevan, B., Drummond, R. J., Maycock, W. d'A., Capps, R. B., and Bennett, A. M.: The carrier state in viral hepatitis, J.A.M.A. 154:1059, 1954.

374. Stokes, J., Jr., Blanchard, M., Neefe, J. R., Gellis, S. S., and Wade, G. R.: Methods of protection against homologous serum hepatitis: I. Studies on the protective value of gamma globulin in homologous serum hepatitis SH virus, J.A.M.A. 138:336, 1948.

375. Stokes, J., Jr., Farquhar, J. A., Drake, M. E., Capps, R. B., and Ward, C. S.: Infectious hepatitis: Length of protection by immune serum globulin (gamma globulin) during epidemics, J.A.M.A. 147: 714, 1951.

376. Ström, J.: A comparison between family infections during epidemics of poliomyelitis and hepatitis in Stockholm, Acta med. scand. 165:49, 1959.

377. Strumia, M. M., Burns, M. E., Sample, A. B., and McGraw, J. J., Jr.: The incidence of post-transfusion hepatitis. II. A 13-year survey including 2 years during which blood donors were screened by means of liver function studies, Am. J. Clin. Path. 30:133, 1958.

378. Sultz, H. A.: A study of the role of tissue-penetrations in the transmission of viral hepatitis, Am. J. Pub. Health 54:1263, 1964.

379. Summerskill, W. H. J., and Jones, F. A.: Corticotrophin and steroids in the diagnosis and management of "obstructive" jaundice, Brit. Med. J. 2:1499, 1958.

380. Sundermann, F. W.: Status of clinical hemoglobinometry in the United States, Am. J. Clin. Path. 43:9, 1965.

381. Swift, W. E., Jr., Gardner, H. T., Moore, D. J., Streitfeld, F. H., and Havens, W. P., Jr.: Clinical course of viral hepatitis and the effect of exercise during convalescence, Am. J. Med. 8:614, 1950,

382. Tarshis, I. B.: The cockroach—a new suspect in the spread of infectious hepatitis, Am. J. Trop. Med. Hyg. 11:705, 1962.
383. Taylor, A. R., Rightsel, W. A., Boggs, J. D., and McLean, I. W., Jr.: Tissue culture of hepatitis virus, Am. J. Med. 32:679, 1962.
384. Thompson, J. L., Jr., Sutliff, W. D., Hennessy, T. P., and Norman, S. L.: Transmission of viral hepatitis by dental procedures, J. Med. Ass. Alabama 23:45, 1953.
385. Tigertt, W. D., Berge, T. O., Gerohenoru, W. S., Glesier, C. A., Ereland, W. C., Bruegge, C. V., and Smetena, H. F.: Experimental yellow fever, Trans. N. Y. Acad. Sci. 22:323, 1960.
386. Tisdale, W. A.: Clinical and pathologic features of subacute hepatitis, Medicine 45:557, 1966.
387. ———: Subacute hepatitis, New Engl. J. Med. 268:85, 1963.
388. Toscano, F., and Rossi, G.: Epatopatia in nato da madre affeta da epatite epidemica in gravidanza (studio anatomoclinico), Pediatria 58:209, 1950.
389. Tucker, C. B., Owen, W. H., and Farrell, R. P.: Outbreak of infectious hepatitis apparently transmitted through water, Southern Med. J. 47:732, 1954.
390. Unger, P. N., and Shapiro, S.: The prothrombin response to the parenteral administration of large doses of vitamin K in subjects with normal liver function and in cases of liver disease: a standardized test for the estimation of hepatic function, J. Clin. Invest. 27:39, 1948.
391. Vannfält, K. A.: On the combination diabetes mellitus and acute hepatitis, Acta med. scand. 117:462, 1944.
392. Vellar, O. D.: Acute viral hepatitis in Norwegian track-finders: an epidemiological study in Norway 1962–63, Acta med. scand. 176:651, 1964.
393. Verstraete, M., Vermylen, C., Vermylen, J., and Vandenbroucke, J.: Excessive consumption of blood coagulation components as cause of hemorrhagic diathesis, Am. J. Med. 38:899, 1965.
394. Virchow, R.: Ueber das Vorkommen und den Nachweis des hepatogenen, insbesondere des katarrhabischen Icterus, Virchow's Arch. Path. Anat. 32:117, 1865.
395. Voegt, H.: Zur Aetiologie der Hepatitis epidemica, Münch. med. Wschr. 89:76, 1942.
396. Volwiler, W., and Dealy, J. B., Jr.: Gamma globulin in treatment of chronic phase of epidemic infectious hepatitis, Gastroenterology 12:87, 1949.
397. Volwiler, W., and Elliott, J. A., Jr.: Late manifestations of epidemic infectious hepatitis, Gastroenterology 10:349, 1948.
398. Volwiler, W., Goldsworthy, P. D., MacMartin, M. P., Wood, P. A., Mackay, I. R., and Fremont-Smith, K.: Biosynthetic determination with radioactive sulfur of turn-over rates of various plasma proteins in normal and cirrhotic man, J. Clin. Invest. 34:1126, 1955.
399. Wade, O. L., and Bishop, J. M.: Cardiac Output and Regional Blood Flow, p. 87, Oxford, Blackwell Scientific Publications, 1962.
400. Waldenstrom, J.: Leber, Blutproteine und Nahrungseiweiss Stofwechsen, p. 8, Krh. Sonderband XV, Tagung, Bad Kissingen, 1950.
401. Wallace, D. K., and Owen, E. E.: An evaluation of the mechanism of bilirubin excretion by the human kidney, J. Lab. Clin. Med. 64:741, 1964.
402. Wallace, E. C.: Infectious hepatitis: report of an outbreak, apparently waterborne, Med. J. Australia 1:101, 1958.
403. Wallis, C., Behbehani, A. M., Lee, L. H., and Bianchi, M.: The ineffectiveness of organic iodine (Wescodyne) as a viral disinfectant, Am. J. Hyg. 78:325, 1963.
404. Walz, D. V.: An effective hospital transfusion committee, J.A.M.A. 189:660, 1964.
405. Ward, R., and Krugman, S.: Etiology, epidemiology and prevention of viral hepatitis, Progr. Med. Virol. 4:87, 1962.
406. Ward, R., Krugman, S., Giles, J. P., Jacobs, A. M., and Bodansky, O.: Infective hepatitis: Studies of its natural history and prevention, New Engl. J. Med. 258:407, 1959.
407. Watt, J., and Lindsay, D. R.: Diarrheal disease control studies. I. Effect of fly control in a high morbidity area, Pub. Health Rep. 63:1319, 1948.
408. Webster, W. P., Roberts, H. R., and Penick, G. C.: Hemostasis in factor V deficiency, Am. J. Med. Sci. 248:194, 1964.
409. Wehrle, P. F., and Hammon, W. M.: Absence of active immunization against infectious hepatitis, J.A.M.A. 167:2062, 1958.
410. Weinstein, L., and Davison, W. T.: Neurologic manifestations in the pre-icteric

phase of infectious hepatitis, Ann. Pract. 1:191, 1946.

411. Wenner, H. A., Kamitsuka, P., Lenahan, M., and Archetti, I.: The pathogenesis of poliomyelitis. Sites of multiplication of poliovirus in Cynomolgus monkeys after alimentary infection, Arch. ges. Virusforsch. 9:537, 1959.

412. Wewalka, F.: Zur epidemiologie des Ikterus bei der antisyphilitischen Behandlung, Schweiz. Z. Allg. Path. 16:307, 1953.

413. Whitehead, N. T., and Crouch, H. A.: Infectious jaundice in the Sudan, J. Trop. Med. 29:359, 1926.

414. Willcox, R. G., and Isselbacher, K. J.: Chronic liver disease in young people, Am. J. Med. 30:185, 1961.

415. Williams, R., and Billing, B. H.: Action of steroid therapy in jaundice, Lancet 2:392, 1961.

416. Wood, G. C.: The formation of fibrils from collagen solutions, III; Biochem. J. 75:605, 1960.

417. Woodward, J. J.: Outlines of the Chief Camp Diseases of the United States Armies as Observed During the Present War, p. 193, Philadelphia, Lippincott, 1863.

418. Yoshibumi, H., and Shigemoto, T.: Human experiment with epidemic jaundice, Acta Paediatrica Japonica 47:975, 1941.

419. Yunet, R., and Yunet, W.: Cited by Corelli, F., in Beitrag zum Studium des alsuten Gelenkrheumatismus Bleituhentragung von akutem Gelenkrheumabsumsblut, Z. Rheumaforsch. 4:544, 1941.

420. Zaki, F. G., and Hoffbauer, F. W.: Fatty cirrhosis in the rat, Arch. Path. 80:323, 1965.

421. Zieve, L., Hill, E., Nesbitt, S., and Zieve, B. A.: The incidence of residuals of viral hepatitis, Gastroenterology 25:495, 1953.

422. Zimmerman, H. J., Lowry, C. F., Uyeyama, K., and Reiser, R.: Infectious hepatitis: Clinical and laboratory features of 295 cases, Am. J. Med. Sci. 213:395, 1947.

423. Zimmerman, H. J., Thomas, L. J., and Scherr, E. H.: Fasting blood sugar in hepatic disease with reference to infrequency of hypoglycemia, Arch. Int. Med. 91:577, 1953.

424. Zondek, B., and Bromberg, Y. M.: Infectious hepatitis in pregnancy, J. Mt. Sinai Hosp. 14:222, 1947.

425. Zuckerman, A. J.: Epidemiology of acute hepatitis in the Royal Air Force, Brit. J. prev. soc. Med. 18:183, 1964.

426. ————: The clinical and laboratory features of acute hepatitis in the Royal Air Force, Monthly Bull. Minist. Hlth Lab. Serv. 24:340, 1965.

14

Toxic and Drug-Induced Hepatitis

GERALD KLATSKIN, M.D.

Hepatotoxins, a heterogeneous group of naturally occurring and synthetic chemical agents, produce a variety of lesions in the liver that are classified as forms of toxic hepatitis. Although they may differ in morphology and pathogenesis, all such lesions share a number of features in common. Characteristically, they (1) exhibit a distinctive histologic pattern for any given hepatotoxin, (2) vary in severity in direct relation to the dose, (3) can be elicited in all individuals, (4) are reproducible in experimental animals and (5) appear after a predictable and usually brief latent period following exposure. In many instances, hepatotoxins behave as general protoplasmic poisons and affect not only the liver but also other tissues. Carbon tetrachloride and phosphorus are typical examples in this group.

Many drugs can injure the liver, yet, paradoxically, few are true hepatotoxins. As is shown later, most drugs that produce hepatic damage appear to behave as sensitizing agents rather than hepatotoxins. Accordingly, a distinction must be drawn between drug-induced and toxic hepatitis. The features that characterize the lesions of *drug-induced hepatitis* and serve to distinguish them from those of toxic hepatitis may be summarized as follows: (1) they cannot be reproduced in animals; (2) only a small fraction of exposed individuals are susceptible to this type of hepatic injury; (3) neither the occurrence of such lesions nor their severity can be correlated with the amount of drug consumed; (4) the appearance of the lesions bears no constant temporal relationship to the institution of drug

therapy, the latent period being brief in some individuals and long in others; (5) the histologic pattern of the lesions is more variable, resembling that of extrahepatic biliary obstruction in some instances, and that of viral hepatitis in others; (6) often the lesions are accompanied by extrahepatic manifestations of hypersensitivity, such as fever, rash, arthralgia and eosinophilia.

A few drugs, such as chloroform, are true hepatotoxins and produce the typical lesions of toxic hepatitis. Others, like the organic arsenicals, may behave as sensitizing agents under some conditions and as hepatotoxins under others.

A number of drugs, including some C-17 alpha alkyl substituted steroids and certain agents used for cholecystography, interfere with bile secretion and may give rise to jaundice. However, the functional disorders they produce are not accompanied by hepatic necrosis or inflammation or by evidence of hypersensitivity, so that these drugs are neither true hepatotoxins nor sensitizing agents, and must be considered separately.

Transmission of the hepatitis virus by means of improperly sterilized syringes contaminated with blood constitutes one of the hazards of parenteral drug therapy and has been reported following the administration of a variety of therapeutic agents. This possibility must be borne in mind in evaluating the role of parenterally administered drugs in the etiology of hepatitis, especially when the latter develops during a long course of treatment, or after an extended latent period.

498

TOXIC HEPATITIS

PATHOGENESIS

Several mechanisms have been proposed to account for the actions of hepatotoxins. These include: (1) disturbances in protein synthesis and energy production in the liver resulting from direct injury to hepatic cell membranes, or metabolic alterations in essential constituents of the hepatic cell; (2) impairment of hepatic blood flow, leading to ischemic necrosis, secondary to swelling of the hepatic parenchyma, or to stimulation of the sympathetic nervous system; and (3) alterations in lipid metabolism.

Considering that hepatotoxins differ markedly in chemical structure, it is highly improbable that they all attack the liver in the same way. The uniformity of the biochemical findings in the liver after exposure to hepatotoxins of diverse character suggests that, although these agents probably initiate cellular injury in different ways, the subsequent chain of biochemical events leading to necrosis follows a common pathway.

Several factors, including the nutritional state, alcoholism, pre-existent liver disease and infection, modify the effects of hepatotoxins and are of importance in the pathogenesis of toxic hepatitis (see below).

Some hepatotoxins attack the liver exclusively, though they enter cells elsewhere in the body. The reason for this is not clear. Since many of these agents are degraded or otherwise chemically altered in the liver, it has been proposed that their metabolites are responsible for their specific hepatic actions.[480] Alternative possibilities that must be considered are that agents of this type are concentrated in the liver, or attack enzymes peculiar to the liver.

Direct Effects on Cell Membranes. More than 60 years ago Wells suggested that hepatotoxins produce cellular injury and death by inactivating essential oxidative enzyme systems, leading to cessation of anabolic processes and ultimate dissolution of cytoplasm by autolytic enzymes.[780] The results of more recent studies support this view but attach special importance to enzyme systems concerned with energy production and protein synthesis.

Christie and Judah[135] and others[111, 172] have demonstrated that carbon tetrachloride alters the permeability of the mitochondria of the hepatic cells, resulting in loss of diphosphopyridine nucleotide (DPN) and a decrease in the activity of the DPN-linked dehydrogenases of the Krebs cycle. In addition, there is a concomitant fall in adenosine triphosphate (ATP)[173] and uncoupling of oxidative phosphorylation.[111, 171] Biochemical[135] and electron microscopic[174] studies indicate that the mitochondria of the liver swell and fill with lipid under these conditions. Phosphorus[172] and heliotrine[134] produce similar effects, but whether these occur in other forms of toxic hepatitis is not known.

That carbon tetrachloride can attack the mitochondria directly has been established in *in vitro* experiments.[111, 135] However, anoxia produces similar effects, so that the *in vivo* changes in mitochondrial enzymatic activity observed following carbon tetrachloride poisoning have been attributed by some to ischemia.[516] The latter interpretation is open to question, but there can be little doubt that mitochondrial damage does not constitute the initial event that leads to necrosis, since other histologic,[530, 634] biochemical[598] and electron microscopic[695] changes can be demonstrated much earlier.

Recent studies suggest that the primary site of action of carbon tetrachloride is in the endoplasmic reticulum,[600, 696] a complex of cystoplasmic structures which are the source of the microsomes obtained on centrifugal fractionation of the cells. These play a role in protein synthesis[118] and in certain conjugating systems[355] and possibly in lipid metabolism.[600] Marked dilatation of the cisternae of the endoplasmic reticulum on electron microscopy[696] and inhibition of microsomal enzymatic activities[596] are demonstrable early in the course of carbon tetrachloride poisoning, before morphologic or functional changes in the mitochondria are evident. Interestingly, carbon tetrachloride[696] and other hepatotoxins, such as dimethylnitrosamine,[345] inhibit the *in vitro* incorporation of labeled amino acids into protein by the microsomes of the liver. This supports the view that the inhibition of protein synthesis by hepatotoxins is responsible for the subsequent alterations in mitochondrial morphology and function that ultimately lead to cellular necrosis.[696]

In both carbon tetrachloride[744] and thioacetamide poisoning[250] the calcium content of the hepatic cells increases rapidly. Since high concentrations of calcium produce swelling, loss of potassium and inhibition of respiration and oxidative phosphorylation in mitochondria,[744] it is possible that agents of this type contribute to hepatic injury by altering the permeability of the cell membranes, permitting excess calcium to enter and attack the mitochondria.

Several investigators have suggested that carbon tetrachloride damages the endoplasmic reticulum by enhancing the peroxidation of its structural lipids.[597]

Indirect Metabolic Effects. Diets that are deficient in sulfur-containing amino acids produce massive hepatic necrosis in the rat.[266, 323] According to Himsworth, this effect is dependent upon a specific deficiency of cystine.[322] Moreover, he suggests that lesions of this type are induced not only by dietary restriction but also by a relative deficiency of cystine as a consequence of excessive losses or increased demands. As examples, he cites the hepatic lesions of trinitrotoluene poisoning, which he attributes to the combination of cystine with free nitrous groups, and to the increased demand for cystine imposed by a raised metabolic rate, and the lesions of chronic selenium poisoning, which he believes are also dependent upon a relative deficiency of cystine, created in this instance by the substitution of selenium for sulfur.

The observation that protein deficiency enhances and that supplements of methionine or cysteine inhibit the hepatic necrosis induced by bromobenzene, and the fact that bromobenzene couples with cysteine before it is acetylated and excreted as mercapturic acid,[388] lend support to the hypothesis that hepatotoxins injure the liver by inducing a relative deficiency of sulfur-containing amino acids. According to Drill, a deficiency of this type could lead to hepatic necrosis by interfering with intracellular enzymatic oxidation-reduction systems dependent upon an adequate supply of sulfhydryl groups.[185] However, direct measurements have failed to demonstrate a fall in

the glutathione content of the liver following carbon tetrachloride poisoning.[202] Moreover, it is difficult to reconcile this hypothesis with the observation that a dietary deficiency of sulfur-containing amino acids will not produce hepatic necrosis unless the diet is also deficient in vitamin E[287, 288, 325] and factor 3,[663, 664] a naturally occurring organically bound selenium compound found in many tissues and foods.[665] Indeed, Schwarz has shown that the protective effects of methionine and cystine are dependent not upon their content of sulfhydryl groups but rather upon the presence of trace amounts of selenium.[665]

Ethionine, by trapping adenosine in S-adenosylethionine, depletes the liver of ATP, leading to inhibition of protein synthesis and accumulation of triglyceride.[220] Since all of these effects can be prevented by intraperitoneal injection of ATP or its precursors, the inhibition of protein synthesis is related to the depletion of hepatic ATP. However, this is not the case in carbon tetrachloride poisoning, since ATP injection prevents the decline in hepatic ATP, but does not prevent inhibition of protein synthesis.[351]

Vascular Factors. Alterations in the intralobular circulation may play a role in the pathogenesis of toxic hepatitis. Exposure to carbon tetrachloride, for example, produces an immediate but transient intralobular vasoconstriction, which, as exposure continues, is followed by a more sustained obliteration of the sinusoids, possibly as a consequence of hepatocellular swelling. This has been demonstrated both by the quartz-rod transillumination technic[766] and by intrasplenic India ink injection.[265] Calvert and Brody have attributed the vasoconstriction to stimulation of the central sympathetic areas resulting in a prolonged discharge of the peripheral sympathetic nervous system and increased secretion of epinephrine.[112]

Since the degenerative changes and necrosis produced by carbon tetrachloride and a number of other agents occur in the centrilobular areas where the circulation is most impaired, many investigators have attributed the lesions to ischemia.[265, 766] Evidence in support of this hypothesis has been brought forward by Calvert and Brody.[112]

They reported that cordotomy, a procedure that blocks sympathetic stimuli and prevents hepatic vasoconstriction, fully protects against hepatic necrosis and the alterations in mitochondrial enzymatic activity usually seen following carbon tetrachloride poisoning. However, Plaa and Larson have shown that the protective effect of cordotomy is due to the hypothermia it produces, and that it will not prevent carbon tetrachloride-induced hepatic necrosis if the body temperature is maintained at 36° C.[572]

Interestingly, allyl formate, which causes dilatation of the sinusoids without impairment of circulation, produces peripheral rather than centrilobular necrosis.[633] In this instance the principal point of attack is in the area of maximal concentration of the agent, namely, where it enters the lobule via the portal tract at its periphery. However, the distribution of lesions produced by hepatotoxins may be determined by differences in the susceptibility of the cells in the various zones of the liver rather than by zonal differences in the concentration of hepatotoxin or by circulatory changes. This possibility is suggested by the variations in the biochemical activities of the cells found in different parts of the lobule.[675]

According to Himsworth, ischemia produces hepatic necrosis by limiting the availability of circulating sulfur-containing amino acids.[324] If the hepatic necrosis produced by carbon tetrachloride is the result of ischemia, it is unlikely that a deficiency of sulfur-containing amino acids plays a role, since methionine supplements do not protect against this type of hepatic injury.[184] A low oxygen tension would appear to be a more important factor, inasmuch as anoxemia *per se* can produce similar histologic[490] and biochemical[516] lesions.

On the basis of hepatic blood flow measurements in the intact rat, using the Grayson method of internal thermal conductivity with an implanted thermocouple, Stoner has challenged the concept that ischemia plays a role in the development of central hepatic necrosis following exposure to carbon tetrachloride and other toxic agents.[725] According to this investigator, the impairment of blood flow previously observed by others, using the India ink injection method or the

technic of quartz-rod transillumination, can be attributed to the anesthesia and laparotomy required in such experiments.[726] It is difficult to reconcile Stoner's observations with other indirect evidence pointing to a circulatory disturbance.[112]

A number of agents, including urethane,[180] some senecio alkaloids[630, 670] and massive doses of arsphenamine,[394] appear to produce hepatic lesions by injuring the blood vessels of the liver, leading either to increased vascular permeability and extravasation of blood[180] or to thromboses.[394, 630, 670]

Fatty Infiltration. One of the striking features of the hepatic lesions produced by carbon tetrachloride and a number of other toxic agents is an accumulation of fat within the parenchymal cells. This phenomenon has been variously attributed to (1) mobilization of nonesterified fatty acids from adipose tissue, as a consequence of sympathetic and adrenal medullary stimulation,[112] (2) depression of fatty acid oxidation in the liver due to a reduction in available DPN[172] and ATP[173] that follows mitochondrial damage, and 3) inhibition of the normal mechanism for the transport of triglyceride out of the liver, presumably because of injury to the endoplasmic reticulum.[600]

The concept that carbon tetrachloride mobilizes lipid from the depots by stimulating the sympathetic nervous system and adrenal medulla, and thus produces fatty infiltration of the liver, stems from the observation of Calvert and Brody that adrenalectomy diminishes and cordotomy prevents this effect.[112] More direct evidence indicative of fat mobilization has been obtained in animals whose depot fats were labeled with deuterium prior to carbon tetrachloride administration.[41] The observation that the administration of epinephrine increases the release of nonesterified fatty acids from the isolated epididymal fat pad while carbon tetrachloride does not,[660] and the failure of adrenalectomy to protect against carbon tetrachloride-induced fatty infiltration in some experiments,[10] appear to be inconsistent with the theory that fat mobilization is mediated by sympathetic stimulation and increased epinephrine secretion. However, this does not exclude the possibility that carbon tetrachloride and other hepatotoxins mobilize fatty acids by some other mechanism. Indeed, the elevated levels of free fatty acids found in the plasma following the administration of such agents[351] support this view.

Dianzani has reported that carbon tetrachloride uncouples oxidative phosphorylation and lowers the ATP content of the liver before it produces fatty infiltration.[173] Since ATP is essential in the activation of fatty acid oxidation, he postulates that the accumulation of fat is secondary to a reduction in its rate of oxidation. This view has been disputed by two groups of investigators who have shown that the fat content of the liver rises before there is any uncoupling of oxidative phosphorylation[111, 600] or impairment of octanoate oxidation,[599] and that this effect is not abolished by preventing mitochondrial damage with ethylenediaminetetraacetate.[111]

Carbon tetrachloride, in addition to raising the concentration of lipid in the liver, lowers the plasma level of triglyceride and inhibits the hyperlipema induced by intravenously injected Triton.[600] From this, Recknagel and associates concluded that fat accumulates because of damage to the mechanism normally responsible for the transport of triglyceride out of the liver.[600] Moreover, on the basis of indirect evidence, they have proposed that the most likely locus for this mechanism is the membranous component of the endoplasmic reticulum. Smuckler, Iseri and Benditt, who are in essential agreement with this view, attribute the block in triglyceride transport more specifically to the depressed synthesis of protein required for lipid conjugation.[696] A number of observations support this concept. The most important of these are that on electron microscopy, the earliest findings in the liver following carbon tetrachloride administration are cystic dilatation of the rough endoplasmic reticulum and dislocation of the ribosomes from its membranes,[697] and that these changes are accompanied by an inhibition of ribosomal protein[697] and plasma lipoprotein[667] synthesis.

Nutritional Factors. The susceptibility of animals to hepatotoxins is greatly influenced by their nutritional status. Clinical experience suggests that the same is true of man, but the evidence is not nearly as convincing. In general, starvation and high-fat diets enhance, whereas high-carboydrate and high-protein diets protect against the hepatotoxic effects of these agents. However, in the case of many hepatotoxins the effects of diet are not known. Moreover, the results of changing a single dietary constituent are difficult to interpret, unless due consideration is given to concomitant changes in the other components and caloric value of the diet, and to their effect on net food intake—factors that frequently have been neglected in toxicity studies.

Even a relatively brief period of starvation increases the severity of the hepatic damage produced by carbon tetrachloride[235] and chloroform.[167] High-fat diets enhance their toxicity to an even greater extent.[80, 543] In contrast, carbohydrate appears to protect the liver against injury by these and other agents.[80, 543]

The effects of protein are variable, depending not only on the nature of the hepatotoxin but also on other factors. Thus, protein deficiency increases the susceptibility of the liver to damage by chloroform[506] but not by carbon tetrachloride.[187] Similarly, a surplus of protein protects against the hepatic effects of chloroform[506] but not against those of carbon tetrachloride[187] or many other agents.[185] The protective action of protein also depends in part on the nutritional status. Thus, supplements are far more effective in preventing chloroform injury in the depleted animal than they are in the animal with normal protein stores.[167] The source of protein is another factor that may influence the results. Meat, for example, in contrast with other proteins, actually enhances the toxicity of some agents.[81]

Other dietary constituents are of interest in connection with toxic hepatitis, not only for their possible therapeutic value but also for the clues that they may provide to the mechanisms involved in the actions of hepatotoxins. Of these, choline, methionine, cystine and tocopherol have received the greatest attention.

Choline accelerates the removal of excess fat deposited in the liver as a result of carbon tetrachloride[40] or phosphorus[69] poisoning but does not prevent hepatic necrosis under these conditions. Some investigators have reported that choline partially protects against the mitochondrial injury induced by carbon tetrachloride,[135] but this effect has not been confirmed by others.[111]

Methionine protects against chloroform toxicity both in protein-depleted[507] and stock-fed animals.[103] However, it is not certain that the site of its action is in the liver. At least in protein-depleted animals given carbon tetrachloride, methionine increases the survival time by preventing renal necrosis[289] rather than by protecting against hepatic damage.[184] In conjunction with alpha-tocopherol supplements, methionine also prevents the development of cirrhosis following chronic selenium poisoning.[669] Alpha-tocopherol alone protects against carbon tetrachloride toxicity in rats on low-casein diets. Prolongation of survival in this instance probably is not due to any hepatic effect, since liver damage is not prevented.[341]

Cystine has not been studied as extensively as the other dietary constituents discussed. It affords some protection against the hepatotoxic effects of chloroform in the protein-depleted dog but is inferior to methionine in this respect[506] and has no effect in other forms of toxic hepatitis.[185]

The precise way in which dietary factors affect susceptibility to hepatotoxins is not known, but there is suggestive evidence that indicates that they may do so by altering either the fat content of the liver or the size of its protein stores. In general, susceptibility is enhanced by diets that lead to an increase in hepatic fat or depletion of protein and is reduced by those that produce the reverse changes.[272] The heightened susceptibility associated with fatty infiltration of the liver is thought to depend, in some instances at least, on the solubility of many hepatotoxins in fat.[185, 272] Obviously, this cannot account for increased toxicity of agents that are relatively insoluble. As noted, it has been postulated that some hepatotoxins, and particularly the chlorinated hydrocarbons, produce hepatic necrosis by interacting with sulfur-containing amino acids, thereby in-

ducing a relative deficiency of sulfhydryl groups in essential enzyme systems of the liver.[185] Accordingly, it is believed that low protein diets potentiate the toxic effects of these agents by hastening such depletion. The failure to demonstrate a fall in hepatic glutathione following carbon tetrachloride[202] casts doubt on the validity of this interpretation. An alternative possibility that has received relatively little attention is that protein depletion increases the apparent toxicity of such agents by retarding the regeneration of injured hepatic cells.

At one time, the glycogen concentration of the liver was thought to be the major factor that determined its susceptibility to injury. This concept was responsible for the widespread adoption of high-carbohydrate diets in the therapy of hepatic disease. It is now known that the protective action of carbohydrate depends on its protein-sparing effect and its tendency to reduce hepatic lipids and not on an increase in hepatic glycogen.[272]

Contributory Factors. Ethyl alcohol potentiates the hepatotoxic effects of chloroform,[631] carbon tetrachloride,[409] phosphorus[228] and certain other chlorinated hydrocarbons.[60] Since all of these agents are highly soluble in lipid solvents, it has been suggested that ethanol, by serving as a vehicle, facilitates either their absorption from the intestinal tract or their penetration and storage in cells.[637]

In experimental animals, injection of relatively innocuous bacteria greatly enhances the hepatotoxic effects of chloroform and phosphorus and produces a type of midzonal or massive necrosis that is not seen in uncomplicated poisoning with these agents.[542] It has been proposed that under these conditions the hepatotoxins alter the permeability of the vessels in the liver and thus permit organisms to gain access to the parenchymal cells. Whether or not infection plays a similar role in man is not known.

Anoxia increases the hepatotoxic effects of certain anesthetic agents.[632] This would appear to be an additive rather than a synergistic effect, since anoxemia *per se* can produce serious liver injury.[208, 490]

In experimental animals, antecedent hepatic injury renders the liver more susceptible to further damage by other agents.[60] This may account, in part, for the apparent synergistic effects of chronic alcoholism, infection and anoxia in toxic hepatitis.

PATHOLOGY

The morphologic features of toxic hepatitis vary, depending on the agent, its dose and the route of administration. Usually, the acute hepatic lesions are distributed uniformly throughout the lobules, are arranged in a zonal pattern and show all stages of parenchymal degeneration from simple swelling to acute necrosis, with relatively little inflammatory reaction. Often fatty infiltration is a prominent feature. In the case of many hepatotoxins, the intralobular distribution of the lesions is distinctive. Thus, they characteristically occur in the centrilobular zones in carbon tetrachloride[114] and chloroform[784] intoxication and in the periportal zones in phosphorus poisoning.[324] However, the distribution may vary in some forms of toxic hepatitis. Occasionally, the lesions extend beyond the confines of the individual lobules and give rise to areas of massive necrosis, as, for example, in poisoning with the *Amanita phalloides* toxin[190] and some of the chlorinated naphthalene and diphenyl compounds.[231] Curiously, agents that produce zonal lesions seldom give rise to massive hepatic necrosis, even when large doses are administered. In experimental animals, for example, even lethal doses of carbon tetrachloride or chloroform fail to produce this type of lesion unless they are injected directly into the portal circulation.[116] Carbon tetrachloride poisoning in man may be an exception. The writer has seen two instances of acute poisoning—one by ingestion and the other by inhalation—that were associated with subacute hepatic necrosis and subsequent postnecrotic scarring.

As a rule, acute toxic hepatitis of the zonal type is a self-limited lesion that goes on to complete recovery without residuals. However, if the exposure to a hepatotoxin is continuous or is repeated at intervals that do not permit full recovery on each occasion, a diffuse fibrosis may ensue and terminate in a picture closely resembling Laennec's cirrhosis.[114] When necrosis is zonal, regeneration proceeds in an orderly fashion within the confines of an intact reticulum by proliferation of the remaining viable cells in the same lobule, thereby restoring the normal lobular architecture. However, this is not possible in massive hepatic necrosis, in which regeneration must proceed from distant lobules bordering the zones of necrosis. Large masses of parenchymal cells are formed which compress the intervening necrotic zones, containing intact reticulum, blood vessels and bile ducts, into broad bands. This produces the condition variously described as toxic cirrhosis, postnecrotic scarring with nodular hyperplasia and healed massive or subacute hepatic necrosis.

Prolonged exposure to hepatotoxins, including carbon tetrachloride,[203, 215] selenium[534] and others, induces hepatomas in experimental animals. Although cirrhosis usually precedes the appearance of these tumors, it is not known whether necrosis and regeneration of parenchymal cells are essential for their development.[215] Theoretically at least, hepatotoxins can induce hepatomas in man. However, no authenticated cases have been reported.

CLINICAL FEATURES

Characteristically, the clinical manifestations of hepatic injury do not become evident for a variable interval following exposure to hepatotoxins.

In acute poisoning with agents such as carbon tetrachloride and chloroform, the latent period is relatively brief, usually not exceeding a day or two, and is well correlated with the evolution of the lesion microscopically. Although histologic evidence of hepatocellular injury can be demonstrated within a few hours, necrosis does not reach its peak for a period of 48 hours.[114, 784]

Following repeated exposure to relatively small doses of certain hepatotoxins, there may be a long interval before signs of cirrhosis become clinically evident.[574] This does not constitute a period of true latency, since it is possible to demonstrate the presence of progressive lesions histologically at a very early stage.[114] The delayed appearance of symptoms in this instance is probably related to the fact that the slowly progressive destruction of the parenchyma is accompanied by compensatory hepatocellular regeneration.

Symptoms

Not all of the clinical manifestations in acute toxic hepatitis are the consequence of liver injury, many being related to the extrahepatic pharmacologic and toxic effects of hepatotoxins. In many instances it is difficult to distinguish between the symptoms of hepatic and extrahepatic origin, and occasionally the latter predominate. Signs of renal damage and gastrointestinal irritation are especially common.

The usual clinical picture resembles that of viral hepatitis, except for the absence of preicteric fever and constitutional symptoms. Anorexia, nausea and vomiting are the principal symptoms, and jaundice and hepatomegaly are the major physical findings. In mild cases, jaundice may be absent. Usually, the icterus is accompanied by bilirubinuria, but acholic stools are rare.

In severely poisoned patients with massive or subacute hepatic necrosis, the clinical manifestations tend to be more severe and may include such unusual features as intense abdominal pain, coffee-ground vomitus, a rapid decrease in the size of the liver, ascites, edema, hemorrhagic phenomena, somnolence and coma.

As noted, repeated exposure to hepatotoxins may produce cirrhosis. The clinical course in such cases is variable. In some, there are repeated episodes of acute hepatitis before frank signs of cirrhosis become evident, whereas in others the onset is insidious without antecedent symptoms of acute hepatic injury. Unless the exposure to a hepatotoxin is recognized, the former may be mistaken for relapsing viral hepatitis with posthepatitic cirrhosis, and the latter for Laennec's or some other type of cirrhosis.

Except in the most severely affected cases, recovery from acute toxic hepatitis tends to be more rapid and is less likely to be followed by sequelae than in viral hepatitis. However, the ultimate prognosis depends as much upon the accompanying extrahepatic lesions as upon the state of the liver. Thus, for example, in carbon tetrachloride poisoning, the hepatic lesions may be mild and

heal, while those in the kidney are extensive and lead to progressive renal failure and death.

Laboratory Features

The results of liver function tests are similar to those found in acute viral hepatitis, except that abnormalities of cephalin-cholesterol flocculation and thymol turbidity are less common.[580] This difference may be related to the relative paucity of inflammatory cells in the lesions of toxic hepatitis.

Although liver function tests are of limited value in distinguishing between toxic and viral hepatitis, they can be of great assistance in detecting the early signs of liver injury following known or suspected exposure to hepatotoxins, and in evaluating the severity and the progress of the lesion once it is established. In this connection, the serum transaminase level, because of its sensitivity and the relative ease with which it can be determined, is the most useful single screening test available.

Treatment

If the patient is seen immediately after exposure, an attempt should be made to remove any remaining traces of hepatotoxin from the intestinal tract by lavage and catharsis, or by hyperventilation in the case of toxic vapors. However, such measures are seldom successful once signs of toxic hepatitis are evident, because of the relatively long period of latency between exposure and the appearance of clinical manifestations.

In the case of industrial hepatotoxins, it is important to keep all exposed personnel under close surveillance, preferably with periodic tests of hepatic function, and to remove such individuals from the contaminated environment at the first sign of functional impairment.

Antidotes. A number of chemical agents protect against the injurious effects of hepatotoxins in experimental animals.[185] Only a few have been tested in man, and these have proved to be of no value in the treatment of toxic hepatitis. This is not surprising, since in most experiments these agents have been used prophylactically rather than therapeutically.

BAL (2,3-dimercaptopropanol) would

appear to be an ideal antidote in the early management of toxic hepatitis due to compounds of gold and arsenic, since it combines both with free and tissue-bound metallic ions to form relatively innocuous, soluble thiometal complexes which are excreted readily by the kidneys. However, the results of treatment in man have been disappointing.[196] No doubt this is attributable to the fact that in most instances BAL has been tried in patients with hypersensitivity reactions induced by organic arsenical or gold compounds rather than in those with toxic hepatitis.

Since other chemical agents that protect against hepatotoxins in animals also contain sulfhydryl groups, their effectiveness has been attributed to a sulfhydryl-sparing action in essential enzyme systems. However, some of the nonsulfhydryl analogues of these agents are equally effective,[102] so that their mode of action is unknown.

Reports indicating that antihistamines protect against the hepatotoxic effects of thioacetamide, possibly by preventing mitochondrial swelling,[366] and that adrenergic blocking agents protect against carbon tetrachloride poisoning by preventing hepatic ischemia[112] suggest new approaches to the treatment of toxic hepatitis. Although these agents have not been tried in man, if they do prove to be effective, they will have to be used within a few hours of exposure to the hepatotoxin.

Diet. There are no well-controlled studies establishing the efficacy of dietotherapy in the management of toxic hepatitis in man, the rationale for such treatment being based almost exclusively on the results of animal experiments and on experience with other types of liver disease.

Most experimental studies of the interrelationships between dietary factors and the actions of hepatotoxins have been concerned with the influence of the *antecedent* nutritional status on the incidence and the severity of hepatic injury following intoxication, and not with the effects of diet on the regeneration and the repair of the injured liver—the major considerations in the treatment of toxic hepatitis. This is an important distinction, since it does not follow that a dietary constituent that protects against the hepato-

toxic effects of an agent necessarily facilitates recovery once such injury has occurred.

The effect of *protein* in chloroform poisoning is a case in point. Here there seems to be little doubt that protein depletion enhances toxicity and that protein supplements under these conditions are protective, even if given some hours after exposure.[507] However, there is no evidence to show that such supplements hasten recovery when administered after overt signs of liver disease have appeared. Moreover, the protective action of most dietary constituents, including protein, have been demonstrated in depleted animals, so that no conclusions are warranted regarding their therapeutic value in well-nourished individuals with toxic hepatitis. Also, it cannot be assumed that because a dietary constituent protects against one hepatotoxin it will necessarily do so against all. This is well illustrated in the case of protein, which protects the depleted animal against chloroform[506] but not against carbon tetrachloride[187] intoxication.

Finally, in assessing the results of animal experiments, care must be exercised in distinguishing between the effects of dietary measures on survival and their effects on the liver *per se*, since the former may be related to extrahepatic factors. Thus, in carbon tetrachloride poisoning, methionine increases survival by preventing renal injury but has no effect on liver damage.[289]

The impressive results of dietotherapy in Laennec's cirrhosis have encouraged its adoption in other forms of liver disease, including viral and toxic hepatitis. Although this practice is reasonable, there is no conclusive evidence to indicate that dietary measures are effective in any type of liver injury other than that associated with nutritional deficiency.

In the absence of more precise information regarding the most efficacious form of treatment in toxic hepatitis, it would seem logical to provide a diet rich in protein and carbohydrate on the principle that protein is required for tissue regeneration and is spared when adequate nonprotein calories are provided. Although there is no evidence to indicate that the addition of fat to a well-balanced protein-containing diet is in any way deleterious to the injured liver, fat may be poorly tolerated during the period of anorexia and indigestion in the early stages of hepatitis and has the disadvantage that it is difficult to administer parenterally. Later, however, when the appetite improves, liberal use of fat in the form of milk, cream, cheese and eggs should be encouraged, since it makes for a more palatable diet and facilitates the maintenance of a high caloric intake, thus preventing the weight loss and the debility that so often follow an attack of acute hepatitis.

Obviously, from what has been said, any statements regarding the precise protein and caloric requirements in toxic hepatitis are based on personal opinion and experience rather than on well-documented evidence. With this reservation in mind, it is suggested that 70 to 80 Gm. of protein and 3,000 calories constitute an adequate dietary intake. There is no evidence to indicate that a larger protein intake is more efficacious. Studies in cirrhosis[567] suggest that excessive amounts may actually be harmful in the presence of advanced liver disease, by raising the level of blood ammonia.

In prescribing protein for the patient with toxic hepatitis, due consideration must be given to the status of the kidneys, since hepatotoxins not infrequently produce acute tubular necrosis. In such cases, measures designed to reduce nitrogen retention and to attain a normal internal environment take precedence over the less urgent needs of the liver. Usually this entails omission of dietary protein, provision of sufficient carbohydrate and fat calories to minimize endogenous protein breakdown, and careful regulation of fluid and electrolyte balance. Fortunately, the relatively brief period of protein deprivation usually required does not impede recovery from the associated liver injury. Similarly, individuals with severe anorexia and vomiting who require parenteral feedings do not appear to suffer any ill effects when protein is omitted for a number of days. Although parenterally administered amino acids can be utilized in the face of severe hepatic injury,[199] often they are poorly tolerated, so that their use is not recommended unless the situation demands long-term parenteral feeding.

From a practical standpoint, it is often difficult to achieve an intake of 3,000 calories during the first few days of an acute hepatitis, even if the diet is supplemented with parenterally administered glucose. This need not cause concern, since the easily attainable level of 2,000 calories usually suffices to tide the patient over this acute phase without compromising his chances of recovery or leading to any significant degree of malnutrition.

When all or most of the calories must be administered by the parenteral route, there is an advantage in using relatively concentrated solutions of glucose. Provided that the infusion rate is slow, concentrations of 15 per cent can be infused over long periods of time without significant losses of glucose in the urine or the development of thrombophlebitis.

In experimental animals, vitamin B_{12} given *prophylactically* protects the liver against carbon tetrachloride injury.[581] However, there is no evidence to indicate that vitamins administered *following* toxic injury to the liver facilitate recovery. Therefore, there would appear to be no rationale for supplementing the diet in the treatment of toxic hepatitis, except possibly in instances where the antecedent diet has been deficient, or where prolonged parenteral feedings of vitamin-free glucose may precipitate an acute deficiency state.

The effects of methionine and choline in experimental animals have encouraged the use of these agents in the treatment of toxic hepatitis.[48, 201] However, there is no convincing clinical evidence to show that these dietary supplements have any therapeutic value in well-nourished individuals.

The principles governing the management of the cirrhosis that occasionally follows toxic hepatitis are essentially the same as those for Laennec's cirrhosis and therefore require no further discussion. However, the response to dietotherapy is likely to be far less impressive in the toxic type, since nutritional factors are either lacking or are of subsidiary importance in its pathogenesis.

Bed Rest. Although the importance of bed rest has not been established, it is recommended that the patient with acute toxic hepatitis be kept in bed until hepatic function returns to normal on the principle that immobilization may facilitate repair of the injured liver by enhancing its blood flow and by reducing the metabolic demands made upon it.

DRUG-INDUCED HEPATITIS

CLASSIFICATION

Most drugs that injure the liver appear to do so by inducing a hypersensitivity reaction, but a few behave as true hepatotoxins. Methyltestosterone and a number of other substituted derivatives of testosterone comprise a special category whose actions are difficult to classify. The features that distinguish between these three groups of drugs are discussed at the beginning of this chapter.

The morphologic changes and the clinical manifestations in drug-induced hepatitis may be predominantly those of hepatocellular injury or those of cholestasis, but in many instances features of both types are evident. The synthetic androgens and anabolic agents also produce cholestasis, but the lesions differ in some respects from those seen in other forms of drug-induced hepatitis.

PATHOGENESIS

Surprisingly little is known about the mechanisms responsible for the development of drug-induced hepatitis, chiefly because the lesions are not reproducible in animals. Studies in man have been limited in scope, being largely concerned with the clinical, functional and morphologic features of the established lesion rather than with the fundamental disturbances that provoke hepatic injury.

Hepatocellular Injury. As pointed out, the few drugs that qualify as true hepatotoxins, such as chloroform, behave like other hepatotoxins in that they injure the liver in all individuals given sufficiently large doses, exhibit the same effects in experimental animals and produce a distinctive type of zonal hepatic necrosis following a predictable and usually brief latent period. Characteristically, the extent of the lesions varies with the dose. In contrast, most other drugs that affect the liver produce a type of hepatic

injury (1) that cannot be induced in all individuals, (2) that is not reproducible in animals, (3) whose morphologic features are more variable and less distinctive than in toxic hepatitis, (4) in which neither the occurrence nor the extent of the lesions can be correlated with the amount of drug consumed, and (5) in which the latent period is variable and unpredictable.

The sporadic nature of the susceptibility to drug-induced hepatitis and the frequency with which the hepatic lesions are accompanied by manifestations of hypersensitivity, such as fever, rash and eosinophilia, suggest that drug reactions of this type are allergic in nature. Longcope[454] and Chase[132] have emphasized the similarities between drug reactions and serum sickness and have proposed that both represent forms of acquired hypersensitivity, a view that is supported by the observations of Landsteiner,[411, 412, 413] Rich[612, 614] and others.[733, 777] Of particular interest in this connection is the fact that simple chemical compounds can serve as antigens and induce hypersensitivity,[412, 733] and that the tissue changes in drug reactions closely resemble those of experimental anaphylaxis.[311, 615]

Although the theory of acquired hypersensitivity is based on an impressive body of evidence, some aspects of drug reactions appear to be inconsistent. These include the rarity with which circulating antibodies and skin hypersensitivity can be demonstrated, the inconstancy of the interval between the first exposure to a drug and the development of a reaction, and the variable character of the clinical manifestations. In contrast, the anaphylactic type of hypersensitivity seen in serum sickness and under experimental conditions in animals is characterized by readily demonstrable circulating antibodies and skin sensitivity, an immediate reaction to the antigen in the sensitized host, and a response that is distinctive for the species.[613]

Even in the delayed or tuberculin type of hypersensitivity, the interval between the injection of an antigen and the appearance of a reaction in a sensitive host is usually not longer than 24 to 48 hours, and skin hypersensitivity can be demonstrated with great regularity. At present, our knowledge of drug reaction is too fragmentary to account for these discrepancies, although several possibilities may be considered. Since simple chemical compounds require conjugation with protein before they can serve as antigens,[411, 413, 777] it is conceivable that variations in the length of the latent period are related to differences in the speed with which such conjugates are formed, and that failure to demonstrate circulating antibodies and skin sensitivity may be due to the use of inappropriately conjugated antigens in testing.

Differences in the metabolic pathways followed by drugs may determine the readiness with which antigens are produced and hence account for variations in individual susceptibility. Although drug reactions occur more frequently in individuals with an allergic background, differences in susceptibility cannot be attributed to hereditary constitutional factors alone, since the vast majority of reactions occur in individuals with no such background.

The feature of drug hypersensitivity most difficult to explain is the extreme variability of its manifestations. Why such hypersensitivity is expressed as a fever and a rash in one individual, as hepatitis in another, and as a depression of myelopoiesis in a third, or why some drugs produce one or another of these manifestations more frequently than any of the others is completely unknown. Certainly, in experimental anaphylactic hypersensitivity, there is far less individual variation, and the nature of the sensitizing agent plays no significant role in determining the character of the reaction. Since the lesions are thought to be the consequence of an antigen-antibody reaction on or within cells,[311] it has been suggested that the manifestations of hypersensitivity depend on the distribution of antibody within the tissues.

Closely related to this problem is the question of how the hepatic lesions are produced in drug reactions. Buckley[105] and Follis[233] have presented convincing evidence to show that the hepatic cells do not participate in experimental anaphylactic reactions, and that the focal necrosis and inflammation seen in the liver under such conditions[308, 453] are the consequence of vascular injury. Although vascular lesions can be demonstrated in some cases of drug hypersensitivity,[243]

often the nature of the lesions suggests direct injury to the hepatic parenchymal cells. This raises the question of whether drug reactions may not be more closely related to the delayed tuberculin type of hypersensitivity, the type usually induced by infection, and characterized by sensitization of the tissues generally and by the absence of demonstrable circulating antibodies. Chase, who has studied this problem, believes that both the immediate anaphylactic and delayed tuberculin types of hypersensitivity may play a role in drug reactions.[132] However, this has not been established, so that, for the present at least, drug reactions must be considered a unique form of hypersensitivity.

Some drugs, such as iproniazid, produce hepatic lesions that are indistinguishable from those of viral hepatitis.[577] The possibility that agents of this type enhance the susceptibility to intercurrent infection with the hepatitis virus or light up latent infection in carriers has been considered but has not been investigated.

In differentiating between hepatotoxic and sensitizing drugs, and in evaluating the potential hazards of therapy with such agents, two generalizations are worth bearing in mind. First, if a drug produces hepatic injury in man but fails to do so in other species, it is likely to prove to be a sensitizing agent and may be expected to produce other manifestations of hypersensitivity. Second, if it gives rise to extrahepatic manifestations of hypersensitivity in some individuals, it can be predicted that sooner or later it will produce hepatitis in others.

Cholestasis. Many drugs, such as chlorpromazine, produce a type of hepatitis, generally classified as cholestatic, in which the clinical and the laboratory features resemble those of extrahepatic biliary obstruction. Characteristically, the liver shows evidence of bile stasis but few signs of hepatocellular injury. An inflammatory reaction in the portal triads is a constant feature, except in the type of cholestatic jaundice produced by methyltestosterone and other substituted derivatives of methyltestosterone.

Drug-induced cholestatic hepatitis has been variously attributed to (1) subtle toxic injury to the hepatic parenchymal cells, leading to increased viscosity of the bile and occlusion of the canaliculi[712] or to swelling of the parenchyma and compression of the canaliculi[441]; (2) toxic injury to the canalicular membranes of the parenchymal cells, resulting in effacement or distortion of their microvilli, secondary stasis and inspissation of bile, and ultimate dilatation and rupture of the canaliculi into the spaces of Disse[647, 648]; and (3) a hypersensitivity reaction with injury to both the parenchymal cells and small bile ducts.[807] In support of the view that drugs of this type may be hepatotoxic, it has been demonstrated that in the rat chlorpromazine depresses Bromsulphalein excretion[25] and enhances the hepatotoxic effects of ethionine.[579] However, direct measurements have failed to demonstrate any alterations in bile flow,[683] and administration of massive doses of chlorpromazine for periods up to 6 months has not produced significant hepatic lesions or jaundice in such animals.[579] These observations taken together with the fact that patients may recover from cholestatic hepatitis while still taking the offending drug,[655] or may develop the disorder a week or two after discontinuing its use,[354] appear to be inconsistent with the interpretation that these agents are hepatotoxic. As in hepatocellular type of drug-induced hepatitis, many features of the cholestatic type point to an underlying hypersensitivity reaction. These include its sporadic occurrence in patients receiving such drugs, the immunity of animals and the frequency of its association with fever,[373] rash[141] and eosinophilia.[176]

The mode of action of methyltestosterone and other substituted derivatives of testosterone would appear to differ fundamentally from that of other drugs that produce cholestatic hepatitis. Although jaundice develops only sporadically following large doses of methyltestosterone[781] or norethandrolone,[194, 649] the regular occurrence of Bromsulphalein retention in man[313, 398] and of reduced bile flow[23] and alterations in the electron microscopic appearance of the canaliculi[650] in the rat suggest that these compounds behave more like hepatotoxins than sensitizing agents. Consistent with this

interpretation is the fact that they do not provoke an inflammatory reaction in the liver or produce clinical manifestations of hypersensitivity, such as fever, rash or eosinophilia. However, they differ from most hepatotoxins in that they do not produce hepatic necrosis. Available evidence suggests that they interfere with bile excretion by some unknown mechanism.

Since the plasma levels of conjugated bilirubin and alkaline phosphatase are invariably elevated, it is generally agreed that regurgitation of bile is the major factor responsible for the development of jaundice in cholestatic hepatitis. Several mechanisms have been invoked to account for the reflux of bile under these conditions: (1) occlusion of the canaliculi by inspissated bile,[712] (2) dilatation and ultimate rupture of the canaliculi into the spaces of Disse,[647] (3) obstruction of the small bile radicles in the portal triads by inflammatory exudate[711] and (4) increased permeability of the cholangioles.[329] Since each parenchymal cell is drained by several canaliculi and all canaliculi are arranged in a complex network of intercommunicating channels, it is highly improbable that the scattered bile thrombi seen in cholestatic hepatitis obstruct the flow of bile significantly.

Although the possibility of rupture of the canaliculi into the spaces of Disse cannot be excluded with certainty, electron microscopic studies have failed to demonstrate such communications even under conditions of complete biliary obstruction.[298]

Occlusion of the cholangioles by inflammatory exudate is often cited as an important factor in the pathogenesis of drug-induced cholestasis. However, this has not been established histologically and appears unlikely, since the inflammatory reaction in the portal triads usually is less intense than in the hepatocellular type of drug-induced hepatitis and is totally absent in some cases.

Except in rare instances in which actual necrosis of the cholangioles has been demonstrated,[807] there is no direct evidence that these structures are abnormally permeable under conditions of cholestasis.

One possibility that has received insufficient attention is that drugs may produce cholestasis by affecting the bilirubin transport system and permeability of the hepatic parenchymal cells, thus permitting the reflux of conjugated bilirubin from the cells and/or the canaliculi into the lymph spaces and the sinusoids. That cellular disturbances of this type can occur in the absence of histologic abnormalities is evident from the elegant *in vivo* studies of bile secretion carried out by Hanzon, using direct microscopy of the liver following the injection of uranin, a fluorescent dye that is excreted in the bile.[302] Similarly, reflux of bile from the canaliculi into the lymph spaces via the cytoplasm of the parenchymal cells has been confirmed by electron microscopy.[298] More direct evidence suggestive of altered permeability of the hepatic cells in cholestatic hepatitis is the rise in the serum transaminase level that often occurs in the absence of overt hepatic necrosis.

Of interest are studies on the pathogenesis of "geel-dikkop," a naturally occurring form of cholestatic hepatitis seen in South African sheep that feed on the poisonous plant *Lippia rehmanni*.[620] Rimington and associates have shown that in the rabbit, icterogenin, a triterpene acid derivative of this plant, suppresses bile secretion and blocks the excretion of intravenously injected conjugated and unconjugated bilirubin without producing histologic abnormalities in the liver.[618] They interpret these observations as evidence of a defect in the transport of bilirubin through the hepatic cells and suggest that icterogenin may alter cell permeability, permitting regurgitation of bile from the canaliculi.

PATHOLOGY

Drugs may give rise to a variety of lesions, depending on their mode of action. True hepatotoxins, such as chloroform, produce parenchymal necrosis, degeneration and fatty infiltration with a distinctive zonal pattern in the lobules, and little or no inflammatory reaction. In contrast, sensitizing drugs give rise to hepatocellular and/or cholestatic lesions that differ from those seen in toxic hepatitis.

In the hepatocellular type, produced by agents like the sulfonamides,[243] the liver shows scattered foci of parenchymal necrosis and a diffuse inflammatory reaction that usually is most intense in the portal triads. Bile stasis is an inconstant but common feature, whereas deposition of fat is rare. Occasionally, the portal triads contain granulomata, some of which may involve vessel walls.[243, 517] Some drugs, such as iproniazid and cinchophen, cause lesions that are indistinguishable from those of viral hepatitis and occasionally involve large masses of parenchyma, producing the picture of subacute or massive hepatic necrosis.[577] A fatal outcome is relatively common in this group; in survivors, healing of the liver may be accompanied by scarring and the development of postnecrotic cirrhosis.

Many sensitizing drugs, such as chlorpromazine, produce hepatic lesions in which bile stasis, particularly in the pericentral bile canaliculi, is the predominant feature. Usually, the portal triads are infiltrated to a variable degree with mononuclear, polymorphonuclear and eosinophilic leukocytes. The absence of hepatocellular necrosis and intralobular inflammation is generally emphasized as a characteristic feature of drug-induced cholestatic hepatitis. However, careful study of biopsy specimens frequently reveals such changes, although not to the same extent as in the hepatocellular type.[383, 807] In the writer's experience no sharp distinction can be drawn between the lesions of cholestatic and hepatocellular hepatitis. Although cholestasis may predominate in the one and parenchymal damage in the other, most cases show evidence of both. The hepatitis produced by some drugs may be of the cholestatic type in some individuals and of the hepatocellular type in others.

Usually, recovery from cholestatic hepatitis is relatively prompt and without residuals. However, the disease may run a prolonged course with persistent jaundice and hepatomegaly, occasionally accompanied by splenomegaly, hypercholesterolemia[301] and xanthomatosis.[70, 529, 724] This syndrome has been reported following hypersensitivity reactions to the arsphenamines[301, 724] sulfanilamide,[62] thiouracil,[253] neocinchophen[70] and chlorpromazine.[529] Although ultimate recovery without significant residuals occurs and is said by some[594] to be the rule, there are well-documented instances of slowly progressive periportal inflammation and fibrosis leading ultimately to the development of biliary cirrhosis.[62, 70, 383, 529] Both the clinical and the histologic findings in such cases bear a remarkable resemblance to those described in primary biliary cirrhosis. This suggests the interesting possibility that, in some instances, unrecognized reactions to drugs are important in the pathogenesis of this otherwise obscure disease.

The hepatic lesions produced by methyltestosterone and other substituted derivatives of testosterone are characterized by pericentral canalicular bile stasis and thus resemble those of drug-induced cholestatic hepatitis. However, they differ in that they show no significant hepatocellular damage or inflammatory reaction.[649, 781] Rarely, drugs of this type produce peliosis hepatis,[274, 378] an unusual disorder that may be fatal in which the parenchyma of the liver is studded with blood-filled cystic spaces lined by endothelial or hepatic parenchymal cells. Focal necrosis, vasculitis and agonal congestion have been invoked as possible factors in the pathogenesis of this lesion.

CLINICAL FEATURES

The interval between the first exposure to a drug and the onset of a reaction involving the liver tends to be longer and is less predictable than in toxic hepatitis. Reactions of this type are seen most commonly between the 2nd and 5th week, but may occur as early as the 1st day or only after many months of drug administration. Occasionally, the reaction appears as long as a week or two after cessation of therapy.[329]

Variations in the period of latency appear to be dependent on host factors rather than on the nature of the agent involved. In previously exposed individuals, readministration of a drug may provoke a reaction following the first dose, presumably because of antecedent sensitization. However, similar immediate reactions are seen occasionally in individuals with no history of previous exposure.[426] It is difficult to account for such cases on the basis of hypersensitivity unless it is assumed that inadvertent contact with the drug or with some chemically related compound has occurred in the past.

SYMPTOMS

Not infrequently, the onset of drug-induced hepatitis is heralded by the abrupt appearance of constitutional manifestations of hypersensitivity, such as fever, chills, a morbilliform or urticarial rash, pruritus and arthralgia. Often these are accompanied by anorexia and nausea, and less commonly by vomiting and abdominal pain. Jaundice and dark urine become evident within a few days and usually are accompanied by enlargement and tenderness of the liver. Splenomegaly is seen occasionally but is less common than in viral hepatitis. Acholic stools and pruritus are frequent findings in cholestatic hepatitis but are inconstant features in the hepatocellular type.

In some cases the onset of jaundice is insidious without antecedent or accompanying constitutional symptoms. This is the rule in the type of cholestatic hepatitis produced by methyltestosterone and other substituted derivatives of testosterone and may be seen in other forms of drug-induced hepatic injury.

Liver damage may occur in the absence of jaundice. This is illustrated by the frequency with which Bromsulphalein retention,[419] rises in the serum levels of alkaline phosphatase[383] and transaminase,[649] and histologic changes in the liver[383] can be demonstrated in the course of drug reactions unaccompanied by jaundice or other overt clinical signs of hepatic involvement.

Usually, prompt withdrawal of the offending drug is followed within a few days by subsidence of fever and other constitutional manifestations. However, the signs of hepatitis clear more slowly, usually requiring 2 to 3 weeks for full resolution. Occasionally, they persist for many weeks or even months.

Protracted cholestatic jaundice may be accompanied by progressive enlargement of the liver and the spleen, intractable pruritus and xanthomatosis,[62, 70, 529] features indistinguishable from those of so-called primary biliary cirrhosis. In a few instances, cirrhosis has been demonstrated histologically,[62, 70, 529] but in others the inflammatory reaction and fibrosis in the liver have been less extensive, and apparent clinical recovery has occurred.[594] The ultimate outcome in the latter group is uncertain, since the histologic abnormalities and the raised levels of serum alkaline phosphatase and cholesterol usually persist despite clearing of the jaundice and xanthomatosis. In cases with documented cirrhosis, the disease tends to run a more benign course than in other forms of biliary cirrhosis.

Drugs such as iproniazid, pyrazinamide and cinchophen, which give rise to lesions that resemble those of viral hepatitis, occasionally produce subacute or massive hepatic necrosis. As might be expected, the clinical manifestations under these circumstances are usually more severe than in uncomplicated acute hepatitis, and may include such unusual features as intense abdominal pain, coffee-ground vomitus, a rapid decrease in the size of the liver, ascites, edema, hemorrhagic phenomena, somnolence and coma. Occasionally, the clinical course is deceptively benign, apparent recovery taking place despite the occurrence of postnecrotic scarring and nodular hyperplasia. If the liver is not examined histologically, the true nature of the lesion in such cases may not become evident until signs of cirrhosis appear months or even years later. Usually, however, the course is more prolonged and is characterized by signs of hepatic decompensation. Death may ensue in a few weeks or months and usually is due to hepatic failure, hemorrhage from esophageal varices or intercurrent infection.

LABORATORY FEATURES

In the heptocellular type of drug-induced hepatitis, the results of liver function tests are identical with those seen in acute viral hepatitis, with the exception that high levels of serum alkaline phosphatase are more common.

The typical biochemical pattern in the cholestatic type of hepatitis resembles that of extrahepatic biliary obstruction, except for the occurrence of high levels of serum transaminase early in the course of the disease. Characteristically, there is an increase in serum bilirubin involving the conjugated fraction predominantly, excretion of bilirubin in the urine, a decrease in the output of urobilinogen in the feces, and a sharp rise in the serum levels of alkaline phosphatase and cholesterol. With few exceptions, thymol turbidity and cephalin-cholesterol flocculation remain normal. In the protracted form of cholestatic hepatitis, particularly in cases complicated by xanthomatosis, the concentration of cholesterol rises to high levels, often above those seen in extrahepatic biliary obstruction or primary biliary cirrhosis.[594] Studies with acetate-1-^{14}C indicate that the rate of cholesterol and phospholipid synthesis under these conditions is greatly increased.[529] Both the serum alkaline phosphatase and cholesterol attain high levels relatively early in the disease, a point that may help to distinguish between drug-induced cholestasis and biliary obstruction.

Eosinophilia is an inconstant feature of drug reactions but, when present, may be an important clue to the etiology in drug-induced hepatitis. Usually, the leukocyte count is normal or moderately elevated, but leukopenia and agranulocytosis are seen occasionally.[636]

TREATMENT

Prompt withdrawal of the offending agent is of prime importance in the management of drug-induced hypersensitivity reactions, since this alone may abort the reaction and prevent serious injury to the liver and the bone marrow. However, once provoked, reactions of this type may run a fulminant and even fatal course despite the absence of further exposure to the drug.

Although ACTH and adrenal cortical steroids are useful in other allergic diseases, their efficacy in drug-induced hepatitis has not been established. Nevertheless, since favorable results have been reported in a few instances,[159, 712] it would appear reasonable to employ these agents in severe drug-induced hepatitis that does not respond to drug withdrawal and simple supportive measures, or when continued administration of the offending drug is urgently needed.

Since a serious reaction may follow even a single small dose, it is unwise to readminister drugs that have previously provoked manifestations of hypersensitivity unless the indications are urgent. Successfull desensitization with graded doses has been reported,[765, 772] but it is difficult to evaluate the efficacy of this procedure, since drug reactions may subside spontaneously despite continued administration of the offending agent[354, 655, 689] or may fail to recur when drug therapy is resumed following recovery.[765] If desensitization is attempted, concomitant steroid therapy early in the course may help prevent reactions.[765]

In general, the principles of treatment are the same as for toxic hepatitis and are discussed elsewhere.

In the protracted form of cholestatic hepatitis, special measures may be required to control intractable pruritus, diarrhea and the tendency to decalcification of the bones. Methyltestosterone and norethandrolone relieve the pruritus,[594] but may intensify the jaundice. Although there is no conclusive evidence to indicate that this retards ultimate recovery, it is probably wiser to use cholestyramine, a resin that binds bile acids and prevents their reabsorption from the intestinal tract.[122] Because of the malabsorption that usually accompanies the impairment of bile flow in prolonged cholestasis, vitamin D deficiency and decalcification of the bones may ensue. Accordingly, supplements of vitamin D and calcium should be prescribed to avoid this complication. Diarrhea related to malabsorption of fat may be partially alleviated by reducing the fat content of the diet, but this is done only if the diarrhea is troublesome, since it may lead to wasting.

Prophylaxis

Since the potential hazard of sensitization cannot be evaluated in animals, all new drugs must be considered suspect until proved to be otherwise by prolonged trial in man. If a drug gives rise to any of the manifestations of hypersensitivity, one can be reasonably confident that sooner or later it will produce hepatitis.

Although it is not possible to predict the susceptibility to drug reactions, the hazard appears to be somewhat greater in individuals with an allergic background, particularly those with a history of a previous reaction to other drugs. Indeed, during a reaction, patients may exhibit hypersensitivity to a wide variety of unrelated agents. For that reason it is best to stop all medications until the reaction subsides and then, if necessary, resume their use one at a time.

Patients receiving sensitizing drugs should be watched carefully for early signs of a reaction. If fever, rash or pruritus occur, the medication should be stopped immediately. at least until other possible causes can be excluded. In the case of patients given agents known to produce serious reactions involving the liver, the serum alkaline phosphatase and transaminase should be tested at weekly intervals during the first 2 months, the period of greatest risk.

SPECIAL FEATURES OF AGENTS CAPABLE OF PRODUCING LIVER INJURY

Hepatotoxins comprise such a heterogeneous group with respect to their chemical structure and mode of action that they are difficult to classify in any logical or orderly manner. For convenience, therefore, the following section is arranged alphabetically. The agents selected for discussion by no means constitute a complete inventory of substances that can injure the liver, but most of those known to produce toxic hepatitis in man are included.

ACCIDENTAL AND INDUSTRIAL POISONING

Beryllium

Inhalation of beryllium compounds may provoke either an acute pneumonitis or a chronic granulomatous reaction in the lung. The former, which is more common, follows exposure to most of the beryllium dusts and fumes encountered in industry, appears after a relatively brief incubation period, is characterized pathologically by an exudation of mononuclear cells into the alveoli and usually resolves completely within 4 months.

In contrast, the chronic disease develops chiefly following exposure to beryllium oxide, appears after a relatively long latent period, ranging from a month to 15 years,[303] is characterized pathologically by a diffuse granulomatous reaction that closely resembles sarcoidosis and runs a chronic progressive course that often terminates fatally.[718, 759] Not infrequently, the disease is accompanied by hepatosplenomegaly, a raised level of serum gamma globulin, a negative tuberculin reaction, hypercalcuria and renal stones,[303] features that may make the differentiation from sarcoidosis exceedingly difficult.

Although acute and chronic berylliosis are considered distinct clinical and morphologic entities, it has been suggested, on the basis of autopsy studies, that the chronic granulomatous lesion represents a late development in the evolution of the acute pneumonic process.[195] This view is difficult to reconcile with the observation that, while the inhalation of beryllium compounds provokes an acute pneumonitis, neither inhalation[722] nor parenteral administration[666] of such agents produces granulomas in the lungs of experimental animals.

Several features of the granulomatous reaction suggest that it results from sensitization to beryllium. These include its sporadic occurrence in exposed individuals, the long period of latency, the disparity between the amount of beryllium found in the lungs and the severity of the lesions[718] and the immunity of experimental animals. The fact that patch tests with beryllium salts provoke a granulomatous inflammatory reaction in the skin of affected individuals[170, 701] lends support to the sensitization theory. However, the possibility that beryllium can provoke a granulomatous reaction in the lung by some direct action cannot be excluded with certainty, since subcutaneous injections of beryllium produce granulomas both locally[281, 686] and in regional lymph nodes.[281]

Berylliosis may be acquired in any occupation involving the handling of beryllium or its compounds. Metal workers who machine beryllium or alloys high in beryllium content, and manufacturers of ceramics, radio tubes and neon signs are the principal victims.[702] The use of beryllium phosphorus in fluorescent bulbs was discontinued in 1949, so that this no longer constitutes the hazard it once did.[303] Individuals who live within a 3-mile radius of a beryllium plant may acquire the disease as a consequence of prolonged exposure to low concentrations of beryllium-containing dust and fumes emitted from smoke stacks.[133, 169] Inadvertent intoxication occurs also in individuals who come in contact with the contaminated clothing of beryllium workers.[169, 303]

A variety of hepatic lesions are found in fatal cases of both forms of pulmonary berylliosis. These do not occur with any degree of regularity, nor do they give rise to overt signs of liver disease. In the acute pneumonic type, centrilobular necrosis is the principal finding.[195, 759] Hepatic necrosis also occurs in animals after intravenous injections of beryllium compounds.[666] However, the lesions produced tend to be midzonal in location and do not occur when the beryllium is administered by the respiratory route.[722] Therefore, the centrilobular necrosis in man may be due not to the local toxic action of beryllium but rather to the passive congestion and anoxia that occur terminally in acute beryllium pneumonitis.

In the delayed form of chronic beryllium intoxication, small granulomata, similar to those in the lung, are often found scattered throughout the liver.[133, 169, 759] These are indistinguishable from the lesions seen in sarcoidosis and a number of other related diseases.[385] Chronic passive congestion of the liver secondary to cor pulmonale and heart failure is another abnormality found with some frequency. In rare instances the liver may exhibit central and midzonal necrosis,[169] severe parenchymatous degeneration[169] and a diffuse fibrosis.[195] Whether or not these are directly related to the effects of beryllium is not known.

Both the clinical features and the histologic findings in berylliosis may be indistinguishable from those of sarcoidosis. Usually, a history of exposure to beryllium suffices for differentiation, but in doubtful cases a patch test may be required for confirmation. In this test a small gauze square moistened with a 1 or 2 per cent solution of beryllium sulfate or nitrate is applied to the skin for 48 hours. On removal of the patch, patients with berylliosis exhibit an area of erythema, induration and scaling which may persist for a number of weeks. Biopsy of the skin late in the course of the reaction shows sarcoid-like granulomas with small zones of central necrosis.[701] From the evidence available, this test appears to be sensitive and specific.[170, 701]

CARBON TETRACHLORIDE

Because of its widespread use as a solvent, fire-extinguisher and cleaning agent, carbon tetrachloride is an important cause of toxic hepatitis. Poisoning usually follows inhalation of the vapor in a poorly ventilated enclosed space but also occurs after its ingestion. It is not known whether it is absorbed significantly through the skin. It has been suggested on the basis of autopsy[690] evidence that liver injury is more common after ingestion than after inhalation of carbon tetrachloride. However, this has not been borne out in all studies.[514]

Susceptibility. In animals, as little as 0.02 ml. of carbon tetrachloride/kg. can produce histologically demonstrable hepatic lesions. On the basis of experiments carried out on criminals awaiting execution,[178] it would appear that only slightly larger doses (5 ml.), well within the antihelminthic therapeutic range, occasionally produce similar lesions in man. Although these are usually not detectable clinically, there are marked individual differences in susceptibility, so that even small doses of carbon tetrachloride occasionally inflict serious injury. Fatal intoxication has been reported after the ingestion of as little as 1.5 ml.,[437] yet recovery has followed poisoning with amounts in excess of 100 ml.[423]

With respect to the toxic level of carbon tetrachloride in the atmosphere, it is obviously a function not only of the concentration but also of the duration of exposure. On the basis of animal experiments it has been estimated that a concentration in excess of 0.01 per cent in air is required to produce clinically detectable intoxication in individuals chronically exposed to carbon tetrachloride vapor in their work.[698] The time-dose relationships under other conditions have not been worked out.

Alcohol Ingestion. Clinical and experimental evidence indicates that alcohol greatly increases the susceptibility to carbon tetrachloride. In one autopsy series,[514] for example, 11 of 12 fatal cases of accidental poisoning occurred in alcoholics. Similarly, of 34 individuals being treated for hookworm infestation with small doses of carbon tetrachloride, the only 2 instances of toxicity were encountered in alcoholics.[691] Results of animal experiments confirm these clinical observations.[409]

The mechanism underlying this synergism is not known, but it has been suggested that alcohol, by virtue of its solvent properties, enhances the absorption of carbon tetrachloride from the intestinal tract[409] and facilitates its penetration and storage in cells,[631] or it renders the liver more susceptible to injury by increasing its fat content.[514] Another possibility is that carbon tetrachloride is oxidized to phosgene and then undergoes condensation with ethanol to form ethylchloroformate, a compound allegedly more toxic than carbon tetrachloride.[283]

None of these theories alone, however, accounts for the fact that alcohol enhances the toxicity of both ingested and inhaled carbon tetrachloride, that it increases the severity of injury in both the liver and kidney, and that the increased susceptibility is seen in chronic alcoholics who have not been drinking immediately prior to poisoning.[514] Moreover, whereas alcohol enhances the acute toxic effects of carbon tetrachloride, it does not increase the severity of the hepatic lesions in chronic poisoning.[410]

Nutritional Status. Susceptibility to carbon tetrachloride also appears to depend on the nutritional status. In animals, inanition[235] and high-fat diets[80] increase the toxicity of carbon tetrachloride, whereas, surprisingly, low-protein diets do not.[187] The importance of these factors in man has not been investigated.

Pathologic changes in fatal cases of carbon tetrachloride poisoning[514] closely resemble those described in experimental animals.[114]

The *hepatic lesions* are characterized by diffuse fatty degeneration and necrosis of the centrilobular parenchyma, collapse of reticulum, hemorrhage and leukocytic infiltration. Regeneration occurs early and proceeds from intact cells at the periphery of the lobule. In animals cytologic changes are evident within a few hours and reach a maximum in 24 to 48 hours; regeneration is active by the 3rd day, and histologic recovery is complete by the 14th day. However, the hepatic cells continue to exhibit an increased susceptibility to further injury long after their microscopic appearance has returned to normal.[331] Individuals who have succumbed to renal failure as long as 18 days following intoxication still show signs of liver injury,[514] which suggests that healing may occur more slowly in man.

Massive hepatic necrosis is rare. It will be recalled that the same is true in animals, unless the carbon tetrachloride is injected directly into the portal vein.[116] The writer has seen two instances of subacute hepatic necrosis following a single exposure to carbon tetrachloride.[383] Although these patients recovered clinically, residual postnecrotic scarring was evident on biopsy.

Renal lesions are invariably present in fatal cases and may be the cause of death. The principal findings include degenerative changes in the tubules, the presence of heme and cellular casts, cellular infiltration of the supporting connective tissue, and signs of active regeneration in the tubular epithelium.[514]

The *pulmonary findings* in carbon tetrachloride poisoning are of considerable interest and are seen with great regularity in individuals who survive for longer than 8 days. Characteristically, the alveoli exhibit a fibrinous exudate with pseudomembrane formation, fibroblastic thickening of their walls, and proliferation of their epithelial lining cells.[754] These appear to be related to renal insufficiency and are identical with those seen in other forms of acute renal failure. In addition, the lungs frequently show edema, hemorrhage, congestion and bronchopneumonia, features that are thought to be the result of shock, infection and other factors unrelated to the direct effects of carbon tetrachloride. Often, right-sided dilatation of the heart accompanies these pulmonary changes.

Areas of atypical focal *pancreatitis* may be seen.[514] These too appear to be related to the kidney damage, since they have been observed in other types of acute renal failure.[28] As a rule, the lesions are limited in extent and severity and do not give rise to overt symptoms.

Clinical manifestations of acute carbon tetrachloride poisoning relate to (1) the general toxic and pharmacologic effects of the agent, (2) liver damage or (3) renal injury. Although any of these may predominate, careful examination usually discloses evidence of all three. Often the three groups of symptoms overlap, so that it may be impossible to specify their origin.

The general *toxic* and *pharmacologic effects* of the poison are the first to become evident. Usually, they appear within a few hours but may be delayed for as long as a day. With large oral doses and, more commonly following inhalation of toxic fumes, the onset may be immediate. The most frequent symptoms during this period include dizziness, headache, nausea and vomiting. In more severe cases, there may be confusion, abdominal cramps, diarrhea, generalized muscle pain and vasomotor collapse. Occasionally, exposure to a high concentration of fumes results in a deep but transient narcosis due to the anesthetic properties of the agent. Death seldom occurs during this initial period. Occasionally, even fatal doses of carbon tetrachloride do not produce immediate symptoms, so that the first signs of intoxication are delayed until hepatic or renal involvement becomes evident some days later.

Clinical signs of *liver involvement* appear 2 to 4 days after intoxication, or a day or two after the maximum injury demonstrable histologically. Jaundice and hepatomegaly are the principal clinical manifestations; however, it is evident from autopsy findings[514] that extensive hepatic necrosis may occur without producing either. Therefore, it is important to check the functional stasis of the liver in evaluating the severity of carbon tetrachloride intoxication. The gastrointestinal symptoms which appear shortly after exposure usually increase as the signs of liver damage become evident. In general, the severity of the poisoning is correlated with the depth of jaundice. However, death from renal failure may occur with little or no clinical evidence of hepatic injury.[514, 690, 796]

Autopsy studies indicate that the *kidneys*

are involved about as frequently as the liver, and in many cases renal failure dominates the clinical picture.[514, 690] It has been suggested that there is an inverse relationship between the severity of the lesions in the kidneys and the liver.[514] Most deaths attributable to hepatitis occur during the 1st week, whereas those due to renal failure occur in the 2nd and 3rd weeks.[754] However, as indicated, usually there is evidence of both hepatic and renal injury in all cases. Even in mild intoxication, the urine usually contains albumin and casts during the first few days. In more severe cases, oliguria appears between the 2nd and 4th days and then may progress to complete anuria.

Azotemia is common and occasionally is accompanied by hypertension. During the period of oliguria the specific gravity tends to become fixed at a level of 1.010, and often the urine contains a significant number of red blood cells and polymorphonuclear leukocytes. In some cases, however, the urine shows little, other than a reduced volume and a low specific gravity, despite the presence of severe azotemia. The close resemblance of the clinical picture to that in other forms of acute tubular necrosis has been emphasized.[796] However, dehydration due to fluid losses from the intestinal tract often plays an important role in the development of azotemia and must be taken into consideration in planning therapy.

Not infrequently peripheral and pulmonary *edema* supervene as the azotemia progresses. While cardiac failure may be responsible for this complication in some cases, often faulty regulation of fluid and electrolyte balance is the cause. The dyspnea, cyanosis and signs of consolidation that appear terminally are due usually to the pulmonary lesions associated with azotemia described previously. Occasionally, acute pulmonary edema is seen immediately following exposure to carbon tetrachloride. This is thought to be the result of the direct irritant effect of the agent on the alveoli.

Prognosis. It is difficult to predict the outcome in any given case of carbon tetrachloride poisoning. In general, the outlook is favorable if jaundice is mild and the signs of renal impairment are minimal or absent.

However, the prognosis should be guarded early in the course of mild hepatitis, since the appearance of renal failure may be delayed for a number of days and then terminate fatally. If the patient survives the 1st week he is not likely to die of hepatic failure. Similarly, if azotemia is not evident by the end of the 1st week it is unlikely to develop later, so that the outlook for recovery is excellent.

If the initial effects of acute carbon tetrachloride poisoning are survived, the signs of hepatitis usually subside in 2 to 4 weeks, a period slightly longer than that required for morphologic restitution of the liver in experimental animals.[114] As a rule, there are no residuals, but in occasional cases healing of extensive lesions is followed by postnecrotic scarring.[383] Recovery from renal injury is somewhat slower but is always complete. Occasionally, cirrhosis follows repeated exposure to subclinical toxic doses of carbon tetrachloride,[574] as in experimental animals.[114] The clinical picture in such cases does not differ significantly from that in other types of cirrhosis, so that the diagnosis depends almost entirely on the history of exposure. Early recognition of this condition is important, since the cirrhotic lesion may be reversible in its early stages if further exposure to the toxin is prevented.[114]

Treatment. The general principles of treatment are outlined on pages 505-508. As mentioned, there is no evidence to indicate that supplements of protein, methionine or choline exert any *therapeutic* effect in the well-nourished individual. However, it is possible that they may be of benefit in malnourished individuals if given immediately after intoxication.

A wide variety of chemically unrelated substances, including tocopherol,[340] glutathione,[102] sodium thiomalate,[102] sodium malate,[102] sodium thioglycollate,[102] sodium glycocollate,[102] vitamin B_{12}[581] and adrenergic blocking agents[112] reportedly protect animals against the toxic effects of carbon tetrachloride when given *prophylactically*. However, they have not been tried as therapeutic agents, and their mode of action is not understood.

Hemodialysis is effective in the management of severe renal failure due to carbon tetrachloride poisoning.[283]

CHLORINATED NAPHTHALENES AND DIPHENYLS

Because of their unique physical properties, the chlorinated naphthalenes and the diphenyls make ideal materials for the insulation of electrical wire and condensers. However, they are such potent hepatotoxins that they are no longer widely used in industry. The commercial product employed most frequently, and known as Halowax, consists of a mixture of chlorinated naphthalenes and at one time contained carbon tetrachloride as a solvent. Experimentally, it has been shown that the toxicity of the naphthalenes and the diphenyls is related directly to their degree of chlorination and is enhanced greatly by the presence of small amounts of carbon tetrachloride and alcohol.[60]

Although ingestion of these compounds may lead to poisoning,[60] most cases follow inhalation of fumes given off by the molten agent during the soldering of condensers or the coating of wires.[279] The type of hepatitis produced is unusually severe and often terminates fatally in subacute hepatic necrosis or postnecrotic cirrhosis.[231, 279, 727] Characteristically, the onset is insidious with the development of general debility, anorexia and nausea and usually follows prolonged exposure to the toxin. Occasionally, it is heralded by the appearance of an acneform rash (chloracne), one of the well-recognized signs of toxicity in handlers of the chlorinated naphthalenes. Jaundice and hepatomegaly appear a week or two later and then are followed by a decrease in the size of the liver, ascites and edema. The disease runs a chronic downhill course and usually terminates in hepatic coma and death within a few months.

Occasionally, the lesion is more fulminant, and death due to massive necrosis of the liver supervenes within 2 weeks. Severe abdominal pain is a characteristic feature in such cases. Whether this is due to hepatic necrosis or to the associated acute pancreatitis described by several authors[231, 727] is not known.

Few cases of nonfatal hepatitis have been reported, and no follow-up studies are available to indicate whether recovery without residuals is possible. The remarkable toxicity of the chlorinated naphthalenes and the diphenyls for the liver has also been observed in animals, who show the same tendency toward massive necrosis seen in man.[60]

In contrast with carbon tetrachloride, the chlorinated naphthalenes do not produce renal lesions in animals.[60] However, nephrosis has been reported as an occasional complication in man.[727]

COPPER

Acute copper sulfate poisoning may follow its ingestion with suicidal intent,[136] or its application as a topical astringent and antiseptic agent in the treatment of wounds, dermatitis or burns.[337] Doses of 10 or 15 mg. may produce signs of toxicity, and as little as 1 Gm. may be fatal, although the usual lethal dose is approximately 10 Gm. The principal lesions produced by copper sulfate include an erosive, hemorrhagic gastritis and enteritis, centrilobular hepatic necrosis with bile stasis, and renal tubular necrosis. In addition, it frequently produces severe intravascular hemolysis.

Soon after ingesting copper sulfate, patients note a metallic taste and experience epigastric pain, nausea, vomiting and diarrhea. In severe poisoning, hypotension and shock may ensue. Not infrequently, jaundice appears on the 2nd or the 3rd day, and may be due to either hepatocellular necrosis or hemolysis, or both. The hepatocellular type of jaundice tends to be severe, and usually is accompanied by enlargement and tenderness of the liver, and significant abnormalities of hepatic function. As a rule, hemolytic jaundice is mild, even when hemolysis is severe and associated with hemoglobinuria. Many patients exhibit transient oliguria, hemoglobinuria and microscopic hematuria, but in some, renal failure is severe and progressive.

In one large series, the mortality rate was approximately 15 per cent.[136] Deaths within the first 24 hours usually are attributable to shock, whereas those that occur later are due to hepatic or renal failure, or both.

As might be anticipated, the concentration of copper is increased in the serum, but is even greater in whole blood, due to the unusual avidity of red cells for copper. In at least one case, the level of ceruloplasmin in the serum was greatly elevated.[337] Penicillamine therapy in this case enhanced the urinary excretion of copper, reduced the concentrations of serum copper and ceruloplasmin, and appeared to alleviate the clinical manifestations of toxicity. Corticosteroids also are alleged to be effective in the management of acute copper sulfate poisoning.[284]

The possibility that *chronic* copper poisoning plays a role in the pathogenesis of the hepatic lesions in Wilson's disease is suggested by the high concentrations of copper found in the liver. However, with few exceptions,[486] attempts to produce cirrhosis in animals by the chronic administration of copper salts have failed.[232]

DDT and Other Insecticides

DDT (2,2bis[p-chlorophenyl]-1,1,1-trichlorethane) can produce central necrosis of the liver in animals,[533] and is thus generally regarded as a potential hepatotoxin in man. However, despite its widespread use as an insecticide, it has rarely been reported as a cause of toxic hepatitis. In one instance, the accidental ingestion of 120 ml. of a 5 per cent solution in kerosene produced hepatomegaly, gastrointestinal bleeding, oliguria, coma and death.[693] Autopsy revealed extensive central necrosis and periportal fatty infiltration of the liver and severe tubular degeneration and necrosis of the kidneys. Since DDT alone does not produce renal damage,[533] it was suggested that the kerosene used as a solvent was an important factor in the pathogenesis of the lesions.

In another case, exposure to DDT used as an insecticide produced jaundice in an individual with an underlying cirrhosis.[437]

Rarely, DDT serves as a sensitizing agent. In one such case, it produced periarteritis nodosa.[321] At autopsy, the liver showed enlargement due to congestion, periportal fatty infiltration and a large, thrombosed vein.

A number of other chlorinated hydrocarbons used as insecticides, such as chlordane, dieldrin, lindane and toxaphene, produce characteristic alterations in the cytoplasm of

hepatic cells in the rat when administered at low-dose levels for long periods of time.[547] However, overt hepatic injury has not been reported in man.

Dimethylnitrosamine

Severe toxic hepatitis can follow exposure to dimethylnitrosamine, an agent once used to inhibit corrosion. In the 2 cases reported by Freund, daily exposure to the fumes produced massive hepatic necrosis after 1 month and 12 days, respectively.[245] The onset was abrupt with abdominal cramps, nausea, vomiting and jaundice and was followed within 2 weeks by the appearance of ascites. The less severely ill patient apparently recovered after a prolonged course, but jaundice recurred in 16 months, and the liver remained large and indurated, which suggests that postnecrotic cirrhosis developed. The other patient died in the 6th week following an acute illness characterized by deepening jaundice, intractable ascites and progressive enlargement of the liver and the spleen. Postmortem examination revealed extensive hepatocellular necrosis, a diffuse inflammatory reaction with a predominance of round cells and histiocytes, and periportal hemorrhages.

Dimethylnitrosamine exhibits the same propensity for producing massive hepatic necrosis and ascites in experimental animals, both when it is administered by inhalation[245, 358] and when it is given orally[39] or intraperitoneally.[30, 39] The lesions, which are characterized by extensive centrilobular and midzonal eosinophilic necrosis, resemble those of carbon tetrachloride poisoning but are more sharply circumscribed, show more hemorrhage and are devoid of hydropic or other slightly damaged cells.[39] Small doses given over a long period produce a fatal form of cirrhosis in the rat.[39] In addition, they may give rise to tumors in the liver, kidney and lung.[481]

Although evidence indicates that following its administration dimethylnitrosamine is uniformly distributed through the body water and enters all cells freely, its toxic actions are limited to the liver exclusively.[480] This, taken together with the fact that it exhibits no *in vitro* effects on the metabolic activities of the liver,[30, 345] suggests that the selective hepatotoxic actions of di-methylnitrosamine may depend upon some metabolite formed in the liver.[30, 345, 480, 482]

IRON

Accidental poisoning with compounds of iron is an important problem in young children, who not infrequently ingest coated tablets of ferrous sulfate in the mistaken belief that they are candies.[338, 357, 415, 457]

In fatal cases, the principal autopsy findings are congestion and ulceration of the stomach and small intestine, and striking periportal parenchymal necrosis and mild fatty infiltration in the liver.[457] Similar lesions may be produced in animals.[457]

Vomiting and diarrhea, occasionally accompanied by melena, occur soon after poisoning. In severe cases, shock, acidosis, coma and death follow in rapid succession. Occasionally, mild jaundice is observed in patients who survive.

Prompt lavage of the stomach with sodium bicarbonate and the administration of deferoxamine, by both the gastric and intravenous routes, are effective in the treatment of acute ferrous sulfate poisoning.[357]

There appears to be no doubt that a prolonged excessive intake of iron leads to hemosiderosis of the liver. However, the question of whether or not it can give rise to hemochromatosis remains unresolved. Although prolonged iron administration produces hemochromatosis in choline-deficient rats, it does not do so in animals maintained on an adequate diet.[465] Several instances of hemochromatosis have been reported in individuals who have taken large amounts of iron therapeutically,[573] but in such cases, the possibility cannot be excluded that chronic anemia and other factors play an important role in the development of cirrhosis. Similarly, the increased incidence of hemochromatosis in the South African Bantu,[87] whose dietary intake of iron is excessive,[769] may be attributable to such factors as malnutrition and alcoholism, since the principal source of iron excess is home-brewed beer.[88]

MANGANESE

Industrial workers exposed to manganese dioxide dust and fumes are subject to pneu-monia[217] and a highly characteristic neurologic disorder that closely resembles the progressive lenticular degeneration of Wilson's disease.[119, 131, 217] Because of the possible relationship of the neurologic changes in Wilson's disease to the associated cirrhosis, it has been suggested that a similar hepatic lesion may be responsible for the neurologic disorder in chronic manganese poisoning.[131] The observation that repeated injections of soluble manganese salts produce cirrhosis in animals supports this hypothesis.[226, 346] However, a complete review of all the reported cases of manganese poisoning in man[217, 763] discloses only one instance in which a biliary cirrhosis is said to have been demonstrated.[125] Therefore, it is highly improbable that the type of chronic manganese poisoning encountered in industry produces liver injury.

PHOSPHORUS

With the legal prohibition of the use of elemental yellow phosphorus in the manufacture of matches in this country, acute phosphorus poisoning has become relatively rare. Currently, most cases are due to ingestion of roach paste[408, 474] or rat poison.[408] In the Orient, where yellow phosphorus matches are still in use, the incidence of poisoning is high. As might be expected, the victims are often children.

As little as 15 mg. of yellow phosphorus can produce signs of toxicity, and 60 mg. has caused death.[273] Some roach pastes contain more than 1 Gm.% of phosphorus,[474] so that the ingestion of as little as 5 Gm. may be fatal. The severity of the poisoning in the average case is well illustrated by the mortality rate of 75 per cent among 16 cases reported from the Charity Hospital in New Orleans.[408]

Red phosphorus, another form of the element, is relatively nontoxic apparently because it is insoluble and nonvolatile. Yellow phosphorus is also poorly soluble but is readily dispersed into an aqueous colloidal solution and is volatile.[273]

Although the hepatic manifestations of phosphorus poisoning are of special interest, phosphorus is a potent general protoplasmic poison and may be lethal within 10 hours, even before characteristic tissue changes can be demonstrated histologically.[408]

Symptoms. The initial symptoms, including nausea, vomiting, epigastric burning, abdominal pain and diarrhea, usually occur immediately following the ingestion of phosphorus or within a few hours. These are due to the local action of the poison in the gastrointestinal tract. However, when symptoms do not appear for hours or days, they are related to the systemic effects of absorbed phosphorus.

Shortly after phosphorus is ingested, the breath has a garlic-like odor, and the feces are luminescent in the dark, features that may be of great diagnostic importance.

In severe poisoning, shock and coma follow the initial symptoms in rapid succession, and death may ensue within 48 hours. More commonly, however, the systemic effects are evident 1 to 3 days after phosphorus is ingested, and death occurs during the 1st week. Although it is highly probable that no tissue is wholly exempt, the liver and the kidneys suffer the most severe injury and manifest the most striking structural and functional changes. As in other severe intoxications, tissue damage is so widespread that often it is difficult to determine the site of origin of any given symptom.

The manifestations of systemic intoxication include intractable vomiting, often with blood-streaked material, diarrhea, abdominal cramps and severe prostration. Signs of severe liver injury can always be demonstrated, although hepatomegaly and jaundice may not develop. Jaundice seldom appears before the 4th day and may be delayed for over a week. The prognosis is somewhat better when jaundice appears late. As in other forms of severe hepatitis, the urine contains bilirubin, and the feces tend to become pale, which indicate that bile secretion is suppressed. Not infrequently, hemorrhages occur into the skin and the mucous membranes, presumably due to the associated fall in the prothrombin and fibrinogen levels of the plasma. Other features of severe hepatic failure can occasionally include edema, hypoglycemia, tyrosinuria and an increase in serum amino nitrogen. Usually the kidneys are affected equally severely. Oliguria and azotemia are common, and the urine usually contains albumin, casts and red blood cells.

The latter part of the course is characterized by coma, delirium and vasomotor collapse and, as indicated, death occurs toward the end of the 1st week.

Occasionally, even severely poisoned individuals appear to recover completely. However, one such case, followed by serial biopsies of the liver over a period of 3 months, showed evidence of incomplete healing and progressive fibrosis, a lesion similar to that seen in animals with chronic phosphorus poisoning.[485] How often this type of postnecrotic fibrosis and cirrhosis follows acute phosphorus poisoning in man is not known.

Pathology. At autopsy the liver is enlarged and exhibits extensive periportal fatty infiltration and degenerative changes in the parenchymal cells, occasionally accompanied by a mild inflammatory reaction in the portal triads. In one case seen by the writer, marked periportal bile stasis and pseudoduct formation were outstanding features late in the course of the disease. Massive necrosis of the parenchyma is said to occur[437] but is exceedingly rare. The lesion in experimental phosphorus poisoning[485] is similar, but cellular necrosis is a more prominent feature. The renal tubules and the myocardium also show degenerative changes and fatty infiltration.

Treatment. Gastric lavage with a dilute solution of copper sulfate (0.25 Gm. in a glass of water) and a magnesium sulfate purge are recommended to rid the intestinal tract of any remaining traces of phosphorus. Unfortunately, these are effective only if given within the first few hours.

Treatment is largely supportive, as outlined previously. Choline hastens the removal of fat from the liver in phosphorus poisoning.[69] However, its therapeutic value would appear to be negligible, since it does not prevent hepatic injury.

SELENIUM

In areas where the selenium content of the soil is high, livestock develop "alkali disease," a chronic illness characterized by emaciation, loss of hair, lameness and sloughing of the hoofs.[523] At autopsy, the principal findings are cirrhosis of the liver and myocarditis. Glomerulonephritis, adrenal hemorrhages, erosion of the joint surfaces and ulceration of the intestinal tract are also seen in some instances. The disease is due to ingestion of selenium-containing grain, forage or vegetation, and can be reproduced in experimental animals by adding selenium salts to the diet.

A more acute form of poisoning, known as the "blind staggers," is seen in animals whose feed is unusually high in selenium content. Myocarditis, ulceration of the intestine and erosion of the long bones are the principal findings. Usually, the liver is congested and shows focal areas of necrosis, but frank cirrhosis is rare.

In some strains of rats, the chronic ingestion of seleniferous grain produces not only hepatic necrosis and fibrosis but also adenomas and low-grade carcinomas.[534]

Himsworth has emphasized the similarity between the hepatic lesions in chronic selenium poisoning and those of experimental dietetic massive necrosis and has suggested that the former may be the consequence of an induced deficiency of sulfur-containing amino acids related to the replacement of sulfur by selenium in plant protein.[322] The protective action of casein and methionine in animals fed selenium would appear to support this hypothesis. However, the fact that cystine does not prevent liver damage in such experiments casts doubt on this interpretation.

Of special interest to the clinician is the question of whether or not the ingestion of seleniferous grain leads to hepatic damage in man. Individuals living in seleniferous areas excrete appreciable amounts of selenium in the urine, which indicates that significant exposure has occurred. However, to date none of these has shown evidence of hepatic or other disease.[692]

SENECIO AND RELATED ALKALOIDS

A number of plants belonging to the genera *Senecio, Crotalaria* and *Heliotropium* contain pyrrolizidine alkaloids that are hepatotoxic. In South Africa, Australia, Central Asia and Norway outbreaks of severe liver disease are encountered in sheep, cattle and horses that feed on these plants. Depending upon the degree and the duration of exposure, affected animals exhibit signs of either acute hepatic necrosis or cirrhosis. Similar lesions are reproducible in experimental animals.[591, 658, 671] Occasionally, humans fall victim to this type of poisoning, but in man the senecio alkaloids produce an unusual form of liver disease in which the clinical and pathologic features resemble those of the Chiari syndrome.[670] Both in animals[671] and in man,[670] protein deficiency enhances the toxicity of these agents.

In South Africa, senecio poisoning has been reported in poorly nourished white Europeans who consume bread made of imperfectly winnowed wheat contaminated with the seeds of *Senecio ilicifolius* and *burchelli*, two weeds commonly known as ragwort.[670, 792] A similar form of toxic hepatitis affects natives of Central Asia who eat cereal grains contaminated with the seeds of *Heliotropium lasiocarpine*.[106] Evidence suggests that the use of native "bush teas" containing extracts of *Senecio* and *Crotalaria retusia* for medicinal purposes may be responsible for the development of veno-occlusive disease of the liver in Jamaican children.[730] A similar explanation has been invoked to account for the common occurrences of cirrhosis in the children of West Bengal and Madras, India.[360] However, in this instance, there is contradictory evidence pointing to the hepatitis virus as the responsible agent.[3]

Pathologic Findings. In fatal cases of senecio poisoning, the principal findings are enlargement of the liver, widespread fibrous occlusion of the central and the sublobular veins, and intense congestion and destruction of the centrilobular parenchyma. Usually, the stroma is uninvolved, and there is little or no inflammatory reaction. Organized thrombi may be demonstrable in the larger hepatic veins. In more chronic cases, there is, in addition, fibrosis and round cell infiltration of the portal zones, giving rise to the picture of cirrhosis.[670, 792] It is generally agreed that the primary lesion is in the vessels, and that the parenchymal changes are secondary to intense congestion. However, there is uncertainty whether the fibrous occlusion of the central and sublobular veins follows a proliferative endophlebitis or is the end-result of thrombosis and organization. Similar lesions have been described in the veno-occlusive disease of the liver seen in Jamaica.[93]

The hepatic changes induced by senecio alkaloids in experimental animals are more variable than in man. Although some investigators have demonstrated alterations in the blood vessels with secondary congestion, atrophy and fibrosis of the parenchyma,[318, 630, 792] others have shown that these agents may provoke acute centrilobular necrosis and cirrhosis by a direct action.[106, 134, 658] In the more chronic lesion, there is striking enlargement of the hepatic cells, a feature thought to be characteristic of senecio poisoning, and indicative of a metabolic defect which prevents cellular division and thus leads to loss of cells and ultimate fibrosis.[106] Of particular interest is the fact that in the rat a single small dose of senecio alkaloid may, after a latent period of several weeks during which no necrosis is evident, give rise to a chronic progressive hepatic lesion terminating in a picture resembling postnecrotic cirrhosis.[658, 659]

Clinical Features.[670, 792] In acute senecio poisoning, the onset is sudden with gnawing and colicky epigastric pain, followed within a few days by a rapidly developing ascites. The liver enlarges and within a few weeks becomes firm. Jaundice is an inconstant feature and, in one series at least, occurred in only 2 of 12 cases.[670] Vomiting and diarrhea are present in about a third of cases. Splenomegaly appears to be unusual despite the obvious development of portal hypertension. Occasionally, there is low-grade fever late in the disease. In severe poisoning, there may be early vasomotor collapse, followed later by hematemesis and melena.

Usually, the clinical course is prolonged and is characterized by rapid reaccumulation of ascites, recurrent attacks of abdominal pain, and cachexia. Hypoproteinemia is common, but edema is an inconstant finding. In approximately half the cases, death occurs within 1 to 3 months. Despite the apparent progressive downhill course in the remaining patients, clinical recovery ultimately takes place over a period of several months up to 2 years. Whether or not healing of the hepatic lesions is complete

in such cases is not known, since reports of long-term follow-up biopsy studies are not available.

Mild cases of intoxication probably occur, but have not been described in the literature.

The clinical picture of veno-occlusive disease in children resembles that of senecio poisoning.[93, 730] However, an acute onset is not nearly as common, hepatosplenomegaly and other signs of cirrhosis appearing insidiously in many cases. Also splenomegaly and jaundice are seen more frequently. The mortality rate is high; hepatocellular failure and hematemesis account for most deaths.

Treatment. No specific therapy is available, so that treatment is supportive and directed at maintaining nutrition and controlling the ascites.

TETRACHLORETHANE

Of all the chlorinated hydrocarbons, tetrachlorethane is by far the most toxic. During World War I it was used widely as a solvent for cellulose acetate, chiefly in the "dope" used in varnishing the canvas surfaces of airplanes and, to a lesser extent, in the manufacture of rayon and lacquers. However, it proved to be so toxic that it was abandoned as soon as a suitable substitute (amyl acetate) was found. During World War II it was used again, since it was the only satisfactory solvent for impregnating clothing with materials that neutralized poisonous gases.[286] Despite the imposition of stringent engineering and hygienic controls, signs of toxicity were encountered once again in a high proportion of workers exposed to the agent. However, the control measures prevented serious intoxication, so that no fatalities resulted.[285]

Intoxication usually follows inhalation of the agent but may occur also following its absorption from the skin or the intestinal tract. For reasons that are not entirely clear, females are more susceptible than males, and in both sexes intoxication is more common after the age of 30.[286] The toxic level of tetrachlorethane in the atmosphere is estimated to be in excess of 10 parts per million for individuals exposed for long periods. The odor, which closely resembles that of carbon tetrachloride, is readily detectable at a concentration of 25 parts per million.[285]

Pathologic Findings. The principal pathologic finding in fatal cases is a subacute or massive hepatic necrosis with preservation of the stroma, marked fatty infiltration of surviving parenchymal cells, absence of hepatocellular regeneration, and active proliferation of bile ducts.[707] The early lesions in nonfatal cases have not been described. Fatty degenerative changes are also seen in the renal tubules and myocardium. Essentially the same lesions have been observed in rats exposed to tetrachlorethane vapor.[707, 789]

Symptoms. The early symptoms of tetrachlorethane intoxication are of two types: gastrointestinal and neurologic.[285] Following exposure to low concentrations of the vapor for a number of weeks, there is an insidious onset of anorexia, nausea and vomiting, or of headache, giddiness, drowsiness and paresthesias. These may occur singly or in combination and often are associated with hepatomegaly and impairment of liver function. Jaundice is also present in approximately 10 per cent of such individuals. Occasionally, jaundice appears before other symptoms develop. Prompt cessation of exposure to the contaminated environment at this stage results in rapid recovery, usually within a period of less than a month. Of possible diagnostic significance in early toxicity is the tendency for the absolute and relative number of large monocytes in the peripheral blood to increase.[509]

In more heavily exposed individuals, the onset is similarly delayed and gradual, but gastrointestinal symptoms, hepatomegaly and jaundice are constant findings and usually are associated with tenderness of the liver and weight loss. Not infrequently, the jaundice is intense and persists for weeks and even months following the last exposure to tetrachlorethane. Recovery is possible at this stage,[509] but some individuals run a progressive downhill course, develop ascites and die of hepatic failure.[789] These are the cases that, at autopsy, show subacute hepatic necrosis and postnecrotic scarring.

Prognosis. Before the toxicity of tetrachlorethane was fully understood and ap-

propriate protective measures instituted, the exposure tended to be heavy and often was continued long after signs of intoxication had appeared. As a result, the hepatitis produced was unusually severe. In one such series of 70 cases, for example, the mortality rate was 17 per cent.[420] In contrast, no fatalities were seen in a more recently studied group of 55 cases encountered in a carefully supervised plant. Moreover, the disease was so mild that only 6 of the 55 developed jaundice.[285]

TOLUENE

This aromatic hydrocarbon derived from coal tar is widely used in industry, especially in the manufacture of paints and lacquers. Although it shares the excellent solvent properties of its homologue benzene, it is far less toxic. In individuals exposed to the high concentrations usually encountered during spray painting, toluene appears to exert no significant ill-effects. Hepatomegaly and mild macrocytic anemia are relatively frequent findings, but no instances of frank toxic hepatitis or aplastic anemia have been reported.[278] The nature of the hepatic enlargement has not been investigated. However, in animals exposed to similar concentrations of toluene, both the liver and kidneys show mild degenerative changes.[699]

TRINITROTOLUENE (TNT)

Munition workers exposed to TNT are subject to a number of toxic manifestations of which hepatitis and aplastic anemia are the most important.[448, 492, 551] Functional disturbances of the gastrointestinal, circulatory and central nervous systems, and local irritation of the respiratory tract and the skin are often troublesome but rarely give rise to serious difficulty. Absorption is chiefly from the skin and, to a lesser extent, from the mucous membranes.[38, 420] The presence on the skin of oil and grease, in which TNT is soluble, enhances absorption and increases the chances of intoxication.[38, 515] It is generally stated that inhalation of the fumes is without danger,[515] but this view is not shared by some authorities.[492]

Clinical Features. The hepatitis produced

by TNT has many unusual features, few of which have been adequately explained. Among these are the following: (1) Only a small proportion of individuals exposed to TNT develop hepatitis.[492] (2) Signs of hepatic damage usually appear only after many weeks of exposure[492] or, in some instances, not until several months after cessation of exposure.[788] (3) The disease is almost always severe, being characterized by a prolonged course and a high fatality rate. (4) Massive and subacute necrosis of the liver occur far more frequently and resemble the lesions of idiopathic acute yellow atrophy far more closely than almost any other known type of toxic hepatitis.[324, 719] [720] (5) It is difficult to reproduce the lesion in animals,[322] an unusual circumstance for an agent presumed to be a true hepatotoxin.

In many respects these unusual features are reminiscent of the hypersensitivity type of hepatitis produced by drugs such as cinchophen. However, the chemical structure of TNT and its failure to produce other manifestations of hypersensitivity make it highly improbable that it is a sensitizing agent.

Himsworth has suggested that the long latent period, the occurrence of massive hepatic necrosis, and the failure to reproduce the lesion in animals on normal diets may indicate that TNT injures the liver indirectly by inducing a relative deficiency of sulfur-containing amino acids.[322] In support of this hypothesis, he has pointed out that TNT raises the metabolic rate and thus increases the demand for protein, that at least 2 of its 3 isomers combine with amino acids and make them unavailable, and that by reducing the protein content of the diet it is possible to reproduce TNT hepatitis in experimental animals. However, the isomer of TNT that does not combine with amino acids also produces toxic hepatitis, and a low-protein intake favors the development of hepatic necrosis in experimental animals only when the diet is high in fat. The latter observation suggests the possibility that the peculiarities of TNT toxicity may be related to the fat solubility of the agent.

Possibly dietary fat enhances the absorption of TNT from the intestinal tract and favors its retention in the liver at high concentrations by producing fatty infiltration. Similarly, the enhanced absorption of TNT from the skin in the presence of grease[38, 515] may account for the sporadic occurrence of intoxication in groups of apparently equally exposed individuals. As for the long latent period, it does not necessarily point to an induced nutritional deficiency, as indicated, but may reflect a slow cumulative intoxication with an agent that is absorbed relatively slowly. In cases where the signs of liver disease appear weeks or months after the last exposure to TNT, it is possible that the initial injury incurred during exposure is asymptomatic, and that the lesion produced is progressive.

Symptoms. Usually, the onset of symptoms is insidious, with anorexia, nausea and vomiting. Jaundice appears within 2 weeks and often is followed by hepatomegaly. In severe cases, abdominal pain is a prominent feature, and the liver may be small. The course tends to be prolonged and often is complicated by the development of ascites and hemorrhagic phenomena. Occasionally, there is an associated disturbance of the hemopoietic system, as evidenced by severe leukopenia,[719] macrocytic anemia[719] or aplastic anemia.[551] Both hyperplastic[719] and aplastic[492] bone marrows have been described, suggesting that the changes in the peripheral blood may be due to a maturation arrest in some cases.

Prognosis. The outcome is unpredictable. In most cases reported in the literature death has occurred within a few weeks of acute massive necrosis of the liver[324, 492] or after prolonged hepatic failure resulting from postnecrotic cirrhosis.[720, 788] However, some individuals with TNT hepatitis recover. Unfortunately, little is known about the nature of the lesion in this group or its ultimate fate. In one 3-year follow-up study of 17 such cases,[720] there were no clinical residuals, which suggests that the initial lesion was zonal rather than massive. However, reports of postnecrotic cirrhosis becoming evident as long as 10 years after apparent recovery from TNT hepatitis[324, 788] illustrate that the scarred postnecrotic liver may be difficult to recognize clinically and may decompensate unexpectedly years after its inception. It is highly probable that such lesions can be recognized much earlier by the use of sensitive tests of hepatic function and especially by needle biopsy of the liver.

VOMITING SICKNESS OF JAMAICA

Native Jamaican children, usually from the age of 2 to 5 years are subject to an unusual disease characterized by a sudden onset of severe vomiting, followed soon thereafter by convulsions and coma. Death ensues within 2 or 3 days in 80 per cent of cases. The principal findings at autopsy include fatty infiltration of the liver and kidneys, hyperemia and petechial hemorrhages in the liver, spleen, heart, lungs and brain, and degenerative changes in the renal tubules. The etiology is unknown. However, Hill has reviewed evidence suggesting that malnutrition and the toxic effects of the ackee fruit, cassava and yams may play an important role in its pathogenesis.[317]

This disease is of particular interest because of its striking resemblance to the Reye syndrome (encephalopathy with fatty degeneration of the viscera) first described in 1965.[608] In the many reports, the possibility of intoxication has been considered, but in none has a specific hepatotoxin been implicated. A recent review suggests that the disease is of infectious origin, and possibly attributable to a variety of viruses, including those of chicken pox, measles and mumps.[127]

ANESTHETIC AGENTS

In evaluating the role of an anesthetic agent in the pathogenesis of postoperative hepatitis, due consideration must be given to the nature of the underlying disease, the degree of anoxia attained during anesthesia and the presence of such complicating factors as shock and infection, since each of these alone can produce liver injury.

CHLOROFORM

Chloroform has the well-deserved reputation of being a dangerous hepatotoxin. Although largely supplanted by other less toxic anesthetic agents, it is still used to some extent in various parts of the world for obstetric and minor surgical procedures. Most fatalities have followed prolonged anesthesia, especially during parturition, but deaths have occurred also after as little as ½ ounce of chloroform.[258] Women undergoing prolonged labor appear to be peculiarly susceptible to this type of anesthetic death. This has been ascribed to the malnutrition and the infection which so frequently accompany such labors,[637] a hypothesis consistent with the experimental observation in animals that malnutrition[272, 507] and infection[542] enhance the hepatotoxic effects of chloroform.

From the paucity of reports dealing with nonfatal cases of chloroform hepatitis, it is easy to gain the erroneous impression that chloroform either injures the liver seriously or not at all. However, in animals even a 30-minute period of chloroform anesthesia causes significant impairment of hepatic function, which may persist for as long as 8 days.[632]

Clinical Features. The clinical manifestations of severe chloroform intoxication follow a uniform pattern.[258, 637, 709] Characteristically, the onset of symptoms is delayed for 24 to 72 hours following recovery from anesthesia. Drowsiness and vomiting then appear and are soon followed by jaundice. Vomiting is copious and often becomes coffee-ground in nature. By the 4th day the drowsiness usually progresses to coma, and in approximately half the cases is followed by convulsions. Despite the regular occurrence of severe hepatic damage, jaundice fails to develop in some cases.[709] Fever is unusual, except terminally. Azotemia and acidosis occur early and tend to increase in severity. Although these are usually associated with oliguria and albuminuria, in occasional cases the urinary volume and the urea content are high,[258] suggesting that the azotemia is related in part to the rapid breakdown of protein, rather than to renal failure and dehydration alone.

Prognosis. Most severely intoxicated individuals die in 3 to 8 days, but an occasional patient survives and goes on to complete recovery. Residuals are unlikely in such cases, since the characteristic lesions seen at autopsy are zonal in type. Complete recovery without scarring also occurs in animals exposed to nonfatal doses of chloroform.[784]

Individuals who are exposed to repeated doses of chloroform at frequent intervals occasionally develop cirrhosis. In one such case described by Wilcox, small amounts of chloroform were inhaled daily over a period of 6 months, at the end of which time jaundice and hepatomegaly developed.[789] Subsequently, ascites and other signs of cirrhosis appeared, and death ensued in 18 months.

Pathology. At autopsy the liver is of normal size but may be small. Hepatocellular necrosis is invariably centrilobular in distribution and never massive. Varying fractions of the lobule are destroyed, but a small rim of intact cells is always present around the portal triads. The necrotic cells break up into hyalinized fragments and undergo lysis, while the intact cells peripherally show marked fatty infiltration. As in other types of toxic hepatitis, the reticulum is not destroyed and usually is infiltrated with a number of phagocytic mononuclear cells at the sites of necrosis. The remaining hepatic cells show little evidence of regeneration. Almost identical hepatic lesions have been described in the dog.[784]

The changes in the kidney are less conspicuous than in carbon tetrachloride poisoning and usually consist of fatty infiltration of the convoluted tubules.

Susceptibility. During the past decade considerable attention has been directed to the interrelationships between the hepatotoxic effects of chloroform and certain dietary factors. In brief, starvation,[272] protein-depletion[507] and a high fat intake[543] increase the susceptibility to hepatic damage by chloroform, and diets rich in protein[272] and carbohydrate[272] are protective when given *prophylactically*. Moreover, protein, methionine and, to a lesser extent, cystine protect protein-depleted animals against chloroform toxicity if given from 24 hours before to as late as 4 hours after anesthesia.[506, 507] The theoretical implications of these observations are discussed elsewhere. None of these experimental observations is concerned with the therapeutic effects of these supplements when administered *following*

the development of toxic hepatitis, so that they do not provide a sound basis for treatment.

CYCLOPROPANE

Transient alterations in hepatic function have been observed following cyclopropane anesthesia. Usually, these are relatively minor, but in patients with liver disease they may be more severe.[242] Changes of similar magnitude are seen following anesthesia with ethyl ether. Since the degree of functional impairment bears little relation to the duration of anesthesia, it is highly probable that such hepatic injury is the result of circulatory changes and trauma incidental to surgery rather than of cyclopropane toxicity.

DIVINYL ETHER

Because divinyl ether can produce centrilobular necrosis in dogs,[271] it is generally regarded as a potential hepatotoxin in man. In the dog, the severity of the hepatic damage produced is closely correlated with the duration of anesthesia, the nutritional status and the degree of oxygenation.[270, 271] Accordingly, certain precautions have been recommended. These include administration of carbohydrate preoperatively, limitation of the duration of anesthesia to 1 hour, use of oxygen whenever the period of anesthesia is to exceed ½ hour, and avoidance of divinyl ether in patients with liver disease.[592] Under these conditions, no instances of hepatic injury have been encountered in an extensive clinical experience with this agent.[592] Although it would be unwise to abandon this cautious attitude toward divinyl ether, it should be recognized that its hepatotoxicity for man has not been proved, and that the human liver may be as resistant to it as the monkey's.[271]

ETHER (DIETHYL ETHER)

There are no clinical reports of toxic hepatitis following ether anesthesia. However, experimental evidence indicates that, in the dog at least, ether can produce mild liver injury[270] and transient impairment of hepatic function.[632] Bromsulphalein retention[144] and other functional derangements[242] have been reported following ether anesthesia in man also, but such observations are difficult to interpret in terms of toxicity, since circulatory disturbances and alterations in hepatic structure incidental to surgical manipulation may also affect hepatic function.

HALOTHANE (FLUOTHANE) AND METHOXYFLURANE (PENTHRANE)

In contrast to many other halogenated hydrocarbons, halothane (2-bromo-2-chloro-1,1,1-trifluoroethane) does not produce hepatic necrosis in animals[364] and, hence, cannot be considered an hepatotoxin. Nevertheless, cases of hepatic necrosis have been encountered in man following its use as an anesthetic.[107, 108, 128, 440] Such lesions have been variously ascribed to halothane toxicity or hypersensitivity, to intercurrent infection with the hepatitis virus, or to coincidental factors unrelated to halothane.

In a review based on an analysis of 41 well-documented cases of halothane-associated hepatic necrosis, the writer has presented convincing evidence that halothane is a sensitizing agent, and is capable of producing hepatitis and other manifestations of hypersensitivity in a few uniquely susceptible individuals.[382] Judging from the number of cases of hepatic necrosis that could not be attributed to shock, cardiac failure or sepsis,[27] and making allowance for the incompleteness of the autopsy data and the fact that the mortality rate in halothane-induced hepatitis is approximately 50 per cent,[382] it may be estimated from the data of the National Halothane Study,[734] that the risk of halothane-induced hepatitis is approximately 1 in 10,000.

As in the hepatocellular type of hepatitis induced by other sensitizing drugs, such as iproniazid, pyrazinamide and zoxazolamine,[582] the hepatic lesions seen following halothane anesthesia are indistinguishable from those of viral hepatitis, and cannot be reproduced in animals. Extensive hepatocellular necrosis, an intense inflammatory reaction and a high fatality rate are characteristic. That the hepatitis is attributable to a sensitization reaction rather than to intercurrent infection with the hepatitis virus is strongly suggested by the narrow limits of the latent period between exposure to halothane and the onset of symptoms, the striking increase in the incidence of hepatitis following multiple exposures, the frequency with which the hepatitis is accompanied by other manifestations of hypersensitivity, such as chills, high fever, rash and eosinophilia, and, of particular significance, the regularity with which the hepatitis recurs following re-exposure to halothane.[382]

Characteristically, the onset of halothane-induced hepatitis is abrupt, with moderate to high fever, often accompanied by chills, and occasionally by rash, arthralgia and eosinophilia. In patients exposed to halothane for the first time, the average interval between anesthesia and the onset of symptoms is approximately 7 days, with a range of 1 to 12 days. Following multiple exposures, the latent period is shorter, averaging 3 days (1 to 10 days). Jaundice appears 3 or 4 days after the onset of fever, and usually deepens rapidly. Anorexia, nausea and vomiting are prominent features. Occasionally, there is severe abdominal pain. Coffee-ground vomitus, ascites, edema, somnolence and coma usually indicate a fatal outcome, which occurs in approximately half the cases.

In contrast to viral hepatitis, the leukocyte count tends to be high. Biochemical studies reveal abnormalities indicative of hepatocellular jaundice. However, significant elevations of serum alkaline phosphatase, negative cephalin-cholesterol flocculation reactions and normal thymol turbidity values are more common than in viral hepatitis.

In the writer's experience, prednisone therapy has appeared to be effective when instituted before the onset of hepatic coma, but has failed to prevent a fatal outcome in those with hepatic coma, even when used in massive doses in conjunction with exchange transfusions. However, the number of patients so treated is small, so that insufficient data are available to assess the therapeutic value of corticosteroids and exchange transfusions.

Halothane has a number of advantages over other anesthetic agents, not the least of which is that it is associated with a lower overall postoperative mortality rate follow-ing middle- and high-risk surgical proce-dures.[734] Since the degree to which halo-thane lowers the postoperative mortality from other causes is significantly greater than the estimated 0.005 per cent risk of fatal halothane-induced massive hepatic ne-crosis, continued use of halothane as an anesthetic for such procedures would ap-pear to be both reasonable and desirable. However, every effort should be made to reduce the risk of this complication by avoiding, whenever possible, the use of halothane in low-risk surgical procedures, in planned serial operations and in individ-uals who have experienced an unexplained bout of fever or jaundice following a previ-ous exposure to halothane. In this connec-tion, it should be emphasized that the risk of halothane-induced hepatitis is twice as great following multiple exposures as it is following a single exposure.[382]

Methoxyflurane (Penthrane, 2,2-dichloro-1,1-difluoroethyl methyl ether), a closely related halogenated ether, also may give rise to hepatic necrosis in susceptible indi-viduals,[386, 442] presumably by a similar mechanism, and may provoke a serious re-action in patients previously sensitized to halothane.[440] Accordingly, one agent can-not be substituted for the other once sensi-tization has occurred.

Evidence suggests that halothane may constitute an occupational hazard for occa-sional, uniquely susceptible anesthetists or other operating-room personnel exposed to low concentrations of the agent in the course of their daily work. A recent report describes a young physician who experi-enced an attack of acute hepatitis after hav-ing served as an anesthetist for several months.[53] Following full recovery, he was anesthetized with halothane for a few min-utes to test his reaction to the agent. Within 5 hours he had shaking chills and fever fol-lowed later by the appearance of eosino-philia and biochemical evidence of acute hepatitis. Another case seen by the writer involved an anesthetist who had had recur-rent attacks of acute hepatitis that led to cirrhosis over a 5-year period.[383] Almost all of the relapses had been ushered in by chills and fever that appeared within a few hours

of the patient's return to work following prolonged convalescence and ultimate re-covery from a preceding attack. Challenge with a non-anesthetic dose of halothane for 5 minutes produced chills and fever within 5 hours, and, within 4 hours, evidence of acute hepatitis, which was documented both biochemically and histologically.

TRIBROMOETHANOL (AVERTIN)

As a member of the halogenated hydro-carbon group, Avertin might be expected to behave as a potent hepatotoxin. Actually, however, it produces only slight liver dam-age in dogs[89] and never has been implicated as a cause of toxic hepatitis in man. Never-theless, it is generally assumed that liver disease contraindicates its use as an anes-thetic agent, since the Bromsulphalein re-tention that usually follows Avertin anes-thesia, both in man[144] and in experimental animals,[89] is significantly enhanced in the presence of hepatic damage. A more urgent reason for exercising caution in the patient with liver disease is the danger of delayed recovery from anesthesia related to a de-crease in the rate of Avertin detoxification.[89]

ANTIARTHRITIC AGENTS

CINCHOPHEN

Hepatitis is by far the most serious com-plication of cinchophen therapy and is largely responsible for the decline in the use of this agent over the past 3 decades. Al-though it occurs in less than 0.1 per cent of patients under treatment,[703] the mortality rate is close to 50 per cent.[550] This has encouraged a search for less toxic deriva-tives of cinchophen, but these have proved to be no safer than the parent substance. Included in this group are neocinchophen (the ethyl ester of methyl cinchophen), farastan (mono-iodo-cinchophen), biloptin (di-iodo-cinchophen), oxiliodide (cincho-phen hydroiodide) and guphen (the guaiacol ester of cinchophen).

Clinical Features. A number of features strongly suggest that the hepatitis produced by cinchophen is a manifestation of drug hypersensitivity. These include the follow-ing:

1. Frequently, the hepatitis is associated with other symptoms suggestive of an allergic reaction, such as pruritus, rash, fever, arthralgia and edema.[586, 682]

2. The ingestion of cinchophen sometimes is followed by sudden vasomotor collapse, respiratory distress and syncope, a syndrome closely resembling an anaphylactic reaction.[42, 586, 682]

3. Usually, there is a long latent period between the onset of drug therapy and the appearance of symptoms.[51, 778]

4. The reactions are particularly likely to occur in individuals previously exposed to the drug.[166]

5. Neither the incidence nor the severity of the hepatitis can be correlated with the amount of cinchophen ingested.

6. There is a remarkable tendency for the lesion to progress after withdrawal of the drug.[550]

7. Even lethal doses of cinchophen fail to produce significant hepatic lesions in experimental animals.[344, 421, 605]

Skin tests for hypersensitivity are positive only occasionally,[593, 682] and the results of attempted passive transfer of antibody by the Prausnitz-Küstner technic and of precipitin tests are uniformly negative.[586, 682] However, as indicated, these are seldom positive in other types of drug hypersensitivity.

Usually, hepatitis appears after prolonged cinchophen therapy, often weeks or months following its institution. In occasional instances, however, liver damage is not evident for as long as 6 months following cessation of drug ingestion.[550] It is this long period of latency and the frequent occurrence of massive hepatic necrosis that have led to the suggestion that the injury to the liver may be based on an induced nutritional deficiency.[324] No clinical evidence supports this hypothesis; indeed, the restriction of protein and methionine in the diet does not overcome the natural resistance of animals to hepatic injury by cinchophen.[344] Other possible interpretations of the significance of prolonged latency are discussed elsewhere.

Attempts have been made to correlate the development of cinchophen hepatitis with antecedent liver disease[436] or impaired hepatic function,[436, 593] on the theory that they may render the liver more susceptible to injury, or lead to the production of abnormal toxic metabolites. However, in animals, previous damage with toxic agents, such as chloroform and phosphorus, does predispose the liver to injury by cinchophen,[421, 605] and as yet no toxic metabolites of cinchophen have been isolated.

Pathologic Findings. The high mortality rate in this form of hepatitis is related to the frequent development of acute and subacute massive necrosis of the liver. Almost invariably postmortem examination reveals a small liver without significant nodulation, even when the patient has survived for a number of months.[51, 426, 450, 560, 604] This reflects the fact that usually the destruction is extensive, and unaccompanied by hepatocellular regeneration. Most of the parenchymal cells have either undergone lysis or show severe degenerative changes, including fatty infiltration, vacuolization and hyaline necrosis. The inflammatory reaction is variable, being minimal in some cases and intense in others. As in other types of acute massive hepatic necrosis, the reticulum framework is collapsed and condensed and the bile ducts show active regeneration. In older lesions, the areas of collapse are the site of connective tissue proliferation.

Except for the frequent occurrence of degenerative changes in the epithelium of the renal tubules, and certain alterations to be expected as secondary manifestations of severe hepatic failure, there are no other morphologic signs of cinchophen toxicity.

The nature of the hepatic lesions in nonfatal cases is not known, but there is no reason to believe that it differs fundamentally from that seen at autopsy, except possibly in extent. This raises the question of whether or not restoration of the normal architecture is possible following recovery. Of 3 such cases studied at the Mayo Clinic, 1 exhibited a nodular liver at operation, and 2 had relapses subsequently that proved to be fatal.[778] Therefore, it is possible that postnecrotic scarring is more frequent than is generally recognized.

Symptoms. Usually, the onset is sudden, with anorexia, nausea and vomiting. These may be accompanied by chills and fever, pruritus or urticaria. Jaundice usually follows within a few days but may be delayed for weeks or even months.[778] Anicteric hepatitis has been described[586, 778] but is rare. The jaundice increases in intensity, usually reaching its maximum in a few days and then persists.

As might be expected from the nature of the hepatic lesion, bilirubinuria and pale or clay-colored stools are seen early. Albuminuria, cylindruria and oliguria are common, but severe renal failure is rare. The subsequent course is variable.[778]

Prognosis. In fulminant cases, the patient lapses into coma and dies of hepatic failure within the first few weeks. This is by far the most common type of death. Other cases run a chronic course, occasionally interrupted by clinical remissions; ultimately ascites and edema develop and the patient dies within 6 months of hepatic failure or bleeding from esophageal varices. The most favorable cases improve slowly and go on to apparent recovery in 6 to 8 weeks. As indicated, the prognosis in this group must be guarded, since relapse and evidence of progression may appear at a later date.

In a recent report "cholangiolitic" cirrhosis with xanthomatosis, allegedly due to intrahepatic biliary obstruction, appeared 18 years following neocinchophen therapy.[70] There was no immediate reaction to the drug, but it was considered possible that an anicteric hepatitis had occurred and then progressed at a subclinical level for a number of years. This is a reasonable interpretation, in the light of experience with other drug reactions, although it is difficult to exclude alternative possibilities.

DESACETYLMETHYLCOLCHICINE (COLCEMIDE, DEMECOLCINE)

Desacetylmethylcolchicine, an alkaloid with antimitotic activity, is an effective therapeutic agent in acute gout and chronic myelogenous leukemia. It produces fewer gastrointestinal symptoms than colchicine. However, serious side reactions, including bone marrow depression, alopecia, fever, rash, stomatitis and jaundice, have been reported.[177]

Hepatic involvement is relatively uncommon and usually is of the cholestatic type.[761]

Although massive doses of desacetylmethylcolchicine can produce hepatic congestion and necrosis in rabbits,[761] the character of the hepatic lesions and the associated symptoms seen in man suggest that they are due to drug sensitization.

GOLD

The gold compounds used in rheumatoid arthritis frequently produce manifestations of toxicity. These fall into two groups: (1) anaphylactoid and febrile responses immediately following an injection and (2) delayed reactions involving the skin, mucous membranes, gastrointestinal tract, liver, kidneys and hemopoietic system.[21, 157] It is not known whether these are due to drug intoxication or to sensitization, but the latter is generally considered more likely.

Hepatitis is one of the less common complications of gold therapy and is said to be clinically indistinguishable from the viral type.[307] Since many of the cases reported have occurred in individuals undergoing group therapy in large outpatient clinics,[307] it is possible that they represent instances of syringe-transmitted viral hepatitis. Unfortunately, no epidemiologic or histologic data are available to substantiate this. Massive hepatic necrosis is said to occur rarely,[189] but in no reported cases has the diagnosis been established by postmortem examination. In the few fatalities that have been investigated,[21] the changes in the liver were nonspecific, and no lesions suggestive of a hypersensitivity reaction have been described.

BAL is of some value in the treatment of dermal reactions following gold therapy.[488] Although it is worth a trial in all cases, it is not known whether it affects the course of more serious reactions involving the liver, kidney and hemopoietic system.

INDOMETHACIN (INDOCIN)

Indomethacin [1-(p-chlorobenzoyl)-5-methoxy-2-methylindole-3-acetic acid], rarely produces hepatitis. In one reported fatal case, that of a 12-year-old Negro boy, profuse rectal bleeding and deep jaundice appeared after 5 or 6 months of treatment with prednisone and indomethacin for severe juvenile arthritis.[374] The liver was enlarged and tender, and laboratory studies revealed marked hyperbilirubinemia, increased levels of serum transaminase, a positive cephalin-cholesterol flocculation reaction, prolongation of the prothrombin time and marked leukocytosis. Jaundice deepened progressively, and the patient died 10 days later. Postmortem examination of the liver revealed extensive centrilobular zonal necrosis with bile stasis, small-droplet fatty infiltration of the parenchyma and a minimal inflammatory reaction.

In a second, nonfatal case, jaundice, hepatomegaly and abdominal pain were noted 3 weeks after the onset of indomethacin therapy for chronic rheumatoid arthritis.[224] An unusual feature was the presence in the serum and urine of biliverdin in sufficiently high concentrations to render them green in color. The skin too had a distinct greenish hue. The serum levels of bilirubin and transaminase were only moderately elevated, but those of alkaline phosphatase and cholesterol were high. Liver biopsy revealed centrilobular degeneration and swelling, mild fatty infiltration, bile stasis and an intense mononuclear and neutrophilic inflammatory reaction in both the parenchyma and the portal zones. Because the serum transaminase level continued to rise, prednisone therapy was begun in the 4th week of the disease. The patient was fully recovered 6 weeks later. There was no satisfactory explanation for the biliverdinemia in this case, although the authors suggested that indomethacin inhibited the activity of biliverdin reductase in the liver and spleen, or, alternatively, that a congenital partial deficiency of the enzyme was brought to light by the development of hepatitis.

It would appear from these two reports that indomethacin can give rise to either hepatocellular or cholestatic hepatitis. Although the mechanism has not been established, it is highly probable that hepatitis is attributable to a sensitization reaction, since indomethacin is known to produce other manifestations of hypersensitivity, such as rash, angioneurotic edema, asthma, leukopenia and thrombocytopenia.

PHENYLBUTAZONE (BUTAZOLIDIN)

The high incidence of untoward reactions to phenylbutazone limits its usefulness as an antiarthritic agent. [715, 717] Many of these, including rash, fever, agranulocytosis, thrombocytopenia, lymphadenopathy and swelling of the salivary glands, appear to be manifestations of drug hypersensitivity. However, others, such as edema and peptic ulcer,[400, 680] are probably based on other mechanisms.

Hepatitis is a relatively uncommon complication of phenylbutazone therapy.[213, 494, 713, 715, 721] When it occurs, it is almost always accompanied by other manifestations indicative of drug sensitization. It is seen most frequently during the first 6 weeks of therapy but may occur as long as 10 days after the drug is withdrawn.[213]

Usually, the clinical and the laboratory features are those of acute hepatocellular disease with jaundice and hepatomegaly, but rare instances of anicteric hepatitis have been reported.[721] Histologically, the liver shows scattered parenchymal degeneration and necrosis and a polymorphonuclear and mononuclear inflammatory reaction in the portal triads.[213] Although most patients recover without residuals within 3 months, extensive hepatocellular necrosis with subsequent postnecrotic cirrhosis may be seen occasionally.[213] Rarely, the clinical and laboratory picture is that of cholestatic hepatitis, but even in cases of this type the liver shows evidence of significant hepatocellular involvement.[213] Several fatalities have been reported,[213, 494, 713] but in only one of these was death clearly attributable to the hepatic lesion.[213]

PROBENECID (BENEMID)

Fever, rash and other manifestations of drug sensitization occur in about 2 per cent of patients who receive probenecid and are seen almost exclusively in those given the drug intermittently.[610] Hepatic involvement is rare, but one fatal case has been reported.[610] In this instance, mild hepatitis followed a 2-year course of intermittent probenecid therapy in a patient with an allergic background. Recovery followed withdrawal of the drug, but when it was readministered a month later it promptly produced asthma and rash followed by progressive jaundice, clay-colored stools, hepatomegaly, coma and ultimate death on the 27th day. Postmortem examination revealed massive hepatic necrosis involving the central and the midzonal areas predominantly, and a sparse portal inflammatory reaction without evidence of vasculitis.

ANTIBIOTICS

Some antibiotics can injure the liver, either directly by a toxic action or indirectly by inducing a hypersensitivity reaction. However, many of the infections for which they are used also produce hepatitis, so that often it is difficult to evaluate the role of antibiotics when this complication occurs. Moreover, in prolonged therapy the possibility of syringe-transmitted viral hepatitis must be considered. It has also become apparent that broad-spectrum antibiotics favor the development of disseminated mycotic infections and the emergence of resistant strains of staphylococci, both of which may produce an acute suppurative focal hepatitis.

Chloramphenicol (Chloromycetin)

A small proportion of individuals on chloramphenicol therapy develop severe blood dyscrasias related to toxic depression of the bone marrow.[304, 433] In at least two instances, jaundice has been reported as a complication; in one of these it appeared after aplastic anemia developed and was due to an infection of the liver with staphylococci and candida, so that the drug was implicated only indirectly.[611] In the other, an individual with a history of penicillin sensitivity in the past, nausea, vomiting and vertigo developed immediately following a second course of chloramphenicol.[304] Jaundice appeared on the third day and then cleared promptly. Signs of aplastic anemia did not become evident for 2 months. At autopsy 2 weeks later the liver was normal. Possibly the jaundice in this case was the result of a hypersensitivity reaction involving the liver. This would be consistent with the observation that chloramphenicol does not injure the liver in animals[694] or in patients with hepatitis.[296] Routine biopsies in individuals without hepatic disease also have failed to demonstrate changes in the liver following chloramphenicol therapy.[802]

Chloramphenicol should be used with caution in patients with severe liver disease, since they are unusually prone to bone marrow depression.[731] Their enhanced susceptibility to this complication appears to be related to the high levels of free chloramphenicol that occur in the serum as a result of impaired conjugation in the liver and the slow rate at which the unconjugated form of the drug is excreted by the kidneys.

Erythromycin

Although erythromycin is relatively innocuous so far as the liver is concerned, one of its esters, propionyl erythromycin ester of lauryl sulfate (Ilosone), produces typical cholestatic hepatitis in a small proportion of exposed individuals.[389] Since the hepatitis not infrequently is accompanied by eosinophilia and cannot be reproduced in experimental animals, it is reasonable to assume that it is due to drug sensitization. The occasional occurrence of urticaria and other rashes is consistent with this view.

In most cases, jaundice appears between the 2nd and the 21st days of medication and often is accompanied by abdominal distress, which may be colicky in nature.[221] Characteristically, thymol turbidity and cephalin-cholesterol flocculation are normal, while the serum bilirubin, alkaline phosphatase and transaminase levels rise. The signs and symptoms of liver disease promptly subside when the drug is withdrawn, but usually recur if it is administered a second time.

Griseofulvin

In mice, chronic administration of large doses of griseofulvin leads to the development of hepatic and erythropoietic porphyria accompanied by enlargement of the liver, focal hepatocellular necrosis, ductular proliferation and deposition of pigment in Kupffer cells and bile ducts.[168] The hepatic lesions have been ascribed by some investigators to a direct toxic effect of griseofulvin,[37] and by others to overproduction and increased biliary excretion of protoporphyrin, leading to its deposition in parenchymal and Kupffer cells and its precipitation within the small intrahepatic bile radicles, resulting in biliary obstruction and secondary parenchymal changes.[347] Rats, guinea pigs and rabbits are not susceptible to these effects of griseofulvin.

Many patients receiving therapeutic doses of griseofulvin for tinea infections also show increased protoporphyrin and coproporphyrin in their feces and red blood cells.[619] However, they do not exhibit other biochemical evidence of hepatic injury.[444, 619] Several individuals with acute intermittent porphyria given therapeutic doses of griseofulvin during a remission have experienced a relapse.[64, 601] In one of these, acute porphyria was accompanied by mild Bromsulphalein retention and an increase in serum transaminase.[601]

Griseofulvin may serve as a sensitizing agent and give rise to reactions characterized by fever, rash, urticaria and angioneurotic edema.[268, 710] In at least one instance, cholestatic hepatitis resulted.[95]

NOVOBIOCIN

Therapeutic doses of novobiocin tend to raise the level of unconjugated bilirubin in the serum,[59] and occasionally give rise to overt jaundice,[154] especially in neonates.[736] Since hemolysis does not appear to be the factor responsible for this effect, it is highly probable that the unconjugated hyperbilirubinemia is attributable, at least in part, to a defect in the hepatic uptake or conjugation of bilirubin. Attempts to establish the precise mechanism involved have been unsuccessful. In some strains of rats, novobiocin inhibits the uptake of bilirubin by the liver, but in others it does not.[4] The fact that the hyperbilirubinemia seen in man usually is associated with abnormal retention of Bomsulphalein[154] suggests that there is a defect in bile secretion in addition to impairment of bilirubin uptake or conjugation. Since the hyperbilirubinemia occurs in the absence of detectable changes in hepatic morphology,[736] it would appear to be related to a functional disorder of pigment metabolism rather than to toxic injury.

Not infrequently, novobiocin induces hypersensitivity reactions characterized by fever, rash, pruritus and eosinophilia.[98] Rarely, these may be accompanied by hepatitis. One such patient had massive hepatic necrosis and died on the 13th day following the onset of symptoms.[98] The morphologic changes in the liver were indistinguishable from those seen in fulminant viral hepatitis.

OXACILLIN (PROSTAPHLIN)

The semisynthetic penicillin, sodium oxacillin, produces allergic reactions characterized by fever, rash, urticaria and eosinophilia in approximately 3 per cent of patients. In one such patient, the reaction was accompanied by typical cholestatic hepatitis that resolved in little over 3 months.[742]

Oxacillin therapy occasionally is accompanied by moderate elevation of serum glutamic oxalacetic transaminase.[498] Since no details are available on the circumstances under which this occurs, it is not clear whether such alterations in serum transaminase are due to drug toxicity or sensitization, or to the underlying infection for which the drug is used.

PENICILLIN

In 1 or 2 per cent of individuals given penicillin, manifestations of hypersensitivity develop.[427] Urticaria and other benign types of skin rash predominate, but fatal cases of anaphylactic shock,[767, 791] exfoliative dermatitis[587] and acute vasculitis[65] also have been reported.

Acute hepatitis is a relatively rare complication, usually seen in association with exfoliative dermatitis.[587, 757] In one such nonfatal case, the serum bilirubin and alkaline phosphatase levels were moderately elevated, whereas cephalin-cholesterol flocculation and thymol turbidity remained normal.[757] Biopsy of the liver revealed multiple foci of necrosis, diffuse infiltration of the parenchyma with histiocytes and neutrophils, proliferation of the reticuloendothelium, and portal exudates containing monocytes, eosinophils and neutrophils. Dubin has reported one instance of prolonged penicillin-induced cholestatic hepatitis in which recovery occurred in one and a half years.[191] That the hepatitis provoked by penicillin is due to sensitization and not to hepatotoxicity is evident not only from the other manifestations of hypersensitivity with which it is associated, but also by the fact that the lesions are not reproducible in animals.[16, 299]

RIFAMYCIN SV

Large doses of rifamycin given intravenously produce a transient increase in serum bilirubin and interfere with the excretion of Bromsulphalein.[6] Most of the bilirubin is in the unconjugated form, but at the peak of the rise 25 per cent may be conjugated.[4] In rats, rifamycin reduces the Tm for both conjugated and unconjugated bilirubin, and increases their concentration in the liver, which suggests that rifamycin competes with bilirubin for excretion.[5] However, since the bilirubin retained in the serum is predominantly unconjugated, it is highly probable that the drug also impairs the hepatic uptake of bilirubin.

STREPTOMYCIN

A variety of drug reactions may occur during streptomycin therapy.[607] Some, such as disturbances of the 8th nerve and its nuclei, are clearly toxic in origin, whereas others, such as rash, fever and eosinophilia, are almost certainly manifestations of drug sensitization. The pathogenesis of the renal failure and the bone marrow depression that occur occasionally is not known.

Several instances of jaundice have been reported following streptomycin therapy.[607] Unfortunately, insufficient data are available to state whether these were due to an incidental infection with the hepatitis virus, a toxic reaction or the development of hypersensitivity. However, animal experiments[512] and studies of hepatic function[607] and morphology[802] in man suggest that streptomycin is not a hepatotoxin, and that if jaundice occurs during treatment it is likely to be due to a hypersensitivity reaction, or to syringe-transmitted viral hepatitis.

TETRACYCLINES

Chlortetracycline (Aureomycin). Therapeutic doses of *orally* administered chlortetracycline frequently produce a fine fatty vacuolization of the hepatic parenchyma that is readily reversible on stopping the drug.[643, 645, 802] However, the drug appears to have little effect on hepatic function, even in patients with antecedent liver disease,[143, 674] so that the lesion probably has no clinical importance.

Intravenous chlortetracycline, on the other hand, can produce significant liver damage, as evidenced by impairment of function, clinical jaundice and hepatomegaly.[45, 428, 642] This is most likely to occur in individuals who have received excessively large doses intravenously in addition to oral medication,[45, 428] but significant injury has been observed also after as little as 1 Gm. intravenously for 3 days.[642] Conceivably, hepatitis in such cases is due to the associated infection. However, the same type of injury has been produced experimentally in both man[45] and animals,[429] so that there is little reason to doubt that intravenous chlortetracycline is potentially hepatotoxic. Histologically, the liver shows the same type of fine fatty vacuolization seen after the oral administration of chlortetracycline, but the centrilobular cells tend to undergo autolysis and fragmentation, and bile thrombi are common.[45, 428]

In animals, inactivation of chlortetracycline by heat does not abolish its toxicity for the liver, which suggests that the hepatic lesions are due to a direct chemical effect and not to an indirect action related to chlortetracycline's antibiotic activity.

Of special interest is the observation that chlortetracycline protects animals against the massive hepatic necrosis produced by low-sulfhydryl, low-tocopherol diets, an effect thought to be related to inhibition of the intestinal flora and a reduction in the formation of hypothetical hepatotoxic bacterial metabolites.[290] On the principle that similar bacterial factors may be of importance in the pathogenesis of hepatic coma, chlortetracycline has been recommended as a therapeutic agent in that condition.[222] On the whole, the results of this form of treatment have been disappointing.

Large doses of chlortetracycline also protect against the hepatic and the renal effects of choline deficiency in rats.[47] The mechanism of this action is not known but appears to be related to the antibacterial properties of the drug.

Oxytetracycline (Terramycin). Fine fatty vacuolization of the hepatic parenchyma occurs with great regularity following therapeutic doses of oxytetracycline given either orally or parenterally over a period of several days.[645] The lesion appears to have no clinical significance, since it is readily reversible following withdrawal of the drug and gives rise to neither symptoms nor significant impairment of hepatic function, even in patients with pre-existent liver disease.[383] Similar lesions have been observed in mice and dogs[429] but not in rats.[350]

Severe reactions resembling serum sickness are known to occur in individuals receiving oxytetracycline,[361] so that the occasional development of drug hypersensitivity hepatitis is to be anticipated. However, as yet no such cases have been reported.

Tetracycline (Achromycin). *Orally* administered tetracycline in doses up to 2 Gm. daily occasionally produces fatty infiltration of the liver, but has no adverse effect on hepatic function.[219]

Large doses of tetracycline, especially when given *intravenously* to pregnant women with complicating pyelonephritis, may give rise to severe hepatic injury.[405, 565, 661, 783] In such women, both the clinical and morphologic features mimic those of the acute fatty liver of pregnancy. Most cases occur 3 to 5 days after the onset of intravenous treatment with doses of tetracycline exceeding 2 Gm. daily. However, it has been reported after doses as small as 1 Gm. daily given either intravenously[661] or orally.[783] Although women in the third trimester of pregnancy are the principal victims of this complication, it may occur in the postpartum period and is seen occasionally in nonpregnant women[565] and children[181] and rarely in adult males. The disease is fatal in approximately 80 per cent of cases.

At postmortem examination, most of the parenchymal cells of the liver are distended with fine vacuoles, giving them a foamy appearance. Although foci of necrosis and inflammation are not seen, the number of hepatocellular nuclei is reduced and the Kupffer cells contain large amounts of phagocytosed debris and pigment, indicating antecedent necrosis and loss of parenchyma.[405] In many cases, the kidneys show fatty vacuolization of the renal tubules and foci of cortical necrosis, unrelated to underlying pyelonephritis, and in a high proportion there is evidence of acute pancreatitis.[405]

Inordinately high levels of tetracycline have been found in the serum of patients with tetracycline-induced toxic hepatitis.[783] Accordingly, it has been suggested that impairment of renal function related to pyelonephritis and diminished extracellular fluid volume may be important factors in the pathogenesis of this complication. In addition, the possibility has been considered that pregnancy, by enhancing the uptake and diminishing the excretion of tetracycline by the liver, as it does in the case of Bromsulphalein, leads to an unusually high concentration of the drug in the liver and thus renders it susceptible to toxic injury.[783]

The principal clinical manifestations are nausea, vomiting, abdominal pain and jaundice. Not infrequently the vomitus is coffee-ground in character. Evidence of renal failure is common, and in some cases there are signs of acute pancreatitis. Remarkably, the recovery rate was 80 per cent in one series of 5 cases treated vigorously for acute pancreatitis. In fatal cases, the patient lapses into coma and dies within a few days. Fetal death occurs in 70 per cent of women who die, and in 40 per cent of those who survive.[405]

Laboratory studies reveal leukocytosis, azotemia, evidence of acidosis, and a moderate elevation of the serum levels of bilirubin, alkaline phosphatase and transaminase. Usually, thymol turbidity is normal, but the cephalin-cholesterol flocculation reaction tends to be strongly positive. In many cases, the serum levels of amylase and lipase are increased.

The occurrence of a Fanconi-like syndrome and features simulating disseminated lupus erythematosus have been reported following the use of degraded tetracycline.[732] These have not been accompanied by evidence of hepatic injury.

The hepatotoxic properties of tetracycline have been confirmed in the rat.[508] However, in this species pregnancy does not appear to increase the susceptibility to hepatic injury.

Triacetyloleandomycin (Cyclamycin)

A high proportion of individuals receiving triacetyloleandomycin in a dose of 1 Gm. daily for 2 to 4 weeks show variable alterations in hepatic function, including Bromsulphalein retention, cephalin-cholesterol flocculation, increased thymol turbidity or a raised serum level of transaminase, alkaline phosphatase or bilirubin.[223, 748, 749] Occasionally, these are associated with clinically detectable jaundice, anorexia and mild discomfort in the epigastrium or right upper quadrant of the abdomen. Liver biopsy in patients with drug-induced jaundice reveals moderate cholestasis, foci of hepatocellular degeneration, acidophilic bodies and a portal mononuclear inflammatory reaction. Histologic changes in anicteric drug-induced hepatitis are similar but less striking. Functional abnormalities clear in a few weeks following withdrawal of the drug, but recovery from structural changes in the liver is much slower. Usually, there is a prompt relapse on subsequent challenge with the drug.

When given in doses of less than 1 Gm. daily and for periods of less than 2 weeks, triacetyloleandomycin appears to have no ill effects on the liver.

The pathogenesis of the hepatic lesions induced by this agent is unknown. The frequency with which functional abnormalities are produced, and their apparent dose dependence suggest that triacetyloleandomycin is a hepatotoxin. However, the morphologic features of the hepatic lesions and the promptness with which they recur following challenge are more consistent with drug sensitization. In this connection, it may be of significance that this drug is known to produce other types of allergic reaction.

ANTICONVULSANTS, MUSCLE RELAXANTS AND SEDATIVES

Dilantin (Diphenylhydantoin Sodium)

Approximately 15 per cent of epileptics maintained on Dilantin therapy for prolonged periods develop drug reactions.

Those relating to the gums, the central nervous system and the gastrointestinal tract are almost certainly of toxic origin and usually can be controlled by adjusting the dose. On the other hand, skin reactions, which often are accompanied by fever and other constitutional symptoms, appear to be manifestations of drug hypersensitivity and are far more serious. Although they often subside despite continued drug administration, they occasionally give rise to exfoliative dermatitis[129, 487, 760] or hemorrhagic erythema multiforme[621] and terminate fatally.

Several instances of Dilantin-induced hepatitis have been reported.[129, 156, 193, 306] Without exception, these have occurred in association with other manifestations of hypersensitivity, such as rash, fever, lymphadenopathy and eosinophilia. Occasionally such reactions are accompanied by hepatosplenomegaly without jaundice.[32, 487] In most cases, the clinical and biochemical features are those of hepatocellular jaundice with varying degrees of cholestasis. On biopsy, the liver shows evidence of diffuse injury, with foci of necrosis, acidophilic bodies, infiltration of both the parenchyma and portal triads with many mononuclear cells and eosinophils, and bile stasis.[306] Occasionally, hepatic necrosis is submassive in character and leads to hepatic coma and death.[156] In one fatal case of Dilantin-induced exfoliative dermatitis, there was, in addition to hepatic necrosis, necrosis of arterioles and granuloma formation that involved many tissues, including the liver.[760]

Mesantoin
(3 methyl-5,5-ethylphenylhydantoin)

Mesantoin, a compound closely related to Dilantin, may give rise to fever, rash, lymphadenopathy and aplastic anemia,[255] features that are generally regarded as manifestations of drug hypersensitivity. Minor alterations in hepatic function may be observed under such conditions, but frank hepatitis has not been encountered.[13] At least one instance of acquired hemolytic jaundice has been reported.[700]

Nirvanol
(Phenylethylhydantoin)

Nirvanol, a compound closely related to

Dilantin, was once widely used as a sedative and in the treatment of chorea.[211] It regularly produces a typical sensitization reaction, characterized by fever, rash and eosinophilia, in 1 to 2 weeks. Occasionally, the reaction is severe and terminates fatally, so that the drug has been abandoned in this country. Agranulocytosis and autopsy evidence of liver injury have been described, but no instances of clinically detectable hepatitis have been reported.

PHENOBARBITAL

A review of the literature records only 17 fatalities as a result of reactions to therapeutic doses of phenobarbital.[468] Since tons of the drug have been consumed since it was introduced into clinical medicine, the danger of serious reaction must be small. No doubt mild reactions are relatively common and attract little attention. The other barbiturates appear to produce reactions less frequently. However, none of them is used as widely as phenobarbital, so that the apparent difference in their toxicity may have no significance.

The principal clinical features of phenobarbital reactions are fever and rash. In more severe cases, there may be exfoliative dermatitis, renal failure, signs of hepatitis, and bleeding from the skin and the mucous membranes. It is highly probable that these are manifestations of drug hypersensitivity, although it is held by some that phenol derivatives, liberated during an abnormal type of metabolism in susceptible individuals, are responsible for tissue damage.

The cases of hepatitis reported have all occurred in association with dermal reactions.[468, 776] In one of these,[468] the liver showed extensive midzonal and periportal necrosis, with vacuolization of the remaining cells. However, the hepatocellular changes in other fatal cases[790] have been less striking. In the one nonfatal case reported,[776] moderately severe jaundice, clay-colored stools and dark urine occurred in association with a morbilliform and bullous eruption. Complete recovery followed within 3 weeks.

The writer has seen one instance of chronic hepatitis following a phenobarbital reaction in a 7-year-old child. The onset was with rash, fever and splenomegaly. The rash subsided, except for residual pigmentation, but was followed by arthritis, lymphadenopathy, anemia and progressive hepatosplenomegaly. Biopsy of the liver at the end of 2 years revealed fibrosis of the portal tracts with an intense inflammatory exudate, composed of large reticulum cells, monocytes and plasma cells, and evidence of myeloid metaplasia. Death occurred 2½ years after onset. Unfortunately, permission for autopsy was not obtained.

PHENURONE (PHENACETYLUREA)

Of all the antiepileptic drugs, Phenurone is the one most likely to produce hepatitis.[163, 259] One survey indicates that this complication occurs in approximately 2 per cent of patients under treatment, and that in approximately 10 per cent the disease is fatal.[753] Bone-marrow depression[753] and renal failure[259, 432] are equally serious complications. Fever and rash occur somewhat more frequently but do not appear to be as lethal. Many clinical features suggest that these reactions are manifestations of drug hypersensitivity, which is consistent with the observation that Phenurone does not produce hepatic, renal or hemopoietic injury in animals.[617] As in the case of Dilantin, Phenurone may give rise to signs of true toxicity in the gastrointestinal tract and the central nervous system.[259, 753]

Careful screening of patients may reveal alterations in liver function before clinical signs of hepatitis appear.[1] Therefore, it is probably wise to check the status of the liver with some simple test, such as the serum transaminase level, at frequent intervals, and to stop treatment if any abnormality is detected. As with other types of drug sensitivity, symptoms may appear as early as the first week of therapy, or not until many months have elapsed,[124] so that close supervision is essential for as long as treatment is continued.

The pathologic changes found in fatal cases of hepatitis are not constant.[163, 432] In general, however, there is extensive non-zonal degeneration or necrosis of parenchymal cells with little inflammatory reaction. Occasionally, the renal tubules also show severe degenerative changes.[432]

TRIDIONE (TRIMETHADIONE)

A high proportion of individuals receiving Tridione develop rash, leukopenia, or a characteristic type of visual disturbance.[425] Rarely, hepatitis,[417] nephrosis[785] and fatal aplastic anemia[477] may occur. In one patient with hepatitis,[417] jaundice and exfoliative dermatitis appeared 4 weeks after the onset of Tridione therapy and were associated with a leukemoid reaction in the bone marrow. Uneventful recovery took place in approximately 1 month.

Except for the visual disturbances, which may be of toxic origin, it is generally believed that the side-effects of Tridione are due to drug hypersensitivity, an opinion consistent with the observation that the drug does not produce visceral lesions in animals.[616]

ZOXAZOLAMINE (FLEXIN)

Zoxazolamine (2-amino-5-chlorobenzoxazole) was introduced as a muscle relaxant and later found to be an effective uricosuric agent. Occasionally it produces a form of acute hepatocellular necrosis characterized by clinical and morphologic features indistinguishable from those of acute viral hepatitis.[123, 330, 359] Of the cases reported, most have terminated fatally with signs of massive hepatic necrosis.[123, 330, 456]

Usually, the hepatitis appears following a period of drug administration that may be as short as 1 week or as long as 2 months. The onset is abrupt, with anorexia, nausea, vomiting and abdominal pain, which are followed within a few days by jaundice, dark urine and light stools. Fever is uncommon. Enlargement and tenderness of the liver may be evident early in the course of the disease, but in severe cases, the liver soon shrinks in size and often is not palpable. The laboratory findings are those of severe hepatocellular disease, although high levels of serum alkaline phosphatase may be seen.[359] In fatal cases, there is rapid deepening of the jaundice, fever and the development of hepatic coma with death in 2 or 3 weeks. Prednisone and cortisone have proved to be ineffective in such cases.[123, 330] Full recovery within a period of 3 months has been reported in a patient with a less severe form of zoxazolamine-induced hepatitis who was treated with ACTH.[359]

The pathogenesis of this type of hepatitis is not known. Since zoxazolamine occasionally produces a skin rash, the possibility of drug hypersensitivity must be considered. This is supported by the report that eosinophils predominated in the inflammatory exudate seen in the liver in one fatal case.[123] However, in none of the other reported cases have there been any clinical or morphologic features indicative of a sensitization reaction. A direct hepatotoxic action appears unlikely, since zoxazolamine does not produce hepatic lesions in animals.

CHEMOTHERAPEUTIC AGENTS USED IN INFECTION

ANTIMONY

Although the inorganic compounds of antimony can injure the liver in animals,[273] they do not appear to produce hepatitis in workers exposed to them in industry.[267]

Toxic doses of both the trivalent and the pentavalent organic antimonials induce fatty degeneration of the liver, kidneys and heart in patients undergoing treatment for kala-azar.[728] However, frank hepatitis has been reported only in connection with the pentavalent group.[531, 532] Almost without exception, the jaundice in such cases has appeared a month or two following completion of a course of intravenous injections. Therefore, these may represent instances of syringe-transmitted viral hepatitis. However, neither the clinical features nor the pathologic findings have been described in sufficient detail to permit definite conclusions regarding their etiology.

Antimony dimercaptosuccinate (Astiban), a trivalent antimonial used in the treatment of schistosomiasis, frequently raises the serum level of glutamic oxalacetic transaminase, and less commonly that of alkaline phosphatase.[708, 775] Since the occurrence of these changes appears to be correlated with the total dose employed, it is assumed that they are manifestations of hepatotoxicity. However, biopsy studies of the liver in several patients undergoing treatment have failed to demonstrate significant lesions.[708] No cases of overt hepatitis have been encountered in patients receiving this drug.

It has been suggested that impairment of hepatic function during the treatment of schistosomiasis with antimonials is the result of an allergic reaction to products released from killed ova and worms, and that this can be prevented by concomitant administration of prednisone.[804] Consistent with this possibility is the observation that antimonial treatment of schistosomiasis not infrequently leads to an increase in eosinophilia and the appearance of fever and pruritus.[708]

ARSENIC

At one time it was thought that all types of arsenical hepatitis had a common pathogenesis. However, arsenic can produce liver injury by: (1) a direct toxic action, (2) inducing a hypersensitivity reaction or (3) serving as a vehicle for the accidental transmission of the hepatitis virus.

In animals, massive doses of arsenic, in the form of either the organic compounds once used in the therapy of syphilis[394, 651] or inorganic salts,[762] produce acute necrosis of the liver. Depending on the circumstances, the lesions may be massive,[394] centrilobular[651] or focal[762] in distribution. The counterpart of this type of liver injury is not seen when intermittent therapy with small doses of the arsphenamines is used in the treatment of syphilis, but is common after short-term massive arsenotherapy.[210, 424] Jaundice occurs in 1 to 4 per cent of patients on the latter regimen and, as might be expected, frequently is associated with other manifestations of acute arsenic toxicity, including fever, rash and cerebral symptoms. Usually recovery is rapid and complete.

In contrast, healing of the lesions produced by the inorganic arsenates in animals often is followed by postnecrotic scarring and the picture of cirrhosis.[762] A similar sequence is seen occasionally in individuals who have received potassium arsenite (Fowler's solution) for prolonged periods.[239] Usually, the signs of cirrhosis in such cases develop insidiously without any recognizable antecedent episode of acute hepatitis.

A small proportion of individuals who are given small doses of the arsphenamines intermittently develop a reaction known as "erythema of the 9th day," or Milian's syndrome.[301, 624, 644] Usually, it appears several hours after the 2nd or 3rd injection (8th to 10th day of treatment) and is characterized by fever, rash, arthralgia and eosinophilia and, in some instances, by hepatitis, purpura and renal injury. The latter are particularly prone to occur if treatment is continued after the initial symptoms appear or is resumed following their subsidence. Although the reaction was once thought to be of toxic origin,[624, 704] it is now generally agreed that it is due to drug sensitization.[301, 644]

The hepatitis associated with Milian's syndrome is of the classic cholestatic type. Characteristically, jaundice appears on the 2nd or 3rd day of the reaction and usually is associated with anorexia, nausea and vomiting. The liver tends to enlarge, the spleen may be palpable, and itching is common. As the jaundice deepens, the stools become clay-colored, and the urine dark. The results of liver function tests, especially if carried out late in the disease, are more suggestive of extrahepatic biliary obstruction than they are of hepatocellular damage. Thus, the serum alkaline phosphatase and the cholesterol levels tend to be high, while the cephalin-cholesterol flocculation reaction usually is negative. Liver biopsy at this stage reveals pericholangitis and bile stasis, with little or no evidence of parenchymal injury.

The course of Milian's syndrome is variable. Although uneventful recovery may occur within a few weeks, often it is delayed for many months. Rarely, it is complicated by the development of hepatic fibrosis and xanthomatosis of the skin,[724] a syndrome difficult to distinguish from other types of biliary cirrhosis.

By far the most common type of hepatitis seen in individuals receiving any of the arsphenamines occurs 3 to 18 months after the onset of treatment.[49, 704] There is now unequivocal experimental,[460] histologic[175] and epidemiologic[644] evidence to show that the liver injury in this instance is due not to drug toxicity but rather to accidental syringe-transmission of the hepatitis virus.

No doubt most reported cases of massive hepatic necrosis[256] and postnecrotic cirrhosis[34, 175] following arsenotherapy also fall into this group.

In animals, high-protein and high-carbohydrate diets given *prophylactically* appear to protect against the hepatotoxic effects of arsenic.[155, 503] However, claims for the therapeutic efficacy of cysteine and methionine supplements in postarsphenamine jaundice are based on unconvincing clinical evidence.[564] Moreover, there would appear to be little logic in attempting to "detoxify" arsenic in this situation, since the jaundice is usually due to viral hepatitis or to a sensitization reaction.

The results of treatment with BAL have been equivocal.[196] Since BAL fixes and facilitates the removal of arsenic, it would appear to be a useful agent in the management of true arsenic intoxication, such as occurs after massive arsphenamine therapy, and conceivably may be of value in sensitization reactions when traces of the drug still remain. However, it obviously has no place in the treatment of postarsphenamine jaundice due to the hepatitis virus. No doubt the inclusion of many such cases in treated groups has made the evaluation of therapy difficult.

Inhalation of *arsine* (AsH_3, arsenuretted hydrogen) usually is followed by the development of jaundice, an effect due to an acute hemolytic reaction.

Several instances of hepatitis following *carbarsone* therapy have been reported.[535, 588] These have been attributed to the hepatotoxic effects of the drug itself or one of its hydrolytic products, arsanilic acid, presumably formed during its storage or manufacture.[588] However, the hepatitis usually comes on abruptly following a relatively brief period of carbarsone administration at a low dose level, is typically cholestatic in type, almost always is accompanied by fever, and occasionally is associated with exfoliative dermatitis, features that strongly suggest that the drug is a sensitizing agent rather than an hepatotoxin.

ATABRINE

Prolonged administration of small doses of atabrine occasionally gives rise to skin reactions. Rarely, these are accompanied by fulminant hepatitis, aplastic anemia or agranulocytosis.[445] Similar reactions have been reported following intermittent therapeutic doses.[11] It is not known whether these are due to a toxic effect or to drug sensitization. Since patch tests may be positive,[11] and since large doses do not ordinarily impair hepatic function[109] a sensitization reaction is a distinct possibility. However, a direct toxic action cannot be excluded, since large doses of atabrine can produce hepatic necrosis in dogs.[109]

BISMUTH

The only instances of hepatitis reported following exposure to bismuth compounds have occurred in syphilitics given repeated injections over a long period of time. Descriptions of the clinical features and certain epidemiologic data in these cases suggest syringe-transmission of the hepatitis virus.

ETHIONAMIDE

Ethionamide (alpha-ethyl-thioisonicotinamide), an effective agent in the treatment of tuberculosis, occasionally gives rise to acute hepatitis.[147, 418, 520, 561, 569] The incidence of this complication is estimated to be 5 per cent.[147] Diabetics appear to be particularly susceptible.[147] Of the 18 cases reported up until 1964, 2 resulted in death from extensive hepatic necrosis.[147] Occasionally, this form of drug-induced hepatitis is unaccompanied by jaundice.[147] In addition, ethionamide therapy may lead to alterations in hepatic function without producing clinical signs of hepatitis.[418]

The onset, which occurs 1 to 8 months after starting treatment with ethionamide, is characterized by anorexia, nausea and vomiting, followed within a few days by dark urine and jaundice. Occasionally, these are accompanied by fever and rash. Usually, the signs of hepatitis regress following withdrawal of the drug, and recur when it is administered at a later date.[520, 561] However, hepatic functional abnormalities, in the absence of clinical signs of acute hepatitis, may subside despite continued drug administration.[418]

In addition to hyperbilirubinemia, high

levels of SGOT are the rule. Increased thymol turbidity, positive cephalin-cholesterol flocculation reactions and relatively high values of serum alkaline phosphatase are less constant features. In a few patients, eosinophilia occurs.

The histologic features found on liver biopsy[147] resemble those seen in viral hepatitis.

The occurrence of fever, rash and eosinophilia in some patients, the character of the hepatic lesions and the prompt recurrence usually provoked by drug challenge suggest that ethionine-induced hepatitis is a manifestation of a hypersensitivity reaction. This view is not shared by some authorities, who attribute this complication to intercurrent infection with the hepatitis virus.

Isoniazid

Izoniazid (isonicotinic acid hydrazide, Rimifon, Pyrizidin, Nydrazid), an agent widely used in the treatment of tuberculosis, is a potential hepatotoxin. In animals, prolonged administration of large doses (17.5 to 25.0 mg./kg. for 4 to 5 weeks) produces fatty degeneration of the liver and overt jaundice.[639] The much smaller doses used in man (2 to 10 mg./kg.) do not appear to affect hepatic function.[212, 625] Occasionally, however, they induce hypersensitivity and produce fever, rash and, less commonly, hepatitis.[67, 142, 291, 502, 590, 609] Almost without exception, the hepatitis has been reported in individuals who have received other sensitizing drugs, and particularly para-aminosalicylic acid (PAS), in addition to isoniazid. Although evidence of sensitivity to isoniazid has been established in such cases by provoking an exacerbation of the hepatitis or fever with a test dose following recovery, the possibility cannot be excluded that initial sensitization was induced by PAS. In several reported cases in which isoniazid alone appeared to produce hepatitis, there was a history of an antecedent reaction to PAS.[67, 609]

The clinical and laboratory features of the hepatitis produced by isoniazid resemble those of viral hepatitis. As a rule, full recovery follows withdrawal of the drug. However, at least two fatal cases have been reported.[142, 502] In one instance, drug therapy was reinstituted 1 month after a reaction accompanied by jaundice. This provoked an exacerbation which was followed several months later by a fatal massive hemorrhage from esophageal varices. Postmortem examination revealed postnecrotic cirrhosis thought to be related to the antecedent drug reactions.[502]

In the second case, a patient being treated for sarcoidosis with prednisolone and isonicotinic acid, acute hepatitis with clinical, laboratory and histologic features undistinguishable from those of viral hepatitis, appeared on the 30th day of treatment.[142] Following withdrawal of the drug, full recovery occurred within 2 months. Isoniazid was restarted 10 days later, and the patient continued to take prednisolone. On the 45th day of treatment there was a recurrence of acute hepatitis with rapidly deepening jaundice followed by hepatic coma and death on the 21st day. Autopsy revealed a small liver (900 Gm.) and signs of submassive hepatic necrosis.

Although the hepatitis tends to recur when isoniazid therapy is resumed, oral desensitization has been successful in a number of cases[67]

The closely related isopropyl derivative of isonicotinic acid, iproniazid (Marsilid), was abandoned as an antituberculosis agent soon after it was introduced, since it proved to be more toxic than isoniazid. However, its potential for producing serious hepatocellular injury was not fully appreciated until it was reintroduced as an antidepressant. The features of this type of hepatitis are described in the section on Psychopharmacologic Agents.

Nitrofurantoin (Furadantin)

Nitrofurantoin, when given in large doses, often produces gastric irritation with nausea and vomiting. Less commonly, it gives rise to sensitization reactions characterized by fever, rash, angioneurotic edema, hemolytic anemia or leukopenia. In at least one instance, such a reaction was accompanied by cholestatic hepatitis.[214] The patient, a female, experienced fever and rash during her second course of treatment with nitrofurantoin. On resuming treatment 2 months later, she had an exacerbation of fever,

maculopapular rash, pruritus and eosinophilia within 24 hours, and 4 days later was
found to be jaundiced. The liver was enlarged and tender, and tests of hepatic function were typical of cholestasis with moderate elevation of serum bilirubin, high
alkaline phosphatase and cholesterol, mild
elevation of serum transaminase and negative flocculation reactions. Liver biopsy revealed severe centrolobular bile stasis, foci
of parenchymal necrosis and inflammation,
and enlargement of the portal tracts with
ductular proliferation and an exudate containing numerous neutrophils, eosinophils
and lymphocytes. Full recovery, except for
mild residual Bromsulphalein retention, occurred within 7 weeks.

Para-aminosalicylic Acid (PAS)

Both toxic and allergic reactions may
complicate the course of PAS therapy. Toxic
reactions, which are due to the local irritant
action of the drug in the gastrointestinal
tract, are common but seldom necessitate
interruption of treatment. Allergic reactions,
which are far more serious, occur in approximately 2 to 5 per cent of patients. Usually, such reactions appear between the 3rd
and 6th weeks of medication and are characterized by fever, rash, eosinophilia and
lymphadenopathy.[435, 688, 772] Other less common manifestations of hypersensitivity include hepatitis,[158, 435, 473, 688] Loeffler's syndrome,[772] neutropenia,[435] atypical lymphocytosis[435] and renal damage.[158] A history of
antecedent allergy is relatively common.[688]

As a rule, the onset of hepatitis is preceded by other manifestations of PAS sensitivity, such as fever and rash. The principal clinical features include jaundice, dark
urine and enlargement and tenderness of
the liver. Occasionally, hepatosplenomegaly
occurs without jaundice.[435] Most cases show
a marked increase in serum alkaline phosphatase and abnormalities in the cephalin-
cholesterol flocculation and thymol turbidity reactions.[435] Usually, recovery ensues in
4 to 5 weeks. Histologically, the liver shows
scattered foci of hepatocellular necrosis,
bile stasis and an inflammatory reaction
that is most intense in the portal triads.[688]
A few fatal cases have been reported.[54, 549,
688] In these, death has occurred in 2 to 7

weeks with clinical and morphologic signs
of massive hepatic necrosis.

Occasionally, patch tests are positive,[158]
which supports the view that PAS-induced
hepatitis is due to hypersensitivity. Of interest in this connection, is the report of
positive L.E. tests in the serum of a 32-year-
old patient who had a severe reaction to
PAS characterized by fever, urticaria, lym-
phadenitis, anicteric hepatitis and acute
myocardial infarction.[71]

Although successful desensitization has
been reported in a few instances,[158, 548, 772]
it is difficult to exclude the possibility of
spontaneous desensitization in such cases.[772]
Moreover, reinstitution of drug therapy
often is followed by prompt recurrence of
symptoms.

As pointed out, reactions to PAS not infrequently are associated with or followed
by the development of sensitivity to other
drugs.[140, 688] It is not clear whether these
are indicative of cross-sensitization or of
multiple independent sensitizations.

Pyrazinamide (Aldinamide)

In combination with isoniazid, pyrazinamide is one of the most effective agents
used in the treatment of tuberculosis. However, its usefulness is limited by its tendency to produce hepatitis when administered alone[568] or in combination with other
drugs.[117, 464, 518, 662] A review of the literature indicates that jaundice occurs in approximately 3 per cent of patients receiving a daily dose of 40 mg./kg. of body
weight. Evidence suggests that smaller
doses are less likely to affect the liver.[518]

Usually, the hepatitis occurs late in the
course of treatment, most commonly during
the 6th month, but occasionally as early as
the 2nd. Its duration and severity are variable; some patients develop mild jaundice
and recover within a week, whereas others
run a severe and protracted course. Several
fatalities have been reported.[464]

The clinical and laboratory features are
those of acute hepatocellular disease. Rarely,
in nonfatal cases of unusual severity, the
jaundice is accompanied by ascites.[464] Biopsy in such cases reveals a marked inflammatory reaction involving both the parenchyma and the portal triads, focal areas of

hepatocellular necrosis and marked bile stasis.[383] In a fatal case in which death occurred on the 8th day of illness,[464] there was massive hemorrhagic necrosis of the liver on portmortem examination.[383]

Alterations in hepatic function may be demonstrable during the course of pyrazinamide therapy.[464, 568] It is wise to interrupt therapy as soon as such abnormalities are discovered. Serum transaminase determinations are particularly useful in this connection. Indeed, it has been reported that if treatment is stopped as soon as the transaminase level rises, hepatitis can be avoided.[518]

It is not known whether pyrazinamide produces hepatitis by a direct toxic action or by inducing a sensitization reaction. Since massive doses of the drug can produce hepatic necrosis in dogs,[623] and since the drug is not known to produce other signs of hypersensitivity, a toxic action appears likely. However, the histologic features of the hepatic lesion are more consistent with a sensitization reaction.

STILBAMIDINE

The 4,4'-diamidino derivatives of stilbene (stilbamidine), diphenyl ether (phenamidine), diphenoxypropane (propamidine) and diphenoxypentane (pentamidine), agents once used exclusively in the treatment of trypanosomiasis[22] and leishmaniasis,[379] are of value in the management of multiple myeloma,[22] actinomycosis,[505] blastomycosis[657] and tic douloureux. Because they produce lesions in the liver and the kidneys of animals,[787] there has been concern over their possible toxic effects in man.

Transient vasomotor and gastrointestinal symptoms are common immediately following the first few injections of stilbamidine. Usually, these subside within a few minutes and may be avoided by injecting the drug slowly.[90, 379] Of greater importance is the dissociated sensory disturbance over the distribution of the trigeminal nerve that frequently follows prolonged therapy.[22, 379] The neuropathy appears from 2 to 3 months following cessation of the medication and is due to toxic degeneration of the principal sensory nucleus of the 5th cranial nerve.

Therapeutic doses of stilbamidine (2 to 3 mg./kg. daily or every other day in amounts up to 6.0 Gm.) do not ordinarily cause any significant depression of hepatic or renal function in man.[22] However, in experimental animals, larger doses have produced severe fatty infiltration of the liver, degeneration of the convoluted tubules of the kidneys, and renal failure.[787]

Similar lesions were observed at autopsy in a 7-year-old girl with systemic blastomycosis who received 7.65 Gm. of 2-hydroxy-stilbamidine intravenously over a 36-day period.[538] Each injection was followed by headache, nausea and fever. Twenty-four hours after her last dose of 450 mg., which in retrospect was considered excessive, she had a convulsion, followed by fever and enlargement of the liver. Death occurred on the 4th day. At the height of the reaction the serum bilirubin was 1.4 mg./100 ml.; cephalin-cholesterol flocculation, 4+; and thymol turbidity, 9 units.

A number of years ago a fulminant type of hepatitis was observed in patients undergoing stilbamidine therapy for kala-azar in the Sudan.[379] Characteristically, the symptoms occurred from 1 to 3 months following cessation of therapy. At autopsy, the outstanding findings were extensive centrilobular necrosis and fatty infiltration of the liver. In some cases, the lesions closely resembled those of acute yellow atrophy. The hepatitis was attributed to an increase in the toxicity of the drug related to its storage and exposure to light.

Subsequently, the increase in the toxicity of stilbamidine on exposure to light was confirmed in animals.[36, 247] However, in none of the experiments reported were the long latent period and centrilobular hepatic necrosis reproduced. In retrospect, these deaths were probably due to syringe-transmitted viral hepatitis, especially since the disease was prevalent in the Sudan at the time.

SULFONAMIDES

The sulfonamides fall into the category of drugs that can produce hepatic injury, both by direct toxic action and by the induction of a hypersensitivity reaction. From a clinical point of view, however, only the latter gives rise to serious consequences.

Prolonged administration of sulfonamides to animals leads to the development of focal inflammatory, degenerative and necrotic lesions in liver, kidneys, myocardium and lungs.[164, 244] Similar lesions have been observed in a high proportion of individuals who have received sulfonamides shortly before death.[244, 501] These are thought to be manifestations of true drug intoxication. The depression in hepatic function,[18, 774] and the occasional occurrence of hepatitis in individuals without other signs of hypersensitivity[773] have also been attributed to the toxic effects of the drug. However, the fact that these can seldom be correlated with the amount of drug ingested raises the question of whether they may not be related to some other factor, such as infection or sensitization.

A variable proportion of individuals, depending on the particular sulfonamide derivative employed, develop a reaction characterized by fever, rash, and signs of visceral and bone marrow injury. Although the clinical manifestations often suggest involvement of a single organ, postmortem examination usually reveals widespread inflammatory and necrotic lesions in many of the viscera and blood vessels.[243, 517] Occasionally, identical lesions are found in individuals who have received sulfonamides but have not had clinical manifestations of a drug reaction.[243] The clinical and morphologic features of such reactions resemble those of serum sickness so closely that it is difficult to escape the conclusion that they are allergic in nature,[294, 454, 612] even though attempts to demonstrate specific antibodies have been unsuccessful.[294]

Acute hepatitis occurs in about 0.6 per cent of patients undergoing sulfanilamide therapy,[62, 130, 138, 229, 254, 294, 452, 517, 641] and somewhat less frequently in individuals who receive sulfathiazole,[130] sulfadiazine,[130, 314] sulfamethoxypyridine (Kynex),[750] sulfamethoxazole (Gantanol),[192] sulfadimethoxine (Madribon),[216] and other sulfonamide derivatives. The incidence and severity of the hepatitis cannot be correlated with the amount of drug administered. In most instances, the onset is within the first 2 weeks but may be delayed until the 6th week of therapy, or even later.[641] Rarely, hepatitis and other manifestations of sensitization do not become evident until a number of weeks have elapsed following cessation of medication.[254] Approximately one quarter of these reactions occur in individuals who have been exposed previously to the drug.

Usually, the onset of symptoms is sudden, with fever, anorexia, nausea and vomiting; they may be accompanied by a rash. Jaundice appears on the 3rd to 6th day but may be delayed for as long as 2 weeks. The liver enlarges and often is tender. Occasionally, there is splenomegaly. Dark urine and acholic stools are the rule, at least early in the course. The laboratory features, which are those of hepatocellular damage, are not distinctive, except that the serum alkaline phosphatase level may be very high.[254, 750] Most cases go on to slow recovery, but a few patients lapse into coma and die of hepatic failure.[62, 138, 254, 314, 517, 641] Death may occur as early as the 5th day[314] or may be delayed for several months.[62] Often, ascites is present when the course is chronic.

In mild cases of sulfonamide-induced hepatitis, a diffuse inflammatory reaction involves all portions of the liver, with scattered foci of hepatocellular necrosis[750] and bile stasis. Occasionally, granulomata are seen.[216] In fatal cases, the liver is small and shows evidence of massive necrosis of the parenchyma, collapse of the stroma and an inflammatory reaction in the portal triads.[62, 138, 314, 517] Individuals who die of more generalized reactions show scattered areas of hepatic necrosis, foci of inflammatory cells, and spotty necrosis of vessels. The exudate, which is composed of large mononuclear cells, is predominantly perivascular and periportal in location.[243, 517] Similar lesions may be found in the myocardium, kidneys, bone marrow, skin and other tissues.

It has been suggested that pre-existent hepatic disease renders the liver more susceptible to further injury by the sulfonamides.[130, 773] Autopsy experience does not bear this out. Moreover, there is no clinical evidence that sulfonamides increase hepatic dysfunction in such individuals.[566] However, cirrhotics appear to be peculiarly susceptible to the *other* toxic effects of sulfonamides, particularly in the kidney.[406, 566] Therefore, it is probably wise to avoid their use in liver disease.

Acute hemolytic reactions occasionally follow the ingestion of the sulfonamides and give rise to jaundice, which may be mistaken for a manifestation of hepatitis. These occur early in the course of treatment and especially after sulfanilamide and sulfapyridine administration.[452]

The etiology of the renal complications of sulfonamide therapy is complex. Lesions may be due to the mechanical effects of precipitated drug crystals, the toxic action of the drug or to sensitization reactions. The last type is most often associated with drug hepatitis.

TIBIONE
(Amithiozone, p-Acetylaminobenzaldehyde thiosemicarbazone)

Tibione, used in the treatment of tuberculosis, is generally regarded as a potential hepatotoxin. Although minor alterations in hepatic function[165] and fatty infiltration of the liver[218] have been described as toxic effects, there have been no reports of acute hepatitis. The other manifestations of toxicity, which include nausea, vomiting, rash[165] and agranulocytosis,[585] suggest that the drug may be a sensitizing agent. This is consistent with the observation that even massive doses fail to produce parenchymatous or bone marrow lesions in animals.[585, 706]

Similar alterations in hepatic function and symptoms of sensitization have been observed following the administration of Myvizone (p-formylacetanilide thiosemicarbazone), a compound closely related to Tibione.[687]

CYTOTOXIC AND IMMUNO-SUPPRESSIVE AGENTS

ANTIMETABOLITES

Azathioprine (Imuran). Azathioprine, a purine antagonist, has the same therapeutic actions as 6-mercaptopurine (6-MP), from which it is derived, but is more effective as an immunosuppressive agent.[526] Although

it is metabolized to 6-MP,[206] it appears to be less toxic.[640] In dogs, doses of 3.5 to 5.0 mg./kg. daily for periods up to 60 days raise the serum levels of alkaline phosphatase and transaminase, and produce minor degrees of focal hepatocellular necrosis and degeneration, increased mitotic activity, central congestion, bile stasis and, in some cases, cholangitis, pericholangitis and periportal fibrosis.[729]

Several instances of apparent hepatotoxicity have been reported in man. In a series of 46 patients given azathioprine for a variety of "autoimmune" diseases, one case of biopsy-documented cholestatic hepatitis was encountered in a patient who had received the drug for 178 days in doses up to 350 mg. daily.[150] The relationship of the hepatitis to azathioprine in this case was uncertain, because the patient had also taken prochlorperazine, a known cholestatic agent. In another group of 3 patients being treated with azathioprine for active chronic hepatitis, jaundice was encountered in one, a young girl who had received 4 mg./kg.[476] The hyperbilirubinemia in this case was unaccompanied by other biochemical evidence of hepatocellular injury, and subsided despite continued drug administration.

6-Mercaptopurine (6-MP, Purinethol). A significant number of patients with leukemia treated with 6-MP in doses exceeding 2.5 mg./kg. daily exhibit manifestations of hepatotoxicity.[204, 469] These may appear as early as 2 weeks or as late as 2 years after treatment is begun.

Usually, signs of hepatic injury appear abruptly, with jaundice, dark urine, light stools and enlargement and tenderness of the liver. Often these are associated with other manifestations of drug toxicity, especially oral lesions and leukopenia. The serum levels of bilirubin, alkaline phosphatase and transaminase are elevated, and, occasionally, thymol turbidity and cephalin-cholesterol flocculation are abnormal. The jaundice tends to clear rapidly when drug administration is discontinued. Usually, reinstitution of 6-MP therapy provokes a recurrence.[204] Rarely, the hepatitis is progressive and terminates fatally.

Patients with active chronic liver disease

appear to be peculiarly susceptible to the hepatotoxic effects of 6-MP. In one such case, a dose of only 1.5 mg./kg. given daily for 3 weeks produced fatal hepatic necrosis and marked cholestasis accompanied by hepatic coma, renal failure and terminal shock.[402] Of 12 other patients with active chronic hepatitis, most of whom were given 1.5 to 2.5 mg./Kg. of 6-MP daily, half exhibited jaundice within 2 to 4 weeks.[476] An unusual feature in this group was the fact that the hyperbilirubinemia was unaccompanied by other biochemical evidence of hepatocellular injury, and cleared spontaneously despite continued administration of the drug.

In a nonfatal case seen by the writer, liver biopsy revealed enlargement of the portal triads with marked ductular proliferation, an intense neutrophilic and lymphocytic inflammatory reaction, marked bile stasis and many periportal acidophilic bodies. Postmortem examination of the liver in a personally studied fatal case revealed extensive loss of parenchyma, marked pleomorphism of the remaining hepatocytes, gross distortion of the parenchymal plate pattern, pseudoduct formation and marked bile stasis.

Experiments in animals confirm that 6-MP is an hepatotoxin.[137] However, the doses required to produce hepatic lesions in the rat and the dog are considerably higher on a weight basis than those in man.

Methotrexate (Amethopterin). Methotrexate, an antagonist of folic acid metabolism widely used in the treatment of leukemia, lymphoma, ocular inflammatory disease and psoriasis, frequently produces biochemical evidence of hepatic injury,[316] and occasionally gives rise to overt clinical signs of liver disease.[145, 545, 738, 741] The functional abnormalities, the severity of which appears to be dose related, are reversible if detected early.[316] However, drug treatment, if continued, may give rise to progressive hepatic injury leading to the development of cirrhosis.[145, 738, 741] Formerly the hepatic fibrosis seen under such conditions was attributed to resolution of leukemic infiltrates in the portal triads with secondary collapse.[145] However, this is unlikely since similar lesions have been reported in a patient with psoriasis who had received methotrexate in-

termittently over a 2 year period.[545] Children given the drug for acute leukemia appear to be more susceptible to severe hepatic injury than adults.

In a series of 10 patients with acute leukemia receiving intermittent intensive treatment with methotrexate, increased serum transaminase and Bromsulphalein retention were observed in 9, and hyperbilirubinemia in 2, functional abnormalities that were maximal following completion of each 5-day course of treatment, and tended to regress during drug-free periods.[316] There were no accompanying signs or symptoms of hepatic injury, but liver biopsy revealed infiltration of the portal and periportal zones with neutrophils and mononuclear cells, occasional binucleate hepatocytes, and, less commonly, bile stasis, fatty infiltration and portal fibrosis. Similar but less severe functional and histologic abnormalities were encountered in 8 of 12 patients with ocular inflammatory disease treated less intensively with methotrexate every 4th day for 6 weeks.[316]

Of 7 children with acute leukemia treated with methotrexate by Colsky and associates,[145] all 5 who had a satisfactory remission and remained under treatment for 6 to 14 months developed hepatomegaly and ascites; at postmortem examination portal fibrosis was extensive, and in 3 instances it had progressed to cirrhosis. Jaundice was not a prominent feature, but hyperbilirubinemia was present in all cases.

In another group of 32 children given methotrexate for acute leukemia, 7 developed anorexia, vomiting, hepatosplenomegaly, ascites and edema after 3 to 10 months of treatment.[738] Jaundice was observed in only one. Liver biopsy in 4 of the children revealed swelling and pleomorphism of the parenchymal cells, evidence of regeneration activity, acidophilic necrosis of some cells, and portal fibrosis with ductular proliferation and round cell infiltration. When cyclophosphamide was substituted for methotrexate, fluid retention and hepatosplenomegaly regressed.

ALKYLATING AGENTS

Chlorambucil (Leukeran). Evidence suggests that chlorambucil, a derivative of nitrogen mustard, is hepatotoxic in man. In one series of patients with chronic lymphatic leukemia and lymphoma, 6 exhibited jaundice after having received 6 to 15 mg. of the drug daily for periods of 18 to 75 days.[17] At postmortem examination, the livers in this group showed varying degrees of hepatocellular necrosis, degenerative changes, bile stasis and portal fibrosis. In 2, the picture was that of postnecrotic cirrhosis.

Rarely, chlorambucil serves as a sensitizing agent and gives rise to an allergic type of hepatitis. In one such case, a young man with chronic lymphatic leukemia, a morbilliform rash appeared on the 15th day of treatment, and was followed by nausea, vomiting, abdominal pain and jaundice which lasted for 3 weeks.[392] When chlorambucil therapy was resumed 2 months later, the rash, abdominal pain and hepatomegaly recurred promptly, and subsided when the drug was withdrawn.

Nitrogen Mustard (Mechlorethamine). In the cat, nitrogen mustard produces focal areas of hepatic necrosis, but in most other animals the liver is not affected.[276] There is some uncertainty regarding the possible hepatotoxic effects of the drug in man. In one study, 3 of 50 patients with Hodgkin's disease treated with nitrogen mustard showed miliary foci of hepatic necrosis at autopsy, and 2 of the 4 cases with jaundice appeared to get worse under treatment —effects that were attributed to drug toxicity.[160] However, in another investigation, tests of hepatic function and needle biopsy of the liver failed to show any evidence of injury that could be ascribed to chemotherapy.[809] Moreover, the clinical and functional status of the liver appeared to improve in those cases with antecedent hepatic involvement.

Obviously, it is difficult to interpret the histologic and functional changes in a liver that is already the site of lymphomatous infiltration. Although the possibility of a hepatotoxic action cannot be excluded, the benefits to be derived from nitrogen mustard outweigh its possible dangers, so that the presence of hepatic lesions is not a contraindication to therapy.

A recent report of a hypersensitivity reaction to nitrogen mustard leading to appearance of erythema multiforme,[94] suggests the possibility that, rarely, the drug gives rise to an allergic type hepatitis.

To date there have been no reports of hepatic injury following the use of *triethylenemelamine (TEM)*.

Urethane (Ethyl Carbamate)

Occasionally, patients undergoing prolonged therapy with urethane develop fatal massive hepatic necrosis, manifested clinically with jaundice, ascites and hepatomegaly.[230, 312, 496, 541] Careful study of urethane toxicity in experimental animals suggests that the hepatocellular changes are secondary to vascular injury, with resultant extravasation of edema fluid and blood between the sinusoids and the parenchymal cells.[180]

In one reported case, an elderly woman with suspected multiple myeloma, signs of decompensated cirrhosis appeared after 6 years of continuous daily treatment with urethane.[365]

FOOD POISONING

Aflatoxin

A large number of deaths associated with hepatic lesions have been encountered in turkey poults and other farm animals fed peanut (groundnut) meal contaminated with the fungus *Aspergillus flavus*.[162] The agent responsible for the hepatic lesions has been identified as aflatoxin, a product of the fungus. The lesions have been reproduced in a wide variety of experimental animals.[479, 737] Protein deficiency enhances the hepatotoxic effects of aflatoxin. The hepatic lesions are characterized by focal hepatocellular necrosis, fatty infiltration, striking ductular proliferation and centrilobular endophlebitis. Prolonged administration of aflatoxin may give rise to cirrhosis or hepatoma.

As yet, aflatoxin has not been implicated in human disease, but on the basis of experience with animals, it has been suggested that contamination of food crops by *A. flavus*, and possibly other fungi, plays a role in the pathogenesis of cirrhosis and hepatoma, particularly in malnourished populations.[162]

Epping Jaundice

Occasionally, foodstuffs are contaminated during handling and shipment. A good example is the epidemic of jaundice reported from Epping, England, which was traced to the ingestion of bread baked with flour contaminated with 4,4'-diaminodiphenylmethane, an aromatic amine used as a hardener for epoxy resin.[395] The flour had been contaminated during shipment in a van carrying a broken container of the amine.

In most of the 84 patients involved, the onset was sudden with intermittent, severe abdominal pain that resembled biliary colic. This was followed 2 or 3 days later by rigors and an obstructive-like jaundice, pruritus and hepatomegaly. Usually, jaundice cleared in 4 to 6 weeks; in several patients, it persisted for 3 or 4 months. The biochemical changes were variable, suggesting biliary obstruction in some, and hepatocellular disease in others. Moderate eosinophilia was present in half the cases, but the total leukocyte count remained normal.

The principal histologic features in the liver were portal inflammation with numerous eosinophils, cholangitis, cholestasis and minimal hepatocellular necrosis. In more prolonged jaundice, the picture resembled that of viral hepatitis. Minimal portal scarring was observed following recovery.

There were no deaths in the group.

Mushroom Poisoning (Mycetismus)

Some 70 or 80 species of mushrooms are known to be toxic for man, but only one, *Amanita phalloides*, affects the liver. The others produce gastroenteritis, muscarinic effects, acute hemolysis and disorders of the central nervous system. The unusual toxicity of *A. phalloides* is attested by the 50 per cent mortality rate which follows its ingestion.[237]

Types of Toxin. Two types of toxin isolated from *A. phalloides* are: phallin, a thermolabile glucoside with hemolytic properties, and amanitatoxin, a thermostable agent which characteristically produces fatty degeneration and necrosis of the liver, kidneys and myocardium.[236]

Since phallin is destroyed readily by cooking and during ingestion, it probably plays little role in human poisoning, although its effects can be easily demonstrated in animals when administered by the parenteral route.[236] There is general agreement, therefore, that all of the manifestations of *A. phalloides* poisoning are due to amanitatoxin, which has been identified as a mixture of cylic polypeptides.[786]

Phallin and amanitatoxin are antigenic and can produce specific antibodies in animals.[236] However, the antigenicity of amanitatoxin is weak, so that it has not been possible to develop a potent antiserum for use in treatment.

Pathologic Changes. The principal pathologic changes in fatal cases are found in the liver, kidneys and central nervous system.[190, 758] As a rule, the liver is small and exhibits massive hepatocellular necrosis, intralobular hemorrhage and an acute inflammatory exudate. The parenchymal cells are heavily infiltrated with fat droplets and do not undergo the type of rapid autolysis seen in many other forms of massive hepatic necrosis.

The kidneys show varying degrees of swelling, degeneration and fatty infiltration of the tubular epithelium and congestion of the glomeruli.

The principal findings in the central nervous system include widespread toxic swelling of the cerebral ganglion cells, scattered small punctate hemorrhages and perivascular lymphocytic exudates.

Not infrequently, the myocardium also shows fatty infiltration and degeneration.

Symptoms. Characteristically, the onset of symptoms following the ingestion of *A. phalloides* is delayed for 6 to 15 hours. In contrast, most other poisonous mushrooms produce symptoms within the first few hours. Nausea, vomiting, severe abdominal cramps and diarrhea appear in rapid succession and usually are followed within 24 hours by severe prostration, signs of dehydration and vasomotor collapse. In severe cases, coma supervenes, and death ensues in 3 to 8 days. Usually jaundice appears on the 3rd day[758] but may be absent, even in individuals who survive for several days and then succumb to severe hepatic necrosis.[190]

Enlargement and tenderness of the liver

and splenomegaly are inconstant findings. Signs of renal injury are always present. Early in the course, the urine contains albumin, casts and red blood cells; later, oliguria and azotemia supervene. Clonic spasms and convulsions may develop terminally. These are generally attributed to the central nervous system lesions found postmortem,[190] but evidence based on dog experiments suggests that severe hypoglycemia is a factor in some instances. Hemorrhagic phenomena and anemia are far less common than hepatorenal and neural symptoms but do occur occasionally.

Prognosis. Even the most gravely ill patients with signs of severe hepatic and renal injury may recover,[758] so that it is difficult to predict the outcome in any given case. Nevertheless, vasomotor collapse, increasing azotemia and signs of central nervous system involvement usually denote an unfavorable prognosis. The recovery period is variable, in some instances being as short as 10 days, and in others as long as 6 weeks.[758] Few long-term follow-up studies have been carried out, so that it is not known whether the recovery from hepatic injury is usually complete. However, hepatic fibrosis has been reported as a sequela in several instances,[322] so that residual damage may occur more frequently than is generally recognized.

Therapy. Although there is no specific treatment for *A. phalloides* poisoning, general supportive measures are of the greatest importance in tiding the patient over the initial critical period of dehydration and vasomotor collapse, and the subsequent development of hepatic and renal failure. These include careful regulation of fluid and electrolyte balance, transfusion of whole blood, and the provision of sufficient parenterally administered glucose to meet the caloric requirements and to prevent hypoglycemia. Gastric lavage and saline purges rid the gastrointestinal tract of possible remaining traces of mushroom; however, these procedures are of doubtful value, since usually there is a long interval between the ingestion of mushrooms and the onset of symptoms. However, they may be of value prophylactically in individuals who have partaken of a bad lot of mushrooms, but are not yet ill.

HORMONAL AND METABOLIC AGENTS

ANDROGENS AND RELATED ANABOLIC AGENTS

Methyltestosterone, norethandrolone and a number of other C-17 alpha alkyl substituted steroids occasionally produce an unusual form of cholestatic jaundice. Characteristically, there are no accompanying clinical signs of hypersensitivity or histologic evidence of an inflammatory reaction in the liver, features usually seen in most other forms of drug-induced cholestatic hepatitis. Since Bromsulphalein retention can be demonstrated in a high proportion of individuals given large doses, it is generally believed that agents of this type interfere with the excretion of bile, probably as the result of a direct toxic action. Norethandrolone produces these effects more readily than any other steroid in this group.[489] Neither testosterone and its esters, such as the phenylproprionate,[313] nor the closely related compound, norandrolone,[799] exhibit any adverse effect on the liver.

Most of the substituted derivatives of testosterone stimulate the synthesis of creatine and increase the urinary excretion of creatinine.[489] Although this effect parallels Bromsulphalein retention, the correlation in individual cases is not close. Neither the mechanism of increased creatine synthesis nor its relationship to altered hepatic function is known.

Methyltestosterone. Considering the frequency with which methyltestosterone is prescribed and the small number of cases of cholestatic jaundice reported,[97, 238, 781] it is evident that the incidence of this complication is relatively low. However, when used as an antipruritic agent in obstructive jaundice, it invariably raises the level of serum bilirubin.[449] Daily doses of 30 to 100 mg. for periods of 1 to 5 weeks produce significant Bromsulphalein retention without other signs of hepatic dysfunction in a high proportion of normal subjects and patients without evidence of antecedent liver disease.[313, 489] Much of the Bromsulphalein retained in the serum is in the conjugated form.[121] This has been interpreted as evidence that methyltestosterone interferes with the excretion but not with the conjugation of the dye. However, studies of Bromsulphalein clearance in individuals receiving norethandrolone show that the uptake of dye by the liver also is impaired, so that the effects of steroids of this type may not be limited to impairment of dye transport out of the hepatic cells.[419]

In patients who develop jaundice, the liver shows marked centrilobular bile stasis with little or no evidence of parenchymal damage or inflammatory reaction. In one reported case with prolonged jaundice, biopsy of the liver showed simple cholestasis at the end of 3 weeks, and signs of early biliary cirrhosis, confirmed by gross inspection of the liver, at 11 weeks.[15]

Usually, symptoms appear between the 2nd and 5th months of medication but may be seen as early as the 8th day. The onset is characterized by malaise, nausea and other gastrointestinal disturbances. Jaundice follows within a few days to 4 weeks and is accompanied by dark urine, acholic stools and hepatomegaly. Splenomegaly and pruritus are seen in some cases. Usually, the serum alkaline phosphatase level is significantly elevated, but this is an inconstant finding. In contrast, the serum cholesterol level, the cephalin-cholesterol flocculation reaction and thymol turbidity tend to remain within normal limits.

Often, the jaundice is intense, but usually complete recovery ensues within 3 months. One fatality has been reported.[399] In this case, jaundice appeared after 7 weeks of methyltestosterone therapy at a dose level of 30 mg. daily. The jaundice persisted and was complicated by progressive dehydration and metabolic acidosis which resulted in death at the end of 2 months. Postmortem examination revealed centrilobular hepatocellular degeneration with marked bile stasis.

Norethandrolone (**17α-ethyl-19-nortestosterone, Nilevar**). The effects of norethandrolone on the liver are essentially the same as those produced by methyltestosterone but tend to be more intense. In a high proportion of individuals receiving this drug in daily doses of 25 to 60 mg., impairment of Bromsulphalein excretion can be demonstrated in 1 to 3 weeks, depending on the dose.[398, 649] Less commonly, there may be an increase in serum alkaline phosphatase[398] and glutamic oxalacetic transaminase.[649]

Much of the Bromsulphalein retained in the serum is conjugated,[120] which has been cited as evidence in support of the concept that norethandrolone interferes with the excretion rather than with the conjugation of the dye.[489] In the rat, a similar defect in bilirubin excretion can be demonstrated.[23]

Since electromicroscopic studies of the liver in both man and the rat have shown that norethandrolone regularly produces dilatation of the canaliculi and effacement of their microvilli without any concomitant change in the appearance of the cytoplasm, it has been proposed that these anatomic alterations are responsible for the cholestasis and the impairment of Bromsulphalein excretion induced by this drug.[650] However, clearance studies in man[419] indicate that norethandrolone interferes with both the excretion and uptake of Bromsulphalein by the liver. This suggests that the action of the drug is not limited to the canalicular membranes. The resulting functional derangement is selective and does not affect indocyanine-green clearance.[419]

Only a few instances of overt cholestatic jaundice have been reported,[194, 274, 649] but from the relatively high incidence observed in some series,[194, 649] one may anticipate that many more cases will be encountered as norethandrolone is used more widely, and that they will be seen more frequently than in the case of methyltestosterone therapy. The interval between the onset of norethandrolone administration and the appearance of jaundice is unpredictable and may range from 2 weeks[649] to 10 months.[274] Usually, the jaundice is accompanied by an increase in serum alkaline phosphatase,[194, 274, 649] and not infrequently there is a rise in the serum glutamic oxalacetic transaminase level[649] and a positive cephalin-cholesterol flocculation reaction.[274, 649] In some cases, the jaundice is intense and resolves relatively slowly.[194, 649] Histologically, the liver shows centrilobular bile stasis with bile thrombi in the canaliculi, bile staining of the Kupffer cells and secondary feathery degeneration of the parenchymal cells.[649] Similar changes of lesser degree, occasionally accompanied by lymphocytosis of the portal triads, focal hepatocellular necrosis and nuclear changes indicative of regenerative activity, have been encountered in non-icteric individuals receiving norethandrolone.[398]

At least two fatalities have been reported. Both patients died of hepatic failure following a prolonged course of norethandrolone and at autopsy exhibited marked cholestasis, varying degrees of hepatocellular necrosis and peliosis hepatis. Because of the extensive character of the necrosis in one case, it was assumed that a complicating infection with the hepatitis virus was involved, but the evidence presented in support of this interpretation is not convincing.

Other Substituted Derivatives of Testosterone. Bromsulphalein retention has been observed following the administration of *methandrostenolone* (17α-methyltestosterone, methandienone, Dianabol),[799] *fluoxymesterone* (9α-fluoro-11β-hydroxy-17α-methyltestosterone, Halotestin)[369] and the progestational agents, *norethindrone* (17α-ethinyl-19-nortestosterone, Norlutin), and *norethynodrel* (17α-ethinyl-17β-hydroxy-5 (10)estren-3-one norethisterone).[553] In addition, methandrostenolone frequently raises the serum level of glutamic oxalacetic transaminase.[489] Of interest in connection with the problem of jaundice in the newborn is the observation that most of the natural and synthetic progestational steroids inhibit glucuronide transferase activity in the liver.[342]

Cholestatic jaundice resembling that seen after methyltestosterone therapy has been reported in patients receiving *norethindrone*[752] and *methylestrenalone* (17α-methyl-19-nortestosterone).[563]

ANTITHYROID DRUGS

Methimazole (1-methyl-2-mercaptoimidazole, Tapazole) produces rash and urticaria in approximately 5 per cent of patients,[43] and for that reason is thought to be a sensitizing agent. Less commonly, it gives rise to agranulocytosis and cholestatic hepatitis[628, 681] or cholestatic hepatitis alone.[491]

Propylthiouracil. Rare instances of fatal generalized periarteritis with secondary involvement of the liver[463] and transient hepatocellular jaundice in association with fever and neutropenia[446] have been reported. Presumably, such reactions are due to hypersensitivity.

Thiouracil. Fever, rash, arthralgia, lymphadenopathy, agranulocytosis and swelling of the salivary glands—features suggestive of sensitization—have been observed in patients receiving thiouracil.[248, 253, 336, 557] Less commonly, this drug produces hepatitis.[253, 336, 557] The latter may be of the cholestatic type,[253] but in at least one case which proved to be fatal the liver was greatly reduced in size and showed focal and central hepatocellular necrosis and bile stasis.[336]

Thiourea produces fever, rash, leukopenia and other manifestations of drug sensitization more frequently than does thiouracil.[557] Rarely, it gives rise to periarteritis nodosa. In one such case, the manifestations of generalized vascular disease were accompanied by deep jaundice, which at autopsy appeared to be related to intrahepatic arteritis.[260]

CORTICOSTEROIDS

In experimental animals, large doses of cortisone produce scattered foci of hepatocellular necrosis, and enhance the hepatotoxic effects of carbon tetrachloride.[743] In addition, they give rise to fatty infiltration of the liver, an effect attributable to increased mobilization of fatty acids from adipose tissue depots.[320]

Fatty infiltration of the liver has been observed following the administration of therapeutic doses of cortisone in man.[714] In a child given large doses of prednisone and hydrocortisone for 11 weeks, marked fatty infiltration of the liver was associated with massive fat embolism which resulted in sudden death.[319]

DINITROPHENOL

Occasionally, small doses of dinitrophenol produce an acute cholestatic hepatitis.[685] Although it has not been possible to demonstrate skin sensitivity or the presence of circulatory antibodies in such cases,[493] it is highly probable that the hepatitis is due to drug hypersensitivity. The reasons for believing so include the following: (1) hepatitis may be associated with an urticarial rash,[685] (2) the clinical and laboratory features closely resemble those seen in the hypersensitivity type of arsenical hepatitis,[685] (3) even fatal doses of dinitrophenol do not produce significant alterations in the liver, either in experimental animals[739] or in man,[576, 740] and (4) other common manifestations of drug hypersensitivity, including angioneurotic edema, neutropenia, renal injury and arthritis, have been reported.[20, 459]

Large doses of dinitrophenol often stain the tissues yellow, due to the color of the drug itself. This must be distinguished from true icterus.

ESTROGENIC AND PROGESTATIONAL AGENTS

Natural Estrogens. Both estradiol and its metabolite estriol, when given in relatively large doses, produce abnormal Bromsulphalein retention, an effect attributable primarily to a defect in the transport of dye out of the hepatic cell.[524] In addition, estradiol raises the serum level of alkaline phosphatase, but has no effect on serum bilirubin or other parameters of hepatic function, and does not alter the microscopic appearance of the liver.[525]

It has been suggested that the alterations in hepatic function that occur late in pregnancy are related to the accompanying marked increase in estrogen production.

Natural Progestins. In contrast to the natural estrogens, neither progesterone nor its metabolite pregnanediol impairs hepatic function, as judged by Bromsulphalein clearance in the rat.[251]

Synthetic Estrogens, Progestins and Oral Contraceptives. As in the case of the synthetic androgens, a wide variety of synthetic estrogens and progestins impair the hepatic excretion of Bromsulphalein, possibly by interfering with the uptake and transport of the dye in the liver.[251] If given in sufficiently large doses, they may produce other biochemical and histologic evidence of hepatic injury and cholestasis.[723] The 17-alpha alkyl 19-nor-steroids interfere most

with bile secretion,[646] but other steroids in this group also affect the liver.

In animals, massive doses of stilbestrol (diethylstilbestrol), a nonsteroidal synthetic estrogen, produce hepatic necrosis,[495] whereas small doses impair Bromsulphalein excretion,[251] as in the case of the steroidal estrogens. However, there is no evidence that the therapeutic doses used in man are hepatotoxic.[241, 458, 495]

Most oral contraceptives contain a mixture of a synthetic progestin and a synthetic estrogen, usually in a ratio of approximately 10:1 or greater. Not infrequently, both components are C-17 alpha alkyl substituted 19-nor-steroids. The agents most commonly employed include the progestins, *norethindrone* (norethisterone, 17α-ethinyl-19-nortestosterone, Norlutin), *norethynodrel* (17α-ethinyl-5[10]-estraeneolone), *ethynodiol diacetate* (17α-ethinyl-4-estraenediol diacetate), or *lynestrenol* (ethinylestranol; 17β-hydroxy-17α-ethinyl-estr-4-ene) in doses of 1 to 10 mg. and the estrogens, *ethinyl estradiol* or its 3-methyl ether, *mestranol,* in doses of 0.05 to 0.15 mg.

As might be anticipated from the behavior of their constituents in animals, oral contraceptives give rise to alterations in hepatic function in a significant number of healthy women, the principal abnormality, mild Bromsulphalein retention, occurring in 20 to 40 per cent of individuals tested.[539] The serum alkaline phosphatase is elevated far less frequently. That the action of the oral contraceptives on the liver is not always limited to inhibition of bile secretion is evident from the fact that occasionally they raise the level of serum transaminase, an effect that suggests hepatocellular injury.[86] Menopausal women may be more susceptible to this type of reaction, although in most cases reported the dose employed has been larger than that used for contraception.[205, 723] With large doses, the serum transaminase level rises with regularity, and may be accompanied by hyperbilirubinemia; liver biopsy in such individuals reveals centrilobular necrosis, either with or without cholestasis.[723]

Almost 100 cases of jaundice have been reported in women receiving oral contraceptives.[539, 544] However, considering the widespread use of these agents, the incidence of this complication must be exceedingly low. Genetic or other constitutional factors may be of importance in determining susceptibility to this form of jaundice. This is suggested by the observation that, in approximately 40 per cent of cases, previous pregnancies have been accompanied by manifestations of cholestasis,[539, 544] a complication of pregnancy that may have a hereditary basis.[293] In this connection, it is noteworthy that the largest number of cases of contraceptive-induced jaundice have been reported from Scandinavia[416, 747] and Chile,[544] areas where the incidence of the cholestasis of pregnancy also is relatively high.

The initial symptoms of contraceptive-induced cholestasis—malaise, anorexia and nausea—appear after 2 weeks to several months of medication. Jaundice, pruritus, dark urine and pale stools follow within a few days to 2 weeks. These are unaccompanied by fever, rash or adenopathy. In a few cases, the liver enlarges, but the spleen does not. Usually, the serum levels of bilirubin and transaminase are only moderately elevated, but deep jaundice and levels of transaminase in excess of 1,000 units have been reported.[544, 747] Often, the serum alkaline phosphatase remains normal, but in some cases it rises significantly.[544] On biopsy, the liver shows centrilobular canalicular and intracellular bile stasis, focal hepatocellular degeneration and necrosis, and a scanty parenchymal and portal inflammatory reaction.[544, 747] Cessation of contraceptive therapy is followed by gradual recovery over a period of several weeks. Relapses have been reported following resumption of such therapy.[747]

Impairment of hepatic function and jaundice have been reported following the use of most oral contraceptives, including Enovid (norethynodrel 2.5–10 mg. + mestranol 0.075–0.15 mg.), Lyndiol (ethinylestrenol 5 mg. + mestranol 0.15 mg.), Anovlar (norethindrone acetate 2.5 mg. + ethinylestradiol 0.05 mg.), Ortho-Novum (norethindrone 2 mg. + mestranol 0.1 mg.)

and Ovulen (ethynodiol diacetate 1 mg. + mestranol 0.1 mg.).

Available evidence suggests that the estrogenic component is responsible for the jaundice produced by oral contraceptives. Thus, following recovery from such jaundice, challenge with mestranol provokes a relapse, whereas administration of such progestational components as norethynodrel or lynestrenol does not.[8, 756] In contrast to the synthetic estrogens, the natural estrogen estradiol does not induce jaundice in such cases, although it may raise the level of serum transaminase and cause bromsulphalein retention.[756]

The other manifestations of hepatic dysfunction encountered in women receiving oral contraceptives also appear to be due primarily to the synthetic estrogens contained in these agents.[86, 205] However, at high dose levels, synthetic progestins may be even more injurious to the liver than the estrogens.[723] Also, there is some evidence that the estrogens and progestins in oral contraceptives act synergistically in producing hepatic dysfunction.[723]

Since mestranol produces jaundice and other manifestations of hepatic dysfunction much more readily than norethynodrel, at least at the dose levels found in oral contraceptives, though both agents are C 17 alpha alkyl substituted steroids, alkylation at the C-17 position cannot be the only structural determinant of hepatotoxicity in this group of compounds. As further evidence of this, estradiol, a nonalkylated steroid, also impairs hepatic function.[524, 756] In addition to alkylation at the C-17 position, the presence of a phenolic A ring appears to be a factor in determining the potential of C-18 steroids for blocking Bromsulphalein excretion, and may account for mestranol's unusual activity in this respect.[251] It has been suggested that hypersensitivity plays a role in the case of synthetic estrogens and progestins that produce signs of hepatocellular injury.[646] This appears highly improbable, since large doses of lynestrenol, particularly when fortified with mestranol, produce such injury with regularity.[723]

Although some estrogenic and progestational steroids inhibit hepatic glucuronyl transferase *in vitro*,[343] there is no evidence that they play a role in the biliary excretory defects induced by oral contraceptives. However, pregnane-3(alpha),20-(beta)-diol, an unusual metabolite of progesterone secreted only rarely in human breast milk, inhibits glucuronyl transferase *in vitro*, and gives rise to severe and prolonged unconjugated hyperbilirubinemia in young infants fed such milk.[24]

Oral contraceptives appear to enhance the susceptibility to thromboembolic disease,[499a] and several instances of the Budd-Chiari syndrome have been reported in young women who have used these agents for periods ranging from 2 weeks to 2 years.[138a, 276a, 635a, 705a, 718a] Usually, the disease has proved fatal, but in one case recovery followed withdrawal of the drug.[705a]

HYPOGLYCEMIC AGENTS

Biguanidines. Synthalin (decamethylene-diguanidine), one of the first oral hypoglycemic agents to be used in the treatment of diabetes mellitus, was abandoned soon after its introduction because it produces severe hepatic injury both in animals and in man.[339] Other compounds of this type in current use do not appear to share this property and have not been implicated as etiologic factors in drug hepatitis.[401] These include *phenethylformamidinyliminourea* (*phenformin, DBI*), *amylformamidinyliminourea* (*DBB*) and *isoamylformamidinyliminourea* (*DBC*).

Carbutamide (1-butyl-3-sulfonylurea, BZ-55). Of the several sulfonylureas introduced as hypoglycemic agents in the treatment of diabetes mellitus, carbutamide is the least desirable because of the frequency with which it evokes reactions. These are of the same type produced by the closely related sulfonamides, and include fever, rash, agranulocytosis, hemolytic anemia and hepatitis, manifestations suggestive of drug sensitization.[380]

Several fatalities have been reported, death being due to acute myocarditis,[225] hepatitis,[113] exfoliative dermatitis[380] and bone marrow depression.[380] The most striking finding in these cases has been the presence of foci of necrosis with miliary

granulomata scattered through the viscera, of the type seen in patients with sulfonamide reactions.[243] In one of these cases, the biochemical findings were those of cholestatic hepatitis, but hepatic failure ensued, and autopsy revealed a diffuse hepatitis with numerous areas of hepatocellular necrosis and bile stasis.[113] Similar but less extensive changes have been observed in nonfatal cases.[113]

Chlorpropamide (1-propyl-3-([p-chloro-benzenesulfonyl])urea, Diabinese). One of the chief drawbacks to the use of chlorpropamide as a hypoglycemic agent is the frequency with which it produces cholestatic hepatitis.[100, 292, 297, 603] The incidence of this complication has been estimated to be approximately 0.5 per cent.[603] However, in some series, transient but significant elevations of the serum alkaline phosphatase level have been observed in as many as 25 per cent of patients under treatment with this drug.[755]

Usually, after 2 to 6 weeks of chlorpropamide therapy, the hepatitis is ushered in with anorexia, nausea and vomiting. Soon thereafter dark urine, jaundice and clay-colored stools appear. Fever, rash, pruritus, eosinophilia and hepatomegaly are common but inconstant findings. Although the regular occurrence of hyperbilirubinemia with high serum levels of alkaline phosphatase and cholesterol indicates a cholestatic form of jaundice, it is evident from the rise in SGOT[603] and the positive cephalin-cholesterol flocculation reactions[292, 603] seen in some cases that the cholestasis may be accompanied by significant hepatocellular injury, as in many other forms of cholestatic hepatitis. Histologic studies of the liver bear this out. Characteristically, there is centrilobular bile stasis with bile-staining of the hepatic and Kupffer cells, plus an inflammatory reaction in the portal triads with polymorphonuclear leukocytes, eosinophils and monocytes.[100, 292, 297, 603] However, not infrequently the parenchyma shows feathery degeneration,[603] small foci and necrosis[603] and evidence of increased hepatocellular regenerative activity.[297]

Full recovery is to be anticipated in 1 to 3 months.

The sporadic occurrence of the hepatitis

in patients given the drug, the frequency with which the jaundice is accompanied by fever and eosinophilia, and the failure of the drug to produce hepatic lesions in animals[387, 656] suggest that chlorpropamide is a sensitizing agent rather than a hepatotoxin. In some instances, readministration of the drug following recovery from an attack of chlorpropamide-induced hepatitis does not provoke a relapse.[292] This does not necessarily exclude a sensitization mechanism but may be indicative of spontaneous desensitization.

Of practical importance is the fact that diabetics who recover from chlorpropamide jaundice do not relapse when given tolbutamide.[297, 603]

Metahexamide (N-[3-amino-4-methylbenzenesulfonyl]-N[1]-cyclohexylurea, Euglycin), another of the sulfonureas, produces jaundice in approximately 1 per cent of patients,[755] and at least 2 fatalities from progressive hepatic failure have been reported.[540]

The clinical features of the hepatitis are of the hepatocellular type in some cases[475, 540, 755] and of the cholestatic type in others.[179, 300] Histologically, the liver shows foci of hepatocellular necrosis, predominantly centrilobular in distribution, and, in some instances, an inflammatory reaction in the portal triads and evidence of bile stasis.[179, 300, 540] This combination of hepatocellular injury and cholestasis is reflected in the results of laboratory tests which often show, in addition to hyperbilirubinemia, significantly elevated serum levels of transaminase[300, 475] and alkaline phosphatase[300, 475, 755] and a strongly positive cephalin-cholesterol flocculation reaction.

In fatal cases, the clinical and pathologic picture is that of subacute hepatic necrosis.[540] One apparent recovery from this type of lesion has been reported.[540] In another it was responsible for the development of postnecrotic cirrhosis.[755]

It is not clear whether metahexamide injures the liver by a direct toxic action or by the induction of a hypersensitivity reaction. The sporadic occurrence of the hepatitis and the occasional development of fever and rash in patients receiving the drug[755] are consistent with the latter. However, the fact that large doses produce hepatic lesions in experimental animals[35] suggests that, under some circumstances, metahexamide may behave as a hepatotoxin.

Tolbutamide (l-butyl-3-([p-tolylsulfonyl])-urea, Orinase). Of the sulfonylureas used as hypoglycemic agents tolbutamide appears to evoke drug reactions least frequently.

In an early report on 400,000 patients receiving this agent, no instances of drug-induced hepatitis or alterations in hepatic function are recorded.[179] However, since then, several cases have been encountered.

In one series of 1,500 patients given tolbutamide, 4 instances of liver injury were encountered.[91] One of these, a patient with pre-existent cirrhosis, had a 2-week episode of jaundice following 3 months of drug therapy. In another, death from hepatic failure occurred after 12 months of treatment; postmortem examination revealed mild portal cirrhosis with superimposed acute hepatitis. In the 2 remaining cases, the outstanding features were fever, thrombocytopenic purpura, hepatosplenomegaly, Bromsulphalein retention and elevation of the serum alkaline phosphatase level. These appeared 1 and 6 months, respectively, after treatment was started. Biopsy of the liver in one of the cases revealed fatty infiltration. Recovery followed withdrawal of the drug in one case and administration of hydrocortisone in the other.

Several instances of typical cholestatic hepatitis have been encountered in individuals who have received tolbutamide for periods ranging from 1 to 24 months.[31, 280] Prompt recovery has followed withdrawal of the drug. In one case, continued administration of tolbutamide for 2 months after jaundice appeared resulted in chronic cholestasis with the development of clinical and functional features and histologic changes in the liver that closely resembled those seen in primary biliary cirrhosis.[280] On histologic examination, the liver showed cholestasis, destructive cholangitis and cholangiolitis, and disappearance of the interlobular ducts. Exploratory laparotomy, to exclude biliary obstruction, was followed by massive bleeding from gastric and esophageal microsal ulcerations, hepatic coma and death.

Since tolbutamide occasionally gives rise to allergic reactions, it is possible that the hepatitis it produces also is a manifestation of hypersensitivity. However, in none of the cases reported has the hepatitis been accompanied by fever, rash or eosinophilia.

METABOLIC DISTURBANCES

HYPERTHERMIA

Sustained elevation of the body temperature at a high level often produces severe liver damage. Approximately 20 per cent of individuals subjected to an artificially induced fever of 41.5° C. (106.7° F.) for 7 hours develop clinical jaundice,[466] and an even higher proportion exhibit an increase in serum bilirubin.[771] Similar evidence of hepatic damage is seen also in association with the hyperpyrexia of heatstroke[315, 798] and other febrile diseases.

Hyperpyrexia of sufficient severity and duration may be fatal.[92, 275, 798] The principal findings at autopsy include hemorrhages into the skin, mucous membranes and serosal surfaces, and severe degenerative changes and necrosis in the liver, kidneys and adrenals.[275] All patients who die later than the 2nd day exhibit jaundice and severe centrilobular hepatic necrosis. Superficially, the lesions resemble those in fulminant viral hepatitis. However, there is little or no inflammatory reaction, and the hepatic cells do not show the characteristic rapid and complete autolysis seen in that disease. Cases that run a more prolonged course may show evidence of hepatocellular and bile duct proliferation. Usually, the changes in the liver are the predominant lesion after the first 48 hours, so that they probably have an important bearing on the fatal outcome. In patients that die sooner, the hepatic parenchyma shows cloudy swelling, hydropic vacuolization and fatty infiltration and may be more seriously injured functionally than is evident histologically. This is suggested by the observation that the serum bilirubin invariably rises within 4 hours of the onset of hyperpyrexia.[771]

Pathogenesis of the hepatic injury in hyperpyrexia is not well understood. It is generally believed that anoxia and alterations in essential enzymatic reactions are the major factors responsible for tissue injury.[275] The importance of anoxia has been disputed on the grounds that continuous oxygen administration does not prevent liver damage.[466] However, this is not a valid objection, since oxygen therapy does not overcome the anoxemia of hyperpyrexia.[771] Shock and dehydration may be additional factors in some instances but are certainly not the essential ones.

Clinical manifestations of the hepatitis[466] are difficult to distinguish from those due to the other effects of hyperthermia. Nausea and vomiting occur early and usually are followed on the 2nd or 3rd day by jaundice and hepatomegaly. There is an early increase in the urinary excretion of urobilinogen, and later the urine contains bile. Only occasionally, however, are the stools acholic. In severe cases, there may be central nervous system disturbances, vasomotor collapse and signs of renal failure. Purpuric manifestations have been emphasized, particularly in heatstroke,[798] although they may occur in other types of hyperpyrexia.[275] These appear to be related to the combined effects of a low prothrombin level, a reduction in platelets and an increase in capillary fragility.[798] Pleural effusions, ascites and edema are not rare in fatal cases.[92, 275]

Recovery without residual liver damage occurs in the vast majority of cases. The appearance of shock, anasarca, renal failure and neurologic disturbances are omens of a fatal outcome.

HYPERTHYROIDISM

A high proportion of individuals with hyperthyroidism show evidence of liver damage. In fatal cases, the incidence of significant hepatic lesions may be as high as 90 per cent,[50] and in those who survive the frequency of functional impairment is equally great. In both instances, the severity of the abnormalities correlates closely with the intensity and duration of the underlying thyroid disease. Nevertheless, it is by no means certain that the changes in the liver are due to the direct effects of the thyroid hormone; indeed, other possible interpretations are held to be more likely.

A variety of hepatic lesions occur in patients who die of thyrotoxicosis and its complications.[50, 115, 519, 673] These include: (1) fatty metamorphosis, (2) hepatocellular necrosis, usually focal or central, but occasionally massive, as in acute yellow atrophy, (3) atrophy of the parenchyma, as evidenced by a decrease in the weight of the liver, (4) venous congestion and (5) cirrhosis. Except for cirrhosis and atrophy, similar changes are seen in animals given massive doses of thyroid extract or thyroxine.[257, 310] Nevertheless, some investigators maintain that most of the lesions are nonspecific, and that only the cirrhosis can be attributed to the hyperthyroid state.

Weller describes the characteristic lesion as a patchy lymphocytic inflammatory reaction in the portal triads, which is followed by proliferation of connective tissue and the development of cirrhosis.[779] Moschcowitz, on the other hand, believes that the primary lesion is venous congestion at the periphery of the lobules due to a disturbance in the normal pressure relationships between the branches of the hepatic artery and the portal vein.[519] Accordingly, the cirrhosis that follows resembles that seen in chronic congestive failure, except that the fibrosis is centered around the interlobular septa instead of the central veins. Few pathologists subscribe to either of these interpretations, and most regard the fibrosis as a consequence of fatty infiltration and necrosis of hepatic cells.[115]

Almost every test of liver function that has been investigated, including the concentration of serum bilirubin, the excretion of Bromsulphalein and hippuric acid, the tolerance for galactose and levulose, and the prothrombin level, is abnormal in a significant number of individuals with hyperthyroidism.[295, 470, 478] Similar functional disturbances have been demonstrated in animals with experimentally induced hyperthyroidism.[188] The decrease in galactose and levulose tolerance may be due to alterations in carbohydrate metabolism or absorption, but there is little reason to doubt that the other abnormalities are indicative of liver damage.

The pathogenesis of the hepatic lesions found in hyperthyroidism is a controversial subject. The close relationship between the severity of the hepatic damage and the intensity and the duration of the hyperthyroidism suggests that excessive amounts of thyroid hormone are hepatotoxic.[50] However, studies based on liver biopsy material indicate that, in the absence of complications, even severe hyperthyroidism may not produce significant alterations in hepatic structure or function.[522, 571] This has led some to the conclusion that the lesions found at autopsy are either coincidental or the result of complications.

Although there is little doubt that infection, shock and cardiac failure are responsible for liver damage in many instances, the incidence of these factors in nonfatal cases appears to be too low to account for the frequency with which hepatic involvement can be demonstrated. For that reason many investigators regard liver injury as a manifestation of hyperthyroidism but attribute the deleterious effect of the thyroid hormone to some indirect action. Experimental evidence indicates that hyperthyroidism increases the susceptibility of the liver to injury by anoxia,[471] infection[668] and toxic agents.[472] At one time these effects were thought to depend on a fall in liver glycogen.[139, 803] However, more recent studies indicate that these effects cannot be attributed to changes in hepatic glycogen.[472]

Another interpretation is that hyperthyroidism induces a relative nutritional deficiency by increasing the demands for certain essential dietary constituents.[183, 322] Although this might lead to fatty infiltration and cirrhosis, it would not account for the zonal and focal hepatic necrosis seen in hyperthyroidism. No one mechanism accounts satisfactorily for all the types of liver injury encountered in hyperthyroidism.

The clinical significance of these hepatic lesions is difficult to evaluate. Ordinarily, they give rise to no overt signs of liver disease, except for occasional hepatomegaly, but in approximately 20 per cent of fatal cases they produce jaundice.[50] Therefore, it would seem reasonable to assume that extensive lesions contribute to a fatal outcome. At one time, it was believed that they were responsible for thyrotoxic crises. However, this view has been abandoned for lack of supporting evidence.[470]

PSYCHOPHARMACOLOGIC AGENTS

A wide variety of drugs used as tranquilizers and antidepressants give rise to reactions, some of which affect the liver. The lesions produced may be either cholestatic or hepatocellular in type, depending on the nature of the agent, but in both instances the process appears to be due to drug sensitization rather than to any direct hepatotoxic effect. In dealing with agents of this type, the physician should recognize that, while alterations in chemical structure may reduce the frequency with which certain drugs produce hepatitis, they rarely, if ever eliminate this hazard completely. Accordingly, all newly introduced substituted derivatives of drugs known to provoke reactions involving the liver should be considered suspect, at least until prolonged experience proves them to be innocuous.

PHENOTHIAZINE DERIVATIVES

Cholestatic hepatitis has been reported more frequently after chlorpromazine (Thorazine) than any of the other phenothiazine derivatives used as tranquilizing agents. However, it is difficult to compare the hazards of the drugs in this group, since few of the newer phenothiazine derivatives have been used as extensively as chlorpromazine.

Chlorpromazine (Thorazine) Hydrochloride. Published statistics indicate that the incidence of cholestatic hepatitis in patients given chlorpromazine is 1 to 2 per cent.[141, 354, 451] However, the findings on serial biopsy of the liver and the results of serial determinations of serum alkaline phosphatase and glutamic oxalacetic transaminase suggest that the incidence of anicteric reactions involving the liver is 20 to 50 per cent.[176, 676, 765] Since the occurrence of such reactions is not dependent on the dose, and since the hepatic changes are not reproducible in animals,[579, 695] chlorpromazine cannot be classified as a true hepatotoxin. Schnack has reported that chlorpromazine reduces the biliary excretion of BSP in rats, and interprets this as evidence of hepatotoxicity.[654] However, others have not confirmed this observation.[198] Moreover, it has been found that, in the rat, chlorpromazine does not inhibit the biliary secretion of indo-cyanine green or bilirubin,[305] reduce the rate of bile flow,[683] or raise the pressure within the common hepatic duct.[683]

Frequently, reactions are accompanied by fever, rash and eosinophilia[141, 451] and less commonly by agranulocytosis[451] and a positive patch test.[434] Taken together with the fact that the drug can produce contact dermatitis,[434] these features strongly suggest that chlorpromazine is a sensitizing agent. However, as in many other drug reactions, attempts to demonstrate circulating antibody to chlorpromazine,[83] or to establish the presence of other immunologic abnormalities[431] have met with failure.

According to some reports antecedent liver disease predisposes to the development of cholestatic hepatitis.[373] However, this has not been borne out in other studies.[176] As in the case of many other drug reactions, females appear to be more susceptible than males.

Usually, chlorpromazine jaundice appears between the 2nd and 4th week of therapy. Although it is uncommon in patients who have received the drug for less than a week, it has been reported following 1 day of therapy[794] and even after a single dose.[735] In such cases, and occasionally in others,[207, 354] the onset of jaundice may be delayed for as long as 2 weeks following withdrawal of the drug. Only rarely are reactions of this type seen after the 5th week of drug administration.[373] In patients who have recovered from chlorpromazine-induced hepatitis, re-administration of the drug produces a prompt relapse in some[44, 407, 500] but not in others.[44, 407] Moreover, recovery from chlorpromazine hepatitis may ensue despite continued administration of the drug,[655, 689] a course of events generally attributed to spontaneous desensitization.

In most cases, the onset of chlorpromazine hepatitis is abrupt with fever and mild constitutional symptoms, which are followed in 1 to 4 days by jaundice, dark urine and clay-colored stools.[354, 373, 451, 782] Occasionally, the fever is accompanied by a rash and by chilly sensations or frank shaking chills. Pruritus may precede the appearance of jaundice and often is a troublesome late manifestation. Anorexia, nausea, vomiting and abdominal pain are common but seldom are severe. Hepatic enlargement and tenderness are inconstant findings. Rarely, the spleen is enlarged.

Characteristically, the urine contains bile, and the serum shows a sharp rise in the levels of bilirubin, cholesterol, alkaline phosphatase and transaminase. In contrast, the thymol turbidity and cephalin-cholesterol flocculation reactions remain normal. Rarely, the latter are abnormal, and the serum globulins are increased.

The principal histologic findings in the liver are bile stasis with intra-canalicular bile thrombi and bile-staining of the parenchymal and Kupffer cells in the centrilobular zones and a portal inflammatory exudate, consisting of polymorphonuclear leukocytes, monocytes and eosinophils.[782, 807] Although the features of cholestasis have been emphasized, not infrequently the hepatic parenchyma shows scattered foci of necrosis and evidence of increased regenerative activity.

The intensity and duration of jaundice are variable. Often, jaundice is mild and clears without residuals in 2 to 8 weeks. However, a significant number of cases with intense and prolonged jaundice have been reported.[83, 329, 348, 373, 391, 529, 594, 700] The duration of the disease in these individuals has ranged from 4 months to 5 years. Several have exhibited portal fibrosis histologically,[348, 373, 529, 594] and have had clinical features suggestive of biliary cirrhosis, such as persistent pruritus and xanthomatosis.[83, 348, 391, 529, 770] According to Read and associates,[594] lesions of this type are reversible and never give rise to full-blown cirrhosis even though histologic abnormalities and raised levels of serum alkaline phosphatase and cholesterol may persist. However, this is not borne out by the course of events in the cases reported by Myers et al.[529] and by Walker and Combes.[770] In Myers' patient, portal hypertension and bleeding from esophageal varices developed 5 years after onset. At laparotomy for portacaval shunt, the liver was found to be cirrhotic.[528] A similar case of chlorpromazine-induced biliary cirrhosis of 5-years' duration has been studied by Walker and Combes.[770] The writer has had the privilege of examining serial biopsy sections of the liver from

both of these patients and can vouch for the development of unequivocal advanced biliary cirrhosis.

Several fatalities have been attributed to chlorpromazine hepatitis.[77, 354, 626] However, in the 2 cases in which postmortem examination was carried out, unrelated complicating factors could have played an important role in the fatal outcome. The patient described by Boardman had mitral stenosis, severe congestive failure and a terminal purulent pericarditis.[77] Sections of liver, which the writer has had the privilege of examining, show marked passive congestion and bile stasis. In Rodin and Robertson's case, death occurred on the 40th day of jaundice, following an unexplained episode of shock.[626] The liver showed extensive centrilobular parenchymal necrosis with some degree of bile stasis. Whether the necrosis was attributable to the chlorpromazine reaction or to the terminal episode of shock is not evident from the published protocol.

Because of the possible hazards involved, it is unwise to continue chlorpromazine therapy once the signs of a reaction appear or to resume such therapy following recovery from a reaction. Allegedly, cross-sensitization reactions between chlorpromazine and other phenothiazines are rare.[334] However, promazine occasionally produces cholestatic hepatitis in patients previously sensitized to chlorpromazine. Accordingly, once a reaction has occurred, caution should be exercised in substituting one phenothiazine for another.

The effectiveness of cortisone in the management of chlorpromazine-induced hepatitis is in doubt. Favorable results have been reported in some cases[159, 712] but not in others.[765]

Mepazine (Pacatal). Mild jaundice has been observed in a few patients receiving mepazine.[511] Prompt recovery has followed withdrawal of the drug. Presumably, the underlying lesion in such cases is a cholestatic hepatitis of the type produced by chlorpromazine. However, neither the histopathology nor the clinical features have as yet been reported. Although the incidence of this complication appears to be low, in one series of 76 patients given mepazine, jaundice developed in 2, an incidence of 5.4 per cent.[511]

Perphenazine (Trilifon). At least two instances of perphenazine-induced cholestatic hepatitis have been reported. In one, jaundice appeared after 56 days of drug administration, and cleared within 3 weeks.[148] In the other, the latent period was 60 days, and the duration of the hepatitis was longer, but full recovery occurred ultimately.[63]

Prochlorperazine Maleate (Compazine). Cholestatic hepatitis with clinical and histologic features indistinguishable from those produced by chlorpromazine has been observed in patients receiving prochlorperazine.[497, 705] In addition, several cases of fatal drug-induced massive hepatic necrosis have been reported,[148, 467] illustrating the fact that sensitizing agents that produce cholestasis occasionally give rise to serious hepatocellular disease. The hepatitis in one of these cases was accompanied by agranulocytosis and thrombocytopenia.[467]

Promazine Hydrochloride (Sparine). This agent has no adverse effects on the liver in most individuals,[397] but, rarely, it may give rise to cholestatic hepatitis. In 2 of the cases reported the patients had previously received chlorpromazine. In one, the latter drug had induced hepatitis,[764] whereas in the other it had been well tolerated.[375] Although cross-sensitization may have been a factor in both cases, there are instances in which promazine has failed to provoke a reaction in patients previously sensitized to chlorpromazine.[764]

Several fatalities have been attributed to promazine-induced agranulocytosis.[264, 797] In one such case, the agranulocytosis was accompanied by jaundice.[797] Death occurred on the 4th day, at which time the liver was infiltrated with fat. It is not clear from the published protocol whether the hepatic lesions were attributable to the promazine reaction or were produced by the antibiotics and cortisone used for several days prior to death.

Thioridazine Hydrochloride (Mellaril). At least one case of cholestatic hepatitis and two instances of pruritus accompanied by raised levels of serum transaminase and alkaline phosphatase have been reported in patients receiving thioridazine hydrochloride.[606] In two of these individuals there was evidence of an antecedent hepatic reaction to chlorpromazine. In the third patient, the serum transaminase and alkaline phosphatase levels returned to normal despite continued drug administration.

Trifluoperazine Hydrochloride (Stelazine). Although this agent has been administered to over a million patients, only 2 cases of cholestatic hepatitis have been reported.[29, 390] One had a history of another drug reaction and chlorpromazine had been administered just prior to the use of trifluoperazine.[29] Cholestatic jaundice appeared after 3 days of therapy and persisted for more than 6 months. The other patient recovered in 3 weeks.[390]

The writer has seen a patient with the typical features of early "primary" biliary cirrhosis, in whom the onset with pruritus and jaundice followed several months of intermittent trifluoperazine therapy.[383] Whether or not the drug was responsible for the liver disease in this case is unknown.

MONOAMINE OXIDASE INHIBITORS

A number of monoamine oxidase inhibitors, including iproniazid, isocarboxazid, nialamide, phenelzine and tranylcypromine (Parnate, Parstellazine) are widely used in the treatment of mental depression. All of these agents, with the exception of tranylcypromine, are hydrazine derivatives and produce a severe and often fatal form of hepatitis in a small number of uniquely susceptible individuals. Since tranylcypromine is not a hydrazine derivative and does not affect the liver, it has been suggested that the propensity of the other drugs in this group to produce hepatic injury may be related to their hydrazine content rather than to their capacity to inhibit monoamine oxidase activity. For reasons discussed below, it is highly probable that the hepatic lesions produced are attributable to drug sensitization rather than to a direct hepatotoxic action. In this connection, it is important to note that patients may react to several of the drugs in this group,[333] so that it is hazardous to substitute one for the other once any of them has produced hepatitis.

Iproniazid (1-isonicotinoyl-2-isopropylhy-

drazine, Marsilid). Iproniazid was introduced as a chemotherapeutic agent in the treatment of tuberculosis but was soon abandoned because it proved to be more toxic than the closely related and equally effective compound, isoniazid (isonicotinic acid hydrazide). Some years later its use was revived when it was found to be a potent antidepressant. Only then was its potential for producing serious hepatic injury fully appreciated.

Characteristically, iproniazid gives rise to a form of hepatitis that both clinically and morphologically is indistinguishable from that produced by the hepatitis virus.[577, 578, 629] Moreover, like pyrazinamide, cinchophen and zoxazolamine, it not infrequently gives rise to massive or subacute hepatic necrosis that often proves fatal.[240, 577, 578, 629, 677]

The reported incidence of hepatitis in patients receiving iproniazid is approximately 1.4 per cent.[629] Although estimates based on total sales of the drug are considerably lower,[629] serial studies demonstrating minor increases in serum bilirubin[372] and glutamic oxalacetic transaminase[552] in a significant number of patients suggest that if iproniazid therapy were not controlled carefully, the incidence of overt hepatitis would be considerably higher.

Since hepatitis appears to occur independently of either the dose of iproniazid or the duration of its administration[577, 629] and cannot be reproduced in experimental animals,[61] it is difficult to classify iproniazid as an hepatotoxin. The sporadic occurrence of the hepatitis, the frequency with which it appears after a latent period of several days to weeks following withdrawal of the drug,[629] and its occasional association with a rash[369, 808] suggest that the drug may be a sensitizing agent. However, the rarity of fever and eosinophilia appears to be contradictory. Because of the remarkable resemblance between viral- and iproniazid-induced hepatitis, the possibility has been considered that the drug either enhances susceptibility to intercurrent infections or lights up latent infections with the hepatitis virus. A report indicating that a third of affected individuals exhibited a positive hemagglutination reaction[396] appears to lend some support to this hypothesis. However,

this observation has not been confirmed by others.[383]

If hepatitis is to develop, it does so most commonly after the 4th week of iproniazid therapy, but the interval may be as short as 4 days or as long as 6 months.[629] In almost 20 per cent of cases, it appears 1 to 4 weeks after the cessation of drug administration. The onset may be abrupt, but more often it is insidious, with anorexia, weakness and malaise, occasionally accompanied by pruritus. In contrast with viral hepatitis, there is no fever during the preicteric phase. Darkening of the urine is noted within a day or two and is followed by overt jaundice which appears within 3 to 11 days of the onset.[369] The stools become clay-colored in a high proportion of cases. Jaundice deepens rapidly, reaching a peak in 2 to 4 weeks and usually is more intense than in viral hepatitis. Early enlargement and tenderness of the liver are common and may be accompanied by splenomegaly. In fatal cases, the liver shrinks in size and can seldom be palpated after the 1st week. Concomitantly, the jaundice deepens progressively and often is associated with ascites, gastrointestinal bleeding, fever and terminal hepatic coma. Death may occur as early as the 2nd week or not until several weeks later.

In nonfatal cases, the course tends to be prolonged, often exceeding 3 months. Although no cases of postnecrotic cirrhosis have been reported, subacute hepatic necrosis has been observed in a number of nonfatal cases.[577] On the basis of experience with lesions of this type, it can be predicted that some patients who apparently have recovered from an attack of iproniazid hepatitis will ultimately exhibit clinical or morphologic evidence of postnecrotic cirrhosis.

Characteristically, the concentration of serum bilirubin rises markedly, usually to levels higher than those seen in most cases of viral hepatitis. Although serum glutamic oxalacetic transaminase activity is greatly increased, levels over 500 units are less common than in viral hepatitis. A strongly positive cephalin-cholesterol flocculation reaction and increased thymol turbidity are common but inconstant findings. Raised levels of serum alkaline phosphatase are seen more frequently than in viral hepatitis and in many cases reach the heights seen in cholestatic hepatitis. In fatal cases, the serum concentrations of albumin and cholesterol tend to fall, while that of globulin rises. Often prothrombin activity is greatly depressed in such cases.

As noted, the morphology of the liver in Marsilid-induced hepatitis is indistinguishable from that in viral hepatitis, except that subacute and massive hepatic necrosis are more common.

The mortality rate is approximately 20 per cent.[629] Attempts to stem the downhill course in patients with massive hepatic necrosis by administering corticosteroids or ACTH have generally met with failure.[677, 808] However, they appear to have been more successful in less seriously ill patients with subacute hepatic necrosis.[58, 383] Whether or not cases of this type would have recovered spontaneously is unknown. Moreover, as pointed out, no data are available on the biopsy findings following recovery, so that the question of residual postnecrotic scarring in such patients is unsettled.

Isocarboxazid (Marplan). Although an analogue of iproniazid, this agent produces far fewer undesirable side reactions and thus far has caused only one case of hepatocellular jaundice.[57] In this instance, symptoms suggestive of an upper respiratory infection appeared 4 weeks after the institution of isocarboxazid administration. The preicteric phase was characterized by pruritus, a distaste for cigarettes and intermittent right flank pain. Although jaundice did not become clinically evident until the 3rd week, dark urine and light stools were noted as early as the 3rd day. The jaundice was moderate and cleared within 3 weeks. Serum bilirubin, alkaline phosphatase and transaminase showed modest increases, while the level of cholesterol was depressed. Thymol turbidity was increased, and the cephalin-cholesterol flocculation reaction was strongly positive.

Phenelzine (Nardil). Severe hepatitis has been encountered in patients given phenelzine for periods of 18 days to 5 months.[148, 332, 362] As in hepatitis induced by iproniazid, the clinical features and the histologic findings in the liver are indistinguishable from those of severe viral hepatitis. Death from massive hepatic necrosis within 3 weeks has occurred in 5 of 7 reported cases. Repeated exchange transfusions in one case,[362] begun 12 hours after onset of coma, failed to relieve the coma or to prevent death.

Pheniprazine (beta-phenylisopropyl-hydrazine, Catron, Cavodil). Several instances of severe hepatitis have been reported in patients receiving pheniprazine for periods of 2 weeks to 7 months.[52, 63, 277, 333] In all respects, the clinical, laboratory, and morphologic features have resembled those of iproniazid-induced hepatitis. Two of 6 reported cases terminated fatally with massive hepatic necrosis.[52, 333] One of the patients with nonfatal hepatitis had previously had a mild attack of jaundice while taking iproniazid.[333] In another, following recovery from pheniprazine-induced hepatitis, administration of the monoamine oxidase inhibitor, nialamide (Niamid), provoked a relapse.[333]

Although the paucity of reports suggests that the incidence of hepatitis is low, in one series of 37 patients given pheniprazine for periods of 8 to 40 weeks, one developed severe hepatitis and 4 others showed a significant rise in SGOT.[277]

OTHER PSYCHOPHARMACOLOGIC DRUGS

Chlordiazepoxide Hydrochloride (Librium). Typical cholestatic hepatitis has been encountered in at least 2 patients receiving chlordiazepoxide for 5 and 35 days, respectively.[2, 110] In addition, elevations of SGOT in the absence of jaundice have been observed.[335]

Another closely related benzodiazepine derivative, *diazepam (Valium)*, has been implicated in at least one nonfatal case of severe hepatic necrosis.[148] However, since the patient involved has also received phenoxypropazine, the role played by diazepam is uncertain.

Ectylurea (Nostyn). In the only reported case of hepatic injury induced by ectylurea, both the clinical and the histologic features were those of a mild cholestatic hepatitis.[328] The onset was sudden, with anorexia, nausea and right upper abdominal pain, on the 14th day of therapy. Dark urine, pruritus and faint icterus were noted a few days later. There was a modest increase in serum bilirubin and glutamic oxalacetic transaminase and a marked rise in the alkaline phosphatase level. In contrast, the serum cholesterol concentration, thymol turbidity and cephalin-cholesterol flocculation reaction remained normal. All symptoms subsided within 5 days. When a single 300-mg. dose of ectylurea was given on 2 successive days approximately 3 weeks later there was an immediate relapse of jaundice, pruritus and anorexia, which cleared within a week.

Imipramine Hydrochloride (Tofranil). Jaundice is a relatively uncommon complication of imipramine therapy, and usually subsides promptly following withdrawal of the drug.[19, 151, 327, 422, 484] In the few reported cases in which the clinical features are described, jaundice appeared between the 7th[19] and 110th[484] days of treatment, and was accompanied by fever[19, 327] and biochemical changes suggestive of cholestasis.[19, 327] The one available biopsy specimen of the liver is said to have shown slight, nonspecific inflammation in the parenchyma.[19] In one series of 85 patients receiving imipramine, 19 exhibited a transient rise in serum transaminase unaccompanied by jaundice.[19]

The desmethyl analogue of imipramine, *desipramine hydrochloride (Norpramin, Pertofrane)*, also may give rise to jaundice.[152] Unfortunately, details of the illness in such cases are lacking.

From available data, it appears that both imipramine and desipramine usually produce a cholestatic type of hepatitis. However, in at least one instance, these agents produced massive hepatic necrosis that was fatal.[584] The patient involved noted the onset of rash 2 weeks after starting treatment with imipramine. Substitution of desipramine at this point aggravated the dermatitis, so that drug treatment was discontinued 2 days later. Jaundice, fever and mild eosinophilia appeared 6 weeks after the onset of rash. The jaundice deepened rapidly, the rash become exfoliative in character, and ulcerations of the mucous membranes appeared. Death occurred 2 weeks after the onset of jaundice and approxi-

mately 8 weeks after the appearance of rash. Autopsy revealed massive destruction of the hepatic parenchyma, collapse of reticulin, numerous lipofuscin-filled macrophages and a mixed portal exudate of neutrophils, lymphocytes and histiocytes with occasional plasma cells and eosinophils, features seen in other forms of massive hepatic necrosis produced by reactions to drugs.

Considering the clinical features in this case, and the fact that imipramine and desipramine produce rash, fever, eosinophilia, thrombocytopenia and agranulocytosis, it is highly probable that the hepatic lesions they produce are attributable to drug sensitization.

Meprobamate (Miltown, Equanil). This agent, one of the most widely used tranquilizers, produces a variety of allergic reactions, including rash, fever, angioneurotic edema, arthralgia and thrombocytopenic purpura.[66, 334] Although hepatic involvement in such reactions has not been reported, the writer has seen 2 instances of cholestatic jaundice in patients receiving meprobamate and has heard of 2 others.

MISCELLANEOUS

APIOL DERIVATIVES

Apiol, a camphoraceous material derived from parsley and an important constituent of many illegal proprietary abortifacients, produces hepatic injury in animals and occasionally has been implicated as a hepatotoxic agent in humans.[455] However, in most such cases, complicating factors such as sepsis, hemolysis and shock have made it difficult to assess the role of apiol in the pathogenesis of the hepatic necrosis demonstrated at autopsy.

BURNS AND TANNIC ACID

A variety of hepatic lesions have been observed in individuals with extensive burns.[56, 262, 795] Animal experiments show that most of these can be attributed to tannic acid therapy and possibly to infection.[33, 234, 309] In dogs, extensive burns of the skin, if left untreated, are usually accompanied by central congestion and atrophy of the hepatic parenchyma. However, if infection supervenes, or if tannic acid dressings are applied, central necrosis of the liver ensues.[309] The presence of a burn is not essential for this effect for the same lesions occur when tannic acid is injected subcutaneously into normal animals.[33, 234, 309]

It seems unlikely that burns give rise to hepatic necrosis by reducing blood flow through the liver, since in dogs hepatic oxygen uptake is not reduced following burns.[263]

Severe liver damage, occasionally accompanied by jaundice and ascites, is also seen in patients with fatal burns that have been treated with tannic acid. The midzonal necrosis and the Councilman bodies found in such cases closely resemble those of yellow fever.[56] In contrast, untreated cases show only minor alterations in the staining quality of the parenchymal cells, varying degrees of fatty infiltration and centrilobular atrophy without necrosis.[262] Impairment of hepatic function also has been reported following burns.[795] However, the data do not indicate whether this occurs in the absence of infection and tannic acid therapy.

CARBAMAZEPINE (TEGRETOL)

Carbamazepine (5-carbamyl-5H-dibenzazepine) is chemically related to imipramine (Tofranil) and is used in the treatment of epilepsy and trigeminal neuralgia. It is a sensitizing agent, having produced rash, the Stevens-Johnson syndrome and fatal aplastic anemia in a number of cases.[589] In addition, it has been responsible for at least 2 instances of cholestatic hepatitis on the 7th and 20th day of drug administration.[589]

CHLOROTHIAZIDE

Rarely, chlorothiazide gives rise to cholestatic hepatitis.[182, 349] In one case, itching was noted after only three 0.5 Gm. doses given at daily intervals.[182] The drug was taken intermittently for an additional 2 weeks, at the end of which time jaundice appeared. Except for pruritus, there were no associated symptoms. The histologic and laboratory features were consistent with cholestatic hepatitis; but, because of uncertainty about the diagnosis, exploratory laparotomy was carried out, revealing

a normal biliary tree. Full recovery occurred by the end of 2 months.

In a second case, the jaundice was protracted, and was associated with a lesion resembling biliary cirrhosis.[349] The patient involved took chlorothiazide daily for more than 2 years without ill effects. Two and one-half months after resuming therapy with chlorothiazide she noted the onset of low grade fever, pruritus, anorexia and jaundice. She continued taking the drug for 5 weeks. Liver function studies suggested obstructive jaundice, so that exploratory laparotomy was carried out in the 8th week. The biliary tract proved to be normal. Wedge biopsy of the liver revealed expanded portal tracts with numerous neutrophils and eosinophils, granulomata, atypical ductular proliferation and periportal parenchymal necrosis, bile stasis and early fibrosis. Jaundice and pruritus persisted for several months and then cleared. However, the serum alkaline phosphatase level remained high. The patient died of a cerebrovascular accident 16 months after the onset of jaundice, and, at autopsy, the liver was nodular with portal fibrosis, nodular regeneration and a mononuclear reaction in the triads and septa.

CHOLECYSTOGRAPHY DYES

Bunamiodyl (Orabilex). In a high proportion of individuals given bunamiodyl, a tri-iodophenyl compound, there is a transient increase in the indirect-reacting (unconjugated) fraction of serum bilirubin by the next morning.[82] The rise in total serum bilirubin, which at its peak reaches levels of 1.5 to 2.0 mg./100 ml., returns to normal within 24 hours. Concomitantly, there is a transient increase in Bromsulphalein retention.[684]

Although bunamiodyl inhibits bilirubin conjugation by rat liver *in vitro*, other experimental evidence suggests that the retention of unconjugated bilirubin in the serum is due primarily to competitive inhibition of bilirubin excretion in bile,[72] or impairment of bilirubin uptake by the liver.[68] With respect to Bromsulphalein retention, animal studies suggest that bunamiodyl impairs the hepatic uptake of dye.[68]

Iopanoic Acid (Telepaque) and Iodipamide (Cholografin), two other iodinated compounds used for cholecystography, also produce transient mild hyperbilirubinemia[72] and Bromsulphalein retention,[72, 504] presumably by the same mechanisms involved in the case of bunamiodyl. In addition, *in vitro* studies with iopanoic acid suggest that inhibition of the Bromsulphalein-glutathione conjugating system is a factor in the dye retention produced by this agent.[513]

Rarely, orally administered cholecystography dyes produce reactions that appear to be allergic in nature. In one such case seen by the writer, the temperature rose sharply several hours after 3 Gm. of iopanoic acid was administered. Chills and fever continued for 6 days. A morbilliform rash and eosinophilia were noted in the 3rd day. At the height of the jaundice the liver was enlarged but not tender, serum bilirubin rose to 4.8 mg.%, serum alkaline phosphatase was 26 Bodansky units, thymol turbidity was 7 units, and the SGOT level was 60 units. The cephalin-cholesterol flocculation reaction remained normal. Biopsy at this time revealed a diffuse mononuclear inflammatory reaction involving all portions of the lobules and some of the central veins, and extensive centrilobular and periportal necrosis. Repeat biopsy 2 months after the reaction revealed normal liver tissue. However, full clinical and functional recovery did not occur for another 3 months.

ETHYL ALCOHOL

As pointed out, alcohol enhances the hepatotoxic effects of agents such as carbon tetrachloride, chloroform and phosphorus. In addition, it appears to play a role in the pathogenesis of Laennec's cirrhosis. This raises the question of whether or not alcohol is a hepatotoxin. According to many authorities, alcohol has no direct effect on the liver, but, when imbibed in excessive amounts, encourages a reduction in food consumption that leads to malnutrition, hepatic injury and, ultimately, to Laennec's cirrhosis.

However, experimental studies in animals indicate that, apart from its effects on food consumption, alcohol raises the choline requirement,[384] increases fatty acid synthesis,[438] mobilizes fat from the depots to the liver[595] and potentiates the development of nutritional cirrhosis.[384] Moreover, even in healthy nonalcoholic individuals maintained on a high protein diet, alcohol administration leads to fatty infiltration of the liver, raises the serum transaminase level and produces ultrastructural changes suggestive of toxic injury.[638] Whether or not these effects are implicated in the pathogenesis of Laennec's cirrhosis remains to be established.[202] For a more complete review of this subject see References 356 and 381.

MALE FERN

Male fern extract, widely used in the treatment of tapeworm infestation, regularly raises the level of the indirect-reacting (unconjugated) fraction of bilirubin in the serum and increases Bromsulphalein retention.[537] These changes, which appear within 24 hours, are unaccompanied by alterations in serum alkaline phosphatase or transaminase, and subside within a few days. Usually, the alterations in serum bilirubin and Bromsulphalein are slight, but, occasionally, overt jaundice or a high degree of Bromsulphalein retention may be produced.

It has been suggested that male fern interferes with the hepatic uptake of bilirubin and Bromsulphalein. However, the mechanism involved has not been adequately investigated.

METHYLDOPA (ALDOMET)

Abnormalities of hepatic function, including Bromsulphalein retention, and raised levels of serum transaminase and alkaline phosphatase, occur in a small but significant number of patients receiving methyldopa in the treatment of hypertension.[153] Those that appear within the first 10 days may be accompanied by fever and malaise, but more often they occur insidiously and without symptoms during the first few months of therapy. As a rule, such functional abnormalities promptly revert to normal when the drug is withdrawn. Liver biopsy in several patients has revealed foci of necrosis considered compatible with drug hypersensitivity.

In a few instances, the hepatic functional abnormalities produced by methyldopa have been accompanied by mild jaundice that has cleared promptly on discontinuing medication.[499] However, one instance of severe hepatitis has been reported.[805] In this case, the clinical features and the histologic findings in the liver were indistinguishable from those of viral hepatitis or those produced by drugs like iproniazid. The serum levels of bilirubin, glutamic oxalacetic transaminase and alkaline phosphatase reached peak values of 30 mg./100 ml., 1120 units and 25 K-A units, respectively. On withdrawal of the drug, the hepatitis subsided, but the serum bilirubin level was still elevated on the 45th day.

Considering that methyldopa can give rise to drug fever, agranulocytosis, thrombocytopenia[153] and Coombs' positive hemolytic anemia,[55] and that such reactions may be accompanied by a positive L.E. test and the appearance of rheumatoid factor in the serum,[679] it is highly probable that the hepatic lesions produced by this agent are due to drug hypersensitivity.

NICOTINIC ACID

A significant number of patients on prolonged nicotinic acid therapy for hypercholesteremia show minor degrees of Bromsulphalein retention and slight elevations of serum transaminase, lactic dehydrogenase, and alkaline phosphatase.[555] Raised levels of serum bilirubin are less common.[554] Withdrawal of the drug is followed by prompt recovery. Evidence suggests that preparations designed to provide slow release of the drug may produce hepatic dysfunction more frequently than pure nicotinic acid.[554] Liver biopsy studies in patients maintained on the drug for at least a year have revealed no abnormalities.[556] Although several patients with altered hepatic function have shown a variety of histologic changes in the liver, their relationship to nicotinic acid therapy is uncertain since other etiologic factors have been involved.[555]

At least two instances of apparent nicotinic acid-induced cholestatic hepatitis have been reported. In one, pruritus was noted after 13 months of drug therapy.[622] Treatment was interrupted for a month and then was resumed. Three months later there was

a relapse of pruritus, accompanied this time by jaundice. There were no associated gastrointestinal or constitutional symptoms. The liver was enlarged but nontender, and serum bilirubin was increased to a level of 7.4 mg./100 ml., only 1.0 mg. of which was of the direct-reacting type. There were elevations of serum alkaline phosphatase to 45 K-A units and SGOT to 91 units; thymol turbidity and cephalin-cholesterol flocculation were normal. The drug was stopped, and jaundice cleared in 3 weeks.

In the second case, pruritus appeared several weeks after a 15 month course of nicotinic acid had been discontinued.[554] Jaundice followed 8 days later, but there was no associated anorexia, nausea, vomiting, or hepatomegaly. Serum bilirubin rose to 7.0 mg./100 ml., with a direct-reacting fraction of 5.4 mg., SGOT to 200 units, and serum alkaline phosphatase to 50 K-A units; thymol turbidity remained normal. Drug therapy was discontinued and jaundice cleared in 4 days.

The pathogenesis of the hepatic dysfunction produced by nicotinic acid is not clear. Considering the absence of features suggestive of an allergic reaction, it is unlikely that drug hypersensitivity is involved. Although the occurrence of Bromsulphalein retention, the occasional development of pruritus and jaundice, and the absence of histologic changes in the liver suggest the type of functional cholestasis produced by agents like methyltestosterone, the frequency of raised levels of serum transaminase is atypical and suggests a mild hepatotoxic action.

PHENINDIONE (PHENYLINDANDIONE, HEDULIN, DANILONE)

Phenindione, a widely used anticoagulant, occasionally gives rise to reactions that appear to be allergic in nature. These are characterized by fever, rash, granulocytopenia and/or eosinophilia and may be accompanied by a cholestatic type of hepatitis,[99, 197, 363, 483, 583] and rarely by nephritis.[99] As a rule, the onset is abrupt during the 3rd or 4th week of drug administration, but may occur as early as the 10th day and as late as the 9th week. Rarely, the reaction appears a few days after withdrawal of the drug.[483] Usually, resumption of therapy following recovery provokes a prompt relapse.[99, 483]

Usually, hepatitis subsides following withdrawal of the drug. In some cases, ACTH and corticosteroids have appeared to hasten recovery.[99, 197, 483]

Although some patients with allergic reactions to phenindione can tolerate other anticoagulants, such as ethyl biscoumacetate,[73] relapses or exacerbations have been reported following resumption of treatment with acenocoumarin (nicoumalone, Sintrom).[583] It is probably unwise, therefore, to use any agent in this group once a reaction has occurred.

PHENYLHYDRAZINE

The jaundice seen during phenylhydrazine therapy for polycythemia vera is due primarily to the rapid hemolysis of erythrocytes. It has been suggested that prolonged or excessive treatment also results in liver injury. This is based on the observation that massive doses produce fatty degeneration and centrilobular necrosis of the liver in rabbits,[79] and that following repeated courses of treatment occasional patients develop cirrhosis.[430] However, even prolonged administration of therapeutic doses does not impair hepatic function, either in man[101] or in animals,[261] and following such treatment the liver shows no change other than mild hemosiderosis.[14] There is no reason to implicate phenylhydrazine as the etiologic factor in cirrhosis, since the lesion occurs spontaneously in untreated cases of polycythemia vera.

POLYVINYL PYRROLIDONE (PVP)

The intravenous administration of PVP, a synthetic plasma expander, is followed within a few months by the appearance in the Kupffer cells of globular basophilic deposits thought to be macromolecules of PVP.[249] At least up to a year, the amount of phagocytized material appears to increase with time. Occasionally, a mild inflammatory reaction is associated with the deposition of PVP, but there is no fibrosis or evidence of hepatocellular dysfunction. In animals given repeated injections of PVP, aggregates of PVP-filled histiocytes accumulate in the parenchyma and then extend into the triads.[246]

PRESSOR AGENTS

Although shock alone[208] or shock associated with cardiac failure[376] may produce centrilobular necrosis, the lesions are seldom massive.[104] However, in patients given pressor amines for the control of shock that ultimately proves to be fatal, the liver not infrequently shows large areas of infarction or extensive zones of hemorrhagic necrosis.[104] It has been suggested that the pressor amines are responsible for such lesions by producing ischemia.[104] Consistent with this view is the observation that in healthy dogs infusions of epinephrine, levarterenol, metaraminol, methoxamine, phenylephrine or mephentermine give rise to diffuse hepatic necrosis.[377] However, hemodynamic studies in the dog indicate that, under conditions of hemorrhagic shock, vasopressor drugs like levarterenol increase hepatic arterial blood flow.[149]

Although further study of the problem in man is needed, the latter observations suggest that, under such conditions, pressor amines do not produce hepatic ischemia. However, it is possible that they lead to massive hepatic necrosis indirectly by prolonging survival under conditions of shock and thus permit lesions to develop that otherwise would not become manifest.[104]

PYRIDINE

At one time, pyridine was used in the treatment of convulsive seizures and asthma and still is employed widely in industry as a solvent and as a reagent in the synthesis of certain organic compounds. It can produce severe hepatic and renal injury in man,[575] but the lesions have not been described. In the rat, pyridine produces both fatty infiltration and acute hepatic necrosis and, following prolonged administration, may give rise to cirrhosis.[46] Methionine and choline partially protect against the fatty infiltration and fibrosis but do not prevent the necrosis. Therefore, it has been suggested that pyridine injures the liver, both by a direct toxic action and by producing an intrinsic nutritional deficiency, possibly by diverting methyl groups during its methylation.

QUINETHAZONE (HYDROMOX)

Jaundice has been reported in a patient receiving quinethazone, a nonmercurial diuretic, unrelated to the benzothiadiazines, used in the treatment of hypertension.[350a] In the case involved, asymptomatic mild scleral icterus, slight hepatomegaly and elevation of the serum bilirubin to 3.3 mg./100 ml., with a direct-reacting fraction of 1.5 mg., were noted after 7 weeks of drug therapy. Other tests of hepatic function are said to have been normal. Liver biopsy revealed intracellular bile pigment granules in the centrilobular parenchyma, evidence of increased regenerative activity and infiltration of the portal triads with mononuclear cells and eosinophils. A direct Coombs' test was positive on two occasions. The jaundice cleared rapidly when the drug was withdrawn, but recurred within a week when treatment with quinethazone was resumed.

Since the direct Coombs' test was positive in the case described, and reports indicate that quinethazone occasionally produces rash, it may be a sensitizing agent.

RADIATION

X-ray irradiation of the liver provokes more intense radiation sickness than irradiation over any other area of the body. Although it is clear from both experimental and clinical observations that irradiation can damage the liver, the symptoms of radiation sickness do not appear to be dependent upon hepatic injury, which suggests that they may be due to the indirect effects of irradiation.

In some cases, intensive irradiation over the liver produces severe degeneration and necrosis of the intrahepatic bile ducts while sparing the parenchyma.[126] Thus, the hepatic parenchyma is thought to be relatively resistant to irradiation damage. However, in experimental animals, the parenchymal cells appear to be far more sensitive than the biliary epithelium when massive doses of x-ray are employed, the principal effects being degeneration and necrosis of hepatocytes by a direct action, and varying degrees

of edema, hyperemia and leukocytic infiltration attributable to vascular damage.[26] Smaller doses also affect the hepatic parenchyma, but the changes are more subtle.[447, 793] Similarly, in man, intensive irradiation (3,000 to 6,000 rads) over the liver produces severe damage, giving rise to a syndrome called "radiation hepatitis."[96, 353, 414] Characteristically, ascites and hepatosplenomegaly, occasionally accompanied by abdominal pain and jaundice, appear 2 to 6 weeks following completion of a course of irradiation. The hepatic lesion may heal without residuals, lead to fibrosis of the liver or result in death.

Histologically, the lesion is characterized by progressive fibrosis and obliteration of the central veins, and centrolobular congestion, hemorrhage and atrophy of the parenchyma, features that closely resemble those of the veno-occlusive disease seen in Jamaica and produced by senecio alkaloids.[602] The concept that the vascular lesions precede and are responsible for the congestion and loss of hepatic parenchyma is open to question, since in some studies the parenchymal changes have been observed prior to the appearance of hepatic venous occlusion.[353] There is evidence that, in some cases, the lesions regress or heal without residuals after a period of 4 months.[353, 602] However, marked fibrosis may persist and often is accompanied by terminal jaundice.[96] Rarely, such hepatic lesions may be complicated by stricture of the common duct or fibrosis of the pancreas.[96]

Surprisingly few changes in the liver were observed in *atom bomb casualties*.[439] In individuals who survived for less than 6 weeks, the principal findings were central congestion with atrophy of the hepatic parenchyma, and edema of the central veins. In those who survived longer, the liver exhibited fatty infiltration.

At least two radioactive materials used as therapeutic or diagnostic agents can produce liver injury: *radioactive colloidal gold* and thorium dioxide (*Thorotrast*).

Although there are no clinical reports of liver injury following the use of radioactive colloidal gold, it produces severe midzonal hepatic necrosis in rats.[393] The architecture of the liver is grossly distorted, both by necrosis and by the transformation of the parenchyma to masses of bizarre giant cells. Although the lesion may resemble cirrhosis, there is no fibrosis. Clinically, jaundice and ascites are evident prior to death. Survival varies from a few days to 7 months.

Despite claims to the contrary,[800, 801] there is convincing evidence to show that Thorotrast can produce hepatic injury and give rise to malignancy and certain hemopoietic disorders.

Hepatosplenomegaly with varying degrees of fibrosis and cirrhosis of the liver occurs in a significant number of individuals who have received large doses of colloidal thorium dioxide in the course of hepatosplenography or angiography.[12, 161, 252] Usually, the signs of hepatic disease appear after a latent period of at least 15 years. In animals, large doses of Thorotrast produce foci of hepatic necrosis and fibrosis in a much shorter period of time.[546] A significant number of patients with the disease die of hepatic failure.

A wide variety of malignant tumors have been encountered following Thorotrast administration, usually after a latent period of approximately 20 years.[161, 536, 562] Most often these have involved the liver, and have been of varying histologic types, including hepatoma, cholangiocarcinoma, sarcoma and hemangioendothelioma. Hemangioendotheliomas are particularly frequent.[161] In addition to those found in the liver, carcinomas have been encountered in many other tissues, although their relationship to antecedent Thorotrast administration has been less well defined.[161] Also, instances of both acute and chronic leukemia, lymphoma, aplastic anemia and thrombocytopenic purpura have been reported as late complications of Thorotrast deposits.[161]

All of the injected thorium dioxide is retained in the reticuloendothelium, and especially in the liver and spleen. Over a period of years, some may shift from the liver and the spleen to adjacent lymph nodes, but none is excreted. Although large particles can be demonstrated in the Kupffer cells of the liver and in the reticuloendothelium of the spleen, it is generally believed that the fibrosis that occurs in these organs is due to radioactivity and not to a foreign-body reaction. The 75 ml. dose of 25 per cent thorium dioxide solution required for hepatosplenography has been estimated to possess an alpha ray activity equivalent to that of 1.5 to 3.0 micrograms of radium.[801] In the course of its degradation, a series of other radioactive elements are produced, some of which emit beta and gamma rays in small quantity. Several of these have been identified in the excreta and the expired air many years after the injection of Thorotrast.[716] The carcinogenic potentiality of Thorotrast is also presumed to be related to its radioactivity.

TRANSFUSION REACTIONS

Not infrequently, severe reactions to transfusions of incompatible blood are accompanied by jaundice, a manifestation almost certainly due to acute hemolysis. However, evidence suggests that hepatic injury plays a contributory role. In most fatal cases, the liver shows areas of central necrosis,[85, 269] and similar lesions have been produced in dogs by injecting heterologous hemagglutinins.[559] Healing is followed by diffuse fibrosis in animals that survive, but a similar sequence has not been described in man.

The pathogenesis of the hepatic lesions in transfusion reactions is not well understood. Possibly they are related to shock, which is often present. It has also been suggested that hepatic necrosis results from impaction of the sinusoids with agglutinated erythrocytes.

Jaundice may also follow the transfusion of well-matched blood. This complication, designated by some as "benign postoperative intrahepatic cholestasis,"[652] is seen most commonly during the postoperative course of patients who have been transfused with bank blood.[370, 570, 652, 672] However, it may also occur after transfusions administered to patients with severe trauma or burns.[672] The writer has seen one instance following multiple transfusions in a patient with chronic renal failure who was undergoing periodic hemodialysis. Characteristically, the jaundice appears on the 1st to the 6th postoperative day, increases over the next few days and then clears within a week or two. Both the direct-reacting (conjugated) and indirect-reacting (unconjugated) fractions of serum bilirubin are increased, and are associated with bilirubinuria, but acholic stools and pruritus do not occur. Raised levels of serum alkaline phosphatase and transaminase are common but inconstant findings. Usually, peak values of serum bilirubin are under 10 mg./100 ml., but concentrations of 25 to 40 mg./100 ml. have been reported.[370, 652] Histologically, the liver shows centrilobular bile stasis which, occasionally, is accompanied by focal hepatic necrosis and degenerative changes.[370, 652] In cases with elevated levels of serum alkaline phosphatase, the clinical features may suggest obstructive jaundice. As a rule, the jaundice is asymptomatic and appears to have no adverse effect on the clinical course. Fatalities have been reported in cases of severe postoperative jaundice, but, in these, death has been due primarily to other factors.[370] The possibility that the cholestasis in such cases has played a contributory role cannot be excluded.

The jaundice seen following the transfusion of matched blood is clearly not due primarily to hemolysis. Although not proved, the mechanism involved appears to be related to two factors: first, a disturbance in hepatic secretory function (cholestasis) secondary to impairment of hepatic blood flow related to the effect of surgery, anesthesia, congestive heart failure, shock, trauma or sepsis, and second, a large increase in the load of bilirubin presented to the liver as a result of hemolysis of transfused blood.

TRIMETHOBENZAMIDE HYDROCHLORIDE (TIGAN)

Thus far, only one instance of hepatitis has been attributed to trimethobenzamide hydrochloride, an agent widely used as an antiemetic and for the control of motion sickness.[84] The patient involved noted the onset of jaundice and dark urine, accompanied by epigastric discomfort, anorexia and nausea, on the 5th day of drug administration. The jaundice deepened over the next few days and then began to fade. The results of hepatic function tests were consistent with hepatocellular jaundice, peak values being: serum bilirubin 14.9 mg./100 ml., glutamic oxalacetic transaminase 660

units, glutamic pyruvic transaminase 375 units, alkaline phosphatase 15.3 Sigma units, thymol turbidity 9 units and cephalin-cholesterol flocculation 3+. Biopsy of the liver revealed centrilobular bile stasis, foci of parenchymal necrosis, proliferation of Kupffer cells, enlargement and inflammation of the portal triads and rare acidophilic bodies.

Jaundice cleared rapidly following cessation of drug therapy, but the serum bilirubin was still slightly elevated when last studied at the end of 3 weeks.

Considering that this agent occasionally gives rise to allergic manifestations, such as rash, it is highly probable that the hepatitis described was another manifestation of drug hypersensitivity.

TRIPELENNAMINE (PYRIBENZAMINE) HYDROCHLORIDE

A brief report implicates Pyribenzamine as a cause of cholestatic hepatitis.[74] In the patient involved, an obstructive-like jaundice appeared during the course of treatment with the drug. Exploratory laparotomy failed to demonstrate any evidence of extrahepatic biliary obstruction. On biopsy, the liver showed centrilobular bile thrombi, foci of hepatocellular degeneration and necrosis and an inflammatory reaction. The jaundice persisted for 5 months, but then cleared. Follow-up clinical and biochemical studies several months later revealed no residuals.

REFERENCES

1. Abbott, J. A., and Schwab, R. S.: The serious side effects of the newer antiepileptic drugs; their control and prevention, New Engl. J. Med. 242:943, 1950.
2. Abbruzzese, A., and Swanson, J.: Jaundice after therapy with chlordiazepoxide hydrochloride, New Engl. J. Med. 273: 321, 1965.
3. Achar, S. T., Raju, V. B., and Sriramachari, S.: Indian childhood cirrhosis, J. Pediat. 57:744, 1960.
4. Acocella, G., and Billing, B. H.: Effect of drugs on the hepatic transport of bilirubin in McIntyre, N., and Sherlock, S.: (eds.) Therapeutic Agents and the Liver, p. 1, Oxford, Blackwell Scientific Pub., 1965.

5. ———: The effect of rifamycin SV on bile pigment excretion in rats, Gastroenterology 49:526, 1965.

6. Acocella, G., Nicolis, F. B., and Tenconi, L. T.: The effect of an intravenous infusion of rifamycin SV on the excretion of bilirubin, Bromsulphalein, and indocyanine green in man, Gastroenterology 49:521, 1965.

7. Adams, R. H., and Combes, B.: Viral hepatitis during pregnancy, J.A.M.A. 192:195, 1965.

8. Adlercreutz, H., and Ikonen, E.: Oral contraceptives and liver damage, Brit. Med. J. 2:1133, 1964.

9. Adlercreutz, H., Svanborg, A., and Ånberg, Å.: Recurrent jaundice in pregnancy. II. A study of estrogens and their conjugation in late pregnancy, Am. J. Med. 42:341, 1967.

10. Agostini, C., Perin, A., and Fonnesu, A.: Toxic fatty liver in adrenalectomized rats, Brit. J. Exp. Path. 41:617, 1960.

11. Agress, C. M.: Atabrine as a cause of fatal exfoliative dermatitis and hepatitis, J.A.M.A. 131:14, 1936.

12. Aizawa, M., Kobayashi, H., Maruyama, K., and Hagihara, K.: Two cases of cirrhotic liver associated with Thorotrast, deposit, Acta path. jap. 11:615, 1960.

13. Alexander, H. L.: Reactions with Drug Therapy, p. 167, Philadelphia, Saunders, 1955.

14. Allen, N. W., and Banker, N. W.: Experiments with phenylhydrazine; pathologic anatomy, Ann. Int. Med. 1:683, 1928.

15. Almaden, P. J., and Ross, S. W.: Jaundice due to methyl testosterone therapy, Ann. Int. Med. 40:146, 1954.

16. Ambrus, C. M., Siderin, C. N., Johnson, G. C., and Harrison, J. W. E.: Toxicity of penicillin and Aureomycin in guinea pigs, Antibiot. Chemother. 2:521, 1952.

17. Amromin, G. D., Deliman, R. M., and Shanbrom, E.: Liver damage after chemotherapy for leukemia and lymphoma, Gastroenterology 42:401, 1962.

18. Andersch, M. A.: Hepatic damage associated with sulfonamide therapy in infants and children. II. Changes in liver function test during sulfonamide therapy, Ann. Int. Med. 19:622, 1943.

19. Andersen, H., and Kristiansen, E. S.: Tofranil treatment of endogenous depressions, Acta psychiat. scand. 34:387, 1959.

20. Anderson, H. H., Reed, A. C., and Emerson, G. A.: Toxicity of alpha dinitrophe-

nol; report of a case, JA.M.A. 101:1053, 1933.

21. Anderson, N. L., and Palmer, W. L.: The danger of gold salt therapy; report of a fatal case, J.A.M.A. 115:1627, 1940.

22. Arai, H., and Snapper, I.: The influence of stilbamidine upon kidney function, liver function and peripheral blood in multiple myeloma; neurological sequelae of stilbamidine therapy, New York J. Med. 47:1867, 1947.

23. Arias, I. M.: Effect of norethandrolone on hepatic metabolism of bilirubin by normal and Gunn rats, Clin. Res. 8:367, 1960.

24. Arias, I. M., Gartner, L. M., Seifter, S., and Furman M.: Prolonged neonatal unconjugated hyperbilirubinemia associated with breast feeding and a steroid, pregnane-3(alpha),20(beta)-diol, in maternal milk that inhibits glucuronide formation in vitro, J. Clin. Invest. 43:2037, 1964.

25. Arias, I. M., Jankelson, O. M., and Zamcheck, N.: The effect of chlorpromazine on the excretion of Bromsulphalein (BSP) in human bile, Clin. Res. 4:144, 1956.

26. Ariel, I. M.: The effect of single massive doses of roentgen radiation upon the liver; an experimental study, Radiology 57:561, 1951.

27. Babior, B. M., and Davidson, C. S.: Postoperative massive liver necrosis: a clinical and pathological study, New Engl. J. Med. 276:645, 1967.

28. Baggenstoss, A. H.: The pancreas in uremia: a histopathologic study, Am. J. Path. 24:1003, 1948.

29. Bailey, B. H., and Kay, R. E.: Prolonged phenothiazine hepatitis; report of a case, Am. J. Psychiat. 117:557, 1960.

30. Bailie, M. J., and Christie, G. S.: The acute toxic action of dimethylnitrosamine on liver cells, Biochem. J. 72:473, 1959.

31. Baird, R. W., and Hull, J. G.: Cholestatic jaundice from tolbutamide, Ann. Int. Med. 53:194, 1960.

32. Bajoghli, M.: Generalized lymphadenopathy and hepatosplenomegaly induced by diphenylhydantoin, Pediatrics 28:943, 1961.

33. Baker, R. D., and Handler, P.: Animal experiments with tannic acid suggested by the tannic acid treatment of burns, Ann. Surg. 118:417, 1943.

34. Baldridge, C. W.: The relationship between antisyphilitic treatment and toxic cirrhosis, Am. J. Med. Sci. 188:685, 1934.

35. Bänder, A.: Pharmacological studies of

the sulfonylureas, Ann. N. Y. Acad. Sci. 82:508, 1959.

36. Barber, H. J., Slack, R., and Wien, R.: Increase in toxicity of stilbamidine solution on exposure to light, Nature 151:107, 1943.

37. Barich, L. L., Schwarz, J., Barich, D. J., and Horowitz, M. G.: Toxic liver damage in mice after prolonged intake of elevated doses of griseofulvin, Antibiot. Chemother. 11:566, 1961.

38. Barnes, J. A. P.: Toxic jaundice in munition workers and troops, Brit. Med. J. 1:155, 1917.

39. Barnes, J. M., and Magee, P. N.: Some toxic properties of dimethylnitrosamine, Brit. J. Indust. Med. 11:167, 1954.

40. Barrett, H. M., Best, C H., MacLean, D. L., and Ridout J. H.: The effect of choline on the fatty liver of carbon tetrachloride poisoning, J. Physiol. 97: 103, 1939.

41. Barrett, H. M., Best, C. H., and Ridout, J. H.: A study of the source of liver fat using deuterium as an indicator, J. Physiol. 93:367, 1938.

42. Barron, M.: Cinchophen poisoning: report of a case of severe allergic reaction, J.A.M.A. 82:2010, 1924.

43. Bartels, E. C., and Sjogren, R. W.: 1-Methyl-2-mercaptoimidazole: a new active antithyroid agent, J. Clin. Endocr. 11:1057, 1951.

44. Bartholomew, L. G., Cain, J. C., Frazier, S. H., Petersen, M. C., Foulk, W. T., Soule, E. H., Fleisher, G. E., and Owen, C. A., Jr.: Effect of chlorpromazine on the liver, Gastroenterology 34:1096, 1958.

45. Bateman, J. C., Barberio, J. R., Cromer, J. K., and Klopp, C. T.: Investigation of mechanism and type of jaundice produced by large doses of parenterally administered Aureomycin, Antibiot. Chemother. 3:1, 1953.

46. Baxter, J. H.: Hepatic and renal injury with calcium deposits and cirrhosis produced in rats by pyridine, Am. J. Path. 24:503, 1948.

47. Baxter, J. H., and Campbell, H.: Effects of Aureomycin on renal lesions, liver lipids, and tissue choline in choline deficiency, Proc. Soc. Exp. Biol. Med. 80:415, 1952.

48. Beattie, J., Herbert, P. H., Wechtel, C., and Steele, C. W.: Studies on hepatic dysfunction. I. Carbon tetrachloride poisoning treated with casein digest and methionine, Brit. Med. J. 1:209, 1944.

49. Beattie, J., and Marshall, J.: The aetiology of post-arsphenamine jaundice, Brit. Med. J. 1:547, 1944.

50. Beaver, D. C., and Pemberton, J. DeJ.: The pathologic anatomy of the liver in exophthalmic goiter, Ann. Int. Med. 7:687, 1933.

51. Beaver, D. C., and Robertson, H. E.: Specific character of toxic cirrhosis as observed in cinchophen poisoning; review of five fatal cases, Proc. Mayo Clin. 6:216, 1931.

52. Beer, D. T., and Schaffner, F.: Fatal jaundice after administration of beta-phenylisopropylhydrazine. Report of a case, J.A.M.A. 171:887, 1959.

53. Belfrage, S., Ahlgren, I., and Axelson, S.: Halothane hepatitis in an anesthetist, Lancet 2:1466, 1966.

54. Bellamy, W. E., Jr., Mauck, H. P., Jr., Hennigar, G. R., and Wigod, M.: Jaundice associated with the administration of sodium p-aminosalicylic acid; review of the literature and report of a case, Ann. Int. Med. 44:764, 1956.

55. Belle, M. S., and Mas, I. R.: Methyldopa and positive Coombs' test, J.A.M.A. 200:900, 1967.

56. Belt, T. H.: Liver necrosis following burns, simulating the lesions of yellow fever, J. Path. Bact. 48:493, 1939.

57. Benack, R. T., and Lynch, V.: Jaundice associated with isocarboxazid therapy, New Engl. J. Med. 264:294, 1961.

58. Benaim, S., and Dixon, M. F.: Jaundice associated with administration of iproniazid. Report of two cases, Brit. Med. J. 2:1068, 1958.

59. Benhamou, J. P.: General discussion on drugs and the liver, in McIntyre, N., and Sherlock, S. (eds.): Therapeutic Agents and the Liver, p. 167, Oxford, Blackwell Scientific Publications, 1965.

60. Bennett, G. A., Drinker, C. K., and Warren, M. F.: Morphological changes in the livers of rats resulting from exposure to certain chlorinated hydrocarbons, J. Indust. Hyg. Toxicol. 20:97, 1938.

61. Benson, W. M., Stefko, P. L., and Roe, M. D.: Pharmacologic and toxicologic observations on hydrazine derivatives of isonicotinic acid (Rimifon, Marsilid), Am. Rev. Tuberc. 65:376, 1952.

62. Berger, S. S., and Applebaum, H. S.: Toxic hepatitis due to sulfanilamide; re-

port of a fatal case with histopathologic findings in the liver, J. Lab. Clin. Med. 26:785, 1941.

63. Berkowitz, D., Rotman, M., Greenstein, R. H., and Sloane, N. G.: Occurrence of jaundice during perphenazine and beta-phenylisopropylhydrazine, Am. J. Dig. Dis. 6:160, 1961.

64. Berman, A., and Franklin, R. L.: Precipitation of acute intermittent porphyria by griseofulvin therapy, J.A.M.A. 192:1005, 1965.

65. Berne, R. M.: An unusual sensitivity reaction to penicillin; report of a case with autopsy findings, New Engl. J. Med. 242:814, 1950.

66. Bernstein, C., and Klotz, S. D.: Allergenicity of tranquilizing drugs, J.A.M.A. 163:930, 1957.

67. Berté, S. J., Di Mase, J. D., and Christianson, C. S.: Isoniazid, para-amino-salicylic acid, and streptomycin intolerance in 1,744 patients: an analysis of reactions to single drugs and drug groups plus data on multiple reactions, type and time of reactions, and desensitization, Am. Rev. Resp. Dis. 90:508, 1964.

68. Berthelot, P., and Billing, B. H.: Effect of bunamiodyl on hepatic uptake of sulfobromophthalein in the rat, Am. J. Physiol. 211:395, 1966.

69. Best, C. H., MacLean, D. L., and Ridout, J. H.: Choline and liver fat in phosphorus poisoning, J. Physiol. 83:275, 1935.

70. Bevans, M., and Batchelor, W. H.: Cholangiolitic cirrhosis with intrahepatic biliary tract obstruction and xanthomatosis, Am. J. Med. 9:133, 1950.

71. Bickers, J. N., Buechner, H. A., Hood, B. J., and Alvarez-Chiesa, G.: Hypersensitivity reaction to antituberculosis drugs with hepatitis, lupus phenomenon and myocardial infarction, New Engl. J. Med. 265:131, 1961.

72. Billing, B. H., Maggiore, Q., and Cartter, M. A.: Hepatic transport of bilirubin, Ann. N. Y. Acad. Sci. 111:319, 1963.

73. Bingle, J., and Shine, I.: Phenindione sensitivity, Lancet 2:377, 1959.

74. Bjorneboe, M., Iversen, O., and Olsen, S.: Infective hepatitis and toxic jaundice in municipal hospital during a five-year period, Acta med. scand. 182:491, 1967.

75. Black-Schaffer, B., Johnson, D. S., and Gobbel, W. G., Jr.: Experimental total midzonal hepatic necrosis, Am. J. Path. 26:397, 1950.

76. Boake, W. C., Schade, S. G., Morrissey, J. F., and Schaffner, F.: Intrahepatic cholestatic jaundice of pregnancy followed by Enovid-induced cholestatic jaundice; report of a case, Ann. Int. Med. 63:302, 1965.

77. Boardman, R. H.: Fatal case of toxic hepatitis implicating chlorpromazine, Brit. Med. J. 2:579, 1954.

78. Bodansky, M., Campbell, K., and Ball, E.: Changes in serum calcium, inorganic phosphate and phosphatase activity in pregnant women, Am. J. Clin. Path. 9:36, 1939.

79. Bodansky, M., Marr, W. L., and Brindley, P.: An experimental study of the action of phenylhydrazine hydrochloride and acetylphenylhydrazine (pyrodin) with reference to their use in the treatment of polycythemia vera, Am. J. Clin. Path. 2:391, 1932.

80. Bollman, J. L.: Protective value of foods in experimental cirrhosis, J.A.M.A. 121:1413, 1943.

81. Bollman, J. L., and Mann, F. C.: The physiology of the impaired liver, Ergebn. Physiol. 38:445, 1936.

82. Bolt, R. J., Dillon, R. S., and Pollard, H. M.: Interference with bilirubin excretion by a gall-bladder dye (bunamiodyl), New Engl. J. Med. 265:1043, 1961.

83. Bolton, B. H.: Prolonged chlorpromazine jaundice, Am. J. Gastroent. 48:497, 1967.

84. Borda, I., and Jick, H.: Hepatitis following the administration of trimethobenzamide hydrochloride, Arch. Int. Med. 120:371, 1967.

85. Bordley, J., III: Reactions following transfusion of blood, with urinary suppression and uremia, Arch. Int. Med. 47:288, 1931.

86. Borglin, N. E.: Oral contraceptives and liver damage, Brit. Med. J. 1:1289, 1965.

87. Bothwell, T. H., and Bradlow, B. A.: Siderosis in the Bantu: a combined histopathological and chemical study, Arch. Path. 70:279, 1960.

88. Bothwell, T. H., Seftel, H., Jacobs, P., Torrance, J. D., and Baumslag, N.: Iron overload in Bantu subjects: studies on the availability of iron in Bantu beer, Am. J. Clin. Nutr. 14:47, 1964.

89. Bourne, W., and Raginsky, B. B.: The effect of Avertin upon the normal and impaired liver, Am. J. Surg. 14:653, 1931.

90. Bowesman, C.: A short report on the use

of 4:4'-diamidino stilbene in the treatment of human sleeping sickness, Ann. Trop. Med. *34*:217, 1940.

91. Bradley, R. F.: Role of oral blood sugar-lowering agents in the management of diabetes, Ann. N. Y. Acad. Sci. *82*:513, 1959.

92. Bragdon, J. H.: The hepatitis of hyperthermia; report of a fatal case, New Engl. J. Med. *237*:765, 1947.

93. Bras, G., Jelliffe, D. B., and Stuart, K. L.: Veno-occlusive disease of liver with nonportal type of cirrhosis, occurring in Jamaica, Arch. Path. *57*:285, 1954.

94. Brauer, M. J., McEvoy, B. F., and Mitus, W. J.: Hypersensitivity to nitrogen mustards in the form of erythema multiforme: a unique adverse reaction, Arch. Int. Med. *120*:499, 1967.

95. Breinstrup, H., and Sogaard-Andersen, J.: Intrahepatic cholestasis after griseofulvin therapy, Ugeskr. Laeg. *128*:145, 1966.

96. Brick, I. B.: Effects of million volt irradiation on the gastrointestinal tract, Arch. Int. Med. *96*:26, 1955.

97. Brick, I. B., and Kyle, L. H.: Jaundice of hepatic origin during the course of methyl-testosterone therapy, New Engl. J. Med. *246*:176, 1952.

98. Bridges, R. A., Berendes, H., and Good, R. A.: Serious reactions to novobiocin, J. Pediat. *50*:579, 1957.

99. Brooks, R. H., and Calleja, H. B.: Dermatitis, hepatitis and nephritis due to phenindione (phenylindandione), Ann. Int. Med. *52*:706, 1960.

100. Brown, G., Zoidis, J., and Spring, M.: Hepatic damage during chlorpropamide therapy, J.A.M.A. *170*:2085, 1959.

101. Brown, G. E., and Griffin, H. Z.: The treatment of polycythemia vera (erythremia) with phenylhydrazine, Arch. Int. Med. *38*:321, 1926.

102. Brunschwig, A., Johnson, C., and Nichols, S.: Carbon tetrachloride injury of the liver. The protective action of certain compounds, Proc. Soc. Exp. Biol. Med. *60*:388, 1945.

103. Brunschwig, A., Nichols, S., Bigelow, R. R., and Miles, J.: Sulfhydryl protection of the liver, Arch. Path. *40*:81, 1945.

104. Brunson, J. G., Eckman, P. L., and Campbell, J. B.: Increasing prevalence of unexplained liver necrosis, New Engl. J. Med. *257*:52, 1957.

105. Buckley, J. J., Buckley, S. M., and Gey, M. K.: Tissue culture studies on liver cells of anaphylactically (Arthus) sensitized animals in the presence of the sensitizing antigen, Bull. Johns Hopkins Hosp. *84*:195, 1949.

106. Bull, L. B., and Dick, A. T.: The chronic pathological effects on the liver of the rat of the pyrrolizidine alkaloids heliotrine, lasiocarpine and their N-oxides, J. Path. Bact. *78*:483, 1959.

107. Bunker, J. P., and Blumenfeld, C. M.: Liver necrosis after halothane anesthesia: cause or coincidence? New Engl. J. Med. *268*:531, 1963.

108. Burnap, T. K., Galla, S. J., and Vandam, L. D.: Anesthetic, circulatory and respiratory effects of Fluothane, Anesthesiology *19*:307, 1958.

109. Butt, H. R., Hall, J. E., Watkins, C. H., and Cragg, R. W.: Atabrine dihydrochloride (quinacrine hydrochloride); some observations on its toxicity and on its use in the treatment of malaria, with particular reference to its effect on the liver, Gastroenterology *4*:205, 1945.

110. Cacioppo, J., and Merlis, S.: Chlordiazepoxide hydrochloride (Librium) and jaundice; report of a case, Am. J. Psychiat. *117*:1040, 1961.

111. Calvert, D. N., and Brody, T. M.: Biochemical alterations of liver function by the halogenated hydrocarbons. I. *In vitro* and *in vivo* changes and their modification by ethylenediamine tetraacetate, J. Pharmacol. Exp. Ther. *124*:273, 1958.

112. ———: Role of the sympathetic nervous system in CCl_4 hepatotoxicity, Am. J. Physiol. *198*:669, 1960.

113. Camerini-Davalos, R., Root, H. F., and Marble, A.: Clinical experience with carbutamide (BZ-55); a progress report, Diabetes *6*:74, 1957.

114. Cameron, G. R.: Carbon tetrachloride cirrhosis in relation to liver regeneration, J. Path. Bact. *42*:1, 1936.

115. Cameron, G. R., and Karunaratne, W. A. E.: Liver changes in exophthalmic goitre, J. Path. Bact. *41*:267, 1935.

116. Cameron, G. R., Karunaratne, W. A. E., and Thomas, J. C.: Massive necrosis ("toxic infarction") of the liver following intra-portal administration of poisons, J. Path. Bact. *44*:297, 1937.

117. Campagna, M., Calix, A. A., and Hauser, G: Observations on the combined use of pyrazinamide (Aldinamide) and isoniazid in the treatment of pulmonary tubercu-

losis; a clinical study, Am. Rev. Tuberc. *69*:334, 1954.

118. Campbell, P. N., Greengard, O., and Kernot, B. A.: Studies on the synthesis of serum albumin by the isolated microsome fraction from rat liver, Biochem. J. *74*: 107, 1960.

119. Canavan, M. N., Cobb, S., and Drinker, C. K.: Chronic manganese poisoning; report of a case with autopsy, Arch. Neurol. Psychiat. *32*:501, 1934.

120. Carbone, J. V.: Personal communication to Marquardt, Fisher, Levy and Dowben.[489]

121. Carbone, J. V., Grodsky, G. M., and Hjelte, V.: Effect of hepatic dysfunction on circulating levels of sulfobromophthalein and its metabolites, J. Clin. Invest. *38*:1989, 1959.

122. Carey, J. B., and Williams, G.: Relief of the pruritus of jaundice with a bile-acid sequestering resin, J.A.M.A. *176*:432, 1961.

123. Carr, H. J., Jr., and Knauer, Q. F.: Death due to hepatic necrosis in a patient receiving zoxazolamine. Report of a case and review of the literature, New Engl. J. Med. *264*:977, 1961.

124. Carter, S., Sciarra, R., and Merritt, H. H.: Phenylacetylurea in the treatment of convulsive seizures, Dis. Nerv. Syst. *11*: 139, 1950.

125. Casamajor, L.: Cited by von Oettingen.[763]

126. Case, J. T., and Warthin, A. S.: The occurrence of hepatic lesions in patients treated by intensive deep roentgen irradiation, Am. J. Roentgenol. *12*:27, 1924.

127. Case Records of the Massachusetts General Hospital: Reye's disease, with fatty change and peripheral zonal necrosis of the liver, toxic encephalopathy, and fatty change of renal tubules, New Engl. J. Med. *276*:47, 1967.

128. Chadwick, D. A., and Jennings, R. C.: Massive hepatic necrosis associated with halothane anesthesia, Lancet *1*:793, 1964.

129. Chaiken, B. H., Goldberg, B. I., and Segal, J. P.: Dilantin sensitivity; report of a case of hepatitis with jaundice, pyrexia and exfoliative dermatitis, New Engl. J. Med. *242*:897, 1950.

130. Chaikin, N. W., and Chlenoff, S. O.: Acute hepatitis; Clinical observations in 63 cases, Am. J. Dig. Dis. *12*:151, 1945.

131. Charles, J. R.: Manganese toxaemia; with special reference to the effects of liver feeding, Brain *50*:30, 1927.

132. Chase, M. W.: The allergic state *in* Dubos, R.: Bacterial and Mycotic Infections in Man, ed. 2, p. 168, Philadelphia, Lippincott, 1952.

133. Chesner, C.: Chronic pulmonary granulomatosis in residents of a community near a beryllium plant; three autopsied cases, Ann. Int. Med. *32*:1028, 1950.

134. Christie, G. S.: Liver damage in acute heliotrine poisoning. I. Structural changes, Aust. J. Exp. Biol. Med. Sci. *36*:405, 1958.

135. Christie, G. S., and Judah, J. D.: Mechanism of action of carbon tetrachloride on liver cells, Proc. Roy. Soc. Biol. *142-B*:241, 1954.

136. Chutlani, H. K., Gupta, P. S., Gulati, S., and Gupta, D. N.: Acute copper sulfate poisoning, Am J. Med. *39*:849, 1965.

137. Clarke, D. A., Philips, F. S., Sternberg, S. S., Stock, C. C., Elion, G. B., and Hitchings, G. H.: 6-Mercaptopurine: effects in mouse sarcoma 180 and in normal animals, Cancer Res. *13*:593, 1953.

138. Cline, E. W.: Acute yellow atrophy of the liver following sulfanilamide medication, J.A.M.A. *111*:2384, 1938.

138a. Clubb, A. W., and Giles, C.: Budd-Chiari syndrome after oral contraceptives, Brit. Med. J. *1*:252, 1968.

139. Coggeshall, H. C., and Greene, J. A.: The influence of desiccated thyroid gland, thyroxin, and inorganic iodine, upon the storage of glycogen in the liver of the albino rat under controlled conditions, Am. J. Physiol. *105*:103, 1933.

140. Cohen, A. A., and Lawrence, S. H.: Combined hypersensitivity reaction to sodium para-aminosalicylate and associated antibacterial drug concurrently administered, Ann. Int. Med. *46*:893, 1957.

141. Cohen, I. M., and Archer, J. D.: Liver function and hepatic complications in patients receiving chlorpromazine, J.A.M.A. *159*:99, 955.

142. Cohen, R., Kalser, M. H., and Thomson, R. V.: Fatal hepatic necrosis secondary to isoniazid therapy, J.A.M.A. *176*:877, 1961.

143. Colbert, J. W., Jr., Bungards, L., and Knowlton, M.: Aureomycin, Chloromycetin and Terramycin in treatment of acute viral hepatitis, Proc. Soc. Exp. Biol. Med. *79*:339, 1952.

144. Coleman, F. P.: The effect of anesthesia

on hepatic function, Surgery 3:87, 1938.

145. Colsky, J., Greenspan, E. M., and Warren, T. N.: Hepatic fibrosis in children with acute leukemia after therapy with folic acid antagonists, Arch. Path. 59:198, 1955.

146. Combes, B.: Personal communication.

147. Conn, H. O., Binder, H. J., and Orr, H. D.: Ethionamide-induced hepatitis: a review with a report of an additional case, Am. Rev. Resp. Dis. 90:542, 1964.

148. Cook, G. C., and Sherlock, S.: Jaundice and its relation to therapeutic agents, Lancet 1:175, 1965.

149. Corday, E., and Williams, J. H., Jr.: Effect of shock and of vasopressor drugs on the regional circulation of the brain, heart, kidney and liver, Am. J. Med. 29:228, 1960.

150. Corley, C. C., Jr., Lessner, H. E., and Larsen, W. E.: Azathioprine therapy of "autoimmune" diseases, Am. J. Med. 41:404, 1966.

151. Council on Drugs: Imipramine hydrochloride (Tofranil), J.A.M.A. 178:575, 1961.

152. ————: A new antidepressant—desipramine hydrochloride (Norpramin, Pertofrane), J.A.M.A. 194:82, 1965.

153. ————: A new antihypertensive—methyldopa (Aldomet), J.A.M.A. 186:504, 1963.

154. Cox, R. P., Foltz, E. L., Raymond. S., and Drewyer, R.: Novobiocin jaundice, New Engl. J. Med. 261:139, 1959.

155. Craven, E. B., Jr.: The importance of diet in preventing acute yellow atrophy during arsphenamine treatment, Bull. Johns Hopkins Hosp. 48:131, 1931.

156. Crawford, S. E., and Jones, C. K.: Fatal liver necrosis and diphenylhydantoin sensitivity, Pediatrics 30:595, 1962.

157. Crosby, G. J. V.: The "accidents" of gold treatment in rheumatoid arthritis, Lancet 1:1463, 1936.

158. Cuthbert, J.: Acquired idiosyncrasy to sodium p-aminosalicylate, Lancet 2:209, 1950.

159. Cutts, M.: Chlorpromazine hepatitis treated with cortisone, Ann. Int. Med. 46:1160, 1957.

160. Damashek, W., Weisfuse, L., and Stein, L.: Nitrogen mustard therapy in Hodgkin's disease, Blood 4:338, 1949.

161. daSilva Horta, J., Abbatt, J. D., Cayolla Da Motta, L., and Roriz, M. L.: Malignancy and other late effects following administration of Thorotrast, Lancet 2:201, 1965.

162. Davidson, C. S.: Hepatotoxicity of foods: a consideration of the hepatotoxicity of a few phanerogams and cryptogams; their possible influence in the pathogenesis of cirrhosis and hepatoma, Ann. N. Y. Acad. Sci. 104:1026, 1963.

163. Davidson, D. T., Jr., and Lennox, W. G.: Phenacetylurea—phenurone—in epilepsy, Dis. Nerv. Syst. 11:167, 1950.

164. Davis, H. A., Harris, L. C., Jr., and Schmeisser, H. C.: Tissue changes following prolonged administration of sulfanilamide in rats, Arch. Path. 25:750, 1938.

165. Davis, J. D., Netzer, S., Schwartz, J. A., and Pattison, E. H.: Tibione: laboratory and clinical studies, Dis. Chest 18:521, 1950.

166. Davis, J. S., Jr.: The relation of neocinchophen to the question of cinchophen toxicity, Am. J. Med. Sci. 184:555, 1932.

167. Davis, N. C., and Whipple, G. H.: The influence of fasting and various diets on the liver injury effected by chloroform anesthesia, Arch Int. Med. 23:612, 1919.

168. DeMatteis, F., and Rimington, C.: Disturbance of porphyrin metabolism caused by griseofulvin in mice, Brit. J. Dermat. 75:91, 1963.

169. DeNardi, J. M., Van Ordstrand, H. S., and Carmody, M. G.: Chronic pulmonary granulomatosis; report of 10 cases, Am. J. Med. 7:345, 1949.

170. DeNardi. J. M., Van Ordstrand, H. S., Curtis, G. H., and Zielinski, J.: Berylliosis: summary and survey of all clinical types observed in a twelve-year period, Arch. Indust. Hyg. 8:1, 1953.

171. Dianzani, M. U: Uncoupling of oxidative phosphorylation in mitochondria from fatty livers, Biochim. Biophys. Acta 14:514, 1954.

172. ————: Content and distribution of pyridine nucleotides in fatty livers, Biochim. Biophys. Acta 17:391, 1955.

173. ————: The content of adenosine polyphosphates in fatty livers, Biochem. J. 65:116, 1957.

174. Dianzani, M. U., and Bahr, G. F.: Electron microscope investigation of mitochondria isolated from normal and steatotic livers by differential centrifugation, Acta path. microbiol. scand. 35:25, 1954.

175. Dible, J. H., and McMichael, J.: The pathology of arseno-therapy jaundice, Brit. J. Vener. Dis. 19:102, 1943.

176. Dickes, R., Schenker, V., and Deutsch, L.: Serial liver-function and blood studies in patients receiving chlorpromazine, New Engl. J. Med. 256:1, 1957.

177. Dittman, W. A., and Ward, J. R.: Demecolcine toxicity; a case report of severe hemopoietic toxicity and a review of the literature, Am. J. Med. 27:519, 1959.

178. Dochertz, J. F., and Burgess, E.: The action of carbon tetrachloride on the liver, Brit. Med. J. 2:907, 1922.

179. Dolger, H.: An assessment of oral antidiabetic therapy, Ann. N. Y. Acad. Sci. 82:531, 1959.

180. Doljanski, L., and Rosin, A.: Studies on early changes in the livers of rats treated with various toxic agents, with especial reference to the vascular lesions; histology of the rat's liver in urethane poisoning, Am. J. Path. 20:945, 1944.

181. Dowling, H. F., and Lepper, M. H.: Hepatic reactions to tetracycline, J.A.M.A. 188:307, 1964.

182. Drerup, A. L., Alexander, W. A., Lumb, G. D., Cummins, A. J., and Clark, G. M.: Jaundice occurring in a patient treated with chlorothiazide, New Engl. J. Med. 259:534, 1958.

183. Drill, V. A.: The effect of yeast on the liver glycogen of white rats during hyperthyroidism, J. Nutr. 14:355, 1937.

184. ———: Methionine therapy in experimental liver injury produced by carbon tetrachloride, J. Pharmacol. Exp. Ther. 90:138, 1947.

185. ———: Hepatotoxic agents: mechanism of action and dietary interrelationship, Pharmacol. Rev. 4:1, 1952.

186. Drill, V. A., and Loomis, T. A.: Effect of methionine supplements on hepatic injury produced by carbon tetrachloride, Science 103:199, 1946.

187. Drill, V. A., Loomis, T. A., and Belford, J.: Effect of protein and carbohydrate intake on liver injury produced in dogs by carbon tetrachloride, J. Indust. Hyg. Toxicol. 29:180, 1947.

188. Drill, V. A., and Shaffer, C. B.: Serum cholesterol, serum phosphatase and Bromsulphalein retention in experimental hyperthyroidism, Gastroenterology 1:308, 1943.

189. Driver, J. R., and Weller, J. N.: Untoward results from the use of gold compounds; report of a fatal case, Arch. Derm. Syph. 23:87, 1931.

190. Dubash, J., and Teare, D.: Poisoning by Amanita phalloides, Brit. Med. J. 1:45, 1946.

191. Dubin, I. N.: Unpublished data; cited by Dubin, I. N., Sullivan, B. H., Jr., LeGolvan, P. C., and Murphy, L. C., Am. J. Med. 29:55, 1960.

192. Dujovne, C. A., Chan, C. H., and Zimmerman, H. J.: Sulfonamide hepatic injury: review of the literature and report of a case due to sufamethoxazole, New Engl. J. Med. 277:785, 1967.

193. Duma, R. J., Hendry, C. N., and Donahoo, J. S.: Hypersensitivity to diphenylhydantoin (Dilantin): a case report with toxic hepatitis, Southern Med. J. 59:168, 1966.

194. Dunning, M. F.: Jaundice associated with norethandrolone (Nilevar) administration, J.A.M.A. 167:1242, 1958.

195. Dutra; F. R.: The pneumonitis and granulomatosis peculiar to beryllium workers, Am. J. Path. 24:1137, 1948.

196. Eagle, H., and Magnuson, H. J.: The systemic treatment of 227 cases of arsenic poisoning (encephalitis, dermatitis, blood dyscrasias, jaundice, fever) with 2,3-dimercaptopropanol (BAL), Am. J. Syph. 30:420, 1946.

197. East, E. N., and Beamish, R. E.: Severe sensitivity reaction (hepatitis, dermatitis and pyrexia) attributable to phenylin-danedione, Canad. Med. Ass. J. 77:1028, 1957.

198. Eckardt, E. T., and Plaa, G. L.: The effect of phenothiazine derivatives on the disappearance of sulphobromopthalein from mouse plasma, J. Pharmacol. Exp. Ther. 138:387, 1962.

199. Eckhardt, R. D., Faloon, W. W., and Davidson, C. S.: Improvement of active liver cirrhosis in patients maintained with amino acids intravenously as the source of protein and lipotropic substances, J. Clin. Invest. 28:603, 1949.

200. Eddy, J. H., Jr.: Carbon tetrachloride poisoning; preliminary report on the use of methionine in hepatitis, J.A.M.A. 128:994, 1945.

201. Eden, E., and Harrison, D. D.: Studies in carbon tetrachloride poisoning. III. The possible role of sulphur amino acids

in detoxication, Aust. J. Exp. Biol. Med. Sci. *33*:85, 1955.

202. Editorial: Is alcohol hepatotoxic?, New Engl. J. Med. *278*:905, 1968.

203. Edwards, J. E., and Dalton, A. J.: Induction of cirrhosis of the liver and of hepatomas in mice with carbon tetrachloride, J. Nat. Cancer Inst. *3*:19, 1942.

204. Einhorn, M., and Davidsohn, I.: Hepatotoxicity of mercaptopurine, J.A.M.A. *188*:802, 1964.

205 Eisalo, A., Järvinen, P. A., and Luukkainen, T.: Hepatic impairment during the intake of contraceptive pills: clinical trial with postmenopausal women, Brit. Med. J. *2*:426, 1964.

206. Elion, G. B., Callahan, S., Bieber, S., Hitchings, G. H., and Rundles, R. W.: A summary of investigations with 6-[(1-methyl-4-nitro-5-imidazolyl)thio]purine (B. W. 57-322), Cancer Chemother. Rep. *14*:93, 1961.

207. Elkes, J., and Elkes, C.: Effect of chlorpromazine on the behaviour of chronically overactive psychotic patients, Brit. Med. J. *2*:560, 1954.

208. Ellenberg, M., and Osserman, K. E.: The role of shock in the production of central liver cell necrosis, Am. J. Med. *11*:170, 1951.

209. Ellinger, F.: Response of the liver to irradiation, Radiology *44*:241, 1945.

210. Elliott, D. C., Baehr, G., Shaffer, L. W., Usher, G. S., and Lough, S. A.: An evaluation of the massive dose therapy of early syphilis, J.A.M.A. *117*:1160, 1941.

211. Ellis, F. A.: Reactions to Nirvanol, phenytoin sodium and phenobarbital; report of a case of ectodermosis erosiva pluriorificalis following the ingestion of phenytoin sodium, Southern Med. J. *36*:575, 1943.

212. Elmerdorf, D. F., Jr., Cawthon, W. V., Muschenheim, C., and McDermott, W.: The absorption, distribution, excretion and short-term toxicity of isonicotinic acid hydrazide (nydrazid) in man, Am. Rev. Tuberc. *65*:429, 1952.

213. Engleman, E. P., Krupp, M. A., Rinehart, J. F., Jones, R. C., and Gibson, J. R.: Hepatitis following the ingestion of phenylbutazone, J.A.M.A. *156*:98, 1954.

214. Ernaelsteen, D., and Williams, R.: Jaundice due to nitrofurantoin, Gastroenterology *41*:590, 1961.

215. Eschenbrenner, A. B., and Miller, E.: Liver necrosis and the induction of carbon tetrachloride hepatomas in strain A mice, J. Nat. Cancer Inst. *6*:325, 1946.

216. Espiritu, C. R., Kim, T. S., and Levine, R. A.: Granulomatous hepatitis associated with sulfadimethoxine hypersensitivity, J.A.M.A. *202*: 985, 1967.

217. Fairhill, L. T., and Neal, P. A.: Industrial manganese poisoning, Nat. Inst. Health Bull. No. 182, 1943.

218. Falk, A.: Cited by Davis, J. D., et al.[165]

219. Faloon, W. W., Downs, J. J., Duggan, K., and Prior, J. T.: Nitrogen and electrolyte metabolism and hepatic function and histology in patients receiving tetracycline, Am. J. Med. Sci. *233*:563, 1957.

220. Farber, E., Shull, K. H., Villa-Trevino, S., Lombardi, B., and Thomas, M.: Biochemical pathology of acute hepatic adenosine-triphosphate deficiency, Nature *203*:34, 1964.

221. Farmer, C. D., Hoffman, H. N., II, Shorter, R. G., Thurber, D. L., and Bartholomew, L. G.: Intrahepatic cholestasis associated with the ingestion of erythromycin estolate (Ilosone), Gastroenterology *45*:157, 1963.

222. Farquhar, J. D., Stokes, J., Jr., Whitlock, C. M., Jr., Bluemle, L. W., Jr., and Gambescia, J. M.: Studies on the use of Aureomycin in hepatic disease; a note on Aureomycin therapy in hepatic coma, Am. J. Med. Sci. *220*:166, 1950.

223. Farrar, G. E.: Letter, Wyeth Laboratories, Philadelphia, Pa., Oct. 24, 1961.

224. Fenech, F. F., Bannister, W. H., and Grech, J. L.: Hepatitis with biliverdinaemia in association with indomethacin therapy, Brit. Med. J. *3*:155, 1967.

225. Field, J. B., and Federman, D. D.: Sudden death in a diabetic subject during treatment with BZ-55 (carbutamide), Diabetes *6*:67, 1957.

226. Findlay, G. M.: The experimental production of biliary cirrhosis by salts of manganese, Brit. J. Exp. Path. *5*:92, 1924.

227. Finland, M., and Nichols, R. L.: Novobiocin, Antibiot. Chemother. *4*:209, 1957.

228. Fischler, G.: Über experimentelle erzeugte Lebercirrhose, Dtsch. Arch. klin. Med. *93*:427, 1908.

229. Fitzgibbon, P., and Silver, B.: Toxic necrosis of liver following use of sulfanilamide, Calif. West. Med. *50*:123, 1939.

230. Flanagan, J. F.: Toxic nephrosis and

massive heptic necrosis produced by urethan, Arch. Int. Med. *96*:277, 1955.

231. Flinn, F. B., and Jarvik, N. E.: Liver lesions caused by chlorinated naphthalene, Am. J. Hyg. 27:19, 1938.

232. Flinn, F. B., and von Glahn, W. C.: A chemical and pathologic study of the effect of copper on the liver, J. Exp. Med. *49*:5, 1929.

233. Follis, R. H., Jr.: The metabolism of tissues from anaphylactically hypersensitive animals when antigen is added in vitro, Bull. Johns Hopkins Hosp. 92:371, 1953.

234. Forbes, J. C., and Evans, E. I.: Tannic acid and liver necrosis, Surg. Gynec. Obstet. 76:612, 1943.

235. Forbes, J. C., Leach, B. E., and Outhouse, E. L.: Studies on fat metabolism and susceptibility to carbon tetrachloride, J. Pharmacol. Exp. Ther. 72:202, 1941.

236. Ford, W. W.: The toxicological constitution of *Amanita phalloides,* J. Exp. Med. 8:437, 1906.

237. ————: A new classification of mycetismus (mushroom poisoning), Trans. Ass. Am. Phys. 38:225, 1923.

238. Foss, G. L., and Simpson, S. L.: Oral methyltestosterone and jaundice, Brit. Med. J. *1*:259, 1959.

239. Franklin, M., Bean, W. B., and Hardin, R. C.: Fowler's solution as an etiologic agent in cirrhosis, Am. J. Med. Sci. *219*:589, 1950.

240. Frantz, A. G.: Fatal jaundice associated with iproniazid (Marsilid) therapy; report of a case, J.A.M.A. *167*:987, 1958.

241. Freed, S. C., Rosenbaum, E. E., and Soskin, S.: Alleged hepatotoxic action of stilbestrol, J.A.M.A. *115*:2264, 1940.

242. French, A. B., Barss, T. P., Fairlie, C. S., Bengle, A. L., Jr., Jones, C. M., Linton, R. R., and Beecher, H. K.: Metabolic effects of anesthesia in man. V. Comparison of the effects of ether and cyclopropane anesthesia on the abnormal liver, Ann. Surg. *135*:145, 1952.

243. French, A. J.: Hypersensitivity in the pathogenesis of the histopathologic changes associated with sulfonamide chemotherapy, Am. J. Path. 22:679, 1946.

244. French, A. J., and Weller, C. V.: Interstitial myocarditis following the clinical and experimental use of sulfonamide drugs, Am. J. Path. *18*:109, 1942.

245. Freund, H. A.: Clinical manifestations and studies in parenchymatous hepatitis, Ann. Int. Med. *10*:1144, 1937.

246. Frommer, J.: The pathogenesis of reticuloendothelial foam cells; effect of polyvinylpyrrolidone on the liver of the mouse, Am. J. Path. *32*:433, 1956.

247. Fulton, J. D.: Studies in chemotherapy; toxicity and therapeutic action of certain aromatic diamidines after exposure to light, Ann. Trop. Med. *37*:48, 1943.

248. Gabrilove, J. L., and Kert, M. J.: Sensitivity to thiouracil; report of 3 cases, J.A.M.A. *124*:504, 1944.

249. Gall, E. A., Altemeier, W. A., Schiff, L., Hamilton, D. L., Braunstein, H., Giuseffi, J., Jr., and Freiman, D. G.: Liver lesions following intravenous administration of polyvinyl pyrrolidone (PVP), Am. J. Clin. Path. *23*:1187, 1953.

250. Gallagher, C. H., Gupta, D. N., Judah, J. D., and Rees, K. R.: Biochemical changes in liver in acute thioacetamide intoxication, J. Path. Bact. 72:193, 1956.

251. Gallagher, T. F., Jr., Mueller, M. N., and Kappas, A.: Estrogen pharmacology. IV. Studies on the structural basis for estrogen-induced impairment of liver function, Medicine *45*:471, 1966.

252. Gardner, D. L., and Ogilvie, R. F.: The late results of injection of Thorotrast; two cases of neoplastic disease following contrast angiography, J. Path. Bact. *78*:133, 1959.

253. Gargill, S. L., and Lesses, M. F.: Toxic reactions to thiouracil; report of cases with one fatality, J.A.M.A. *127*:890, 1945.

254. Garvin, C. F.: Toxic hepatitis due to sulfanilamide, J.A.M.A. *111*:2283, 1938.

255. Garvin, J. S., and Gibbs, F. A.: Mesantoin toxicity (a clinical note), Dis. Nerv. Syst. *11*:48, 1950.

256. Gefter, W. I., Turnoff, D., and Schnabel, T. G.: Unusually high icterus index in patient with fatal hepatic necrosis following Mapharsen; case report, Am. J. Syph. 27:629, 1943.

257. Gerlei, F.: Nécrose du foie consécutive à l'empoisonnement par la thyroxine, Ann. anat. path. *10*:555, 1933.

258. Gibberd, G. F.: Delayed chloroform poisoning in obstetric practice, a clinical study, with reports on three cases, Guy's Hosp. Rep. 85:142, 1935.

259. Gibbs, F. A., Everett, G. M., and Richards, R. K.: Phenurone in epilepsy, Dis. Nerv. Syst. *10*:47, 1949.

260. Gibson, P. C., and Quinlan, J. T.: Periarteritis nodosa in thiourea therapy, Lancet 2:108, 1945.

261. Giffin, H. Z., and Allen, E. V.: Experiments with phenylhydrazine; studies on renal and hepatic function and erythropoiesis, Ann. Int. Med. 1:677, 1928.

262. Gillman, J., and Gillman, T.: Structure of the liver in fatal burns, S. Afr. J. Med. Sci. 13:169, 1948.

263. Gilmore, J. P., and Fozzard, H. A.: Liver function following thermal injury, Am. J. Physiol. 198:491, 1960.

264. Glaser, G. L., and Adams, D. A.: Agranulocytosis with promazine administration: report of three cases, Ann. Int. Med. 48:372, 1958.

265. Glynn, L. E., and Himsworth, H. P.: The intralobular circulation in acute liver injury by carbon tetrachloride, Clin. Sci. 6:235, 1948.

266. Glynn, L. E., Himsworth, H. P., and Neuberger, A.: Pathological states due to deficiency of the sulphur-containing amino acids, Brit. J. Exp. Path. 26:326, 1945.

267. Gocher, T. E. P.: Antimony intoxication, Northw. Med. 44:92, 1945.

268. Goldblatt, S.: Severe reaction to griseofulvin: sensitivity investigation, Arch. Dermat. 83:936, 1961.

269. Goldring, W., and Graef, I.: Nephrosis with uremia following transfusion with incompatible blood; report of seven cases with three deaths, Arch. Int. Med. 58:825, 1936.

270. Goldschmidt, S.. Ravdin, I. S., and Lucké, B.: Anesthesia and liver damage; protective action of oxygen against the necrotizing effect of certain anesthetics on the liver, J. Pharmacol. Exp. Ther. 59:1, 1937.

271. Goldschmidt, S., Ravdin, I. S., Lucké, B., Muller, G. P., Johnston, C. G., and Ruigh, W L.: Divinyl ether; experimental and chemical studies, J.A.M.A. 102:21, 1934.

272. Goldschmidt, S., Vars, H. M., and Ravdin, I. S.: The influence of the foodstuffs upon the susceptibility of the liver to injury by chloroform, and the probable mechanism of their action, J. Clin. Invest. 18:277, 1939.

273. Goodman, L., and Gilman, A.: The Pharmacological Basis of Therapeutics, New York, Macmillan, 2d ed., 1955.

274. Gordon, B. S., Walf, J., Krause, T., and Shai, F.: Peliosis hepatis and cholestasis following administration of norethandrolone, Am. J. Clin. Path. 33:156, 1960.

275. Gore, I., and Isaacson, N. H.: The pathology of hyperpyrexia; observations at autopsy in 17 cases of fever therapy, Am. J. Path. 25:1029, 1949.

276. Graef, I., Karnofsky, D. A., Jager, V. B., Krichesky, B., and Smith, H. W.: The clinical and pathologic effects of nitrogen and sulfur mustards in laboratory animals, Am J. Path. 24:1, 1948.

276a. Grayson, M. J., and Reilly, M. C. T.: Budd-Chiari syndrome after oral contraceptives, Brit. Med. J. 1:512, 1968.

277. Greenblatt, I. J., and Kahn, A.: Clinical toxicity studies of a monoamine oxidase inhibitor, Ann. N. Y. Acad. Sci. 80:947, 1959.

278. Greenburg, L., Mayers, M. R., Hermann, H., and Moskowitz, S.: The effects of exposure to toluene in industry, J.A.M.A. 118:573, 1942.

279. Greenburg, L., Mayers, M. R., and Smith, A. R.: The systemic effects resulting from exposure to certain chlorinated hydrocarbons, J. Indust. Hyg. Toxicol. 21:29, 1939.

280. Gregory, D. H., Zaki, G. F., Sarosi, G. A., and Carey, J. B., Jr.: Chronic cholestasis following prolonged tolbutamide administration: associated with destructive cholangitis and cholangiolitis, Arch. Path. 84:194, 1967.

281. Grier, R. S., Nash, P., and Freiman, D. G.: Skin lesions in persons exposed to beryllium compounds, J. Indust. Hyg. Toxicol. 30:228, 1948.

282. Griffith, R. S.: Eli Lilly Bulletin, August 23, 1961.

283. Guild, W. R., Young, J. V., and Merrill, J. P.: Anuria due to carbon tetrachloride intoxication, Ann. Int. Med. 48:1221, 1958.

284. Gupta, P. S., Bhargava, S. P., and Sharma, M. L.: Cited by Holtzman et al.[337]

285. Gurney, R.: Tetrachlorethane intoxication: early recognition of liver damage and means of prevention, Gatsroenterology 1:1112, 1943.

286. ———: Useful procedures in early diagnosis of liver damage following exposure to the chlorinated hydrocarbons, New Jork J. Med. 47:2566, 1947.

287. György, P.: Relation of dietary factors

to liver injury, p. 67, Tr. 6th Liver Injury Conf., New York, Macy, 1947.

288. György, P., and Goldblatt, H.: Further observations on the production and prevention of dietary hepatic injury in rats, J. Exp. Med. 89:245, 1949.

289. György, P., Seifter, J., Tomarelli, R. M., and Goldblatt, H.: Influence of dietary factors and sex on the toxicity of carbon tetrachloride in rats, J. Exp. Med. 83:449, 1946.

290. György, P., Stokes, J., Jr., and Goldblatt, H.: Antimicrobial agents in the prevention of experimental dietary injury of the liver, Trans. Ass. Am. Phys. 64:289, 1951.

291. Haber, E., and Osborne, R. K.: Icterus and febrile reactions in response to isonicotinic acid hydrazine. Report of two cases and review of the literature, New Engl. J. Med. 260:417, 1959.

292. Hadley, W. B., Kachadurian, A., and Marble, A.: Studies with chlorpropamide in diabetic patients, Ann. N. Y. Acad. Sci. 74:621, 1959.

293. Haemmerli, U. P.: Jaundice during pregnancy, with special emphasis on recurrent jaundice during pregnancy and its differential diagnosis, Acta med. scand. Suppl. 444, 1966.

294. Hageman, P. O., and Blake, F. G.: A specific febrile reaction to sulfanilamide; drug fever, J.A.M.A. 109:642, 1937.

295. Haines, S. F., Magath, T. B, and Power, M. H.: The hippuric acid test in hyperthyroidism, Ann. Int. Med. 14:1225, 1941.

296. Hall, L., and Wharton, G. K.: Chloramphenicol (Chloromycetin) in the treatment of viral hepatitis, Gastroenterology 19:69, 1951.

297. Hamff, L. H., Ferris, H. A., Evans, E. C., and Whiteman, H. W.: The effects of tolbutamide and chlorpropamide on patients exhibiting jaundice as a result of previous chlorpropamide therapy, Ann. N. Y. Acad. Sci. 74:820, 1959.

298. Hampton, J. C.: Electron microscopic study of extrahepatic biliary obstruction in the mouse, Lab. Invest. 10:502, 1961.

299. Hamre, D. M., Rake, G., McKee, C. M., and MacPhillamy, H. B.: The toxicity of penicillin as prepared for clinical use, Am. J. Med. Sci. 206:642, 1943.

300. Hamwi, G. J., Skillman, T. G., Kruger, F. A., Roush, W. H., and Freedy, L. R.: Comparative pharmacology and clinical responses to metahexamide, Ann. N. Y. Acad. Sci. 82:547, 1959.

301. Hanger, F. M., and Gutman, A. B.: Postarsphenamine jaundice apparently due to obstruction of intrahepatic biliary tract, J.A.M.A. 115:263, 1940.

302. Hanzon, V.: Liver cell secretion under normal and pathologic conditions studied by fluorescence microscopy on living rats, Acta physiol. scand. 28, Supp. 101, 1952.

303. Hardy, H. L., and Stoeckle, J. D.: Beryllium disease, J. Chron. Dis. 9:152, 1959.

304. Hargraves, M. M., Mills, S. D., and Heck, F. J.: Aplastic anemia associated with administration of chloramphenicol, J.A.M.A. 149:1293, 1952.

305. Hargreaves, T., and Lathe, G. H.: Drugs affecting biliary excretion, in McIntyre, N., and Sherlock, S. (eds.): Therapeutic Agents and the Liver, p. 9, Oxford, Blackwell Scientific Publ., 1965.

306. Harinasuta, U., and Zimmerman, H. J.: Diphenylhydantoin sodium hepatitis, J.A.M.A. 203:1015, 1968.

307. Hartfall, S. J., and Garland, H. G.: Further observations on the gold treatment of rheumatoid arthritis, Lancet 1:1459, 1936.

308. Hartley, G., Jr., and Lushbaugh, C. C.: Experimental allergic focal necrosis of the liver, Am. J. Path. 18:323, 1942.

309. Hartman, F. W., and Romence, H. L.: Liver necrosis in burns, Ann. Surg. 118:402, 1943.

310. Hashimoto, H.: The heart in the experimental hyperthyroidism with special reference to its histology, Endocrinology 5:579, 1921.

311. Hawn, C. V., and Janeway, C. A.: Histological and serological sequences in experimental hypersensitivity, J. Exp. Med. 85:571, 1947.

312. Hazlett, B. E., Taylor, H. E., and Whitelaw, D. M.: Fulminating hepatic necrosis in a patient with multiple myeloma treated with urethane. Report of a case, Blood 10:76, 1955.

313. Heaney, R. P., and Whedon, G. D.: Impairment of hepatic Bromsulphalein clearance by two 17-substituted testosterones, J. Lab. Clin. Med. 52:169, 1958.

314. Herbert, P. A., and Scaricaciottoli, T. M.: Diffuse hepatitis necrosis caused by sulfadiazine, Arch. Path. 40:94, 1945.

315. Herman, R. H., and Sullivan, B. H., Jr.:

Heatstroke and jaundice, Am. J. Med. 27:154, 1959.

316. Hersh, E. M., Wong, V. G., Henderson, E. S., and Freireich, E. J.: Hepatotoxic effects of methotrexate, Cancer 19:600, 1966.

317. Hill, K. R.: The vomiting sickness of Jamaica: a review, West. Ind. Med. J. 1:243, 1952.

318. Hill, K. R., Stephenson, C. F., and Filshie, I.: Hepatic veno-occlusive disease produced experimentally in rats by the injection of monocrotaline, Lancet 1:623, 1958.

319. Hill, R. B., Jr.: Fatal fat embolism from steroid-induced fatty liver, New Engl. J. Med. 265:318, 1961.

320. Hill, R. B., Jr., Droke, W. E., and Hays, A. P.: Hepatic lipid metabolism in cortisone-treated rat, Exp. Molec. Path. 4: 320, 1965.

321. Hill, W. R., and Damiani, C. R.: Death following exposure to DDT, New Engl. J. Med. 235:897, 1946.

322. Himsworth, H. P.: Lectures on the Liver and Its Diseases, Cambridge, Mass., Harvard, 1947.

323. Himsworth, H. P., and Glynn, L. E.: Massive hepatic necrosis and diffuse hepatic fibrosis (acute yellow atrophy and portal cirrhosis): their production by means of diet, Clin. Sci. 5:93, 1944.

324. ———: Toxipathic and trophopathic hepatitis, Lancet 1:457, 1944.

325. Himsworth, H. P., and Lindan, O.: Dietetic necrosis of the liver: the influence of α-tocopherol, Nature 163:30, 1949.

326. Hirsheimer, A.: The synthesis and excretion of hippuric acid in pregnancy, Am. J. Obstet. Gynec. 29:395, 1935.

327. Hoaken, P. C. S.: Jaundice during imipramine treatment, Canad. Med. Ass. J. 90:1367, 1964.

328. Hochman, R., and Robbins, J. J.: Jaundice due to ectylurea, New Engl. J. Med. 259:583, 1958.

329. Hoffbauer, F. W.: Clinical aspects of jaundice resulting from intrahepatic obstruction, J.A.M.A. 169:1453, 1959.

330. Hoffbauer, F. W., Nelson, O. L. N., Wagner, D. J., and Knutsen, A.: Fatal liver necrosis in two patients receiving zoxazolamine, Gastroenterology 34:1048, 1958.

331. Hoffman, J., Himes, M. B., Klein, A., Poulos, V., and Post, J.: Responses of the liver to injury. Effect of previous injury upon the healing pattern after acute carbon tetrachloride poisoning, Arch. Path. 62:96, 1956.

332. Holdsworth, C. D., Atkinson, M., Dossett, J. A., and Goldie, W.: Hepatitis caused by the newer amine-oxidase-inhibiting drugs, Lancet 2:1459, 1961.

333. Holdsworth, C. D., Atkinson, M., and Goldie, W.: Hepatitis caused by the newer amine-oxidase-inhibiting drugs, Lancet 2:621, 1961.

334. Hollister, L. E.: Allergic reactions to tranquilizing drugs, Ann. Int. Med. 49: 17, 1958.

335. Hollister, L. E., Motzenbecker, F. P., and Degan, R. O.: Withdrawal reactions from chlordiazepoxide ("Librium"), Psychopharmacologia 2:63, 1961.

336. Holoubek, J. E., Mathews, W. R., and Hollis, W. J.: Thiouracil hepatitis, Am. J. Med. 5:138, 1948.

337. Holtzman, N. A., Elliott, D. A., and Heller, R. H.: Copper intoxication: report of a case with observations on ceruloplasmin, New Engl. J. Med. 275:347, 1966.

338. Hoppe, J. O., Marcelli, G. M. A., and Tainter, M. L.: A review of the toxicity of iron compounds, Am. J. Med. Sci. 230: 558, 1955.

339. Hornung, S.: Synthalin und Leberschädigung, Klin. Wschr. 7:69, 1928.

340. Hove, E. L.: Interrelation of α-tocopherol and protein metabolism; protective effect of vitamin E and certain nitrogenous compounds against CCl_4 poisoning in rats, Arch. Biochem. 17:467, 1948.

341. Hove, E. L., and Hardin, J. O.: Effect of vitamin E and CCl_4 on fat, respiration and choline oxidase of rat livers, Proc. Soc. Exp. Biol. Med. 78:858, 1951.

342. Hsia, D. Y. Y., Dowben, R. M., Shaw, R., and Grossman, A.: Inhibition of glucuronosyl transferase by progestational agents from serum of pregnant women, Nature 187:693, 1960.

343. Hsia, D. Y., Riabov, S., and Dowben, R. M.: Inhibition of glucuronosyl transferase by steroid hormone, Arch. Biochem. 103:181, 1963.

344. Hueper, W. C.: Toxicity and detoxification of cinchophen; experimental studies, Arch. Path. 41:592, 1946.

345. Hultin, T., Arrhenius, E., Löw, H., and Magee, P. N.: Toxic liver injury. Inhibition by dimethylnitrosamine of incorporation of labelled amino acids into pro-

teins of rat liver preparations *in vitro*, J. Biochem. 76:109, 1960.

346. Hurst, E. W., and Hurst, P. E.: The aetiology of hepato-lenticular degeneration: experimental liver cirrhosis; poisoning with manganese, chloroform, phenylhydrazine, bile and guanidine, J. Path. Bact. 31:303, 1928.

347. Hurst, E. W., and Paget, G. E.: Protoporphyrin, cirrhosis and hepatoma in the livers of mice given griseofulvin, Brit. J. Dermatol. 75:105, 1963.

348. Hurt, P., and Wegmann, T.: Protrahierter Largactilikterus mit Übergang in primäre biliäre Cirrhose, Acta hepatosplen. 8:87, 1961.

349. Huseby, K. O.: Jaundice with persisting pericholangiolitic inflammation in a patient treated with chlorthiazide; report of a case, Am. J. Dig. Dis. 9:439, 1964.

350. Hustead, A. P.: The effects of Terramycin on the rat liver, Thesis, Yale University, 1952.

350a. Hutchison, J. C., Roediger, P. M., and Werblin, M.: Cholestatic jaundice following administration of quinethazone, Current Therap. Res. 6:199, 1964.

351. Hyams, D. E., Taft, E. B., Drummey, G. D., and Isselbacher, K. J.: The prevention of fatty liver by administration of adenosine triphosphate, Lab. Invest. 16:604, 1967.

352. Imhauser, K.: Harnstoffsynthese in der Fettleber, Arch. exp. Path. Pharmak. 145:120, 1929.

353. Ingold, J. A., Reed, G. B., Kaplan, H. S., and Bagshaw, M. A.: Radiation hepatitis, Am. J. Roentgenol. 93:200, 1965.

354. Isaacs, B., Macarthur, J. G., and Taylor, R. M.: Jaundice in relation to chlorpromazine therapy, Brit. Med. J. 2:1122, 1955.

355. Isselbacher, K.: Enzymatic mechanisms of hormone metabolism. II: Mechanism of hormonal glucuronide formation, Recent Progr. Hormone Res. 12:134, 1956.

356. Isselbacher, K. J., and Greenberger, N. J.: Metabolic effects of alcohol on the liver, New Engl. J. Med. 270:351, 402, 1964.

357. Jacobs, J., Greene, H., and Gendel, B. R.: Acute iron intoxication, New Engl. J. Med. 273:1124, 1965.

358. Jacobson, K. H., Wheelwright, H. J., Jr., Clem, J. H., and Shannon, R. N.: Studies on the toxicology of n-nitrosodimethylamine vapor, Arch. Industr. Health 12:617, 1955.

359. Jasper, H.: Jaundice in a patient receiving zoxazolamine (Flexin), Am. J. Gastroent. 34:419, 1960.

360. Jeliffe, D. B., Bras, G., and Mukherjee, K. L.: Veno-occlusive disease of the liver and Indian childhood cirrhosis, Arch. Dis. Child. 32:369, 1957.

361. Johnston, T. G., and Cazort, A. G.: Severe serum sickness reaction with cyanosis following Terramycin, Antibiot. Chemother. 3:481, 1953.

362. Jones, E. A., Clain, D., Clink, H. M., MacGillivray, M., and Sherlock, S.: Hepatic coma due to acute hepatic necrosis treated by exchange blood-transfusion, Lancet 2:169, 1967.

363. Jones, N. L.: Hepatitis due to phenindione sensitivity, Brit. Med. J. 2:504, 1960.

364. Jones, W. M., Margolis, G., and Stephen, C. R.: Hepatotoxicity of inhalation anesthetic drugs, Anesthesiology 19:715, 1958.

365. Jonstam, R.: Urethane-induced hepatic failure, Acta med. scand. 170:701, 1961.

366. Judah, J. D.: Effect of antihistamines on mitochondrial swelling and liver injury, Nature 185:390, 1960.

367. Judah, J. D., and Rees, K. R.: Mechanism of action of carbon tetrachloride, Fed. Proc. 18:1013, 1959.

368. Kahil, M. E., Fred, H. L., Brown, H., and Davis, J. S.: Acute fatty liver of pregnancy; report of two cases, Arch. Int. Med. 113:63, 1964.

369. Kahn, M., and Perez, V.: Jaundice associated with the administration of iproniazid. Report of nine cases, Am. J. Med. 25:898, 1958.

370. Kantrowitz, P. A., Jones, W. A., Greenberger, N. J., and Isselbacher, K.: Severe postoperative hyperbilirubinemia simulating obstructive jaundice, New Engl. J. Med. 276:591, 1967.

371. Karnofsky, D. A., Burchenal, J. J., Armistead, G. C., Southam, C. M., Bernstein, J. L., Craver, L. F., and Rhoads, C. P.: Triethylene melamine in the treatment of neoplastic disease; compound with nitrogen-mustard-like activity suitable for oral and intravenous use, Arch. Int. Med. 87:477, 1951.

372. Katz, R., Klinger, J., Silva, L., Rodriguez, J., and Ducci, H.: Serial hepatic study in patients treated with iproniazid, Ann. N. Y. Acad. Sci. 80:898, 1959.

373. Kelsey, J. R., Jr., Moyer, J. H., Brown,

W. G., and Bennett, H. D.: Chlorpromazine jaundice, Gastroenterology 29: 865, 1955.

374. Kelsey, W. M., and Scharyj, M.: Fatal hepatitis probably due to indomethacin, J.A.M.A. 199:586, 1967.

375. Kemp, J. A.: Jaundice occurring during administration of promazine, Gastroenterology 32:937, 1957.

376. Killip, T., III, and Payne, M. A.: High serum transaminase activity in heart disease. Circulatory failure and hepatic necrosis, Circulation 21:646, 1960.

377. King, W. M.: Cited by Brunson et al.[104]

378. Kintzen, W., and Silny, J.: Peliosis hepatis after administration of fluoxymesterone, Canad. Med. Ass. J. 83:160, 1960.

379. Kirk, R., and Henry, A. J.: Observations on the toxicity of stilbamidine, Ann. Trop. Med. 38:99, 1944.

380. Kirtley, W. R.: Occurrence of sensitivity and side reactions following carbutamide, Diabetes 6:72, 1957.

381. Klatskin, G.: Alcohol and its relation to liver damage, Gastroenterology 41:443, 1961.

382. ———: Mechanisms of toxic and drug-induced hepatic injury, in Fink, B. R. (ed.): Toxicity of Anesthetics, pp. 159–172, Baltimore, Williams & Wilkins, 1968.

383. ———: Unpublished data.

384. Klatskin, G., Krehl, W. A., and Conn, H. O.: The effect of alcohol on the choline requirement, J. Exp. Med. 100:605, 615, 1954.

385. Klatskin, G., and Yesner, R.: Hepatic manifestations of sarcoidosis and other granulomatous diseases, Yale J. Biol. Med. 23:207, 1950.

386. Klein, N. C., and Jeffries, G. H.: Hepatotoxicity after methoxyflurane administration, J.A.M.A. 197:1037, 1966.

387. Knick, B.: Clinical and experimental studies with chlorpropamide in diabetes mellitus, in normal individuals, and in nondiabetics with hepatic disease, Ann. N. Y. Acad. Sci. 74:858, 1959.

388. Koch-Weser, D., de la Huerga, J., and Popper, H.: Hepatic necrosis due to bromobenzene and its dependence upon available sulfur amino acids, Proc. Soc. Exp. Biol. Med. 79:196, 1952.

389. Kohlstaedt, K. G.: Propionyl erythromycin ester lauryl sulfate and jaundice, J.A.M.A. 178:89, 1961.

390. Kohn, N., and Myerson, R. M.: Cholestatic hepatitis associated with trifluoperazine, New Engl. J. Med. 264:549, 1961.

391. Kohn, N. N., and Myerson, R. M.: Xanthomatous biliary cirrhosis following chlorpromazine, Am. J. Med. 31:665, 1961.

392. Koler, R. D., and Forsgren, A. L.: Hepatoxicity due to chlorambucil; report of a case, J.A.M.A. 167:316, 1958.

393. Koletsky, S., and Gustafson, G.: Liver damage in rats from radioactive colloidal gold, Lab. Invest. 1:312, 1952.

394. Kolmer, J. A., and Lucké, B.: A study of the histologic changes produced experimentally in rabbits by arsphenamine, Arch. Derm. Syph. 3:483, 1921.

395. Kopelman, H., Scheuer, P. J., and Williams, R.: The liver lesion of the Epping jaundice, Quart. J. Med. 35:553, 1966.

396. Korn, R. J.: Discussion, Second Marsilid Symposium, May 8, 1958, Chicago, Ill.

397. Korn, R. J., Rock, W., and Zimmerman, H. J.: Studies of hepatic function in patients receiving promazine, Am. J. Med. Sci. 235:431, 1958.

398. Kory, R. C., Bradley, M. H., Watson, R. N., Callahan, R., and Peters, B. J.: A six-month evaluation of an anabolic drug, norethandrolone, in underweight persons. II: Bromsulphalein (BSP) retention and liver function, Am. J. Med. 26:243, 1959.

399. Koszalka, M. F.: Medical obstructive jaundice; report of a death due to methyltestosterone, J. Lancet 77:51, 1957.

400. Krainin, P.: Gastric ulcer with massive hemorrhage following use of phenylbutazone; report of a case, J.A.M.A. 152:31, 1953.

401. Krall, L. P., and Bradley, R. F.: Clinical evaluation of formamidinyliminourea, a new biguanidine oral blood sugar lowering compound: comparison with other hypoglycemic agents, Ann. Int. Med. 50:586, 1959.

402. Krawitt, E. L., Stein, J. H., Kirkendall, W. M., and Clifton, J. A.: Mercaptopurine hepatotoxicity in a patient with chronic active hepatitis, Arch. Int. Med. 120:729, 1967.

403. Kreek, M. J., Sleisenger, M. H., and Jeffries, G. H.: Recurrent cholestatic jaundice of pregnancy with demonstrated estrogen sensitivity, Am. J. Med. 43:795, 1967.

404. Kreek, M. J., Weser, E., Sleisenger, M. H., and Jeffries, G. H.: Idiopathic cholestasis of pregnancy: the response to challenge with the synthetic estrogen, ethinyl estradiol, New Engl. J. Med. 277: 1391, 1967.

405. Kunelis, C. T., Peters, J. L., and Edmondson, H. A.: Fatty liver of pregnancy and its relationship to tetracycline therapy, Am. J. Med. 38:359, 1965.

406. Kuzma, J. F., and Polley, T. Z.: The role of the liver in renal sulfonamide complications, Am. J. Med. Sci. 214:651, 1947.

407. Labhardt, F.: Technique, side effects and complications of Largactil therapy, Schweiz. Arch. Neurol. Psychiat. 73:338, 1954.

408. LaDue, J. S., Schenken, J. R., and Kuker, L. H.: Phosphorus poisoning; report of 16 cases with repeated liver biopsies in a recovered case, Am. J. Med. Sci. 208: 223, 1944.

409. Lamson, P. D., Gardner, G. H., Gustafson, R. K., Maire, E. D., McLean, A. J., and Wells, H. S.: The pharmacology and toxicology of carbon tetrachloride, J. Pharmacol. Exp. Ther. 22:215, 1923.

410. Lamson, P. D., and Wing, R.: Early cirrhosis of the liver produced in dogs by carbon tetrachloride, J. Pharmacol. Exp. Ther. 29:191, 1926.

411. Landsteiner, K.: Anaphylactic shock by azo dyes, J. Exp. Med. 57:633, 1933.

412. Landsteiner, K., and Jacobs, J.: Studies on the sensitization of animals with simple chemical compounds; anaphylaxis induced by arsphenamine, J. Exp. Med. 64:717, 1936.

413. Landsteiner, K., and vander Scheer, J.: Serological reactions with simple chemical compounds (precipitin reactions), J. Exp. Med. 56:399, 1932.

414. Lansing, A. M., Davis, W. M., and Brizel, H. E.: Radiation hepatitis, Arch. Surg. 96:878, 1968.

415. Large, H. L., Jr.: A case of iron intoxication caused by Roncovite with a note on striation of portal blood flow, Am. J. Clin. Path. 35:427, 1961.

416. Larsson-Cohn, U., and Stenram, U.: Liver ultrastructure and function in icteric and non-icteric women using oral contraceptive agents, Acta. med. scand. 181:257, 1967.

417. Leard, S. E., Greer, W. E. R., and Kaufman, I. C.: Hepatitis, exfoliative dermatitis and abnormal bone marrow occurring during Tridione therapy; report of case with recovery, New Engl. J. Med. 240:962, 1949.

418. Lees, A. W.: Toxicity in newly diagnosed cases of pulmonary tuberculosis treated with ethionamide, Am. Rev. Resp. Dis. 88:347, 1963.

419. Leevy, C. M., Cherrick, G. R., and Davidson, C. S.: Observations on norethandrolone-induced abnormalities in plasma decay of sulfobromophthalein and indocyanine green, J. Lab. Clin. Med. 57:918, 1961.

420. Legge, T. M.: Toxic jaundice in munition workers and troops, Brit. Med. J. 1: 155, 1917.

421. Lehman, A. J., and Hanzlik, P. J.: Cinchophen toxicosis; results of experimental subacute and chronic cinchophen poisoning, Arch. Int. Med. 52:471, 1933.

422. Lehmann, H. E., Cahn, C. H., and deVerteuil, R. L.: The treatment of depressive conditions with imipramine, Canad. Psychiat. Ass. J. 3:155, 1958.

423. Lehnherr, E. R.: Acute carbon tetrachloride poisoning; report of a case, Arch. Int. Med. 56:98, 1935.

424. Leifer, W., Chargin, L., and Hyman, H. T.: Massive dose arsenotherapy of early syphilis by intravenous drip method: recapitulation of the data (1933 to 1941), J.A.M.A. 117:1154, 1941.

425. Lennox, W. G.: Tridione in the treatment of epilepsy, J.A.M.A. 134:138, 1947.

426. Lenzer, A. R., Lockie, L. M., and Becker, C. F.: Acute yellow atrophy following cinchophen administration; report of case, New Engl. J. Med. 236:500, 1947.

427. Lepper, M. H., Dowling, H. F., Robinson, J. A., Stone, T. E., Brickhouse, R. L., Caldwell, E. R., Jr., and Whelton, R. L.: Symposium on antibiotics; studies on hypersensitivity to penicillin; incidence of reactions in 1303 patients, J. Clin. Invest. 28:826, 1949.

428. Lepper, M. H., Wolfe, C. K., Zimmerman, H. J., Caldwell, E. R., Jr., Spies, H. W., and Dowling, H. F.: Effect of large doses of Aureomycin on human liver, Arch. Int. Med. 88:271, 1951.

429. Lepper, M. H., Zimmerman, H. J., Carroll, G., Caldwell, E. R., Jr., Spies, H. W., Wolfe, C. K., and Dowling, H. F.:

Effects of large doses of Aureomycin, Terramycin and chloramphenicol on livers of mice and dogs, Arch. Int. Med. 88:284, 1951

430. Levi, E.: Über die Ursache der Lebercirrhose bei Polycythämie Leberschädigung durch Phenylhydrazintherapie, Z. klin. Med. 100:777, 1924.

431. Levine, R. A., Briggs, G. W., and Lowell, D. M.: Chronic chlorpromazine cholangiolitic hepatitis; report of a case with immunofluorescent studies, Gastroenterology 50:665, 1966.

432. Levy, R. W., Simmons, D. J., and Aaronson, S.: Fatal hepatorenal syndrome associated with phenurone therapy, New Engl. J. Med. 242:933, 1950.

433. Lewis, C. N., Putnam, L. E., Hendricks, F. D., Kerlan, I., and Welch, H.: Chloramphenicol (Chloromycetin) in relation to blood dyscrasias with observations on other drugs, Antibiot. Chemother. 2:601, 1952.

434. Lewis, G. M., and Sawicky, H. H.: Contact dermatitis from chlorpromazine. Report of two cases, J.A.M.A. 157:909, 1955.

435. Lichtenstein, M. R., and Cannemeyer, W.: Severe para-aminosalicylic acid hypersensitivity simulating mononucleosis or hepatitis, J.A.M.A. 152:606, 1953.

436. Lichtman, S. S.: Toxic hepatitis ascribed to the use of cinchophen; illustration of the analgesic effect of jaundice in long-standing rheumatoid arthritis, J. Mt. Sinai Hosp. 6:199, 1939.

437. ———: Diseases of the Liver, Gallbladder and Bile Ducts, ed. 2, Philadelphia, Lea & Febiger, 1949.

438. Lieber, C. S., and Schmid, R.: The effect of ethanol on fatty acid metabolism; stimulation of fatty acid synthesis in vitro, J. Clin. Invest. 40:394, 1961.

439. Liebow, A. A., Warren, S., and DeCoursey, E.: Pathology of atomic bomb casualties, Am. J. Path. 25:853, 1949.

440. Lindenbaum, J., and Leifer, E.: Hepatic necrosis associated with halothane anesthesia, New Engl. J. Med. 268:525, 1963.

441. Lindsay, S., and Skahen, R.: Jaundice due to chlorpromazine (Thorazine) therapy. A histological study of the hepatic lesions in five patients, Arch. Path. 61:84, 1956.

442. Lischner, M. W., MacNabb, G. M., and Galambos, J. T.: Fatal hepatic necrosis following surgery: Possible relation to methoxyflurane anesthesia, Arch. Int. Med. 120:725, 1967.

443. Little, D. M., Barbour, C. M., and Given, J. B.: The effects of fluothane, cyclopropane, and ether anesthesias on liver function, Surg. Gynec. Obstet. 107:712, 1958.

444. Livingood, C. S., Brannen, M., Orders, R. L., Kopstein, J. B., and Rebuck, J. W.: Effect of prolonged griseofulvin administration on liver, hematopoietic system, and the kidney, Arch. Dermat. 81:760, 1960.

445. Livingood, C. S., and Dieuaide, F. R.: Untoward reactions attributable to atabrine, J.A.M.A. 129:1091, 1945.

446. Livingston, H. J., and Livingston, S. F.: Agranulocytosis and hepatocellular jaundice; toxic reactions following propylthiouracil therapy, J.A.M.A. 135:422, 1947.

447. Livingston, K. E., and McCallion, D. J.: The immediate effects of severe local X irradiation on the liver of the hamster, Canad. J. Med. Sci. 30:571, 1952.

448. Livingstone-Learmonth, A., and Cunningham, B. M.: Observations on the effects of tri-nitrotoluene on women workers, Lancet 2:261, 1916.

449. Lloyd-Thomas, H. G. L., and Sherlock, S.: Testosterone therapy for the pruritus of obstructive jaundice, Brit. Med. J. 2:1289, 1952.

450. Loewenthal, L. J. A., MacKay, W. A., and Lowe, E. C.: Two cases of acute yellow atrophy of the liver following administration of Atophan, Brit. Med. J. 1:592, 1928.

451. Lomas, J., Boardman, R. H., and Markowe, M.: Complications of chlorpromazine therapy in 800 mental-hospital patients, Lancet 1:1144, 1955.

452. Long, P. H., Haviland, J. W., Edwards, L. B., and Bliss, E. A.: The toxic manifestations of sulfanilamide and its derivatives with reference to their importance in the course of therapy, J.A.M.A. 115:364, 1940.

453. Longcope, W. T.: Cirrhosis of the liver produced by chronic protein intoxication, Trans. Ass. Am. Phys. 28:497, 1913.

454. ———: Serum sickness and analogous reactions from certain drugs, particularly the sulfonamides, Medicine 22:251, 1943.

455. Lowenstein, L., and Ballew, D. H.: Fatal acute hemolytic anemia, thrombocyto-

penic purpura, nephrosis and hepatitis resulting from ingestion of a compound containing apiol, Canad. Med. Ass. J. 78:195, 1958.

456. Lubell, D. L.: Fatal hepatic necrosis associated with zoxazolamine therapy, N. Y. State J. Med. 62:3807, 1962.

457. Luongo, M. A., and Bjornson, S. S.: The liver in ferrous sulfate poisoning: a report of three fatal cases in children and an experimental study, New Engl. J. Med. 251:995, 1954.

458. MacBryde, C. M., Castrodale, D., Loeffel, E., and Freedman, H.: The synthetic estrogen diethylstilbestrol; clinical and experimental studies, J.A.M.A. 117:1240, 1941.

459. MacBryde, C. M., and Taussig, B. L.: Functional changes in liver, heart and muscles, and loss of dextrose tolerance resulting from dinitrophenol, J.A.M.A. 105:13, 1935.

460. MacCallum, F. O.: Transmission of arsenotherapy jaundice by blood: failure of faeces and nasopharyngeal washings, Lancet 1:342, 1945.

461. McCloskey, J. F.: Protective action of chlorophyll on hepatic necrosis in rats, Am. J. Clin. Path. 21:723, 1951.

462. McCloskey, J. F., and McGehee, E. H.: Effect of subcutaneous and intraoral administration of carbon tetrachloride on the liver of the rat, Arch. Path. 49:200, 1950.

463. McCormick, R. V.: Periarteritis occurring during propylthiouracil therapy, J.A.M.A. 144:1453, 1950.

464. McDermott, W., Ormond, L., Muschenheim, C., Deuschle, K., McCune, R. M., Jr., and Tompsett, R.: Pyraxinamide-isoniazid in tuberculosis, Am. Rev. Tuberc. 69:319, 1954.

465. MacDonald, R. A., and Pechet, G. S.: Experimental hemochromatosis in rats, Am. J. Path. 46:85, 1965.

466. MacDonald, R. M.: Toxic hepatitis in fever therapy, Canad. Med, Ass. 51:445, 1944.

467. McFarland, R. B.: Fatal drug reaction associated with prochlorperazine (Compazine), Am. J. Clin. Path. 40:284, 1963.

468. McGeachy, T. E., and Bloomer, W. E.: The phenobarbital sensitivity syndrome, Am. J. Med. 14:600, 1953.

469. McIlvane, S. K., and MacCarthy, J. D.: Hepatitis in association with prolonged 6-mercaptopurine therapy, Blood 14:80, 1959.

470. McIver, M. A.: Liver changes in hyperthyroidism, Surgery 12:654, 1942.

471. ———: Deleterious effects of anoxia on the liver of the hyperthyroid animal, Arch. Surg. 46:171, 1943.

472. McIver, M. A., and Winter, E. A.: Further studies on increased susceptibility to chloroform poisoning produced in the albino rat by injection of crystalline thyroxin, J. Clin. Invest. 21:191, 1942.

473. McKendrick, G. D. W.: Toxic hepatitis from para-aminosalicylic acid, Lancet 2: 668, 1951.

474. McLean, S., MacDonald, A., and Sullivan, R. C.: Acute phosphorus poisoning from the ingestion of roach paste; report of a fatal case in a child, J.A.M.A. 93: 1789, 1929.

475. Mach, B., Field, R. A., and Taft, E. B.: Metahexamide jaundice; report of a case, New Engl. J. Med. 261:438, 1959.

476. Mackay, I. R., Weiden, S., and Ungar, B.: Treatment of active chronic hepatitis and lupoid hepatitis with 6-mercaptopurine and azothioprine, Lancet 1:899, 1964.

477. Mackay, R. P., and Gottstein, W. K.: Aplastic anemia and agranulocytosis following Tridione; a fatal case, J.A.M.A. 132:13, 1946.

478. Maddock, W. G., Pedersen, S., and Coller, F. A.: Studies of the blood chemistry in thyroid crisis, J.A.M.A. 109:2130, 1937.

479. Madhaven, T. V., Suryanarayana Rao, K., and Tulpule, P. G.: Effect of dietary protein level on susceptibility of monkeys to aflatoxin liver injury, Indian J. Med. Res. 53:984, 1965.

480. Magee, P. N.: Toxic liver injury. The metabolism of dimethylnitrosamine, Biochem. J. 64:676, 1956.

481. Magee, P. N., and Barnes, J. M.: Induction of kidney tumours in the rat with dimethylnitrosamine (N-nitrosodimethylamine), J. Path. Bact. 84:19, 1962.

482. Magee, P. N., and Lee, K. Y.: Experimental toxic liver injury by some nitrosamines, Ann. N. Y. Acad. Sci. 104:916, 1963.

483. Makous, N., and Vander Veer, J. B.: Severe drug sensitivity reaction to phenindione (phenylindandione), J.A.M.A. 155:739, 1954.

484. Malitz, S., Wilkens, B., and Esecover,

H.: Preliminary evaluation of Tofranil in a combined in-patient and out-patient setting, Canad. Phychiat. Ass. J. 4:S152, 1959.

485. Mallory, F. B.: Phosphorus and alcoholic cirrhosis, Am. J. Path. 9:557, 1933.

486. Mallory, F. B., and Parker, F., Jr.: Experimental copper poisoning, Am. J. Path. 7:351, 1931.

487. Mandelbaum, H., and Kane, L. J.: Dilantin sodium poisoning report of a case with dermatitis exfoliativa, pyrexia and hepatic and splenic enlargement, Arch. Neurol. Psychiat. 45:769, 1941.

488. Margolis, H. M., and Caplan, P. S.: BAL in treatment of toxicity from gold, Ann. Int. Med. 27:353, 1947.

489. Marquardt, G. H., Fisher, C. I., Levy, P., and Dowben, R. M.: Effect of anabolic steroids on liver function tests and creatine excretion, J.A.M.A. 175:851, 1961.

490. Martin, G. H., Bunting, C. H., and Lovenhart, A. S.: The morphological changes in the tissues of the rabbit as a result of reduced oxidations, J. Pharmacol. Exp. Ther. 8:112, 1916.

491. Martinez-Lopez, J. I., Greenberg, S. E., and Kling, R. R.: Drug-induced hepatic injury during methimazole therapy, Gastroenterology 43:84, 1962.

492. Martland, H. S.: Tri-nitro-toluene poisoning, J.A.M.A. 68:835, 1917.

493. Matzger, E.: Can sensitivity to dinitrophenol be determined by skin tests?, J.A.M.A. 103:253, 1934.

494. Mauer, E. F.: The toxic effects of phenylbutazone (Butazolidin); review of the literature and report of the twenty-third death following its use, New Engl. J. Med. 253:404, 1955.

495. Mazer, C., Israel, S. L., and Ravetz, E.: The synthetic estrogen stilbestrol; experimental and clinical evaluation, J.A.M.A. 116:675, 1941.

496. Meacham, G. C., Tillotson, F. W., and Heinle, R. W.: Liver damage after prolonged urethane therapy, Am. J. Clin. Path. 22:22, 1952.

497. Mechanic, R. C., and Meyers, L.: Chlorpromazine-type cholangitis; report of a case occurring after the administration of prochlorperazine, New Engl. J. Med. 259:778, 1958.

498. Medical Letter on Drugs and Therapeutics, Oxacillin 4:29, 1962.

499. ———: Methyldopa 6:47, 1964.

499a. Medical Research Council: Risk of thromboembolic disease in women taking oral contraceptives: a preliminary communication to the Medical Research Council by a subcommittee, Brit. Med. J. 2:355, 1967.

500. Melrose, A. G., and Roy, J. R.: Late prognosis of chorpromazine jaundice, Brit. Med. J. 1:818, 1959.

501. Menten, M. L., and Andersch, M. A.: Hepatic damage associated with sulfonamide therapy in infants and children; morphologic pathology, Ann. Int. Med. 19:609, 1943.

502. Merritt, A. D., and Fetter, B. F.: Toxic hepatic necrosis (hepatitis) due to isoniazid; report of a case with cirrhosis and death due to hemorrhage from esophageal varices, Ann. Int. Med. 50:804, 1959.

503. Messinger, W. J., and Hawkins, W. B.: Arsphenamine liver injury modified by diet. Protein and carbohydrate protective but fat injurious, Am. J. Med. Sci. 199:216, 1940.

504. Meyer, R. R.: Effect of iopanoic acid on the sulfobromophthalein test, J.A.M.A. 194:343, 1965.

505. Miller, J. M., Long, P. H., and Schoenbach, E. B.: Successful treatment of actinomycosis with "stilbamidine," J.A.M.A. 150:35, 1952.

506. Miller, L. L., Ross, J. F., and Whipple, G. H.: Methionine and cystine, specific protein factors preventing chloroform liver injury in protein depleted dogs, Am. J. Med. Sci. 200:739, 1940.

507. Miller, L. L., and Whipple, G. H.: Liver injury, liver protection, and sulfur metabolism; methionine protects against chloroform liver injury even when given after anesthesia, J. Exp. Med. 76:421, 1942.

508. Miller, S. E. P., MacSween, R. N. M., Glen, A. C. A., Tribedi, K., and Moore, F. M. L.: Experimental studies on the hepatic effects of tetracycline, Brit. J. Exp. Path. 18:51, 1967.

509. Minot, G. R., and Smith, L. W.: The blood in tetrachlorethane poisoning, Arch. Int. Med. 28:687, 1921.

510. Mistilis, S. P., Skyring, A. P., and Goulston, J. M.: Effect of long-term tetracycline therapy, steroid therapy and colectomy in pericholangitis associated with ulcerative colitis, Aust. Ann. Med. 14:286, 1965.

511. Mitchell, P. H., Sykes, P., and King, A.: Effects of "Pacatal" on symptoms in chronic psychotic female in-patients, Brit. Med. J. *1*:204, 1957.

512. Molitor, H., Graessle, O. E., Kuna, S., Mushett, C. W., and Silber, R. H.: Some toxicological and pharmacological properties of streptomycin, J. Pharmacol. Exp. Ther. *86*:151, 1946.

513. Monroe, L. S., and Longmore W. J.: Inhibition of sulfobromophtnalein (BSP) conjugation with gluatathione by iopanoic acid (Telepaque), Gastroenterology *50*:396, 1966.

514. Moon, H. D.: The pathology of fatal carbon tetrachloride poisoning with special reference to the histogenesis of the hepatic and renal lesions, Am. J. Path. *26*:1041, 1950.

515. Moore, B.: Toxic jaundice in munition workers and troops, Brit. Med. J. *1*:155, 1917.

516. Moore, K. E., and Brody, T. M.: Functional changes in liver mitochondria following in situ anoxia, Am. J. Physiol. *198*:677, 1960.

517. More, R. H., McMillan, G. C., and Duff, G. L.: The pathology of sulfonamide allergy in man, Am. J. Path. *22*:703, 1946.

518. Morrissey, J. F., and Rubin, R. C.: The detection of pyrazinamide-induced liver damage by serum enzyme determinations, Ann. Rev. Resp. Dis. *80*:855, 1959.

519. Moschcowitz, E.: Pathogenesis of cirrhosis of the liver occurring in patients with diffuse toxic goitre, Arch. Int. Med. *78*:497, 1946.

520. Moulding, T. S., Jr., and Goldstein, S.: Hepatotoxicity due to ethionamide, Am. Rev. Resp. Dis. *86*:252, 1962.

521. Mount, F. W., Wunderlich, G. S., Murray, F. J., and Ferebee, S. H.: Hepatic toxicity of pyrazinamide used with isoniazid in tuberculous patients. A United States Public Health Service Tuberculosis Therapy Trial, Am. Rev. Resp. Dis. *80*:371, 1959.

522. Movitt, E. R., Gersth, B., and Davis, A. E.: Needle liver biopsy in thyrotoxicosis, Arch. Intern. Med. *91*:729, 1953.

523. Moxon, A. L., and Rhian, M.: Selenium poisoning, Physiol. Rev. *23*:305, 1943.

524. Mueller, M. N., and Kappas, A.: Impairment of hepatic excretion of sulfobromophthalein (BSP) by natural estrogens, Trans. Ass. Am. Phys. *77*:248, 1964.

525. ———: Estrogen pharmacology. I. The influence of estradiol and estriol on hepatic disposal of sulfobromophthalein (BSP) in man, J. Clin. Invest. *43*:1905, 1964.

526. Murray, J. E., Merrill, J. P., Harrison, J. H., Wilson, R. E., and Dammin, G. J.: Prolonged survival of human-kidney homografts by immunosuppressive drug therapy, New Engl. J. Med. *268*:1315, 1963.

527. Muschenheim, C., McDermott, W., McCune, R., Deuschle, K., Ormond, L., and Tompsett, R.: Pyrazinamide-isoniazid in tuberculosis. III. Results in 58 patients with pulmonary lesions one year after the start of therapy, Am. Rev. Tuberc. *70*:743, 1954.

528. Myers, J. D.: Personal communication, Dec., 1961.

529. Myers, J. D., Olson, R. E., Lewis, J. H., and Moran, J. T.: Xanthomatous biliary cirrhosis following chlorpromazine, with observations indicating overproduction of cholesterol, hyperprothrombinemia, and the development of portal hypertension, Trans. Ass. Phyns *70*:243, 1957.

530. Myren, J.: Injury of liver tissue in mice after single injections of carbon tetrachloride, Acta path. microbiol, scand., Supp. 116, 1956.

531. Napier, L. E.: The pentavalent compounds of antimony in the treatment of kala-azar; aminostiburea; an analysis of the treatment in 52 cases, Indian J. Med. Res. *16*:141, 1928.

532. ———: The pentavalent compounds of antimony in the treatment of kala-azar; urea-stibamine; an analysis of the treatment in 70 consecutive cases, Indian J. Med. Res. *16*:901, 1929.

533. Nelson, A. A., Draize, J. H., Woodward, G., Fitzhugh, O. G., Smith, R. B., Jr., and Calvery, H. O.: Histopathological changes following administration of DDT to several species of animals, Pub. Health Rep. *59*:1009, 1944.

534. Nelson, A. A., Fitzhugh, O. G., and Calvery, H. O.: Liver tumours following cirrhosis caused by selenium in rats, Cancer Res. *3*:230, 1943.

535. Nelson, R. S.: Hepatitis due to carbarsone; report of two cases, J.A.M.A. *160*:764, 1956.

536. Nettleship, A., and Fink, W. J.: Neo-

plasms of the liver following injection of Thorotrast, Am. J. Clin. Path. 35:422, 1961.

537. Nosslin, B.: Bromsulphalein retention and jaundice due to unconjugated bilirubin following treatment with male fern extract, Scand. J. Clin. Lab. Invest. 15, Suppl. 69:206, 1963.

538. Oberman, J. W., and Gilbert, E. F.: The toxicity of 2-hydroxystilbamidine: probable fatal toxic reaction during treatment of blastomycosis, Ann. Int. Med. 48: 1401, 1958.

539. Ockner, R. K., and Davidson, C. S.: Hepatic effects of oral contraceptives, New Engl. J. Med. 276:331, 1967.

540. O'Donovan, C. J. O.: Toxicity of Euglycin (metahexamide), Circular letter from the Upjohn Co., Kalamazoo, Mich., May 13, 1959.

541. Ohler, R. L., Houghton, J. D., and Moloney, W. C.: Urethane toxicity; report of a case of hepatic necrosis apparently due to urethane, New Engl. J. Med. 243:984, 1950.

542. Opie, E. L.: On the relation of combined intoxication and bacterial infection to necrosis of the liver, acute yellow atrophy and cirrhosis, J. Exp. Med. 12:367, 1910.

543. Opie, E. L., and Alford, L. B.: The influence of diet upon necrosis caused by hepatic and renal poisons. I. Diet and hepatic lesions of chloroform, phosphorus, or alcohol, J. Exp. Med. 21:1, 1915.

544. Orellana-Alcalde, J. M., and Dominguez, J. P.: Jaundice and oral contraceptive drugs, Lancet 2:1278, 1966.

545. O'Rourke, R. A., and Eckert, G. E.: Methotrexate-induced hepatic injury in an adult: a case report, Arch. Int. Med. 113:191, 1964.

546. Orr, C. R., Popoff, G. D., Rosedale, R. S., and Stephenson, B. R.: A study of the effect of thorium dioxide sol injected in rabbits, Radiology 30:370, 1938.

547. Ortega, P., Hayes, W. J., Jr., and Durham, W. F.: Pathologic changes in the liver of rats after feeding low levels of various insecticides, Arch. Path. 64:614, 1957.

548. Paine, D.: Allergic reactions to para-aminosalicylic acid; report of six cases, Arch. Int. Med. 96:768, 1955.

549. ———: Fatal hepatic necrosis associated with aminosalicylic acid; review

of the literature and report of a case, J.A.M.A. 167:285, 1958.

550. Palmer, W. L., Woodall, P. S., and Wang, K. C.: Cinchophen and toxic necrosis of the liver; a survey of the problem, Trans. Am. Phys. 51:381, 1936.

551. Panton, P. N.: Toxic jaundice in munition workers and troops, Brit. Med. J. 1: 157, 1917.

552. Pare, C. M. B., and Sandler, M.: Acute hepatic necrosis following iproniazid therapy. Value of glutamic-oxaloacetic transaminase estimation in early detection, Lancet 1:282, 1959.

553. Parry, G. R., and West, G. H., Jr.: Cited by Marquardt et al.[489]

554. Parsons, W. B., Jr.: Studies of nicotinic acid use in hypercholesteremia: changes in hepatic function, carbohydrate tolerance and uric acid metabolism, Arch. Int. Med. 107:653, 1961.

555. ———: Use of nicotinic acid to reduce serum lipid levels, J. Am. Geriat. Soc. 10: 850, 1962.

556. Parsons, W. B., Jr., and Flinn, J. H.: Reduction of serum cholesterol levels and beta-lipoprotein cholesterol levels by nicotinic acid, Arch. Int. Med. 103:783, 1959.

557. Paschkis, K. E., Cantarow, A., Rakoff, A. E., Walkling, A. A., and Tourish, W. J.: Thiourea and thiouracil in treatment of thyrotoxicosis, J. Clin. Endocr. 4:179, 1944.

558. Patwardhan, M. V., Ramalingaswami, V., Suramachari, S., and Patwardhan, V. N.: Nutritional factors in toxic liver injury. I. Biochemical and histological study of liver injury produced by carbon tetrachloride in normal rats, Indian J. Med. Sci. 7:533, 1953.

559. Pearce, R. M.: Experimental cirrhosis of the liver, J. Exp. Med. 8:64, 1906.

560. Permar, H. H., and Goehring, H. D.: Cinchophen poisoning; report of two cases with histologic observations, Arch. Int. Med. 52:398, 1933.

561. Pernod, J.: Hepatic tolerance of ethionamide, Am. Rev. Resp. Dis. 92:39, 1965.

562. Person, D. A., Sargent, T., and Isaac, E.: Thorotrast-induced carcinoma of the liver; a case report including results of whole body counting, Arch. Surg. 88: 503, 1964.

563. Peters, J. H., Randall, A. H., Jr., Mendeloff, J., Peace, R., Coberly, J. C., and Hurley, M. B.: Jaundice during adminis-

tration of methylestrenolone, J. Clin. Endocr. *18*:114, 1958.

564. Peters, R. A., Thompson, R. H. S., King, A. J., Williams, D. I., and Nicol, C. S.: The treatment of post-arsphenamine jaundice with sulfur-containing amino-acids, Quart. J. Med. *14*:35, 1945.

565. Peters, R. L., Edmondson, H. A., Mikkelsen, W. P., and Tatter, D.: Tetracycline-induced fatty liver in nonpregnant patients: a report of six cases, Am. J. Surg. *113*:622, 1967.

566. Peterson, O. L., Deutsch, E., and Finland, M.: Therapy with sulfonamide compounds for patients with damage to the liver, Arch. Int. Med. *72*:594, 1943.

567. Phillips, G. B., Schwartz, R., Gabuzda, G. J., Jr., and Davidson, C. S.: The syndrome of impending hepatic coma in patients with cirrhosis of the liver given certain nitrogenous compounds, New Engl. J. Med. *247*:239, 1952.

568. Phillips, S., Larkin, J. C., Jr., Litzenburger, W. L., Horton, G. E., and Haimsohn, J. S.: Observations on pyrazinamide (aldinamide) in pulmonary tuberculosis, Am. Rev. Tuberc. *69*:443, 1954.

569. Phillips, S., and Tashman, H.: Ethionamide jaundice, Am. Rev. Resp. Dis. *87*:896, 1963.

570. Pichmayer, I., and Stich, W.: Der bilirubinostatische Ikterus, eine neue Ikterusform beim Zusammentreffen von Operation, Narkose und Bluttransfusion, Klin. Wschr. *40*:665, 1962.

571. Piper, J., and Poulsen, E.: Liver biopsy in thyrotoxicosis, Acta med. scand. *127*:439, 1947.

572. Plaa, G. L., and Larson, R. E.: Role of body temperature in the protection afforded against CCl_4 hepatotoxicity by cervical cordotomy, Gastroenterology *46*:302, 1964.

573. Pletcher, W. D., Brody, G. L., and Meyers, M. C.: Hemochromatosis following prolonged iron therapy in a patient with hereditary nonspherocytic hemolytic anemia, Am. J. Med. Sci. *246*:27, 1963.

574. Poindexter, C. A., and Greene, C. H.: Toxic cirrhosis of the liver; report of a case due to long continued exposure to carbon tetrachloride, J.A.M.A. *102*:2015, 1934.

575. Pollack, L. J., Finkelman, I., and Arieff,

A. J.: Toxicity of pyridine in man, Arch. Int. Med. *71*:95, 1943.

576. Poole, F. E., and Haining, R. B.: Sudden death from dinitrophenol poisoning, report of a case with autopsy, J.A.M.A. *102*:1141, 1934.

577. Popper, H.: Pathologic findings in jaundice associated with iproniazid therapy, J.A.M.A. *168*:2235, 1958.

578. ———: Hepatic injury in patients who have received iproniazid, Ann. N. Y. Acad. Sci. *80*:928, 1959.

579. Popper, H., Dubin, A., Bruce, C., Kent, G., and Kushner, D.: Effect of chlorpromazine upon experimental hepatic injury, J. Lab. Clin. Med. *49*:767, 1957.

580. Popper, H., and Franklin, M.: Diagnosis of hepatitis by histologic and functional laboratory means, J.A.M.A. *137*:230, 1948.

581. Popper, H., Koch-Weser, D., and Szanto, P. B.: Protective effect of vitamin B_{12} upon hepatic injury produced by carbon tetrachloride, Proc. Soc. Exp. Biol. Med. *71*:688, 1949.

582. Popper, H., Rubin, E., Gardiol, D., Schaffner, F., and Paronetto, R.: Drug-induced liver disease: a penalty for progress, Arch. Int. Med. *115*:128, 1965.

583. Portal, R. W., and Emanuel, R. W.: Phenindione hepatitis complicating anticoagulant therapy, Brit. Med. J. *2*:1318, 1961.

584. Powell, W. J., Jr., Koch-Weser, J., and Williams, R. A.: Lethal hepatic necrosis after therapy with imipramine and desipramine, J.A.M.A. *206*:642, 1968.

585. Preheim, D. V., and Peck, M. E.: Agranulocytosis due to amithiazone therapy, Am. Rev. Tuberc. *65*:339, 1952.

586. Quick, A. J.: The probable allergic nature of cinchophen poisoning, with special reference to the Arthus phenomenon and with precautions to be followed in cinchophen therapy, Am. J. Med. Sci. *187*:115, 1934.

587. Rabinovitch, J., and Snitkoff, M. C.: Acute exfoliative dermatitis and death following penicillin therapy, J.A.M.A. *138*:496, 1948.

588. Radke, R. A., and Baroody, W. G.: Carbarsone toxicity: a review of the literature and report of 45 cases, Ann. Int. Med. *47*:418, 1957.

589. Ramsay, I. D.: Carbamazepine-induced jaundice, Brit. Med. J. *4*:155, 1967.

590. Randolph, H., and Joseph, S.: Toxic

hepatitis with jaundice occurring in a patient treated with isoniazid, J.A.M.A. *152*:38, 1953.

591. Ratnoff, O., and Mirick, G.: Influence of sex upon lethal effects of hepatotoxic alkaloid, monocrotaline, Bull. Johns Hopkins Hosp. *84*:507, 1949.

592. Ravdin, I. S., Eliason, E. L., Coates, G. M., Holloway, T. B., Ferguson, L. K., Gill, A. B., and Cooke, T. J.: Divinyl ether; report of its further use as a general anaesthetic, J.A.M.A. *108*:1163, 1937.

593. Rawls, W. B., Gruskin, B. J., Ressa, A. A., and Gordon, A. S.: The relation between skin sensitivity, liver function, leucopenic index, and toxic effects from cinchophen, J. Lab. Clin. Med. *24*:597, 1939.

594. Read, A. E., Harrison, C. V., and Sherlock, S.: Chronic chlorpromazine jaundice, with particular reference to its relationship to primary biliary cirrhosis, Am. J. Med. *31*:249, 1961.

595. Rebouças, G., and Isselbacher, K. J.: Studies on the pathogenesis of the ethanol-induced fatty liver. I. Synthesis and oxidation of fatty acids by the liver, J. Clin. Invest. *40*:1355, 1961.

596. Recknagel, R. O.: Depression of glucose-6-phosphatase activity in carbon tetrachloride fatty liver, Fed. Proc. *19*:137, 1960.

597. Recknagel, R. O., and Ghoshal, A. K.: Lipoperoxidation as a vector in carbon tetrachloride hepatotoxicity, Lab. Invest. *15*:132, 1966.

598. Recknagel, R. O., and Litteria, M.: Biochemical changes in carbon tetrachloride fatty liver; concentration of carbon tetrachloride in liver and blood, Am. J. Path. *36*:521, 1960.

599. Recknagel, R. O., and Lombardi, B.: Cited by Recknagel et al.[600]

600. Recknagel, R. O., Lombardi, B., and Schotz, M. C.: A new insight into pathogenesis of carbon tetrachloride fat infiltration, Proc. Soc. Exp. Biol. Med. *104*:608, 1960.

601. Redeker, A. G., Sterline, R. E., and Bronow, R. S.: Effect of griseofulvin in acute intermittent porphyria, J.A.M.A. *188*:466, 1964.

602. Reed, G. B., Jr., and Cox, A. J., Jr.: The human liver after radiation injury, a form of veno-occlusive disease, Am. J. Path. *48*:597, 1966.

603. Reichel, J., Goldberg, S. B., Ellenberg, M., and Schaffner, F.: Intrahepatic cholestasis following administration of chlorpropamide; report of a case with electron miscroscopic observations, Am. J. Med. *28*:654, 1960.

604. Reichle, H. S.: Toxic cirrhosis of liver due to cinchophen, Arch. Int. Med. *44*:281, 1929.

605. ———: Cinchophen poisoning: an attempt to produce toxic cirrhosis of the liver in rats, Arch. Int. Med. *49*:215, 1932.

606. Reinhart, M. J., Benson, R. M., Kwass, S. K., and Storey, W. F.: Suggestive evidence of hepatotoxicity concomitant with thioridazine hydrochloride use, J.A.M.A. *197*:767, 1966.

607. Report to Council on Pharmacy & Chemistry, A.M.A.: The effects of streptomycin on tuberculosis in man; preliminary statement, J.A.M.A. *135*:634, 1947.

608. Reye, R. D. K., Morgan, G., and Baral, J.: Encephalopathy and fatty degeneration of the viscera: a disease entity of childhood, Lancet *2*:749, 1963.

609. Reynolds, E.: Isoniazid jaundice and its relationship to iproniazid jaundice, Tubercle *43*:375, 1962.

610. Reynolds, E. S., Schlant, R. C., Gonick, H. C., and Dammin, G. J.: Fatal massive necrosis of the liver as a manifestation of hypersensitivity to probenecid, New Engl. J. Med. *256*:592, 1957.

611. Rheingold, J. J., and Spurling, C. L.: Chloramphenicol and aplastic anemia, J.A.M.A. *149*:1301, 1952.

612. Rich, A. R.: The role of hypersensitivity in periarteritis nodosa as indicated by seven cases developing during serum sickness and sulfonamide therapy, Bull. Johns Hopkins Hosp. *71*:123, 1942.

613. ———: The Pathogenesis of Tuberculosis, Springfield, Ill., Thomas, 1944.

614. ———: Hypersensitivity to iodine as a cause of periarteritis nodosa, Bull. Johns Hopkins Hosp. *77*:43, 1945.

615. Rich, A. R., and Gregory, J. E.: The experimental demonstration that periarteritis nodosa is a manifestation of hypersensitivity, Bull. Johns Hopkins Hosp. *72*:65, 1943.

616. Richards, R. K.: Cited by Lennox, W. G.[425]

617. Richards, R. K., and Everett, G. M.: Cited by Tyler and King.[753]

618. Rimington, C., Heikel, T., Knight, B. C.,

Williams, E. J., and Ritchie, H. D.: Studies on biliary excretion in the rabbit: effect of icterogenin on bile flow and the excretion of bilirubin, phylloerythrin, coproporphyrin, alkaline phosphatase, and Bromsulphalein, Gastroenterology 38:796, 1960.

619. Rimington, C., Morgan, P. N., Nicholls, K., Everall, J. D., and Davies, R. R.: Griseofulvin administration and porphyrin metabolism: a survey, Lancet 2:318, 1963.

620. Rimington, C., Quin, J. I., and Roets, G. C. S.: Studies upon the photosensitization of animals in South Africa. X. The icterogenic factor in geel-dikkop. Isolation of active principles from Lippia rehmanni pears, Onderstepoort J. Vet. Sci. 9:225, 1937.

621. Ritchie, E. B., and Kolb, W.: Reaction to sodium diphenyl hydantoinate (Dilantin sodium); hemorrhagic erythema multiforme terminating fatally, Arch. Derm. Syph. 46:856, 1942.

622. Rivin, A. U.: Jaundice occurring during nicotinic acid therapy for hypercholesteremia, J.A.M.A. 170:2088, 1959.

623. Robinson, H. J., Siegal, H., and Pietrowski, J. J.: Toxicity of pyrazinamide, Am. Rev. Tuberc. 70:423, 1954.

624. Robinson, S. S.: "Erythema of the ninth day"; complicated by acute hepatitis and jaundice on continuation of arsphenamine therapy, Arch. Derm. Syph. 37:1031, 1938.

625. Robitzek, E. H., and Selikoff, I. J.: Hydrazine derivatives of isonicotinic acid (Rimifon, Marsilid) in the treatment of active progressive caseous-pneumonic tuberculosis; preliminary report, Am. Rev. Tuberc. 65:402, 1952.

626. Rodin, A. E., and Robertson, D. M.: Fatal toxic hepatitis following chlorpromazine therapy; report of a case with autopsy findings, Arch. Path. 66:170, 1958.

627. Roman, B.: Acute yellow atrophy of the liver, Arch. Path. 4:399, 1927.

628. Rosenbaum, H., and Reveno, W. S.: Agranulocytosis and toxic hepatitis from methimazole, J.A.M.A. 152:27, 1953.

629. Rosenblum, L. E., Korn, R. J., and Zimmerman, H. J.: Hepatocellular jaundice as a complication of iproniazid therapy, Arch. Int. Med. 105:583, 1960.

630. Rosenfeld, I., and Beath, O. A.: Tissue changes induced by Senecio riddelii, Am. J. Clin. Path. 15:407, 1945.

631. Rosenthal, S. M.: Some effects of alcohol upon the normal and damaged liver, J. Pharmacol. Exp. Ther. 38:291, 1930.

632. Rosenthal, S. M., and Bourne, W.: The effect of anesthetics on hepatic function, J.A.M.A. 90:377, 1928.

633. Rosin, A., and Doljanski, L.: Studies on the early changes in the livers of rats treated with various toxic agents, with especial reference to the vascular lesions; the histology of the rat's liver in allyl formate poisoning, Am. J. Path. 22:317, 1946.

634. ————: Pyroninophilic structures of liver cells in carbon tetrachloride poisoning, Proc. Soc. Exp. Biol. Med. 62:62, 1946.

635. Roth, L. G.: Infectious hepatitis in pregnancy, Am. J. Med. Sci. 225:139 1953.

635a. Rothwell-Jackson, R. L.: Budd-Chiari syndrome after oral contraceptives, Brit. Med. J. 1:252, 1968.

636. Rotstein, J., Frick, P. S., and Schiele, B. C.: Agranulocytosis associated with chlorpromazine therapy, Arch. Int. Med. 96:781, 1955.

637. Royston, G. D.: Delayed chloroform poisoning following delivery, Am. J. Obstet. Gynec. 10:808, 1925.

638. Rubin, E., and Lieber, C. S.: Alcohol-induced hepatic injury in non-alcoholic volunteers, New Engl. J. Med. 278:870, 1968.

639. Rubin, B., Hassert, G. L., Jr., Thomas, B. G. H., and Burke, J. C.: Pharmacology of isonicotinic acid hydrazide (nydrazid), Am. Rev. Tuberc. 65:392, 1952.

640. Rundles, R. W., Laszlo, J., Itoga, T., Hobson, J. B., and Garrison, F. E., Jr.: Clinical and hematologic study of 6-[(1-methyl-4-nitro-5-imidozolvl)thio] purine (B. W. 57-322) and related compounds, Cancer Chemother. Rep. 14:99, 1961.

641. Russell, H.: Acute toxic necrosis of the liver following the use of sulfanilamide, Ann. Int. Med. 14:168, 1940.

642. Rutenburg, A. M., and Pinkes, S.: The hepatotoxicity of intravenous Aureomycin, New Engl. J. Med. 247:797, 1952.

643. Saint, E. G., and Joske, R. A.: A note on fatty change in liver complicating Aureomycin therapy, Med. J. Aust. 1:222, 1953.

644. Salaman, M. H., King, A. J., Williams,

D. I., and Nicol, C. S.: Prevention of jaundice resulting from anti-syphilitic treatment, Lancet *2*:7, 1944.

645. Sborov, V. M., and Sutherland, D. A.: Fatty liver following Aureomycin and Terramycin therapy in chronic hepatic disease, Gastroenterology *18*:598, 1951.

646. Schaffner, F.: The effect of oral contraceptives on the liver, J.A.M.A. *198*:1019, 1966.

647. Schaffner, F., and Popper, H.: Electron microscopic study of human cholestasis, Proc. Soc. Exp. Biol. Med. *101*:777, 1959.

648. ———: Morphologic studies of cholestasis, Gastroenterology *37*:565, 1959.

649. Schaffner, F., Popper, H., and Chesrow, E.: Cholestasis produced by the administration of norethandrolone, Am. J. Med. *26*:249, 1959.

650. Schaffner, F. Popper, H., and Perez, V.: Changes in bile canaliculi produced by norethandrolone: electron microscopic study of human and rat liver, J. Lab. Clin. Med. *56*:623, 1960.

651. Schifrin, A.: Der Einfluss qualitativ verschiedener Ernährungsformen auf die durch Salvarsan hervorgerufenen Lebernekrosen, Virchow's Arch. path. Anat. *287*:175, 1932.

652. Schmid, M., Hefti, M. L., Gatticker, R., Kistler, H. J., and Senning, Å.: Benign postoperative intrahepatic cholestasis, New Engl. J. Med. *272*:545, 1965.

653. Schmidt, H. R., and Herold, L.: Leberfunktionsprufungen bei der Hyperemesis gravidarum, Arch. Gynaek. *156*:463, 1934.

654. Schnack, H.: Zur Aetiologie des Chlorpromazin-Ikterus: Tierexperimentelle und klinische Beobachtungen, Path. Microbiol. *27*:419, 1964.

655. Schneider, E. M., Daugherty, C., and DeVore, J. K.: Chlorpromazine jaundice; the effect of continued chlorpromazine ingestion in the presence of chlorpromazine jaundice, Southern, Med. J. *51*:287, 1958.

656. Schneider, J. A., Salgado, E. D., Jaeger, D., and Delahunt, C.: The pharmacology of chlorpropamide, Ann. N. Y. Acad. Sci. *74*:427, 1959.

657. Schoenbach, E. B., Miller, J. M., Ginsberg, M., and Long, P. H.: Systemic blastomycosis treated with stilbamidine; a preliminary report, J.A.M.A. *146*:1317, 1951.

658. Schoental, R., and Magee, P. N.: Chronic liver changes in rats after a single dose of lasiocarpine, a pyrrolizidine (senecio) alkaloid, J. Path. Bact. *74*:305, 1957.

659. ———: Further observations on the subacute and chronic liver changes in rats after a single dose of various pyrrolizidine (senecio) alkaloids, J. Path. Bact. *78*:471, 1959.

660. Schotz, M. C., and Recknagel, R. O.: Effect of carbon tetrachloride on release of free fatty acids by rat adipose tissue, Proc. Soc. Exp. Biol. Med. *103*:398, 1960.

661. Schultz, J. C., Adamson, J. S., Jr., Workman, W. W., and Norman, T. D.: Fatal liver disease after intravenous administration of tetracycline in high dosage, New Engl. J. Med. *269*:999, 1963.

662. Schwartz, W. S., and Moyer, R. E.: The chemotherapy of pulmonary tuberculosis with pyrazinamide used alone and in combination with streptomycin, para-aminosalicylic acid or isoniazid, Am. Rev. Tuberc. *70*:413, 1954.

663. Schwarz, K.: A hitherto unrecognized factor against dietary necrotic liver degeneration in American yeast (factor 3), Proc. Soc. Exp. Biol. Med. *78*:852, 1951.

664. ———: Casein and factor 3 in dietary necrotic liver degeneration; concentration of factor 3 from casein, Proc. Soc. Exp. Biol. Med. *80*:319, 1952.

665. ———: Factor 3, selenium and vitamin E, Nutr. Rev. *18*:193, 1960.

666. Scott, J. K.: Pathologic anatomy of acute experimental beryllium poisoning, Arch. Path. *45*:354, 1948.

667. Seakins, A., and Robinson, D. S.: The effect of the administration of carbon tetrachloride on the formation of plasma lipoproteins in the rat, Biochem. J. *86*:401, 1963.

668. Sealy, W. C.: The induction of liver necrosis in rabbits by the combination of experimental hyperthyroidism and Shope papilloma, Ann. Surg. *113*:572, 1941.

669. Sellers, E. A., You, R. W., and Lucas, C. C.: Lipotropic agents in liver damage produced by selenium or carbon tetrachloride, Proc. Soc. Exp. Biol. Med. *75*:118, 1950.

670. Selzer, G., and Parker, R. G. F.: Senecio poisoning exhibiting as Chiari's syndrome; report on 12 cases, Am. J. Path. *27*:885, 1951.

671. Selzer, G., Parker, R. G. F., and Sapeika, N.: An experimental study of senecio poisoning in rats, Brit. J. Exp. Path. *32*: 14. 1951.

672. Sevitt, S.: Hepatic jaundice after blood transfusions in injured and burned subjects, Brit. J. Surg. *46*:68, 1958.

673. Shaffer, J. M.: Disease of the liver in hyperthyroidism, Arch. Path. *29*:20, 1940.

674. Shaffer, J. M., Farquhar, J. D., Stokes, J., Jr., and Sborov, V. M.: Studies on the use of Aureomycin in hepatic disease; Aureomycin therapy in acute viral hepatitis, Am. J. Med. Sci. *220*:1, 1950.

675. Shank, R. E., Morrison, G., Cheng, C. H., Karl, I., and Schwartz, R.: Cell heterogeneity within the hepatic lobule (quantitative histochemistry), J. Histochem. Cytochem. *7*:237, 1959.

676. Shay, H., and Siplet, H.: Study of chlorpromazine jaundice, its mechanism and prevention. Special reference to serum alkaline phosphatase and glutamic oxalacetic trasaminase, Gastroenterology *32*:571, 1857.

677. Shay, H., and Sun, D. C. H.: Massive necrosis of the liver following iproniazid, Ann. Int. Med. *49*:1246, 1958.

678. Sheehan, H. L.: The pathology of acute yellow atrophy and delayed chloroform poisoning, J. Obstet. Gynaec. Brit. Emp. *47*:49, 1940.

679. Sherman, J. D., Love, D. E., and Harrington, J. F.: Anemia, positive lupus and rheumatoid factors with methyldopa, Arch. Int. Med. *120*:321, 1967.

680. Shields, W. E., Adamson, N. E., Jr., and MacGregor, J. B.: Peptic ulcer perforation following administration of phenylbutazone, J.A.M.A. *152*:28, 1953.

681. Shipp, J. C.: Jaundice during methimazole ("Tapazole") administration, Ann. Int. Med. *42*:701, 1955.

682. Short, C. L., and Bauer, W.: Cinchophen hypersensitiveness; report of four cases and a review, Ann. Int. Med. *6*:1449, 1933.

683. Shorter, R. G., Bollman, J. L., and Baggenstoss, A. H.: Pressures in common hepatic duct of the rat, Proc. Soc. Exp. Biol. Med. *102*:682, 1959.

684. Shotton, R., Carpenter, M., and Rinehart, W. B.: Bromsulphalein retention due to administration of a gall-bladder dye (bunamiodyl), New Engl. J. Med. *264*:550, 1961.

685. Sidel, N.: Dinitrophenol poisoning causing jaundice: report of a case, J.A.M.A. *103*:254, 1934.

686. Silverman, S. B., and Erickson, C. C.: Subcutaneous beryllium granuloma, Arch. Path. *50*:63, 1950.

687. Simmons, G. Hobson, L. B., Resnick, A., DeNicola, R., and Bennett, R. H.: Human pharmacology of p-formylacetanilide thiosemicarbazone (Mivizone), Am. Rev. Tuberc. *62*:128, 1950.

688. Simpson, D. G., and Walker, J. H.: Hypersensitivity to para-aminosalicylic acid, Am. J. Med. *29*:297, 1960.

689. Skromak, S. J., Schreader, C. J., O'Neill, J. F., and Ciccone, E. F.: Observations of chlorpromazine induced jaundice with continued use of the drug, Am. J. Med. Sci. *234*:85, 1957.

690. Smetana, H.: Nephrosis due to carbon tetrachloride, Arch. Int. Med. *63*:760, 1939.

691. Smillie, W. G., and Pessoa, S. B.: Treatment of hookworm disease with carbon tetrachloride, Am. J. Hyg. *3*:35, 1923.

692. Smith, M. I.: Chronic endemic selenium poisoning; review of the more recent field and laboratory studies, J.A.M.A. *116*:562, 1941.

693. Smith, N. J.: Death following accidental ingestion of DDT; experimental studies, J.A.M.A. *136*:469, 1948.

694. Smith, R. M., Josyln, D. A., Gruhzit, O. M., McLean, I. W., Jr., Penner, M. A., and Ehrlich, J.: Chloromycetin: biological studies, J. Bact. *55*:425, 1948.

695. Smith, Kline and French Laboratories Bulletins (Philadelphia): Thorazine, Nov., Dec., 1954.

696. Smuckler, E. A., Iseri, O. A., and Benditt, E. P.: Studies on carbon tetrachloride intoxication. I. The effect of carbon tetrachloride on incorporation of labelled amino acids into plasma proteins, Biochem. Biophys. Res. Commun. *5*:270, 1961.

697. ———: An intracellular defect in protein synthesis induced by carbon tetrachloride, J. Exp. Med. *116*:55, 1962.

698. Smyth, H. F.: Safe practices in the industrial use of carbon tetrachloride, J.A.M.A. *107*:1683, 1936.

699. Smyth, H. F., and Smyth, H. F., Jr.: Inhalation experiments with certain lacquer solvents, J. Indust. Hyg. *10*:261, 1928.

700. Snapper, I., Marks, D., Schwartz, L., and Hollander, L.: Hemolytic anemia second-

ary to Mesantoin, Ann. Int. Med. 39:619, 1953.

701. Sneddon, I. B.: Berylliosis: a case report, Brit. Med. J. 1:1448, 1955.

702. ———: Beryllium disease, Postgrad. Med. J. 34:262, 1958.

703. Snyder, R. G., Traeger, C. H., Zoll, C. A., Kelly, L. C., and Lust, F. J.: The use of cinchophen in the treatment of chronic arthritis, J. Lab. Clin. Med. 21: 541, 1936.

704. Soffer, L. J.: Postarsphenamine jaundice, Am. J. Syph. 21:309, 1937.

705. Solomon, F. A., Jr., and Compagna, F. A.: Jaundice due to prochlorperazine (Compazine), Am. J. Med. 27:840, 1959.

705a. Somayaji, B. N., Eeles, B. N., Paton, A., and Parker, R. G. F.: Budd-Chiari syndrome after oral contraceptives, Brit. Med. J. 1:53, 1968.

706. Spain, D. M., Childress, W. G., and Fishler, J. S.: The effect of 4-acetylaminobenzal thiosemicarbazone (tibione) on experimental tuberculosis in guinea pigs, Am. Rev. Tuberc. 62:144, 1950.

707. Spillsbury, B. H.: Toxic jaundice in munition workers and troops, Brit. Med. J. 1:156, 1917.

708. Spingarn, C. L., Edelman, M. H., Waye, J. D., Donoso, E., and Gregory, C.: Observations on the treatment of schistosomiasis Mansoni with antimony dimercaptosuccinate (TWSb), Am. J. Med. 34: 477, 1963.

709. Stander, H. J.: Delayed chloroform poisoning, Am. J. Obstet. Gynec. 23:882, 1932.

710. Steagall, R. W., Jr.: Severe reaction to griseofulvin, Arch. Dermat. 88:218, 1963.

711. Steigmann, F., and Popper, H.: Intrahepatic obstructive jaundice, Gastroenterology 1:645, 1943.

712. Stein, A. A., and Wright, A.: Hepatic pathology in jaundice due to chlorpromazine, J.A.M.A. 161:508, 1956.

713. Steinberg, G. L., Bohrod, M. G., and Roodenburg, A. I.: Agranulocytosis following phenylbutazone (Butazolidin) therapy; report of a fatal case, J.A.M.A. 152:33, 1953.

714. Steinberg, H., Welb, W. M., and Rafsky, H. A.: Hepatomegaly with fatty infiltration secondary to cortisone therapy. Case report, Gastroenterology 21:304, 1952

715. Steinbrocker, O., Berkowitz, S., Ehrlich, M. Elkind, M., and Carp, S.: Phenylbutazone therapy of arthritis and other painful musculoskeletal disorders, J.A.M.A. 150:1087, 1952.

716. Stenstrom, W.: Elimination of radioactive elements by patients and rabbits after injection of Thorotrast, Radiology 37:698, 1941.

717. Stephens, C. A., Jr., Yeoman, E. E., Holbrook, W. P., Hill, D. F., and Goodin, W. L.: Benefits and toxicity of phenylbutazone (Butazolidin) in rheumatoid arthritis, J.A.M.A. 150:1084, 1952.

718. Sterner, J. H., and Eisenbud, M.: Epidemiology of beryllium intoxication, Arch. Industr. Hyg. 4:123, 1951.

718a. Sterup, K., and Mosbech, J.: Budd-Chiari syndrome after taking oral contraceptives, Brit. Med. J. 4:660, 1967.

719. Stewart, M. J.: Toxic jaundice in munition workers and troops, Brit. Med. J. 1: 156, 1917.

720. ———: Atrophy of the liver, Brit. Med. J. 2:584, 1920.

721. Stifel, J. L., and Burnheimer, J. C.: Agranulocytosis following administration of phenylbutazone (Butazolidin); report of a case, J.A.M.A. 151:555, 1953.

722. Stokinger, H. E., Sprague, G. F., III, Hall, R. H., Ashenburg, N. J., Scott, J. K., and Steadman, L. T.: Acute inhalation toxicity of beryllium. I. Four definitive studies of beryllium sulfate at exposure concentrations of 100, 50, 10 and 1 mg. per cubic meter, Arch. Industr. Hyg. 1:379, 1950.

723. Stoll, B. A., Andrews, J. T., and Motteram, R.: Liver damage from oral contraceptives, Brit. Med. J. 1:960, 1966.

724. Stolzer, B. L., Miller, G., White, W. A., and Zuckerbrod, M.: Postarsenical obstructive jaundice complicated by xanthomatosis and diabetes mellitus, Am. J. Med. 9:124, 1950.

725. Stoner, H. B.: The mechanism of toxic hepatic necrosis, Brit. J. Exp. Path. 37: 176, 1956.

726. ———: The effect of anaesthesia and laparotomy on the blood-flow through the necrotic liver, Brit. J. Surg. 45:81, 1957.

727. Strauss, N.: Hepato-toxic effects following occupational exposure to Halowax (chlorinated hydrocarbons), Rev. Gastroenterol. 11:381, 1944.

728. Struthers, E. B., Chang, H. H., Lin, L. C., and Ch' en, J. T.: Antimony in the

treatment of kala-azar, and its toxic effects, Chinese Med. J. 47:1421, 1933.

729. Stuart, F. P., Torres, E., Hester, W. J., Dammin, G. J., and Moore, F. D.: Orthotopic autotransplantation and allotransplantation of the liver: functional and structural patterns in the dog, Ann. Surg. 165:325, 1967.

730. Stuart, K. L., and Bras, G.: Veno-occlusive disease of the liver, Quart. J. Med. 26:291, 1957.

731. Suhrland, L. G., and Weisberger, A. S.: Chloramphenicol toxicity in liver and renal disease, Arch. Int. Med. 112:747, 1963.

732. Sulkowski, S. R., and Haserick, J. R.: Simulated systemic lupus erythematosus from degraded tetracycline, J.A.M.A. 189:152, 1964.

733. Sulzberger, M. B., and Simon, F. A.: Asrphenamine hypersensitiveness in guinea pigs; experiments demonstrating (A) the regional geographic variability in susceptibility to sensitization (B) the chemical specificity of the hypersensitivity; and (C) variation in the sensitizing proclivities (sensitization index) of different brands, J. Allergy 6:39, 1934.

734. Summary of the National Halothane Study: Possible association between halothane anesthesia and postoperative hepatic necrosis, J.A.M.A. 197:775, 1966.

735. Sussman, R. M., and Summer, P.: Jaundice following the administration of 50 mg. of chlorpromazine, New Engl. J. Med. 253:499, 1955.

736. Sutherland, J. M., and Keller, W. H.: Novobiocin and neonatal hyperbilirubinemia; an investigation of the relationship in an epidemic of neonatal hyperbilirubinemia, Am. J. Dis. Child. 101:447, 1961.

737. Svoboda, D., Grady, H. J., and Higginson, J.: Aflatoxin B_1 injury in rat and monkey liver, Am. J. Path. 49:1023, 1966.

738. Taft, L. I.: Methotrexate induced hepatitis in childhood leukemia, Israel J. Med. Sci. 1:823, 1965.

739. Tainter, M. L., and Cutting, W. C.: Miscellaneous actions of dinitrophenol; repeated administrations, antidotes, fatal doses, antiseptic tests and actions of some isomers, J. Pharmacol. Exp. Ther. 49:187, 1933.

740. Tainter, M. L., and Wood, D. A.: A case of fatal dinitrophenol poisoning, J.A.M.A. 102:1147, 1934.

741. Talerman, A., and Thompson, R. B.: Hepatic fibrosis in a child possibly due to prolonged methotrexate, J. Clin. Path. 19:81, 1966.

742. Ten Pas, A., and Quinn, E. L.: Cholestatic hepatitis following the administration of sodium oxacillin, J.A.M.A. 191:674, 1965.

743. Tanyol, H., and Rehfuss, M. E.: Hepatotoxic effect of cortisone in experimental animals, Am. J. Dig. Dis. 22:169, 1955.

744. Thiers, R. E., Reynolds, E. S., and Vallee, B. L.: The effect of carbon tetrachloride poisoning on subcellular metal distribution in rat liver, J. Biol. Chem. 235:2130, 1960.

745. Thomas, E. W., Landy, S., and Cooper, C.: Reactions to penicillin therapy for syphilis, J. Invest. Derm. 10:77, 1948.

746. Thomas, S. F., Henry, G. W., and Kapplan, H. S.: Hepatolienography: past, present and future, Radiology 57:669, 1951.

747. Thulin, K. E., and Nermark, J.: Seven cases of jaundice in women taking an oral contraceptive, Anovlar, Brit. Med. J. 1:584, 1966.

748. Ticktin, H. E., and Robinson, M. M.: Effects of some antimicrobial agents on the liver, Ann. N. Y. Acad. Sci. 104:1080, 1963.

749. Ticktin, H. E., and Zimmerman, H. J.: Hepatic dysfunction and jaundice in patients receiving triacetyloleandomycin, New Engl. J. Med. 267:964, 1962.

750. Tisdale, W. A.: Focal hepatitis, fever and skin rash following therapy with sulfamethoxypyridazine, a long-acting sulfonamide, New Engl. J. Med. 258:687, 1958.

751. Tulloch, J. A.: A multiplicity of reactions to carbutamide (BZ-55) therapy; report of a case, Diabetes 7:316, 1958.

752. Tyler, E. T., and Olson, H. J.: Fertility promoting and inhibitory effects of new steroid hormonal substances, J.A.M.A. 169:1843, 1959.

753. Tyler, M. W., and King, E. Q.: Phenacemide in treatment of epilepsy, J.A.M.A. 147:17, 1951.

754. Umiker, W., and Pearce, J.: Nature and genesis of pulmonary alterations in carbon tetrachloride poisoning, Arch. Path. 55:203, 1953.

755. Unger, R. H., Madison, L. L., and Carter, N. W.: Relative effectiveness of newer oral agents in the regulation of diabetic patients imperfectly controlled by tolbutamide studied within the framework of a tentative subclassification of the disease, Ann. N. Y. Acad. Sci. 82: 570, 1959.

756. Urban, E., Frank, B. W., and Kern, F. Jr.: Liver dysfunction with mestranol but not with norethyndrel in a patient with Enovid-induced jaundice, Ann. Int. Med. 68:598, 1968.

757. Valdivia-Barriga, B., Feldman, A., and Orellana, J.: Generalized hypersensitivity with hepatitis and jaundice after the use of penicillin and streptomycin, Gastroenterology 45:114, 1963.

758. Vander Veer, J. B., and Fairley, D. L.: Mushroom poisoning (mycetismus); report of four cases, Arch. Int. Med. 55: 773, 1935.

759. Van Ordstrand, H. S.: Current concepts of beryllium poisoning, Ann. Int. Med. 35:1203, 1951.

760. Van Wyk, J. J., and Hoffman, C. R.: Periarteritis nodosa; a case of fatal exfoliative dermatitis resulting from "Dilantin sodium" sensitization, Arch. Int. Med. 81:605, 1948.

761. Velasco, H. A., and Sokal, J. E.: Cholestatic jaundice in association with desacetylmethylcolchicine. Report of a case, New Engl. J. Med. 260:1280, 1959.

762. VonGlahn, W. C., Flinn, F. B., and Keim, W. F., Jr.: Effect of certain arsenates on the liver, Arch. Path. 25: 488, 1938.

763. von Oettingen, W. F.: Manganese: its distribution, pharmacology and health hazards, Physiol. Rev. 15:175, 1935.

764. Waitzkin, L.: Hepatic dysfunction during promazine therapy, New Engl. J. Med. 257:276, 1957.

765. ———: Probable hepatic allergy to chlorpromazine and deliberate desensitization, Ann. Int. Med. 53:116, 1960.

766. Wakim, K. G., and Mann, F. C.: Effect of experimental cirrhosis on the intrahepatic circulation of blood in the intact animal, Arch. Path. 33:198, 1942.

767. Waldbott, G. L.: Anaphylactic death from penicillin, J.A.M.A. 139:526, 1949.

768. Waldo, J. F., and Tyson, J. T.: Hypersensitivity to penicillin, J. Clin. Invest. 28:1039, 1949.

769. Walker, A. R. P., and Arvidsson, U. B.: Iron intake and haemochromatosis in the Bantu, Nature 166:438, 1950.

770. Walker, C. O., and Combes, B.: Biliary cirrhosis induced by chlorpromazine, Gastroenterology 51:631, 1966.

771. Wallace, J., and Bushby, S. R. M.: Physiological and biochemical changes following hyperthermy treatment, Brit. J. Vener. Dis. 19:155, 1943.

772. Warring, F. C., Jr., and Howlett, K. S.: Allergic reactions to para-aminosalicylic acid; report of seven cases, including a case of Loeffler's syndrome, Am. Rev. Tuberc. 65:235, 1952.

773. Watson, C. J.: The effect of sulfanilamide upon the liver, Surgery 5:616, 1939.

774. Watson, C. J., and Spink, W. W.: Effect of sulfanilamide and sulfapyridine on hemoglobin metabolism and hepatic function, Arch. Int. Med. 65:825, 1940.

775. Waye, J. D., Donoso, E., Spingarn, C. L., and Edelman, M. H.: Cardiotoxic effects of antimony dimercaptosuccinate in schistosomiasis; with special reference to coexistent hepatic dysfunction, Am. J. Cardiol. 10:829, 1962.

776. Weber, F. P.: A case of morbilliform and bullous eruption with jaundice, from Luminal, in a choreic child, Brit. J. Child. Dis. 22:280, 1925.

777. Wedum, A. G.: Immunological specificity of sulfonamide azoproteins, J. Infect. Dis. 70:173, 1942.

778. Weir, J. F., and Comfort, M. W.: Toxic cirrhosis caused by cinchophen, Arch. Int. Med. 52:685, 1933.

779. Weller, C. V.: Hepatic pathology in exophthalmic goiter, Ann. Int. Med. 7: 543, 1933.

780. Wells, H. G.: Delayed chloroform poisoning: allied conditions: a note on the cause of the anatomic and clinical changes observed, J.A.M.A. 46:341, 1906.

781. Werner, S. C., Hanger, F. M., and Kritzler, R. A.: Jaundice during methyl testosterone therapy, Am. J. Med. 8:325, 1950.

782. Werther, J. L., and Korelitz, B. I.: Chlorpromazine jaundice; analysis of twenty-two cases, Am. J. Med. 22:351, 1957.

783. Whalley, P. J., Adams, R. H., and Combes, B.: Tetracycline toxicity in pregnancy: liver and pancreatic dysfunction, J.A.M.A. 189:357, 1964.

784. Whipple, G. H., and Sperry, J. A.: Chloroform poisoning; liver necrosis and repair, Bull. Johns Hopkins Hosp. *20*: 278, 1909.

785. White, J. C.: Nephrosis occurring during trimethadione therapy, J.A.M.A. *139*: 376, 1949.

786. Wieland, T., Schmidt, G., and Wirth, L.: Über die Giftstoffe des Knollenblätterpilzes VIII, Justus Liebig's Ann. Chem. *577*:215, 1952.

787. Wien, R., Freeman, W., and Scotcher, N. M.: The metabolic effects produced by certain aromatic diamidines, Ann. Trop. Med. *37*:19, 1943.

788. Wilcox, W. W.: Toxic jaundice, Lancet *2*:1, 1931.

789. ————: Toxic jaundice, Lancet *2*:57, 1931.

790. Wile, M. J., and Benson, J. A.: Exfoliative dermatitis due to phenobarbital with fatal outcome; report of two cases, Ann. Int. Med. *13*:1243, 1940.

791. Wilensky, A. O.: Fatal delayed anaphylactic shock after penicillin, J.A.M.A. *131*:1384, 1946.

792. Wilmot, F. C., and Robertson, G. W.: Senecio disease, or cirrhosis of the liver due to senecio poisoning, Lancet *2*:848, 1920.

793. Wilson, M. E., and Stowell, R. E.: Cytological changes following roentgen irradiation of the liver in mice, J. Nat. Cancer Inst. *13*:1123, 1953.

794. Woldman, E. E., and Fishman, D.: Intrahepatic obstructive jaundice following the administration of 75 mg. of chlorpromazine, Ann. Int. Med. *47*:332, 1957.

795. Wolff, W. A., Elkinton, J. R., and Rhoads, J. E.: Liver damage and dextrose tolerance in severe burns, Ann. Surg. *112*:158, 1940.

796. Woods, W. W.: The changes in the kidneys in carbon tetrachloride poisoning, and their resemblance to those in the "crush syndrome," J. Path. Bact. *58*:767, 1946.

797. Woodward, D. J., and Solomon, J. D.: Fatal agranulocytosis occurring during promazine (Sparine) therapy, J.A.M.A. *162*:1308, 1956.

798. Wright, D. O., Reppert, L. B., and Cutino, J. T.: Purpuric manifestations of heat stroke; studies of prothrombin and platelets in twelve cases, Arch. Int. Med. *77*:27, 1946.

799. Wynn, V., Landon, J., and Kawerau, E.: Studies on hepatic function during methandienone therapy, Lancet *1*:69, 1961.

800. Yater, W. M., and Coe, F. O.: Ten years' experience with Thorotrast hepatosplenography, Ann. Int. Med. *18*:350, 1943.

801. Yater, W. M., and Whitmore, E. R.: Histopathologic study of tissues of 65 patients injected with thorium dioxide sol for hepatosplenography, with a follow-up study of 10 old cases, Am. J. Med. Sci. *195*:198, 1938.

802. Yesner, R., and Kunkel, P.: Preliminary observations on the effect of Aureomycin, Terramycin, Tibione, combined Tibione and Streptomycin and Chloromycetin on the morphology of the liver in man, Yale J. Biol. Med. *23*:299, 1951.

803. Youmans, J. B., and Warfield, L. M.: Liver injury in thyrotoxicosis as evidenced by decreased functional efficiency, Arch. Int. Med. *37*:1, 1926.

804. Zaky, A., Dorry, L., and Salam, A.: The protective action of prednisone on the liver during tartar emetic treatment of bilharzial cirrhosis, J. Trop. Med. Hyg. *66*:188, 1963.

805. Zarday, Z., Rosenthal, W. S., and Wolff, F. W.: Severe liver toxicity after methyldopa, N. Y. State J. Med. *67*:1897, 1967.

806. Zeffren, J. L., and Sherry, S.: Effects of prolonged tolbutamide therapy on hepatic function and serum cholesterol of adult diabetic patients, Metabolism *6*: 504, 1957.

807. Zelman, S.: Liver cell necrosis in chlorpromazine jaundice (allergic cholangiolitis); a serial study of twenty-six needle biopsy specimens in nine patients, Am. J. Med. *27*:708, 1959.

808. Zetzel, L., and Kaplan, H.: Liver damage concurrent with iproniazid administration, New Engl. J. Med. *258*:1209, 1958.

809. Zimmerman, H. J., Alpert, L. K., and Howe, J. S.: The effect of nitrogen mustard (bis-β-chlorethyl amine) on liver function and structure in patients with neoplastic disease, J. Lab. Clin. Med. *40*:387, 1952.

15

Hepatitis Associated With Systemic Infections

GERALD KLATSKIN, M.D.

Many systemic infections produce structural and functional changes in the liver which occasionally are accompanied by jaundice. Fortunately, these are seldom of sufficient severity to alter the course of the underlying disease or to require special treatment. However, unless their relationship to infection is recognized, they may lead to serious diagnostic errors. Jaundice is particularly likely to be misleading, since it may be misinterpreted as a sign of primary hepatic or biliary tract disease and thus divert attention from the underlying infection and lead to inappropriate treatment.

Although the pathogenesis of hepatic injury in systemic infections is obscure in many instances, the following mechanisms may be of importance in some: (1) direct invasion of the parenchyma by blood-borne or lymph-borne infectious agents, (2) hepatocellular injury by circulating toxins and (3) nonspecific injury to the liver related to hyperpyrexia, malnutrition and anoxemia.

Considering the importance of the liver in clearing the blood of circulating organisms,[23] it might be anticipated that many instances of hepatitis would be the result of direct invasion by infectious agents. Actually, however, organisms seldom can be demonstrated in the liver. This does not preclude the possibility that organisms engulfed by the liver produce hepatocellular injury and then undergo dissolution. The observation that intraportally injected streptococci induce acute hepatitis and then vanish[178] would appear to be consistent with such a mechanism. However, it is generally believed that most instances of hepatic injury associated with infection are of toxic origin. Although circulating toxins have not been demonstrated in such cases, the cell bodies of certain bacteria contain endotoxins capable of producing liver damage.[196]

In evaluating the role of infection in the pathogenesis of hepatic injury, due consideration must be given to the nonspecific effects of fever, anoxemia and malnutrition. These depress hepatic function and may be responsible for some of the lesions found in the liver. However, they seldom give rise to jaundice.

Since many bacteria can hemolyze red cells in culture media, the question arises whether or not hemolysis plays any role in the jaundice associated with infection. In *Clostridium welchii* sepsis, the evidence is clear that hemolysis is the principal factor responsible for jaundice. However, the importance of hemolysis in other infections is in doubt, since the frequency and severity of the jaundice seldom can be correlated with the hemolytic properties of the organism involved.

Occasionally, infection provokes an exacerbation of symptoms in patients with chronic liver disease. The reason for this is not clear, although experimental evidence indicates that the injured liver is unusually susceptible to the toxic effects of infection.[206] Accordingly, it is important to search for signs of antecedent liver disease whenever jaundice appears during the course of an infection.

A great many infections are accompanied by alterations in the serum protein pattern which may affect the results of the thymol turbidity, the cephalin-cholesterol flocculation and other similar reactions often erroneously regarded as specific tests of liver function. Such changes are not necessarily related to hepatic injury, so that the results of turbidity and flocculation tests must be interpreted with caution in the face of infection. A nonspecific effect should be suspected whenever the abnormalities in "liver function" are limited to those dependent on the serum protein pattern.

BACTERIAL INFECTIONS

GRAM-POSITIVE COCCI

Pneumococcus. Most, if not all, patients with lobar pneumonia exhibit impairment of hepatic function,[73, 301] and 3 to 24 per cent develop jaundice.[73, 151, 231, 301] It is highly probable that the hepatocellular injury responsible for these manifestations is due primarily to the toxic effects of the underlying pneumococcal infection, an interpretation consistent with the observation that a similar type of liver damage occurs in pneumococcal peritonitis and sepsis.[16] Fever and anoxemia may be contributory factors, although they seldom can be correlated with the degree of hepatic dysfunction present.[301]

It is reasonable to suppose that the occurrence of jaundice merely signifies a more severe grade of hepatocellular injury than is usually present in pneumonia. However, it has been suggested that increased hemolysis is a factor, an opinion based on the observation that the fecal excretion of urobilinogen is increased.[227] Further studies of urobilinogen excretion by modern methods are needed to confirm this observation. If hemolysis is a factor, it is unlikely that it occurs in the pneumonic lung, as once thought, since the jaundice usually appears during the stage of gray hepatization when most of the red cells have vanished,[227] and since jaundice may occur in the absence of pneumonia, as in pneumococcal peritonitis.[16]

Since the right lung usually is involved in cases with jaundice, a mechanical or anatomic factor has been thought to be involved.[241] This hypothesis has no sound physiologic or pathologic basis.

The factors that predispose to jaundice are not known. The severity and extent of the pneumonia do not appear to be crucial, nor does the presence of bacteremia.[301] Since the jaundice occurs late in the course of the disease, it might be anticipated that delayed or ineffectual treatment would be a factor. However, the introduction of modern antibiotic therapy does not appear to have reduced the incidence of jaundice materially.[301] Suggestive evidence has been presented to show that Type II[73] and Type V[231] pneumococcal infections are particularly likely to produce jaundice, an effect attributed to the severity of the infection in the case of the former and to the unusual hemolytic properties of the organism in the latter. Unfortunately, the data presented do not permit any conclusions regarding the validity of these interpretations. The antecedent status of the liver may be an important factor. This is suggested by the observation that chronic alcoholics with pneumonia are particularly likely to develop jaundice.[301]

The clinical features of the jaundice in pneumococcal pneumonia are not distinctive. Usually, the onset is on the 5th or 6th day of the disease but may occur as early as the second or as late as the twelfth day.[241] Usually, it is associated with bilirubinuria and the excretion of large amounts of urobilinogen. In most cases the hepatitis is mild to moderate in severity and subsides promptly as the pneumonia resolves. Rarely, however, it is sufficiently severe to produce coma.[35] At one time the occurrence of jaundice was regarded as a bad omen, but the results of more recent studies do not bear this out.[73, 241, 301]

The principal pathologic changes in the liver observed at autopsy include basophilic degeneration of the hepatic cells, evidence of active hepatocellular regeneration with frequent mitotic figures, and leukocytic infiltration of the portal triads.[16] The latter is an inconstant finding, according to some pathologists.[227]

Staphylococcus. The liver is seldom involved in staphylococcal bacteremia, although rare instances of hepatic abscess[255] and jaundice[34, 255] have been reported. Unfortunately, the findings in the liver have not been described, so that the pathogenesis of the jaundice in such cases is not known. Although toxic hepatitis would appear to be the most likely cause, hemolysis has been suggested as a factor, since marked anemia often accompanies the jaundice.[255] The demonstration of methemoglobin in the urine of one reported case would appear to be consistent with this interpretation.[34]

Streptococcus. Occasionally, hemolytic streptococcal infections are complicated by jaundice. Most instances occur in association with bacteremia,[144] but a few have been reported as an early manifestation of scarlet fever.[86] The incidence appears to be somewhat lower than in pneumococcal infection, jaundice having been encountered in less than 3 per cent of cases in one series of 246 streptococcal bacteremias.[144] Jaundice may occur also in anaerobic streptococcal sepsis,[34] but this is unusual.

In contrast with the relatively minor changes produced by the pneumococcus, streptococcal infections can seriously injure the liver. Two types of hepatic lesion have been described.[178] The first, presumably due to a circulating toxin, is characterized by centrilobular hepatocellular degeneration and necrosis, and an acute polymorphonuclear inflammatory reaction in the portal zones. The other, due to invasion of the parenchyma by histologically demonstrable streptococci, consists of scattered focal areas of acute nonsuppurative hepatocellular necrosis. In rare instances the process may be diffuse and resemble acute yellow atrophy. Occasionally, the lesions are zonal in distribution but, in contrast to the toxic type, tend to be periportal[178] or midzonal.[206]

Of interest is the question of whether or not streptococci, borne to the liver either by the blood during episodes of transient bacteremia or by the lymph, can provoke chronic hepatitis. At one time it was believed that many cases of cirrhosis were due to such infections, since streptococci could occasionally be demonstrated in the liver.[195, 206] However, the presence of bacteria is now regarded as a complication of cirrhosis and not its cause. Normally, the liver can clear the blood of large numbers of bacteria without becoming infected[23] and is sterile on culture.[239] The diseased liver may be less efficient in this respect and thus permit organisms to gain a foothold. Interestingly, the intravenous injection of streptococci in normal animals does not affect the liver, but when accompanied by a small dose of a hepatotoxin, such as chloroform, produces severe hepatic necrosis.[206]

Streptococci that gain access to the liver via the bile ducts or their lymphatics are said to give rise to a type of chronic hepatitis that terminates in cirrhosis.[178] However, it is difficult to exclude the possibility that the cirrhosis in such cases is secondary to chronic cholangitis.

A curious syndrome, known as cholangitis lenta, has been ascribed to a primary *Streptococcus viridans* infection of the hepatic bile radicles. Clinically, it is characterized by protracted chills and fever, bacteremia, cachexia and anemia. Since jaundice and hepatomegaly are inconstant findings, the hepatic origin of the sepsis may be overlooked. Splenomegaly and ascites are rare. Superficially at least, the syndrome resembles endocarditis lenta (subacute bacterial endocarditis), which accounts for its name. Considerable doubt has been cast on the specificity of the disease, since other bacteria can produce the same clinical picture, and, in carefully investigated cases, an underlying stone or malignancy can often be demonstrated in the biliary tract.[98, 159] However, the possibility of a primary S. *viridans* cholangitis cannot be excluded with certainty, although it must be rare if it occurs at all.

Various types of hepatobiliary disease, especially when accompanied by cholestasis, may raise the antistreptolysin O titer in serum.[106] This appears to be a nonspecific phenomenon related to increased serum beta-lipoprotein, and can be abolished by precipitating the latter with dextran and calcium chloride.

GRAM-NEGATIVE COCCI

Gonococcus. Jaundice is a relatively common complication of gonococcal septicemia due to acute endocarditis[37, 164, 259, 291] and usually is associated with areas of focal necrosis and polymorphonuclear infiltration in the liver.[37, 164] Whether the lesions are due to toxemia or to bacterial invasion is unknown. However, since hepatic abscess occurs occasionally in such cases,[17] bacterial invasion is possible. Presumably the jaundice is due to hepatocellular injury, although histologic changes have not been demonstrable in all cases.[259] Since in some individuals severe anemia develops rapidly and active phagocytosis of erythrocytes in the reticuloendothelial system is evident,[164] hemolysis may be a contributory factor.

Occasionally, the gonococcus produces acute perihepatitis in women with pelvic inflammatory disease.[87, 120, 280] Characteristically, there is a history of gonorrheal infection, and a recent episode, usually within 1 to 2 months, of lower abdominal pain, fever and leukorrhea. The onset is sudden with severe right upper quadrant pain, followed by fever, local tenderness and spasm, and leukocytosis. The pain is aggravated by respiration, coughing and twisting and may radiate to the back or either shoulder. Often a friction rub is audible over the liver. The disease may be mistaken for acute cholecystitis, especially since x-ray studies often reveal a nonfunctioning gallbladder. At operation the characteristic findings are a sharply localized fibrinous peritonitis overlying the liver, and an acute inflammatory reaction in the hepatic capsule. Occasionally, gonococci can be recovered from the fluid drained from the area postoperatively. The fluorescent test for gonococcal antibodies is said to be reliable in identifying the etiology in cases with negative cultures.[280] The symptoms subside spontaneously within a few days to a week. However, treatment with large doses of penicillin is recommended.[280] In many cases of acute inflammatory reaction is followed by the development of "violin-string" adhesions between the anterior surface of the liver and the abdominal wall. As a rule, these are asymptomatic but occasionally they give rise to chronic or intermittent pain.

ENTERIC GRAM-NEGATIVE BACILLI

Escherichia coli. Occasionally, E. coli in-fections give rise to jaundice. This complication is relatively infrequent in adults, occurring only in those with bacteremia,[143] but is relatively common in young infants with severe E. coli urinary tract infections, even in the absence of bacteremia or significant fever.[29, 107] The mortality rate in such infants is high, particularly when the infection appears during the first week of life.[107] Although sepsis is the principal cause of death, hepatic insufficiency may play a contributory role in some cases. Usually, at postmortem examination, the liver shows central bile stasis, focal hepatocellular necrosis, evidence of regenerative activity, including giant-cell transformation of the parenchyma, and a minimal inflammatory reaction in the portal triads.[29, 107] Occasionally, however, no hepatic lesions can be demonstrated.[107] Almost certainly, toxic hepatocellular injury accounts for the jaundice, but hemolysis may be a contributory factor, as suggested by some.[107] Since intravenously injected E. coli do not affect the liver in experimental animals unless accompanied by a small dose of an hepatotoxin, such as chloroform,[206] it is reasonable to assume that some toxic factor is elaborated in human infections complicated by jaundice.

E. coli septicemia is an occasional complication of decompensated Laennec's cirrhosis.[64, 273, 286] Not infrequently there is an accompanying peritonitis. Indeed, it has been suggested that this is invariably the case.[64] Characteristically, there is a sudden onset of chills, fever, abdominal pain, tenderness and signs of ileus, often followed by hypotension and hepatic coma. Despite the severity of the infection and of the underlying liver disease, appropriate antibiotic therapy usually is effective. However, hepatic function often deteriorates leading to death in a month or two.[64] How bacteria gain access to the circulation has not been established. However, it has been suggested that edema and degeneration of the intestinal mucosa, secondary to portal hypertension, hypoproteinemia, diarrhea and alteration in the intestinal bacterial flora induced by the use of antibiotics, lowers local resistance, permitting organisms to enter the portal circulation. Because of hepatic injury and the presence of numerous shunts between the portal and systemic veins, such organisms may escape phagocytosis and destruction in the liver and thus gain access to the general circulation. Infection of the peritoneum may be of hematogenous origin, or may follow transmural migration of bacteria from the intestinal lumen.

Occasionally, ulcerative colitis is complicated by a form of chronic pericholangitis that may progress to biliary cirrhosis. (See Chap. 30.) Recurrent bouts of an obstructive-like jaundice, a persistently elevated level of serum alkaline phosphatase and hepatomegaly are the principal manifestations. As the lesion progresses, splenomegaly, ascites, bleeding from esophageal varices and/or hepatic coma may appear. It has been suggested that this disorder is due to portal bacteremia with either E. coli or Streptococcus fecalis,[39, 43] and that, in some cases, long-term tetracycline therapy may be effective, at least for a time.[222] However, the relationship of hepatobiliary disease in ulcerative colitis to bacterial seeding of the liver via the portal vein, and the efficacy of antibiotics in its treatment, are open to question.[192a]

Salmonella. Two types of hepatitis are seen in association with salmonella infections: one occurs in epidemics and is due to a concurrent infection with the hepatitis virus; the other occurs sporadically and is directly related to the effects of the salmonella.

In some outbreaks of epidemic jaundice members of the salmonella group can be recovered from the blood and feces.[20, 125, 288] During World War I, when such infections were prevalent among troops in the Dardanelles and Mesopotamia, it was not certain whether the jaundice was due to a salmonella cholangitis[20, 125, 288] or to a double infection with both the salmonella and the virus of infectious hepatitis.[184] However, it is now known that, under conditions of crowding and poor sanitation, epidemics of both diseases can occur simultaneously, and that double infections are relatively common. This was demonstrated under experimental conditions by Havens and Wenner, who observed 2 instances of Salmonella choleraesuis bacteremia in a group of 5 in-

dividuals with experimentally induced viral hepatitis living in an institution where salmonella infections were prevalent.[115] In most outbreaks of hepatitis complicated by salmonellosis, members of the paratyphoid group (S. paratyphi and S. schottmüleri) have been implicated. In the Dardanelles and Mesopotamian campaigns previously mentioned, jaundice occurred in 5 per cent of infections with these organisms.[289]

Occasionally, the jaundice that accompanies a salmonella infection is clearly unrelated to an intercurrent viral hepatitis. In paratyphoid fever, for example, it may be the result of an acute suppurative cholangitis, while in food poisoning with S. typhimurium and S. enteritidis it usually is due to a toxic hepatitis.[289] On clinical grounds alone it may be difficult to distinguish between these various types of jaundice. However, viral hepatitis should be suspected when jaundice occurs with great frequency during an epidemic of paratyphoid, and particularly when cases of jaundice begin to appear in individuals without evidence of salmonella infection. Suppurative cholangitis is more likely to be the cause in sporadic cases of paratyphoid. Toxic hepatitis is almost always responsible when jaundice occurs in food poisoning.

Typhoid Fever. Hepatomegaly occurs in approximately 25 per cent of patients with typhoid fever.[265] Usually, it appears during the 2nd or 3rd week of the disease and persists until defervescence. The enlargement is probably related to the presence of the characteristic focal areas of parenchymal necrosis and the portal inflammatory reaction found at autopsy.[180] Occlusion of the sinusoids by proliferation and embolization of endothelial phagocytes[180] and toxic injury[97] have been cited as possible etiologic factors in their pathogenesis. Similar lesions have been produced in experimental animals with an antigenic extract of typhoid bacilli,[196] so that a toxic origin is highly probable.

Jaundice is said to be a relatively rare complication in typhoid fever.[208] However, in one large series it occurred in almost 4 per cent of cases.[265] Usually, it appears at the height of the fever, runs a relatively benign course and is associated with many of the clinical features of viral hepatitis.[265] Although it usually is presumed to be due to a mild cholangitis,[208, 289] there is little or no autopsy evidence to support this. A few instances of suppurative cholangitis, pylephlebitis and solitary hepatic abscess have been reported,[208] but the nature of the lesion in most mild cases is not known. A toxic hepatitis would appear to be the most likely etiology in cases without suppuration of the biliary tract,[265] but morphologic studies are too few to warrant any definite conclusions.

Acute cholecystitis occurs in a small proportion of individuals with typhoid fever and may be a serious complication if suppuration ensues. It probably occurs more often than is recognized clinically[265] and may serve to initiate a chronic cholecystitis and cholelithiasis. Such individuals are particularly likely to become carriers of typhoid bacilli.

Although the carrier state usually is attributed to chronic infection of the gallbladder with *Salmonella typhosa*, there may be a delay of as long as 5 years following cholecystectomy before these organisms are eradicated from the stools.[91] Moreover, there is evidence that, in some cases, the infection involves the intrahepatic bile ducts,[81, 175] and will not respond to either cholecystectomy or antibiotic therapy.[175] T-tube drainage, in addition to cholecystectomy, appears to be effective in such cases.[81] Of interest is a report that carriers with infections of the intrahepatic bile ducts may experience recurrent bouts of cholangitis with jaundice that occasionally give rise to biliary cirrhosis.[81]

Shigella. As in salmonella infections, epidemic bacillary dysentery occasionally is accompanied by a high incidence of jaundice,[227] a complication not seen in sporadic cases. On epidemiologic grounds it is highly probable that the coincidence of jaundice and dysentery in such epidemics is due to double infections with shigella and the hepatitis virus. It is unlikely that acute cholangitis is a cause of the jaundice, since the lesion has not been observed in autopsy studies.

OTHER GRAM-NEGATIVE BACILLI

Brucellosis. Biopsy studies indicate that hepatic granulomata occur with great regularity in active brucellosis.[138, 258] In addition, the liver may show portal fibrosis and lymphocytosis and necrosis of parenchymal cells. The granulomatous lesions, which are composed of masses of epithelioid cells, and a few lymphocytes, giant cells and plasma cells, closely resemble those seen in tuberculosis and other granulomatous diseases.[149] Caseation does not occur, but other types of necrosis are common. Identical lesions have been observed in mice and guinea pigs infected with *Br. abortus*, and evidence has been presented to show that the proliferation of epithelioid cells, which are derived from Kupffer cells, is a reaction to the intracellular growth of organisms and is a sign of a good defense mechanism.[41] Animals infected with the more invasive *Br. suis* develop suppurative lesions, which has been interpreted as evidence of low resistance.

Most hepatic granulomata demonstrated by needle biopsy have occurred in *Br. abortus* infections.[149, 258] Hepatic lesions are said to be rare in human infections with *Br. suis* and *melitensis*.[258] However, instances of both acute hepatitis[204] and abscess of the liver and spleen[257] have been reported as complications of *Br. suis* infections. The clinical course in patients with abscess has been characterized by recurrent bouts of chills and fever for periods up to 25 years, the presence in the liver or spleen of calcific deposits, and recovery following surgical drainage of liver abscesses, or splenectomy in the case of splenic abscesses.

Many patients with brucellosis exhibit hepatomegaly and/or splenomegaly,[61, 138] but only a few develop jaundice. Positive cephalin-cholesterol flocculation reactions and elevations of serum alkaline phosphatase are common,[138, 148] but, occasionally, the results of these and other tests of liver function are normal even in the presence of hepatic lesions.[258]

Occasionally, Brucella organisms can be cultured from liver biopsy specimens at a time when the blood is sterile,[62] so that cultures of this type may be helpful diagnostically. As indicated, the liver or spleen may exhibit calcific deposits on roentgenographic examination in patients with long-standing infections. Characteristically, those in the spleen tend to be large and numerous, resembling snowflakes, and can be distinguished from the small uniform calcifications of tuberculosis and the densely outlined foci seen in histoplasmosis.[298]

Although brucellosis does not produce hepatic scarring in experimental animals,[41] it may give rise to cirrhosis in man.[61, 78, 138, 172, 173, 182, 233] At one time, the causal relationship between brucellosis and cirrhosis was doubted, particularly because the liver in such cases rarely if ever showed granulomata. However, in several well-documented cases the progression from acute necrotizing granulomatous hepatitis to cirrhosis has been demonstrated by serial biopsies.[138, 148] Of particular interest in these cases has been the disappearance of granulomata and the development of a lesion indistinguishable from that of postnecrotic cirrhosis.

Granuloma Inguinale. Occasionally, the Donovan body, believed to be a gram-negative bacillus, produces a disseminated infection which involves the joints, bones and viscera. The liver in such cases may be studded with miliary abscesses filled with foamy mononuclear cells containing Donovan bodies.[170]

Tularemia. During its dissemination, *Pasteurella tularensis* frequently invades the liver, among other organs, and produces characteristic focal lesions.[90] In one autopsy series, these were present in 10 of 12 cases.[220] The acute lesions, which are seen during the first 2 weeks of the disease, are characterized by areas of focal necrosis infiltrated with large mononuclear cells. Later, they become granulomatous and exhibit a central zone of necrosis, which, occasionally, is caseous, surrounded by radially arranged epithelioid cells and fibroblasts and a peripheral collar of lymphocytes and giant cells.[90] Clinical manifestations of hepatic involvement are unusual. In one series, overt hepatitis was evident in only 4 of 600 cases.[89] However, the incidence has been somewhat higher in fatal cases, which invariably are associated with a disseminated infection.[220] Jaundice and hepatosplenomegaly are the usual findings and occasionally are associated with peritonitis and ascites.[89]

GRAM-POSITIVE BACILLI

Clostridia. In *C. welchii* (*perfringens*) bacteremia, an intense jaundice and severe anemia develop due to the hemolytic action of the exotoxin produced. The serum contains free hemoglobin, methemalbumin, methemoglobin and hematin, in addition to increased amounts of bilirubin.[34] Although the jaundice is primarily of hemolytic origin, hepatic injury almost certainly is a factor in some cases, since the organisms tend to invade the liver and give rise to extensive gas formation.

The other clostridia involved in gas bacillus infections produce similar hemolytic exotoxins and may induce jaundice in the same manner.

The relationship of clostridial infections to infarction of the liver is of interest. In dogs, occlusion of the arterial circulation to the liver is invariably fatal within 96 hours. This is attributable to the development of clostridial bacteremia and massive hepatic necrosis, and can be prevented by the administration of large doses of penicillin or chlortetracycline.[54, 183] Apparently, since oxygen tension in the liver is reduced, anaerobes grow rapidly, which leads to bacteremia and massive hepatic necrosis. Although massive hepatic necrosis and death may follow hepatic artery ligation in man,[27, 134] clostridial infections do not appear to be responsible. This species difference probably is related to the fact that clostridia are normally present in the dog's liver[54, 239] but not in man's.[239]

MYCOBACTERIAL INFECTIONS

TUBERCULOSIS

The results of autopsy,[168, 232, 278] biopsy[38, 103, 149, 156, 181, 187, 224, 238] and functional[124, 156, 238] studies show that the liver is affected in a high proportion of individuals with tuberculous infections. Two types of hepatic lesions are seen: (1) granulomata due to hematogenous spread of tubercle bacilli from other sites, and (2) nonspecific alterations in the hepatic parenchyma and stroma, such as fatty infiltration, fibrosis, amyloidosis and congestion, attributable to the effects of prolonged infection, malnutrition, anoxia and cardiac failure.

In most tuberculous infections, the associated hepatic lesions produce few if any symptoms. Occasionally, however, the liver is severely affected and gives rise to significant clinical manifestations. In some cases, the liver bears the brunt of the infection, while the initial focus is inconspicuous. This produces a clinical picture sometimes called "primary" miliary tuberculosis of the liver.[269] Closely related to this disorder is the syndrome of splenic tuberculosis[123, 292] in which the spleen appears to be the principal organ involved.

Most tuberculous lesions in the liver are miliary in character. Occasionally, however, the tubercles coalesce to form large abscess-like masses known as tuberculomas, or spread diffusely along the walls of the intrahepatic bile ducts, giving rise to so-called "tubular" tuberculosis or tuberculous cholangitis.

Early in its development, the miliary tubercle, which is just visible to the naked eye, consists of a compact mass of epithelioid cells, often surrounded and infiltrated by lymphocytes. As the tubercle matures, giant cells and small foci of central eosinophilic necrosis appear. Ultimately, the lesion heals by scarring, but occasionally, it resolves without a trace. Frank caseation is relatively uncommon in the liver except when the granulomata coalesce. Despite some reports to the contrary, there does not appear to be any consistency about the distribution of the lesions, some being found in the parenchyma, others in the portal triads.[149] Acid-fast bacilli are surprisingly difficult to demonstrate. In one large autopsy series, for example, they were found in only 38 per cent of the hepatic granulomata examined.[278] Even fewer organisms have been encountered in specimens of liver obtained by needle biopsy.[103, 149, 156, 181, 187] This is an important point, since in the absence of acid-fast bacilli and caseation, it is impossible to differentiate the lesions of tuberculosis from those seen in other granulomatous diseases.[149]

Although several investigators[42, 153] have reported that the presence of acid-fast bacilli in tissues can be demonstrated more readily by fluorescence microscopy than by standard staining technics, this has not been borne out in the writer's experience with liver biopsy material.[148] Of greater significance is a recent report indicating that tubercle bacilli can be detected in stained smears and by guinea pig inoculation or culture of homogenized liver obtained by needle biopsy, even when granulomata cannot be demonstrated histologically.[10]

In guinea pigs, intramuscular injection of Freund's adjuvant produces epithelioid granulomas in the liver.[132] This suggests the interesting possibility that some hepatic lesions in patients with tuberculosis are due to the breakdown products of tubercle bacilli or to an immune reaction rather than to hematogenous spread of the infection.

The frequency with which tubercles are found in the liver depends upon the type of tuberculosis, its extent and degree of activity and the size of the specimen examined. In an extensive study of needle biopsy material, Haex and van Beek demonstrated granulomata in 90 to 100 per cent of cases in all forms of tuberculosis.[103] They attributed their success in large measure to the fact that they studied serial sections of all specimens. However, using the same technic the writer has found that, while the incidence of hepatic granulomata is close to 100 per cent in acute miliary tuberculosis and in "primary" miliary tuberculosis of the liver, it is nearer to 50 per cent in other forms of the disease.[148] Even fewer lesions have been encountered in studies based on single rather than serial sections.[187, 238] As pointed out by Hamperl,[108] one reason for the inordinately high incidence of hepatic granulomas reported by some investigators[103, 156] is their practice of classifying nonspecific foci of reticuloendothelial hyperplasia as tubercles.

Primary Tuberculous Infections. In the few biopsy studies of this form of the disease, granulomata have been found in the liver in approximately 64 per cent of cases.[187] From available reports it would appear that lesions of this type produce no significant symptoms.

In 452 successive autopsies in Cleveland, Reichle and Work found healed granulomata in the liver, spleen and kidneys in 20 per cent of cases and demonstrated the presence of tubercle bacilli by guinea pig inoculation in 3 of the 14 lesions investigated.[224] On the basis of collateral evidence they suggested that lesions of this type are attributable to hematogenous spread of tubercle bacilli during primary infections acquired early in life. Okudaira and associates questioned this interpretation; they presented evidence that, in endemic areas such as Ohio, healed granulomata in the liver and spleen, especially when calcified, are usually due to histoplasmosis.[205] Nevertheless, in view of the bacteriologic findings reported by Reichle and Work,[224] it must be conceded that at least some healed granulomata are of tuberculous origin. If such lesions are indicative of dissemination of tubercle bacilli during primary infections acquired early in life, the interesting possibility must be considered that the clinical syndromes of so-called "primary" tuberculosis of the liver and tuberculous splenomegaly are attributable to activation of such organisms rather than to recent hematogenous spread of tubercle bacilli from other sites.

Acute Miliary Tuberculosis. Almost always the liver is heavily seeded with granulomata in acute miliary tuberculosis, and occasionally lesions of this type give rise to hepatomegaly and jaundice.[72, 103, 144, 149, 181, 284] It is not clear whether the jaundice in such cases is due to granulomatous destruction of the parenchyma, obstruction of intrahepatic bile ducts, or toxic hepatocellular injury. Possibly, multiple mechanisms are involved.

Needle biopsy of the liver is a useful diagnostic procedure in this disease. Characteristic granulomata can be demonstrated in most cases, particularly if serial sections are examined, and sometimes even before pulmonary lesions are detectable radiographically.[60, 68, 149, 181] However, caution must be exercised in interpreting such lesions as conclusive evidence of tuberculosis, unless acid-fast bacilli can be demonstrated, which is not always possible.[149] Nevertheless, taken together with the presenting clinical features, the finding of miliary granulomata often is all that is needed to confirm a tentative diagnosis in cases of obscure fever.

Chronic Tuberculosis. Discrete miliary granulomata are demonstrable in the liver in a high proportion of fatal cases of chronic tuberculosis, the incidence being as high as 99 per cent in some autopsy series[168] and seldom less than 79 per cent in others.[237, 278] Their occurrence has been correlated with the presence of intestinal lesions by some investigators,[168] but not by others,[237] suggesting that tubercle bacilli reach the liver not only by way of the portal vein but also via the hepatic artery. Although the hepatic lesions found at autopsy may be indicative of terminal dissemination of tubercle bacilli, experience with biopsy material suggests that similar hematogenous spread can occur at any stage of the disease.[103, 149, 279] According to Haex and van Beek, the number, lobular distribution and histologic features of the hepatic lesions correlate with the clinical course of the underlying tuberculosis.[103, 279]

The hepatic granulomata in chronic tuberculosis seldom produce symptoms. However, it has been reported that in 80 per cent of fatal cases extensive terminal dissemination of tubercles to the liver gives rise to jaundice.[284] In at least one nonfatal case, active pulmonary tuberculosis was complicated by abdominal pain, obstructive jaundice and melena. Surgical exploration revealed massive hemorrhage into the biliary tree. Presumably the hemobilia was attributable to tuberculous involvement of the bile ducts, since caseating granulomata and acid-fast bacilli were demonstrated in the liver, and prompt recovery followed institution of specific chemotherapy.[2]

Occasionally, the tubercles in the liver and the spleen are calcified and are demonstrable roentgenographically. This occurs most commonly in children with chronic miliary tuberculosis.[198]

"Primary" Miliary Tuberculosis of the Liver. Occasionally, the liver is invaded massively by tubercle bacilli while the remaining tissues, with the exception of the spleen, are either spared or affected only minimally.[269] In untreated cases, the infection ultimately spreads to other tissues. Obviously, the infection is never "primary" in the liver, but often it is difficult to demonstrate the initial focus. The term *pylephlebogenous tuberculosis* has been applied to cases in which seeding of the liver has occurred via the portal vein from an infected site in the abdomen.[221, 284, 293] Similarly the syndrome of *Typhobacillosis of Landouzy*, described by European clinicians as a form of disseminated tuberculosis characterized by high fever and the absence of localizing signs, probably belongs in the category of "primary" hepatic tuberculosis, since the liver in such cases invariably contains numerous tubercles.[103]

The principal clinical features are chills, fever, sweats, prostration and weight loss. Abdominal pain and hepatosplenomegaly are common but inconstant findings. Occasionally, jaundice or ascites is present. Although overt localizing signs of extrahepatic tuberculosis or roentgenographic evidence of miliary pulmonary lesions are rare, peripheral adenopathy and calcification of abdominal lymph nodes are not unusual.

In cases with splenomegaly, particularly when accompanied by leukopenia and anemia, two features commonly seen in this disease, the clinical picture merges with that of splenic tuberculosis. Fundamentally, there is no difference between these two disorders, since in both, the liver and spleen are affected, and only rarely is it possible to establish which organ was involved first. Nevertheless, it is helpful clinically to distinguish between "primary" hepatic and splenic tuberculosis, since their presenting features differ somewhat.

Before the era of specific chemotherapy, the disease usually ran a fulminant course, terminating fatally within a few weeks or months. More recent experience indicates that infections of this type often respond to treatment with isoniazid, para-aminosalicylic acid and streptomycin.[269]

Splenic Tuberculosis. Miliary tubercles are found in the spleen in most cases of acute disseminated tuberculosis and, less commonly, in other forms of the disease. Rarely, the infection appears to be limited to the spleen, although, as pointed out, the liver also is affected in most cases. As in "primary" tuberculosis of the liver, it may

be difficult to demonstrate the initial focus of infection. Occasionally, the signs of splenic infection appear following apparent recovery from acute miliary tuberculosis.[189, 275]

In acute splenic tuberculosis, the principal features are splenomegaly and severe constitutional symptoms, including chills, fever, sweats, prostration and weight loss.[59, 292] In the chronic form, constitutional symptoms are less prominent, and the characteristic manifestations are splenomegaly and a variety of hemopoietic disorders, including anemia,[80, 123, 219] neutropenia,[53, 219] polycythemia,[88, 101] pancytopenia,[130] myelofibrosis[8] and granulocytic leukemia.[8] It is not clear whether the tuberculosis in such cases gives rise to the blood dyscrasia, is totally unrelated, or merely reflects an enhanced susceptibility to infection attributable to either the hemopoietic disease itself or to the agents used in its treatment. Although the relationship remains obscure, the fact that tuberculous infections in experimental animals may incite massive splenomegaly, pancytopenia and myelofibrosis suggests that, at least in some cases, tuberculosis is responsible for the development of myeloproliferative disorders in man.[8]

Although tubercles may be present in other tissues, simple splenectomy not infrequently effects an apparent cure in both the acute[59] and chronic[219] forms of the disease. The value of splenectomy in cases with polycythemia has been questioned.[88, 101] Since the operation is attended by a high mortality in all forms of splenic tuberculosis, it would seem reasonable to employ specific chemotherapy before resorting to splenectomy.

Tuberculomas. Rarely, large caseating masses or abscesses of tuberculous origin are found in the liver. Usually, a primary focus is demonstrable in the mesenteric nodes, intestine or lungs, but occasionally none can be found.[119] The suggestion that lesions of this type are produced by lymphogenous spread of tubercle bacilli, appears unlikely in view of the fact that the drainage of lymph in the liver is from within outward.

Tuberculomas, which may be single or multiple, give rise to chills, fever, enlargement and tenderness of the liver and, less commonly, splenomegaly and jaundice.[197] Usually, death ensues within a few months, but recovery has been reported following surgical drainage.[119] The effectiveness of specific chemotherapy has not been investigated.

Tuberculous Cholangitis ("Tubular" Tuberculosis of the Liver). This form of the disease is exceedingly rare and is said to occur chiefly in children and in races peculiarly susceptible to tuberculosis.[232] Spread of the infection to the biliary tract always follows rupture of a caseating tuberculoma or abscess into the bile ducts. Although tuberculous lesions are found in the intestine or the adjacent mesenteric nodes in most cases,[232, 284] there is no evidence to indicate that the cholangitis is due to an ascending infection. The lesions may be limited to one area or may extend along the entire course of the ducts.

Clinically, the principal features are a septic temperature, pain in the right upper quadrant, and cachexia. Jaundice and clay-colored stools occur when the larger ducts are involved[284] but are not seen in all cases.[232] Usually, the course is rapidly downhill and terminates fatally within a few months. However, in no case reported has specific chemotherapy been employed.

Nonspecific Changes in the Liver. The liver is fatty in a high proportion of individuals who die of tuberculosis; the incidence is 34 to 42 per cent in most autopsy series.[136, 168, 237, 278] It is said to be somewhat higher in tuberculous enteritis,[136] but this has not been borne out in all studies.[237] Malnutrition and chronic alcoholism appear to be the principal factors responsible for this change. Fatty infiltration is the most common cause of hepatomegaly in patients with tuberculosis and probably accounts for many of the alterations in hepatic function observed in such individuals.

Cirrhosis is found in 1 to 6 per cent of fatal cases.[168, 237, 278] Although healing of granulomata may result in focal scarring, there is no evidence that it produces cirrhosis. In most cases, the latter complication appears to be the result of associated malnutrition and chronic alcoholism.

At autopsy, many livers exhibit focal portal fibrosis, lymphocytosis, and proliferation of bile ducts,[168, 237] changes apparently unrelated to the presence of tubercles. The pathogenesis of these lesions is uncertain, although it has been suggested, on the basis of insufficient evidence, that they are due to the toxic products of the tubercle bacillus.[237] Possibly, they represent an early stage of alcoholic cirrhosis in some instances and healed granulomatous lesions in others.

Amyloidosis is far less common than fatty infiltration, occurring in only 5 to 10 per cent of fatal cases of pulmonary and osseous tuberculosis.[136, 278] The amyloid is deposited primarily between the sinusoidal endothelium and the parenchymal cells, causing atrophy of the latter as it accumulates. Clinically, the liver is enlarged and firm when amyloidosis is extensive, and often there is accompanying splenomegaly. Despite the parenchymal atrophy, there is remarkably little impairment of hepatic function. Jaundice is so rare that, when it occurs, it almost always is due to some other cause. Albuminuria, indicative of renal involvement, is present in most cases. Ascites occurs occasionally but seldom is due to amyloidosis alone.

Several authors have commented on the frequency of passive congestion of the liver in fatal cases of tuberculosis.[168, 278] In one series it was present in 94 per cent of cases and was attributed to right-sided heart failure secondary to advanced pulmonary disease.[278]

Liver Function in Tuberculosis. A high proportion of patients with active tuberculosis exhibit alterations in hepatic function.[124, 156] The rise in serum alpha and gamma globulin[245] and the abnormal cephalin-cholesterol flocculation reactions[156] in such individuals appear to be related to infection rather than to the presence of hepatic lesions. In patients with extensive granulomatous involvement of the liver, high levels of serum alkaline phosphatase may be seen. Bromsulphalein retention may be due to any of the hepatic lesions described. As indicated, jaundice and hyperbilirubinemia are rare, except in patients with tuberculous cholangitis and in a few with tuberculomas or miliary tuberculosis of the liver. Occasionally, the prothrombin level is depressed and is said to be a contributory factor in the pathogenesis of hemoptysis.[163]

LEPROSY

Approximately half the cases of lepromatous leprosy that come to autopsy exhibit miliary granulomata in the liver.[210, 272] These cannot be distinguished from the lesions seen in sarcoidosis and other granulomatous diseases. Often the liver also contains amyloid.

LEPTOSPIRAL AND SPIROCHETAL INFECTIONS

LEPTOSPIROSIS

Definition. Characteristically, *Leptospirae* that are pathogenic for man invade the blood stream and produce an acute febrile illness of relatively brief duration. Some of the more virulent strains induce acute inflammatory lesions, especially in the liver, kidneys, meninges, muscles and eyes, which not only prolong the disease but also give rise to some of its most striking clinical manifestations.

The term "Weil's disease" is somewhat ambiguous, since it is used both as a general designation for any type of leptospirosis that produces jaundice and as a synonym for infections with *L. icterohaemorrhagiae* specifically. The former interpretation is undesirable, since a classification of the leptospiroses based on the presence or the absence of jaundice overemphasizes the importance of an inconstant secondary manifestation of a systemic disease and necessitates an arbitrary distinction between icteric and nonicteric infections with the same organism. However, the latter interpretation is no easier to defend, since several strains of *Leptospirae* can produce the same clinical picture first described by Weil. The term "leptospirosis," qualified wherever possible by the strain and the special tissues involved, is more informative and less confusing but is more cumbersome.

Other terms used to describe infections with special strains of *Leptospirae* include canicola fever (*L. canicola*), mud fever (*L. grippotyphosa*), autumnal fever (*L. au-* *tumnalis*), swineherd's disease (*L. pomona*) and others. Some strains produce jaundice about as frequently as *L. icterohaemorrhagiae*, whereas others do so rarely or not at all.

Etiology. A large number of serologically distinct strains of pathogenic leptospirae have been identified,[100, 283] but only 5 account for the bulk of infections encountered in the United States: *L. icterohaemorrhagiae*, *L. canicola*,[229, 230] *L. pomona*,[25, 240, 267] *L. grippotyphosa*[32, 256] and *L. autumnalis*.[94] In all, some 22 serotypes have been identified in this country.[116]

Most leptospiral infections in this country are due to *L. icterohaemorrhagiae*, and some to *L. canicola*, strains that often produce jaundice. *L. grippotyphosa*, recently recovered from a jaundiced case in Texas,[256] causes mud fever or summer influenza, a mild nonicteric illness common in Eastern Europe.[283] *L. autumnalis* is the etiologic agent in Fort Bragg fever, a mild febrile disease characterized by fever, splenomegaly and pretibial rash without jaundice.[94] In Japan the same organism, or a closely allied variant, produces autumnal fever, a mild illness frequently accompanied by jaundice. *L. pomona* has been implicated in several nonicteric infections in this country.[25, 240, 267] In Europe, it produces swineherd's disease, which is characterized by a biphasic fever, rash, meningitis and gastroenteritis, and occasionally by jaundice.[99]

Although the various strains of leptospirae differ in antigenic structure and virulence, they exhibit identical morphologic features. Characteristically, they are long, slender structures, measuring 6 to 9 μ in length and 0.25 μ in breadth, with sharp pointed ends that are hooked either in the same or opposite directions. Tightly coiled minute spirals running their length give them a beaded appearance under darkfield illumination. Despite the absence of flagellae or undulating membranes, they are capable of a variety of undulating, twisting and propulsive movements. Apparently, minute forms occur, since Berkefeld filtrates, which contain no visible leptospirae, can infect guinea pigs.[128] In liquid media leptospirae are demonstrated best by means of darkfield illumination. Although it is possible to stain them in dried, thick films by the Giemsa technic, silver stains are required for their demonstration in tissues.

Leptospirae may be cultivated at 25 to 30° C. in a variety of media containing guinea-pig kidney, whole blood or serum, and may be grown on the chorioallantoic membrane of the chick embryo. However, it is more common to propagate them in susceptible animals. Young guinea pigs are used most widely, but since they may be resistant to such strains as *L. canicola*[229] and *L. grippotyphosa*,[256] hamsters and white mice often are employed. A wide variety of other rodents are also susceptible to experimental infections.

Coincidental with the disappearance of organisms from the blood stream in leptospiral infections, there is a rapid rise in the titer of specific serum agglutinins. Although cross-agglutination with other leptospirae is common, the titer usually is significantly higher with the specific strain involved. Therefore, serologic tests are reasonably reliable in distinguishing between various leptospiral infections, although it is not certain that all the strains identified in this way are distinct species. For the most accurate identification of leptospiral strains, absorption and neutralization tests are needed.

Epidemiology. Human infections with leptospirae invariably are the consequence of close contact with animals or their excreta. The animals that constitute the natural reservoir of these infections do not necessarily suffer any ill effects from the organisms they harbor, as in the case of the rat. However, some species, such as the dog, develop an acute illness which may closely resemble that seen in man.

As the principal vector of *L. icterohaemorrhagiae*, the rat is responsible for most cases of Weil's disease. The dog can transmit the disease to man but this is infrequent.[190, 193] *L. icterohaemorrhagiae* have been recovered from a variety of other animals, including field mice, cats, pigs, horses and foxes,[13, 31] but these do not appear to be responsible for infections in man.

In the rat, leptospirae are found in the kidney and urine, but not in the blood, liver or other tissues.[127] The infection is transmitted from rat to rat by ingestion of urine-contaminated food and water, and possibly through sexual intercourse.[31] A high proportion of the rat population has been found infected in all parts of the world where surveys have been carried out.[127, 243] In the United States the incidence in urban areas is 25 to 35 per cent.[190, 193]

Considering the opportunities for infection, it is noteworthy that only 67 cases of Weil's disease were reported in this country up until 1941,[13] an incidence well below that of Holland and England where rat leptospirosis is no more common. No doubt this reflects a failure on our part to recognize the disease. This is borne out by the rapid increase in the number of cases reported since clinicians have become aware of the prevalence of the disease and diagnostic laboratory facilities have become more generally available. Reports of 20 to 80 cases from a single city have become commonplace,[118, 194] and there is reason to believe that this trend will continue as interest in the disease grows and public health authorities provide more facilities for serologic testing.

With few exceptions, human infections with *L. icterohaemorrhagiae* can be traced to contact with contaminated rat urine. Occasionally, the disease is acquired as a result of rat-bite,[127] accidental contact with live cultures in the laboratory[243] or handling of infected rat tissues, as in the case of ratcatchers. Man-to-man and intra-uterine fetal infections are said to be rare,[13] and at least one instance of probable venereal transmission has been reported.[243] The abraded skin and the intact mucous membranes, especially of the conjunctival sac, nose, mouth and throat, serve as the usual portals of entry. There is considerable doubt that leptospirae can penetrate the intact skin,[243] and it is unlikely that they gain entry through the stomach and the upper intestinal tract, since they are destroyed readily in an acid medium. However, the guinea pig can be infected experimentally by feeding leptospirae or by instilling them into the rectum.[128]

Although Weil's disease may be acquired in any rat-infested environment, certain occupations provide peculiarly favorable conditions for infection, so much so, indeed, that some states now recognize leptospirosis as a compensable occupational disease.[31] In this country, fish cutters and cleaners, butchers, miners, ratcatchers, sewer workers, plumbers, tunnel diggers, garbage handlers and dock workers are particularly subject to the disease.[13, 31, 194] As might be expected, infected dogs constitute a special hazard for veterinarians and other dog handlers.[190] In other parts of the world, especially in tropical and semitropical areas, the disease is particularly likely to affect sugarcane cutters[212] and rice-field workers who are obliged to work in contaminated irrigated fields. During warfare soldiers not infrequently become infected in poorly drained trenches.

Another important way in which Weil's disease may be acquired is by swimming or by accidental immersion in stagnant bodies of water. The latter is particularly common in the canals of Holland.[283] Although swimming is said to be somewhat less hazardous than accidental immersion, outbreaks have been reported among swimmers both in this country[114] and abroad.[228, 283]

The environmental factors that favor the transmission of Weil's disease and account for many of its epidemiologic features include dampness, a temperature of 22° to 25° C., and a neutral or slightly alkaline medium[127] in which leptospirae may survive for as long as 3 weeks.[31] Although most cases in this country are said to occur during the summer months,[13] in one large series reported from Detroit[194] no seasonal variation in incidence was observed. In view of the occupations that predispose to infection, it is not surprising to find that 90 per cent of the cases occur in adult males, and that the disease is relatively rare in children.[194]

L. canicola infections follow close contact with dogs or their excreta.[229, 230] On the basis of serum agglutinin studies in healthy animals, it would appear that the incidence of leptospirosis is high, varying from 4 to 34 per cent in different areas.[190, 229] The relative frequency of *L. canicola* and *L. icterohaemorrhagiae* infections in dogs varies, but in general the former greatly outnumber the latter.[190] Both strains produce a severe illness in the dog which terminates fatally in 50 to 80 per cent of cases. The disease may be manifested by jaundice, a severe hemorrhagic gastroenteritis, or both.[229] Following recovery, the animal may excrete leptospirae in the urine for a number of months, due to the development of a chronic nephritis.

Since *L. canicola* survives in neutral stagnant water, as does *L. icterohaemorrhagiae*, human infections occasionally follow bathing in contaminated water. More often, however, they are the consequence of other types of direct or indirect contact with urine.

The relative infrequency of *L. canicola* infections in man, despite a high incidence in dogs, has been attributed to the following: the dog (1) is only a temporary shedder of leptospirae; (2) seldom contaminates the environment to the same extent as the rat; and (3) has acid urine, which does not permit long survival of leptospirae.[229]

In the swampy areas of eastern Europe, *L. grippotyphosa* is carried by the vole and the wood mouse, which contaminate the soil and the water with their urine and thus transmit the infection to man. In the only cases reported in this country[32, 256] the source of infection was not determined.

The animal vector of the *L. autumnalis* strain responsible for Fort Bragg fever is not known.[94] However, the closely related type strain *Akiyami A*, which produces autumnal fever in Japan, is carried by the field mouse.[283]

In some parts of Europe, swine are asymptomatic carriers of *L. pomona* and serve as the intermediate host in swineherd's disease.[99] In this country, the same organism is responsible for recurrent iridocyclitis in horses and recently has been identified in cattle,[95] swine[240] and mules.[240] Of the cases reported in this country, one outbreak occurred in a group of individuals who swam in a creek in which several dead hogs had been seen,[240] one followed the handling of raw beef and pork in an abattoir,[25] and the last occurred in an individual who had been in contact with young pigs.[267] Since *L. pomona* has not been found in rats,[240] it is highly probable that the infection in these individuals was acquired from swine.

Pathogenesis. Following an incubation period of 7 to 13 days (extreme 4 to 19),[243] and coincidental with the onset of symptoms, *L. icterohaemorrhagiae* which have gained access to the body appear in the blood in large numbers and soon are disseminated to many, if not all, tissues.[128] By the end of a week, however, the leptospirae usually have vanished from the blood and seldom can be found in any tissue except the kidney and occasionally the liver.[112, 128, 179] Rarely, a few degenerate leptospirae are demonstrable in the adrenals, lymph nodes, myocardium, spleen, testis, lung, pancreas, intestine, gallbladder, central nervous system and skin as late as the 16th day of the disease.[128] It is generally assumed that the disappearance of organisms from both the blood and tissues is related to the development of immune bodies,[128] although diagnostically significant titers usually cannot be demonstrated until several days to a week later.

Clinical manifestations related to the involvement of the liver, kidney and other special tissues do not become evident until the end of the 1st week, or even later, when leptospiremia is diminishing or actually has ceased. Since most fatalities occur in the 2nd and 3rd week of the disease,[13, 128] little is known about the early lesions in man. However, the autopsy findings in several cases that have died on the 5th or 6th day[112, 179, 249] suggest that tissue injury may occur during the stage of leptospiremia and before localizing symptoms become evident. In experimental animals, leptospirae may be demonstrable in the liver before they appear in the blood.[12]

The liver, kidneys, muscles and blood vessels are the tissues most frequently involved in leptospirosis *icterohaemorrhagiae*, but many others may be affected in individual cases.

Liver. One of the striking features of Weil's disease is the remarkable discrepancy between the severity of jaundice and the extent of hepatic lesions found at autopsy. The histologic changes observed usually include: (1) dissociation of the hepatic cells and disorganization of the centrilobular architecture, (2) active hepatocellular regeneration, as evidenced by the presence of binucleate cells and mitoses, (3) minimal degenerative changes in the cytoplasm and the nuclei of the parenchymal cells, (4) bile stasis, especially in the centrilobular canaliculi and (5) a predominantly mononuclear infiltration of the portal zones.[9, 13, 179, 249]

In the most severe cases, small areas of focal necrosis occur, and, rarely, massive hepatic necrosis has been reported.[251]

However, necrosis is distinctly unusual, and the liver may show no changes whatever in severe cases with deep jaundice.[249]

It is difficult to account for the unusual regenerative activity of the parenchyma which is such a striking feature in this disease. It would seem reasonable to suppose that it represents a response to antecedent cellular necrosis. However, serial studies of the liver in experimentally infected animals do not support this interpretation, mitotic activity being demonstrable in the absence of necrosis, as in man.[12] Nevertheless, the hepatic cells show cytoplasmic ultrastructural changes suggestive of toxic injury.[236] These include dilatation of the endoplasmic reticulum and Golgi apparatus, swelling of the mitochondria, and an increase in lysosomes.

Leptospirae can be demonstrated in the liver in only half the cases that come to autopsy. Usually, they overlie the parenchymal cells but do not appear to penetrate them.[12]

Almost certainly the jaundice in Weil's disease is due to hepatocellular injury. Since it may occur in the absence of necrosis,[249] it must be assumed that morphologically intact cells suffer a functional impairment of bilirubin excretion. There is no evidence of extrahepatic biliary obstruction, and the presence of bile thrombi in the canaliculi is probably the consequence of cellular injury and bile stasis, rather than of intrahepatic biliary obstruction. Phagocytosis of erythrocytes occurs in the liver, spleen and sites of hemorrhage,[12] so that an increased rate of hemoglobin breakdown may contribute to the development of jaundice. However, it is never severe enough to account for the depth of jaundice usually encountered in Weil's disease.

Since nonicteric leptospirosis is rarely fatal, it is not known whether it produces changes in the liver. Abnormalities of hepatic function have been observed in some cases,[230] but not in others.[145]

Kidneys. In general, the renal lesions in Weil's disease[13, 133, 249] are more impressive than those in the liver, and leptospirae are demonstrable more frequently. When present, the latter are found both in the tubules and the interstitial tissue.[13, 110]

Usually, the kidneys are enlarged and moderately bile-stained. Microscopically, they show: (1) degeneration and necrosis of the convoluted tubules; (2) a diffuse inflammatory reaction in the interstitial tissue characterized by an infiltrate of lymphocytes, monocytes and occasional polymorphonuclear and eosinophilic leukocytes; (3) numerous granular casts, and cellular debris in the distal convoluted and collecting tubules; and (4) small hemorrhages into the capsule, the interstitial tissue and the tubules. Usually, the glomeruli are intact, but occasionally they show changes resembling those in acute glomerular nephritis.[13]

The lesions in the kidney are probably due to the invasion of leptospirae and not to the associated hepatic failure. As might be expected from their localization, they frequently produce a type of renal insufficiency that closely resembles that seen in acute tubular necrosis due to other causes.

Muscles. Highly characteristic lesions can be demonstrated in the skeletal muscles in most *L. icterohaemorrhagiae* infections, and their number can be correlated with the severity of the disease.[250] It is possible that they are responsible for the myalgia which is such a striking clinical feature. Early in the disease individual fibers show localized areas of vacuolization with loss of striations and multiplication of adjacent sarcolemma nuclei. Later, sarcolemma cells invade these necrotic foci and remove any remaining debris. In mild cases, new myofibrils appear within these cells, whereas in more severe cases the foci are infiltrated with lymphocytes and plasma cells and undergo fibrosis. Leptospirae have not been demonstrated in any of these lesions, although they have not been studied before the 8th day of the disease. The absence of hemorrhage and vascular lesions serves to distinguish them from

Zenker's degeneration and the lesions seen in rickettsial disease.

Blood Vessels. Frequently the serosal surfaces, the mucous membranes and many of the viscera exhibit petechial hemorrhages. In more severe cases, there may be purpura of the skin and gross bleeding into the gastrointestinal tract, pulmonary tree or urinary tract. Since the platelet count is not reduced and the bleeding and coagulation times are not prolonged, it is generally believed that the hemorrhages are due to capillary injury.[13] Usually the prothrombin concentration is only slightly to moderately decreased,[246] but occasionally it falls to very low levels in severely jaundiced cases[31] and thus may contribute to the hemorrhagic tendency.

Central Nervous System.[13] Often, the meninges are the site of a low-grade lymphocytic and plasmocytic inflammatory reaction. Usually, this is accompanied by pleocytosis of the cerebrospinal fluid. Degenerative changes are seen in the neurons, but there is no inflammatory reaction in the substance of the brain or the spinal cord.

Heart. A variety of lesions may occur in the heart, including (1) hemorrhages into the epicardium and endocardium, (2) round-cell infiltration and degenerative changes in the myocardium resembling those seen in skeletal muscle[31] and (3) rarely, acute vegetative endocarditis.[13]

Clinical Manifestations.[13, 133, 246] The clinical manifestations of leptospirosis *icterohaemorrhagiae* emerge in two phases. Early in the disease, there are severe constitutional symptoms related to the presence of leptospirae in the blood. Later, localizing signs appear, pointing to invasion of the specialized tissues, especially the liver, kidneys and meninges. The two phases overlap to some extent, and in some cases localizing signs never develop. In classic Weil's disease, hepatic and renal manifestations dominate the latter half of the clinical course. Occasionally, these are accompanied by signs of an inflammatory reaction in the meninges, eyes, myocardium or other tissues. Although these are generally considered complications of the disease, they are, in fact, evidence of the same type of leptospiral invasion that occurs in the liver and the kidney. Occasionally, the liver is spared, and the major localizing manifestations are limited to other specialized tissues. This is particularly likely to occur in mild infections with *L. icterohaemorrhagiae*, or with some of the other strains that ordinarily do not induce jaundice.

Characteristically, the onset of symptoms in leptospirosis *icterohaemorrhagiae* is sudden, with fever, muscular pain, headache and severe prostration. The lumbar muscles and the calves are particularly involved and may be tender. Chilly sensations are common, and occasionally a shaking chill ushers in the disease. Usually, marked conjunctival infection is present and is a helpful diagnostic sign. As the disease progresses, hemorrhagic herpes labialis, gastrointestinal symptoms, nuchal rigidity and cough may appear. Morbilliform and scarlatiniform rashes are seen occasionally but are unusual. At this stage, leptospirae can be demonstrated in the blood, but physical signs, other than those of a severe infection, may be completely lacking. Leukocytosis is common and often the cerebrospinal fluid contains an increased number of cells.

Toward the end of the 1st week, as the leptospirae are disappearing from the blood, the temperature falls, but the general condition worsens. Although muscular aching and many of the other constitutional symptoms diminish, prostration, anorexia and gastrointestinal complaints increase, and at the same time the characteristic signs of hepatic and renal involvement appear. Jaundice, which usually is noted on the 6th or 7th day, rapidly increases in intensity, reaching a peak within a few days. Generally it is accompanied by enlargement and tenderness of the liver, bilirubinuria and, occasionally, clay-colored stools, pruritus and bradycardia. Splenomegaly occurs in less than 10 per cent of cases.

During the initial febrile period, the urine often contains a small amount of albumin, a few cells and casts. However, as the typical renal lesion develops, the urinary output falls, albuminuria increases, casts, leukocytes and erythrocytes appear in increasing numbers, the specific gravity tends to become fixed at 1.010, and, in the most severe cases, azotemia and anuria ensue. The blood pressure tends to fall to a low level, and a number of other cardiovascular abnormalities may be noted. Epistaxis and other hemorrhagic phenomena often occur at this time. Central nervous system manifestations are also common, especially in seriously ill patients.

In favorable cases, clinical improvement becomes evident as early as the end of the 2nd week. Convalescence may be delayed until the 3rd or 4th week in severe infections. Usually, recovery is slow, convalescence being marked by asthenia and anemia. Relapses occur in approximately 20 per cent of cases. These are characterized by a brief recrudescence of fever and mild constitutional symptoms which appear between the 3rd and 5th week. Rarely, there are several such episodes.

Most deaths occur on the 9th to 16th day, although fatalities have been reported as early as the 5th and as late as the 21st day.[179] Renal and hepatic failure account for most of these, but cardiac decompensation, massive hemorrhage and terminal pneumonia may be important complicating factors. The mortality rate in *L. icterohaemorrhagiae* infections varies in different parts of the world. Differences in strain virulence, individual susceptibility and environmental factors probably account for some of these variations, but the frequency with which mild infections are recognized would appear to be an important factor, especially since the mortality rate in nonicteric cases is negligible. In this country the rate is approximately 25 per cent, which is somewhat higher than in parts of Europe where there is a greater awareness of the disease.[243]

Fever. Characteristically the temperature rises abruptly to 102° to 104° F., runs an irregular remittent course and falls to normal by rapid lysis in 4 to 7 days. Occasionally, fever is more prolonged, but it rarely exceeds 12 days.[126] Although a sudden onset is highly characteristic, it is not seen in all cases. Severe shaking chills are relatively uncommon. The brevity of the fever and the absence of recurrent chills are of great importance in differential diagnosis.

Jaundice. The onset of jaundice is variable but rarely if ever occurs before the 3rd or after the 10th day of disease. Characteristically, it reaches a maximum within a few days and then subsides over a period of a week to 10 days. The intensity of the jaundice is variable, depending on the severity of the infection but, in general, tends to be mild to moderate.[118] Tests of liver function usually reveal the typical pattern of hepatocellular injury.[56, 261] On the basis of current statistics, it is estimated that one third of infections with *L. icterohaemorrhagiae* are unaccompanied by jaundice.[31] It has been suggested that the liver is not completely spared in such cases, since hepatomegaly[246] and impairment of liver function are common.[230]

Renal Manifestations. All gradations of renal injury are seen in Weil's disease. In approximately 15 per cent of cases, the kidney appears to be spared.[283] This is apt to occur in patients without jaundice. However, severe renal failure has been reported in nonicteric Weil's disease and has been termed leptospiral nephritis.[262] Despite its severity, the renal lesion appears to be reversible and goes on to complete recovery in nonfatal cases. Often, leptospirae can be demonstrated in the urine between the 13th and 15th days and occasionally as early as the 6th day.[128] Usually, they disappear by the 40th day but, rarely, may persist for many months.[262]

Meninges and Central Nervous System. Spinal-fluid pleocytosis and xanthochromia are seen in approximately 90 percent of patients with Weil's disease.[50] Usually, the cell count is under 100 but may be as high as 3,000/cu. mm. Lymphocytes predominate, but in the first week of the disease as many as 50 per cent of the cells may be polymorphonuclear. The nature of the pigment is not known. Although it is assumed to be bilirubin, often there is a discrepancy between the small amount that can be determined chemically and the depth of the color observed visually.[58] The protein content is increased in only half the fluids with pleocytosis and seldom is high. Only half the cases with abnormal spinal fluid findings develop clinical signs of meningitis. Occasionally, meningismus occurs in the absence of spinal fluid abnormalities. Leptospirae may be demonstrable in the fluid during the first week of the disease.[133]

Meningitis is seen also in nonicteric infections with *L. icterohaemorrhagiae*[24, 48] and may be readily confused with other forms of lymphocytic meningitis due to neurotropic viruses. Certain clinical and epidemiologic features suggest that there are some fundamental differences between this type of leptospiral meningitis and that seen in classic Weil's disease. The former occurs in males under the age of 30, chiefly late in the summer, and usually is associated with a normal leukocyte count and little or no muscle tenderness.[24] It is particularly apt to occur following bathing or accidental immersion in infected waters and often is accompanied by pharyngitis, suggesting that the portal of entry is in the nasopharynx or possibly the conjunctivae.[48] Characteristically, the clinical course is benign, and the patients are rarely severely ill. An identical type of meningitis is seen frequently in swineherd's disease due to *L. pomona*.[99]

A variety of other central nervous system manifestations in seriously ill patients with leptospirosis include delirium, hallucinations, restlessness, apathy, convulsions and loss of consciousness. Since morphologic changes seldom can be demonstrated, it must be assumed that they are due to functional disturbances related to the toxemia of infection, renal insufficiency and hepatic failure.

Hemorrhage. Epistaxis and small conjunctival petechiae are relatively common in Weil's disease. In severe cases, hemorrhages occur with great regularity.[126] These may take the form of purpura in the skin and mucous membranes, melena, hematemesis, hemoptysis or hematuria. Rarely, massive hemorrhage into the adrenals may produce the Waterhouse-Friderichsen syndrome.[131]

Ocular Manifestations. Iridocyclitis, a late sequel of Weil's disease, occurs in approximately 10 per cent of patients.[13] It may appear during convalescence or not until a number of months have elapsed following recovery. The same complication has been reported recently following an *L. pomona* infection in this country.[25] Optic neuritis and hemorrhages into various portions of the ocular globe also occur but are unusual.

Gastrointestinal Symptoms. Anorexia, nausea, vomiting, constipation and abdominal pain are frequent complaints in Weil's disease. The pain is of particular importance, since it may lead to errors in diagnosis and needless surgical exploration for acute appendicitis or cholecystitis.[118]

Cardiovascular Manifestations. In addition to hypotension and tachycardia, which are common in many other severe infections, patients with Weil's disease are particularly subject to disturbances in cardiac function. Dilatation of the heart, gallop rhythm, conduction defects, arrhythmias and electrocardiographic abnormalities occur.[31] These probably can be related to the presence of myocardial lesions, although functional disturbances due to renal failure, hemorrhage and toxemia may play a role in many cases. Pericarditis also occurs occasionally.[58] All of these abnormalities appear to be reversible and leave no residuals following recovery. Rarely, leptospirae are responsible for an acute vegetative endocarditis.[13] Of interest is a report of myocarditis and arthritis due to an *L. pomona* infection which simulated rheumatic fever.[267]

Respiratory. Almost half the patients with Weil's disease develop cough and sputum, and occasionally these are accompanied by signs of a patchy pneumonitis.[31, 246]

Canicola Fever. Infections with *L. canicola* produce a clinical picture that is almost identical with that of classic Weil's disease due to *L. icterohaemorrhagiae.* However, the symptoms tend to be somewhat less severe, jaundice is less frequent, and death is rare.[229, 230]

Laboratory Features. HEMATOLOGIC.[13, 31, 228, 246] Usually, the leukocyte count is 12,000 to 20,000, but may be as high as 30,000/cu. mm. The percentage of polymorphonuclear cells is increased, and occasionally myelocytes can be demonstrated in the peripheral blood smear. The bleeding and clotting times and the platelet count are usually normal. A microcytic hypochromic anemia, probably due to hemorrhage, often is present late in the disease.

Liver Function Tests. In jaundiced cases the results of liver function tests are consistent with hepatocellular injury. There is an increase in serum bilirubin, thymol turbidity, serum alkaline phosphatase, Bromsulphalein retention and urine urobilinogen, and a decrease in prothrombin and serum cholesterol. The cephalin-cholesterol flocculation reaction is positive.[56] Bile is present in the urine, and the stools may be clay-colored.[246] The prompt direct-reacting fraction of bilirubin in the serum is increased.[261] On electrophoretic analysis, the serum shows an increase in alpha-2 and gamma globulin and a decrease in albumin.[261]

Demonstration of Leptospirae. Leptospirae are present in the blood during the 1st week of the disease but not thereafter. Usually, they appear in the urine toward the end of the 2nd week and may persist for 30 days or more.[128] Occasionally, they can be demonstrated in the spinal fluid during the period of leptospiremia.[133]

Methods used to detect leptospirae in these fluids include (1) darkfield examination, (2) animal inoculation and (3) culture. On the whole, inoculation of susceptible animals, especially young guinea pigs, mice and hamsters, is most satisfactory. Cultural technics are probably equally effective, but few routine laboratories are prepared to carry them out. Darkfield examination of blood is the least reliable method, except in the hands of an expert, since fibrin strands are readily mistaken for leptospirae. However, the procedure may be of value in demonstrating leptospirae in the urine.

Guinea pigs, weighing approximately 175 Gm., are injected intraperitoneally with 3 to 5 ml. of defibrinated blood or plasma, or the spun sediment of freshly passed neutral urine suspended in saline. The animal usually exhibits jaundice on the 7th or 8th day and dies on the 10th to 12th. At autopsy, the characteristic findings are bile staining of the tissues, and hemorrhages into the pleura and the peritoneum. Leptospirae are readily demonstrable in the blood and peritoneal fluids by darkfield examination or culture. Often, it is possible to recover the organisms earlier by examining aspirated peritoneal fluid when the animal's temperature rises on the 4th or 5th day.

Serologic Tests. Specific agglutinins appear in the serum during the 2nd week. Rarely, they can be detected as early as the 6th day,[133] but diagnostic titers of 1:300 usually are not found before the 14th day.[13] The titer continues to rise during convalescence, often exceeding 1:20,000, and not infrequently remains elevated for many years.[209] The most reliable results are obtained with a freshly prepared antigen of suspended formalinized leptospirae.[243]

Specific lysins and complement-fixing antibodies are also present in the serum. The latter appear somewhat earlier than the agglutinins and lysins, occasionally as early as the 2nd day.[96]

Diagnosis. During the first few days, Weil's disease may be confused with a number of febrile illnesses, including influenza, typhus, trichinosis, brucellosis and sepsis of various types. As localizing signs develop in the liver, kidneys and meninges, it must be differentiated from viral hepatitis, obstructive jaundice, acute nephritis and acute bacterial and viral meningitis.

The occupational history, or other opportunity for exposure to a rat-contaminated environment or to dogs, the abrupt onset, early prostration, muscle pain and prominent conjunctival injection should alert the clinician to the possibility of Weil's disease early in the course. Later, the combination of jaundice with signs of nephritis and/or meningitis is highly suggestive of the diagnosis. Spinal-fluid xanthochromia and pleocytosis are particularly important clues, since the combination is seldom seen in any type of jaundice other than leptospiral. In severe viral hepatitis and decompensated cirrhosis with jaundice, the spinal fluid may contain a small amount of bilirubin and an increased concentration of protein, but the cell count remains normal.[7] Rarely, biliary obstruction is associated with spinal-fluid xanthochromia, but only when the jaundice is intense and of long duration. In contrast, Weil's disease often produces xanthochromia when the jaundice is mild and of very short duration.[50] The brevity of the febrile period, usually less than a week and

rarely as long as 12 days, is another important feature which serves to distinguish Weil's disease from many of the other conditions which simulate it.

The most difficult cases to recognize are those in which jaundice does not develop. These may present as acute fevers without localizing signs, or as cases of primary meningitis or nephritis. Except in the mildest infections, the clinical features are identical with those of the leptospiremic stage of Weil's disease.

Of prime importance in the diagnosis is the need for a more general awareness of the wide distribution of the disease and its protean manifestations. Once Weil's disease is considered as a possibility, laboratory confirmation is relatively simple. During the 1st week an attempt should be made to isolate leptospirae from the blood by guinea-pig inoculation. At the same time, a specimen of blood should be examined for leptospiral agglutinins. Since these usually are not demonstrable in significant titer until the end of the 2nd week, the first determination merely serves as a baseline for subsequent determinations, which should be carried out at weekly intervals. A titer of 1:300 is generally considered diagnostic. If there is no rise in titer by the end of a month, the diagnosis of Weil's disease can be excluded. Muscle biopsy and spinal-fluid examination are important adjuncts, since they make it possible in many cases to establish a presumptive diagnosis before the results of guinea-pig inoculation can be obtained, or before the rise in agglutinins can be demonstrated.

Treatment. Of all the specific therapeutic agents that have been tried in Weil's disease, only immune serum of animal origin [13, 128, 228] and transfusions of convalescent whole blood and plasma[13, 118, 128, 212] are effective and then only if given before jaundice appears. Unfortunately, antileptospiral serum is not available in this country, and, only under the most unusual circumstances, is a convalescent donor at hand.

The results of antibiotic therapy have been equivocal. Penicillin is lethal for leptospirae in cultures and protects guinea pigs against death if given within 18 hours of infection; however, it is not effective if administered after symptoms appear.[6] There are reports of excellent results in patients treated on the 1st day of disease,[212] and failures in cases whose treatment was begun after jaundice appeared.[126]

In a group of 67 cases studied in Puerto Rico, penicillin, chlortetracycline, oxytetracycline, chloramphenicol and streptomycin had no effect on the duration of fever and failed to prevent or ameliorate hepatic and renal involvement.[105] Interestingly, the antibiotics frequently failed to eradicate leptospiremia and prevent relapses.[31] However, the treatment was not begun until an average of 6.7 days had elapsed, and 44 per cent of cases were jaundiced.

In view of its *in vitro* action on leptospirae and its effectiveness in protecting animals against fatal infections,[6] it would seem reasonable to employ massive doses of penicillin early in the course of Weil's disease, at least until the results of antibiotic therapy have been evaluated more fully.

The general management of Weil's disease is much like that of any other acute systemic infection. However, there is, in addition, an urgent need for a close watch on kidney function, and, when renal insufficiency supervenes, for judicious regulation of fluid, electrolyte and nitrogen balance. As in other types of acute renal failure characterized by severe oliguria and azotemia, the aim is to maintain the internal chemical environment as close to normal as possible. This is accomplished by limiting the intake of fluid and electrolytes to measured or estimated losses and maintaining a low-protein intake while providing sufficient carbohydrate and fat to meet caloric demands. Frequent determinations of blood and urine electrolytes greatly facilitate such regulation but are not always essential.

Often, blood loss is an important consideration in severe infections and should be replaced.

There is no evidence that diet affects the hepatic lesion in leptospirosis. The high-protein intake often recommended in liver disease may be distinctly harmful if renal insufficiency is present.

Prophylaxis. Vaccines prepared from heat-killed or phenol-treated leptospirae are effective immunizing agents.[283] They are used to some extent in areas where the disease is prevalent, as in Japan, and in laboratory workers who are heavily exposed to infection.

RELAPSING FEVER

Often the liver and spleen are enlarged in relapsing fever and, in severe cases, there may be jaundice.[57, 294] The latter is not accompanied by other signs of hepatic failure and fades promptly when the fever subsides. Presumably, the jaundice is due to hepatocellular injury, although, as in Weil's disease, necrosis is unusual. In fatal infections, which invariably are accompanied by jaundice, the liver is enlarged and intensely congested. The Kupffer cells are swollen and contain phagocytized red blood cells, spirochetes and pigment, and the portal zones show a moderate inflammatory reaction.[11]

SYPHILIS

Congenital Syphilis. *Treponema pallidum* infections of the fetus tend to be severe, and frequently cause fetal death resulting in abortion or stillbirth. Severely infected infants who survive may appear normal at birth, but usually exhibit evidence of widespread syphilitic involvement of the tissues within a few weeks. In those with less severe infections, manifestations of congenital syphilis, usually of more limited distribution, may not appear until several years later.[263]

Many infants with congenital syphilis exhibit hepatosplenomegaly. Frank jaundice is relatively uncommon, but, when present at birth and accompanied by anemia, may simulate erythroblastosis.[93] However, other stigmata of syphilis, such as osteochondritis, periostitis or skin lesions and a positive serologic test for syphilis are always present, so that diagnosis is seldom difficult. Hypoproteinemia and edema are seen in some cases. Hepatosplenomegaly and jaundice recede following penicillin therapy.[93]

In fatal cases of congenital hepatic syphilis, the liver shows a fine diffuse fibrosis that extends from the portal triads into the lobules, enclosing the parenchymal plates, a diffuse round-cell inflammatory reaction involving both the septa and parenchyma, small granulomatous lesions within the septa, and evidence of arteritis. In Levaditi silver-stained sections, numerous treponemata can be demonstrated within connective tissue trabeculae, the walls of small vessels and the parenchymal cells.[177]

Early Acquired Syphilis. Rarely, the rash, mucosal lesions and lymphadenopathy of secondary syphilis are accompanied by an *acute hepatitis* with jaundice that clears promptly following institution of specific antiluetic therapy.[51, 104] The clinical features in such cases are said to be indistinguishable from those of viral hepatitis. On microscopic examination, the hepatic parenchyma shows numerous miliary granulomata and a diffuse, round-cell inflammatory reaction.[104] This type of hepatitis, which is limited to patients with untreated, early active syphilis, must be distinguished from the cholestatic hepatitis induced by drug-sensitization early in the course of treatment with organic arsenicals,[109] the toxic hepatitis produced by massive arsenotherapy,[162] and intercurrent viral hepatitis acquired in the course of intravenous therapy with improperly sterilized equipment.[235]

Late Syphilis. The characteristic hepatic lesion of late syphilis is the *gumma*, a focal granuloma that tends to undergo central caseous necrosis followed by encapsulation and fibrosis, ultimately giving rise to a contracted stellate scar. The lesions vary in size from microscopic to grossly visible, large nodules, and usually are multiple in number and irregular in distribution. When the gummas are numerous, scarring distorts the normal architecture of the liver, producing the picture of *hepar lobatum*, which, superficially at least, may resemble a coarsely nodular postnecrotic cirrhosis.[104, 268] Occasionally, amyloidosis of the liver is an accompanying feature.[268]

In most cases, hepatic gummas are asymptomatic. Occasionally, however, they give rise to abdominal pain and fever, which respond to antiluetic therapy.[104] When the lesions are multiple and associated with extensive scarring (hepar lobatum), jaundice, ascites and signs of portal hyperten-

sion may appear.[104, 268] The liver may be enlarged and tender, and, occasionally, nodules can be palpated. Splenomegaly is relatively uncommon.

The diagnosis of hepatic syphilis may be exceedingly difficult in patients with serologic and other evidence of syphilis who present with overt signs of liver disease. Not infrequently the latter prove to be manifestations of nonsyphilitic lesions, the most common being Laennec's cirrhosis. Liver biopsy is helpful in such cases.

MYCOTIC INFECTIONS

ACTINOMYCOSIS[65]

In abdominal actinomycosis, the liver not infrequently is infected via portal radicles draining involved segments of the intestinal tract or by direct extension from contiguous viscera. In disseminated infections, organisms may reach the liver by way of the hepatic arteries. Occasionally, the disease appears to be primary in the liver, but, obviously, infections of this type must arise in an inconspicuous lesion somewhere in the distribution of the portal vein. In rare instances, the gallbladder appears to be the primary focus. It has been suggested that in cases of this type the organisms invade the gallbladder via the bile ducts.

On reaching the liver, *Actinomyces bovis* induce a granulomatous reaction and fibrosis. As the lesions extend, they undergo central necrosis, giving rise to characteristic thick-walled multiloculated abscesses. Often these reach the surface of the liver and extend into the abdominal wall, the diaphragm or the adjacent viscera.

The signs of hepatic involvement may be overlooked when there are more extensive lesions in the other intra-abdominal viscera. Usually, however, the liver is enlarged and tender and may exhibit localized swellings on its surface. Irregular fever, sweats, leukocytosis and anemia are the usual concomitant findings.

Diagnosis depends on the demonstration of *A. bovis* in aspirated pus or tissue sections. Until the organisms are found, differentiation from amebic abscess, malignancy and gumma may be difficult.

BLASTOMYCOSIS

The primary lesion in *Blastomyces dermatitidis* infections is either in the skin or the lungs. In the pulmonary type, general dissemination is not uncommon, and the liver is one of the organs frequently involved.[185] The lesions produced are usually suppurative but occasionally are granulomatous and closely resemble those in tuberculosis.

Brazilian blastomycosis,[46] a closely related disease due to *Paracoccidioides brasiliensis*, usually starts in the mouth and spreads to the adjacent lymph nodes. In some cases the organisms are disseminated to the liver, spleen and bone marrow. The principal clinical manifestations, which include fever, anemia, eosinophilia, adenopathy and splenomegaly, often suggest Hodgkin's disease.

In the liver the organisms are localized chiefly in the periportal tissues, where they incite a granulomatous reaction characterized by a nodular infiltration of lymphocytes, eosinophils and foreign-body giant cells. Later, these areas undergo fibrosis, giving rise to a cirrhosis-like picture.

COCCIDIOIDOMYCOSIS

Coccidioides immitis gives rise to two types of infection: (1) an acute benign, self-limited, influenza-like disease, known as "San Joaquin Valley Fever" and (2) a chronic progressive coccidial granulomatosis which often is fatal. The former represents a primary infection of the lung and often is associated with hilar adenopathy and erythema nodosum. The latter is the result of a wide-spread dissemination of the organisms from a primary site, usually in the lung, to many of the tissues including the liver, where they produce isolated granulomas and abscess-like foci.[244]

Occasionally, the disseminated form of the disease mimics sarcoidosis. In one such case, the principal features included fever, weight loss, peripheral and hilar adenopathy, uveitis, arthritis and epididymitis.[15] Biopsy sections of the epididymis and a peripheral node revealed noncaseating granulomata indistinguishable from those of sarcoidosis. Recovery followed treatment with amphotericin B.

CRYPTOCOCCOSIS (TORULOSIS)

Cryptococcus neoformans, a yeast commonly found in soil and in the excreta of pigeons, is pathogenic for man.[166] If dust containing these organisms is inhaled, granulomatous pneumonitis results. It often runs a benign, self-limited course and may be asymptomatic. Dissemination of the infection to other tissues, and particularly the central nervous system, bone and skin, is a serious, and often fatal, complication seen most commonly in patients with underlying lymphomatous disease. Occasionally, dissemination is limited to the meninges, a type of infection that occurs especially in individuals exposed to pigeons.

The tissues invaded by cryptococci show a granulomatous reaction accompanied by little necrosis.[166] Occasionally, both the lesions and the clinical features resemble those of sarcoidosis.[252]

Although disseminated cryptococcal infections frequently are accompanied by hepatosplenomegaly and the presence in the liver of small granulomata, they seldom give rise to overt clinical manifestations of hepatic disease. Only two instances of extensive hepatocellular necrosis leading to hepatic failure and death have been reported.[234] In both cases, the zones of necrosis contained numerous cryptococci, suggesting an etiologic relationship. However, the possibility that the organisms were secondary invaders in an underlying viral or drug-induced hepatitis could not be excluded.

Amphotericin B appears to be effective in the treatment of disseminated cryptococcosis, although relapses are common in cases with central nervous system involvement.[166]

HISTOPLASMOSIS

There is growing evidence that histoplasmosis is a relatively common disease in this country, especially in the Mississippi Valley.[22] Most infections are asymptomatic and are manifested by benign pulmonary lesions or skin sensitivity to histoplasmin.

Occasionally, however, *Histoplasma capsulatum* gives rise to serious lung disease, ulcerative lesions in the mucosa of the oropharynx and larynx, or widely disseminated lesions in the liver, spleen, visceral lymph nodes, bone marrow, kidneys, adrenals, endocardium and other tissues.[211] Patients with lymphomatous disease appear to be peculiarly susceptible to this type of infection.[200]

The characteristic lesion is a granuloma composed of epithelioid and giant cells. The organisms, which are present in large numbers engulfed in epithelioid and other phagocytic reticuloendothelial cells, may be difficult to demonstrate in routine sections, unless stained by the Hotchkiss-McManus technic.[129, 214]

The close resemblance between the clinical and histologic features in histoplasmosis and sarcoidosis has been emphasized repeatedly.[129, 214, 225] Even the Schaumann bodies and the asteroids, so characteristic of the lesion in sarcoidosis, may be seen in histoplasmosis.[214] Differentiation between the two diseases depends upon the presence or absence of histoplasma in the tissues and skin sensitivity to histoplasmin. On clinical grounds, histoplasmosis should be suspected when ulcerative lesions are found in the oropharynx and larynx, or when the adrenals are involved extensively. In many instances death is due to adrenal insufficiency.[214] Not infrequently the central portions of the granuloma undergo caseation necrosis, in which case the disease may be mistaken for tuberculosis.[214]

In endemic areas, healed and calcified granulomata of the liver and spleen are demonstrable in a high proportion of individuals examined postmortem, and *H. capsulatum* can be identified in many such lesions.[205]

Hepatomegaly and splenomegaly occur in more than half the cases with the disseminated form of the disease.[211, 253] As a rule, these give rise to no localizing symptoms, but occasionally are accompanied by jaundice and ascites. Fever, anemia and weight loss are the more usual associated symptoms.

Since the liver is involved frequently, needle biopsy may be of value in establishing the diagnosis of histoplasmosis, especially when more superficial lesions are not available for histologic study. However, the lesions of histoplasmosis cannot be distinguished from those of sarcoidosis, tuberculosis and other granulomatous diseases on histologic grounds alone,[149] so that a careful search for organisms in appropriately stained sections, a histoplasmin skin test and complement-fixation tests for histoplasmosis are indicated whenever hepatic granulomata are encountered.

MONILIASIS AND ASPERGILLOSIS

Occasionally, small abscesses are found in the liver in cases of disseminated moniliasis[148] and aspergillosis.[69] Although they may produce jaundice, often they are silent, the principal clinical manifestation being related to the involvement of the lung, heart valves and central nervous system. The number of disseminated *Candida* infections appears to be increasing, due to the widespread use of antibiotics, which encourage the growth of these organisms.[152] Drug addicts, who use the intravenous route, are also peculiarly susceptible to this type of infection.[135, 302]

MUCORMYCOSIS

Most fungi of the order *Mucorales* are saprophytes found on decaying vegetable matter and in the soil. However, some members of the group, particularly those of the genus *Rhizopus*, are pathogenic for man. Characteristically, these organisms invade the blood vessels of the brain, lungs and gastrointestinal tract, and occasionally of other tissues, resulting in thrombosis and septic infarction of tissue. Diabetes mellitus, lymphoma, a wide variety of other diseases, including hepatitis and cirrhosis, and therapy with antibiotics, steroids and folate antagonists predispose to such infections.

In at least one instance of disseminated mucormycosis, chills, fever, abdominal pain and deep jaundice were the principal features.[171] Surgical biopsy of the liver revealed foci of central necrosis without significant inflammatory reaction, which were interpreted as evidence of toxic injury.

PROTOZOAN INFECTIONS

MALARIA

Liver function studies suggest that *naturally acquired* malaria produces a mild form of hepatic injury rather frequently.[121, 147, 191, 242] However, not all of the functional disturbances observed can be attributed to the direct effects of the plasmodium; nor are they all necessarily indicative of hepatocellular damage.

Bromsulphalein retention, for example, which occurs with great regularity at the height of an attack, is due, in part at least, to the nonspecific effects of fever,[175] while the increase in serum bilirubin and urine urobilinogen, which frequently are accompanied by a significant fall in hemoglobin,[121] are in a large measure the result of increased hemolysis. Characteristically, the serum albumin level tends to fall, while the globulin level rises. This is particularly striking in *therapeutic* malaria, when the patient is permitted to experience a number of paroxysms of fever before therapy is instituted.[154, 155] A sharp fall in serum cholesterol, especially in the esterified fraction, is also seen in these cases.[102, 155] It is reasonable to suppose that the changes in serum protein and lipid are the consequence of impaired hepatic function, although other factors may be contributory.

The cephalin-cholesterol flocculation reaction is almost invariably strongly positive,[223] even in attacks of relatively brief duration.[165] Since it occurs with regularity and often is unaccompanied by other signs of hepatic involvement, it has been suggested that flocculation may be due to nonspecific changes in the serum proteins related to infection, rather than to hepatocellular injury.[223]

Alterations in galactose tolerance and hippuric acid synthesis have also been observed in some cases.[165] Characteristically, hepatic function promptly returns to normal following recovery from an attack of malaria, although occasionally minor abnormalities persist for many weeks.[165] However, even repeated relapses do not lead to any permanent impairment of function.[165, 277]

Hepatomegaly can be demonstrated during an acute attack in approximately half the cases of malaria.[147] Almost invariably it is accompanied by splenomegaly, and occasionally it is associated with tenderness. Following recovery, the liver returns to its normal size within a few days. However, after repeated relapses it may remain enlarged for a long time.[277]

Clinically detectable jaundice occurs in less than 1 per cent of cases and, when present, is usually mild.[121, 147] It appears on about the 4th day of illness and usually lasts for about a week. Only half the cases are associated with hepatomegaly.

There appear to be two distinct types of jaundice: one, very mild, and almost certainly hemolytic in origin; the other, somewhat more severe and probably due to a combination of hemolysis and hepatocellular damage. The former is characterized by a slight elevation in total serum bilirubin, without a concomitant increase in the prompt direct fraction, or the presence of bile in the urine. In the latter, both the direct and the indirect reacting fractions of serum bilirubin are increased, and the urine contains both bile and increased amounts of urobilinogen. *Plasmodium falciparum* infections are particularly likely to produce jaundice, whereas quartan malaria rarely does so.[121]

Studies of liver biopsy material obtained during acute attacks of malaria have revealed a number of histologic changes.[66] These include: (1) swelling of the parenchymal cells with alterations in cytoplasmic staining, (2) a marked increase in hepatocellular mitotic activity, with hyperchromatism and variability in the size of the nuclei, (3) compression of the sinusoids, and infiltration with lymphocytes and monocytes, (4) occasional small foci of necrosis and (5) hyperplasia of the Kupffer cells. At autopsy, cases of chronic malaria show hemosiderosis of the parenchymal cells, infiltration of the Kupffer cells with hemozoin pigment, and centrilobular atrophy and necrosis.[121, 147, 264] Not infrequently, there is also a diffuse fibrosis of the liver, which is generally regarded as an unrelated complication of malaria.[264] Nonspecific hepatic granulomas occur occasionally; these have been described by at least two groups of workers.[66] Their significance and pathogenesis are not known.

The type of liver damage seen in *therapeutic* malaria differs from that in the *naturally acquired* disease in that it tends to be more severe, is occasionally fatal[186] and often occurs late in the disease or even following recovery.[52, 155] The reasons for these differences are: (1) in many cases the hepatic lesions are due to an intercurrent infection with the hepatitis virus acquired during the inoculation of malarial blood[52] and (2) the course of the malaria is not interrupted by therapy until the patient has had a large number of paroxysms. In both instances the hepatic injury produced tends to be more severe than in naturally acquired malaria. This is well illustrated by the serum albumin concentration, which almost invariably falls to a low level in inoculation malaria and often is accompanied by edema,[154] rare features in the naturally acquired disease.

TOXOPLASMOSIS

The infantile form of toxoplasmosis, an infection with the protozoa *Toxoplasma gondii*, presumably acquired *in utero* from a mother with no overt signs of the disease, characteristically produces encephalomyelitis, hydrocephalus and chorioretinitis, and terminates fatally. Almost half the cases develop hepatomegaly and jaundice, but morphologic changes in the liver are rare.[49] Only 1 of the 18 cases reported up to 1946 exhibited significant hepatic lesions (severe parenchymatous degeneration, distortion of the lobular architecture and extramedullary hematopoiesis), and in only one other were *Toxoplasma* demonstrable in the liver. Accordingly, no satisfactory explanation can be offered for either the hepatomegaly or the jaundice. In a few instances, jaundice has been associated with the presence of nucleated red blood cells in the peripheral blood and splenomegaly, leading to a clinical diagnosis of erythroblastosis fetalis. However it is generally believed that, usually, both the hematologic changes and the jaundice are related in some way to the underlying infection.[49]

Rarely, toxoplasmosis gives rise to a fatal rickettsial-like disease in adults, characterized by chills, fever, rash and signs of pneumonitis, myocarditis and/or encephalitis.[141, 247] Except for functional impairment in some cases,[141] there are no clinical signs of hepatic involvement. However, on postmortem examination the liver usually shows focal areas of inflammation and hepatocellular necrosis.

More commonly, the adult form of toxoplasmosis presents as a nonfatal infection that resembles infectious mononucleosis and is characterized clinically by fever, rash, lymphadenopathy and hepatosplenomegaly.[44] Rarely, such infections are accompanied by jaundice and other manifestations of an acute hepatitis.[281] The clinical and laboratory features resemble those of viral hepatitis, but, usually, the preicteric phase of the disease is longer, and lymphadenopathy is more prominent. Histologically, the liver shows scattered foci of hepatocellular necrosis, a diffuse mononuclear inflammatory reaction that involves both the triads and the parenchyma, swelling of Kupffer cells, and the presence, in Giemsa-stained sections, of *Toxoplasma* within reticuloendothelial and hepatic cells. Confirmation of the diagnosis depends on the demonstration of a rising titer of antibody by the Sabin dye, indirect hemagglutination, complement fixation or slide flocculation test.[281]

RICKETTSIAL DISEASE

Q FEVER

Rickettsial infections due to *Coxiella burneti* and known as Q fever give rise to chills, fever and signs of pneumonitis. Often, these are accompanied by hepatosplenomegaly and alterations in hepatic structure and function, and in 5 per cent of cases overt clinical jaundice develops.[218] In a high proportion of cases, the results of liver function tests are similar to those seen in viral hepatitis, although high levels of serum alkaline phosphatase are somewhat more common, whereas the levels of serum transaminase seldom exceed 200 units.

Occasionally, the hepatitis is unaccompanied by pneumonia,[3] in which case the disease is clinically indistinguishable from viral hepatitis, differentiation depending on the demonstration of a rising titer of complement-fixing antibody or the isolation of *C. burneti* by guinea pig inoculation. Rarely, the clinical features and findings in the blood suggest infectious mononucleosis.[82]

On biopsy, the liver usually shows focal areas of hepatocellular necrosis and an inflammatory reaction in the portal triads.[218] In some cases, the zones of necrosis are infiltrated with polymorphonuclear and mononuclear cells,[218] but in others they are replaced by circumscribed granulomata composed of epithelioid cells and multinucleated giant cells.[213] Diffuse hepatocellular inflammation and necrosis have been reported in fatal cases.[274] According to some authorities, focal eosinophilic necrosis of the sinusoidal walls with swelling and proliferation of Kupffer cells that fill the sinusoidal lumen is said to be characteristic of the disease.[30]

VIRAL INFECTIONS

ADENOVIRUSES

Not infrequently, adenoviruses can be recovered from individuals with few or no symptoms. When resistance is reduced, this agent may give rise to severe bronchopulmonary lesions. There is a report of a 10-month-old boy with thymic alymphoplasia (Swiss type of agammaglobulinemia) who died of a terminal disseminated adenovirus type 2 infection associated with necrosis of the liver, bile ducts, pancreas, bronchopulmonary tree and lymph nodes.[287] The hepatic parenchyma contained numerous confluent, sharply circumscribed zones of coagulation necrosis. Adjacent hepatic cells contained intranuclear inclusions, sometimes surrounded by a clear halo, that resembled those of cytomegalic inclusion disease. The bile ducts also showed foci of coagulation necrosis and intranuclear inclusions.

Several strains of adenovirus have been recovered on tissue culture of blood obtained from patients with acute viral hepatitis.[113, 199] It is doubtful that any of these agents is the etiologic factor responsible for viral hepatitis, but their significance remains to be elucidated.

COXSACKIE B VIRUSES

Infections with Group B strains of the Coxsackie virus may be accompanied by a wide variety of clinical manifestations, including aseptic meningitis, pleurodynia, myocarditis, pericarditis and meningoencephalitis. Rarely, they give rise to acute hepatitis.[207, 266]

Characteristically, the onset of illness is abrupt with chills and fever, followed within a few days by jaundice and hepatomegaly, moderate elevations of serum bilirubin, transaminase, alkaline phosphatase and thymol turbidity, and a positive cephalin-cholesterol flocculation reaction. Almost always, there are other manifestations of Coxsackie B infection, such as aseptic meningitis, pleurodynia or myocarditis. In cases with meningitis, the clinical features may be mistaken for those of Weil's disease. More often, however, the disease resembles viral hepatitis.

Biopsy of the liver in one case revealed intense infiltrations of the portal triads with mononuclear cells, a few neutrophils and occasional eosinophils, foci of similar inflammatory cells in the periportal parenchyma, inflammatory cells within the walls of the portal veins and marked swelling of the central parenchymal cells, many of which contained bile droplets.[266]

Diagnosis depends on culturing the virus from the feces or demonstrating a significant rise in neutralizing antibody titer in the serum. Since Coxsackie infections tend to occur in epidemics during the summer months, the possibility of this etiologic factor should be considered in all cases of hepatitis appearing at that time, particularly when accompanied by other features suggestive of Coxsackie infection.

CYTOMEGALIC INCLUSION DISEASE

The agent responsible for cytomegalic inclusion disease in man, a member of the salivary gland virus group, is species specific. Neutralization tests suggest that several closely related strains are involved.[285] The incidence of complement-fixing antibodies is high in newborn infants, falls between the ages of 6 months and 2 years, and then rises steadily, reaching a peak of approximately 80 per cent in individuals over 35 years of age.[71] Considering that clinically apparent cytomegalic inclusion disease is relatively uncommon, especially in adults, it is apparent that most infections must be asymptomatic. Moreover, since the cytomegalovirus not infrequently attacks individuals with underlying disease, its etiologic importance in the pathogenesis of many lesions is difficult to establish.

Disseminated cytomegalic inclusion disease in the newborn[71, 285] is characterized by the appearance soon after birth of jaundice, ascites, edema, hepatosplenomegaly, hemolytic anemia and thrombocytopenic purpura. Not infrequently, microcephaly, mental retardation, motor disability, chorioretinitis and cerebral calcifications become apparent in infants who survive. The cytomegalovirus has been recovered from the mothers of such infants, so that, almost certainly, the infection is acquired *in utero*.[188] Half the infants affected are premature. Other predisposing factors include interstitial pneumonitis due to *Pneumocystis carinii*, a variety of other infections, cretinism and various visceral and skeletal malformations. Characteristically, the liver shows numerous foci of hepatocellular necrosis, giant cell transformation of surviving parenchymal cells, bile stasis, mononuclear and neutrophilic infiltration of the portal triads, and the presence within enlarged epithelial cells of large homogeneous, amphophilic intranuclear inclusions surrounded by a clear halo that are pathognomonic of cytomegalovirus infection. The latter seldom are numerous, and are found most frequently in bile duct epithelium, but may occur in hepatic or Kupffer cells. It has been suggested that most cases of neonatal hepatitis are due to cytomegalic inclusion disease.[285] However, no evidence of such infection has been found in those unaccompanied by the other features of congenital cytomegalic inclusion disease.[188] It has been reported that in a group of apparently healthy children shown to be passing the virus in their urine, a significant number exhibited hepatomegaly and alterations in hepatic function, and that the incidence of viruria in children with evidence of liver disease was significantly higher than in their controls.[110] Whether the cytomegalovirus played a role in the pathogenesis of the hepatic abnormalities encountered in this group or was a secondary invader was not established. The fact that the authors of this report recovered the virus from a patient with Wilson's disease favors the latter interpretation.

Rarely, disseminated cytomegalic inclusion disease affects adults. In most cases, such infections are complications of debilitating disease of the hemopoietic and reticuloendothelial system,[296] neoplasm,[79] immunosuppressive therapy[296] or infections with *Pneumocystis carinii*[290] or toxoplasma.[117] Almost any tissue, including the liver, may be involved in such cases, but the two most common lesions are a necrotizing fibrinous pneumonia and necrosis of the adrenals.

Occasionally, previously healthy adults infected with cytomegalovirus exhibit protracted fever and a blood picture indistinguishable from that of infectious mononucleosis.[150, 160] Characteristically, there is no accompanying pharyngitis or lymphadenopathy, or any rise in the heterophile antibody titer. Hepatic functional abnormalities are common, and, in some cases, jaundice and hepatomegaly appear.[160] The course of the disease in such cases is benign.

Although the presence of typical inclusions in biopsy material may establish the diagnosis, often they cannot be found even after careful search. Usually confirmation of the diagnosis depends on isolation of the virus from urine, saliva, cerebrospinal fluid or tissue in tissue cultures of human fibroblasts or on the demonstration of a rising titer of complement-fixing or neutralizing antibodies.[71, 285]

HERPES SIMPLEX

Disseminated infections with the herpes simplex virus are limited to the newborn infants of the few mothers who have no circulating antibody to the virus[36, 176] and to children under the age of 5 years whose titer of maternally-acquired antibody has fallen to a low level and who have not yet been exposed to the virus and developed their own.[276] The portal of entry is not known, but contact with an actively infected adult can usually be established.[36]

In contrast to the dermal and mucosal localization of the virus in adults, disseminated herpes simplex infections in infants characteristically produce necrotic lesions in the liver, adrenals and esophagus, usually without involving the skin or mucous membranes.

The illness starts abruptly with low grade fever and respiratory symptoms, and is followed within a few days by jaundice, hepatomegaly, increasing lethargy and gastrointestinal bleeding. Death invariably ensues within a week or two.

Characteristically, the liver shows extensive hepatocellular necrosis, usually diffusely distributed, but occasionally centrolobular or midzonal, sparse inflammatory cells, numerous multinucleated hepatocytes, and the presence within surviving parenchymal cells of pathognomonic intranuclear eosinophilic inclusion bodies.

Infectious Mononucleosis

The etiology of infectious mononucleosis is uncertain. However, recent serologic evidence suggests that the E B virus, a herpestype virus associated with cell lines derived from Burkitt lymphomas, or a closely related agent, is implicated.[202]

Histologic evidence confirms the impression gained from functional studies that the liver is almost invariably involved in infectious mononucleosis.[4, 19, 140, 142, 282, 300] The outstanding morphologic feature is an intense inflammatory reaction involving the portal triads and sinusoids. Various types of mononuclear cells, including lymphocytes, large monocytes, epithelioid cells and plasma cells, predominate, but a few polymorphonuclear cells and eosinophils are seen in some cases. In addition, there is proliferation and swelling of the Kupffer cells in the sinusoids, where in conjunction with other monocytic cells, they tend to form small aggregates which resemble granulomata. Although most authorities minimize the importance of hepatocellular necrosis, careful study usually reveals scattered acidophilic bodies[148] and significant loss of parenchymal

cells around the enlarged portal triads; moreover, at least two instances of fatal hepatic necrosis have been reported.[5]

Usually, there is striking evidence of regenerative activity, even when hepatic necrosis is minimal or absent. Mitoses, variations in cell size, hyperchromatism and binucleate cells are common. Bile stasis may be evident in cases with jaundice. Some degree of collapse and condensation of the reticulum may be seen around the portal triads, but frank fibrosis does not occur. In severe cases, the central veins may show a striking endophlebitis.[148] Usually, the bile ducts are not altered, but in some cases proliferation is evident.[74, 148] The extent and the severity of the inflammatory reaction and the relative paucity of the necrosis in most cases serve to differentiate the lesions of infectious mononucleosis from those of viral hepatitis. However, often the two lesions are indistinguishable.[148]

Inflammatory lesions similar to those found in the liver have been described in the lymph nodes, bone marrow, kidneys, heart, lungs and many other tissues,[4] indicating that the hepatic lesions represent only one facet of a generalized reaction involving the reticuloendothelial system.

The results of liver function tests are abnormal in most, if not all, cases of infectious mononucleosis.[45, 63, 77, 84, 92, 137] However, these are not necessarily indicative of hepatocellular injury in all instances. Since they are not closely correlated with the histologic changes in the liver,[4, 282] and may remain abnormal long after recovery,[26, 77, 137] some of the abnormalities, such as the cephalin-cholesterol flocculation and thymol turbidity reactions, are perhaps due to nonspecific serum protein changes related to the underlying infection.

Characteristically, the serum albumin level falls while the gamma globulin rises.[260] Occasionally, there is also a less-pronounced increase in alpha-1 and beta globulin. Although the heterophile agglutinins are found chiefly in the gamma-globulin fraction, they do not appear to be responsible for the distorted electrophoretic pattern.[260] Cephalincholesterol flocculation reactions are strongly positive and thymol turbidity is increased in at least 80 per cent of cases, the number depending on the frequency with which the tests are repeated. Often, the serum alkaline phosphatase level is markedly elevated, even in the absence of jaundice.[70]

Bromsulphalein retention, an increase in serum transaminase and urinary urobilinogen and a decrease in serum cholesterol esters and prothrombin are less constant findings. The serum bilirubin level is increased in 10 to 30 per cent of cases.[26, 137, 140] Bilirubinuria is said to occur in the absence of hyperbilirubinemia in some cases.[63]

Clinical manifestations of liver disease are relatively uncommon. Jaundice occurs in 5 to 10 per cent of cases,[1, 26, 92, 137] and hepatomegaly slightly more frequently.[28] In general, the jaundice tends to be mild and subsides in less than a month, but in occasional instances it is intense and persists for several months.[1] Moreover, as indicated, fatal massive hepatic necrosis may ensue.[5] The appearance of jaundice may precede or coincide with the inset of lymphadenopathy, and occasionally occurs without lymphadenopathy. Usually, there is little difficulty in recognizing that the jaundice is due to hepatocellular injury; however, differentiation from viral hepatitis may be exceedingly difficult, especially since atypical lymphocytes may be found in both diseases. The diagnosis depends on the demonstration of a significant rise in the heterophile agglutinin titer, which usually occurs in the 2nd week; rarely, the rise does not occur until the 7th or 8th week.[18] The results of liver function tests are usually consistent with some type of hepatocellular injury but in exceptional cases[137] may suggest an obstructive jaundice.

The clinical significance of the morphologic and the functional changes in the liver in nonicteric cases is a matter of dispute. Some authors take the extreme view that they are responsible for the constitutional symptoms in infectious mononucleosis, and that diets high in protein, carbohydrate and vitamins hasten recovery.[63] Although the degree of hepatic dysfunction may be correlated with the intensity of the symptoms, the two do not appear to be related causally. Indeed, both reflect the severity of the infection. Most investigators have failed to confirm the alleged effectiveness of dietotherapy in shortening the course of the disease.[77]

The results of liver function tests usually return to normal by the end of the second month.[77, 137] Occasionally, however, abnormalities persist for as long as 2 years,[26] which has led to concern over the possibility that chronic hepatitis and cirrhosis may follow an attack of infectious mononucleosis. One alleged case of postinfectional cirrhosis has been reported,[161] but chronic alcoholism and malnutrition were present and could not be excluded as the responsible etiologic factors. In the opinion of most investigators[45, 142] there is no convincing histologic or clinical evidence that infectious mononucleosis gives rise to any type of chronic liver disease. However, premature ambulation in patients with significant liver damage may prolong convalescence and aggravate postinfectional asthenia. For that reason, it would seem reasonable to enforce bed rest, at least until jaundice and hepatic tenderness have subsided. Persistent abnormalities in cephalin-cholesterol flocculation and thymol turbidity, unaccompanied by other signs of active liver disease, are not an indication for continued restriction of activity.

Corticosteroid therapy appears to be of benefit in patients severely ill with infectious mononucleosis.[70, 254] The efficacy of chloroquine, which has been recommended by some,[67] is in doubt.[203]

PSITTACOSIS

The psittacosis virus, which is responsible for a naturally occurring disease of birds, is occasionally transmitted to man as a consequence of direct contact with infected birds or inhalation of air-borne virus particles. In man, the virus produces a serious, often fatal infection characterized by fever, severe constitutional symptoms and pneumonitis. Not infrequently, the liver and the spleen are enlarged, and, rarely, in severe cases the disease is complicated by hepatitis with overt jaundice.[299] The principal histologic findings in the liver include scattered foci of hepatocellular necrosis, a variable mononuclear reaction in the portal triads, and proliferation of the Kupffer cells, often accompanied by erythrophagocytosis and cytophagocytosis.

REOVIRUS

The pathogenicity of reoviruses for man has not been established beyond doubt. However, evidence suggests that they cause some forms of summer diarrhea and certain febrile illnesses accompanied by rash seen in children.

A report of hepatitis and encephalitis in 3 infants with reovirus infections is of particular interest, since similar lesions are encountered in experimentally infected infant mice.[139] In all 3 cases, reovirus was recovered from the feces at the height of the disease, and, in one that died, the virus was isolated from the brain at autopsy. Fever and signs of encephalitis dominated the clinical picture. Although jaundice and hepatomegaly were not noted in the infant who died, autopsy on the fifth day of illness revealed numerous small foci of centrilobular and midzonal hepatocellular degeneration and necrosis, occasional acidophilic bodies and sparse mononuclear inflammatory cells. The two survivors exhibited hepatomegaly and high levels of serum transaminase. Only one of these became mildly jaundiced.

RUBELLA

Approximately 20 per cent of infants born of mothers infected with the rubella virus during the first trimester of pregnancy exhibit a syndrome characterized by cataracts, deafness, congenital anomalies of the heart and mental retardation, often accompanied by microcephaly.[157, 215, 216] Disorders of the liver, blood, bone, lungs and blood vessels are common but less frequent manifestations. The rubella virus, which remains viable for several months in such infants, can be readily recovered from the nasopharynx, body fluids and tissues.

A high proportion of infants with the congenital rubella syndrome exhibit hepatosplenomegaly.[157] Usually this recedes in a few days, but may persist for several weeks. In some cases, hepatomegaly is accompanied by jaundice and other manifestations of acute hepatitis. The hepatic lesions in such infants vary in severity, ranging from a fatal form indistinguishable from neonatal giant cell hepatitis to a mild hepatitis characterized by cholestasis, periportal inflammation and minimal hepatocellular necrosis.[83] The rubella virus can be recovered from the liver with regularity in such cases. Reportedly the hepatitis described occasionally gives rise to cirrhosis.[157]

The relative importance and frequency of rubella and cytomegalovirus infections in the pathogenesis of neonatal hepatitis have not yet been established.

DISEASES OF PRESUMED INFECTIOUS ORIGIN

SARCOIDOSIS

Sarcoidosis is a generalized granulomatous disease of unknown etiology. Although clinical manifestations of hepatic involvement are relatively uncommon, the liver often contains granulomata. Indeed, of all tissues affected, the liver stands second only to lymph nodes and lungs. In one series of autopsied cases collected from the literature,[40] the incidence of hepatic granulomata was 66.5 per cent. Needle biopsy studies of the liver indicate that the incidence is equally high in less severely ill, nonfatal cases.[47, 149, 187, 248] Considering the frequency with which granulomata are demonstrated in such small specimens, it is apparent that, in most cases, the lesions are numerous and uniformly distributed.

The characteristic sarcoidal lesion in the liver is a sharply circumscribed, discrete, round or oval compact mass of epithelioid cells, giant cells and a few lymphocytes embedded in a fine reticular mesh.[149] The lesion may be found anywhere within the lobule, but is most common in the portal triads and in the centrilobular parenchyma. Occasionally, the granulomata contain minute foci of fibrinoid necrosis, but they never undergo caseation necrosis. Schaumann bodies and asteroid inclusions are rare in hepatic lesions. As a rule, the granulomata tend to remain discrete, but, in occasional cases, they coalesce to form large masses that replace the parenchyma, destroying the normal lobular architecture, and giving rise to a picture that resembles cirrhosis.[40, 149, 217] Not infrequently, granulomata can be demonstrated in the walls of the central and portal veins, and, occasionally, they partially occlude their lumens.[47] Lesions of this type may play a role in the pathogenesis of the ascites and portal hypertension seen in some cases.[40, 55, 158, 192, 217] As sarcoidal granulomata mature, they are enveloped in a capsule of collagen and ultimately undergo diffuse fibrosis and hyalinization.

The granulomata of sarcoidosis can seldom be distinguished from those of tuberculosis, berylliosis and other systemic granulomatous diseases on histologic grounds alone. Accordingly, all other known causes of granulomatous reactions must be excluded by appropriate bacteriologic, serologic and clinical studies before such lesions are accepted as evidence of sarcoidosis.

Nonspecific hepatic granulomata, which closely resemble those of sarcoidosis, are seen, not infrequently, in association with a wide variety of other hepatic lesions.[47, 148] This occurs most frequently in primary biliary cirrhosis, but is seen in other forms of cirrhosis and in both viral and drug-induced hepatitis. Since available evidence suggests that sarcoidosis is always a generalized disease, the diagnosis should not be made on the basis of granulomata found in the liver when other manifestations of the disease are lacking, particularly when the granulomata are associated with other hepatic lesions, such as hepatitis or cirrhosis.

Few patients with hepatic granulomata due to sarcoidosis exhibit overt signs of liver disease. Slight enlargement of the liver is relatively common, but tenderness, induration and nodularity are rare. Significant enlargement, induration and tenderness of the liver indicate massive granulomatous involvement, but often are attributable to cor pulmonale and congestive failure secondary to advanced pulmonary disease. Splenomegaly occurs in approximately half the patients with significant hepatomegaly, and may be due to granulomatous infiltration, congestion or both.

Several instances of jaundice have been reported.[40, 75, 122, 149, 201, 217] In some, it has been obstructive in character and associated with clinical, functional and histologic features suggestive of granulomatous biliary cirrhosis.[40, 75, 122] In one such case[270] there was a high titer of mitochondrial antibodies in the serum, suggesting that the patient may have had two unrelated diseases, sarcoidosis and primary biliary cirrhosis. In another case on record, jaundice was attributable to obstruction of the common bile duct by enlarged granulomatous lymph nodes.[111]

Ascites is uncommon and usually occurs in association with jaundice and extensive granulomatous infiltration of the liver.[40, 122, 201, 217] However, in one well-documented case, surgical exploration revealed that the ascites was attributable to widespread granulomatous involvement of the parietal and visceral peritoneum.[295]

Portal hypertension, often accompanied by hemorrhage from esophageal varices, is a well known but relatively uncommon complication of hepatic sarcoidosis. Although it has appeared to be a sequela of granulomatous cirrhosis in some cases,[149, 201] more often it has been encountered in patients with only modest or no hepatic fibrosis.[55, 158, 192, 217] Moreover, in at least 2 instances, wedged hepatic vein pressure has been normal in the face of raised splenic pulp pressure,[158, 192] suggesting a presinusoidal block. It is highly probable that the portal hypertension in such cases is attributable to granulomatous invasion and compression of the small portal veins in the triads. As indicated, the writer has documented the occurrence of such lesions in biopsy material (see Reference 47, Fig. 14), although he has not had the opportunity to correlate them with measurements of portal pressure.

Occasionally, sarcoidosis of the liver gives rise to progressive hepatic failure that leads to death.[40, 201]

Minor alterations in hepatic function can be demonstrated in a high proportion of individuals with sarcoidosis.[149] Some of these, such as increases in serum bilirubin, serum alkaline phosphatase and Bromsulphalein retention, appear to be related to the presence of hepatic granulomata, but others, including an increase in serum globulin, thymol turbidity and cephalin-cholesterol flocculation or a fall in serum albumin, may be due, in part at least, to extrahepatic factors. The hyperglobulinemia is closely correlated with the extent and activity of the lesions generally and, therefore, is a useful index in following the course of the disease. The high serum alkaline phosphatase levels occasionally seen in sarcoidosis are due to extensive hepatic involvement, although granulomatous infiltration of the bones may play a role in some cases. Although the impairment of hepatic function parallels the extent of the lesions in the liver, it is generally less severe than in cirrhosis and other types of chronic hepatitis.

Liver disease seldom is suspected in cases of sarcoidosis with scattered hepatic granulomata. However, when the liver is greatly enlarged, and especially when accompanied by splenomegaly, it may be exceedingly difficult to differentiate sarcoidosis from cirrhosis, chronic hepatitis due to other causes, Hodgkin's disease and other forms of malignant lymphoma.

Needle biopsy of the liver is a particularly valuable diagnostic procedure in sarcoidosis, not only in cases with overt signs of liver disease, but also in those with predominantly extrahepatic lesions. Since histologic confirmation is always essential, the procedure may provide the only means of establishing the diagnosis when more accessible lesions in the skin and the peripheral lymph nodes are not available for examination.

ERYTHEMA NODOSUM

Erythema nodosum is generally regarded as a manifestation of hypersensitivity to a variety of agents, including bacteria, viruses, fungi and chemical compounds.[85] Occasionally, the skin lesions, which are the most striking feature of the disease, are accompanied by hilar adenopathy, pulmonary infiltrates and eye lesions.[146] In such cases, the liver often contains miliary granulomata.[149] It is evident from Löfgren's work[167] that, at least in tuberculin-negative cases, early sarcoidosis is responsible for most instances of erythema nodosum accompanied by hilar adenopathy and other disseminated lesions.

The writer has found hepatic granulomata in patients with erythema nodosum associated with tuberculosis but not in the type associated with drug reactions.[148]

REFERENCES

1. Abrams, H. L.: Infectious mononucleosis with intense jaundice of long duration, New Engl. J. Med. 238:295, 1948.
2. Agrawal, H. S., Benson, J. W., and Major, J. J.: An unusual case of hemobilia: hepatic tuberculosis with hemorrhage, Arch. Surg. 95:202, 1967.
3. Alkan, W. J., Evenchik, Z., and Eschar, J.: Q fever and infectious hepatitis, Am. J. Med. 38:54, 1965.
4. Allen, F. H., Jr., and Kellner, A.: Infectious mononucleosis; autopsy report, Am. J. Path. 23:463, 1947.
5. Allen, U. R., and Bass, B. H.: Fatal hepatic necrosis in glandular fever, J. Clin. Path. 16:337, 1963.
6. Alston, J. M., and Broom, J. C.: The action of penicillin on leptospira and on leptospiral infections in the guinea pig, Brit. Med. J. 2:718, 1944.
7. Amatuzio, D. S., Weber, L. J., and Nesbitt, S.: Bilirubin and protein in the cerebrospinal fluid of jaundiced patients with severe liver disease with and without hepatic coma, J. Lab. Clin. Med. 41:615, 1953.
8. Andre, J., Schwartz, R., and Dameshek, W.: Tuberculosis and myelosclerosis with myeloid metaplasia; report of three cases, J.A.M.A. 178:1169, 1961.
9. Arean, V. M.: The pathologic anatomy and pathogenesis of fatal human leptospirosis (Weil's disease), Am. J. Path. 40:393, 1962.
10. Arm, H. G., LeColvan, P. L., Sabour, M., Shehata, E., and Salib, M.: Microbiologic study of liver biopsies in chronic pulmonary tuberculosis cases in Egypt, U. S. Navy Research Report NM 72 01 03.12.01 (undated).
11. Ash, J. E., and Spitz, S.: Pathology of Tropical Diseases, An Atlas, Philadelphia, Saunders, 1945.
12. Ashburn, L. L., and Packchanian, A.: Histogenesis of experimental icterohemorrhagic spirochetosis in albino American deer mice (Peromyscus maniculatus gambeli), Am. J. Trop. Med. 23:607, 1943.
13. Ashe, W. F., Pratt-Thomas, H. R., and Kumpe, C. W.: Weil's disease; complete

review of American literature and an abstract of the world literature; seven case reports, Medicine 20:145, 1941.

14. Ashton, N.: A case of multiple tuberculomata of the liver, J. Path. Bact. 58: 95, 1946.

15. Bacharach, T., and Zalis, E. G.: Sarcoid syndrome associated with coccidioidomycosis, Am. Rev. Resp. Dis. 88:248, 1963.

16. Baehr, G., and Klemperer, P.: Degenerative and diffuse inflammatory diseases of liver; correlation of pathology and clinical medicine as illustrated by cases from clinical-pathological conferences of Mount Sinai Hospital, New York, Int. Clin. 2:107, 1929.

17. Baker and Carter: Cited by Blumer and Nesbit.[37]

18. Bakst, H., and Leibowitz, S.: Infectious mononucleosis; report of a case with first appearance of significant numbers of heterophile antibodies and abnormal lymphocytes ("virocytes") in seventh week of illness, Am. J. Med. 13:235, 1952.

19. Bang, J., and Wanscher, O.: The histopathology of the liver in infectious mononucleosis complicated by jaundice, investigated by aspiration biopsy, Acta med. scand. 120:437, 1945.

20. Barker, L. F., and Sladen, F. J.: A small epidemic of jaundice with symptoms of gastro-intestinal catarrh, Bull. Johns Hopkins Hosp. 20:310, 1909.

21. Barondess, J. H., and Erle, H.: Serum alkaline phosphatase activity in hepatitis of infectious mononucleosis, Am. J. Med. 29:43, 1960.

22. Beadenkopf, W. G., and Loosli, C. G.: Histoplasmosis, tuberculosis, coccidioidomycosis, J.A.M.A. 146:621, 1951.

23. Beeson, P. B., Brannon, E. S., and Warren, J. V.: Observations on the sites of removal of bacteria from the blood in patients with bacterial endocarditis, J. Exp. Med. 81:9, 1945.

24. Beeson, P. B., and Hankey, D. D.: Leptospiral meningitis, Arch. Int. Med. 89:575, 1952.

25. Beeson, P. B., Hankey, D. D., and Cooper, C. F., Jr.: Leptospiral iridocyclitis; evidence of human infection with Leptospira pomona in the United States, J.A.M.A. 145:229, 1851.

26. Bennett, H. D., Frankel, J. J., Bedinger, P., and Baker, L. A.: Infectious mono-

nucleosis with hepatitis, Arch. Int. Med. 86:391, 1950.

27. Berman, J. K., and Hull, J. E.: Hepatic, splenic and left gastric arterial ligations in advanced portal cirrhosis, Arch. Surg. 65:37, 1952.

28. Bernstein, A.: Infectious mononucleosis, Medicine 19:85, 1940.

29. Bernstein, J., and Brown, A. K.: Sepsis and jaundice in early infancy, Pediatrics 29:873, 1962.

30. Bernstein, M., Edmundson, H. A., and Barbour, B. H.: The liver lesion in Q fever, clinical and pathologic features, Arch. Int. Med. 116:491, 1965.

31. Bertucci, E. A., Jr.: Leptospirosis, Am. J. Med. Sci. 209:86, 1945.

32. Bigham, R. S., Jr.: Benign aseptic meningitis due to Leptospira grippotyphosa, Arch. Int. Med. 92:587, 1953.

33. Bingel: Cited by Moon.[195]

34. Bingold, K.: Über septischen Ikterus, Z. klin. Med. 92:140, 1921.

35. Birch, C. A.: Jaundice complicating pneumonia, with special reference to jaundice with cholaemia and its treatment, Lancet 1:1046, 1937.

36. Bird, T., Ennis, J. E., Wort, A. J., and Gardner, P. A.: Disseminated herpes simplex in newborn infants, J. Clin. Path. 16:423, 1063.

37. Blumer, G., and Nesbit, R. R.: A case of gonococcal septicaemia with endocarditis and hepatitis, Int. Clin. 4:44, 1936.

38. Bock, H. E., Olderhausen, H. F. v., and Tellesz, A.: Was leistet die Leberpunktion bei der Tuberkulose? Verh. deutsch. Ges. inn. Med. 59:351, 1953.

39. Boden, R. W., Rankin, J. G., Goulston, S. J. M., and Morrow, W.: The liver in ulcerative colitis. The significance of raised serum-alkaline-phosphatase levels, Lancet 2:245, 1959.

40. Branson, J. H., and Park, J. H.: Sarcoidosis—hepatic involvement: presentation of a case with fatal liver involvement, including autopsy findings and review of the evidence for sarcoid involvement of the liver as found in the literature, Ann. Int. Med. 40:111, 1954.

41. Braude, A. I.: The evolution and significance of the hepatic granuloma in experimental brucellosis, J. Clin. Invest. 29:799, 1950.

42. Braunstein, H., and Adriano, S. M.: Fluorescent stain for tubercle bacilli

in histologic sections. I. Diagnostic efficiency in granulomatous lesions of lymph nodes, Am. J. Clin. Path. 36:37, 1961.

43. Brooke, B. N., and Slaney, G.: Portal bacteremia in ulcerative colitis, Lancet 1:1206, 1958.

44. Brown, J., and Jacobs, L.: Adult toxoplasmosis; report of a case due to laboratory infection, Ann. Int. Med. 44:565, 1956.

45. Brown, J. W., Sims, J. L., White, E., and Clifford, J. E.: Liver function during infectious mononucleosis, Am. J. Med. 6:321, 1949.

46. Büngeler, W.: Über die brasilianische Blastomykose und den histologischen Nachweis der Paracoccidioides brasiliensis, Virchows Arch. path. Anat. 309:76, 1942.

47. Bunim, J. J., Kimberg, D. V., Thomas, L. B., Van Scott, J., and Klatskin, G.: Syndrome of sarcoidosis, psoriasis, and gout. Combined clinical staff conference at the National Institutes of Health, Ann. Int. Med. 57:1018, 1962.

48. Buzzard, E. M., and Wylie, J. A. H.: Meningitis leptospirosis, Lancet 2:417, 1947.

49. Callahan, W. P., Jr., Russell, W. O., and Smith, M. G.: Human toxoplasmosis. A clinicopathologic study with presentation of five cases and review of the literature, Medicine 25:343, 1946.

50. Cargill, W. H., Jr., and Beeson, P. B.: The value of spinal fluid examination as a diagnostic procedure in Weil's disease, Ann. Int. Med. 27:396, 1947.

51. Chaikin, N. W., and Chlenoff, S. O.: Acute hepatitis; clinical observations in 63 cases, Am. J. Dig. Dis. 12:151, 1945.

52. Chalmers, T. C., Jr.: The occurrence of jaundice in therapeutic and natural malaria, J. Clin. Invest. 26:1055, 1947.

53. Chapman, A. Z., Reeder, P. S., and Barker, L. A.: Neutropenia secondary to tuberculous spenomegaly; report of a case, Ann. Int. Med. 41:1225, 1954.

54. Chau, A. Y. S., Goldbloom, V. C., and Gurd, F. N.: Clostridial infection as a cause of death after ligation of the hepatic artery, Arch. Surg., 63:390, 1951.

55. Cheitlin, M. D., Sullivan, B. H., Myers, J. E., Jr., and Hench, R. F.: Portal hypertension in hepatic sarcoidosis, Gastroenterology 38:60, 1960.

56. Chinn, A. B., Roth, H. P., and Moore, R. D.: Hepatic function tests in Weil's disease, Am. J. Med. Sci. 222:530, 1951.

57. Chung, H., and Chang, F. C.: Relapsing fever; clinical and statistical study of 337 cases, Chin. Med. J. 55:6, 1939.

58. Clapper, M., and Myers, G. B.: Clinical manifestations of Weil's disease with particular reference to meningitis, Arch. Int. Med. 72:18, 1943.

59. Coffee, H. D., and Lipton, S.: Primary tuberculosis of the spleen; report of a case, Arch. Surg. 47:478, 1943.

60. Cohen, A. G., and Giges, B.: Punch biopsy of liver in detection of hematogenous tuberculosis, J.A.M.A. 146:1416, 1951.

61. Cohen, E. B., Brucellosis at the State of Wisconsin General Hospital, Wisconsin M. J. 45:847, 1946.

62. Cohen, F. B., Robins, B., and Lipstein, W.: Isolation of Brucella abortus by percutaneous liver biopsy, New Engl. J. Med. 275:228, 1957.

63. Cohn, C., and Lidman, B. I.: Hepatitis without jaundice in infectious mononucleosis, J. Clin. Invest. 25:145, 1946.

64. Conn, H. O.: Spontaneous peritonitis and bacteremia in Laennec's cirrhosis caused by enteric organisms: a common but rarely recognized syndrome, Ann. Int. Med. 60:568, 1964.

65. Cope, Z.: Actinomycosis, p. 133, London, Oxford, 1938.

66. Corcoran, T. E., Hegstrom, G. J., Zoeckler, S. J., and Keil, P. G.: Liver structure in nonfatal malaria, Gastroenterology 24:53, 1953.

67. Cowley, R. G., and Myers, J. E., Jr.: Chloroquine in the treatment of infectious mononucleosis, Ann. Int. Med. 57:937, 1962.

68. Craddock, C. G., and Meredith, H. C., Jr.: Punch liver biopsy in the diagnosis of miliary tuberculosis; report of a case, New Engl. J. Med. 241:527, 1949.

69. Crawley, E. P.: Aspergillosis and the aspergilli; report of a unique case of the disease, Arch. Int. Med. 80:423, 1947.

70. Creditor, M. C., and McCurdy, H. C.: Severe infectious mononucleosis, Ann. Int. Med. 50:218, 1959.

71. Crome, L.: Cytomegalic inclusion body disease, World Neurology 2:447, 1961.

72. Cruice, J. M.: Jaundice in tuberculosis, Am. J. M. Sci. 147:720, 1914.

73. Curphey, T. J., and Solomon, S.: Studies

on liver function in pneumococcus pneumonia, Am. J. Med. Sci. *196*:348, 1938.

74. Custer, R. P., and Smith, E. B.: The pathology of infectious mononucleosis, Blood *3*:830, 1948.

75. Dagradi, A. E., Sollod, N., and Friedlander, J. H.: Sarcoidosis with marked hepatosplenomegaly and jaundice: a case report with biopsy findings, Ann. Int. Med. *36*:1317, 1952.

76. Dawson, B., Hume, W. E., and Bedson, S. P.: Infective jaundice, Brit. Med. J. *2*: 345, 1917.

77. DeMarsh, Q. B., and Alt, H. L.: Hepatitis without jaundice in infectious mononucleosis, J. Lab. Clin. Med. *32*:320, 1947.

78. Diehl, F., and Roth, F.: Hepatolienale Syndrome bei Bangscher Krankheit, Dtsch. Arch. klin. Med. *178*:271, 1935.

79. Duvall, C. P., Casazza, A. R., Grimley, P. M., Carbone, P. P., and Rowe, W. P.: Recovery of cytomegalovirus from adults with neoplastic disease, Ann. Int. Med. *64*:531, 1966.

80. Engelbreth-Holm, J.: A study of tuberculous splenomegaly and splenogenic controlling of the cell emission from the bone marrow, Am. J. Med. Sci. *195*:32, 1938.

81. Erlik, D., and Reitler, R.: Intrahepatic typhoid infection as a cause of the carrier state, Lancet *1*:1216, 1960.

82. Eschar, J., Waron, M., and Alkon, W. J.: Syndromes of Q fever, J.A.M.A. *195*: 390, 1966.

83. Esterly, J. R., Slusser, R. J., and Ruebner, B. H.: Hepatic lesions in the congenital rubella syndrome, J. Pediat. *71*: 676, 1967.

84. Evans, A. S.: Liver involvement in infectious mononucleosis, J. Clin. Invest. *27*: 106, 1948.

85. Favour, C. B., and Sosman, M. C.: Erythema nodosum, Arch. Int. Med. *80*:435, 1947.

86. Fishbein, W. N.: Jaundice as an early manifestation of scarlet fever. Report of three cases in adults and review of the literature, Ann. Int. Med. *57*:60, 1962.

87. Fitz-Hugh, T., Jr.: Acute gonococcic peritonitis of the right upper quadrant in women, J.A.M.A. *102*:2094, 1934.

88. Fitzpatrick, W. J., and Schwartz, S. O.: Polycythemia secondary to tuberculosis of the spleen; report of a case, Am. Rev. Tuberc. *60*:660, 1949.

89. Foshay, L.: Tularemia: a summary of certain aspects of the disease including methods for early diagnosis and the results of serum treatment in 600 patients, Medicine *19*:1, 1940.

90. Francis, E.: A summary of present knowledge of tularemia, Medicine *7*:411, 1928.

91. Freitag, J. L.: Treatment of chronic typhoid carriers by cholecystectomy, Public Health Rep. *79*:567, 1964.

92. Gall, E. A.: Serum phosphatase and other tests of liver function in infectious mononucleosis, Am. J. Clin. Path. *17*: 529, 1947.

93. Gellis, S. S.: Jaundice present at birth, Med. Clin. N. Amer. *31*:1185, 1947.

94. Gochenour, W. S., Jr., Smadel, J. E., Jackson, E. B., Evans, L. B., and Yager, R. H.: Leptospiral etiology of Fort Bragg fever, Public Health Rep. *67*:811, 1952.

95. Gochenour, W. S., Jr., Yager, R. H., and Wetmore, P. W.: Antigenic similarity of bovine strains of leptospirae (United States) and *Leptospira pomona*, Proc. Soc. Exp. Biol. Med. *74*:199, 1950.

96. Gochenour, W. S., Jr., Yager, R. H., Wetmore, P. W., and Hightower, J. A.: Laboratory diagnosis of leptospirosis, Am. J. Public Health *43*:405, 1953.

97. Goodpasture, E. W.: Concerning the pathogenesis of typhoid fever, Am. J. Path. *13*:175, 1937.

98. Greene, L. N.: Common duct stone simulating "cholangitis lenta," J. Mt. Sinai Hosp. *7*:144, 1941.

99. Gsell, O.: Leptospirosis Pomona, die Schweinehüterkrankheit, Schweiz. med. Wschr. *76*:237, 1946.

100. ———: Klinik der Leptospirenerkrankungen (Leptospirosen in Europa mit Ausnahme der L. icterohaemorrhagiae), Ergebn. inn. Med. Kinderheilk. *1*:367, 1949.

101. Guild, A. A., and Robson, H. N.: Polycythemia vera with tuberculous splenomegaly; report of a case, Edinburgh M. J. *57*:145, 1950.

102. Guttman, S. A., Potter, H. R., Hanger, F. M., Moore, D. B., Pierson, P. S., and Moore, D. H.: Significance of cephalin-cholesterol flocculation test in malarial fever, J. Clin. Invest. *24*:296, 1945.

103. Haex, A. J. Ch., and van Beek, C.: Tu-

berculosis and aspiration liver biopsy; its clinical significance *in* Diagnosis and Therapy, Haarlem, DeErven F. Bohn N. V., 1955.

104. Hahn, R. D.: Syphilis of the liver, Am. J. Syph. 27:529, 1943.

105. Hall, H. E., Hightower, J. A., Rivera, R. D., Byrne, R. J., Smadel, J. E., and Woodward, T E.: Evaluation of antibiotic therapy in human leptospirosis, Ann. Int. Med. 35:981, 1951.

106. Hällen, J.: Non-specific streptolysin O inhibition in diseases of the liver and biliary system, Acta path. microbiol. scand. 57:301, 1963.

107. Hamilton, J. R., and Sass-Kortsak, A.: Jaundice associated with severe bacterial infection in young infants, J. Pediat. 63: 121, 1963.

108. Hamperl, H.: Über Retothelknötchen in Leberpunktaten von Tuberkulosekranken, Klin. Wschr. 31:681, 1953.

109. Hanger, F. M., and Gutman, A. B.: Postarsphenamine jaundice apparently due to obstruction of intrahepatic biliary tract, J.A.M.A. 115:263, 1940.

110. Hanshaw, J. B., Betts, R. F., Simon, G., and Boynton, R. C.: Acquired cytomegalovirus infection: association with hepatomegaly and abnormal function tests, New Engl. J. Med. 272:602, 1965.

111. Haroutunian, L. M., Fisher, A. M., and Smith, E. W.: Tuberculosis and sarcoidosis, Bull. Johns Hopkins Hosp. 115:1, 1964.

112. Harris, W. H., Jr.: Comparison of pathologic observations in Weil's disease and in yellow fever, Arch. Path. 34:663, 1942.

113. Hartwell, M. V., Love, G. I., and Eidenbock, M. P.: Adenovirus in blood clots from cases of infectious hepatitis, Science 152:1390, 1966.

114. Havens, W. P., Jr., Bucher, C. J., and Reimann, H. A.: Leptospirosis: a public health hazard; report of a small outbreak of Weil's disease in bathers, J.A.M.A. 116:289, 1941.

115. Havens, W. P., Jr., and Wenner, H. A.: Infectious hepatitis complicated by secondary invasion with salmonella, J. Clin. Invest. 25:45, 1946.

116. Heath, C. W., Jr., Alexander, A. D., and Galton, M. M.: Leptospirosis in the United States. Analysis of 483 cases in man 1949–1961, New Engl. J. Med. 273:857, 1965.

117. Hemsath, F. A., and Pinkerton, H.: Disseminated cytomegalic inclusion disease and disseminated toxoplasmosis in an adult with myeloid metaplasia; report of a case, Am. J. Clin. Path. 26:36, 1956.

118. Heringman, E. C., and Phillips, J. H.: Weil's disease; a report of twenty-three cases, New Engl. J. Med. 273:471, 1947.

119. Herrell, W. E., and Simpson, W. C.: Recurrent hyperpyrexia due to solitary tuberculoma of the liver, with review of the literature, J.A.M.A. 111:517, 1938.

120. Hertz, C. S.: Acute gonococcic perihepatitis, Proc. Staff Meet., Mayo Clin. 13: 577, 1938.

121. Hills, A. G.: Malarial jaundice, Am. J. Med. Sci. 212:45, 1946.

122. Holtzman, I. N.: Sarcoidosis followed by biliary cirrhosis and xanthomatosis, New York State J. Med. 61:1757, 1961.

123. Howells, L.: Tuberculosis splenomegaly, Brit. J. Tuberc. 33:178, 1939.

124. Hurst, A., Maier, H. M., and Lough, S. A.: Studies of hepatic function in pulmonary tuberculosis, Am. J. Med. Sci. 214:431, 1947.

125. Hurst, A. F.: Infective jaundice at Gallipoli, Brit. Med. J. 1:527, 1917.

126. Hutchison, J. H., Pippard, J. S., and White, M. H. G.: Outbreak of Weil's disease in the British Army in Italy. I. clinical study, Brit. Med. J. 1:81, 1946.

127. Ido, Y., Hoki, R., Ito, H., and Wani, H.: The rat as a carrier of Spirochaeta icterohaemorrhagiae, the causative agent of Weil's disease (spirochaetosis icterohaemorrhagica), J. Exp. Med. 26:341, 1917.

128. Inada, R., Ido, Y., Hoki, R., Kaneko, R., and Ito, H.: The etiology, mode of infection, and specific therapy of Weil's disease (spirochaetosis icterohaemorrhagica), J. Exp. Med. 23:377, 1916.

129. Israel, H. L., DeLamater, E., Sones, M., Willis, W. D., and Mirmelstein, A.: Chronic disseminated histoplasmosis; an investigation of its relationship to sarcoidosis, Am. J. Med. 12:252, 1952.

130. Iversen, O. H., and Ofstad, E.: Acute disseminated tuberculosis with hematological symptoms and corticosteroid therapy, Acta med. scand. 166:291, 1960.

131. Jackson, H., and Oleesky, S.: An unusual case of Weil's disease, Brit. Med. J. 2: 813, 1946.

132. Jahiel, R. I., and Koffler, D.: Hepatic granulomas induced in guinea pigs by Freund's adjuvant with and without ho-

mologous liver, Brit. J. Exp. Path. *42*: 338, 1961.

133. Jehgers, H. J., Houghton, J. D., and Foley, J. A.: Weil's disease; report of a case with postmortem observations and review of recent literature, Arch. Path. *20*:447, 1935.

134. Jennings, W. K.: Discussion, Arch. Surg. *65*:26, 1952.

135. Joachim, H., and Polayes, S. H.: Subacute endocarditis and systemic mycosis (monilia), J.A.M.A. *115*:205, 1940.

136. Jones, J. M., and Peck, W. M.: Incidence of fatty liver in tuberculosis with special reference to tuberculosis enteritis, Arch. Int. Med. *74*:371, 1944.

137. Jordan, W. S., Jr., and Albright, R. W.: Liver function tests in infectious mononucleosis, J. Lab. Clin. Med. *35*:688, 1950.

138. Joske, R. A., and Finckh, E. S.: Hepatic changes in human brucellosis, M. J. Aust. *1*:266, 1955.

139. Joske, R. A.: Keall, D. D., Leak, P. J., Stanley, N. F., and Walters, M. N. I.: Hepatitis-encephalitis in humans with reovirus infection, Arch. Int. Med. *113*: 811, 1964.

140. Kalk, H., and Ulbricht, J.: Klinische Beobachtungen bei der infektiösen Mononucleose, Z. klin. Med. *148*:265, 1951.

141. Kass, E. H., Andrus, S. B., Adams, R. D., Turner, F. C., and Feldman, H. A.: Toxoplasmosis in the human adult, Arch. Int. Med. *89*:759, 1952.

142. Kass, E. H., and Robbins, S. L.: Severe hepatitis in infectious mononucleosis; report of a case with minimal clinical manifestations, and death due to rupture of the spleen, Arch. Path. *50*:644, 1950.

143. Keefer, C. S.: Jaundice—its clinical significance, Med. Clin. N. Amer. *15*:929, 1932.

144. Keefer, C. S., Ingelfinger, F. J., and Spink, W. W.: Significance of hemolytic streptococcic bacteremia; a study of two hundred and forty-six patients, Arch. Int. Med. *60*:1084, 1937.

145. Kennedy, C. C., Crozier, T. H., and Houston, A. C.: Canicola fever; a human case in Northern Ireland, Brit. Med. J. *1*:197, 1953.

146. Kerley, P.: The etiology of erythema nodosum, Brit. J. Radiol. *16*:199, 1943.

147. Kern, R. A., and Norris, R. F.: Liver involvement in malaria, U. S. Nav. M. Bull. *43*:847, 1944.

148. Klatskin, G.: Unpublished data.

149. Klatskin, G., and Yesner, R.: Hepatic manifestations of sarcoidosis and other granulomatous diseases. A study based on histological examination of tissue obtained by needle biopsy of the liver, Yale J. Biol. Med. *23*:207, 1950.

150. Klemola, E., and Kääriäinen, L.: Cytomegalovirus as a possible cause of a disease resembling infectious mononucleosis, Brit. Med. J. *2*:1099, 1965.

151. Klemperer, P.: Pathology of icterus, New York J. Med. *33*:1309, 1933.

152. Kligman, A. M.: Are fungous infections increasing as a result of antibiotic therapy?, J.A.M.A. *149*:979, 1952.

153. Koch, M. L., and Cote, R. A.: Comparison of fluorescence microscopy with Ziehl-Neelsen stain for demonstration of acid-fast bacilli in smear preparations and tissue sections, Am. Rev. Resp. Dis. *91*:283, 1965.

154. Kopp, I., and Solomon, H. C.: The relationship of hypoalbuminemia to the edema of malaria, Am. J. Med. Sci. *202*: 861, 1941.

155. ————: Liver function in therapeutic malaria, Am. J. Med. Sci. *205*:90, 1943.

156. Korn, R. J., Kellow, W. F., Heller, P., Chomet, B., and Zimmerman, H. J.: Hepatic involvement in extrapulmonary tuberculosis; histologic and functional characteristics, Am. J. Med. 27:60, 1959.

157. Korones, S. B.: Congenital rubella syndrome: advances and new concepts, G. P. *35*:78, 1967.

158. Kreel, L., and Williams, R.: Arteriovenography of portal system, Brit. Med. J. *2*:1500, 1964.

159. LaManna, C.: Über die sogenannte Cholangitis lenta, Virchows Arch. path. Anat. *298*:515, 1936-1937.

160. Lamb, S. G., and Stern, H.: Cytomegalovirus mononucleosis with jaundice, Lancet *2*:1003, 1966.

161. Leibowitz, S., and Brody, H.: Cirrhosis of the liver following infectious mononucleosis, Am. J. Med. *8*:675, 1950.

162. Leifer, W., Chargin, L., and Hyman, H. T.: Massive dose arsenotherapy of early syphilis by intravenous drip method; recapitulation of the data (1933 to 1941), J.A.M.A. *117*:1154, 1941.

163. Levy, S.: Vitamin K in tuberculosis, with special reference to pulmonary hemorrhage, Am. Rev. Tuberc. *45*:377, 1942.

164. Lichtman, S. S.: Gonococcal endocardi-

tis with jaundice, J. Mt. Sinai Hosp. 4:72, 1937.

165. Lippincott, S. W., Ellenbrook, L. D., Hesselbrock, W. B., Gordon, H. H., Gottlieb, L., and Marble, A.: Liver function tests in chronic relapsing vivax malaria, J. Clin. Invest. 24:616, 1945.

166. Littman, M. L.: Cryptococcosis (torulosis); current concepts and therapy, Am. J. Med. 27:976, 1959.

167. Löfgren, S.: Primary pulmonary sarcoidosis, Acta med. scand. 145:424, 1953.

168. Lorentz, F. H.: Die Leber in ihrem Verhalten zur Tuberkulose und Cirrhose, Ztschr. Tuberk. 20:232, 1913.

169. Lowbeer,, L.: Discussion, J.A.M.A. 134: 678, 1947.

170. Lyford, J., III, Johnson, R. W., Jr., Blackman, S., and Scott, R. B.: Pathologic findings in a fatal case of disseminated granuloma inguinale with miliary bone and joint involvement, Bull. Johns Hopkins Hosp. 79:349, 1946.

171. McBride, R. A., Corson, J. M., and Dammin, G. J.: Mucormycosis, two cases of disseminated disease with cultural identification of Rhizopus; review of literature, Am. J. Med. 28:832, 1960.

172. McCoy, C. C.: A fatal case of undulant fever complicated by cirrhosis of the liver, Clin. Misc., Mary I. Bassett Hosp. 2:109, 1935.

173. McCullough, N. B., and Eisele, C. W.: Brucella hepatitis leading to cirrhosis of the liver, Arch. Int. Med. 88:793, 1951.

174. McDougal, R. A., Beamer, P. R., and Hellerstein, S.: Fatal herpes simplex hepatitis in a newborn infant, Am. J. Clin. Path. 24:1250, 1954.

175. McFadzean, A. J. S., and Ong, G. B.: Intrahepatic typhoid carriers, Brit. Med. J. 1:1567, 1966.

176. Machella, T. E., Fine, R., and Burgoon, D. F.: The relationship of Bromsulphalein retention to the fever of natural P. falciparum malaria, Am. J. Med. Sci. 213:81, 1947.

177. McIntosh, J.: The occurrence and distribution of the Spirochaeta pallida in congenital syphilis, J. Path. Bact. 13:239, 1909.

178. MacMahon, H. E., and Mallory, F. B.: Streptococcus hepatitis, Am. J. Path. 7:299, 1931.

179. McNee, J. W.: Spirochaetal jaundice; the morbid anatomy and mechanism of production of jaundice, J. Path. Bact. 23:342, 1919-1920.

180. Mallory, F. B.: A histological study of typhoid fever, J. Exp. Med. 3:611, 1898.

181. Mansuy, M. M., and Seiferth, W. J.: Miliary tuberculosis of the liver: liver biopsy as an adjunct to diagnosis, Am. J. Med. Sci. 220:293, 1950.

182. Markoff, N. G.: Zur Frage der Leberschädigung bei Bang'scher Krankheit, Zbl. inn. Med. 58:993, 1937.

183. Markowitz, J., Rappaport, A., and Scott, A. C.: Prevention of liver necrosis following ligation of hepatic artery, Proc. Soc. Exp. Biol. Med. 70:305, 1949.

184. Martin, C. J.: Concerning the pathology and etiology of the infectious jaundice common at the Dardanelles, 1915, Brit. Med. J. 1:445, 1917.

185. Martin, D. S., and Smith, D. T.: Blastomycosis (American blastomycosis, Gilchrist's disease); report of 13 new cases, Am. Rev. Tuberc. 39:488, 1939.

186. Materna, A.: Leberschädigung durch Impfmalaria, Wien. klin. Wschr. 44: 1331, 1931.

187. Mather, G., Dawson, J., and Hoyle, C.: Liver biopsy in sarcoidosis, Quart. J. Med. 24:331, 1955.

188. Medearis, D. N., Jr.: Observations concerning human cytomegalovirus infection and disease, Bull. Johns Hopkins Hosp. 114:181 1964.

189. Meredith, H. C., Jr., Early, J. Q., and Becker, W.: Tuberculous splenomegaly with hypersplenism syndrome; a case report, Blood 4:1367, 1949.

190. Mever, K. F., Stewart-Anderson, B., and Eddie, B.: Epidemiology of leptospirosis, Am. J. Public Health 29:347, 1939.

191. Mirsky, I. A., von Brecht, R., and Williams, L. D.: Hepatic dysfunction in malaria, Science 99:20, 1944.

192. Mistilis, S. P., Green, J. R., and Schiff, L.: Hepatic sarcoidosis with portal hypertension, Am. J. Med. 36:1470, 1964.

192a. Mistilis, S. P., Skyring, A. P., and Goulston, S. J. M.: Effect of long-term tetracycline therapy, steroid therapy and colectomy in pericholangitis associated with ulcerative colitis, Australasian Ann. Med. 14:286, 1965.

193. Molner, J. G., and Meyer, K. F.: Jaundice in Detroit, Am. J. Public Health 30:509, 1940.

194. Molner, J. G., Meyer, K. F., and Raskin,

H. A.: Leptospiral infections; survey, J.A.M.A. *136*:814, 1948.

195. Moon, V. H.: Experimental cirrhosis in relation to human cirrhosis, Arch. Path. *18*:381, 1934.

196. Morgan, H. R.: Pathologic changes produced in rabbits by a toxic somatic antigen derived from Eberthella typhosa, Am. J. Path. *19*:135, 1943.

197. Morris, E.: Tuberculosis of the liver, Am. Rev. Tuberc. *22*:585, 1930.

198. Morrison, J. B.: Calcified miliary tuberculosis of the spleen, Tubercle *35*:38, 1954.

199. Muirhead, E. E., Schneider, H., and McCaughey, R. S.: Candidate viruses in hepatitis, Transfusion *3*:443, 1963.

200. Nelson, N. A., Goodwin, H. L., and Oster, H. L.: The association of histoplasmosis and lymphoma, Am. J. Med. Sci. *233*:56, 1957.

201. Nelson, S., and Schwabe, A. D.: Progressive hepatic decompensation with terminal hepatic coma in sarcoidosis; report of a case, Am. J. Dig. Dis. *11*:495, 1966.

202. Niederman, J. C., McCollum, R. W., Henle, G., and Henle, W.: Infectious mononucleosis: clinical manifestations in relation to EB virus antibodies, J.A.M.A. *203*:205, 1968.

203. Norfleet, R. G., and Rickenbach, H. F.: Infectious mononucleosis treated with chloroquine; a double blind study of 25 cases, Arch. Int. Med. *113*:412, 1964.

204. Nushan, H., and Bailey, A. A.: Acute hepatitis due to brucellosis, Ann. Int. Med. *39*:915, 1953.

205. Okudaira, M., Straub, M., and Schwarz, J.: The etiology of discrete splenic and hepatic calcifications in an endemic area of histoplasmosis, Am. J. Path. *39*:599, 1961.

206. Opie, E. L.: On the relation of combined intoxication and bacterial infection to necrosis of the liver, acute yellow atrophy and cirrhosis, J. Exp. Med. *12*:367, 1910.

207. O'Shaughnessey, W. J., and Buechner, H. A.: Hepatitis associated with a coxsackie B5 virus infection during late pregnancy, J.A.M.A. *179*:71, 1962.

208. Osler, W.: Hepatic complications of typhoid fever, Johns Hopkins Hosp. Rep. *8*:373, 1899-1900.

209. Packchanian, A., and Tom, N.: Persis-
tence of Leptospira antibodies in the circulating blood of patients recovered one to over twenty years from Weil's disease, J. Immun. *46*:263, 1943.

210. Pardo-Costello, V., and Tiant, F. R.: Leprosy; correlation of its clinical, pathologic, immunologic and bacteriologic aspects, J.A.M.A. *121*:1264, 1943.

211. Parsons, R. J., and Zarafonetis, C. J. D.: Histoplasmosis in man; report of 7 cases and a review of 71 cases, Arch. Int. Med. *75*:1, 1945.

212. Patterson, H. M.: Weil's disease; observations in sixty-one cases with special reference to the use of penicillin in six cases, J.A.M.A. *134*:1077, 1947.

213. Picchi, J., Nelson, A. R., Waller, E. E., Razavi, M., and Clizer, E. E.: Q fever associated with granulomatous hepatitis, Ann. Int. Med. *53*:1065, 1960.

214. Pinkerton, H., and Iverson, L.: Histoplasmosis; three fatal cases with disseminated sarcoid-like lesions, Arch. Int. Med. *90*:456, 1952.

215. Plotkin, S. A., Cochran, W., Lindquist, J. M., Cochran, G. G., Schaffer, D. B., Scheie, H. G., and Furukawa, T.: Congenital rubella syndrome in late infancy, J.A.M.A. *200*:435, 1967.

216. Plotkin, S. A., Oski, F. A., Hartnett, E. M., Hervada, A. R., Friedman, S., and Gowing, J.: Some recently recognized manifestations of the rubella syndrome, J. Pediat. *67*:182, 1965.

217. Porter, G. H.: Hepatic sarcoidosis: a cause of portal hypertension and liver failure; review, Arch. Int. Med. *108*:482, 1961.

218. Powell, O. W.: Liver involvement in "Q" fever, Aust. Ann. Med. *10*:52, 1961.

219. Price, A. E., and Jardine, R. L.: Primary tuberculosis of the spleen: its clinical resemblance to Banti's disease; with a report of 3 cases, Ann. Int. Med. *4*:1574, 1931.

220. Pullen, R. L., and Stuart, B. M.: Tularemia; analysis of 225 cases, J.A.M.A. *129*:495, 1945.

221. Randolph, B. M.: Acute miliary tuberculosis; case report, Am. Rev. Tuberc. *22*:593, 1930.

222. Rankin, J. G., Boden, R. W., Goulston, S. J. M., and Morrow, W.: The liver in ulcerative colitis; treatment of pericholangitis with tetracycline, Lancet *2*:1110, 1959.

223. Read, H. S., Kaplan, L. I., Becker, F. T., and Boyd, M. F.: An analysis of complications encountered during therapeutic malaria, Ann. Int. Med. 24:444, 1946.

224. Reichle, H. S., and Work, J. L.: Incidence and significance of healed miliary tubercles in the liver, spleen and kidneys, Arch. Path. 28:331, 1939.

225. Reimann, H. A., and Price, A. H.: Histoplasmosis resembling sarcoidosis, Trans. Ass. Am. Phys. 62:112, 1949.

226. Rheingold, J. J., and Spurling, C. L.: Chloramphenicol and aplastic anemia, J.A.M.A. 149:1301, 1952.

227. Rich, A. R.: The pathogenesis of the forms of jaundice, Bull. Johns Hopkins Hosp. 47:338, 1930.

228. Robertson, K.: Weil's disease: a rare condition?, Brit. Med. J. 2:810, 1946.

229. Rosenbaum, H. D.: Canicola fever; case report and review of literature, Arch. Int. Med. 78:531, 1946.

230. Rosenberg, B. L.: Canicola fever; review with report of two cases, Am. J. Med. 11:75, 1951.

231. Rosenblüth, M. B., and Block, M.: Pneumonia due to type V pneumococcus, Arch. Int. Med. 60:567, 1937.

232. Rosenkranz, K., and Howard, L. D.: Tubular tuberculosis of the liver, Arch. Path. 22:743, 1936.

233. Rothenberg, R. C.: Undulant fever: a fatal case, Ann. Int. Med. 6:1275, 1933.

234. Sabesin, S. M., Fallon, H. J., and Andriole, V. T.: Hepatic failure as a manifestation of cryptococcosis, Arch. Int. Med. 111: 661, 1963.

235. Salaman, M. H., King, A. J., Williams, D. I., and Nicol, C. S.: Prevention of jaundice resulting from antisyphilitic treatment, Lancet 2:7, 1944.

236. Sandborn, E. B., Côté, M. G., and Viallet, A.: Electron microscopy of a human liver in Weil's disease (leptospirosis icterohaemorrhagica), J. Path. Bact. 92:369, 1966.

237. Saphir, O.: Changes in the liver and in the pancreas in chronic pulmonary tuberculosis with special reference to the islets of Langerhans, Arch. Path. 7:1026, 1929.

238. Sarin, L. R., Samuel, K. C., and Bhargava, R. K.: Hepatic derangement in pulmonary tuberculosis, Am. Rev. Tuberc. 76:410, 1957.

239. Sborov, V. M., Morse, W. C., Giges, B., and Jahnke, E. J., Jr.: Bacteriology of the human liver, J. Clin. Invest. 31:986, 1952.

240. Schaefer, M.: Leptospiral meningitis. Investigation of a water-borne epidemic due to L. pomona, J. Clin. Invest. 30: 670, 1951.

241. Schiff, L.: Serum bilirubin in health and in disease, Arch. Int. Med. 40:800, 1927.

242. Schneider, L. A., and Shallenberger, P. L.: A study of hepatic function in acquired malaria, Am. J. Med. Sci. 214: 80, 1947.

243. Schüffner, W.: Recent work on leptospirosis, Trans. Roy. Soc. Trop. Med. Hyg. 28:71, 1934.

244. Schwartz, J., and Muth, J.: Coccidioidomycosis: a review, Am. J. Med. Sci. 221:89, 1951.

245. Seibert, F. B., and Nelson, J. W.: Electrophoresis of serum; serum proteins in tuberculosis and other chronic diseases, Am. Rev. Tuberc. 47:66, 1943.

246. Senekjie, H. A.: The clinical manifestations of leptospirosis in Louisiana, J.A.M.A. 126:5, 1944.

247. Sexton, R. C., Eyles, D. E., and Dillman, R. E.: Adult toxoplasmosis, Am. J. Med. 14:366, 1953.

248. Shay, H., Berk, J. E., Sones, M., Aegerter, E. E., Weston, J. K., and Adams, A. B.: The liver in sarcoidosis, Gastroenterology 19:441, 1951.

249. Sheehan, H. L.: Outbreak of Weil's disease in the British Army in Italy. II. Post-mortem and histological findings, Brit. Med. J. 1:83, 1946.

250. Sheldon, W. H.: Lesions of muscle in spirochetal jaundice (Weil's disease; spirochetosis icterohemorrhagica), Arch. Int. Med. 75:119, 1945.

251. ———: Personal communication.

252. Shields, L. H.: Disseminated cryptococcosis producing a sarcoid type of reaction; the report of a case treated with amphotericin B, Arch. Int. Med. 104: 763, 1959.

253. Silverman, F. N., Schwarz, J., and Lahey, M. E.: Histoplasmosis, Am. J. Med. 19: 410, 1955.

254. Simonsen, E., and Christiansen, K.: Mononucleosis infectiosa, a 5 year material with special reference to the effect of prednisolone treatment, Acta med. scand. 180:729, 1966.

255. Skinner, D., and Keefer, C. S.: Significance of bacteremia caused by Staphylococcus aureus; a study of one hundred

and twenty-two cases and a review of the literature concerned with experimental infection in animals, Arch. Int. Med. 68:851, 1941.

256. Spain, R. S., and Howard, G. T.: Leptospirosis due to Leptospira grippotyphosa, J.A.M.A. 150:1010, 1952.

257. Spink, W. W.: Host-parasite relationship in human brucellosis with prolonged illness due to suppuration of the liver and spleen, Am. J. Med. Sci. 247:129, 1964.

258. Spink, W. W., Hoffbauer, F. W., Walker, W. W., and Green, R. A.: Histopathology of the liver in human brucellosis, J. Lab. Clin. Med. 34:40, 1949.

259. Steiner, W. R., and Walton, L. L.: Gonorrheal endocarditis with bilateral parotitis and toxic jaundice as additional complications, Ann. Int. Med. 11:1464, 1938.

260. Sterling, K.: The serum proteins in infectious mononucleosis. Electrophoretic studies, J. Clin. Invest. 28:1057, 1949.

261. ———: Hepatic function in Weil's disease, Gastroenterology 15:52, 1950.

262. Stiles, W. W., Goldstein, J. D., and McCann, W. S.: Leptospiral nephritis, J.A.M.A. 131:1271, 1946.

263. Stokes, J. H.: Modern Clinical Syphilology, pp. 993–1067, Philadelphia, Saunders, 1927.

264. Strong, R. P.: Sitt's Diagnosis, Prevention and Treatment of Tropical Diseases, ed. 6, p. 55, New York, Blakiston, 1942.

265. Stuart, B. M., and Pullen, R. L.: Typhoid; clinical analysis of three hundred and sixty cases, Arch. Int. Med. 78:629, 1946.

266. Sun, N. C., and Smith, V. C.: Hepatitis associated with myocarditis: unusual manifestation of infection with coxsackie Group B, type 3, New Engl. J. Med. 274:190, 1966.

267. Sutliff, W. D., Shepard, R., and Dunham, W. B.: Acute Leptospira pomona arthritis and myocarditis, Ann. Int. Med. 39:134, 1953.

268. Symmers, D., and Spain, D. M.: Hepar lobatum. Clinical significance of the anatomic changes, Arch. Path. 42:64, 1946.

269. Terry, R. B., and Gunnar, R, M.: Primary miliary tuberculosis of the liver, J.A.M.A. 164:150, 1957.

270. Thompson, R. P. H., and Williams, R.: Treatment of chronic intrahepatic cholestasis with phenobarbitone, Lancet 2:646, 1967.

271. Thorne, F. C., and Estabrook, J. S.: The association of bacillary dysentery and infectious jaundice, with special reference to epidemiology and bacteriologic control, J.A.M.A. 117:89, 1941.

272. Tilden, I. L.: Lepromatous leprosy; a reticuloendothelial disease; histopathologic aspects, Am. J. Clin. Path. 15:165, 1945.

273. Tisdale, W. A.: Spontaneous colon bacillus bacteremia in Laennec's cirrhosis, Gastroenterology 40:141, 1961.

274. Tonge, J. I., and Derrick, E. H.: A fatal case of "Q" fever associated with hepatic necrosis, M. J. Aust. 1:594, 1959.

275. Ts'ui-Ting, H., and Tsung-Hua, L.: Tuberculosis of the spleen treated by splenectomy; report of a case, Chin. Med. J. 74:287, 1956.

276. Tucker, E. S., III, and Scofield, G. F.: Hepatoadrenal necrosis: fatal systemic herpes simplex infection; review of literature and report of two cases, Arch. Path. 71:538, 1961.

277. Tumulty, P. A., Nichols, E., Singewald, M. L., and Lidz, T.: An investigation of the effects of recurrent malaria; an organic and psychological analysis of 50 soldiers, Medicine 25:17, 1946.

278. Ullom, J. T.: The liver in tuberculosis, Am. J. Med. Sci. 137:694, 1909.

279. vanBeek, C., Haex, A. J., and Smit, A.: Liver biopsies in diagnosis of acute hematogenic tuberculosis, Ned. geneesk. 93:2708, 1949.

280. Vickers, F. N., and Maloney, P. J.: Gonococcal perihepatitis; report of three cases with comments on diagnosis and treatment, Arch. Int. Med. 114:120, 1964.

281. Vischer, T. L., Bernheim, C., and Engelbrecht, E.: Two cases of hepatitis due to Toxoplasma gondii, Lancet 2:919, 1967.

282. Wadsworth, R. C., and Keil, P. G.: Biopsy of the liver in infectious mononucleosis, Am. J. Path. 28:1003, 1952.

283. Walch-Sorgdrager, B.: Leptospiroses, Bull. Health Organ., League of Nations 8:143, 1939.

284. Warthin, A. S.: The occurrence of icterus in tuberculosis, Int. Clin. (21st Series) 1:89, 1911.

285. Weller, T. H., and Hanshaw, J. B.: Virologic and clinical observations on cytomegalic inclusion disease, New Engl. J. Med. 256:1234, 1962.

286. Whipple, R. L., Jr., and Harris, J. F.: B. coli septicemia in Laennec's cirrhosis of the liver, Ann. Int. Med. 33:462, 1950.

287. Wigger, H. J., and Blanc, W. A.: Fatal hepatic and bronchial necrosis in adenovirus infection with thymic alymphoplasia, New Engl. J. Med. 275:870, 1966.

288. Willcox, W. H.: The epidemic jaundice of campaigns, Brit. Med. J. 1:297, 1916.

289. Willcox, W.: Toxic jaundice, Lancet 2:1 1931.

290. Williams, G., Stretton, T. B., and Leonard, J. C.: Cytomegalic inclusion disease and Pneumocystis carinii infection in an adult, Lancet 2:951, 1960.

291. Williams, R. H.: Gonococcic endocarditis; study of twelve cases, with ten postmortem examinations, Arch. Int. Med. 61:26, 1938.

292. Winternitz, M. C.: Tuberculosis of the spleen, Arch. Int. Med. 8:680, 1912.

293. Wolf, G. A., Jr., and Flory, C. M.: Miliary tuberculosis of the liver, Am. Rev. Tuberc. 51:553, 1945.

294. Wolff, B. P.: Asiatic relapsing fever; report of 134 cases treated with Mapharsen, Ann. Int. Med. 24:203, 1946.

295. Wong, M., and Rosen, S. W.: Ascites in sarcoidosis due to peritoneal involvement, Ann. Int. Med. 57:277, 1962.

296. Wong, T., and Warner, N. E: Cytomegalic inclusion disease in adults. Report of 14 cases with a review of the literature, Arch. Path. 74:403, 1962.

297. Woodward, T. E., Hall, H. E., Hightower, J. A., and Pons, E.: Antibiotic therapy of leptospirosis with discussion of effects on leptospiremia, J. Clin. Invest. 30:683, 1951.

298. Yow, E. M., Brennan, J. C., Nathan, M. H., and Israel, L.: Calcified granulomata of the spleen in long-standing Brucella infection. A report of a case of twenty-five years' duration, Ann. Int. Med. 55:307, 1961.

299. Yow, E. M., Brennan, J. C., Preston, J., and Levy, S.: The pathology of psittacosis: a report of 2 cases with hepatitis, Am. J. Med. 27:739, 1959.

300. Ziegler, E. E.: Infectious mononucleosis; report of a fatal case with autopsy, Arch. Path. 37:196, 1944.

301. Zimmerman, H. J., and Thomas, L. J.: The liver in pneumococcal pneumonia: observations in 94 cases on liver function and jaundice in pneumonia, J. Lab. Clin. Med. 35:556, 1950.

302. Zimmerman, L. E.: Candida and Aspergillus endocarditis, with comments on the role of antibiotics in dissemination of fungus disease, Arch. Path. 50:591, 1950.

16

Active Chronic Hepatitis

STEVEN PAUL MISTILIS, M.B., B.S., M.R.A.C.P.

Active chronic hepatitis was first described by Waldenstrom in 1950.[180] He drew attention to a form of chronic liver disease in young women characterized by moderate jaundice, acne, amenorrhea, hepatosplenomegaly and hyperglobulinemia. In 1951, Kunkel reported preliminary observations on a similar disorder[100] and in 1956, with Bearn and Slater, published a detailed account of chronic liver disease in 26 young women.[15] He emphasized the high incidence of amenorrhea, hirsutism, obesity, acne, pigmented abdominal striae, Cushingoid facies, arthritis, febrile episodes, hypergammaglobulinemia and a coarse nodular cirrhosis.

In 1955 Joske and King reported the presence of the lupus erythematosus (L.E.) cell phenomenon in some patients with active chronic hepatitis.[91] In the following year Mackay, Taft and Cowling applied the term "lupoid hepatitis" to this association,[109] over 100 cases of which had been reported by 1965.[3, 6, 8, 12, 13, 18, 65, 71, 75, 91, 94, 99, 106, 109, 113, 158, 169, 177, 185] This focused attention on the possible role of immune factors in etiology and pathogenesis. Many workers have compared the clinical, biochemical and pathologic changes in patients with and without the L.E. cell phenomenon without finding any significant differences.[3, 4, 115, 131, 154, 188] There appears to be no justification for the continued use of the term lupoid hepatitis.

Active chronic hepatitis was initially thought to occur only in young women. However, in 1961 Willocx and Isselbacher found that it also affects males and produces clinical features identical with those encountered in females.[188] Read and coworkers in 1963 introduced the term active "juvenile" cirrhosis to emphasize the prevalence of the disorder in young people.[154] However, Page and Good described the disease in children[142-144] and Cattan[30] and Reynolds[156] reported the same disorder in postmenopausal women. It is evident that the disease affects both sexes in all age groups.

There is considerable confusion over the definition of active chronic hepatitis as a disease entity for many reports have been concerned with a particular age group or sex, or with a group of patients having in common some of the more unusual or florid manifestations. This has given rise to many terms including chronic liver disease in young women,[15] plasma cell hepatitis,[142-144] active juvenile cirrhosis[154] chronic liver disease in young people,[188] progressive hepatitis,[9, 22] lupoid hepatitis,[5, 53, 85, 87, 109, 110, 114, 136, 156] autoimmune hepatitis[111] and liver disease in young women with hyperglobulinemia.[90] Most cases so reported are in fact variants of the one disorder. It is likely that *some* of the cases reported by Dible as cryptogenic cirrhosis,[44] by Klatskin as subacute hepatic necrosis,[95] by Logan as chronic hepatitis in children,[105] by Havens as chronic viral hepatitis,[74] by Gall as posthepatitic cirrhosis,[59] by Tisdale as subacute hepatitis,[175] by Kelsall as subacute and chronic hepatitis,[92] and by Bjørneboe as subchronic atrophy of the liver[21] are examples of active chronic hepatitis.

Terminology is thus confusing and in some instances it has focused attention on unproved etiologic factors. The term *ac-*

tive chronic hepatitis is now widely accepted,[63, 86, 115, 124, 127, 131, 168] for it embodies 2 of the essential features of this disorder, namely, established chronic progressive liver disease and superimposed episodes of active disease. Although this is a generalized disease affecting many organs other than the liver, the term "active chronic hepatitis" directs attention to the major organ involved. It is probably desirable to retain this descriptive term until the cause or causes of the disease are known.

In 1957, Gajdusek found that the serum of patients with active chronic hepatitis fixed complement when added to human liver extract, and the reaction became known as the autoimmune complement fixation test.[55] This serologic reaction was initially considered to be highly significant but it has since been shown that the serum of patients with numerous unrelated diseases also fixes complement when added to various tissue extracts.[10, 14, 25, 42, 45, 46, 64, 108, 135, 149, 153] A number of other abnormal serologic reactions have been subsequently described by Doniach and others in active chronic hepa-

titis, cryptogenic cirrhosis and primary biliary cirrhosis.[25, 46, 68, 80, 89, 181, 184] Certain patterns of antibody formation have emerged, but it remains impossible to relate the lack of organ specificity of these antibodies to a disorder that affects mainly the liver. Specific antibodies against liver tissue have not yet been isolated in active chronic hepatitis or in any other chronic liver disease,[46] and the fundamental nature of the disorder remains unknown. Various theories have been advanced but the relevance of these to the etiology and pathogenesis of the disease constitutes a basis for continuing controversy.

CLINICAL FEATURES

AGE AND SEX (FIG. 16–1)

Although active chronic hepatitis may occur in either sex, it is much commoner in women; 80 per cent of a recent series were females.[131, 154, 168] The disease may appear in any age group. Cases have been reported in children and in adults over the age of 50,

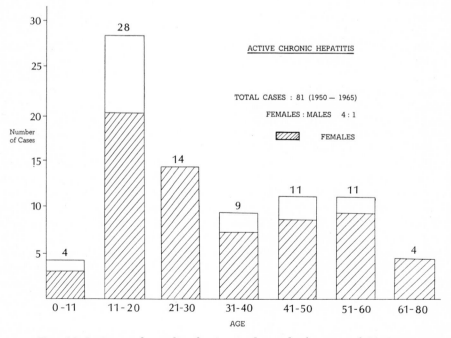

FIG. 16–1. Age and sex distribution in the author's series of 81 patients with active chronic hepatitis.

TABLE 16–1. ACTIVE CHRONIC HEPATITIS:
FEATURES DURING ONSET (82 PATIENTS)

I. ABRUPT (Identical to Acute Viral Hepatitis)	32%
II. INSIDIOUS (Period of 6 Months)	68%

INSIDIOUS GROUP (68%)   Features in 56
Patients.*

	PER CENT OF PATIENTS
Slowly progressive jaundice	61
Severe anorexia	46
Asymptomatic hepatomegaly	36
Abdominal pain	35
Epistaxis	21
Acne	19
Persistent fever	11
Arthralgia	11

* Most patients presented with 2 or more of these features.

the oldest patient being 76 years. However, in approximately 50 per cent of cases the onset of the disease occurs between the ages of 10 and 30 years. This is in contrast to other forms of chronic liver disease such as primary biliary cirrhosis, alcoholic liver disease, hemochromatosis and cryptogenic cirrhosis, in which the peak incidence occurs between the ages of 30 and 60 years.[168]

ONSET

Presenting Features (Table 16–1). In approximately one-third of the patients, the onset is abrupt with features indistinguishable from acute infectious hepatitis. However, in active chronic hepatitis, the illness persists and, over a period of months, the patients develop manifestations rarely encountered in acute infectious hepatitis.

More commonly, the onset is insidious with progressive changes over a period of months. Patients often give a history of weakness and fatigue, anorexia and weight loss, vague abdominal pain, amenorrhea, troublesome acne, mild chronic diarrhea, various skin rashes, fever, arthralgia or slowly progressive jaundice. In any individual, a combination of 2 or more of these features is often seen.

In some patients, liver disease may be totally unsuspected, for extrahepatic manifestations such as ulcerative colitis, pleurisy, arthritis and skin rashes initially dominate the clinical picture. Some patients may present with severe abdominal pain or obscure and prolonged fever. Patients are sometimes referred at the outset to various special departments because of amenorrhea, possible Cushing's disease, arthritis, acne or one of a number of skin lesions.

Physical Signs (Table 16–2). Despite the various manifestations patients often look healthy and well nourished. Jaundice is usually moderate and may be confined to the sclerae. About 20 per cent of patients are not jaundiced at any stage of the disease.

Other signs commonly encountered at the onset include hepatomegaly, splenomegaly, spider nevi, palmar erythema, acne, fever and skin rashes. Occasionally patients present with all the features of hypercorticism such as pigmented abdominal striae, moon facies, obesity and hirsutism. Spider nevi are prominent and may appear singly on the face, back and upper limbs or as a conglomerate diffuse redness at the base of the neck. Signs of portal hypertension or hepatic encephalopathy are rarely encountered early in the course of the disease.

Hepatomegaly may be significant, and in approximately one-third of the cases the liver extends 6 to 12 cm. below the right costal margin. In 25 per cent of cases the

TABLE 16–2. ACTIVE CHRONIC HEPATITIS:
SIGNS AT ONSET (82 PATIENTS)

	PER CENT OF PATIENTS
Jaundice	80
Hepatomegaly	75
Splenomegaly	49
Spider nevi	45
Palmar erythema	33
Hepatic tenderness	30
Acne	21
Rash	9
Hepatic encephalopathy	9
Ascites	9
Hirsutism	8
Arthritis	8
Abdominal striae; "moon facies"	6

liver is not palpable. The liver is tender in about 30 per cent of cases, and this often persists for many weeks and may be associated with continuous abdominal discomfort which may last for months.

The spleen is enlarged early in the course of the disease in almost half the cases and is occasionally tender to palpation. Splenomegaly may be found in the absence of other clinical manifestations of portal hypertension. In this situation it may be part of a diffuse lymphoid-reticular hyperplasia sometimes associated with generalized lymphadenopathy.

CLINICAL COURSE (Table 16–3)

Recurrent episodes of jaundice, anorexia, vague abdominal pain and malaise frequently punctuate the course of the disease. Episodes of jaundice may last from several weeks to 6 months and some patients may have persistent cholestasis for 1 to 2 years. Fever, bruising, purpura, increasing acne, splenomegaly and an enlarging tender liver may also be present during an episode of activity. The spectrum of severity is considerable and may vary from little more than weakness and malaise with moderate elevation of the serum glutamic oxaloacetic transaminase (SGOT) to jaundice with hepatic

TABLE 16–3. ACTIVE CHRONIC HEPATITIS: FEATURES DURING THE COURSE (82 PATIENTS)

	PER CENT OF PATIENTS
Jaundice	
Episodic (1 to 6 months)	56
Persistent (1 to 2 years)	24
Hepatic coma	
Spontaneous	17
Precipitated	14
Hematemesis	31
Hypersplenism*	41
Ascites	41
Hepatomegaly	73
Splenomegaly	49
Esophageal varices	42
Spider nevi	21

* Defined as patients with platelet counts below 100,000/c.mm. with or without leukopenia.

failure. Episodes of active disease do not appear abruptly in most cases, but develop insidiously over some weeks. They may develop spontaneously, but frequently appear to follow undue exertion or intercurrent infection. In the untreated patient, an episode of active liver disease may persist for weeks or months. The course of the disease is unpredictable and many patients make a good clinical recovery from acute episodes of severe jaundice with grossly impaired hepatic function.

Ascites or *signs of hepatic encephalopathy* may occur. Although hepatic coma is commonly a terminal event, episodes may be reversible. Coma may be precipitated by gastrointestinal bleeding, septicemia, drug administration or heart failure, but in 50 per cent of cases it appears spontaneously when the liver disease is most active. Hepatic insufficiency in such cases is probably due to extensive liver necrosis. In general, if spontaneous episodes of hepatic failure or ascites develop the prognosis is poor.

In *no* case has return of the liver to normal been documented. However, the disease ultimately becomes inactive in approximately 40 per cent of cases. By this time cirrhosis is established, the liver becomes smaller, the spleen increases in size and episodes of gastrointestinal bleeding, ascites and hypersplenism dominate the clinical picture. One should never assume that bleeding arises from esophageal varices, for it may be due to peptic ulcer or erosive gastritis. The latter should be considered in patients with a history of excessive salicylate intake for relief of joint symptoms. Thrombocytopenia may be a significant factor if bleeding persists.

Signs of portal hypertension may be transient and reversible early in the disease. This is not a situation unique to active chronic hepatitis, for transient portal hypertension may occur in other forms of acute hepatic injury such as viral hepatitis, severe fatty liver and alcoholic hepatitis.[70, 103, 145, 146, 155] Portal hypertension in this situation is due to extensive parenchymal necrosis and inflammation producing a critical obstruction to portal venous blood flow. This possibility should always be borne in mind, for attempts to relieve the increased portal pressure by a portacaval shunt carry a high mortality.

INVOLVEMENT OF OTHER ORGANS
(Table 16–4)

Active chronic hepatitis appears to be a multisystemic disease, for about half the patients have associated conditions apparently unrelated to the liver. Those commonly seen include arthralgia or arthritis, skin rashes, ulcerative colitis, pleurisy, pericarditis, glomerulonephritis, myocarditis, thrombocytopenic purpura, thyroiditis and diabetes. Patients may also have generalized lymphadenopathy, severe hemolytic anemia and various pulmonary and neurologic abnormalities.

These extrahepatic manifestations may precede clinical liver disease, coincide with the onset of the liver disease or, more frequently, follow it. They usually appear singly during the course of the illness or less commonly in combination. The severity of the systemic manifestations varies considerably but, in general, liver disease dominates the clinical picture.[115, 131, 154, 188]

Arthralgia and Arthritis. Arthritis or arthralgia usually affects the wrist and other large joints. It may be confined to a single joint but often involves several joints. The joint manifestations are commonly migratory and are often accompanied by fever. They usually consist of arthralgia but occasionally there is arthritis with joint swelling. All the features of rheumatoid arthritis may be seen, but most cases are completely resolved without permanent joint deformity. Arthralgia and arthritis may recur, and this usually coincides with episodes of active liver disease.

Skin Lesions.[115, 131, 154] Skin rashes may be transient. The commonest is an erythematous lesion of the face. Less frequently encountered are a maculopapular rash, nodular lesions simulating erythema nodosum, vitiligo, impetigo and purpura. Some patients may have multiple chronic indolent leg ulcers or a diffuse and intense pigmentation. Rarely lesions on the face are indistinguishable from those of systemic lupus erythematosus.

Ulcerative Colitis. The incidence of ul-

TABLE 16–4. ACTIVE CHRONIC HEPATITIS: SYSTEMIC MANIFESTATIONS (82 PATIENTS)

	PER CENT OF PATIENTS
Chronic diarrhea (including colitis)	28
Skin lesions	20
Polyarthralgia ± Arthritis	18
L.E. cell phenomenon	15
Ulcerative colitis	11
Pleurisy ± Pericarditis	11
Chronic glomerulonephritis	7
Diabetes	6
Myocarditis	4
Thyroiditis	4
One or more of the above	41

cerative colitis varies considerably and has been reported in up to 10 per cent of cases.[131] This is probably a conservative estimate. Mild, chronic diarrhea has been reported in approximately 30 per cent of patients with active chronic hepatitis,[131] due possibly to mild colitis. This can be diagnosed only by serial examinations of the rectum and sigmoid during an attack of diarrhea. Barium enema frequently reveals few or no significant changes in early or mild cases or where the disease is confined to the rectosigmoid region.

Ulcerative colitis is usually severe with involvement of the entire colon and in most cases appears before the onset of clinical liver disease.[69, 79, 81, 96, 123, 125, 129, 131, 132, 139, 154, 176, 188] Colitis may dominate the clinical picture and the diagnosis of liver disease may be overlooked. Occasionally corticosteroid therapy directed to the colitis suppresses the clinical manifestations of active liver disease. The diagnosis will not be missed if liver biopsy is performed in all cases of colitis with hepatomegaly. For patients with both ulcerative colitis and active chronic hepatitis, prognosis is probably less favorable than for patients with active chronic hepatitis not complicated by ulcerative colitis.

Renal Disease.[115, 131, 154, 172] The kidney is involved in less than 10 per cent of reported cases.[115, 131, 154] Renal involvement has probably been underestimated, for some patients can be shown to have extensive renal pathology in the absence of functional changes.[154, 172] Renal biopsy may reveal a membranous or proliferative glomerulonephritis in the absence of proteinuria, abnormal findings in the urine or elevated blood urea and serum creatinine.[154, 172]

The clinical manifestations of renal disease, when present, are chronic glomerulonephritis or the nephrotic syndrome. Renal disease rarely dominates the clinical picture and symptoms and signs of overt renal failure are uncommon. Varying degrees of renal insufficiency may occur in terminal liver failure.

Other Changes. Reported abnormalities of the thyroid gland include thyrotoxicosis, Hashimoto's disease, diffuse goiter and myxedema with thyroid atrophy.[131,154] The incidence of thyroid abnormalities appears greater than the expected frequency in the general population.

A high incidence of pulmonary disease has been noted in one large series of 81 cases.[154] Lobar pneumonia, hilar gland enlargement, primary pulmonary hypertension,[35] transient opacities on the chest radiograph,[33] and lobar collapse have all been seen. Acute pulmonary changes occur when the liver lesion is most active.[154] Furthermore, recurrent lung infections sometimes seem to provoke a relapse of jaundice.

Abnormalities of the nervous system include polyneuritis, epilepsy, psychoses and cerebral vasculitis with hemiplegia. These changes were recorded in 2 series but involved only a few patients.[115, 154] It is uncertain whether this is a chance association or whether there is an increase in incidence of these neurologic lesions.

ENDOCRINE MANIFESTATIONS
(Table 16-5)

The endocrine changes seen in order of decreasing frequency include amenorrhea, acne, hirsutism, pigmented striae of the skin, gynecomastia in males, obesity and Cushingoid facies. These changes are usually found in the adolescent and young adult group. A combination of 2 or more of these features in one patient is seen in only 20 per cent of cases. Furthermore, florid signs of hyper-

TABLE 16-5. ACTIVE CHRONIC HEPATITIS: ENDOCRINE FEATURES BEFORE AND DURING STEROID THERAPY (82 PATIENTS)

	PER CENT OF PATIENTS	
	Before Steroids	During Steroids°
Amenorrhea	38	38
Acne	21	44
Hirsutism	8	21
Pigmented skin striae	6	16
Cushingoid facies	6	29
Gynecomastia (males)	11	11
Two or more of the above	22	

° Additional changes during steroid therapy include repeated infections (osteomyelitis, meningitis, septicemia, moniliasis, staphylococcal abscesses, pyelitis) in 5 patients, severe diabetes in 2 patients and severe hypertension, marked muscle wasting and osteoporosis with vertebral collapse in one patient.

corticism resembling Cushing's syndrome occur in less than 10 per cent of patients.[131]

Acne usually affects the face, may extend to the chest and back and has no particular distinguishing features. Troublesome acne, resistant to therapy, may be present for some time before the underlying liver disease becomes obvious. Acne is often more extensive and severe during an active episode of the disease.

Endocrine manifestations become more florid during corticosteroid therapy. Severe hypertension, marked obesity, severe muscle wasting, edema, diabetes and osteoporosis with vertebral body collapse may develop. Some of these changes may occur after even a relatively short course of treatment and thus may limit the use of these drugs.

Metabolism of steroids such as cortisol, estradiol, estrone, bile acids and aldosterone is impaired in most forms of chronic liver injury.[23, 41, 48] It is assumed that the rate of cortisol synthesis is not increased and that the manifestations of hypercorticism reflect an impairment of its metabolic clearance.[48]

MORBIDITY AND PROGNOSIS
(Fig. 16-2)

Patients often require repeated hospitalization and long periods of complete bed rest for spontaneous episodes of active liver disease or the complications of cirrhosis. Time spent in the hospital is 6 to 30 per cent of the total duration of the disease.[131] This morbidity is considerable and few patients return to a full and active life. The mortality rate is significantly greater early in the illness when the disease is most active. Patients who survive this critical period have an appreciably better prognosis. Few patients however live longer than 10 years from the time of diagnosis.[131, 154]

Certain factors appear to influence mortality and morbidity. In the author's series,[131] mortality was greater in patients with an abrupt hepatitis-like onset, persistent cholestasis, ulcerative colitis, episodes of spontaneous or precipitated hepatic coma, ascites or extensive necrosis in liver biopsy sections. The presence of L.E. cells, age, sex and involvement of the kidney, joints, thyroid, skin or serous membranes did not appreciably affect the prognosis. Furthermore, mortality was not increased in patients with an SGOT greater than 500 units, a serum bilirubin exceeding 10 mg.%, a zinc sulfate turbidity greater than 20 units or a serum globulin in excess of 6.0 gm.% at any time during the disease. Mortality was significantly lower if the onset was insidious, if jaundice was absent and when the liver disease became active. In the individual patient biochemical changes are not helpful in predicting the outcome. Deep jaundice with grossly deranged liver function tests need not signify a poor prognosis, nor need mild jaundice with compensated liver disease imply a good one.

The chief cause of death is liver cell failure which may be spontaneous[131, 154] or precipitated by gastrointestinal bleeding, septicemia or cardiac failure. Associated ulcerative colitis may be fatal. Renal failure *per se* is an uncommon cause of death, but a combined picture of hepatorenal insufficiency may be seen. Death sometimes results from serious complications of prolonged steroid administration.

Cumulative survival, calculated by the

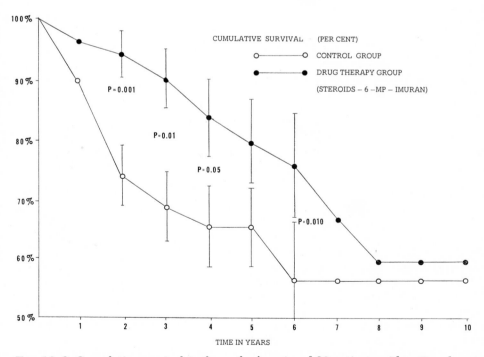

Fig. 16–2. Cumulative survival in the author's series of 82 patients with active chronic hepatitis. Calculations were based on the life table method. Vertical bars indicate standard deviation on either side of the calculated mean values.

life survival method, is the only meaningful expression of survival in chronic disease. This takes into consideration the duration of the disease in both dead and live patients, the mortality in each year and the variable periods during which patients are observed, which in turn depends upon the time at which they enter the study. The cumulative survival for one group of patients with active chronic hepatitis who had not received any specific form of drug therapy was found to be 65 per cent by the end of the fifth year (Fig. 16–2). There was a sharp fall in the curve during the first 2 years due to the many deaths early in the disease. Survival by the end of the fifth year is only slightly better than that reported for a group of patients with cirrhosis from other causes.[37, 61, 140]

LABORATORY FEATURES

HEMATOLOGIC CHANGES

Moderate normocytic, normochromic anemia is common and is probably due to reduced red cell survival from splenic hypersequestration. Patients with esophageal varices or ulcerative colitis may have severe anemia from chronic blood loss.

Thrombocytopenia with a peripheral platelet count consistently below 100,000/c.mm. is found in up to 40 per cent of cases. There may be an associated leukopenia, with a peripheral white cell count below 4,000/c.mm. These changes are probably due to hypersplenism, for restoration of the platelet and white cell count to normal levels has been reported following splenectomy.

Occasionally a polymorphonuclear leukocytosis with white cell counts exceeding 12,000/c.mm. occurs in the absence of infection.[154] In one series, peripheral blood smears showed eosinophils in excess of 5 per cent in a third of the patients at some time during the disease.[186] Both these findings are unexplained.

Hypoprothrombinemia is not nearly so profound as might be expected, for only 8 of 82 patients in my series had values below 50 per cent of normal.

However, other coagulation factors may be severely depressed.

LIVER FUNCTION TESTS (Table 16–6)

Serum Bilirubin and Serum Alkaline Phosphatase. Marked hyperbilirubinemia is distinctly uncommon. Serum bilirubin levels rarely exceed 20 mg.% and average 5 to 8 mg.%. For a number of patients, serum bilirubin may be below 2 mg.% at the onset, and for some clinical jaundice does not develop during the entire illness. Hyperbilirubinemia is usually found when the disease is active.

Serum alkaline phosphatase is usually elevated at the onset and during episodes of active liver disease. The level is usually below 35 K.A. units but in some cases is extremely high.

Serum Glutamic Oxaloacetic Transaminase (SGOT). SGOT usually increases during the active stage of the disease but there is little correlation between the level of SGOT and the degree of liver necrosis seen histologically. SGOT appears to be the best biochemical index of activity, and in the individual case serial estimations are of value in assessing the effect of therapy.

Increase in SGOT rarely approaches the levels seen in acute infectious hepatitis. Values above 1,000 units have been reported in the occasional case[156] but in general the levels do not exceed 800 units/ml., and average 200 to 300 units/ml.[131, 154]

Serum Globulins. Hyperglobulinemia is common in active chronic hepatitis but extreme values are rare. Globulin levels exceeding 7.0 gm./100 ml. were found in only 9 of the 82 patients I studied[131] and 6 of the 81 patients reported by Read.[154] Some patients may have normal globulin levels[131, 154] and the disease has even been reported in patients with agammaglobulinemia.[67] Serum globulin levels in other forms of cirrhosis are generally lower, but Reynolds reported globulin levels exceeding 6.0 gm.% in alcoholic cirrhosis[156] and half of Armas-Cruz' patients with portal cirrhosis had a globulin level above 4.0 gm.%.[7] The diagnostic value of this test in active chronic hepatitis has probably been overstressed.

TABLE 16–6. LIVER FUNCTION TESTS DURING COURSE:
MEAN* OF HIGHEST AND LOWEST VALUES

TEST	NO. OF PATIENTS TESTED†	MEAN HIGHEST	MEAN LOWEST
Serum bilirubin (mg.%)	78	7.5	1.2
Serum alkaline phosphatase (K.A. units)	78	37	16
Zinc sulfate turbidity (units)	77	29	13
Serum proteins (Gm.%)	73	8.6	7.0
Serum albumin (Gm.%)	59	3.3	3.1
Serum globulin (Gm.%)	59	5.5	3.7
Bromsulphalein retention (45 min.) (%)	44	29	—
Prothrombin time (% normal)	68	—	72
SGOT (units)	56	237	55

* The highest and lowest values in each individual patient were recorded and the mean calculated for the overall group.

† Only patients in whom serial liver function tests were done are included. In most of these over 15 tests were done during the course of the disease.

Hyperglobulinemia is due to an increase in all the immunoglobulin fractions (IgG, IgM, IgA) with a diffuse broad-based pattern on paper electrophoresis.[115] There appears to be no correlation between the degree of hypergammaglobulinemia and the intensity of the plasma cell infiltration in the liver.[66] The highest globulin levels occur during active disease and hyperglobulinemia may persist for many months after the serum bilirubin and SGOT return to normal. There is a good correlation between the changes in the zinc sulfate turbidity and the hypergammaglobulinemia.

Serum Albumin and Bromsulphalein Retention (BSP). Persistent hypoalbuminemia and abnormal BSP retention are consistently present during the cirrhotic stage of the disease and are the best biochemical indices of chronicity. Both may be transient, however, occurring during an active stage of the disease. Serial estimations of BSP retention may be useful in evaluating the effect of therapy.

SEROLOGIC TESTS (Table 16–7)

Numerous abnormal serologic reactions have been reported in patients with active chronic hepatitis. These include the L.E. cell phenomenon, antinuclear factors,[25, 46, 80] latex and sheep cell agglutination,[11, 64, 82] various complement fixing reactions,[10, 14, 42, 45, 46, 56, 64, 107, 108, 135, 149] biologically false-positive reactions for syphilis,[8, 13, 99, 114] and antibody fixing reactions to gastric mucosal cells, smooth muscle, thyroid, renal tubular epithelial cells and hepatic parenchymal cells.[46, 68, 89, 184] Localization of antibodies to various cell constituents such as the mitochondria and nuclei has also been reported.[46]

Lupus Erythematosus Cell Phenomenon (L.E. Cell). L.E. cells in the peripheral blood have been found in a large number of patients,[3, 6, 8, 12, 13, 18, 65, 71, 75, 91, 94, 99, 106, 109, 113, 158, 169, 177, 185] but the incidence has been extremely variable and the clinical significance of this test in active chronic hepatitis is unknown. Mackay and Wood found that

TABLE 16–7. INCIDENCE OF ANTIBODY REACTIONS IN PATIENTS
WITH VARIOUS FORMS OF LIVER DISEASE

DIAGNOSIS	No. PATIENTS TESTED	C.F.T.	A.N.F.	S.M.A.	MITOCHONDRIAL ANTIBODIES
Active chronic hepatitis	43	30%	56%	67%	28%*
Primary biliary cirrhosis	41	85%	31%	50%	98%
Cryptogenic cirrhosis	32	31%	16%	28%	31%
Alcoholic cirrhosis	14	0	7%	0	0
Extrahepatic obstruction	28	0	0%	0	7%
Infective hepatitis	25	8%	0%	8%	4%
Drug hepatitis	12	$\frac{1}{12}$	0%	—	$\frac{3}{12}$
Colitis with pericholangitis	5	0	—	—	0
Controls	200 to 850	3%	0%	3%	2%

(Doniach, D., Roitt, I. M., Walker, J. G., and Sherlock, S.: Clin. Exp. Immun. *1*, 1966.)
C.F.T., Complement fixation test
A.N.F., Antinuclear factor (titre of $\frac{1}{120}$ or higher)
S.M.A., Smooth muscle antibodies
* The actual pattern of fluorescence is not completely identical to that obtained using sera of patients with primary biliary cirrhosis. (Doniach and Roitt: Personal communication.)

positive tests were associated with a greater frequency of splenomegaly and systemic manifestations and occurred preponderantly in women.[114] In a number of subsequent series no significant clinical, biochemical or pathologic differences were found between patients with and without L.E. cells. A positive reaction, however, is more likely to be found when the disease is active.[131, 154]

Antinuclear Factor (A.N.F.). A high incidence of A.N.F., varying from 42 to 77 per cent, has been reported in active chronic hepatitis,[25, 46, 80] and is frequently found in patients with a negative L.E. cell reaction. Patients with active chronic hepatitis and a positive A.N.F. do not differ from patients with a negative reaction. The A.N.F. titre does not correlate with the clinical activity as measured by the SGOT levels but apparently the A.N.F. titre and the serum globulin levels correlate somewhat.[46]

Complement Fixing Reactions. In 1957 Gajdusek found that sera of patients with active chronic hepatitis and primary biliary cirrhosis fixed complement when added to human liver extract,[55] and positive reactions were for some time considered to be specific for these 2 forms of liver disease. Since then, positive reactions have been detected in a number of unrelated disorders, and it is now evident that this test is not specific for any disease or pathologic process.[10, 14, 25, 42, 45, 46, 64, 108, 135, 149, 153] Furthermore, there appears to be no correlation between the titre of complement fixing reactions and the level of gamma globulin in active chronic hepatitis.

Fluorescent Antibody Tests. Doniach recently reported a high incidence of antinuclear, antimitochondrial ("M") and smooth muscle antibodies (S.M.A.) in a large series of patients with active chronic hepatitis, cryptogenic cirrhosis, primary biliary cirrhosis and various collagen diseases.[46] Only 2 of the 28 patients with extrahepatic biliary obstruction and one of the 25 patients with acute infectious hepatitis gave positive results and then only in a low titre. Uniformly negative results for S.M.A. and "M" antibodies were obtained in alcoholic cirrhosis. These antibody reactions show a predilection for certain diseases[46, 68, 89, 181, 184] and not all forms of infection or liver injury in man can induce this type of antibody formation. The tests are relatively simple to perform[183] and may find a place in the routine diagnosis of liver disease.

PATHOLOGY

A liver biopsy is often essential to establish the diagnosis of active chronic hepatitis and may help in assessing its severity and in evaluating therapy. Findings vary with the stage at which the biopsy is obtained. The characteristic features are best seen in liver biopsy sections obtained early in the course or during an active phase of the disease.

ACTIVE STAGE (FIGS. 16–3 to 16–6)

The most characteristic feature in the active stage is *perilobular* parenchymal degeneration and necrosis with inflammatory cell infiltration (Figs. 16–3, 16–4). The degree of hepatitis varies markedly not only within a single lobule but also from lobule to lobule. It is not uncommon to encounter completely unaffected lobules adjacent to those which are severely involved. This variable degree of perilobular hepatitis has been described as "piecemeal necrosis."[148, 150]

There is a striking accumulation of lymphocytes, plasma cells and histiocytes in the portal tracts, interlobular septa and adjacent peripheral portions of the lobule. Parenchymal cells degenerate, individual hepatocytes are lost, collagen fibers proliferate and bile ductules increase. This perilobular hepatitis leads to an erosion of the limiting plate with replacement fibrosis. Collagen deposition surrounding and isolating single cells or groups of degenerating hepatocytes is a characteristic early finding. Later fibrosis is more obvious.

Other changes less frequently seen in the active stage include discrete foci of inflammation within the lobule, acidophilic degeneration of parenchymal cells, Kupffer cell proliferation and pericentral or peripheral bile stasis. Fat is striking in its absence although minor degrees of steatosis are occasionally found in patients given large doses of steroids. Parenchymal regeneration with binucleate hepatocytes and cords of double cell thickness are often evident at this stage, and occasionally giant multinucleate hepatocytes are found.

The *parenchymal cells* at the limiting plate (Fig. 16–5) vary considerably in size and shape, and large balloon-shaped cells with hypochromatic vacuolated cytoplasm are frequently present. Nuclear size and staining vary. These abnormal parenchymal cells are commonly found in small aggregates surrounded by fine strands of fibrous tissue. Occasional parenchymal cells are smaller than normal with condensed, homogenous eosinophilic cytoplasm. Some of these cells resemble those found in acute viral hepatitis.[116]

Although the changes are often confined to

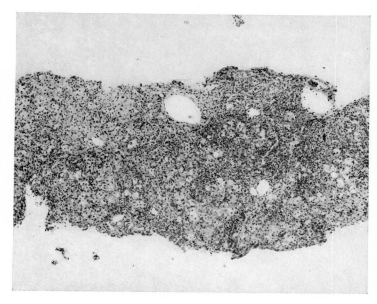

FIG. 16–3. Active chronic hepatitis— needle biopsy specimen 8 months after onset. There is intense inflammatory cell infiltration in the portal tracts, septa and adjacent hepatic lobules. There has been parenchymal cell fallout in the perilobular region and surviving cells show vacuolization and degenerative changes. The degree of change is variable from one part of the section to another. There is some fibrosis in the portal tracts and septa but the architecture is intact and there is no evidence of cirrhosis.

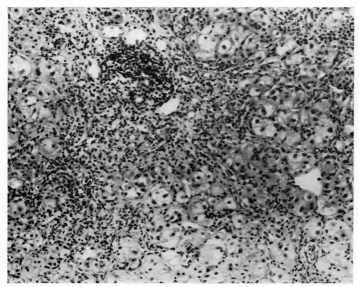

FIG. 16–4. Active chronic hepatitis—needle biopsy specimen 8 months after onset. Inflammatory cells have accumulated in and about the portal tract. The parenchymal cells are variable in size and swollen, and the cytoplasm shows varying degrees of hypochromasia. Groups of parenchymal cells are surrounded by fine strands of fibrous tissue. The degree of inflammatory cell infiltration and degenerative change in parenchymal cells at the lobular periphery is variable ("piecemeal necrosis").

the limiting plate, the entire lobule, or 2 or more consecutive lobules, may be involved. The involvement of many lobules may produce a picture similar to that of fulminant hepatitis (Fig. 16–6). Extensive "necrosis" with stromal collapse may account for episodes of spontaneous hepatic coma during the course of the disease and for the broad bands of fibrous tissue encountered histologically in the later stages.

Cellular infiltration is present to some degree in most portal tracts but is concentrated at the lobular periphery spreading into the lobule and interlobular septa. The cell types seen in decreasing order of frequency are lymphocytes, plasma cells and histiocytes with an occasional eosinophil and polymorph.

Deposition of *collagen tissue* around parenchymal cells at the periphery of the lobule is a characteristic feature of the disease. Fine fibrous strands extend from the limiting plate for varying distances into the lobule. The progressive loss of parenchymal cells at the

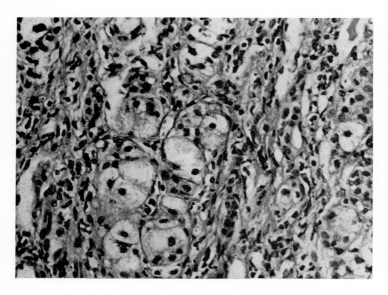

FIG. 16–5. Active chronic hepatitis— needle biopsy specimen. An area of piecemeal necrosis in a zone adjacent to an interlobular septum. The parenchymal cells show the typical degenerative changes. A mild degree of fibrosis, ductular proliferation and mononuclear cell infiltration is also evident.

FIG. 16–6. Submassive necrosis in a patient with active chronic hepatitis—second needle biopsy section 2 years after onset. There has been extensive parenchymal cell fallout of several entire consecutive lobules. Numerous central veins and portal tract structures can be seen in the area of lobular collapse. The changes may be contrasted with the small area of surviving parenchyma. The first needle biopsy section in this patient showed perilobular hepatitis with piecemeal necrosis.

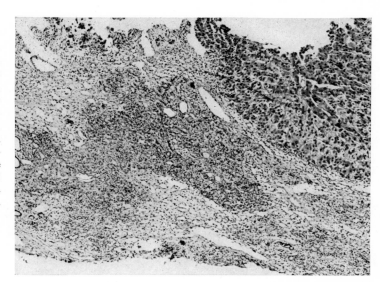

limiting plate is accompanied by varying degrees of portal, septal and perilobular fibrosis. Cirrhosis is inevitable but in the first year of the disease architecture is preserved in two-thirds of cases.

The changes in the active stage of the disease can be readily distinguished from those in acute viral hepatitis. The picture of pericentral necrosis, with restriction of the inflammatory cell infiltration to the portal tracts, and discrete foci of necrosis within the lobule, intense sinusoidal cellular infil-

tration, preservation of the limiting plate and the absence of significant perilobular necrosis and fibrosis is rarely seen in active chronic hepatitis.

INACTIVE STAGE (FIGS. 16–7, 16–8)

The inflammation has subsided although complete resolution is not always found and minor degrees of cellular infiltration in the portal tracts may be present. The junction of the hepatic lobule and portal tract (limiting plate) is now clearly defined but may be

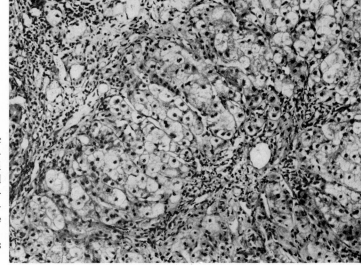

FIG. 16–7. Inactive chronic hepatitis—needle biopsy section. Fibrosis is established and extends from the portal tracts and septa into the lobule. Cords and groups of parenchymal cells of double plate thickness (regeneration) are surrounded by fine strands of fibrous tissue.

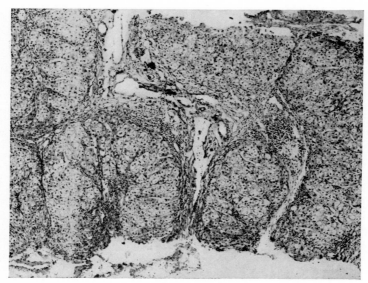

FIG. 16–8. Cirrhosis following active chronic hepatitis—needle biopsy section. There is loss of lobular architecture. Strands of fibrous tissue surround and dissect the hepatic lobules. The lobular pattern is distorted considerably and cords of parenchymal cells appear encased in the fibroblastic change. Some residual activity is still evident with inflammatory cellular change in the periphery of two lobules.

uneven with some discontinuity from the loss of parenchymal cells. The degree of fibrosis depends on both the duration of the disease and the extent of the previous necrosis and varies throughout the liver. The architecture may be preserved, fibrosis in these cases being periportal, septal or perilobular with extension of septate strands into the lobule.

Extension of fibrosis with lobular dissection leads to cirrhosis (Fig. 16–8). Although cirrhosis is present in only one-third of cases early in the disease, it develops rapidly and is present in most cases 2 years after the onset. Features of posthepatitic, portal and postnecrotic cirrhosis in the one case is the picture most commonly seen. Regenerative nodules range in size from small groups of cells encased in fibrous tissue to the large nodules typical of postnecrotic cirrhosis.

Pathologically the disease may be conveniently classified as being inactive or active, but changes are often combined. Sequential biopsies in the one patient are likely to show different patterns including active chronic hepatitis, inactive chronic hepatitis or established cirrhosis with or without inflammation and necrosis.

ETIOLOGY

The cause of the disease is not known. Two currently held theories are those of a viral infection or a basic disturbance of immunity. However, a virus has *not* been isolated and, as yet, *no direct* evidence supports an autoimmune disturbance.

DISTURBANCE OF IMMUNITY

Altered immune reaction in active chronic hepatitis is suggested by the following findings:

1. L.E. cells and antinuclear factors.
2. Many abnormal serologic reactions.
3. Associated hypergammaglobulinemia.
4. Plasma cell infiltration in the liver biopsy.
5. Dramatic clinical and biochemical response to steroids and immunosuppressive drugs.
6. Frequent association with other diseases in which an autoimmune process has been postulated, such as glomerulonephritis, myocarditis, ulcerative colitis, Hashimoto's thyroiditis[78, 118, 154] and Sjögrens syndrome.[99]
7. Abnormal immunoglobulin synthesis in one family with active chronic hepatitis.[31]
8. Striking resemblance of a few cases to disseminated lupus erythematosus, in which a disturbance of immunity is more firmly established.
9. Similarity of histologic changes in the liver to immunologically-induced chronic liver injury in animals.[147]
10. Changes such as Coombs' posi-

tive hemolytic anemia, glomerulonephritis, plasma cell infiltration in the liver, antinuclear factors and abnormal immunoglobulins in New Zealand Black mice in which the disease is considered to be due to an autoimmune process.[19, 50, 76, 77, 84, 120, 137]

Serologic Reactions. A positive complement fixation reaction in active chronic hepatitis was initially marshalled as evidence to support an autoimmune basis for the disease.[106, 113] It is now evident that these antibodies are neither disease specific nor even species specific,[14, 46, 149] and probably represent an immunologic phenomenon only in terms of an *in vitro* test.[149] However, true antibodies are present in active chronic hepatitis, for immunofluorescence can also be obtained with purified IgG prepared from the serum of these patients.[46]

In postulating a causal relationship between immune process and active chronic hepatitis, it has been difficult to relate the nonorgan specificity of these antibodies to a disorder that mainly affects the liver. However, in view of the demonstration of several liver specific antigens,[1, 122] the possible coexistence of organ and nonorgan specific antibodies cannot be completely discarded.

Effect of Immunosuppressive Drugs (6-MP and Azathioprine). In 1958, Schwartz reported that 6-mercaptopurine inhibited antibody production and later described favorable clinical results in treating acquired hemolytic anemia and lupus erythematosus with this agent.[43, 165] Its use in active chronic hepatitis was first reported by Page and Good[143] and a good clinical response to this drug has been confirmed.[63, 112, 127, 142, 144] Patients do not usually show any improvement for 3 or 4 weeks. Since 6-MP affects antibody production immediately[141] a rapid response to therapy would be expected; the delay suggests an alternate biological action, and experiments in the rabbit have shown that it strongly inhibits the cellular response to inflammation.[141]

Several workers investigated a number of immunologic reactions in man and demonstrated that 6-MP had no effect on *established* natural antibody levels (isohemagglutinins, antibodies against gram-negative infections, etc.), on *established* delayed hypersensitivity (P.P.D., *Candida*, dermato-

phytin), or on gamma globulin levels.[104, 142] They concluded that 6-MP would not be expected to suppress an autoimmune process, for this probably represents an *established* delayed hypersensitivity reaction.

6-MP has been shown to prevent viral replication *in vitro*[161] and its anti-inflammatory effect in active chronic hepatitis may reflect a suppression of a chronic viral infection.[142] In any case there is no evidence, as yet, that 6-MP in *the dose used* for the treatment of active chronic hepatitis has any effect on established abnormal immune reactions,[104, 142] and the term "immunosuppressive" in this context may be misleading.

VIRAL ETIOLOGY

Although a virus has *not* been isolated in active chronic hepatitis, the possibility cannot be discarded. Indeed, the lack of viral serology makes even the diagnosis of acute epidemic "viral" hepatitis uncertain. A virus may not only be the initiating factor but its continued presence might explain the persistent destruction of the liver.[142] The plausible progression of acute viral hepatitis to active chronic hepatitis remains controversial.

Considerable *indirect* evidence suggests the presence of a virus in this disease. This is based on the following findings:

1. A clinical picture identical to and indistinguishable from acute infectious hepatitis in a significant number of cases seen early in the course of the disease.[131, 154, 168]

2. Similarity of many histologic changes in the liver *early* in the disease to those of acute infectious hepatitis.[95, 124]

3. A history, in some patients, of contact at or near the onset of the disease with persons who have acute infectious hepatitis.[131]

4. An increasing number of reports show transition of alleged acute viral hepatitis to postnecrotic cirrhosis.[20, 88, 98, 101, 152, 157, 163, 166, 174]

5. The recent demonstration that acute viral hepatitis is a multisystemic disease with significant pathologic changes in many organs other than the liver (e.g., kidney, bone marrow, small intestine, stomach).[38-40]

6. Isolation of a slow-growing virus in an increasing number of animal and human diseases (scrapie, visna, Aleutian disease of

mink, NZB mice disease, kuru) hitherto considered fundamentally genetic, or, like active chronic hepatitis, immunologic in nature.[16, 28, 32, 51, 57, 58, 72, 121, 134, 170, 171] These findings should stimulate increased efforts to isolate a slow-growing virus in other diseases in man such as active chronic hepatitis.

DIAGNOSIS

The following criteria are helpful in the diagnosis of active chronic hepatitis and in its differentiation from closely related disorders:

Liver Biopsy Changes of Both Acute and Chronic Hepatitis. These include perilobular parenchymal cell necrosis and degeneration, inflammatory cell infiltration and varying degrees of periportal and intralobular fibrosis. For some cases a diagnosis can be made without histology, but for others it is essential. Liver biopsy is important in differentiating closely related disorders.

Clinical and/or biochemical evidence of active liver disease such as jaundice, anorexia, malaise, fatigue, weight loss, recent spider nevi and acne, bruising, fever, hepatosplenomegaly, florid changes of hypercorticism, hepatic tenderness and the signs of hepatic encephalopathy. Laboratory features include elevation of the SGOT, serum bilirubin, serum alkaline phosphatase, zinc sulfate turbidity and serum globulins and depression of the prothrombin time. Fluctuation in the severity of these changes over a period of 2 to 6 months is a valuable index of activity.

Clinical Evidence of Established Chronic Liver Disease. This is indicated by the presence of portal hypertension, ascites, persistent hepatosplenomegaly, mild chronic jaundice, persistent spider nevi, and long-standing acne, amenorrhea and hirsutism. The important changes in liver function tests include *persistent* hyperglobulinemia, hypoalbuminemia, hypoprothrombinemia and BSP retention. Assessment of chronicity in many cases requires observation for 6 months.

Features that are *often* seen in active chronic hepatitis but are *not* essential for the diagnosis include:

1. *Endocrine changes* such as amenorrhea, acne, hirsutism, pigmented abdominal striae, gynecomastia in males and Cushingoid facies.

2. *Multi-organ involvement* such as arthritis, skin rashes, ulcerative colitis, pleurisy, glomerulonephritis, pericarditis, thyroiditis, myocarditis, thrombocytopenic purpura and Coombs' positive hemolytic anemia.

3. *Liver biopsy changes of cirrhosis* in the first 2 years of the disease or dominance of plasma cells in the inflammatory exudate.

4. *Specific age group and sex*: the disease may affect males and females in all age groups.

5. *Jaundice*: the course may be anicteric and serum bilirubin may not be elevated at the onset.

6. *Marked hypergammaglobulinemia*: in many cases the levels may not exceed 2 gm% and in some cases there may be hypogammaglobulinemia.

7. *Presence of abnormal serologic phenomena* such as L.E. cells, antinuclear factors, complement fixing antibodies, false-positive tests for syphilis, sheep red cell or latex agglutination and antibodies to smooth muscle, parietal cells, thyroid and mitochondria.

DIFFERENTIAL DIAGNOSIS

A clinical picture superficially resembling active chronic hepatitis may be seen in primary biliary cirrhosis, persistent or recurrent hepatitis, systemic lupus erythematosus, alcoholic liver disease, pericholangitis with ulcerative colitis, cryptogenic cirrhosis with hepatic decompensation, drug-induced hepatitis, sclerosing cholangitis and benign recurrent intrahepatic cholestasis.

Primary Biliary Cirrhosis.[2, 29, 54, 151, 159, 160, 167, 186] Both active chronic hepatitis and primary biliary cirrhosis occur predominately in females and are of unknown etiology. The peak incidence of primary biliary cirrhosis is between 40 and 60 years, and it is rarely encountered before the age of 30 years.[2, 68, 167, 168] In active chronic hepatitis the onset in 50 per cent of patients is between 11 and 30 years. The presence of intense pruritus early in the disease, marked skin pigmentation, extreme hypercholesterolemia, xantho-

mata, steatorrhea, severe hypoprothrombinemia and marked elevation of the serum
alkaline phosphatase in a patient who is surprisingly free of symptoms is characteristic
of primary biliary cirrhosis[2, 29, 160] and is not
seen in active chronic hepatitis. Patients with
primary biliary cirrhosis do not usually have
distinct episodes of active liver disease with
periods of remission. The course is slow and
unremitting.

In both disorders there may be extreme
hyperglobulinemia, marked elevation of zinc
sulfate turbidity and splenomegaly early in
the course of the disease. The incidence of
L.E. cells, smooth muscle antibodies, antinuclear factors and antimitochondrial antibodies is similar in both disorders.

Pathologically, the changes *early* in the
course of primary biliary cirrhosis are diagnostic.[29, 54, 151, 160, 186] Inflammation is confined to the portal tracts and is most concentrated around biliary ducts. There is early
ductular destruction with portal fibrosis, and
in one-third of cases granulomas with giant
cells may be found. Perilobular parenchymal
necrosis and inflammation is usually not
striking. Differentiation from active chronic
hepatitis may be difficult in the later stages
of the disease when perilobular parenchymal
necrosis is present and cirrhosis is established.

Acute Viral Hepatitis (Table 16–8). Active chronic hepatitis may begin abruptly
with a clinical picture indistinguishable from
acute infectious hepatitis. Even in cases with
an insidious onset, the features more closely
resemble acute viral hepatitis than any other
liver disease. Differentiation of these 2 disorders early in the disease becomes even
more difficult if a patient with active chronic
hepatitis has a history of contact with a
jaundiced person.

Most cases of acute viral hepatitis do not
persist beyond 6 weeks and resolution is usually complete. A few patients may have
a relapse and in others the illness may last
for more than 6 months. In *persistent* or *recurrent hepatitis*[126, 173, 179] the stigmata of
chronic liver disease do *not* develop and in
most cases the clinical features, liver function tests and histologic changes in the liver
are *identical* to those seen with the first at-

tack or during the stage of resolution. Furthermore, signs of hypercorticism and
chronic irreversible changes in other organs
are rarely encountered. Fibrosis or cirrhosis
is not extensive and perilobular necrosis, if
present, is usually mild.

**Disseminated Lupus Erythematosus
(D.L.E.).** Features common to both lupus
erythematosus and active chronic hepatitis
include arthralgia, pleurisy, pericarditis,
skin rashes, pulmonary infiltrates, glomerulonephritis, pyrexia, splenomegaly, lymphadenopathy, myocarditis, L.E. cells, anemia,
hypergammaglobulinemia, thrombocytopenia and various abnormal serologic reactions.
Both diseases show a predilection for females
with a similar peak age incidence.

Liver involvement, however, is distinctly
uncommon in classic D.L.E.[73, 97] Liver
changes, if present, consist of cellular infiltration in the portal tracts. Other hepatic manifestations characteristic of active chronic
hepatitis are rarely encountered.

Pericholangitis and Ulcerative Colitis
(Table 16–9). Pericholangitis is the commonest hepatic lesion associated with ulcerative colitis;[24, 47, 117, 123, 125, 129, 132, 133, 178] active chronic hepatitis is probably next in
frequency. These 2 hepatic diseases can be
readily differentiated, for they have distinct
clinical, laboratory and pathologic features.
Occasionally both lesions coexist in the one
aspiration biopsy section. The clinical findings in these circumstances are usually those
of active chronic hepatitis.

TREATMENT

Long periods of bed rest are often required
during episodes of activity which punctuate
active chronic hepatitis. Although the overall
prognosis is grave, any drug therapy that
will control the active phase of the liver disease, and thus shorten hospitalization and
morbidity, warrants a trial. To this extent
corticosteroids, 6-mercaptopurine and Azathioprine are most rewarding.

CORTICOSTEROIDS

Corticosteroids are effective in the "control" of this disease and in the many reported
series the results are comparable.[93, 106, 111,]

TABLE 16–8. DIFFERENTIAL DIAGNOSIS OF ACTIVE CHRONIC
HEPATITIS AND ACUTE VIRAL HEPATITIS

	ACUTE INFECTIOUS HEPATITIS	ACTIVE CHRONIC HEPATITIS
CLINICAL FEATURES		
Age	Children, adults 10–30 yrs. (90%)	All ages 10–30 yrs. (50%)
Sex	Equal incidence	Females 70–80%
History of contact	Common	5–10%
Abrupt onset (weeks)	90%	30%
Insidious onset (months)	Rare	70%
Anorexia	Weeks	Months
Jaundice	Deep	Mild
Spider nevi	Occasional	40–50%
Fever	Days	Weeks
Splenomegaly	10–15%	50%
Acne	Uncommon	20%
Amenorrhea	Occasional	30–40%
Cushingoid facies	Rare	5–10%
Glomerulonephritis	± Acute	Chronic
Skin lesions	5%	20%
Ulcerative colitis	Nil	10–15%
Arthralgia	Occasional	20%
Pleurisy, myocarditis, thyroiditis	Rare	10%
Episodic jaundice	Uncommon	60%
Recurrent episodes	Rare	Common
Cholestasis (1–2 years)	Rare	25%
Hepatic coma	Rare	30%
Portal hypertension	± Transient	40–50% Persistent
Recovery	95% +	Nil
LABORATORY FEATURES		
Anemia	Transient; mild	50%; moderate
Thrombocytopenia	Occasional	40% below 100,000/c.mm.
Leukopenia	Transient	Persistent
Elevated E.S.R.	Weeks	Months
Bilirubin	Above 10 mg.% (80%)	Below 10 mg.% (80%)
SGOT 1,000	Common	Uncommon
Hyperglobulinemia	Uncommon	Common
Elevated $ZnSO_4$ turbidity	Transient (Weeks)	Persistent (months)
Hypoalbuminemia	Uncommon	Common
BSP retention	Transient	Persistent
Low prothrombin time	Occasional (Transient)	Often (persistent)
L.E. cells	Rare	10–15%
Antinuclear factor	3–5%	70–80%
Smooth muscle antibodies	0	70–90%
Thyroid, gastric antibodies	Rare	Common
Mitochondrial antibodies	0	70–90%
PATHOLOGY		
Uniformity	100%	50%
Portal triaditis	100%	Common
Sinusoidal infiltration	Common	Uncommon

TABLE 16–8 Continued

	ACUTE INFECTIOUS HEPATITIS	ACTIVE CHRONIC HEPATITIS
Perilobular inflammation	Uncommon	100%
Bile stasis	Pericentral	Pericentral, periportal
Limiting plate	Intact	Involved
Parenchymal necrosis	Focal; pericentral	Perilobular (piecemeal)
Panlobular necrosis	Rare	20%
Councilman bodies	Common	Variable
Balloon cells	Occasional: focal	Marked (perilobular)
Duct proliferation	Rare	Present
Kupffer cells	Occasionally prominent	Often enlarged
Fibrosis	±Mild; periportal	Marked (periportal, septal intralobular)
Cirrhosis	Rare	Common
Regeneration	Cellular	Rosettes, micro-macronodular

[113-115, 127, 130, 138, 143, 154, 162, 164, 187, 188] They relieve symptoms with an increased sense of well-being, improve fatigue and weakness, relieve anorexia, decrease jaundice, control arthralgia and in most cases reduce fever. Serum bilirubin and SGOT are often affected dramatically but hyperglobulinemia may persist. Corticosteroids often shorten the period of hospitalization and the most gratifying results are obtained in patients who are obviously ill and severely jaundiced.

A high initial daily dose of 60 mg. of prednisone for 2 to 3 weeks is necessary in most cases. The dose is reduced gradually over a period of months to a level between 5 to 20 mg./day. The maintenance dose varies in each case and the ideal dose can be determined only after a period of trial and error. Once symptoms are relieved, the serial changes in the biochemical tests of hepatic function provide the best means of following the process of the disease. Patients should be seen at regular intervals and the dosage adjusted, depending upon the levels of SGOT and serum bilirubin. In this regard, even minor changes in these 2 tests are significant. Biochemical remission is not always complete but suppression is adequate in most cases.

Every 6 months, drug withdrawal should be attempted, but in some cases this often proves impossible. Any attempt should be gradual with a daily dose reduction of only 2.5 to 5.0 mg. of prednisone followed by an observation period of at least 2 to 3 weeks.

A more drastic or rapid reduction in dosage may lead to a further exacerbation of the disease.

Steroid therapy does not induce permanent remission and episodes of active liver disease may develop even after a long course of therapy. In these cases the steroid dosage should be increased and complete bed rest may also be needed. Patients should be kept in the hospital for several weeks after the SGOT and serum bilirubin return to near normal levels. Short periods of bed rest followed by rapid return to a full active life should be avoided, for relapses are common in these circumstances.

In many cases, long-term steroid therapy in a dose necessary to control the activity of the disease is attended by serious complications. Since endogenous hypercorticism may be a prominent feature in untreated cases, it is not surprising that patients are sensitive to even small doses of steroids. Complications to long-term steroid therapy include obesity and moon facies, severe acne, hirsutism, pigmented abdominal striae, serious infections, alopecia, muscle wasting, osteoporosis and diabetes. In some patients, serious complications or unpleasant cosmetic effects may necessitate a drastic reduction of steroid dosage at the expense of adequate control.

Although steroids do not appear to increase overall survival,[127, 131, 154, 168] they reduce *early* mortality. This is consistent with the symptomatic improvement, reduction in the total period of hospitalization needed

TABLE 16–9. DIFFERENTIAL DIAGNOSIS OF ACTIVE CHRONIC HEPATITIS AND
PERICHOLANGITIS ASSOCIATED WITH ULCERATIVE COLITIS

	ACTIVE CHRONIC HEPATITIS	PERICHOLANGITIS
Sex	Predominantly females	Equal incidence
Jaundice	Common (80%)	50%
Spider nevi	Common	Uncommon
Involvement of joints, kidney, skin	Common	Uncommon
Hypercorticism	Common	Rare
Liver failure	Common	Uncommon
Portal hypertension	Para- and pre-sinusoidal	Pre-sinusoidal
Globulins	Elevated	Normal
Serum alkaline phosphatase (50 + K.A.)	Uncommon	Common
Cholesterol	Normal	Elevated
L.E. cells	Positive	Negative
Tissue antibodies (S.M.A., A.N.F., "M")	70 − 80%	0%
Colitis	Severe	Moderate
Prognosis	Poor	Good
Liver death	Common	Uncommon
Inflammation	Perilobular	Periductular
Piecemeal necrosis	Marked	± Minimal
Parenchymal degeneration	100%	Occasional
Therapy	Steroids, 6-MP, Azathioprine	Antibiotics, Cholestyramine

A.N.F., antinuclear factor
"M", antimitochondrial antibodies
S.M.A., smooth muscle antibodies

and control of the biochemical indices of activity seen with this drug therapy. However, corticosteroids do not arrest fibrosis or prevent the development of cirrhosis[124, 154, 156] and these findings are consistent with the unaltered overall survival.

AZATHIOPRINE (IMURAN) AND 6-MERCAPTOPURINE (PURETHANOL)

The use of 6-mercaptopurine in the treatment of diseases of presumed autoimmune etiology was pioneered by Dameshek and Schwartz in 1960.[43, 165] Subsequently several workers have supported the initial impression that purine analogs (6-MP and Azathioprine) are of value in the treatment of active chronic hepatitis. However, only a small number of patients have been treated with these drugs,[9, 112, 127, 128, 142] and their use in the long-term management of this disease is limited to a few reports.

6-MP is a hepatotoxin.[27, 119, 127] Jaundice has been reported in a number of patients given 6-MP in a dose of 2.5 to 5.0 mg./kg. for the treatment of leukemia.[119] Some of these were shown to have intrahepatic cholestasis, centrilobular necrosis or fatty metamorphosis.[27, 34, 52] The drug also produces bone marrow suppression with leukopenia and thrombocytopenia. The toxic effects appear to be dose-related and can be consistently reproduced in man and animals.

It is not surprising that severe toxic reactions including anorexia, jaundice, hepatic coma, thrombocytopenia, leukopenia and purpura were encountered initially with the use of 6-MP in the treatment of active chronic hepatitis.[112, 128] Although the dose used (1.5 mg./kg./day) is less than that which produces toxicity in other diseases, it appears to be excessive in some patients with this liver disease.

The toxic nature of the drug probably accounts for the reluctance of many workers to use it. However, encouraging results have been reported when a smaller dose (0.5 to 1.0 mg./kg./day) of 6-MP was used. At this dose level no toxic reactions were encountered when 6-MP or Azathioprine were given for periods of up to 4 and a half years.[127, 128]

Azathioprine or 6-MP should be given if the disease cannot be controlled adequately by or complications occur from steroid therapy. Indeed, these drugs are in many ways superior to corticosteroids because control of the clinical and biochemical indices of activity is more sustained and adequate.[127, 128] Furthermore, the time spent in the hospital is markedly reduced and the patient can lead a more normal existence. However, improvement in the progressive histologic changes in the liver cannot be demonstrated and further periods of observation are required to evaluate the effect of these drugs on overall survival.

Azathioprine is almost completely converted to mercaptopurine, and because it is slowly released from the liver, it has been thought to be superior to 6-MP and less toxic. A daily maximum dose of 1.0 to 1.5 mg./kg. of Azathioprine controls the disease in most cases. It is probably safer to begin with small doses and gradually increase the levels until the desired control is achieved. In this way toxic reactions may be avoided and the maximum dose a patient can safely tolerate can be determined. Caution should be exercised in a severely jaundiced patient or if there is severe thrombocytopenia or leukopenia. In these cases an initial course of steroids should be given. In the occasional case activity of the disease is best controlled by a *combination* of steroids and Azathioprine.

REFERENCES

1. Abelev, G. I.: Antigenic structure of chemically-induced hepatomas, Progr. Exp. Tumor Res. 7:104, 1965.
2. Ahrens, E. H., Payne, M. A., Kunkel, H. G., Eisenmenger, W. J., and Blondheim, S. H.: Primary biliary cirrhosis, Medicine 29:299, 1950.
3. Alarcon-Segovia, D., Bartholomew, L. G., Cain, J. C., and Baggenstoss, A. H.: Significance of the lupus erythematosus cell phenomenon in older women with chronic hepatic disease, Proc. Mayo Clin. 40:193, 1965.
4. Alfrey, C. P., Jr., Bartholomew, L. G., Cain, J. C., and Baggenstoss, A. H.: Chronic disease of the liver in young women: an evaluation of patients with a negative clot test for lupus erythematosus, Gastroenterology 43:532, 1962.
5. Anderssen, N., and Skjaeggestad, O.: Lupoid hepatitis, Acta med. scand. 171:385, 1962.
6. Appelbaum, J. J., Job, H., and Kern, F., Jr.: Hepatitis associated with disseminated lupus erythematosus, Gastroenterology 40:766, 1961.
7. Armas-Cruz, R., Yazigi, R., Lopez, O., Montero, E., Cabello, J., and Lobo, G.: Portal cirrhosis: an analysis of 208 cases with correlations of clinical, laboratory and autopsy findings, Gastroenterology 17:327, 1951.
8. Aronson, A. R., and Montgomery, M. M.: Chronic liver disease with a "lupus erythematosus-like syndrome," Arch. Int. Med. 104:544, 1959.
9. Arter, W. J., Perkins, K. W., and Blackburn, C. R. B.: Experience with the use of 6-mercaptopurine and "Imuran" in the treatment of progressive hepatitis (active chronic hepatitis), Aust. Ann. Med. 15:222, 1966.
10. Asherson, G. L., and Broberger, O.: Incidence of heamagglutinating and complement fixing antibodies, Brit. Med. J. 1:1429, 1961.
11. Atwater, E. C., and Jacox, R. F.: The latex-fixation test in patients with liver disease, Ann. Int. Med. 58:419, 1963.
12. Bartholomew, L. G., Cain, J. C., Baggestoss, A. H., and Hagedorn, A. B.: Further observations on hepatitis and cirrhosis in young women with positive clot tests for lupus erythematosus, Gastroenterology 39:730, 1960.
13. Bartholomew, L. G., Hagedorn, A. B., Cain, J. C., and Baggenstoss, A. H.: Hepatitis and cirrhosis in women with positive clot tests for lupus erythematosis, New Engl. J. Med. 259:947, 1958.
14. Beall, G. N., and Ohanian, S. H.: The nature of the complement fixing antigen in normal human liver extracts, J. Lab. Clin. Med. 61:67, 1963.
15. Bearn, A. G., Kunkel, H. G., and Slater, R. J.: The problem of chronic liver dis-

ease in young women, Am. J. Med. *21*: 3, 1956.

16. Beck, E., Daniel, P. M., Alpers, M., Gajdusek, D. C., and Gibbs, C. J., Jr.: Experimental kuru in chimpanzees: pathological report, Lancet *2*:1056, 1966.

17. Berman, L., Axelrod, A. R., Goodman, H. L., and McClaughry, R. I.: So-called "lupus erythematosus inclusion phenomenon" of bone marrow and blood, Am. J. Clin. Path. *20*:403, 1950.

18. Bettley, F. R.: The "L. E. cell" phenomenon in active chronic viral hepatitis, Lancet *2*:724, 1955.

19. Bielschowsky, M., Helyer, B. J., and Howie, J. B.: Spontaneous haemolytic anaemia in mice of the NZB/BL strain, Proc. Univ. Otago Med. Sch. 37:9, 1959.

20. Bjørneboe, M.: Panel discussion on therapy, course and prognosis, *in* Hartman, F. W., et al. (eds.): Hepatitis Frontiers, Henry Ford Hosp. Int. Symposium, pp. 563–569, Boston, Little, Brown, 1957.

21. Bjørneboe, M., and Raaschou, F.: The pathology of sub-chronic atrophy of the liver; a comparison with cirrhosis hepatis Laennec, Acta med. scand. (Supp.) *234*:41, 1949.

22. Blackburn, C. R. B.: Infectious hepatitis, Med. J. Aust. *1*:219, 1961.

23. Blum, M., and Spritz, N.: The metabolism of intravenously injected isotopic cholic acid in Laennec's cirrhosis, J. Clin. Invest. *45*:187, 1966.

24. Boden, R. W., Rankin, J. G., Goulston, S. J. M., and Morrow, W.: The liver in ulcerative colitis: the significance of raised serum alkaline phosphatase levels, Lancet *2*:245, 1959.

25. Bouchier, I. A. D., Rhodes, K., and Sherlock, S.: Serological abnormalities in patients with liver disease, Brit. Med. J. *1*:592, 1964.

26. Brandriss, M. N.: Current studies on the effect of antimetabolites on nonneoplastic disease, Ann. Int. Med. 59:398, 1963.

27. Burchenal, J. H., and Ellison, R. R.: Symposium on the experimental pharmacology and clinical use of antimetabolites. IX. The pyrimide and purine antagonists, Clin. Pharm. Ther. *2*:523, 1961.

28. Burger, D., and Hartsough, G. R.: Encephalopathy of mink. II, Experimental and natural transmission, J. Infect. Dis. *115*:393, 1965.

29. Cameron, R., and Hou, P. C.: Biliary Cirrhosis, London, Oliver and Boyd, 1962.

30. Cattan, R., Vesin, P., and Bodin, H.: Cirrhoses dysprotéinémiques d'origine inconnue chez la femme, Bull. Soc. Med. hôp., Paris 73:608, 1957.

31. Cavell, B., and Leonhardt, T.: Hereditary hyperglobulinaemia and lupoid hepatitis, Acta med. scand. *177*:751, 1965.

32. Chandler, R. L.: Encephalopathy in mice produced by inoculation with scrapie brain material, Lancet *1*:1378, 1961.

33. Chrispin, A. R., and Lessof, L.: The chest radiograph in juvenile cirrhosis (active chronic hepatitis), Brit. J. Radiol. 38:685, 1965.

34. Clark, P. A., Hsia, Y. E., and Huntsman, R. G.: Toxic complications of treatment with 6-mercaptopurine: two cases with hepatic necrosis and intestinal ulceration, Brit. Med. J. *1*:393, 1960.

35. Cohen, N. M., and Mendelow, H.: Concurrent active "juvenile" cirrhosis and "primary pulmonary hypertension," Am. J. Med. 39:127, 1965.

36. Conley, C. L.: The L. E. cell test, J. Chron. Dis. 5:275, 1957.

37. Conn, H. O., and Lindenmuth, W. S.: Prophylactic portacaval anastomosis in cirrhotic patients with esophageal varices, New Engl. J. Med. 272:1255, 1965.

38. Conrad, M. E.: Conjoint clinic on infectious hepatitis, J. Chron. Dis. *19*:199, 1966.

39. Conrad, M. E., Hartman, R. S., and Astaldi, G.: The gastrointestinal lesion in viral hepatitis, Ann. Int. Med. *60*: 723, 1964.

40. Conrad, M. E., Schwartz, F. D., and Young, A. A.: Infectious hepatitis—a generalized disease; a study of renal, gastrointestinal and hematologic abnormalities, Am. J. Med. 37:789, 1964.

41. Coppage, N. S., Jr., Island, D. P., Cooner, A. E., and Liddle, G. W.: Metabolism of aldosterone in normal subjects and in patients with hepatic cirrhosis, J. Clin. Invest. 41:1672, 1962.

42. Cruickshank, B.: Auto-allergic reactions of brain, testes, liver, pancreas and skeletal muscle, *in* Gell, P. G. H., and Coombs, R. R. A. (eds.): Clinical Aspects of Immunology, p. 663, Blackwell's Scientific Publications, Oxford, Blackwell, 1963.

43. Dameshek, W., and Schwartz, R.: Treatment of certain "autoimmune" diseases with antimetabolites; a preliminary re-

port, Trans. Ass. Am. Physicians 73:113, 1960.

44. Dible, J. H.: Degeneration, necrosis and fibrosis in the liver, Brit. Med. J. 1:833, 1951.

45. Diecher, H. R. G., Holman, H. R., and Kunkel, H. G.: Anticytoplasmic factors in the sera of patients with systemic lupus erythematosus and certain other diseases, Arthr. & Rheum. 3:1, 1960.

46. Doniach, D., Roitt, I. M., Walker, J. G., and Sherlock, S.: Tissue antibodies in primary biliary cirrhosis, active chronic (lupoid) hepatitis, cryptogenic cirrhosis and other liver diseases and their clinical implications, Clin. Exp. Immun. 1:237, 1966.

47. Dordal, E., Glagov, S., and Kirsner, J.: Hepatic lesions in chronic inflammatory bowel disease, Gastroenterology 52:239, 1967.

48. Drucker, W. D., and Christy, N. P.: The metabolism of steroid hormones in hepatic disease, Med. Clin. N. Amer. 47:663, 1963.

49. Dustan, H. P., Taylor, R. D., Corcoran, A. C., and Page, I. H.: Rheumatic and febrile syndrome during prolonged hydralazine treatment, J.A.M.A. 154:23, 1954.

50. East, J., de Sousa, M. A. B., and Parrott, D. M. U.: Immunopathology of New Zealand Black (NZB) mice, Transplantation 3:711, 1965.

51. East, J., Prosser, P. R., Holborow, E. J., and Jaquet, H.: Autoimmune reactions and virus-like particles in germ-free NZB mice, Lancet 1:755, 1967.

52. Einhorn, M., and Davidsohn, I.: Hepatotoxicity of mercaptopurine, J.A.M.A. 188:802, 1964.

53. Fischer, D. A.: The "Lupoid hepatitis" syndrome: report of a case followed by serial liver biopsies, Ann. Int. Med. 57:988, 1962.

54. Foulk, W. T., Baggenstoss, A. H., and Butt, H. R.: Primary biliary cirrhosis: re-evaluation by clinical and histological study of 49 cases, Gastroenterology, 47:354, 1964.

55. Gajdusek, D. C.: An "autoimmune" reaction against human tissue antigens in certain chronic diseases, Nature 179:666, 1957.

56. ————: An "autoimmune" reaction against human tissue antigens in certain acute and chronic diseases. I. Serological investigations, Arch. Int. Med. 101:9, 1958.

57. ————: Slow-virus infections of the nervous system, New Engl. J. Med. 276:392, 1967.

58. Gajdusek, D. C., Gibbs, C. J., Jr., and Alpers, M.: Experimental transmission of kuru-like syndrome to chimpanzees, Nature 209:794, 1966.

59. Gall, E.: Posthepatic, postnecrotic and nutritional cirrhosis; a pathologic analysis, Am. J. Path. 36:241, 1960.

60. Gallagher, N. D., and Goulston, S. J. M.: Persistent acute viral hepatitis, Brit. Med. J. 1:906, 1962.

61. Garceau, A. J., and Chalmers, T. C.: The Boston inter-hospital liver group: the natural history of cirrhosis. I. Survival with esophageal varices, New Engl. J. Med. 268:469, 1963.

62. Gausewitz, P. L., Jones, F. S., and Worley, G.: Fatal generalized moniliasis, Am. J. Clin. Path. 21:41, 1951.

63. Geenen, J. E., Hensley, G. T., and Winship, P. H.: Chronic active hepatitis treated with 6-mercaptopurine, Ann. Int. Med. 65:1277, 1966.

64. Gökcen, M.: Autoimmunity in liver disease; serologic investigations with clinical correlations, J. Lab. Clin. Med. 59:533, 1962.

65. Goldgraber, M. B., and Kirsner, J. B.: The use of adrenal steroids in subacute and chronic cholangiolitic hepatitis; a clinicopathologic correlation, Arch. Int. Med. 103:354, 1959.

66. Goldstein, G., and Mackay, I. R.: Lupoid hepatitis: computer analysis defining "hepatitis" and "cirrhosis" phases and relationships between hepatocellular damage and immune reactions in the liver, Aust. Ann. Med. 16:62, 1967.

67. Good, R. A., and Page, A. R.: Fatal complications of virus hepatitis in two patients with agammaglobulinemia, Am. J. Med. 29:804, 1960.

68. Goudie, R. B., MacSween, R. N. M., and Goldberg, D. M.: Serological and histological diagnosis of primary biliary cirrhosis, J. Clin. Path. 19:527, 1966.

69. Gray, N., Mackay, I. R., Taft, L. I., Weiden, S., and Wood, I. J.: Hepatitis, colitis, and lupus manifestations, Am. J. Dig. Dis. 3:481, 1958.

70. Green, J., Mistilis, S. P., and Schiff, L.: Acute alcoholic hepatitis; a clinical study

of 50 cases, Arch. Int. Med. *112*:113, 1963.

71. Green, P., and Rubin, L.: Amenorrhea as a manifestation of chronic liver disease, Am. J. Obstet. Gynec. 78:141, 1959.
72. Hartsough, G. R., and Burger, D.: Encephalopathy of mink. I. Epizoologic and clinical observations, J. Infect. Dis. *115*: 387, 1965.
73. Harvey, A. M., Shulman, L. E., Tumulty, P. A., Conley, C. L., and Schoenrich, E. H.: Systemic lupus erythematosus: review of the literature and clinical analysis of 138 cases, Medicine 33:291, 1954.
74. Havens, W. P.: Liver disease and antibody formation, Int. Arch. Allergy and Appl. Immunol. *14*:75, 1959.
75. Heller, R., Zimmerman, H. J., Rosenvaig, S., and Singer, K.: The L.E. cell phenomenon in chronic hepatic disease, New Engl. J. Med. *254*:1160, 1956.
76. Helyer, B. J., and Howei, J. B.: Spontaneous autoimmune disease in NZB/BL mice, Brit. J. Haemat. *9*:119, 1963.
77. Hicks, J. D., and Burnet, F. M.: Renal lesions in the autoimmune mouse strains NZB and FI NZB × NZW, J. Path. Bact. *91*:467, 1966.
78. Hijmans, W., Doniach, D., Roitt, I. M., and Holborow, E. J.: Serological overlap between lupus erythematosus, rheumatoid arthritis and thyroid autoimmune disease, Brit. Med. J. *2*:909, 1961.
79. Hoffbauer, F. W., McCartney, J. S., Dennis, C., and Karlson, E. L.: The relationship of chronic ulcerative colitis and cirrhosis, Ann. Int. Med. *39*:267, 1953.
80. Holborow, E. J., Asherson, G. L., Johnson, G. D., Barnes, R. D. S., and Carmichael, D. S.: Antinuclear factor and other antibodies in blood and liver diseases, Brit. Med. J. *1*:656, 1963.
81. Holdsworth, C. D., Hall, E. W., Dawson, A. M., and Sherlock, S.: Ulcerative colitis in chronic liver disease, Quart. J. Med. *34*:211, 1965.
82. Holley, H. L., Hammack, W. J., and Douglas, C.: The application of the sensitized sheep cell test to sera of patients with non-rheumatic diseases and false positive serological reactions for rheumatoid arthritis, Am. J. Med. Sci. *242*:331, 1961.
83. Holman, H. R., Deicher, H. R. G., and Kunkel, H. G.: The L.E. cell and the

L. E. serum factors, Bull. N. Y. Acad. Med. *35*:409, 1959.
84. Holmes, M. C., and Burnet, F. M.: The natural history of autoimmune disease in NZB mice: a comparison with the pattern of human autoimmune manifestations, Ann. Int. Med. 59:265, 1963.
85. Hutchings, H. E., and Wigley, R. A. D.: Lupoid hepatitis, New Zealand Med. J. 58:12, 1959.
86. Ichida, F.: Clinico-pathological studies of active chronic hepatitis in Vandenbroucke, J., De Groote, J., and Standaert, L. O. (eds.): Advances in Hepatology, p. 28, New York, Karger, 1965.
87. Jackson, W. B.: Lupoid hepatitis, New Zealand Med. J. 61:302, 1962.
88. Jersild, M.: Infectious hepatitis, with subacute atrophy of the liver; an epidemic in women after the menopause, New Engl. J. Med. 237:8, 1947.
89. Johnson, G. D., Holborow, E. J., and Glynn, L. E.: Antibody to smooth muscle in patients with liver disease, Lancet 2: 878, 1965.
90. Jones, W. A., and Castleman, B.: Liver disease in young women with hyperglobulinemia, Am. J. Path. 40:315, 1962.
91. Joske, R. A., and King, W. E.: The L. E. cell phenomenon in active chronic viral hepatitis, Lancet 2:477, 1955.
92. Kelsall, A. R., Stewart, A., and Witts, L. J.: Subacute and chronic hepatitis, Lancet 1:195, 1947.
93. Kern, F., Vinnik, I., Struthers, J. E., and Hill, R. B.: Treatment of chronic hepatitis with adrenal cortical hormones, Am. J. Med. 35:310, 1963.
94. King, J. D.: Lupoid hepatitis with advanced atrophic cirrhosis: review of the literature and report of a case, A.M.A. Arch. Path. 68:669, 1959.
95. Klatskin, G.: Subacute hepatic necrosis and post necrotic cirrhosis due to anicteric infections with the hepatitis virus, Am. J. Med. 25:333, 1958.
96. Kleckner, M. S., Stauffer, M. H., Bargen, J. A., and Dockerty, M. B.: Hepatic lesions in the living patient with chronic ulcerative colitis as demonstrated by liver biopsy, Gastroenterology 22:13, 1952.
97. Kofman, S., Johnson, G. C., and Zimmerman, H. J.: Apparent hepatic dysfunction in lupus erythematosus, Arch. Int. Med. 95:669, 1955.
98. Krarup, N. B., and Roholm, K.: The de-

velopment of cirrhosis of the liver after acute infectious hepatitis elucidated by aspiration biopsy, Acta med. scand. *108*: 306, 1941.

99. Krook, H.: Liver cirrhosis in patients with a lupus erythematosus-like syndrome, Acta med. scand. *169*:713, 1961.

100. Kunkel, H. G., Ahrens, E. H., Eisenmenger, W. J., Bongiovanni, A. M., and Slater, R. J.: Extreme hyperglobulinemia in young women with liver disease of unknown etiology, J. Clin. Invest. *30*:654, 1954.

101. Kunkel, H. G., and Labby, D. H.: Chronic liver disease following infectious hepatitis. II. Cirrhosis of the liver, Ann. Int. Med. *32*:433, 1950.

102. Lee, S. L., Michael, S. R., and Vural, I. L.: The L. E. (lupus erythematosus) cell, Am. J. Med. *10*:446, 1951.

103. Leevy, C. M., Zinke, M., Baber, J., and Chey, W. Y.: Observations on the influence of medical therapy on portal hypertension in hepatic cirrhosis, Ann. Int. Med. *49*:837, 1958.

104. Levin, H., Landy, M., and Frei, E.: The effect of 6-mercaptopurine on immune response in man, New Engl. J. Med. *271*:16, 1964.

105. Logan, G. B.: Prognosis of chronic hepatitis in children, Proc. Mayo Clin. *25*: 299, 1950.

106. Mackay, I. R.: The problem of persisting destructive disease of the liver, Gastroenterology *40*:617, 1961.

107. Mackay, I. R., and Gajdusek, D. C.: An "autoimmune" reaction against tissue antigens in certain acute and chronic diseases. II. Clinical correlations, Arch. Int. Med. *101*:30, 1958.

108. Mackay, I. R., and Larkin, L.: The significance of the presence in human serum of complement-fixing antibodies to human tissue antigens, Aust. Ann. Med. 7:251, 1958.

109. Mackay, I. R., Taft, L. I., and Cowling, D. C.: Lupoid hepatitis, Lancet 2:1323, 1956.

110. ———: Lupoid hepatitis and the hepatic lesions of systemic lupus erythematosus, Lancet *1*:65, 1959.

111. Mackay, I. R., Weiden, S., and Hasker, J.: "Autoimmune hepatitis," Ann. N. Y. Acad. Sci. *124*:767, 1965.

112. Mackay, I. R., Weiden, S., and Ungar, B.: Treatment of active chronic hepatitis

and lupoid hepatitis with 6-mercaptopurine and Azathioprine, Lancet *1*:899, 1964.

113. Mackay, I. R., and Wood, I. J.: Autoimmunity in liver disease, *in* Popper, H., and Schaffner, F. (eds.): Progress in Liver Disease, p. 39, New York, Grune & Stratton, 1961.

114. ———: Lupoid hepatitis: a comparison of 22 cases with other types of chronic liver disease, Quart. J. Med. *31*:485, 1962.

115. MacLachlan, M. J., Rodnan, G. P., Cooper, W. M., and Fennell, R. H.: Chronic active ("lupoid") hepatitis, Ann. Int. Med. *62*:425, 1965.

116. Mallory, T. B.: The pathology of epidemic hepatitis, J.A.M.A. *134*:655, 1947.

117. McCarthy, C. F., and Read, A. E.: Bleeding esophageal varices in ulcerative colitis, Gastroenterology *42*:325, 1962.

118. McConkey, B., and Callaghan, P.: Thyroiditis and cirrhosis of the liver, Lancet *1*:939, 1960.

119. McIlvanie, S. K., and MacCarthy, J. D.: Hepatitis in association with prolonged 6-mercaptopurine therapy, Blood *14*:80, 1959.

120. Mellors, R. C.: Autoimmune disease in NZB/BL mice. I, Pathology and pathogenesis of a model system of spontaneous glomerulonephritis, J. Exp. Med. *122*:25, 1965.

121. Mellors, R. C., and Huang Chen Ya: Immunopathology of NZB/BL mice. V, Virus-like (filterable) agent separated from lymphoma cells and identifiable by electron microscopy, J. Exp. Med. *124*: 1031, 1966.

122. Milgrom, F., Tuggac, Z. M., and Witebsky, E.: Organ-specific antigens of liver, testicle and pituitary, J. Immun. *94*:157, 1965.

123. Mistilis, S. P.: Pericholangitis and ulcerative colitis. I, Pathology, etiology and pathogenesis, Ann. Int. Med. *63*:1, 1965.

124. ———: Natural history of active chronic hepatitis. II. Pathology, pathogenesis and clinico-pathological correlation, Aust. Ann. Med. *17*:Nov., 1968.

125. ———: Active chronic hepatitis and ulcerative colitis, Submitted for publication, 1968.

126. ———: Persistent hepatitis: clinicopathological study, In preparation, 1968.

127. Mistilis, S. P., and Blackburn, C. R. B.:

The treatment of active chronic hepatitis with 6-Mercaptopurine and Azathioprine, Aust. Ann. Med. *16*:305, 1967.

128. Mistilis, S. P., Blackburn, C. R. B., and Fung, W. P.: The use of 6-mercaptopurine and Imuran in the treatment of active chronic hepatitis, Gastroent., Suppl. 106 (Liver Research), 478, 1967.

129. Mistilis, S. P., and Goulston, S. J. M.: Liver and ulcerative colitis, *in* Badenoch, J., and Brooke, B. N. (eds.): Recent Advances in Gastroenterology, London, Churchill, Boston, Little-Brown, 1965.

130. Mistilis, S. P., and Schiff, L.: Steroid therapy in chronic hepatitis, Arch. Int. Med. *113*:54, 1964.

131. Mistilis, S. P., Skyring, A. P., and Blackburn, C. R. B.: Natural history of active chronic hepatitis. I. Clinical features, course, diagnostic criteria, morbidity, mortality and survival, Aust. Ann. Med. *17*:214, 1968.

132. Mistilis, S. P., Skyring, A. P., and Goulston, S. J. M.: Pericholangitis and ulcerative colitis. II. Clinical aspects, Ann. Int. Med. *63*:17, 1965.

133. ———: Effect of long term tetracycline therapy, steroid therapy and colectomy in pericholangitis associated with ulcerative colitis, Aust. Ann. Med. *14*:286, 1965.

134. Morris, J. A., and Gajdusek, D. C.: Encephalopathy in mice following inoculation of scrapie sheep brain, Nature *197*:1084, 1963.

135. Muschel, L. H., Simonton, L. A., Wells, P. A., and Fife, E. H., Jr.: Occurrence of complement-fixing antibodies reactive with normal tissue constituents in normal and disease states, J. Clin. Invest. *40*:517, 1961.

136. Naish, J. M.: Autoclastic (lupoid) hepatitis, Brit. J. Clin. Pract. *14*:749, 1960.

137. Norins, L. C., and Holmes, M. C.: Antinuclear factors in mice, J. Immun. *93*:148, 1964.

138. O'Brien, E. N., Goble, A. J., and Mackay, I. R.: Plasma transaminase activity as an index of effectiveness of cortisone in chronic hepatitis, Lancet *1*:1245, 1958.

139. Olhagen, L.: Ulcerative colitis in cirrhosis of the liver, Acta med. scand. *162*:143, 1958.

140. Orloff, M. J., Halasz, N. A., Lipman, C., Schwabe, A. D., Thompson, J. C., and Weidner, W. A.: The complications of cirrhosis of the liver, Ann. Int. Med. *66*:165, 1967.

141. Page, A. R., Condie, R. M., and Good, R. A.: Effect of 6-mercaptopurine on inflammation, Am. J. Path. *40*:519, 1962.

142. ———: Suppression of plasma cell hepatitis with 6-mercaptopurine, Am. J. Med. *36*:200, 1964.

143. Page, A. R., and Good, R. A.: Plasma cell hepatitis with special attention to steroid therapy, Am. J. Dis. Child. *99*:288, 1960.

144. ———: Plasma cell hepatitis, Lab. Invest. *11*:351, 1962.

145. Palmer, E. D., and Brick, I. B.: Esophageal varices in non-cirrhotic patients, Am. J. Med. *17*:641, 1954.

146. ———: Varices of the distal esophagus in the absence of portal and superior caval hypertension, Am. J. Med. Sci. *230*:515, 1955.

147. Paronetto, F., and Popper, H.: Aggravation of hepatic lesions in mice by in vivo localization of immune complexes (Auer hepatitis), Am. J. Path. *47*:549, 1965.

148. Paronetto, F., Rubin, E., and Popper, H.: Local formation of gamma globulin in the diseased liver and its relation to hepatic necrosis, Lab. Invest. *11*:150, 1962.

149. Pasnick, K. J., Beall, G. N., Van Arsdel, P. P., and Stevens, S. R.: Complement fixing reactions with liver tissue in human disease, Am. J. Med. *33*:774, 1962.

150. Popper, H.: What is chronic hepatitis? Gastroenterology *50*:444, 1966.

151. Popper, H., Rubin, E., and Schaffner, F.: Editorial: The problem of primary biliary cirrhosis, Am. J. Med. *33*:807, 1962.

152. Post, J., Gellis, S., and Lindenauer, H. J.: Studies on the sequel of acute infectious hepatitis, Ann. Int. Med. *33*:1378, 1950.

153. Prasad, P.: Autoimmune antibodies in infantile cirrhosis, Brit. Med. J. *2*:1031, 1962.

154. Read, A. E., Sherlock, S., and Harrison, C. V.: Active "juvenile" cirrhosis considered as part of a systemic disease and effect of corticosteroid therapy, Gut *4*:378, 1963.

155. Reichman, S., and Davis, W. D., Jr.: The splenic approach to the portal circulation; intrasplenic and intrahepatic pressure measurements in acute and convalescent hepatitis, Gastroenterology *33*:609, 1957.

156. Reynolds, T. B., Edmondson, H. A., Peters, R. L., and Redeker, A.: Lupoid

hepatitis, Ann. Int. Med. *61*:650, 1964.

157. Richardson, W., and Castleman, B.: Discussion of Case 36011, Weekly Clinicopathological exercises; case records of the Massachusetts General Hospital, New Engl. J. Med. *242*:26, 1950.

158. Robson, M. D.: Systemic lupus erythematosus complicating chronic liver disease, Guy's Hosp. Rep. *108*:438, 1959.

159. Rubin, E.: Interpretation of the liver biopsy, Gastroenterology *45*:400, 1963.

160. Rubin, E., Schaffner, F., and Popper, H.: Primary biliary cirrhosis, Am. J. Path. *46*: 387, 1965.

161. St. Geme, J. W., Jr.: The inhibitory effect of 6-mercaptopurine on the in vitro replication of animal viruses, Presented at Midwest Society for Pediatric Research, Cincinnati, Ohio, October, 1962.

162. Sborov, V. M., Bluemle, L. W., Neefe, J. R., and Gyorgy, P.: The clinical usefulness of cortisone and ACTH in liver disease, Gastroenterology *28*:745, 1955.

163. Schaefer, J. W., Schiff, L., Gall, E. A., and Oikawa, Y.: Progression of acute hepatitis to post-necrotic cirrhosis, Am. J. Med. *42*:348, 1967.

164. Schiff, L.: The use of steroids in liver disease, Medicine *45*:565, 1966.

165. Schwartz, R., Stack, J., and Dameshek, W.: Effect of 6-mercaptopurine on antibody production, Proc. Soc. Exp. Biol. Med. *99*:164, 1958.

166. Sherlock, S.: Post-hepatitis cirrhosis, Lancet *1*:817, 1948.

167. ————: Primary biliary cirrhosis (chronic intrahepatic obstructive jaundice), Gastroenterology *37*:574, 1959.

168. ————: Waldenstrom's chronic active hepatitis, Acta med. scand. *179*:(Supp. 445), 1966.

169. Shipton, E. A.: A contribution to the study of collagen disease and the L. E. cell phenomenon, Med. J. Aust. *1*:911, 1957.

170. Sigurdsson, B., Palsson, P. A., and Grimsson, H.: Visna, demyelinating transmissible disease of sheep, J. Neuropath. Exp. Neurol. *16*:389, 1957.

171. Sigurdsson, B., Thormar, H., and Palsson, P. A.: Cultivation of visna virus in tissue culture, Arch. ges. Virusforsch. *10*:368, 1960.

172. Silva, H., Hall, E., Hill, K. R., Shaldon, S., and Sherlock, S.: Renal involvement in active "juvenile" cirrhosis J. Clin. Path. *18*:157, 1965.

173. Smetana, H. F.: The histopathology of acute non-fatal hepatitis, Bull. N. Y. Acad. Med. *28*:482, 1952.

174. Sun, S. C., Chuong, S. M., and Fresh, C. D. R.: A viral hepatitis study on Taiwan, Arch. Int. Med. *115*:261, 1965.

175. Tisdale, W. A.: Subacute hepatitis, New Engl. J. Med. *268*:85; 138, 1963.

176. Tumen, H. J., Monaghan, J. F., and Jobb, E.: Hepatic cirrhosis as a complication of chronic ulcerative colitis, Ann. Int. Med. *26*:542, 1947.

177. Upjohn, C.: L. E. cell phenomenon associated with chronic hepatitis, Proc. Roy. Soc. Med. *51*:742, 1958.

178. Vinnick, L. E., Kern, F., Jr., and Corley, W. D.: Serum 5-nucleotidase and pericholangitis in patients with chronic ulcerative colitis, Gastroenterology *45*:492, 1963.

179. Volwiler, W., and Elliott, J. A.: Late manifestations of epidemic infectious hepatitis, Gastroenterology *10*:349, 1948.

180. Waldenstrom, J.: Leber, Blutproteine und Nahrungseiweiss Stoffwechsel, Sonderband XV, p. 8, Tanung, Bad Kissingen, 1950.

181. Walker, J. G., Doniach, D., Roitt, I. M., and Sherlock, S.: Serological tests in diagnosis of primary biliary cirrhosis, Lancet *1*:827, 1965.

182. Walshe, J. R., and Zimmerman, H. J.: The demonstration of the "L.E." phenomenon in patients with penicillin hypersensitivity, Blood *8*:65, 1953.

183. Weller, T. H., and Coons, A. H.: Fluorescent antibody studies with agents of varicella and herpes zoster propagated in vitro, Proc. Soc. Exp. Biol. Med. *86*:789, 1954.

184. Whittingham, S., Irwin, J., Mackay, I. R., and Smalley, M.: Smooth muscle auto-antibody in "autoimmune hepatitis," Gastroenterology *51*:449, 1966.

185. Wilkinson, M., and Sacker, L. S.: The lupus erythematosus cell and its significance, Brit. Med. J. *2*:661, 1957.

186. Williams, G. E. G.: Pericholangiolitic biliary cirrhosis, J. Path. Bact. *89*:23, 1965.

187. Williams, R.: The place of steroid therapy in the treatment of liver disease, Med. Clin. N. Amer. *47*:801, 1963.

188. Willocx, R. G., and Isselbacher, K. J.: Chronic liver disease in young people, Am. J. Med. *30*:185, 1961.

17

Fatty Liver: Biochemical and Clinical Aspects

KURT J. ISSELBACHER, m.d., and *DAVID H. ALPERS*, m.d.

The accumulation of excessive lipid in the liver has been referred to by a variety of terms including fatty infiltration, fatty metamorphosis and fatty degeneration of the liver. By chemical criteria, a fatty liver usually is synonymous with the hepatic accumulation of triglyceride. In the normal liver, triglyceride is not readily evident by light microscopy, but if special lipid stains are used one may see small lipid droplets in the hepatocytes. However under conditions of hepatic triglyceride accumulation, lipid droplets appear surrounded by membranes. Recently these membrane-enclosed lipid droplets have been referred to as liposomes. Increasing accumulation of fat in the liver also forms so-called liposomes.[76]

In the normal liver approximately 5 per cent of the weight is due to fat. The major hepatic lipids include phospholipids, triglycerides, fatty acids, cholesterol and cholesterol esters. Under conditions of fat accumulation, 40 to 50 per cent of its weight may be due to lipid, mostly in the form of triglyceride. Numerous chemical or pharmacologic agents cause the production of a fatty liver as one of their main toxic effects. However, in most clinical situations in which a fatty liver is found, it is usually only one facet of a broader metabolic derangement which often includes necrosis.

Perhaps the most common occurrence of fatty liver in the United States is associated with alcoholism. For this reason, in this review the biochemical and clinical aspects of alcohol-induced fatty liver are emphasized.

The major aspects of normal lipid metabolism are discussed, followed by a consideration of the many mechanisms that may lead to triglyceride accumulation in the liver.

LIPID METABOLISM AND THE LIVER

Fatty Acid Metabolism. In fatty liver the major lipid fractions that increase in amount are the fatty acids and triglycerides. Phospholipids, cholesterol and cholesterol esters usually increase only to a limited degree. Figure 17–1 shows a scheme of fatty acid and triglyceride metabolism. Dietary fats consist primarily of triglycerides which are hydrolyzed in the intestine to monoglycerides and fatty acids. The latter are then absorbed, and resynthesized in the intestinal cell to triglycerides. The triglycerides interact with protein, cholesterol and phospholipid in the intestinal cell to form chylomicrons. These then enter the lymph after which they reach the bloodstream and the liver.

There is considerable debate as to the mechanism of hepatic uptake of chylomicrons and the triglyceride which they contain. It has not been established whether the triglyceride enters the liver cell as such and is subsequently hydrolyzed within the cell,[55, 85] or whether the lipid is first trapped in the spaces of Disse, hydrolyzed there and then enters the liver cell as fatty acids.[21] Whichever is correct, it is clear that triglycerides presented to the liver are hydrolyzed to glycerol and fatty acids. The fatty acids

Fig. 17–1. Uptake and release of triglycerides (TG) and fatty acids (FA) by the liver.

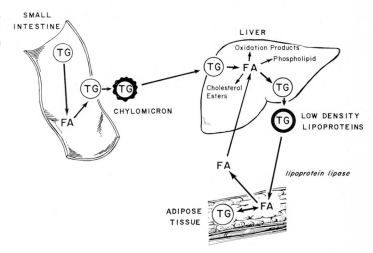

may then (1) be oxidized and used for energy; (2) be utilized for resynthesis of triglyceride; (3) be converted to phospholipids; or (4) lead to the formation of cholesterol esters. Lipids leave the liver in the form of lipoproteins. In the case of triglyceride, this is in the form of low density or beta-lipoproteins.

In the nonhepatic tissues—and especially in adipose tissue—the uptake of the triglycerides—(beta-lipoproteins) again requires hydrolysis. This appears to be mediated by a lipase located on the surface of endothelial or tissue cells.[67] This lipase is considered to be similar to or identical to that activated or liberated by heparin administration (i.e., postheparin lipoprotein lipase). Evidence suggests that this postheparin lipoprotein lipase is important in removing chylomicrons from the blood after the ingestion of a fatty meal.[17] The fatty acids are then converted again to triglyceride which is stored in adipose tissue. When needed for energy the adipose tissue triglycerides are once more hydrolyzed to fatty acids and released into the bloodstream. These considerations lead to the following conclusions:

1. Transport of triglycerides from one tissue to another involves hydrolysis to fatty acids followed by resynthesis to triglycerides.

2. Serum triglycerides are predominantly of dietary and hepatic origin.

3. In the fasting state, the serum fatty acids that reach the liver are primarily derived from adipose tissue; in the postprandial state, the serum free fatty acids are of both exogenous and endogenous origin.

Fatty Acid Mobilization. Mobilization of fatty acids from adipose tissue is subject to numerous regulatory mechanisms that determine the rate at which free fatty acids enter the bloodstream. Table 17–1 lists some of these factors. As is outlined below, influx of fatty acids to the liver is an important factor

TABLE 17–1. SOME FACTORS THAT AFFECT MOBILIZATION OF FATTY ACIDS FROM ADIPOSE TISSUE

FACTORS	INCREASED MOBILIZATION	DECREASED MOBILIZATION
Nutritional	Low glucose availability	High glucose availability
Hormonal	Glucagon Corticosteroids Growth hormone Thyroid	Insulin
Nervous	Sympathetic stimulation	Cordotomy Sympathetic blocking agents
Chemical	Epinephrine Norepi- nephrine	Nucleotides Nicotinic acid Salicylates Tranquilizers Adenosine triphosphate Chlorphenoxy- isobutyrate (Atromid)

in the production of fatty liver of diverse etiologies. Fatty liver can occur in the absence of hepatic damage, if the rate at which fatty acids are brought to the liver exceeds the ability of the liver to metabolize and re-secrete the fatty acids into the circulation in the form of triglycerides.[20]

Hepatic availability of glucose may be one factor in the formation of a fatty liver since many of the clinical conditions in which hepatic fat is seen are characterized by starvation. When blood glucose is reduced a reciprocal increase in plasma fatty acids tends to occur due to mobilization from adipose tissue. Corticosteroids, catecholamines and sympathetic stimulation likewise increase the rate at which fatty acids are released from adipose tissue.[61] Thus, parenteral administration of epinephrine and norepinephrine can lead to an increased lipid deposition in the liver.[20] Catecholamines have been indirectly implicated in many experimental models of fatty liver, most noticeably those produced by carbon tetrachloride and ethanol.[8] However, it is not clear whether their role in the production of a fatty liver is clinically important.

Other chemicals, notably adenosine triphosphate, appear to decrease the fat accumulation produced by agents such as ethionine, carbon tetrachloride and ethanol (Table 17–1).[34] Administration of ATP leads to a decrease in circulating free fatty acids, which appears to be secondary to the relative hypothermia which follows ATP injections. Numerous other chemicals, including salicylates and tranquilizers, decrease fatty acid mobilization.[9]

Recently, chlorphenoxyisobutyrate (Atromid) has been used to induce hypolipidemia. In animals this drug causes a decrease in plasma triglycerides and inhibits the release of newly formed triglycerides from the liver.[24] This decreased rate of secretion of hepatic triglyceride has been confirmed in isolated perfused livers.[15] However, in the intact animal the liver does not become fatty, presumably because plasma free fatty acid levels decrease also.

Fatty Acid Uptake and Utilization by Liver. Fatty acids liberated from adipose tissue are carried in the bloodstream bound to albumin. Approximately one third of the circulating free fatty acids are removed by the liver, a third by skeletal muscle and the rest by other tissues, especially myocardium.[60, 77]

In considering the transport, synthesis and metabolism of fatty acids, it must be kept in mind that these include the essential fatty acids, such as linoleic acid, which cannot be synthesized by the mammalian organisms. When tissues such as liver are called upon to synthesize fatty acids from 2 carbon precursors, the main products are saturated long-chain fatty acids such as palmitic acid.

The mechanism of uptake of fatty acids by the liver is not well understood but agents such as norepinephrine have been shown to diminish fatty acid uptake by the isolated perfused liver.[30] Following hepatic uptake, fatty acids may be metabolized (i.e., oxidized) or re-esterified to triglycerides, phospholipids and cholesterol esters. Quantitatively most of the fatty acids reaching the liver are re-secreted into the bloodstream as triglycerides in the form of low density (beta) lipoproteins. Hepatic triglyceride formation or accumulation is greatly affected by the rate at which fatty acids are presented to the liver[83] but undoubtedly other factors affect this also.[86] As indicated above, although fatty acids are incorporated into phospholipids and cholesterol esters, when a fatty liver is produced the predominant lipid that accumulates is triglyceride.

Synthesis and Release of Triglycerides. After the re-esterification of fatty acids to triglycerides by enzymes located in the smooth endoplasmic reticulum of the liver cell, the triglycerides interact with protein (apoprotein, lipid-acceptor protein) cholesterol and phospholipid to form lipoprotein.[19] This protein is synthesized by the rough endoplasmic reticulum but it may also be liberated as an apoprotein into the bloodstream.[68] Little is known about the mechanism whereby protein and triglyceride interact to form lipoproteins. It is not clear whether the secretion of lipoprotein into the plasma requires energy or is mediated by enzymes. Lombardi has suggested that the rate at which triglycerides are secreted is proportional to the rate at which they are synthesized.[51]

MECHANISMS IN THE PRODUCTION OF FATTY LIVER

The number of theories for the pathogenesis of fatty liver are based on the normal physiology outlined above. These are graphically depicted in Figure 17–2. Singly or in combination any of these factors might be involved. An increased supply of fatty acids might result from increased hepatic synthesis of fatty acids or from decreased oxidation or utilization of fatty acids by the liver. In addition, the secretion of triglycerides might be impaired either secondary to diminished lipoprotein formation or to impaired release of complete lipoproteins. Although there are no definitive data concerning the relative importance of these mechanisms, some are undoubtedly more important than others, depending on the agent directly responsible for the production of a fatty liver. Some of these pharmacologic or toxic agents for which a mechanism has been proposed are discussed below.

Increased Fatty Acid Supply. The data on fatty livers produced *acutely* by a number of agents suggest that much of the lipid that accumulates in the liver is derived from adipose tissue. This is not surprising since most acute studies have been performed on fasting animals, and under these conditions the plasma free fatty acids are predominantly those released from peripheral lipid depots. Many of the hormonal and experimental manipulations that interfere with the mobilization of fatty acids from adipose tissue are also effective in blocking a fatty liver. This emphasizes that by varying the supply of fatty acids to the liver one can influence directly the extent or degree of hepatic fat accumulation. Thus if the rate of fatty acids influx is reduced, the liver will contain less fat.

There is no evidence for an increased *rate* of uptake of fatty acids as a cause of a fatty liver. Recknagel recently reviewed the data describing fatty acid flux in CCl_4 induced fatty liver.[65] He concluded that the fatty acids being supplied to the liver accounted for all the fat accumulation in the liver.

Increased Triglyceride Formation. As indicated above, a significant amount of the fatty acids presented to the liver are normally esterified to triglyceride. One could postulate that, given a certain supply of fatty acids, factors would lead to (1) direct stimulation of this enzymatic esterification mechanism or (2) decreased incorporation of fatty acids into phospholipid and cholestrol ester and hence indirectly lead to increased triglyceride formation. In some experimental situations (e.g., alcohol-induced fatty liver), the former appears to be the case.[74]

Decreased Synthesis or Release of Lipoproteins. A scheme depicting the synthesis and release of lipoproteins from the liver cell is shown in Figure 17–2. Sites are also

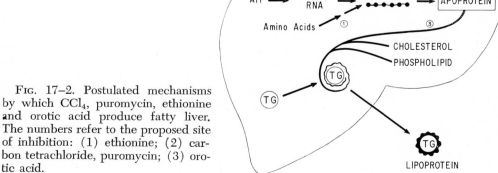

Fig. 17–2. Postulated mechanisms by which CCl_4, puromycin, ethionine and orotic acid produce fatty liver. The numbers refer to the proposed site of inhibition: (1) ethionine; (2) carbon tetrachloride, puromycin; (3) orotic acid.

shown at which interference in this process has been experimentally suggested using specific hepatotoxins. Obviously the first possible block would be a decrease in the synthesis of protein from amino acids, a process known to occur on ribosomes and the rough endoplasmic reticulum. Indeed many of the experimental toxins used to produce a fatty liver inhibit protein synthesis.

In the case of carbon tetrachloride one of the earliest lesions noted microscopically is at the level of the endoplasmic reticulum, and biochemically protein synthesis is dramatically decreased.[81] This is associated with a breakdown of polyribosomes (needed for protein synthesis) to single ribosomes.[80] Peroxidation of lipids, including microsomal lipids, is increased following CCl_4, and it is possible that microsomal membrane function is affected by this process.[64]

Ethionine interferes with protein synthesis and leads to a fatty liver. This drug lowers hepatic ATP levels, leads to a decrease in polyribosomes, diminished protein and phospholipid synthesis.[18] The timing of events after ethionine administration is consistent with the notion that inhibition of protein synthesis alone accounts for the accumulation of fat in the liver. Protein synthesis is affected 2 hours after the drug is given, but fat accumulation does not begin for 1 to 2 hours thereafter. Since the half-life of the apoprotein portion of low density lipopro-

teins has been estimated to be about 1 to 2 hours in the rat,[1, 56] the interval between inhibition of protein synthesis and the accumulation of fat after ethionine is consistent with the time needed for the turnover of existing apoproteins. Puromycin, phosphorus and tetracycline are additional examples of agents that by a variety of mechanisms interfere with protein synthesis and thus induce fatty liver.

Administration of orotic acid to animals also leads to fatty liver.[84] This is readily counteracted or reversed by the administration of adenine. Orotic acid interferes with the formation of lipoproteins but not by the mechanism of impaired protein synthesis.[90] Roheim et al. have suggested that orotic acid somehow interferes with the interaction of the apoprotein and triglyceride.[69] However, the actual mechanism whereby proteins (i.e., apoproteins) and lipids combine to form lipoproteins remains to be elucidated.

FATTY LIVER OF THE ALCOHOLIC—METABOLIC AND CLINICAL ASPECTS

BIOCHEMICAL MECHANISMS

Fatty liver can follow either acute or chronic administration of alcohol in laboratory animals and in man. All of the mechanisms postulated in Figure 17–2 have at some time been proposed for the alcoholic

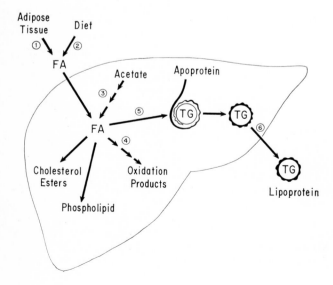

FIG. 17–3. Possible mechanisms by which alcohol produces fatty liver: (1) increased mobilization after acute intoxication; (2) dietary fat utilized if available; (3) increased hepatic synthesis of fatty acids; (4) decreased hepatic oxidation of fatty acids; (5) increased esterification to triglyceride; (6) decreased hepatic release of lipoprotein at high doses. FA, fatty acids; TG, triglycerides.

fatty liver by various investigators. Although there is still no definitive answer about the exact mechanism, it is clear that alcohol affects a number of processes that affect triglyceride accumulation in the liver (Fig. 17–3). It is perhaps simplest at first to emphasize those parameters of lipid metabolism that alcohol apparently does not affect, i.e., intestinal absorption of lipids, hepatic chylomicron uptake, hepatic protein synthesis or lipoprotein formation. It does, however, affect influx of fatty acids to the liver, synthesis and oxidation of fatty acids, triglyceride formation and release of lipoproteins from the liver.[35]

In reviewing the many studies on alcohol effects on lipid metabolism, numerous reports on first inspection appear to give conflicting results and to be contradictory. Many of the discrepancies however are readily explained by the fact that the effects of alcohol vary with a variety of experimental or clinical conditions. Thus results of *acute* experiments performed with large doses of alcohol and no other sources of calories differ from those of *chronic* experiments when alcohol is given in smaller amounts and other dietary nutrients are provided. Sex is also important, since the female animal is much more susceptible to hepatic fat accumulation than the male.

Fatty Acid Mobilization. Most of the current evidence suggests that the fatty acids present in hepatic triglycerides after alcohol administration are derived from the bloodstream and hence are of extrahepatic origin. Under fasting conditions, during acute alcohol intoxication, most of the plasma fatty acids that reach the liver are derived from adipose tissue. On the other hand, when alcohol and food are administered chronically the fatty acids in the plasma to a large extent reflect the fatty acids present in the triglycerides absorbed from the intestinal tract.[50]

When alcohol is highly concentrated in the bloodstream (i.e., greater than 250 mg./100 ml.), the free fatty acids in the serum increase markedly.[73] However, at lower blood levels (i.e., 80 to 100 mg./100 ml.) no significant changes in serum free fatty acids are detected.[47] Since a fatty liver may develop under these latter conditions with prolonged alcohol administration, Lieber has suggested that *increased* mobilization of fatty acids to the liver is not important as a primary mechanism for the development of the fatty liver.[45]

Nevertheless, in acute experiments with single large doses of alcohol, the fatty acid composition of the liver suggests that much of the lipid is derived from extrahepatic sources.[46, 74] When mobilization of fatty acids from adipose tissue is interfered with, as by adrenalectomy, cordotomy, hypophysectomy and adrenergic blocking agents, the amount of fat which accumulates in the liver after alcohol is markedly reduced.[63]

In chronic experiments in rats and man, where alcohol plus food is administered, the fatty acids in the liver tend to reflect the lipids in the diet.[46, 50] These acute and chronic experiments are not contradictory but simply reflect the importance of hepatic influx of fatty acids and the relationship of lipid that accumulates to the plasma composition. The latter is in turn influenced by whether the animal or subject is fasting or is ingesting fat. Therefore, while mobilization of free fatty acids may *increase* only with very high blood alcohol levels, influx of fatty acids to the liver must be *normal* for significant hepatic fat accumulation to occur.

Increased Hepatic Fatty Acid Synthesis. Lieber and Schmid observed that ethanol stimulates hepatic fatty acid synthesis *in vivo* and *in vitro*.[49] They postulated that the increased hepatic DPNH levels found after alcohol ingestion account for this increased synthesis. Ethanol is largely metabolized in the liver (90 to 98 per cent) and hepatic alcohol dehydrogenase converts DPN to DPNH as ethanol is metabolized to acetaldehyde. However, in the *de novo* synthesis of fatty acids from acetate, TPNH rather than DPNH is required. Some fatty acids are produced by elongation, and recent observations indicate that DPNH as well as TPNH may serve as hydrogen donors in the elongation of fatty acid chain lengths and in the conversion of saturated to unsaturated fatty acids.[6, 33] Thus, the results of Lieber and Schmid may be related to these latter 2 processes. Rebouças and Isselbacher also noted increased fatty acid synthesis in the liver after ethanol ingestion, but considered this effect nonspecific.[63]

Glucose and sorbitol were also found to increase fatty acid synthesis without the concomitant formation of a fatty liver. Moreover, in cordotomized rats ethanol increased hepatic fatty acid synthesis, but did not produce a fatty liver. Thus, while ethanol may, under certain conditions, increase hepatic fatty acid synthesis, it is unclear whether this is a major factor in the production of the alcohol-induced fatty liver.

Decreased Fatty Acid Oxidation. In man, ingestion of alcohol decreases oxidation of lipids under conditions which do not affect carbohydrate or protein metabolism.[3] Lieber and co-workers have shown that oxidation of long-chain fatty acids after ethanol ingestion is impaired to a greater extent than that of medium-chain fatty acids, and have suggested that this difference accounts for the greater accumulation of long-chain fatty acids after ethanol ingestion.[48] Under normal circumstances, however, medium-chain fatty acids are more rapidly metabolized than are long-chain fatty acids. The evidence that decreased oxidation is an important or major factor in the alcoholic fatty liver must be examined further. *In vitro*, ethanol can decrease oxidation of lipids, but so can other substances that do not lead to the development of a fatty liver (glucose, sorbitol, xylitol and nicotinamide).[63] Thus, although this mechanism has been suggested recently as the most likely cause of fatty liver produced by ethanol,[45] further evidence is needed.

Increased Esterification of Fatty Acids to Triglycerides. As indicated above, normally when fatty acids are presented to the liver they are readily esterified to triglycerides but also yield phospholipids and cholesterol esters. Conceivably alcohol could lead to increased conversion of fatty acids to triglycerides either directly or indirectly by inhibiting their incorporation into phospholipids and cholesterol esters. While not much is known about the factors that regulate hepatic triglyceride synthesis, experiments with acute alcohol administration to rats have shown alterations in the esterifying system in liver microsomes. Scheig and Isselbacher demonstrated that microsomes isolated from rats 16 hours after an acute alcohol load showed a four-fold increase in the conversion of ^{14}C-palmitate to triglyceride.[74] No studies have been performed with chronic alcohol administration and thus the action of alcohol on enhancing triglyceride formation requires further study.

Decreased Hepatic Release or Secretion of Triglycerides. There has been no demonstrated effect of alcohol on protein synthesis. No experiments have been carried out to date to indicate that it influences the interaction of lipid and apoprotein to form lipoprotein, as has been demonstrated in orotic acid fatty liver. As indicated above, many toxic agents leading to a fatty liver cause a decreased synthesis of protein and lipoprotein, and as a consequence decreased release of lipid into the bloodstream. In the case of CCl_4 and ethionine, the plasma triglycerides decrease. When alcohol is administered to man, plasma triglycerides initially increase.[73] However, when blood alcohol reaches high levels (i.e., greater than 250 mg./100 ml.), plasma triglycerides *decrease*, together with an increase in plasma free fatty acids. Thus, there is nothing to suggest an interference in hepatic lipid secretion except at high alcohol levels. Such a decreased release has been shown in isolated rat liver perfusions at a perfusate alcohol level of 400 mg./100 ml.[72] Since hepatic lipid must accumulate at lower levels of blood alcohol, and since at these levels decreased hepatic lipid release has not been demonstrated, one must assume that this mechanism is not a primary one but possibly a contributory factor.

In summary, alcohol administration both acutely and chronically affects many aspects of lipid metabolism. Some of these actions may be primary or major in regard to production of a fatty liver. Others may be minor or serve only to contribute to or affect the extent of the fatty liver. The principal mechanism whereby alcohol induces fatty liver is unclear.

PATHOLOGY OF FATTY LIVER OF THE
ALCOHOLIC

Grossly the liver is extremely enlarged, often weighing up to 6,000 Gm. The external and cut surfaces are smooth and pale yellow. Microscopically the liver cells are filled with fat vacuoles. Alcoholic hyalin or Mallory bodies are often seen. They are nearly specific for alcoholic liver disease, with or without fat, but have been seen in the livers of malnourished children in India,[79] and in some other nonalcoholic induced liver disorders.[53] By light microscopy these bodies are eosinophilic, coarsely granular, usually perinuclear in distribution and always intracellular. On electron microscopy these bodies have been claimed by some to represent strands of endoplasmic reticulum,[4] and by others, altered mitochondria.[59]

In alcohol damaged livers pathologic findings range from only fat in the liver to marked necrosis with polymorphonuclear infiltration and bile stasis, with only moderate fat in hepatocytes. These are most likely different manifestations of the same toxic injury induced by alcohol, since both extremes may be seen in the same patient at various stages of his illness. In addition, many patients who present with acute alcoholism have not eaten for days, and some of the hepatic fat may be related to starvation.

Recently the morphologic changes induced by alcohol in man have been studied by electron microscopy.[71] Within days after alcohol ingestion Rubin and Lieber noted vacuolization of the endoplasmic reticulum, distorted mitochondrial cristae, an increase in free polyribosomes and autophagic vacuoles. The exact significance of these changes is not clear.

CLINICAL AND LABORATORY FEATURES

Alcoholic Fatty Liver. The clinical features found in patients with fatty liver tend to be similar, but the best descriptions are those associated with ethanol ingestion.[23, 43] In the majority of patients there is hepatomegaly, often of striking proportions. About one half of the patients have pain and hepatic tenderness. A small percentage have jaundice, ascites, peripheral edema or signs of vitamin deficiency. The more severe the hepatic fat accumulation, the more likely is vitamin deficiency. Splenomegaly is uncommon unless hepatic fibrosis or frank cirrhosis are present.[43] If alcohol is withheld, splenomegaly may be reversible as may the early fibrotic changes.

The most characteristic laboratory finding is elevated BSP retention. The serum albumin is frequently low and the globulin elevated. Hyperbilirubinemia is seen in about 25 per cent of cases and levels in general do not exceed 20 mg./100 ml.[43] The transaminase (SGOT) is usually less than 100 units, and rarely exceeds 300 units. The prothrombin time is prolonged in about half the patients. Alkaline phosphatase is elevated in only about 15 per cent and usually only modestly (up to 10 Bodansky units). However, the laboratory findings and clinical features depend very much on whether fatty liver alone is present or whether there is also some degree of necrosis or intrahepatic cholestasis. Moreover, the amounts of fat and necrosis in the liver usually vary independently. Therefore, the amount of fat in the liver may not correlate well with the degree of abnormality in liver function tests.[28]

Alcoholic Hepatitis. This entity is referred to as "florid cirrhosis," "toxic hepatitis" and "acute alcoholic hepatitis," but it is not a syndrome separate from alcoholic fatty liver. Necrosis is merely another manifestation of hepatic injury related to alcohol. Pathogenetically the lesions may be similar, but the experimental study of ethanol-induced hepatic necrosis is rudimentary. On liver biopsy one sees much fat, and in addition diffuse cell dropout with polymorphonuclear infiltration and occasionally acidophil bodies. The inflammatory reaction is diffuse but often more marked around the portal vein.

When this pathologic picture is seen, patients present with hepatomegaly and abdominal pain just as they do with a fatty liver alone. However anorexia, nausea, vomiting, fever and jaundice tend to be more frequent. Anemia and leukocytosis are usually present, and the alkaline phosphatase is more frequently elevated, but in most cases only up to 10 Bodansky units. Usually this syndrome is found after a prolonged bout of drinking.

Phillips and Davidson first noted the importance of necrosis occurring with the fatty liver of alcohol,[57] but the largest and best studied group is that reported by Green et al.[25] Most of the reported patients have had a history or past evidence of chronic liver disease. Bilirubin and SGOT levels are elevated in most patients. Despite the necrosis seen on liver biopsy, transaminase is usually not above 100 units. This condition is a frequent cause of undiagnosed fever in alcoholic liver disease. While the fatty liver of the alcoholic may be associated with a variable degree of necrosis, necrosis is not seen in the absence of fat. Although the degree of necrosis does not correlate well with the amount of fat or with liver function tests, in general, the more severe the necrosis, the more serious the clinical course.

Acute Fatty Liver with Cholestasis. Rarely, alcoholic fatty liver presents as obstructive jaundice.[2] Typically these patients have a history of *marked* alcohol ingestion. The presenting symptoms are frequently identical to those seen in alcoholic hepatitis—in fact, acute inflammatory changes in the liver can complicate this form of fatty liver. The liver is very large and tender and liver function tests indicate the presence of cholestasis. Alkaline phosphatase is 2 to 8 times normal. Serum cholesterol may be above 500 mg.%. The cephalin flocculation test may be negative, and about half the patients have jaundice. Grossly the liver is large and yellow and microscopically practically every liver cell is filled with fat. Cholestasis may be difficult to detect because of the severe fatty changes.

These patients are often thought to have biliary tract disease because of fever, right upper quadrant pain and obstructive liver chemistries. A large tender liver may be a clue to the correct diagnosis. Since surgical intervention may be fatal, the possibility of fatty liver must be considered beforehand.

Zieve's Syndrome. Zieve has pointed out the association of hyperlipemia and hemolytic anemia in alcoholic disease.[91] However, indiscriminate use of the term Zieve's syndrome has obscured the fact that each component can occur separately, and that more than one mechanism may exist for each. Hyperlipemia may occur with ingestion of large amounts of alcohol, as outlined above, or may be associated with pancreatitis. In addition, serum triglycerides, phospholipids, free fatty acids and free cholesterol increase in both hepatocellular and obstructive liver disease.[58] Mild hemolytic anemia is common in liver disease, regardless of whether or not hyperlipemia is present.[37] Furthermore, a causal relationship between hyperlipemia

and hemolytic anemia has not been demonstrated.[5] Thus, hyperlipemia, hemolytic anemia, liver disease and pancreatitis all occur to varying degrees in alcoholism. In our opinion, the term "Zieve's syndrome" although useful in bringing these manifestations of alcoholism to clinical attention, is of limited usefulness.

DIAGNOSIS AND TREATMENT

All of the acute changes induced by ethanol (fatty liver, alcoholic hepatitis and acute fatty liver with cholestasis) are reversible. The diagnosis can be suspected clinically, but is best made by needle biopsy.

The acute hepatic lesions associated with ethanol sometimes cannot be clearly separated pathologically from each other. Although the lesions are reversible, the change may occur very slowly. It is not unusual for recovery to begin after only 2 to 3 weeks of hospitalization, and total recovery to require months. Treatment is supportive. The mainstay of therapy is abstinence from ethanol.

OTHER CLINICAL DISORDERS CHARACTERIZED BY FATTY LIVER

Starvation. Many studies have confirmed the fact that during starvation, serum free fatty acids increase, and the turnover of these fatty acids is enhanced.[10] This can be associated with a moderate increase in liver fat. The mechanism seems to be related to the lack of availability of glucose, increase in growth hormone and heightened sympathetic nervous activity, all of which mobilize free fatty acids from adipose tissue. Liver function tests are usually normal, except for BSP retention, which has been reported to be as high as 44 per cent during starvation.[70]

Kwashiorkor. There seems to be agreement that the syndrome known as kwashiorkor is a distinct clinical entity, consisting of edema, skin changes, impaired growth and a fatty liver. This condition is seen mainly in young children following consumption of a protein free diet which often has a high carbohydrate content. Much evidence suggests that kwashiorkor is world-wide, but it occurs rarely in the United States.

Fatty liver is only one aspect of the syndrome. The liver is enlarged and yellow, and there is a striking degree of fatty infiltration. The earliest deposition of fat is in the cells at the periphery of the lobules, but as the condition progresses, the cells of the middle and central areas of the lobules become involved.[62] When a high protein diet is administered, fat disappears first from the center of the liver lobule, and last from the peripheral cells. The condition does not progress to cirrhosis, which suggests that fat alone is an insufficient stimulus for the formation of fibrosis.

The serum-free fatty acids are increased, which suggests that increased mobilization of fat is important. One theory to explain this fact suggests that plasma glucose may fall as the result of inability to mobilize liver glycogen.[44] The plasma fatty acid increase would then be a compensation for the relative hypoglycemia. The rate of albumin synthesis is diminished and it has been suggested that lipoprotein synthesis is also affected, impairing the release of triglyceride from the liver. Some factor other than increased mobilization must be operative, because the plasma-free fatty acid levels are as high in marásmus as in kwashiorkor, yet fatty liver does not develop in marasmus.[22]

Obesity. Mild degrees of fatty infiltration have been reported in obese persons. The majority of these patients have had abnormal glucose tolerance tests, but are not severely diabetic. BSP retention is the most frequently abnormal liver function test. Liver biopsy has revealed, in addition to fat, inflammation of the portal triads.[89] It is not clear whether obesity itself caused portal inflammation or whether these patients had concomitant liver disease. The fatty infiltration can be reversed by weight reduction.

Diabetes Mellitus. Fatty infiltration of a striking degree can be seen in uncontrolled diabetes, frequently in children with ketoacidosis. The liver may be swollen and tender, and the BSP elevated. Reversal is rapid following control of the diabetes. The mechanism is unclear, but may be related to the marked mobilization of fatty acids from adipose tissue during uncontrolled diabetes.

Many reports suggest that in adult type, stable diabetes fatty liver may develop. Two separate studies have suggested that approximately 40 per cent of diabetics have moderate fatty infiltration, with or without cirrhosis.[40, 42] However, no clear distinction has been made between primary liver disease with secondary diabetes and primary diabetes mellitus. Certainly if fat in the liver is significant in a stable, adult diabetic, causes other than the diabetes should be sought.

Fatty liver of pregnancy. This syndrome often cannot be easily differentiated clinically from fulminant viral hepatitis. However, the laboratory features and pathology are clearly not the same as those in hepatitis. Forty cases have been reported and reviewed recently by Haemmerli.[26] In this series the age at onset was 16 to 42 years. Almost all reported cases involve patients during their first pregnancy. The syndrome begins with the sudden onset of vomiting and abdominal pain, usually during the 36th to 40th week of pregnancy. There is a rapid progression to jaundice, hematemesis, tachycardia, premature labor, oliguria, coma, convulsions and death. The total illness usually lasts 1 to 2 weeks. Only 6 of the 40 reported cases survived. In some of these surviving cases early cesarean section was performed. Therefore, the syndrome might be reversible if recognized early enough.

Laboratory results suggest obstructive jaundice. The bilirubin is usually above 10 mg.%, alkaline phosphatase is increased, but the cephalin flocculation is negative. Azotemia is a frequent finding. Pathologically the liver is yellow and soft. Microscopically the fat is deposited, first centrally, then spreads to involve the entire lobule. The cells often show fine fat vacuoles. It is usually stated that there is no necrosis or inflammation, although at least one case of hepatic necrosis has been reported.[13] Bile thrombi can be present. Acute pancreatitis is sometimes present and fat can be found in the pancreas, brain and kidneys. When recovery has occurred, it is noted first at the periphery of the lobule. Haemmerli claims that in this condition there is always a rim of intact cells in the periphery of each lobule, but this was not found in the 6 cases reported by Kunelis et al.[41] The mechanism of fatty infiltration during pregnancy is unknown.

Tetracycline-induced Fatty Liver. The administration of large intravenous doses (>2

Gm./day) of tetracycline and its derivatives is associated with a fine fatty vacuolization of the liver. This has been seen in nonpregnant as well as pregnant patients, but, in either case, the pathology is similar to that seen in fatty metamorphosis of pregnancy. A number of cases of fatty liver have been reported in association with tetracycline administration during pregnancy.[14] The fatty liver was reversible when tetracycline was discontinued.

However, approximately 75 per cent of the reported patients have died. In a typical case, 3 to 12 days after tetracycline has been given, there is an abrupt onset of jaundice, nausea and vomiting, spontaneous delivery, coma and finally death 1 to 2 weeks after the first dose of tetracycline. The laboratory findings and pathology in tetracycline-induced fatty liver are similar to those in fatty metamorphosis of pregnancy, except that jaundice is not so common. Some patients have recovered, but only when the tetracycline administration was stopped. Tetracycline inhibits protein synthesis when used in large doses, but it has not yet been established that fatty liver occurs by this mechanism.

A few cases have been reported using parenteral doses of only 1 Gm./day, so that during pregnancy an upper limit of 1 Gm./day should be used.[11] It is not clear whether in the pregnant woman the tetracycline-induced fatty liver is an entity distinct from fatty metamorphosis of pregnancy. However, tetracycline hepatotoxicity is reported rarely in the absence of pregnancy.

Corticosteroid Administration. In Cushing's syndrome moderate to severe fatty infiltration of the liver is reportedly not uncommon.[82] Fatty liver has been reported in patients receiving high doses of exogenous steroids over a period of weeks. Two reports have documented that upon withdrawal of steroids, fat embolism occurred in the absence of trauma. The mechanism of steroid-induced fatty liver is unknown.

In animals, plasma free fatty acids increase when cortisol is given.[32] This has been interpreted as suggesting that increased mobilization of fatty acid is involved. However, recently it has been suggested that with low doses of steroids all the increase in fatty acids can be accounted for by a decreased esterification of fatty acids in the liver.[38] Lipolysis in adipose tissues does occur with high doses, and clinically fatty liver occurs only with high doses of steroids. Steroids given during viral hepatitis in the dose of 30 to 40 mg. of prednisone/day, can result in a moderate fatty infiltration which is never seen in hepatitis in the absence of steroids. Systemic fat embolism has been reported after abrupt cessation of steroid therapy[31, 39] and fatty liver has been implicated as a possible source.

Carbon Tetrachloride. CCl_4 has attracted more attention in recent years as an experimental hepatotoxin than as a cause of fatty liver in man. However, its presence in fire extinguishers and cleaning fluids makes it available for toxicity in humans. Norwood has suggested that the incidence of CCl_4 poisoning is greatly underestimated.[54] In a population of 30,000 people in 1 year he documented 58 cases of CCl_4 poisoning; 51 of them were mild, 7 severe including 2 fatalities. Fatalities have been reported with 1.5 ml., whereas recovery has occurred after ingestion of 20 ml. Individual variation seems to be great. However, ingestion of 15 to 20 ml. is usually fatal in man.[88]

CCl_4 is absorbed via the GI tract or the lungs. It has been claimed that hepatotoxicity is more common after ingestion than inhalation, and that renal damage is more common after inhalation, but this distinction is not always true. Previous ingestion of alcohol, inanition and high fat diets seem to enhance toxicity. It is unclear how alcohol increases liver damage by CCl_4, whether by increasing the absorption of CCl_4 or by making the liver more susceptible to CCl_4. Most of the CCl_4 absorbed is excreted via the lungs within 2 days.[88] CCl_4 can be detected in the blood or expired air during this time period.

Clinically CCl_4 often produces dizziness, nausea, vomiting and headache as early symptoms. The time of onset depends on the dose. A burning sensation in the mouth, esophagus and stomach is often present very early after ingestion. Subsequently, abdominal cramps, confusion, decreased consciousness, delirium, restlessness, choreiform movements, muscle pain, diarrhea, vasomotor collapse and even coma may ensue. Characteristically, jaundice, hepatomegaly and ascites occur in severe poisoning by the third day, and death in the first week is usually due to hepatic necrosis. However, neither jaundice nor hepatomegaly need occur, even after ingestion, and deaths have been reported without much evidence of liver failure. When death occurs in the second or third week, renal failure is the usual cause.

Laboratory data usually reveal elevated transaminases, prolongation of the prothrombin time, positive cephalin flocculation and normal or slightly elevated alkaline phosphatase. Hepatic pathology shows marked fatty change, with centrilobular necrosis. The fat seems to begin centrilobularly and spreads to involve the entire lobule. Many acute inflammatory cells are present, especially in the centrilobular areas. The fat may be present in cells as fine vacuoles or large cysts. Treatment is only supportive, but should include gastric lavage, since CCl_4 greatly delays gastric emptying. Therefore, some CCl_4 may remain in the stomach for hours after ingestion.

Recknagel has recently reviewed the mechanism of CCl_4 hepatotoxicity.[65] It seems clear that diminished protein synthesis with decrease in lipoprotein synthesis and release from the liver is an important factor in producing fatty liver. The exact mechanism whereby this occurs is unknown. Recknagel has suggested that in some way CCl_4 forms peroxides of lipids which then damage cellular membranes. Although this idea has attractive features, it remains only a theory. None of the many agents used to prevent CCl_4-induced fatty liver or necrosis in animals (adrenergic blocking agents, antihistamines, antioxidants) has proved useful clinically, since they must all be given before the toxin is administered.

Phosphorus. Of the 3 forms of elemental phosphorus, only yellow phosphorus is toxic appreciably to the liver. It is a common component of many roach and rat poisons. After ingestion, frequently a burning sensation is felt in the mouth and throat. Abdominal pain and vomiting of violent nature follow. Within 1 or 2 days jaundice appears, and death occurs fairly rapidly. A fatal dose for man is about 60 mg.

Pathologically the liver shows periportal necrosis and fat at early times with the center of the lobule relatively spared. With severe poisoning the entire liver is rapidly involved. Gastric lavage is the treatment of choice.

Reye's Syndrome. In 1963 Reye et al.[66] described a syndrome which has since been reported with increasing frequency.[7, 16, 36] The syndrome consists of encephalopathy with fatty degeneration of the viscera, and often follows an antecedent viral infection. Both sexes are affected. The disorder has been reported in children from infancy to adolescence.

The syndrome begins with a mild prodromal illness. There is often a history of varicella in the patient or evidence of other viral illness in the family. After a 2 to 3 day period of improvement from the viral illness, intractable vomiting begins together with abdominal pain. There is a rapid progression, often within hours, to delirium, psychotic behavior, then stupor with spasticity and decerebrate posturing and finally to coma, with or without convulsions. There are no focal neurologic signs. The majority of the reported patients have died, but when recovery occurs it is rapid, again, often within hours or several days. Hepatomegaly appears during the rapid progression to coma, and may revert to normal even when encephalopathy persists.

Laboratory studies show some leukocytosis, normal findings on lumbar puncture and an elevated transaminase (SGOT). Transaminase levels as high as 3,200 units have been observed. Jaundice is usually not present, but most cases have a positive cephalin flocculation and a prolonged prothrombin time. Many of the fatal cases have had hypoglycemia. Pathology reveals a large liver if death has occurred early. Fatty change is marked and generalized. There is usually some neutrophilic infiltration, without generalized necrosis. Other viscera (kidneys, heart, pancreas) may show fatty infiltration. To date the brain has been normal morphologically. The mechanism for this syndrome is totally obscure, except that it always follows a clinical infection, usually of a viral nature. However, to date all viral cultures and complement fixation tests have failed to reveal a specific etiologic agent.

Familial Metabolic Disorders Associated

with Increased Hepatic Lipid. Certain inherited metabolic disorders can be associated with a fatty liver, but this is usually merely incidental. However, since the presence of fat often raises questions of alcohol ingestion or some other causes for the production of a fatty liver, small amounts of fat (usually clinically insignificant) may occur in these diseases. These disorders include Down's syndrome, galactosemia, hereditary fructose intolerance, the early stages of Wilson's disease, Refsum's syndrome, familial hyperlipemia (Type I of Frederickson), abetalipoproteinemia and glycogen storage disease, Type I. It should be kept in mind that since these patients often have nausea and vomiting and hence decreased caloric intakes, some of the lipid accumulation may be due in part to the effects of starvation. Recently, Schiff and co-workers reported a case of cirrhosis with a very high hepatic content of cholesterol esters rather than triglycerides, and a suspicion of similar involvement in a sister and brother.[75]

FATTY LIVER AND CIRRHOSIS

The role of fat *per se* in the production of cirrhosis has been discussed extensively in the literature. Most of the evidence in favor of this hypothesis stems from experiments utilizing the choline-deficient rat as a model. Hartroft has demonstrated that choline deficiency in a person with a low protein diet leads to cirrhosis.[29] That the 2 conditions might be related was further supported by the fact that both fatty change and fibrosis began centrilobularly. However, Handler and Dubin noted that choline deficiency could produce fatty liver which could be maintained for months without the production of cirrhosis.[27] One explanation for this discrepancy is that only cells with large amounts of fat lead to cirrhosis, perhaps by causing pressure on adjacent cells.[52] On the other hand, severe choline deficiency leads to necrosis. Thus, the more severe amounts of fat would be associated with the most necrosis. Not surprisingly, this lesion could progress to cirrhosis. When another animal model is examined that produces fatty liver without necrosis (orotic acid feeding), no cirrhosis is seen, even after prolonged feeding.[78]

The clinical counterpart to choline deficiency is kwashiorkor, and cirrhosis is rare in kwashiorkor. The fatty liver is not present for many years, most patients recover spontaneously and protein deficiency may retard experimental cirrhosis.[62] However, it seems remarkable that a liver as fatty as that in kwashiorkor is not associated with an increased incidence of cirrhosis, and would support the concept that fat *per se* has nothing to do with cirrhosis. Only 2 adequate long-term follow-up studies of patients with kwashiorkor included liver histology.[12, 87] In neither of these was cirrhosis found, although the cases investigated had been treated. Nevertheless, it is possible that kwashiorkor, if untreated for prolonged periods of time, may lead to cirrhosis.[62] Many of the other clinical conditions associated with fatty liver are so regularly accompanied by necrosis that the relation of fatty liver alone to cirrhosis cannot be demonstrated. Conditions that are most often seen with necrosis (alcohol, CCl_4) most often lead to cirrhosis. On the other hand, tetracycline-induced fatty liver and fatty liver of pregnancy, although sometimes fatal, rarely lead to hepatic necrosis and when there is recovery do not appear to have resulted in cirrhosis. Thus there is no evidence that hepatic fat accumulation by itself leads to cirrhosis. It seems more likely that the accumulation of fat is merely the most obvious manifestation of the pathologic process which eventually proceeds to cirrhosis.

REFERENCES

1. Avigan, J., Eder, H. A., and Steinberg, D.: Metabolism of the protein moiety of rabbit serum lipoproteins, Proc. Soc. Exp. Biol. Med. 95:429, 1957.
2. Ballard, H., Bernstein, M., and Farrar, J. T.: Fatty liver presenting as obstructive jaundice, Am. J. Med. 30:196, 1961.
3. Barnes, E. W., Cooke, N. J., King, A. J., and Passmore, R.: Observations on the metabolism of alcohol in man, Brit. J. Nutr. 19:485, 1965.
4. Biava, C.: Mallory alcoholic hyalin: a heretofore unique lesion of hepatocellular ergastoplasm, Lab. Invest. 13:301, 1964.

5. Blass, J. P., and Dean, H. M.: The relation of hyperlipemia to hemolytic anemia in an alcoholic patient, Am. J. Med. *40:* 283, 1966.

6. Bloomfield, D. K., and Bloch, K.: The formation of $\triangle^9$-unsaturated fatty acids, J. Biol. Chem. *235:*337, 1960.

7. Bradford, W. D., and Latham, W. C.: Acute encephalopathy and fatty hepatomegaly, Am. J. Dis. Child. *114:*152, 1967.

8. Brodie, B. B., and Maikel, R. P.: Role of the sympathetic nervous system in drug-induced fatty liver, Ann. N. Y. Acad. Sci. *104:*1049, 1963.

9. Carlson, L. A., and Bally, P. R.: Inhibition of lipid mobilization, *in* Adipose Tissue, Handbook of Physiology, vol. 5, p. 557 (Am. Physiol. Soc., Washington, D.C.), Baltimore, Williams & Wilkins, 1965.

10. Carlson, L. A., Boberg, J., and Hogstedt, B.: Some physiological and clinical implications of lipid mobilization from adipose tissue, *in* Adipose Tissue, Handbook of Physiology, vol. 5, p. 625 (Am. Physiol. Soc., Washington, D.C.,) Baltimore, Williams & Wilkins, 1965.

11. Clinicopathological conference, Am. J. Med. *43:*274, 1967.

12. Cook, G. C., and Hutt, M. S. R.: The liver after kwashiorkor, Brit. Med. J. *3:*454, 1967.

13. Czernobilsky, B., and Bergnes, M. A.: Acute fatty metamorphosis of the liver in pregnancy with associated liver cell necrosis, Obstet. & Gynec. *26:*792, 1965.

14. Dowling, H. F., and Lepper, M. H.: Hepatic reactions to tetracycline, J.A.M.A. *188:*307, 1964.

15. Duncan, C. H., Best, M. M., and Despopoulos, A.: Inhibition of hepatic secretion of triglycerides by chlorophenoxyisobutyrate (CPIB) (Abstr.), Circulation *30:* Suppl. 3, 1964.

16. Dvorackova, I., Vortel, V., and Hroch, M.: Encephalitic syndrome with fatty degeneration of the viscera, Arch. Path. *81:*240, 1966.

17. Engelberg, H.: Heparin lipemia clearing reaction and fat transport in man, Am. J. Clin. Nutr. *8:*21, 1960.

18. Farber, E., Shull, K. H., Villa-Trevino, S., Lombardi, B., and Thomas, M.: Biochemical pathology of acute hepatic adenosine-triphosphate deficiency, Nature *203:*34, 1964.

19. Farber, E.: On the pathogenesis of fatty liver, Gastroenterology *50:*137, 1966.

20. Feigelson, E. B., Pfaff, W. W., Karmen, A., and Steinberg, D.: The role of plasma free fatty acids in development of fatty liver, J. Clin. Invest. *40:*2171, 1961.

21. Felts, J. M., and Mayes, P. A.: Lack of uptake and oxidation of chylomicron triglycerides to carbon dioxide and ketone bodies by the perfused rat liver, Nature *206:*195, 1965.

22. Fletcher, K.: Observations on the origin of liver fat in infantile malnutrition, Am. J. Clin. Nutr. *19:*170, 1966.

23. Goldberg, M., and Thompson, C. M.: Acute fatty metamorphosis of the liver, Ann. Int. Med. *55:*416, 1961.

24. Gould, R. G., Swyryd, E. A., Coan, B. J., and Avoy, D. R.: Effects of chlorphenoxyisobutyrate on liver composition and triglyceride synthesis, J. Atheroscl. Res. *6:* 555, 1966.

25. Green, J., Mistilis, S., and Schiff, L.: Acute alcoholic hepatitis: a clinical study of 50 cases, Arch. Int. Med. *112:*67, 1963.

26. Haemmerli, U. P.: Jaundice during pregnancy, Acta med. scand. *179:* Suppl. 444, p. 1, 1966.

27. Handler, P., and Dubin, I. N.: The significance of fatty infiltration in development of hepatic cirrhosis due to choline deficiency, J. Nutr. *31:*141, 1946.

28. Harinasuta, U., Chomet, B., Ishalk, K., and Zimmerman, H. J.: Steatonecrosis—Mallory body type, Medicine *46:*161, 1967.

29. Hartroft, W. S. Experimental reproduction of human hepatic disease, *in* Popper, H., and Schaffner, F. (eds.): Progress in Liver Disease, vol. 1, p. 68, New York, Grune & Stratton, 1961.

30. Heimberg, M., and Fizette, N. B.: The action of norepinephrine on the transport of fatty acids and triglycerides by the isolated perfused rat liver, Biochem. Pharm. *12:*392, 1963.

31. Hill, R. B., Jr.: Fatal fat embolism from steroid-induced fatty liver, New Engl. J. Med. *265:*318, 1961.

32. Hill, R. B., Jr., Droke, W. E., and Hays, A. P.: Hepatic lipid metabolism in the cortisone treated rat, Exp. & Molec. Path. *4:*320, 1965.

33. Holloway, P. W., Peluffo, R., and Wakil, S. J.: On the biosynthesis of dienoic fatty acids by animal tissues, Biochem. Biophys. Res. Commun. *12:*300, 1963.

34. Hyams, D. E., Taft, E. B., Drummey, G. D., and Isselbacher, K. J.: The prevention of fatty liver by administration of adenosine triphosphate, Lab. Invest. 16:604, 1967.

35. Isselbacher, K. J., and Greenberger, N. J.: Metabolic effects of alcohol on the liver, New Engl. J. Med. 270:351, 402, 1964.

36. Jabbour, J. T., Howard, P. H., Jr., and Jaques, W. E.: Encephalopathy and fatty degeneration of the liver and kidneys, J.A.M.A. 194:1245, 1965.

37. Jandl, J. H.: The anemia of liver disease: observations on its mechanisms, J. Clin. Invest. 34:390, 1955.

38. Jeanrenaud, B.: Effect of glucocorticoid hormones on fatty acid mobilization and reesterification in rat adipose tissue, Biochem. J. 103:627, 1967.

39. Jones, J. P., Jr., Engleman, E. P., and Najarian, J. S.: Systemic fat embolism after renal homotransplantation and treatment with corticosteroids, New Engl. J. Med. 273:1453, 1965.

40. Kalk, H.: The relationship between fatty liver and diabetes mellitus, Germ. Med. Mth. 5:81, 1960.

41. Kunelis, C. T., Peters, J. L., and Edmondson, H. A.: Fatty liver of pregnancy and its relationship to tetracycline therapy, Am. J. Med. 38:359, 1965.

42. Leevy, C. M.: Diabetes mellitus and liver dysfunction, Am. J. Med. 8:290, 1950.

43. ———: Fatty liver: a study of 270 patients with biopsy proven fatty liver and a review of the literature, Medicine 41:249, 1962.

44. Lewis, B., Hansen, J. D. L., Wittman, W., Krut, L. H., and Stuart, F.: Plasma free fatty acids in kwashiorkor and the pathogenesis of fatty liver, Am. J. Clin. Nutr. 15:161, 1964.

45. Lieber, C. S.: Metabolic derangements induced by alcohol, Ann. Rev. Med. 18:35, 1967.

46. Lieber, C. S., Jones, D. P., and DeCarli, L. M.: Effects of prolonged ethanol intake: production of fatty liver despite adequate diets, J. Clin. Invest. 44:1009, 1965.

47. Lieber, C. S., Leevy, C. M., Stein, S. W., George, W. S., Cherrick, G. R., Abelmann, W. H., and Davidson, C. S.: Effect of ethanol on plasma free fatty acids in man, J. Lab. Clin. Med. 59:826, 1962.

48. Lieber, C. S., Lefèvre, A., Spritz, N., Feinman, L., and DeCarli, L. M.: Difference in hepatic metabolism of long and medium chain fatty acids, J. Clin. Invest. 46:1451, 1967.

49. Lieber, C. S., and Schmid, R.: The effect of ethanol on fatty acid metabolism; stimulation of hepatic fatty acid synthesis in vitro, J. Clin. Invest. 40:394, 1961.

50. Lieber, C. S., and Spritz, N.: Effects of prolonged ethanol intake in man: role of dietary, adipose, and endogenously synthesized fatty acids in the pathogenesis of the alcoholic fatty liver, J. Clin. Invest. 45:1400, 1966.

51. Lombardi, B.: Considerations on the pathogenesis of fatty liver, Lab. Invest. 15:1, 1966.

52. MacDonald, R. A., Schmid, R., and Mallory, G. K.: Regeneration in fatty liver and cirrhosis, Arch. Path. 69:175, 1960.

53. Meister, H. P., and Szanto, P. B.: Occurrence of Mallory's bodies (alcoholic hyaline) in acute symptomatic and asymptomatic hepatitis (Abstr.), Gastroenterology 44:484, 1963.

54. Norwood, W. D., Fuqua, P. A., and Scudder, B.C.: Carbon tetrachloride poisoning, Arch. Industr. Hyg. 1:90, 1950.

55. Olivecrona, T., and Belfrage, P.: Mechanisms for removal of chyle triglyceride from the circulating blood as studied with [^{14}C] glycerol and [^{3}H] palmitic acid labelled chyle, Biochim. Biophys. Acta 98:81, 1965.

56. Oncley, J. C.: Plasma lipoproteins, in Page, I. H. (ed.): Chemistry of Lipides as Related to Atherosclerosis, p. 114 Springfield, Ill., Thomas, 1958.

57. Phillips, G. B., and Davidson, C. S.: Acute hepatic insufficiency of the chronic alcoholic, Arch. Int. Med. 94:585, 1954.

58. Phillips, G. B.: The lipid composition of serum in patients with liver disease, J. Clin. Invest. 39:1639, 1960.

59. Porta, E. A., Hartroft, W. S., and de la Iglesia, F. A.: Hepatic changes associated with chronic alcoholism in rats, Lab. Invest. 14:1437, 1965.

60. Quarfordt, S. H., and Goodman, DeW. S.: Metabolism of doubly-labelled chylomicron cholesteryl esters in rat, J. Lipid Res., 8:264, 1967.

61. Raben, M. S.: Regulation of fatty acid release with particular reference to pituitary factors, in Adipose Tissue, Handbook

of Physiology, vol. 5, p. 331 (Am. Physiol. Soc., Washington, D.C.), Baltimore, Williams & Wilkins, 1965.

62. Ramalingaswami, V.: Perspectives in protein malnutrition, Nature *201*:546, 1964.

63. Rebouças, G., and Isselbacher, K. J.: Studies on pathogenesis of ethanol-induced fatty liver. I. Synthesis and oxidation of fatty acids by liver, J. Clin. Invest. *40*:1355, 1961.

64. Recknagel, R. O., and Ghoshal, A. K.: Lipoperoxidation as a vector in carbon tetrachloride hepatotoxicity, Lab. Invest. *15*:132, 1966.

65. Recknagel, R. O.: Carbon tetrachloride hepatotoxicity, Pharm. Rev. *19*:145, 1967.

66. Reye, R. D. K., Morgan, G., and Baral, J.: Encephalopathy and fatty degeneration of viscera: a disease entity in childhood, Lancet *2*:749, 1963.

67. Robinson D. S., and French, J. E.: Heparin, the clearing factor lipase, and fat transport, Pharm. Rev. *12*:241, 1960.

68. Roheim, P. S., Miller, L., and Eder, H. A.: The formation of plasma lipoproteins from apoprotein in plasma, J. Biol. Chem. *240*: 2994, 1965.

69. Roheim, P. S., Switzer, S., Girard, A., and Eder, H. A.: Alterations of lipoprotein metabolism in orotic acid-induced fatty liver, Lab. Invest. *15*:21, 1966.

70. Rozental, P., Biava, C., Spender, H., and Zimmerman, H. J.: Liver morphology and function tests in obesity and during total starvation, Am. J. Dig. Dis. *12*:198, 1967.

71. Rubin, E., and Lieber, C. S.: Early fine structural changes in the human liver induced by alcohol, Gastroenterology *52*: 1, 1967.

72. Schapiro, R. H., Drummey, G. D., Shimizu, Y., and Isselbacher, K. J.: Studies on the pathogenesis of the ethanol-induced fatty liver. II. Effect of ethanol on palmitate-1-C^{14} metabolism by the isolated perfused rat liver, J. Clin. Invest. *43*:1338, 1964.

73. Schapiro, R. H., Scheig, R. L., Drummey, G. D., Mendelson, J. H., and Isselbacher, K. J.: Effect of prolonged ethanol ingestion on the transport and metabolism of lipids in man, New Engl. J. Med. *272*: 610, 1965.

74. Scheig, R., and Isselbacher, K. J.: Pathogenesis of ethanol-induced fatty liver. III.

In vivo and *in vitro* effects of ethanol on hepatic fatty acid metabolism in rat, J. Lipid Res. *6*:269, 1965.

75. Schiff, L., Schubert, W. K., McAdams, A. J., Spiegel, E. L., and O'Donnell, J. F.: Hepatic cholesterol ester storage disease, a familial disorder. I. Clinical aspects, Am. J. Med. *44*:538, 1968.

76. Schlunk, F. F., and Lombardi, B.: Liver liposomes. I. Isolation and chemical characterization, Lab. Invest. *17*:30, 1967.

77. Shapiro, B.: Lipid metabolism, Ann. Rev. Biochem. *36*:247, 1967.

78. Sidransky, H., and Verney, E.: Chronic fatty liver without cirrhosis induced in the rat by dietary orotic acid, Am. J. Path. *46*: 1007, 1965.

79. Smetana, H. G., Hadley, G. G., and Sirsat, S. M.: Infantile cirrhosis: An analytical review of the literature and a report of 50 cases, Pediatrics *28*:107, 1961.

80. Smuckler, E. A., and Benditt, E. P.: Studies on carbon tetrachloride intoxication. III. A subcellular defect in protein synthesis, Biochemistry *4*:671, 1965.

81. Smuckler, E. A., Iseri, O. A., and Benditt, E. P.: An intracellular defect in protein synthesis induced by carbon tetrachloride, J. Exp. Med. *116*:55, 1962.

82. Soffer, L. J., Iannaccone, A., and Gabrilove, J. L.: Cushing's syndrome, a study of 50 patients, Am. J. Med. *30*:129, 1961.

83. Spitzer, J. J., and McElroy, W. T., Jr.: Some hormonal effects on uptake of free fatty acids by the liver, Am. J. Physiol. *199*:876, 1960.

84. Standerfer, S. B., and Handler, P.: Fatty liver induced by orotic acid feeding, Proc. Soc. Exp. Biol. Med. *90*:270, 1955.

85. Stein, Y., and Shapiro, B.: Uptake and metabolism of triglycerides by the rat liver, J. Lipid Res. *1*:326, 1960.

86. Steinberg, D., and Vaughan, M.: Release of free fatty acids from adipose tissue *in vitro* in relation to rates of triglyceride synthesis and degradation, *in* Adipose Tissue, Handbook of Physiology, vol. 5, p. 335 (Am. Physiol. Soc., Washington, D.C.), Baltimore, Williams & Wilkins, 1965.

87. Suckling, P. V., and Campbell, J. A. H.: A five year follow-up of coloured children with kwashiorkor in Cape Town, J. Trop. Pediat. *2*:173, 1956.

88. Von Oettingen, W. F.: The Halogenated Hydrocarbons of Industrial and Toxico-

logical Importance, p. 107, Amsterdam, Elsevier, 1964.

89. Westwater, J. O., and Fainer, D.: Liver impairment in the obese, Gastroenterology 34:686, 1958.

90. Windmueller, H. G., and Levy, R. I.: Total inhibition of hepatic β-lipoprotein production in the rat by orotic acid, J. Biol. Chem. 242:2246, 1967.

91. Zieve, L.: Jaundice, hyperlipemia and hemolytic anemia: a heretofore unrecognized syndrome associated with alcoholic fatty liver and cirrhosis, Ann. Int. Med. 48:471, 1958.

18

Portal Cirrhosis (Laennec's Cirrhosis)

ARTHUR J. PATEK, JR., M.D.

Hepatic cirrhosis is characterized by chronic, diffuse inflammation of the liver, accompanied by proliferation of connective tissue, by degenerative and regenerative changes in liver cells, resulting in distortion of hepatic architecture. Many clinicians and pathologists have regarded cirrhosis of the liver as a disease entity or they have believed that differentiation of separate types was not feasible on the basis of anatomic differences. Others, notably Mallory,[149] Karsner,[115] and Rössle[211] believed such differentiation was possible. In recent years distinguishing features of certain types have become clear, and with time further delineation will become possible. Thus it seems proper to differentiate from portal cirrhosis certain types on the basis of known etiology, and anatomic and clinical characteristics. These include *postnecrotic cirrhosis, cirrhosis of hemochromatosis, of hepatolenticular degeneration,* and *primary biliary cirrhosis.*

The term "portal cirrhosis" is a repository, a name applied to several diseases that result in diffuse inflammation and fibrosis of the liver. Since the liver, like any other organ, can react to injury in a limited number of ways, there is little wonder that the final pathology from a variety of insults may appear to be similar. As shown by Himsworth and others, repeated, sublethal injury with a poison such as carbon tetrachloride may produce a finely diffuse cirrhosis of the portal type, whereas the same agent in greater dosage may produce the anatomic lesions of postnecrotic cirrhosis.[98] Therefore, anatomic classifications provide limited information. Ideal groupings should be made according to etiology. Here, too, this is not possible, since causative agents are not entirely established. Because of these limitations a mixed type of classification is retained, employing more or less conventional terms.

This and the following chapter deal with 2 of the commoner types of cirrhosis: (1) Diffuse portal cirrhosis commonly associated with alcoholism and malnutrition—*Laennec's cirrhosis.* (2) *Postnecrotic cirrhosis,* a coarsely nodular variety, seen at times as a sequel to infectious hepatitis. The clinical and pathologic differentiation of these types is by no means clearcut. Occasionally, the lesions are mixed in type and defy classification. In certain instances the liver of a patient presumed to have died of posthepatitic cirrhosis shows morphologic changes of Laennec's cirrhosis, and in other instances postnecrotic cirrhosis is discovered in a patient whose clinical course suggested alcoholic (Laennec's) cirrhosis.

It is not possible to prove whether these exceptions are real or apparent. Because of our limited knowledge it seems more helpful to emphasize the distinguishing features rather than the confusion. In the ensuing chapters the more characteristic features of the 2 types are stressed. The classification in Table 18–1, although not entirely satisfactory, serves as a framework for the material to be presented.

INCIDENCE OF LAENNEC'S CIRRHOSIS

Laennec's cirrhosis is world-wide in distribution, affecting all races and nationalities. In the Orient it is encountered particularly in China, India, Java and the Malay States.

TABLE 18–1. CLASSIFICATION

A. Portal cirrhosis
   1. Laennec's (alcoholic; nutritional; septal; atrophic; hypertrophic)
   2. Undetermined etiology
   3. Florid cirrhosis (acute fatty cirrhosis; alcoholic hepatitis)
B. Postnecrotic cirrhosis (toxic, posthepatitic; healed yellow atrophy; subacute yellow atrophy; multiple nodular hyperplasia).
C. Mixed or unclassified cirrhosis.

In South Africa, East Africa and in the Caribbean Islands a "nutritional" type of cirrhosis, similar in many respects to Laennec's cirrhosis, is widespread and constitutes one of the challenging public health problems of these areas. The relation of this type of cirrhosis to kwashiorkor is not fully established. In Western Europe and North and South America cirrhosis is associated commonly with chronic alcoholism. Descriptions of the disease vary somewhat from area to area. It appears likely that the differences are related to complicating conditions, such as malnutrition and intercurrent infections. Nutritional deficiency generally involves multiple factors which differ in separate regions of the world according to the staple foods available. The patients suffer from various deficiency diseases in addition to cirrhosis. In South Africa, for example, the livers contain a high degree of iron pigment not encountered elsewhere. In other areas amebiasis, malaria and parasitic infestations are commonplace. In these countries the patients suffer from multiple diseases; indeed, in many instances the hepatic lesions appear to be mixed or unclassifiable. That is, they present features of both portal and postnecrotic cirrhosis.

Some observers believe that the relation of malnutrition to cirrhosis, as seen in the Bantu, is not well established.[97] Indeed, they suggest that cirrhosis in this region is postnecrotic in type. This is controversial. Therefore, it may be questioned whether the term "Laennec's cirrhosis" should embrace these variants from classic descriptions of the disease. However, on the basis of clinical descriptions and pathologic findings it appears that the most prevalent cirrhosis associated with or following kwashiorkor corresponds to Laennec's cirrhosis.[50]

Since cirrhosis of the liver is not a reportable disease, the clinical incidence cannot be determined. The lack of standard nomenclature also renders figures from mortality data unreliable, as pointed out by Karsner.[115] In surveys of autopsy statistics by Rowntree,[212] De Jong,[53] Ratnoff and Patek[198] there was considerable variability within the same country.

De Jong, in a compilation of 585,963 autopsies from various parts of the world, found the incidence of cirrhosis to be less than 3 per cent in 254,525; 2 to 3 per cent in 209,037; greater than 3 per cent in 122,401. Despite the limitations of such data, it is clear that the relative incidence is high in certain areas. In China,[269] Ceylon[247] and India[241] figures vary from 4 to 7 per cent or more. In East Africa an incidence of 6.7 per cent[251] and in Chile 8.5 per cent[3] have been reported.

Rowntree found that in Europe the death rate from cirrhosis was highest in Italy and lowest in Norway.[212] Other reports suggest unusually high rates in Switzerland (3.6 to 12 per cent) when compared with those from Germany, Holland, Sweden and the U.S.S.R.[198] Rolleston and McNee have indicated that death rates from cirrhosis in England and Wales fluctuate in accordance with deaths due to alcoholism.[207] This has been emphasized by Rowntree.[212]

In the United States mortality data on cirrhosis show wide differences. For example, in 4 series of autopsies, incidences of 3 per cent,[149] 6 per cent,[23] 2.2 per cent[163] and 1.2 per cent[64] have been given. The usual range is 2 to 4 per cent of autopsies. On the West Coast, the incidence has been somewhat higher than the average, presumably due to the Asiatic population. In Boston[203] and New York[198] cirrhosis seems to have a predilection for persons of Italian and Irish stock.

In recent years the mortality from cirrhosis appears to have increased. The death rate in the United States from cirrhosis per 100,000 population was 10.8 in 1958 and

13.9 in 1967.* At ages 45 to 64 the only diseases that outrank cirrhosis of the liver as causes of death are heart disease, cancer, and cerebral hemorrhage. Death rates appear to be greater among those in a lower socioeconomic level.†

The widespread occurrence of Laennec's cirrhosis suggests that environmental factors are related to its incidence more significantly than are racial factors.

ETIOLOGY

DIETARY FACTORS

Clinical Observations. Attention was first directed to the possible role of dietary factors in countries where alcoholism is an unimportant feature in the background of the disease. In a report of 84 cases of cirrhosis of the liver in China, Yang in 1928 stated that over 70 per cent were in the laboring group subsisting on coarse carbohydrate foods.[269] In 1933 Rao observed that the diets of patients with cirrhosis of the liver in Southern India were deficient in protein, fat and vitamins, especially A, C and D.[195] In 1934 Yenikomshian reported that patients in Syria with hepatic cirrhosis lived on a diet chiefly of bread and legumes, a diet poor in protein and vitamin A.[270] In 1937 Tyagaraja noted that the diets of patients with cirrhosis in Ceylon had been deficient in nitrogenous foods and vitamins.[247] Although the above authors stressed the poor dietaries in the background of cirrhosis, other factors, such as enteric fevers, malaria and parasitic infestations were considered by them to be of primary etiologic importance. No systematic attempt to influence the course of the disease by dietary means was reported.

In the Western hemisphere more than 50 per cent of patients with Laennec's cirrhosis are chronic alcoholics. The frequent association of chronic alcoholism with deficiency diseases, such as pellagra and beriberi, has been well established by studies of Spies and DeWolf,[230] Strauss[233] and co-workers, Romano[208] and others. Likewise, in patients with "alcoholic" cirrhosis it has been observed that their dietaries have been deficient in protein and dairy foods, and that they frequently showed signs of coexisting deficiency diseases.[110, 175, 224, 258] When such patients were fed a highly nutritious diet, the clinical improvement that followed seemed to be beyond chance expectation.[175, 176]

More recently, extensive surveys of "nutritional" cirrhosis in South Africa,[26, 49] East Africa[243] and Jamaica[256] have indicated that cirrhosis of the liver is widespread in these areas. Although the type of cirrhosis does not conform strictly to Laennec's cirrhosis, there are basic similarities. Moreover, the favorable response to dietary treatment in the form of skimmed milk supplements has been dramatic.

Experimental Observations. On the basis of clinical observations[168, 175, 176] it has been postulated that dietary deficiency plays an etiologic role in Laennec's cirrhosis. This concept has been strengthened greatly by experimental work. In studies concerned with diabetes mellitus,[1] it was observed that depancreatized animals developed fatty livers which, in turn, could be prevented by the feeding of raw pancreas or lecithin.[96] In further experiments conducted by Best and Huntsman,[17, 18] by Tucker and Eckstein[244] and others the feeding of either choline or methionine prevented the excessive deposits of fat in the liver. Du Vigneaud and associates later demonstrated transmethylation in the body.[58] They showed that choline, in the presence of homocystine, can be transformed into methionine. Biologically, therefore, either choline or methionine has this "lipotropic" effect, or the ability to prevent abnormal deposits of fat in the liver.

Fatty liver has long been of interest because it is a common precursor of Laennec's cirrhosis. Chaikoff reported the occurrence of cirrhosis in dogs with chronic fatty livers resulting from pancreatectomy.[31] Intrigued by the relation of choline to fatty liver, other workers suspected that prolonged deficiency of choline brings about not only fatty liver but also cirrhosis. This proved to be so. Reports from 4 laboratories described the production of fatty liver and cirrhosis in the rat by means of diets deficient in

* National Center for Health Statistics, Monthly vital statistics report, vol. 16, No. 13, July 26, 1968.

† Statistical Bulletin, Metropolitan Life Insurance Co. 38:8, 1957 and 49:4, 1968.

choline and methionine.[21, 45, 84, 259] Since these substances are present chiefly in protein-containing foods, the experimental diets were deficient in protein as well. Dietary cirrhosis has been produced in other animals beside the rat, notably in the dog[31] and monkey.[265]

Deficiency of certain amino acids (such as lysine, tryptophan and threonine) may produce fatty changes in the livers of rats.[91, 228, 266] With amino-acid deficiency fatty deposits are periportal, whereas in choline-deficient rats the fatty deposits are chiefly about the central vein. Whether amino-acid deficiency contributes to the development of cirrhosis has not been established.

Other factors, notably the type of fat,[44] can modify the severity of dietary cirrhosis of choline deficiency. In several studies polyunsaturated fats have sharply increased the incidence and severity of cirrhosis,[86, 172, 173] whereas in other reports saturated fats seem to have exerted this effect.[272] Experimental conditions were dissimilar in these studies, so that the differences cannot be reconciled at present. However, it is evident that dietary factors besides choline affect the severity of the disease.

Although experimental dietary cirrhosis and human Laennec's cirrhosis may not be the same disease, the analogy seems close in many respects.

Role of Alcohol (Statistical Data)

The association of alcoholism and cirrhosis has long been known. Vesalius and Fernel are said to have recognized this relationship. Hart (1633), Bailie (1812) and Bright (1827) observed that the disease was seen commonly in those who imbibed spiritous liquors.[223] In general, the incidence of alcoholism in cirrhosis has been higher in clinical series of cases than in those based on postmortem findings. This might be anticipated, since the history of alcoholism usually is not elicited when it is not suspected. In several clinical series reported from Europe and the United States the incidence of alcoholism in cirrhosis has varied from 52 to 86 per cent, with a mean of about 75 per cent; in other series based on postmortem findings the figures ranged from 20

to 75 per cent with a mean incidence of about 50 per cent.[198] The type of alcoholic beverage apparently bears no relation to the severity or the frequency of the disease.

Parallel changes in the incidences of alcoholism and cirrhosis reveal further their close relationship. When the consumption of liquor was curtailed, as during Prohibition in the United States and during World War I, there was a corresponding decline in deaths from cirrhosis. Since the repeal of Prohibition deaths associated with chronic alcoholism in the United States have increased steadily. Higher death rates from cirrhosis of the liver account for most of the increase. The age-adjusted death rate for cirrhosis rose from 9.4 per 100,000 in 1951–53 to 10.9 in 1961–63, an increase of about one sixth. The upward trend is greatest in the nonwhite population, with a rise from 10.2 per 100,000 in 1951–53 to 16.6 in 1961–63, an increase of about two-thirds. Although these figures include all types of cirrhosis, the majority are associated with chronic alcoholism.[232]

The duration of alcoholism preceding the onset of hepatic failure averages about 15 years in our experience. The steady drinker is more likely to acquire the disease than the "spree" drinker, presumably because the steady drinker suffers from chronic malnutrition.

Although alcoholism is a frequent precursor to cirrhosis, the incidence of cirrhosis among alcoholics is relatively low. It has been estimated variously that from 1 to 30 per cent of chronic alcoholics develop cirrhosis.[198] Since alcoholism generally is not reported unless the patient is institutionalized, accurate data are not obtainable. On the basis of autopsy findings, Joliffe and Jellinek estimated that about 8 per cent of chronic alcoholics develop cirrhosis.[109] The incidence is not impressive, and one might infer that alcoholism alone does not produce cirrhosis.

Experimental Evidence. In 1934 Virgil Moon reviewed studies on experimental cirrhosis up to that time. He wrote:

The belief that cirrhosis is caused by alcohol has not received experimental support. Without exception the agents which have produced cirrhosis experimentally were capable of causing hepatic necrosis. Alcohol, even in large amounts and long continued, has caused only parenchymatous degeneration and fatty changes. These have not resulted in necrosis nor in permanent hepatic changes. However, the probability that alcohol acts as a contributing or predisposing factor has received experimental support. Alcohol has been found to accentuate the injurious effects of bacteria, phosphorus, chloroform, and of carbon tetrachloride, upon the livers of animals. It is probable that alcohol may similarly accentuate the effects of injurious agents upon the human liver. By virtue of this property alcohol may be an important contributing factor in the development of human cirrhosis.[153]

In the intervening years many studies have been made of the toxicology of alcohol, revealing widespread interference with several metabolic functions.[102, 136, 261, 262] Metabolism of alcohol is accompanied by reduction of DPN (diphosphopyridine nucleotide) to DPNH in the cytoplasm of the hepatic cell, and this may have far-reaching effects. Of particular interest has been the relation of alcohol toxicity to the development of fatty liver, since the latter regularly precedes the development of alcoholic cirrhosis. Lowry and co-workers reported that in the production of nutritional cirrhosis in the rat on a low casein diet the substitution of 20 per cent alcohol for water intensified the disease.[142] Best and co-workers indicated that this effect might be due to the substitution of added calories, since with isocaloric diets the addition of sucrose had the same effect as alcohol in comparable experiments.[16] Klatskin later presented evidence suggesting that alcohol interferes with the availability of choline, aside from a caloric effect.[123] Other experiments indicate that with larger amounts of alcohol, fatty livers can be produced despite "adequate" intake of protein and choline,[137] although these dietary factors provide partial protection. There appear to be several pathways by which alcoholic fatty liver develops (see Chapter 17, Fatty Liver).

Although fatty liver is a regular precursor to dietary cirrhosis, it is perhaps an associated phenomenon and not causally related. In studies with rats on choline-deficient diets, hepatic triglycerides may increase for months without leading to cirrhosis; the development of dietary cirrhosis bears little or no correlation with the concentration of hepatic triglycerides.[172, 173]

The above observations concern fatty liver produced by choline-deficient diets, and the analogy does not necessarily apply to fatty liver from alcohol. However if the fatty liver from alcohol toxicity should lead to cirrhosis it is doubtful that it will be on the basis of increased content of triglycerides in the liver. In recent studies employing electron microscopy, several investigators have observed changes in endoplasmic reticulum followed by swelling and deformity of mitochondria in rats with alcoholic fatty livers.[101, 120, 190] Chronic injury to these structures might lead to necrosis of liver cells and subsequent cirrhosis.

Clinical Evidence. Zieve and Hill, in a study of 744 well-nourished male army veterans, reported that there were no significant differences in hepatic function between heavy imbibers and occasional imbibers or abstainers.[274] Only a few reports have been made on the effect of administering alcohol to patients with cirrhosis. Patek and Post fed alcohol to 4 hospitalized patients recovering from liver failure.[175] Nine ounces of 40 per cent alcohol (equivalent to 108 cc. absolute alcohol) were fed daily for 6, 6, 14 and 18 months respectively in addition to a nutritious, high-protein diet. Clinical improvement continued. There was no return of ascites or jaundice. Similar experiences have been reported by others in short-term observations.[30, 234, 252]

In more recent studies larger doses of alcohol have been employed. In one study 21 patients with decompensated Laennec's cirrhosis were given 12 ounces of 55 per cent alcohol daily (equivalent to 198 cc. absolute alcohol) for 2 months.[63] When administered with a diet containing 2,400 calories and 100 to 120 Gm. protein, improvement was progressive. However deleterious effects were observed in 4 out of 6 patients placed on diets containing 25 to 30 Gm. protein. In 4 instances the diets were also low in calories (1,480 cal.).

In another study 13 patients with decompensated cirrhosis were given comparable doses of alcohol (3 ml. 95% alcohol/kg. body wt.) together with a high caloric diet containing 55 to 75 Gm. protein.[202] The patients made steady clinical improvement. There were changes in serum bilirubin, serum albumin, and SGOT toward normal values in 2 or 3 months. A second group of 10 patients receiving considerably larger amounts of alcohol made similar improvement. Biopsies performed at the end of alcohol administration did not show signs of increasing fat in the liver.[202]

In general these studies indicate that patients with advanced cirrhosis tolerate substantial amounts of alcohol while receiving a nutritious diet, rest and supportive care in the hospital. With low protein, low caloric diets, alcohol was not so well tolerated. Nevertheless the degree of tolerance in these patients is surprising.

Alcoholism predisposes to Laennec's cirrhosis and is hepatotoxic. However, in the pathogenesis of the disease it is not established whether alcohol acts chiefly by interfering with normal metabolic processes or by furthering nutritional deficiency. On the basis of evidence cited it seems likely that both factors are involved.

Relation to Infectious Hepatitis

Whether or not acute infectious hepatitis leads to Laennec's cirrhosis is an unresolved problem. In several large series of cases, infectious hepatitis was not listed among etiologic factors of Laennec's (or portal) cirrhosis.[23, 32, 64, 122, 255] Presumably, it was not considered or was inconspicuous. In other series, where the possibility was investigated, the incidence of antecedent hepatitis has shown considerable range, with values from 1.4 to 13 per cent. [20, 62, 65, 176, 195, 198, 209]

Two large series are of especial interest because of the relatively high incidence of antecedent hepatitis and because they included control groups of patients.[3, 100] In a study of 100 cases of Laennec's cirrhosis Howard and Watson[100] encountered 17 with a story of previous hepatitis, in contrast with a control hospital group of only 3. This is a significant difference. Armas-Cruz and associates[3] reported an incidence of 25.7 per cent in a series of 208 cases, as compared with 18.3 per cent of corresponding controls. In this series the differences between the 2 groups was not considered

to be significant. The basis for these variations is not evident unless it is related to regional factors. Howard and Watson pointed out that the ratio of females to males was greater, and the incidence of alcoholism lower in their cases than in other reported series, suggesting a somewhat different type of case material.

Analysis of the sequelae of infectious hepatitis also provides diverse results and interpretations. In several large series concerned with chronic or relapsing infectious hepatitis no mention has been made of the development of Laennec's cirrhosis. For example, no instances were cited in 431 cases reported by Barker, Capps and Allen[8]; in 350 cases reported by Kunkel and associates[132]; or in 217 cases reported by Klatskin and Rappaport,[125] nor in 1,293 cases reported by Cullinan, King and Rivers.[43] Likewise, in a selected group of 112 cases, Post and associates[192] described 4 instances of postnecrotic cirrhosis but none of the Laennec type. In a series of 140 cases of hepatitis Fernando and Thanabalasunderam cited several instances of massive necrosis and of postnecrotic cirrhosis (toxic cirrhosis) but none of the Laennec type.[68]

However, there are several reports of cases studied postmortem[19, 54, 112, 257] and numerous reports[4, 55, 129, 130, 209, 227], of cases studied by means of serial biopsies in which the development of portal or Laennec's cirrhosis has been cited. Although the accurate definition of cirrhosis from needle biopsy is often impossible, there is no basis for questioning postmortem findings unless the classification of cirrhosis varies with different observers.

This appears to be the present difficulty, for what one observer might designate Laennec's, another would designate postnecrotic cirrhosis.[76, 200] Baggenstoss and Stauffer throw further light on this subject.[5] They compared 43 autopsied cases of "alcoholic" cirrhosis with 43 cases of "posthepatitic" cirrhosis. The latter comprised patients whose histories strongly suggested infectious hepatitis as the causative agent. Although most of the latter conformed to the description of postnecrotic cirrhosis, in 7 instances the morphology resembled the finely diffuse changes of Laennec's cirrhosis.

This seems reasonable. Experimentally[29, 153] all gradations from massive necrosis and atrophy to a finely diffuse cirrhosis can be produced by hepatotoxins, depending upon the dosage, the agent employed and the chronicity of the injury. If a chronic infectious hepatitis exists, it should produce on occasion a finely diffuse cirrhosis.

Therefore, it appears that a diffuse, portal type of cirrhosis may follow an episode of infectious hepatitis although it is rare. The morphologic features of this cirrhosis at autopsy may be indistinguishable from Laennec's cirrhosis.

Syphilis as a Predisposing Factor

The incidence of syphilis in patients with cirrhosis of the liver appears to be relatively high. In several series it has been reported to occur in 8 to 28 per cent of cases, the figures being based upon serologic or clinical data, or both. The mean value in 10 series comprising 1,429 cases was 14.6 per cent.[23, 64, 65, 70, 176, 198, 221, 222, 225, 270] Because of this frequency it has been suggested that either the spirochete or antisyphilitic therapy may be etiologic factors. The evidence indicates that the only characteristic hepatic lesion of syphilis[87] is that of hepar lobatum, in which deep lobulations result from gummata. There is no doubt that arsphenamine and its derivatives are hepatotoxic, but the incidence of cirrhosis would appear to bear little relation to the extent of arsphenamine therapy. More likely, patients who develop cirrhosis after arsenotherapy have had homologous serum hepatitis, as pointed out by Dible.[55] Certain of these might develop portal cirrhosis, although they would fall more characteristically into the group with postnecrotic cirrhosis.

The concurrence of syphilis and Laennec's cirrhosis raises two further questions, namely, the incidence of cirrhosis in persons with syphilis, and the incidence of syphilis in chronic alcoholics without cirrhosis. Information on the first is not at hand. However, the incidence of syphilis in alcoholics is high,[164] and the association of alcoholism and syphilis in Laennec's cirrhosis is no more frequent than might be expected by chance.[65, 198]

Diabetes Mellitus

It is not known whether diabetes mellitus and Laennec's cirrhosis are significantly related. In several autopsy series of cirrhosis the incidence of diabetes mellitus was low.[198] In at least 2 studies it was concluded that the two diseases were not related significantly.[73, 199] Others, however, disagree. Jaques found that in 177 patients dying of diabetes mellitus, 16.3 per cent had portal cirrhosis as compared to 8.4 per cent of controls.[105] Part of the difficulty of interpretation is due to the definition of diabetes mellitus itself.[12] An abnormal glucose tolerance curve, sometimes encountered in patients with cirrhosis, does not necessarily represent diabetes mellitus. The peak incidence of diabetes mellitus occurs between 45 and 64 years,[61] which corresponds to that of Laennec's cirrhosis.

It is my impression that there is a true increase in the incidence of diabetes mellitus in the presence of cirrhosis. Whether or not this represents a special type of diabetes mellitus has not yet been established.

Other Antecedent Factors

Chemicals such as *carbon tetrachloride, phosphorus* and *chlorinated naphthalenes* are common causes of toxic hepatitis in industry. In certain instances, this appears to have progressed to portal cirrhosis. Workers whose diets have been poor, and especially those who drink alcohol to excess, are prone to poisoning by these agents. However, these "chemical" cirrhoses doubtless comprise a small percentage of the total number of portal cirrhoses.

The incidence of Laennec's cirrhosis is increased in the presence of certain diseases, such as *thyrotoxicosis, malaria* and *bacillary dysentery*. The relation of these diseases to Laennec's cirrhosis appears to be indirect. These same diseases often are complicated by malnutrition, which in turn would enhance hepatic injury.

Constitutional Factors

There is a greater tendency for the male rat to develop hepatic cirrhosis than the female rat, when fed a diet deficient in protein and choline. The basis for this sex difference is unknown. It is stated that the young growing rat develops the disease more readily than the adult. However, there is no difficulty in producing the disease in the adult. There are differences in susceptibility to cirrhosis in various rat strains and in different colonies of the same strain.[171] There are also individual differences. For example, about 75 per cent of young male rats of the Sprague, Dawley strain placed on a standard cirrhosis-producing diet, develop the disease within 5 months, whereas the remainder are relatively resistant. By means of inbreeding experiments,[170] resistance to the disease can be transmitted to successive generations.

It is possible that analogies exist in human Laennec's cirrhosis. There have been reports of familial cirrhosis in which environmental factors did not appear to play a determining role.[144] It has been observed that certain subjects seem to acquire the disease more readily than others, even though their alcohol intake has not been extreme or their food intake unusually poor.[124] Likewise, there is a predisposition of the male over the female to develop the disease. Since this sex ratio parallels the frequency of alcoholism, it does not provide a strong argument.

Doubtless, constitutional factors modify the susceptibility to Laennec's cirrhosis; however, the existence of such factors has yet to be demonstrated.

PATHOGENESIS

All cirrhoses are characterized by destruction of hepatic cells, scar formation and regeneration of parenchyma.[196] In Laennec's cirrhosis cell death appears to be due to either lack of essential substances or a noxious agent (alcohol), or both. It is not established whether the primary lesion involves fatty changes. In experimental dietary cirrhosis, as mentioned, these changes appear to be of secondary importance. This does not exclude the possibility that fatty changes are basic to Laennec's cirrhosis in man. It seems plausible that cells that degenerate and break under stress of fatty infiltration are already injured. Studies based on electron microscopy, histo- and cytochemistry have revealed extensive

changes in the structure of liver cells that have not been evident with light microscopy.[186]

Early signs of hepatocellular injury are widening of pericellular spaces, probably due to change in permeability of the membrane. The microvilli forming the walls of the bile canaliculi may become blunted and the canaliculi dilated or ruptured. Mitochondria are swollen. Endoplasmic reticulum and lysosomes show degenerative changes. The data concerning these complex changes and their relation to cellular function are insufficient to interpret.

Scar formation appears to have two components, namely remnants of reticulum framework from dead parenchymal cells and newly formed connective tissue. Fiber formation usually is associated with mesenchymal irritation or inflammation, presumably from injured liver cells. The stimulus to fibroblastic activity is unknown.

Regenerative changes are seen soon after liver cells are injured. The cells exhibit increased mitoses and become swollen with granular, eosinophilic cytoplasm. While hormones, dietary factors and blood supply affect the rate of cell growth, none of these is a primary stimulus. There is evidence that humoral factors regulate liver regeneration, but they have not been identified.[229]

PATHOLOGY

The liver is diffusely nodular or granular, leathery in texture and of reddish-yellow color, occasionally mottled with green. The size of the organ is variable, with weights ranging from 900 to 3,000 Gm. As a rule, the liver is moderately reduced in volume and weight.[115, 122, 198] Increased size of the liver usually is due to the presence of fat.[39, 64] From clinical observations there appears to be a tendency toward shrinking with progressive hepatic failure. The discoloration depends upon the degree of jaundice, fat, fibrosis and congestion.

The diameter of the nodules varies from less than 1 mm. to more than 1 cm. (Fig. 18–1 A, B). At times larger nodules and broad scars are seen which resemble the gross appearance of postnecrotic cirrhosis.[5, 115] Indeed, in certain instances classifi-

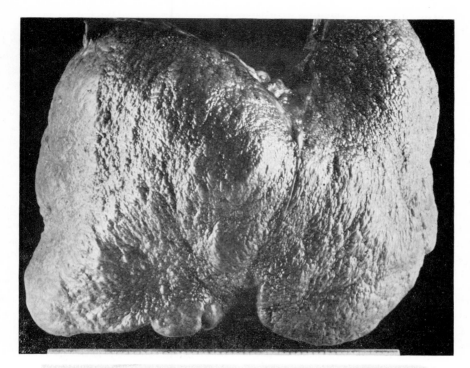

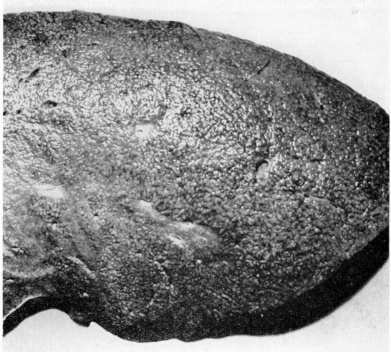

FIG. 18-1. Laennec's cirrhosis. (A, *top*) The liver is large, pale and uniformly finely nodular. (B, *bottom*) Sectioned surface of the cirrhotic liver, demonstrating the comparatively fine nodularity and regularly disposed delicate fibrous tissue.

cation is impossible. Such instances Mallory was inclined to designate as "unclassified" cirrhosis.[149] In general, however, the nodules are diffuse and fine, as revealed especially on the cut surface.

The chief microscopic feature is widespread overgrowth of connective tissue which destroys the normal lobular structure (Fig. 18–2). Early fibroblastic changes are most conspicuous in the peripheral zones in the region of the portal triads.[115] From the portal areas bands of connective tissue extend toward other portal areas. They may invade the cords of liver cells as well. This is somewhat at variance with the findings in experimental nutritional cirrhosis in the rat, in which early changes are seen in the region of the central veins from which the connective tissue projects toward the portal areas. The differences may be more apparent than real, since the developmental stages in human disease are more difficult to establish. The cellular infiltration in the portal triads is predominantly lymphocytic or histiocytic, although polymorphonuclear cells may be present as well. Some observers have described preponderance of the latter cells. Possibly the differences relate to the stage of the cirrhotic process, since death frequently is due to causes other than

hepatic failure. In the region of the triads proliferating bile ducts also may be seen.

Parenchymal liver cells show degenerative changes, in particular fatty vacuolization, hyalin deposits and scattered small foci of necrosis. In other areas there are signs of cellular regeneration. Fatty vacuolization may be extreme in early stages of the disease, whereas in later stages the fat is inconspicuous.

Serial biopsies of the liver have shown that fatty changes may regress within a few weeks in patients fed a nutritious, protein-rich diet.[134, 191, 202, 252] Mallory[149] described hyalin droplets in the liver cells, peculiar degenerative changes that are common to "alcoholic" cirrhosis. These droplets may coalesce into larger masses within the cells.

On the basis of histochemical studies this material appears to be a denatured protein or an insoluble basic protein complex within otherwise viable cells.[162] On the basis of electron microscopy Hartroft considers the Mallory body to be giant mitochondria.[93] Although such changes are encountered far more frequently in Laennec's cirrhosis than in other types they are not pathognomonic of the disease.[152] In scattered areas the cells appear to have lost their nuclei. In others, large cells with deeply stained nuclei—at

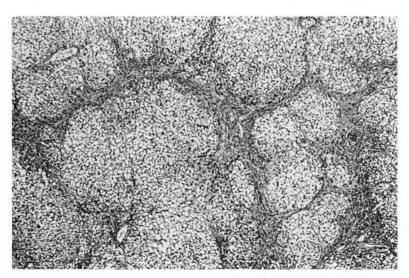

Fig. 18–2. Laennec's cirrhosis. Microphotograph reveals fine fibrosis, micronodulation and pseudolobule formation. Intracellular fat vacuolization is prominent.

times multinucleated—are seen. They may be several times the normal size. Such cells are considered as regenerating cells.

A striking feature is the displacement of vascular channels. Small branches of the portal vein are seen in the connective tissue septa, where they appear to be compressed by the regenerating nodules.[117] The hepatic veins may be unidentifiable or may be displaced eccentrically in the lobule. The extreme degree of change in vascular pattern has been demonstrated by means of injection studies by McIndoe[147] and others.[253] The finer arborizations of the portal tree are lost, and only the stenosed main trunks remain. Whereas the portal venous system transports the major portion of inflow blood of the normal liver (approximately 80 per cent under standard conditions), there is evidence that the hepatic artery assumes a larger burden in the presence of cirrhosis.

Anastomoses between the two inflow systems have been demonstrated in the presence of cirrhosis.[146] It is possible that this admixture increases further the elevated portal venous pressure produced by bands of connective tissue. Engorged tributary veins draining the mesentery, spleen and stomach are commonly seen, as well as many collateral veins over the abdominal wall and along the inner surface of the peritoneum. The most serious consequence of increased portal venous pressure is rupture of veins in the lower esophagus and cardiac end of the stomach, accounting for about 30 per cent of fatal cases.[198]

Splenomegaly occurs in 70 to 85 per cent of cases. The true size and weight of the spleen is doubtless greater than the recorded weight in many instances because of shrinkage from loss of blood at the time of autopsy. Histologic changes vary from simple hyperemia to extensive fibrosis. In the later stages the pulp spaces contain little blood, the trabeculae become larger, the malpighian bodies become smaller, and fibrosis may appear around the central vessels. The term "congestive splenomegaly" implies that the enlargement is due to congestion or stasis, but it seems more likely that it is related to the duration and the intensity of portal vein hypertension.

McMichael and others have pointed out the frequent occurrence of sclerosis of the portal vein and its branches and have suggested that this is related to increased venous pressure. The studies of Thompson,[239] Rousselot and Whipple clearly established that splenomegaly is associated with increased portal venous pressure. No essential differences were detected between the splenomegaly of cirrhosis and that of extrahepatic block in the portal venous system. On this account they concluded that splenomegaly is mechanical in origin.

Others have suggested that toxic or infectious agents play a contributory role in splenomegaly of cirrhosis.[28, 148, 201] Although this possibility cannot be excluded, evidence suggests that increased pressure in the portal vein is primarily responsible. The subject has been reviewed critically by Moschcowitz.[156]

Secondary changes, such as jaundice, ascites and peripheral edema are generally present in fatal cases.

Signs of malnutrition and specific deficiency states are frequent.[176] These include pellagrous changes in the skin, atrophy of the tongue papillae, polyneuritis and degenerative changes in the brain stem.

Signs of hormonal derangement are found, especially in the male.[140] These include atrophy of the testes, gynecomastia and decrease in body hair.

Chronic pancreatitis is seen in about 15 per cent of cases. This lesion is also seen in chronic alcoholism without cirrhosis, and its relation to cirrhosis may be incidental.

Peptic ulcer is seen in 1.8 to 20 per cent of cases and at times causes severe hemorrhage. It is not clear whether this complication is more frequent than the expected incidence of peptic ulcer of a control population.[219] (See Complications.)

Infections are contributory causes of death in about 25 per cent of cases. The most commonly encountered are bronchopneumonia, peritonitis, phlebitis, phlegmonous enteritis, glomerulonephritis and endocarditis. Although tuberculous peritonitis and miliary tuberculosis were formerly frequent complications, these have been encountered rarely in recent years. (See Complications.)

Since patients who enter the hospital in

hepatic failure have a mean age of 50 years, they are prone to certain other diseases that may or may not be related to cirrhosis.[105, 185, 198] The conditions most frequently encountered besides those mentioned above are diabetes mellitus, cholecystitis, heart failure and neoplasm.

LATENT CIRRHOSIS

Cirrhosis of the liver may be asymptomatic. Of 167 cases examined postmortem, Rolleston and McNee found 87 that had been latent during life.[207] McCartney[145] reported that 35 per cent of 245 autopsied cases of portal cirrhosis had been latent during life. In reviewing the charts of 865 patients with the diagnosis of cirrhosis of the liver, Ratnoff and Patek found 386 with adequate clinical signs of the disease and 49 in which the diagnosis was discovered postmortem or at operation.[198] The remaining 430 cases were excluded because of insufficient data.

The average age at death is approximately the same for latent and active cases. The disease is no more advanced in older than in younger patients with latent cirrhosis. From this it has been inferred that the disease can be arrested.[145] Clinical and experimental observations in recent years support this interpretation.

Patients who recover from hepatic failure and lead an exemplary life (i.e., abstain from alcohol and follow a nutritious diet) appear to have a normal life expectancy, even though their livers show considerable damage. However, they seem to be more delicate, more vulnerable to intercurrent illnesses than the average healthy adult. Experience with this group is too limited to permit more than a clinical impression.

CLINICAL FINDINGS

Symptoms

The onset of Laennec's cirrhosis is usually gradual. The early symptoms may be so vague that one cannot ascertain the time of onset. The patient often states that he has had indigestion for years, that he lacked stamina or felt old before his time but was

TABLE 18–2. INITIAL SYMPTOMS AND SIGNS IN 386 CASES OF LAENNEC'S CIRRHOSIS

SYMPTOMS	NUMBER OF CASES	PER CENT OF CASES
Swollen abdomen	107	27.7
Abdominal pain	48	12.4
Hematemesis	39	10.1
Edema of legs	36	9.6
Jaundice	34	8.8
Nausea and vomiting	29	7.5
Weakness	22	5.7
Abdominal distress	17	4.4
Bleeding, epistaxis	15	3.8
Diarrhea	14	3.6
Anorexia	9	2.3

In 46 cases, multiple symptoms were listed at onset.

unaware of actual illness until abdominal swelling, jaundice or hemorrhage supervened.

The initial symptoms and signs of liver failure, as determined from a large group of patients,[198] are listed in Table 18–2.

With the frank development of the disease, symptoms are more pronounced. Table 18–3 includes data from several series of cases. Although differences exist, possibly related to regional factors, the salient features are present with similar frequency in the several series listed.

Anorexia is an early and telltale symptom, often not recognized by the patient so much as by his family. Meals are scanty and haphazard. This history, to be sure, is common to alcoholics without cirrhosis, but the persistent, chronic malnutrition of the steady drinker is particularly typical of the cirrhotic.

Weight loss occurs in about half the patients. Others show surprisingly little change, and it seems evident that alcohol must provide a large share of their caloric intake. Indeed, beer drinkers with cirrhosis are often obese, and this tends to obscure an underlying state of malnutrition.

Nausea, vomiting, gagging, flatulence are frequent symptoms. These have been attributed, in part, to associated alcoholic gastritis.

Gaseous distention of the abdomen may distress patients for months or years preceding the onset of ascites.

TABLE 18–3. SYMPTOMS IN LAENNEC'S CIRRHOSIS (PER CENT INCIDENCE)

	RATNOFF AND PATEK[198]	PATEK ET AL.[176]	DOUGLASS AND SNELL[57]	ARMAS-CRUZ ET AL.[3]	GARCEAU ET AL.[76]
No. of cases	386	124	444	208	471
Average age	50	49		45	53
Males	69	65	77	70	73
Alcoholism	54	77	64	78	89
Weight loss	53	89	22	49	—
Anorexia	35	78	9	86	—
Nausea and vomiting	30	51	4	72	—
Abdominal pain	31	50	23	60	—
Epistaxis	18	40		19	—
Hematemesis	27	34	16	31	41
Weakness	21	—	21	94	—
Diarrhea	20	—		30	—
Nocturia	26	—		—	—

Abdominal pain is of varying degree. It has no peculiar characteristic. It may be mild, dull, sharp, wavelike or steady. It is more apt to occur shortly after meals. It may be confined to the region of the liver or referred to the epigastrium or the lower abdomen. Fairly often it is associated with tenderness of the liver and occasionally with friction rubs over the liver or the spleen. This symptom has been attributed to capsular swelling, perihepatitis, spasm of the biliary ducts or intermittent vascular spasm. It is likely that no single mechanism can account for its variegated pattern. In general, abdominal pain is experienced during active liver failure and abates with improvement. Severe, boring, constant pain radiating to the posterior thorax suggests penetrating peptic ulcer, pancreatitis or superimposed carcinoma of the liver.[264]

Hematemesis. This dreaded symptom is estimated to occur in 8 to 40 per cent of patients with cirrhosis and is one of the chief causes of death. Wang[255] reported an incidence of 8 per cent and Eppinger, 9 per cent.[62] In more recent experience hematemesis has occurred in 24 to 41 per cent of the cases.[3, 76, 176]

Hemorrhage usually arises from rupture of one or more esophageal varices and occasionally from veins in the cardiac portion of the stomach. Prevailing opinion favors use of prompt endoscopy and roentgenography after hematemesis in order to establish the site of the bleeding and to institute appropriate medical or surgical measures.[10, 165] In roentgenographic studies the veins are seen to be greatly enlarged and tortuous, whereas at autopsy they are collapsed and at times so inconspicuous that the site of bleeding cannot be detected.

Occasionally, peptic ulcer or gastritis is the basis for hematemesis. In a series of 76 patients with Laennec's cirrhosis and bleeding from the upper gastrointestinal tract, esophageal varices accounted for 62 per cent, peptic ulcer for 18 per cent and gastric erosions for 5 per cent.[66] In another series of 92 patients varices accounted for 38 per cent, gastritis for 31 per cent and peptic ulcer for 13 per cent.[46] Also, massive blood loss from esophageal or gastric varices can occur without hematemesis, by means of slow leakage into the gastrointestinal tract. Frequently, the patient has a foreboding of the event. He feels weak and anxious and complains of epigastric fullness and nausea. These symptoms may precede vomiting by several hours. However, hematemesis also occurs without warning. With massive bleeding, fever and azotemia are usually seen. It is believed that fever is due to the retention of blood in the intestinal tract. Azotemia is ascribed partly to the retention of blood and also to impaired renal excretion due to shock.[107, 218]

PHYSICAL SIGNS

The chief signs of Laennec's cirrhosis are listed in Table 18–4. These data, derived

Portal Cirrhosis (Laennec's Cirrhosis)

TABLE 18–4. PHYSICAL SIGNS IN LAENNEC'S CIRRHOSIS (PER CENT INCIDENCE)

	RATNOFF AND PATEK[198]	PATEK ET AL.[176]	DOUGLASS AND SNELL[57]	ARMAS-CRUZ ET AL.[3]	GARCEAU ET AL.[76]
No. of cases	386	124	444	208	471
Ascites	78	93	48	74	82
Palpable liver	75	79	71	71	—
Peripheral edema	61	60	35	41	—
Jaundice	65	67	34	70	84
Vascular spiders	15	62	26	45 (?)	66
Collateral veins	24	61	19	63	—
Palpable spleen	44	55	32	31	48
Fever	24	49		30	—
Esophageal varices	—	48		22	52
Glossitis	—	48		—	—
Mental change	—	38		16	64
Polyneuritis	13	36		—	—
Herniae	9	33		8	—
Clubbed fingers	5	18		—	—
Hydrothorax	6	17		9	—

from several series of cases, apply for the most part to hospitalized patients in failure and reflect an advanced stage of the disease. There is fair agreement in these studies with respect to classic features: ascites, jaundice, edema, hepatomegaly, splenomegaly. Less conspicuous signs show wider differences which probably relate to the special interests of the observers. The series cited are only a few of the many reported clinical studies. In addition to those listed, data have been derived from reports by Henrikson[94]; Wang[255]; Chapman, Snell and Rowntree[32]; Eppinger[62]; and several texts, such as Rolleston and McNee[207]; Tumen and Bockus[245], and others.[226, 276]

Studies limited to autopsied cases are not included in the table, since they deal only with fatal cases.

Fever is commonplace. The mechanism is not known. It usually is intermittent with afternoon rises to 100° or 101° F. The white blood cell count is normal or slightly increased. Fever is seen especially when signs of liver failure are present, such as jaundice and ascites. In a series of 124 cases there were 61 patients (49 per cent) with fever. With improvement, fever abated. Subsidence of fever is one of the early, favorable signs of improvement (cf. Fig. 18–6).

In occasional instances of Laennec's cirrhosis, fever is a conspicuous feature. This type of response also may be seen in active phases of the disease, so-called alcoholic hepatitis or *florid cirrhosis*. Jaundice and leukocytosis may be conspicuous in this group (cf. p. 716).

Persistent fever should alert one to the possibility of intercurrent infections, in particular tuberculous pleurisy or peritonitis, which may be present without other features of tuberculosis.[27] In our experience and that of others[242] blood cultures are not positive unless obvious infection is present. However in one report on 155 patients with febrile alcoholic cirrhosis, bacteremia was present in 34 cases.[248] In 17 instances *Escherichia coli* was recovered. This finding merits further study. (see Complications.)

Ascites is probably the most characteristic sign of the disease. Erasistratus is said to have associated ascites with hepatic disease. Morgagni[198] described a patient with ascites, which he attributed in part to impeded blood flow through the vena portae and to the scirrhous state of the liver.[198] In several large series of autopsied cases the incidence of ascites varied from 57 to 85 per cent[53, 76, 128, 207] (see Chap. 11 on ascites).

Edema. The mean incidence of edema, as determined from 11 series of cases, was 61 per cent, with values ranging from 35[57] to 87 per cent.[195, 255] The highest values were reported from the Orient, and they may be due in part to coexisting beriberi. In others, congestive heart failure may be present, but this appears to be an unimportant factor in the large majority of cases.

Edema may appear as an early sign, and it may precede the formation of ascites.[32, 198] Fagin and Thompson recorded edema as the earliest symptom in 13 of 71 patients.[65] Wang stated that about one third of his patients developed edema before ascites; one third, coincident with ascites; and one third, after the appearance of ascites.[255] Almost always it is accompanied by hypoalbuminemia, which in turn has been considered a primary cause for edema. The rapid disappearance of peripheral edema (in contrast with ascites) after the intravenous administration of concentrated human albumin solution lends support to this concept.[240]

In many patients peripheral edema fluctuates with the amount of ascites present. After abdominal paracentesis, for example, edema may decrease sharply. It seems likely that both decreased colloid osmotic pressure from hypoalbuminemia and increased intra-abdominal pressure from ascites play a part in the formation of edema.

Hydrothorax occurs in a significant number of patients with Laennec's cirrhosis, and in almost every recorded instance is associated with ascites. The incidence is generally 10 to 15 per cent. In most instances hydrothorax is discovered by x-ray and causes no respiratory difficulty. Rarely thoracenteses are needed to relieve pressure. The fluid generally has the characteristics of a transudate but frequently shows increased red blood cells microscopically.[81, 249] A few instances of grossly bloody pleural fluid have been reported.[34]

The mechanism is similar to that of Meigs' syndrome, in which hydrothorax is secondary to ovarian tumor. Meigs demonstrated by means of carbon particles that fluid traversed the diaphragm via the lymphatics.[151] With similar technics Johnston and Loo showed that in cirrhosis with ascites fluid passed from the abdominal cavity into the pleural space via lymphatics in the diaphragm.[108]

Jaundice. Clinical jaundice appears in about half the patients at some time in the course of the disease. In 12 series of cases the mean incidence was 52 per cent, with a range of 34 to 67 per cent. The incidence of jaundice would be higher if subclinical icterus were included in the data. Jaundice, in patients with cirrhosis of the liver, indicates activity of the disease. Frequently, it is the presenting sign of hepatic failure. In 208 cases cited by Armas-Cruz et al.[3] jaundice was the initial symptom in 116 cases— a figure somewhat higher than in most studies.[3]

In the large majority of patients jaundice is moderate or mild. Frequently, it is detected only by laboratory test. Jaundice clears with other signs of improvement and tends to increase with other signs of failure. However, it is not an essential companion to hepatic failure. For example, in 217 fatal cases Evans and Gray found only 64 (29.5 per cent) icteric.[64] In the studies recorded by Armas-Cruz et al. 30 per cent had normal values for serum bilirubin at death.

The clinical significance of jaundice in patients with cirrhosis is not popularly understood. The gravity of this sign is shown by an analysis of the duration of life after the onset of jaundice in 245 patients[198] (Fig. 18–3). Of these, 44 per cent lived 6 months after the onset of jaundice; 26 per cent, 1 year; and 23 per cent, 2 years.

The mechanism of jaundice in Laennec's cirrhosis is not established. However, when one considers the vast structural changes, it is to be wondered that jaundice is no more frequent or intense. The chief causes appear to be functional derangement of the liver cells and compression of bile ducts by connective tissue overgrowth. The ability of parenchymal cells to conjugate and transport bilirubin appears to be reduced.[2] This is indicated by impaired bilirubin tolerance tests. In addition, there may be an increased work load created by hemolysis of red cells. Also, it has been suggested that superimposed hepatitis or necrosis may account for the intense jaundice that sometimes appears terminally, but there is little evidence to support this point of view.[175, 198] Studies of autopsied cases show little or no correlation between the presence of jaundice and necrosis.

Hepatomegaly. The liver is palpable in about 75 per cent of the patients. In addition to the size of the liver, palpability depends upon increased hardness and possibly some degree of downward displacement of the organ, as well as thinness and relaxation of the abdominal wall. Indeed, small livers are occasionally palpable. In 1896 Foxwell pointed out that the liver might be felt without being above average weight.[72] Eppinger noted that the liver was palpable in 80 per cent of his series but enlarged in only 50 per cent on pathologic examination.[62] Ratnoff and Patek found only a rough correlation between palpability and size of the liver.[198] The average weight of 73 palpable livers showing cirrhosis was 1,820 Gm., the weights ranging from 695 to 5,100 Gm. In 30 nonpalpable livers with cirrhosis the average weight was 1,370 Gm., the weights ranging from 570 to 2,920 Gm. Similar findings are reported by others.[3]

It is commonly believed that the liver enlarges early in the disease and decreases in size with progression of the disease; that at first it is hypertrophic and later atrophic.

Little evidence supports this opinion. The liver also appears to decrease in size with recovery from the disease. At times rapid shrinking is observed, which suggests that palpability is related to edema and fatty changes as well as to increased density from fibrosis.

Splenomegaly. The spleen is enlarged on physical examination in 30 to 50 per cent of patients and at autopsy in 70 to 80 per cent of cases. This indicates that considerable numbers are overlooked at examination, since the spleen is larger in life than after death.

The demonstration of splenomegaly is important toward establishing the diagnosis of cirrhosis, since it is so constant a feature. Splenomegaly is not encountered in the early, fatty, precirrhotic stage of the disease. When present, it indicates a well-advanced process, for the size of the spleen presumably reflects the height and duration of portal vein hypertension caused by fibrosis (cf. Pathology).

The spleen appears to vary in size from day to day and may shrink greatly after

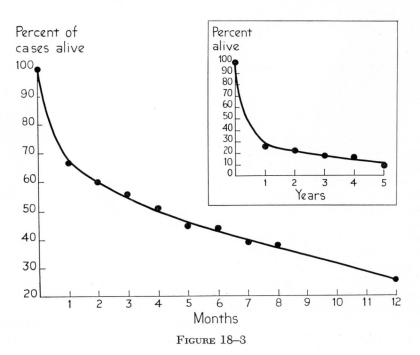

SURVIVAL AFTER ONSET OF JAUNDICE

Figure 18–3

blood loss. If persistent, repeated search is made, a rewardingly high percentage of palpable spleens is found. In doubtful cases, roentgenography may help to reveal the presence of an enlarged spleen.

Vascular Changes. Generalized circulatory changes occur frequently in patients with cirrhosis of the liver.[113, 159, 206, 215] The most conspicuous findings are increased cardiac output, diffuse vasodilatation and increased blood volume. Although alcoholism, anemia and thiamine deficiency may contribute to these changes, they do not fully account for them. The mechanism is not understood. There is evidence of increased venous admixture of arterial blood, which may be related to pulmonary arteriovenous anastomoses or possibly to shunting of portal venous blood into pulmonary veins.

Dilated superficial veins, signs of collateral circulation between the portal and the systemic systems, appear upon the abdomen and the chest in 25 to 60 per cent of recorded cases. Like splenomegaly and esophageal varices, they reflect the degree of obstruction in the portal venous system. With infrared photography the extent of the collateral circulation can be detected earlier than with the naked eye. The *caput medusae,* popularly identified with cirrhosis, is a rarity and was seen in only 4 of 386 patients.[198] This grouping of paraumbilical veins is far more characteristic of obstruction to the inferior vena cava than it is of Laennec's cirrhosis. *Venous hum* is heard occasionally over a large umbilical or paraumbilical vein connecting the portal and the systemic venous system.[238, 268]

Hemorrhoids are commonplace in cirrhosis. However, it is questionable that they occur more frequently in cirrhotics than in others of comparable age.

Vascular Spider. One of the most reliable signs of hepatic cirrhosis is the vascular spider, known also as the spider nevus or angioma (Fig. 18–4). It may be seen in as many as 60 per cent of patients. The spider is a tiny bright-red arteriole, from which radiate hairlike branches for a distance of 0.5 to 1.0 cm. The central core pulsates, and this pulsation can be demonstrated by applying counterpressure over the area with a glass slide; because of their arterial struc-

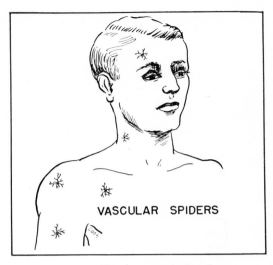

VASCULAR SPIDERS

Fig. 18–4. Extreme example of vascular spiders in a case of hepatic cirrhosis. (Schiff, L.: Clinical Approach to Jaundice, Springfield, Ill., Thomas)

ture they may give rise to spurting hemorrhages.

On histologic section these vessels resemble small arteries or arterioles, and at times they resemble arterial segments of glomus vessels. For reasons unknown they are seen almost exclusively on the face, arms and upper trunk; rarely are they seen over the lower trunk or the legs. In a rough fashion their appearance tends to parallel the course of the disease. They increase in number during failure and decrease with improvement.

Earlier studies have elucidated the arterial nature of these vessels.[78, 141, 177] In a monograph on this subject Bean has suggested that the vascular spider is related to the concentration of circulating estrogens or related steroids.[11] He points out that the only other condition in which these are seen with some frequency is pregnancy—especially between the 2nd and 5th months.

There are several objections to the hypothesis. On measuring urinary excretion of estrogens in cases of cirrhosis two groups of workers found that the occurrence of the vascular spider did not correlate with the amount of urinary estrogen (free or conjugated) excreted.[56, 213] Others have administered excessive amounts of estrogens to patients with metastatic carcinoma but have produced no vascular spiders. However, a related steroid or steroid metabolite may be involved in the pathogenesis of the spider.

Many healthy persons have *congenital spiders* which are indistinguishable from the acquired type and appear to have no relation to hepatic disease.

Esophageal and Gastric Varices. The frequency of these venous dilatations is doubtless greater than is recognized clinically. In one study varices occurred in 59 of 124 patients (48 per cent).[176] This included cases of hematemesis, as well as those demonstrated at autopsy or by roentgenography. Newer refinements in the use of x-rays doubtless will disclose a higher frequency. On direct esophagoscopy about 85 per cent of cases of portal cirrhosis show dilated esophageal veins. An occasional esophageal varix is said to occur in the absence of portal hypertension.

Esophageal varices may vary in size from day to day, according to several observers,[6, 133, 201] and at times may disappear. The size of the varix does not bear a direct relation to its propensity to bleed. Local factors probably play a role inasmuch as other collateral veins seldom rupture, although subjected to the same increased pressure.

Since roughly 30 per cent of patients with Laennec's cirrhosis die from bleeding esophageal varices, the question has been raised as to the value of prophylactic surgery. Palmer and associates have advocated this, and presented data to support their point of view.[166] Child has indicated the difficulties of interpreting the medical literature on this subject.[33] In most surgical experience the case material has been selective. That is, half the patients subjected to surgery have survived one hemorrhage by 6 months. Most patients undergoing this operation have been selected as good risks. The survival period of these patients cannot properly be compared to an unselected series of cirrhotic patients with esophageal hemorrhage.

In a study of the natural history of esophageal varices, Baker and associates observed the course of 115 patients with demonstrated varices for 1 to 6 years (average 3.3 years).[6] In this group 33 patients (28 per cent) bled, but only 11 patients (10 per cent) died from the first hemorrhage. On the basis of their findings prophylactic surgery did not seem justified. Similar conclusions were reached in more recent studies.[38, 77]

Indications for surgery in these patients should vary with the condition of the patient. In patients who show progressive deterioration with jaundice, ascites, stupor and severe functional derangement, esophageal hemorrhage may supervene and be the immediate cause of death. For these patients surgery is useless. However, in the group whose chief difficulty appears to be vascular (bleeding), and who show minimal signs of liver cell failure, surgery may prolong life for many years. Corrective surgery should be carried out after the first hemorrhage in this "good risk" group, provided that the source of bleeding from varices is established. As pointed out by Child, the intermediate group poses the difficult problem of decision. (For detailed discussion, see Chap. 9, Portal Hypertension.)

Liver Palms. This condition is characterized by flushed, mottled, reddening of the thenar and the hypothenar eminences and the fingertips. Often it is seen in conjunction with the vascular spiders and doubtless is related to similar vascular changes. However, liver palms are seen in a variety of other conditions (notably rheumatoid arthritis) and in healthy persons.

Hernia. Abdominal hernia is a common complication of cirrhosis of the liver, presumably due to increased intra-abdominal pressure. Chapman, Snell and Rowntree noted that herniae developed in 6 of 58 patients who had cirrhosis without ascites and in 47 of 112 patients with ascites.[32] These herniae were umbilical in 24, ventral in 7, inguinal in 9 and epigastric in 2 instances.

Tanyol reported somewhat different findings.[236] In a series of 66 cirrhotic patients, 25 (38 per cent) developed herniae. In all but one patient the herniae developed prior to the onset of ascites. Tanyol suggested that both portal cirrhosis and abdominal hernia are related to a constitutional defect in mesenchymal tissue. Although it is an interesting concept, the evidence does not seem to be adequate.

Repair of abdominal hernia may be mandatory because of strangulation, and most patients tolerate the procedure. However, as Yonemoto and Davidson point out, it is important to prepare these patients well with rest and a nutritious diet before surgery.[271] In general, an elective procedure should be deferred until ascites has disappeared.

Of particular interest is the umbilical hernia. The sac may be so thin as to rupture spontaneously.[71] Periumbilical veins surround these herniae. In the course of surgical repair these collaterals are ligated. The sudden occlusion of the venous channels imposes an extra load on the portal circulation. A report on the surgical repair of 15 umbilical herniae in patients with cirrhosis described 5 deaths from hematemesis shortly after operation.[9] The author points out the hazard of repairing umbilical herniae in these patients and ascribes this to the sudden increased load in the portal venous bed.

Sexual and Related Disturbances

Impotence in males is commonplace.[62] Presumably, this is on an organic basis, since testicular atrophy and fibrosis frequently are observed at autopsy. Henschen and Bruce reported testicular fibrosis in 16 of 81 cases of Laennec's cirrhosis and atrophy in 8 instances.[95] Other studies confirm this observation.[13, 16, 140, 155] Urinary androgen has been found to be subnormal.

Although these changes suggest an organic basis for impotence, it should be borne in mind that the majority of the patients are alcoholics, and that the average age of the males is 50 years. Loss of libido in patients with chronic illness in this age group would not be surprising. Data concerning sterility are not at hand.

Gynecomastia, loss of axillary and pubic hair and the appearance of vascular spiders, commonly seen in cirrhotics,[3, 62, 140] have been attributed to failure of the damaged liver to detoxify estrogens. Assays of urine have shown constant decreases in 17-ketosteroids[25] and frequent increases in free and conjugated urinary estrogens.[56, 213] However, corresponding changes in 17-ketosteroids and estrogens are found in cirrhotic patients who lack these clinical features. Correlation between the laboratory changes and these physical signs has not been impressive.[56, 213]

Gynecomastia is seen most commonly in patients with advanced cirrhosis and in conjunction with testicular atrophy, loss of libido, female escutcheon of pubic hair and loss of axillary hair.

However it also is encountered in patients recovering from hepatic failure, during a period of high protein feeding. Breast enlargement and tenderness may be associated in these patients with increase in testicular size and in libido and regrowth of male hair. In contrast to the first group, gynecomastia appears during a period of masculinization and does not appear to be estrogenic in origin. These patients resemble the liberated prisoners of war with "refeeding gynecomastia."[114, 126] Generally this type of gynecomastia is transient.

Recently the incidence of gynecomastia has increased sharply with the use of certain diuretics. It has been seen particularly in patients treated with spironolactone.

Menstrual Disorders. Corresponding studies for the female are less satisfactory because of the relatively few women of premenopausal age with Laennec's cirrhosis. Both increased and decreased menstrual flow have been described in association with cirrhosis.[198] In our experience decreased or absent menstruation is characteristic; indeed, return of normal menses is a sign of recovery from liver failure.[176] In 66 females with Laennec's cirrhosis Armas-Cruz and co-workers reported 39 (59 per cent) with amenorrhea.[3] However, it is not clear from their data how many were of premenopausal age.

Menorrhagia or metrorrhagia is associated more usually with a generalized bleeding diathesis or with local pelvic pathology. There is little information concerning sexual drive, hormonal changes or pathologic changes in the ovaries in this group of patients. Pregnancy apparently can occur in the presence of cirrhosis, as reported by Tenney and King.[237]

HEMORRHAGIC PHENOMENA

Although several blood-clotting factors may be altered in Laennec's cirrhosis, a grave bleeding tendency is unusual. **Epistaxis, purpura and gingival bleeding** are the manifestations most commonly seen.

In childhood and adolescence nosebleeds are experienced by persons who seem to be healthy otherwise. Generally, this tendency is outgrown. However, the appearance of nosebleed in adult life suggests the possibility of cirrhosis of the liver, as well as primary blood dyscrasia.

In a series of 386 cases[198] 70 (18 per cent) had a history of epistaxis and 33 (9 per cent) had purpura; of these 12 had both symptoms. In reviewing 208 cases, Armas-Cruz and associates listed 19.2 per cent with a tendency to epistaxis and purpura.[3] In a series of 124 patients in whom the symptom of epistaxis was inquired into specifically, an incidence of 40 per cent was obtained.[176] It seems probable that epistaxes are related to increased vascularity or to changes in the nasal mucosa, since in most instances there is no generalized bleeding tendency.

Purpura and gingival bleeding (5 to 10 per cent of cases) are seen more often with advanced hepatic disease and with changes in the blood-clotting factors than is the case with epistaxis. Fagin and Thompson observed this tendency only in jaundiced patients.[65] The rare occurrence of hematuria and melena from multiple bleeding points in the intestine also is associated with advanced hepatic failure.

Multiple deficiencies in blood-clotting factors have been described.[41, 69, 92, 135, 160, 197, 260] The degree of change in these factors reflects roughly the severity of hepatic disease. The most pronounced deficiencies involve factors concerned with the conversion of prothrombin to thrombin, or the second phase of coagulation. For practical purposes the measurement of prothrombin time is the most useful aid, inasmuch as changes in other plasma-clotting factors tend to parallel the changes in prothrombin time.[69] In the presence of cirrhosis the administration of vitamin K brings about slight, if any, increase in the concentration of prothrombin.[69]

Most patients with cirrhosis also have thrombocytopenia,[154, 263] which may be moderate or severe. This appears to be due to hypersplenism. The degree of thrombocytopenia does not necessarily parallel changes in blood-clotting factors.

The bleeding tendency in cirrhosis often presents serious problems in the course of surgery. Multiple transfusions depress the blood platelets and thus may accentuate a bleeding tendency.[69] Blood platelets and AC globulin deteriorate rapidly in stored bank blood. Because of this it is desirable to use fresh blood whenever possible. (See Chap. 5 for full discussion of clotting factors.)

ANEMIA

Anemia occurs frequently in Laennec's cirrhosis. The degree of anemia bears only a poor correlation with the severity of the disease. Other conditions often complicate the problem, notably blood loss, malnutrition and possibly toxic effects of alcohol. The degree of anemia may be exaggerated by an expanded plasma volume.[88, 179]

Characteristically the anemia of cirrhosis is either normocytic or macrocytic,[106, 210] the red cells showing little variation in size or shape. Reticulocytosis varying from 2 to 15 per cent has been reported. The bone marrow is normoblastic and shows hyperactivity with extension of red marrow into the shaft of the femur.[15] Urobilinogen excretion is usually increased. The life span of the transfused, tagged red cell is shortened.[111, 225] These changes are consistent with a hemolytic process that has been ascribed to splenic hyperactivity.[103] Coombs' test generally is negative and osmotic fragility is not increased.

The anemia usually does not respond to administration of folic acid or liver extract but gradually improves with recovery from the underlying disease. Schiff and associates demonstrated the presence of antianemic substance (against pernicious anemia) in livers of patients who died from hepatic cirrhosis with macrocytic anemia.[217] Therefore the anemia does not appear to be due to lack of storage of anti-anemic principle.

Occasional cases of macrocytic anemia appear to be due to folic acid deficiency. In 16 cases of alcoholic Laennec's cirrhosis with anemia Jandl and Lear found 4 with megaloblastic bone marrow and abnormal granulocyte precursors characteristic of folic acid deficiency.[104] Hematologic response to folic acid was prompt.

In addition to the above are a group of patients with acute hemolytic anemia occurring typically after alcoholic bouts. These patients have large fatty livers and frequently early changes of cirrhosis. They may have acute abdominal pain, fever and a triad of signs described by Zieve—anemia, hyperlipemia and jaundice.[273, 275] Osmotic fragility may be increased. It is believed that lipemia follows release of lipid from the liver, and that the increased fragility is due to a lysolecithin.

Iron deficiency anemia may result not only from frank blood loss in cirrhosis but also from occult seepage of blood into the gastrointestinal tract. The presence of hypochromic microcytic anemia without obvious cause should alert one to this probability.

In a recent study of 46 patients with chronic liver disease, Kimber and associates demonstrated that multiple factors were involved in most cases of anemia.[121]

LABORATORY CHANGES

Characteristic changes in laboratory tests are shown in Table 18–5. The table indicates findings usually encountered in *advanced* Laennec's cirrhosis. For the most part the tests in common use are of diagnostic value, reflecting the presence or the absence of hepatic damage, but they do not provide an index to the type or the extent of injury. They lack a sufficient degree of sensitivity. A considerable degree of cirrhosis may be present with normal or almost normal laboratory tests.

In following the course of the disease, investigators have found that serial values for several tests have shown a rough correlation between clinical and laboratory changes. These include serum albumin, serum bilirubin, prothrombin time and cholesterol esters.

TREATMENT

REST

Emphasis is placed upon rest, nutritious diet and supportive measures. By the time the patient accepts hospitalization he is usually weak, mentally dulled, distended with ascites and agreeable to rest in bed. With improvement he asks for more freedom, and since convalescence may involve many months, it is not feasible to enforce bed rest indefinitely. For those who are in moderate failure bed rest for at least half the day is advocated. Resumption of activity is allowed gradually as jaundice, fever and ascites subside.

It is better to prescribe a program that is likely to be accepted than one which is too

TABLE 18–5.   CHARACTERISTIC LABORATORY CHANGES IN ADVANCED LAENNEC'S CIRRHOSIS

Serum albumin	Decreased (especially in presence of ascites)
Serum globulin	Increased (chiefly gamma)
Cephalin flocculation	Positive (2 to 4+) in about 75% of cases
Thymol turbidity	Increased in about 50% of cases
Bromosulphalein dye retention	Increased in over 90% of cases
Serum bilirubin	Increased slightly
Urine urobilinogen	Increased
Serum alkaline phosphatase	Normal or moderate increase
Serum cholesterol total	Normal
Serum cholesterol ester	Decreased
Prothrombin time	Increased slightly
Erythrocyte sedimentation rate	Increased
White blood count	Normal or moderately increased
Blood urea nitrogen	Normal (increased in failure)
SGOT and SGPT	Moderate increase (100 to 150)

demanding and sooner or later is rejected. However, this point of view does not apply to the problem of alcoholism. All too frequently patients return to their old habits, undoing in a few weeks the improvement that they made in many months. There should be no compromise with the patient with regard to alcohol, for he seldom is able to restrict his intake within reasonable bounds. Many doctors are too indulgent in treating this fundamental aspect of therapy.

DIET

The dietary management of Laennec's cirrhosis has been subjected to changing fashions. In the early 1900's a popular diet, especially in France, consisted chiefly of milk. Somewhat later, studies on dogs with Eck fistulas indicated that they tolerated meat and fat poorly. Following these reports, diets restricted in meat and fat and relatively high in carbohydrate were advocated for the treatment of liver disease in general. In the 1940's clinical experience with cirrhosis indicated that patients responded favorably to diets which were relatively rich in protein and unrestricted in fat.[175, 176] More recently, with the rediscovery of "ammonia intoxication" as a factor in hepatic coma, the place for protein-rich diets in the treatment of cirrhosis again has been questioned.[182, 231]

The need for a nutritious diet is apparent in most patients. They show signs of tissue wasting and often signs of specific malnutrition, such as polyneuritis. Usually they tolerate a generous, nutritious diet without difficulty. A standard diet employed at the Columbia Research Service, Goldwater Memorial Hospital, Welfare Island, provides 114 Gm. of protein, 365 Gm. of carbohydrate and 175 Gm. of fat. In the opinion of some authorities this diet is unduly high in carbohydrate and fat. Davidson[48] has suggested a more moderate intake, with a diet containing protein 77 Gm., carbohydrate 255 Gm., and fat 126 Gm. The differences between these diets are unimportant, for the chief concern is to make food inviting to a patient whose appetite is meager.

The rationale for administering a protein-rich diet to these patients receives strong support from experimental work.[21, 45, 84, 259, 265] Cirrhosis of the liver, similar in most aspects to Laennec's cirrhosis, has been produced in the rat, dog and monkey by means of diets restricted in protein and relatively rich in carbohydrate and/or fat. Other studies have shown that recovery from this type of cirrhosis is effected by diets that are rich in proteins.[36, 174, 235]

What is the protein requirement of a patient with cirrhosis? This cannot be defined categorically. The normal adult is said to require about 0.5 Gm. protein/kilo body weight under basal conditions. However, the patient in hepatic failure is not normal and is not under basal conditions. There is need for increased dietary protein to compensate for tissue wasting and to facilitate repair and regeneration of the liver.

Although positive nitrogen balance usually is achieved by diets containing 1 Gm. protein/kilo body weight, this does not necessarily imply optimal nutrition. In our clinic a protein intake of about 1.5 Gm./kilo body weight is advised. Most patients tolerate these diets well. However, in view of the increasing prevalence of hepatic stupor or coma, a cautious attitude toward the use of high protein diets is justified. Particularly is this true in patients who have been subjected to portacaval shunt operations[146] and in others with persistently elevated blood ammonia. If there is a tendency to mental confusion or torpor, the protein content of the diet must be reduced sharply to the point where "ammonia intoxication" is controlled. The recognition and treatment of this symptom complex (see Chap. 12) has been an important advance in the management of cirrhosis of the liver. When the intake of protein is reduced drastically the patient must subsist on his own tissue protein. Since these patients are already deficient in protein, a protracted restriction is undesirable, and one should attempt to restore gradually the intake of protein up to tolerance.

Restriction of dietary fat has been a general rule in the care of patients with hepatic disease. This is based largely upon experience with obstructive jaundice, in which there is decreased flow of bile and faulty absorption of fats. Restriction of dietary fat is less necessary in cirrhosis. Although there is a moderate increase in the fat content of the stool[83] we have encountered no ill effects from diets containing 175 Gm. of fat daily. Liver biopsies of patients being fed these diets have shown no increased infiltration with fat. Therefore, the present evidence does not suggest the need for restriction of dietary fat in patients with cirrhosis of the liver.[42]

Carbohydrate should be fed in amounts adequate to satisfy caloric needs and to serve as a protein-sparer. A relatively high carbohydrate intake is indicated in the presence of coma.

Brewer's yeast powder (which contains 50 per cent protein) has been given in divided dosage up to 50 Gm. daily as milk nog. Vitamin B_{12} has been administered by injection in doses of 100 to 300 mcg. weekly. Although there is little scientific basis for these adjuvants, I believe that they help to restore nutrition and a sense of well being. Long-continued use of vitamin mixtures with so-called "therapeutic formula" seems unwise because of the high content of vitamin A. However, when patients exhibit signs of specific malnutrition, such as polyneuritis or Wernicke's encephalopathy, appropriate therapeutic vitamins should be administered.

CONTROL OF ASCITES

Ascites generally can be controlled with careful regulation of sodium and fluid intake and the use of diuretic agents. (See Chap. 11). An unfortunate result of effective control of ascites is premature resumption of physical activity. It is well to insist upon rest periods and limited activity so long as it is necessary to administer diuretics and to maintain sodium restriction.

TREATMENT OF HEPATIC COMA

Coma may be the terminal stage of progressive hepatic failure; it may appear abruptly in the course of intercurrent infection; it may accompany or follow esophageal hemorrhage; it may follow the administration of opiates and other drugs.[158] The outcome depends in large measure upon the precipitating conditions. Hepatic coma is discussed fully in Chapter 12.

TREATMENT OF INTERCURRENT INFECTIONS

Intercurrent infections formerly accounted for about 25 per cent of the deaths from cirrhosis. With the advent of antibiotics the dangers from infection have decreased sharply. Although instances have been cited of hepatic damage produced by sulfonamide drugs, the risk seems justified when continued infection is the alternative. In this regard our experiences[176] confirm that of Peterson and co-workers.[180] Obviously care should be taken to avoid antibiotics with known hepatotoxicity. For example, large doses of tetracycline administered intravenously may be hepatotoxic.[220]

TREATMENT OF HEMATEMESIS

Whole blood should be transfused as soon as possible; delay may result in irreversible shock or coma. Transfusions are continued as long as there is evidence of bleeding. The patient should be sedated only lightly, since he has a tendency to lapse into coma.

Diagnostic measures to ascertain the source of the bleeding should be undertaken promptly (see Chapter 9). The use of esophageal tamponade and the indications for surgery are further discussed also in the same chapter.

SPECIFIC ADJUVANTS

Choline and Methionine. Although choline and methionine prevent experimental nutritional cirrhosis in the rat, there is less evidence that they are effective in the reparative process after cirrhosis has been produced. Dietary protein (apart from its content of methionine) and probably other nutrients appear to play an important role in repair of nutritional cirrhosis.[85, 183]

In dealing with the human disease, where conditions are far less susceptible to control, it has been difficult to assess the value of lipotropic substances.[127, 168, 252] For the most part patients have received highly nutritious diets as well as supplementary choline and methionine. Beneficial effects have been measured by function tests and by serial biopsies of the liver. Comparisons with past experience and with other series of cases have suggested that improvement was the result of "lipotropic" therapy.[74, 214] In the experience of others[119, 134, 191, 252] their therapeutic effect has been unimpressive, and the fatty, cirrhotic liver responds as favorably to bed rest and normal hospital diet as it does to treatment with choline and methionine. The average hospital diet probably supplies adequate amounts of choline and methionine.

Human Serum Albumin Solution. Conflicting opinions have been expressed concerning the value of administering intravenously concentrated human serum albumin solution. Kunkel and associates made studies on 17 patients with severe hepatic disease.[131] In 14 of 15 patients ascites disappeared soon following therapy. Patients with either postnecrotic or Laennec's cirrhosis responded. The improved nutrition and clinical status suggested positive benefit from this therapy. Post and co-workers observed 34 patients critically ill with hepatic cirrhosis.[194] Here, too, substantial benefit was attributed to treatment with intravenous albumin solution. Nine of 16 patients recovered from coma, an unusually high incidence. Dykes reported that 10 of 13 cases with resistant ascites responded well to intravenous albumin infusions.[59]

In contrast, Faloon and his co-workers were unimpressed by this form of medication.[167] Only 4 of 20 patients experienced a prompt diuresis that could be attributed to therapy. In several instances esophageal hemorrhage occurred within a short time of therapy. Pulmonary edema, due to rapid expansion of plasma volume, also is a hazard in patients who have decreased cardiac reserve.

There appears to be a place for treatment with concentrated human serum albumin, not so much for its effect upon ascites formation (as was hoped originally) but as an available and utilizable form of plasma protein. In patients who are critically ill, whose serum albumin is much reduced, this would seem to be a rational form of therapy. Untoward reactions are infrequent if repeated small doses (25 Gm. or less) are administered slowly intravenously.

Cortisone and its Derivatives. In the treatment of severe, progressive hepatitis or chronic hepatitis cortisone may be dramatically effective. However, there is little, if any, evidence that cortisone is indicated in Laennec's cirrhosis. Moreover this drug introduces the hazards of possible bleeding from the gastrointestinal tract, decreased resistance to infection, precipitation of toxic psychosis and other side effects.[24, 217]

RESULTS OF TREATMENT; PROGNOSIS

The outlook for patients with Laennec's cirrhosis has improved considerably in recent years. This is shown statistically by comparing periods of survival in the years 1937 to 1947 with corresponding experience from 1916 to 1938. Figure 18–5 illustrates the period of survival after the onset of ascites (as an index of liver failure) in 2 series. The upper line A refers to patients treated with a nutritious diet (rich in protein) and prolonged hospitalization. The lower line B refers to the control series, also hospitalized but for lesser periods of time. The standard diet for hepatic disease during 1916 to 1938 was high in carbohydrate and low in protein and fat. The more favorable course of the recent series doubtless is due not only to dietary factors and bed rest but also to more effective measures to combat infection and control shock from hemorrhage.

The experience of several clinics has been in general agreement with these findings,[47, 70, 99, 252, 256a] whereas others have questioned whether the prognosis has been improved.[75] Statistics concerning prognosis are difficult to compare because they have not been based on like conditions. The case material and methods of analysis differ in several reported series. Ideally, prognosis would indicate the period of survival from the first symptoms of the disease. Since this is not feasible in cirrhosis, arbitrary points have been selected, such as the duration of life after the onset of ascites or jaundice,[176] or after entry to the hospital.[75] One group of patients, studied in a hospital for chronic disease, obviously did not include those who might have died before transfer from a general hospital. In another study the patient material was limited to those with "unequivocal varices." This resulted in the selection of 471 patients from a total of 950 with the diagnosis of cirrhosis. The duration of hospitalization and the type of patient care also are determining factors in prognosis. From the experience on our medical service there is little doubt that progress has been made in modifying the course of the disease and in improving the prognosis.

The outcome depends greatly upon the stage of the disease at which treatment is started. At an early stage it is possible to achieve fairly complete clinical and histologic recovery. Results are much less satisfactory in those with advanced hepatic failure. In a group of 124 patients 61 (roughly 50 per cent) made sustained significant improvement. These results were possible only because of long-continued hospitalization and dietary care.

Figure 18–6 shows the length of time from the beginning of therapy to the disappearance of certain signs of hepatic failure in the 61 patients who made significant improvement. Although there is individual variation, jaundice and fever tend to disappear more rapidly than ascites and edema. In about 75 per cent of cases these 4 signs disappeared within 3 months. In a few cases it took 6 to 12 months to accomplish this end. Gain in weight and strength, subsidence of epitaxis, return of menses and improved laboratory functions accompanied these changes. Esophageal varices at times may disappear after prolonged medical treatment.[201]

In general, there was considerable lag before the laboratory tests reflected clinical changes. Certain tests, such as the Bromsulphalein dye test, may remain abnormal for years despite sustained clinical improvement. In 40 of 61 patients dye retention decreased; in 21 cases the cephalin flocculation test became negative; in all cases serum albumin increased. The mean value for serum albumin before therapy was 2.8 Gm./100 cc. and after treatment, 4.2

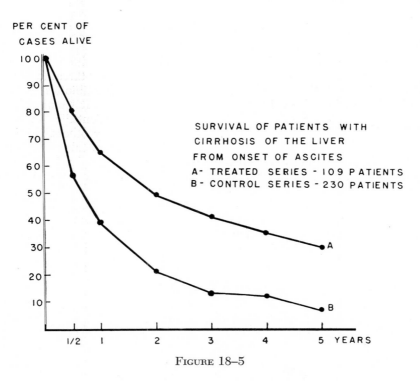

PER CENT OF
CASES ALIVE

SURVIVAL OF PATIENTS WITH
CIRRHOSIS OF THE LIVER
FROM ONSET OF ASCITES
A- TREATED SERIES - 109 PATIENTS
B- CONTROL SERIES - 230 PATIENTS

FIGURE 18–5

DISAPPEARANCE OF SIGNS OF LIVER FAILURE

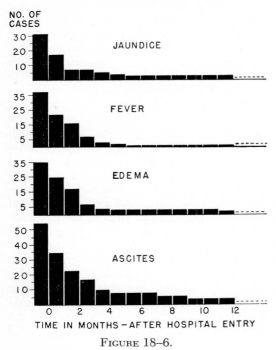

FIGURE 18-6.

TABLE 18-6. INTERCURRENT INFECTIONS IN 386 PATIENTS WITH LAENNEC'S CIRRHOSIS[198]

	NUMBER OF PATIENTS
Bronchopneumonia	17
Nontuberculous peritonitis	12
Lobar pneumonia	5
Bacteremia	4
Erysipelas	3
Phlebitis	3
Tuberculous peritonitis	2
Pyelonephritis	2
Miscellaneous	8

Gm./100 cc. In our experience and that of others serial values for serum albumin correspond fairly closely to clinical changes and thus serve as a useful guide to prognosis.[3, 157] In other hands the serum cholesterol ester has been of similar value.

HISTOLOGIC CHANGES WITH CLINICAL IMPROVEMENT

There is a poor correlation between the clinical or functional changes in Laennec's cirrhosis and the histologic findings obtained at biopsy of the liver or at autopsy.[127, 193, 204, 250] Fat disappears from the liver several weeks after the institution of an adequate diet. Changes in size, shape and staining quality of the liver cells, changes in inflammatory cellular reaction, and particularly in connective-tissue response are unpredictable. In certain cases there appears to be regression at least of the more acute changes, whereas in others dramatic clinical improvement may be observed with little alteration of histologic structure. However, there is disagreement

on this point, some observers reporting a closer correlation between clinical and pathologic changes.[187, 252, 254]

There are few reports of comparative studies made after long periods of treatment. In the rat with experimental cirrhosis almost complete restoration of normal-appearing liver is possible in 10 months by means of a nutritious diet.[38, 174, 235] It seems likely that similar changes can occur in man over a period of years.

COMPLICATIONS AND ASSOCIATED CONDITIONS

Intercurrent infections are frequent, and they were a serious threat to life prior to the introduction of antibiotics. Table 18-6 lists the infections most commonly seen in a series of 386 patients.[198] Similar data have been recorded by others.[145, 207]

In former years tuberculosis was a common complication. In 1920 Blumenau reported that of 126 autopsied cases with cirrhosis, in 10 per cent death was due to tuberculosis. In 1929, Rolleston and McNee stated that "in about 12 to 14 per cent of cases with cirrhosis death is due to pulmonary tuberculosis,"[207] and this apparently was the usual experience at the turn of the century in Europe. In more recent years tuberculosis has been less frequently encountered in cirrhotics. In 1933 McCartney found 3 cases of active tuberculosis in 158 cases of cirrhosis at autopsy.[145] Evans and Grey in 1938 reported 6 cases of active tuberculosis in 217 cases of cirrhosis at autopsy. In the series listed in Table 18-6, tuberculosis was present *clinically* in only 4 of 386 patients. Two had tuberculous peritonitis. However, tuberculous peritonitis may be more prevalent than has been suspected. Burack and Hollister reported 47 cases of tuberculous peritonitis collected over 25 years at the Boston City Hospital; twenty of the 47 cases had cirrhosis of the liver and ascites.[27]

Infections with enteric organisms causing bacteremia and peritonitis are a relatively common but rarely recognized syndrome, according to Conn. These are seen chiefly in debilitated patients with advanced cirrhosis.[37, 118, 248]

In addition to the listed infections, phlegmonous enteritis is encountered in a significant number of cases, apparently intervening shortly before death. This has been observed also in cases of acute yellow atrophy, and it is not specific for Laennec's cirrhosis.[184]

Renal Abnormalities. The term "hepatorenal syndrome" has been abandoned by some writers, since it probably embraces several conditions.[167] Renal failure, or azotemia, is a grave complication and generally is seen only in patients with advanced disease. It is encountered in patients who have had gastrointestinal bleeding. In these it has been attributed to the absorption of nitrogenous products and to impaired renal function from shock. It also can occur abruptly after abdominal paracentesis, due presumably to sudden reduction in extracellular fluid. Formerly, it occurred commonly after surgery on patients with cirrhosis. With modern anesthesia and avoidance of shock, this complication has become infrequent. Drug-induced diuresis occasionally precipitates renal failure but it is not responsible for the majority of cases.[138]

Measurements of renal function usually show decreased renal plasma flow and possibly decreased glomerular filtration. However, the changes often are moderate and usually do not account for the degree of failure. Histologic changes also may show minimal involvement of the tubules. The basis for renal failure (if it is such) is not clear. (For full discussion of this subject see Chap. 11).

Glomerulonephritis as an associated condition was found in 7 per cent of 200 cases of cirrhosis. Both acute and chronic forms were encountered. The pathologic lesions were those of intracapillary glomerulonephritis. Since the usual incidence of glomerulonephritis does not exceed 1 per cent of the hospital population, this association appears to be significant.[178]

Peptic Ulcer. Peptic ulcer is found in 1.8 to 20 per cent of cases of Laennec's cirrhosis.[14, 198, 219] Figures vary both in clinical and autopsied series of cases. In 3 autopsied series the incidences of peptic ulcer were 11.5, 14 and 17 per cent, respectively.[51, 66, 139] Control series of nonhepatic cases showed incidences of 6.6 and 10.6 per cent.[66, 139] The data suggest that there is an increase of peptic ulcer in the presence of cirrhosis, although this is open to question.

When bleeding originates in the upper gastrointestinal tract the possibility of peptic ulcer must be kept in mind. In a series of 76 patients with Laennec's cirrhosis and bleeding from the upper gastrointestinal tract, peptic ulcer accounted for 18 per cent;[66] in another series of 92 patients peptic ulcer accounted for 13 per cent.[46]

There have been occasional reports of the occurrence of peptic ulcer after portacaval shunts.[146] Whether or not the shunting operation was responsible for the ulcers is unknown. Clarke has described studies of his own and of other workers with experimental animals in which diversion of portal blood around the liver resulted in increased gastric acid secretion and predisposed to the formation of ulcer.[35]

Cardiovascular abnormalities have been noted in patients with advanced Laennec's cirrhosis.[159, 206] In many instances the cardiac index is increased. This has been ascribed to increased circulating volume of blood, to arterial oxygen unsaturation and to multiple shunts between the portal and the systemic venous systems. Usually these changes are slight, and it is doubtful that they would produce failure in an otherwise competent heart.

Neurologic Disorders. Hepatic coma is the most common disorder in this category. It is a toxic encephalopathy, metabolic in nature and frequently reversible or transient (see Chap. 12).

In addition to metabolic disorders, degenerative changes in the basal ganglion and brain stem and demyelinating disease of the spinal cord are encountered. As in hepatic coma, an important feature appears to be the portacaval bypass. The lesions, however, are irreversible and are not necessarily associated with coma. Victor, Adams and Cole have described 27 cases that closely resembled Wilson's disease.[250] Pathologic examination disclosed astrocyte hyperplasia and degenerative changes in the cortex, cerebellum and lenticular nucleus. Dayan and Williams have reported demyelinating changes in the peripheral nerves of the legs.[52]

Dupuytren's Contracture. Wolfe, Summerskill and Davidson report the frequent occurrence of Dupuytren's contracture in chronic alcoholics and especially in those patients with Laennec's cirrhosis.[267] The pathogenesis of the lesion is not known. Since it is not encountered, as a rule, in patients with postnecrotic cirrhosis, there is some question as to whether these contractures are related to disturbed hepatic function. There appears to be no correlation between the degree of impairment of liver function and the presence of Dupuytren's contracture.[161]

Thrombosis of the Portal Vein. This relatively rare condition is encountered in roughly 2 per cent of the cases of cirrhosis. When thrombosis is partial there are few distinguishing symptoms. With sudden closure of the vein more severe symptoms occur, such as shock, hematemesis, paralytic ileus, rapid onset of ascites and cholemia. Under these circumstances the condition should be suspected.

Primary Carcinoma of the Liver. This is much less frequent than secondary tumors of the liver. The majority of patients with primary hepatoma have had preceding cirrhosis. The tumor may be hepatocellular or cholangiocellular in type. The incidence of primary hepatomas appears to be greater in patients with postnecrotic cirrhosis than in those with Laennec's cirrhosis. The incidence in the postnecrotic group is 10 to 15 per cent, whereas in Laennec's cirrhosis

the incidence is 2 to 4 per cent. There are pronounced geographic differences in incidence of hepatoma.

Symptoms generally are those of the underlying cirrhosis. The diagnosis is suggested by rapid clinical deterioration associated with enlarging, nodular, tender liver and abdominal pain. Hemoperitoneum is not uncommon. A rise of serum alkaline phosphatase in the absence of obstructive jaundice is highly suggestive of the disease. (For full discussion see Chap. 24.)

CAUSES OF DEATH

Death in Laennec's cirrhosis occurs more frequently from complications of the disease than from hepatic failure. In several series of cases hepatic failure accounted for 15 to 50 per cent of fatalities; hemorrhage, 20 to 40 per cent; intercurrent infections, especially pneumonia and peritonitis, 10 to 25 per cent; and renal shut-down about 10 per cent.[3, 5, 32, 57, 64, 75, 158, 198] Postoperative deaths also were commonplace. They revealed the grave risk of surgery in the presence of hepatic failure. The chief cause of death today undoubtedly is esophageal or gastric hemorrhage.

ACUTE FLORID CIRRHOSIS (ALCOHOLIC HEPATITIS, STEATONECROSIS)

This symptom complex may be seen in conjunction with fatty liver or as an acute episode in Laennec's cirrhosis. Characteristically there is a history of recent heavy imbibing of alcohol coupled with severe malnutrition and sudden onset of hepatic failure. These patients tend to be younger than the average cirrhotic. The illness may appear abruptly with the onset of jaundice, fever, abdominal pain and tenderness, ascites, edema and vascular spiders. Stupor may occur within a few days or weeks.[89, 116, 181, 188, 189]

Laboratory tests indicate hepatocellular damage, as shown by increased bilirubin, altered serum proteins, prolonged prothrombin time and moderately increased transaminase tests. SGOT is generally 100 to 200 units. Often the degree of functional impairment in hepatic tests seems less than the clinical severity of the illness. White blood counts of 15,000 to 25,000 are usual. Anemia is frequent. Rarely a patient presents with signs of obstructive jaundice due to intrahepatic biliary stasis. Signs of obstructive jaundice abate within a few weeks.

The liver is greatly enlarged and fatty. Phillips and Davidson have listed 4 characteristic findings in these cases: hyalin degeneration of Mallory, focal necroses, inflammatory cellular reaction and parenchymal disorganization.[181] Popper and Szanto described similar findings.[188] In addition, they pointed out the frequency of bile stasis in the biliary capillaries, a feature that had been emphasized by Connor.[40] In some cases there is no infiltration with connective tissue, but in most instances fine strands of loose connective tissue extend into the parenchyma. Other cases representing a more mature stage show regenerating nodules and connective tissue septa radiating from portal zones.

A sizable number of patients with acute florid cirrhosis die after a brief illness. Patients with underlying cirrhosis have a more severe disease and a graver outlook. Prognosis is difficult to predict at the time of entry. The presence of asterixis, persistently high serum bilirubin and mounting azotemia are serious omens.[89] In one series of 51 cases[116] there were 8 deaths (16 per cent); in another series of 56 cases[181] there were 18 deaths (32 per cent); and in a more recent series of 50 cases[82] there were 2 deaths (4 per cent). Harinasuta and associates suggest that earlier studies may have been selective and that the mortality probably is considerably lower.[90]

Treatment is similar to that described for Laennec's cirrhosis. Bed rest, a balanced nutritious diet and abstinence from alcohol are emphasized. Steroid therapy does not appear to be effective.

REFERENCES

1. Allan, F. N., Bowie, D. J., MacLeod, J. J. R., and Robinson, W. L.: Behaviour of depancreatized dogs kept alive with insulin, Brit. J. Exp. Path. 5:75, 1924.
2. Arias, I. M.: The transport of bilirubin in the liver *in* Popper. H., and Schaffner, F. (eds.): Progress in Liver Diseases, vol. 1, p. 187, New York, Grune & Stratton, 1961.
3. Armas-Cruz, R., Yazigi, R., Lopez, O., Montero, E., Cabello, J., and Lobo, G.: Portal cirrhosis: an analysis of 208 cases, with correlation of clinical, laboratory and autopsy findings, Gastroenterology 17:327, 1951.
4. Axenfeld, H., and Brass, K.: Klinische und bioptische Untersuchungen über den sogenannten Icterus catarrhalis, Frankfurt. Z. Path. 57:147, 1942.
5. Baggenstoss, A. H., and Stauffer, M. H.: Posthepatitic and alcoholic cirrhosis: clinicopathologic study of 43 cases of each, Gastroenterology 22:157, 1952.
6. Baker, L. A., Smith, C., and Lieberman, G.: Natural history of esophageal varices: Study of 115 cirrhotic patients in whom varices were diagnosed prior to bleeding, Am. J. Med. 26:228, 1959.
7. Ballard, H., Bernstein, M., and Farrar, J. T.: Fatty liver presenting as obstructive jaundice, Am. J. Med. 30:196, 1961.
8. Barker, M. H., Capps, R. B., and Allen, F. W.: Chronic hepatitis in the Mediterranean theater: a new clinical syndrome, J.A.M.A. 129:653, 1945.
9. Baron, H. C.: Umbilical hernia secondary to cirrhosis of the liver. Complications of surgical correction, New Engl. J. Med. 263:824, 1960.
10. Baum, S., Nusbaum, M., Clearfield, H. R., Kuroda, K., and Tumen, H. J.: Angiography in the diagnosis of gastrointestinal bleeding, Arch. Int. Med. 119:16, 1967.
11. Bean, W. B.: Vascular Spiders and Related Lesions of Skin, Springfield, Ill., Thomas, 1958.
12. Beaser, S. B.: Clinical states with decreased glucose tolerance, J.A.M.A. 199:990, 1967.
13. Bennett, H. S., Baggenstoss, A. H., and Butt, H. R.: The testis, breast and prostate of men who died of cirrhosis of the liver, Am. J. Clin. Path. 20:814, 1950.
14. Bergman, F., and van der Linden, W.: The association of peptic ulcer with cirrhosis of the liver; an analysis of an autopsy series, Acta. path. microbiol. scand. 65:161, 1965.
15. Berman, L., Axelrod, A. R., Horan, T. N., Jacobson, S. D., Sharp, E. A., and Vonderheide, E. C.: The blood and bone

marrow in patients with cirrhosis of the liver, Blood 4:511, 1949.

16. Best, C. H., Hartroft, W. S., Lucas, C. C., and Ridout, J. H.: Liver damage produced by feeding alcohol or sugar and its prevention by choline, Brit. Med. J. 2:1001, 1949.

17. Best, C. H., and Huntsman, M. E.: Effects of components of lecithine upon deposition of fat in liver, J. Physiol. 75:405, 1932.

18. ———: Effect of choline on liver fat of rats in various states of nutrition, J. Physiol. 83:255, 1935.

19. Bjørneboe, M., and Raaschou, F.: The pathology of subchronic atrophy of the liver: a comparison with cirrhosis hepatis Laennec, Acta med. scand., Supp. 234, pp. 41-62, 1949.

20. Bloomfield, A. L.: The natural history of chronic hepatitis (cirrhosis of the liver), Am. J. Med. Sci. 195:429, 1938.

21. Blumberg, H., and McCollum, E. V.: Prevention by choline of liver cirrhosis in rats on high fat, low protein diets, Science 93:598, 1941.

22. Blumenau, E.: Über Todesursache bei Lebercirrhose, Arch. Verdauungskr. 27:1, 1920.

23. Boles, R. S., and Clark, J. H.: The role of alcohol in cirrhosis of the liver; a clinical and pathologic study based on four thousand autopsies, J.A.M.A. 107:1200, 1936.

24. Bongiovanni, A. M., Blondheim, S. H., Eisenmenger, W. J., and Kunkel, H. G.: Effects of ACTH in patients with liver disease, J. Clin. Invest. 29:798, 1950.

25. Bongiovanni, A. M., and Eisenmenger, W. J.: Adrenal cortical metabolism in chronic liver disease, J. Clin. Endocr. 11:152, 1951.

26. Brock, J. F., and Autret, M.: Kwashiorkor in Africa, Bull. W.H.O., 5:1, 1952.

27. Burack, W. R., and Hollister, R. M.: Tuberculous peritonitis. A study of forty-seven proved cases encountered by a general medical unit in 25 years, Am. J. Med. 28:510, 1960.

28. Cameron, G. R., and deSaram, G. S. W.: A method for permanently dissociating the spleen from the portal circulation (the "marsupialised" spleen) and its use in the study of experimental liver cirrhosis, J. Path. Bact. 48:41, 1939.

29. Cameron, G. R., and Karunaratne, W. A. E.: Carbon tetrachloride cirrhosis in relation to liver regeneration, J. Path. Bact. 42:1, 1936.

30. Carbone, J., Sborov, V., Fanska, R., and Ringgold, K.: The effect of wine in decompensated hepatic cirrhosis, J. Clin. Invest. 36:878, 1957.

31. Chaikoff, I. L., Connor, C. L., and Biskind, G. R.: Fatty infiltration and cirrhosis of the liver in depancreatized dogs maintained with insulin, Am. J. Path. 14:101, 1938.

32. Chapman, C. B., Snell, A. M., and Rowntree, L. G.: Decompensated portal cirrhosis; report of one hundred and twelve cases, J.A.M.A. 97:237, 1931.

33. Child, C. G.: Shattuck lecture; portal circulation, New Engl. J. Med. 252:837, 1955.

34. Christian, H. A.: Bloody pleural fluid, unusual complication of cirrhosis of liver, Ann. Int. Med. 10:1621, 1937.

35. Clarke, J. S.: Influence of the liver upon gastric secretion, Am. J. Med. 29:740, 1960.

36. Cohen, S. I., Schmatolla, E., Bevans, M., and Patek, A. J., Jr.: Amino acid mixtures in the treatment of experimental dietary cirrhosis in the rat, Arch. Int. Med. 101:291, 1958.

37. Conn, H. O.: Spontaneous peritonitis and bacteremia in Laennec's cirrhosis caused by enteric organisms, Ann. Int. Med. 60:568, 1964.

38. Conn, H. O., and Lindenmuth, W. W.: Prophylactic portacaval anastomosis in cirrhotic patients with esophageal varices, New Engl. J. Med. 272:1255, 1965.

39. Connor, C. L.: The etiology and pathogenesis of alcoholic cirrhosis, J.A.M.A. 112:387, 1937.

40. ———: Fatty infiltration of the liver and the development of cirrhosis in diabetes and chronic alcoholism, Am. J. Path. 14:347, 1938.

41. Cowling, D. C.: Coagulation defects in liver disease, J. Clin. Path. 9:347, 1956.

42. Crews, R. H., and Faloon, W. W.: The fallacy of a low-fat diet in liver disease, J.A.M.A. 181:754, 1962.

43 Cullinan, E. R., King, R. C., and Rivers, J. S.: The prognosis of infectious hepatitis; a preliminary account of a long-term follow-up, Brit. Med. J. 1:1315, 1958.

44. Daft, F. S.: Experimental differentiation between liver necrosis and liver cirrhosis and some dietary factors affecting their

development, Ann. N. Y. Acad. Sci. *57*: 623, 1954.

45. Daft, F. S., Sebrell, W. H., and Lillie, R. D.: Production and apparent prevention of a dietary liver cirrhosis in rats, Proc. Soc. Exp. Biol. Med. *48*:228, 1941.

46. Dagradi, A., Sanders, D., and Stempien, S. J.: The sources of upper gastrointestinal bleeding in liver cirrhosis, Ann. Int. Med. *42*:852, 1955.

47. Davidson, C. S.: Cirrhosis of the liver treated with prolonged sodium restrictions; improvement in nutrition, hepatic function, and portal hypertension, J.A.M.A. *159*:1257, 1955.

48. ———: Medical management of cirrhosis of the liver, J. Chron. Dis. 2:55, 1955.

49. Davies, J. N. P.: Essential pathology of kwashiorkor, Lancet *1*:317, 1948.

50. ———: The pathology of dietary liver disease in tropical Africa, Ann. N. Y. Acad. Sci. *57*:714, 1954.

51. Davis, M. D.: Portal cirrhosis. A study of 100 consecutive autopsied cases, U. S. Armed Forces Med. J. *9*:57, 1958.

52. Dayan, A. D., and Williams, R.: Demyelinating peripheral neuropathy and liver disease, Lancet 2:133, 1967.

53. DeJosselin De Jong, R.: Leberzirrhose, pp. 38-120, Compt. rend. Prem. Conf. Soc. internat. de Path. géograph., Geneva, Kundig, 1931.

54. Dible, J. H.: Degeneration, necrosis, and fibrosis in the liver, Brit. Med. J. *1*:833, 1951.

55. Dible, J. H., McMichael, J., and Sherlock, S. P. V.: Pathology of acute hepatitis: aspiration biopsy studies of epidemic, arsenotherapy and serum jaundice, Lancet 2:402, 1943.

56. Dohan, F. C., Richardson, E. M., Bluemle, L. W., Jr., and Gvörgy, P.: Hormone excretion in liver disease, J. Clin. Invest. *31*:481, 1952.

57. Douglass, B. E., and Snell, A. M.: Portal cirrhosis: an analysis of 444 cases with notes on modern methods of treatment, Gastroenterology *15*:407, 1950.

58. Du Vigneaud, V., Chandler, J. P., Cohn, M., and Brown, G. B.: The transfer of the methyl group from methionine to choline and creatine, J. Biol. Chem. *134*: 787, 1940.

59. Dykes, P. W.: A study of the effects of albumin infusions in patients with cirrhosis of the liver, Quart. J. Med. *30*: 297, 1961.

60. Edmondson, H. A., Glass, S. J., and Soll, S. N.: Gynecomastia associated with cirrhosis of the liver, Proc. Soc. Exp. Biol. Med. *42*:97, 1939.

61. Entmacher, P. S., and Marks, H. H.: Diabetes in 1964: a world survey, Diabetes *14*:212, 1965.

62. Eppinger, H.: Die Leberkrankheiten, Vienna, Springer, 1937.

63. Erenoglu, E., Edreira, J. G., and Patek, A. J., Jr.: Observations on patients with Laennec's cirrhosis receiving alcohol while on controlled diets, Ann. Int. Med. *60*:814, 1964.

64. Evans, N., and Gray, P. A.: Laennec's cirrhosis. Report of 217 cases, J.A.M.A. *110*:1159, 1938.

65. Fagin, I. D., and Thompson, F. M.: Cirrhosis of the liver, an analysis of 71 cases, Ann. Int. Med. *21*:285, 1944.

66. Fainer, D. C., and Halsted, J. A.: Sources of upper alimentary tract hemorrhage in cirrhosis of the liver, J.A.M.A. *157*:413, 1955.

67. Faloon, W. W., Eckhardt, R. D., Murphy, T. L., Cooper, A. M., and Davidson, C. S.: An evaluation of human serum albumin in the treatment of cirrhosis of the liver, J. Clin. Invest. *28*:583, 1949.

68. Fernando, P. B., and Thanabalasunderam, R. S.: Infective hepatitis and cirrhosis of the liver, Quart. J. Med. *20*:403, 1951.

69. Finkbiner, R. B., McGovern, J. J., Goldstein, R., and Bunker, J. P.: Coagulation defects in liver disease and response to transfusion during surgery, Am. J. Med. *26*:199, 1959.

70. Fleming, R. G., and Snell, A. M.: Portal cirrhosis with ascites: an analysis of 200 cases with special reference to prognosis and treatment, Am. J. Dig. Dis. 9:115, 1942.

71. Flood, F. B.: Spontaneous perforation of the umbilicus in Laennec's cirrhosis with massive ascites, New Engl. J. Med. *264*: 72, 1961.

72. Foxwell, A.: Alcoholic cirrhosis of the liver, Brit. J. Med. *1*:393, 1896.

73. Frankel, J. J., Asbury, C. E., Jr., and Baker, L. A.: Hepatic insufficiency and cirrhosis in diabetes mellitus, Arch. Int. Med. *86*:376, 1950.

74. Franklin, M., Salk, M. R., Steigmann, F., and Popper, H.: Clinical, functional, and histologic responses of fatty metamorpho-

sis of human liver to lipotropic therapy, Am. J. Clin. Path. *18*:273, 1948.

75. Garceau, A. J., Chalmers, T. C., and the Boston Inter-Hospital Liver Group, The natural history of cirrhosis. 1. Survival with esophageal varices, New Engl. J. Med. *268*:469, 1963.

76. Garceau, A. J., and the Boston Inter-Hospital Liver Group, The natural history of cirrhosis. II. The influence of alcohol and prior hepatitis on pathology and prognosis, New Engl. J. Med. *271*:1173, 1964.

77. Garceau, A. J., Donaldson, R. M., Jr., O'Hara, E. T., Callow, A. D., Muench, H., and Chalmers, T. C.: A controlled trial of prophylactic portacaval-shunt surgery, New Engl. J. Med.: *270*:496, 1964.

78. Gilbert, A., and Herscher, M.: Des naevi artériels et capillaires dans les maladies du foie et des voies biliares, C. R. Soc. Biol. *55*:167, 1903.

79. Gillman, J., and Gillman, T.: Liver disease in Johannesburg; relation to pellagra, Lancet *1*:169, 1948.

80. Glass, S. J., Edmonson, H. A., and Soll, S. N.: Sex hormone changes associated with liver disease, Endocrinology *27*:749, 1940.

81. Goffart, M.: Étude clinique et biologique des épanchements pleuraux des cirrhotiques, Rev. belge Sci. méd. *10*:341, 1938.

82. Green, J., Mistilis, S., and Schiff, L.: Acute alcoholic hepatitis, Arch. Int. Med.: *112*:67, 1963.

83. Gross, J. B., Comfort, M. W., Wollaeger, E. E., and Power, M. H.: Total solids, fat, and nitrogen in the feces: V. A study of patients with primary parenchymatous hepatic disease, Gastroenterology *16*:140, 1950.

84. György, P., and Goldblatt, H.: Observations on conditions of dietary hepatic injury (necrosis, cirrhosis) in rats, J. Exp. Med. *75*:355, 1942.

85. ———: Treatment of experimental dietary cirrhosis of the liver in rats, J. Exp. Med. *90*:73, 1949.

86. György, P., Goldblatt, H., and Ganzin, M.: Dietary fat and cirrhosis of the liver. Gastroenterology *37*:637, 1959.

87. Hahn, R. D.: Syphilis of the liver, Am. J. Syph. *27*:529, 1943.

88. Hall, C. A.: Erythrocyte dynamics in liver disease, Am. J. Med. *28*:541, 1960.

89. Hardison, W. G., and Lee, F. I.: Prognosis in acute liver disease of the alcoholic patient, New Engl. J. Med.: *275*:61, 1966.

90. Harinasuta, U., Chomet, B., Ishak, K., and Zimmerman, H. J.: Steatonecrosis—Mallory body type, Medicine *46*:141, 1967.

91. Harper, A. E. Monson, W. J., Benton, D. A., and Elvehjem, C. A.: The influence of protein and certain amino acids, particularly threonine, on the deposition of fat in the liver of the rat, J. Nutr. *50*:383, 1953.

92. Harrington, W. J., Manheimer, R. H., Desforges, J. F., Minkel, H. P., Crow, C. B., and Stohlman, F.: The bleeding tendency in hepatocellular and obstructive jaundice, Bull. New Engl. Med. Center *12*:121, 1950

93. Hartroft, W. S. Experimental reproduction of human hepatic disease *in* Popper, H., and Schaffner, F. (eds.): Progress in Liver Disease, vol. 1, p. 68, New York, Grune and Stratton, 1961.

94. Henrikson, E. C.: Cirrhosis of the liver, Arch. Surg. *32*:413, 1936.

95. Henschen, F., and Bruce, T.: Ueber die Häufigkeit und Formen der Lebercirrhose in Stockholm, pp. 237-250, Compt. rend. Prem. Conf. Soc. internat. de Path. géograph., Geneva, Kundig, 1931.

96. Hershey, J. M.: Substitution of lecithin for raw pancreas in the diet of depancreatized dog, Am. J. Physiol. *93*:657, 1930.

97. Higginson, J., Grobbelaar, B. G., and Walker, A. R. P.: Hepatic fibrosis and cirrhosis in man in relation to malnutrition, Am. J. Path. *33*:29, 1957.

98. Himsworth, H. P.: Lectures on the Liver and Its Diseases, Cambridge, Mass., Harvard, 1950.

99. Hoagland, C. L.: The therapy of liver diseases, Bull. N. Y. Acad. Med. *21*:537, 1945.

100. Howard, R., and Watson, C. J.: Antecedent jaundice in cirrhosis of the liver, Arch. Int. Med. *80*:1, 1947.

101. Iseri, O. A., Lieber, C. S., and Gottlieb, L. S.: The ultra structure of fatty liver induced by prolonged ethanol ingestion, Am. J. Path. *48*:535, 1966.

102. Isselbacher, K. J., and Greenberger, N. J.: Metabolic effects of alcohol on the liver, N. Engl. J. Med. *270*:351, 402, 1964.

103. Jandl, J. H.: The anemia of liver disease: observations on its mechanism, J. Clin. Invest. *34*:390, 1955.

104. Jandl, J. H., and Lear, A. A.: Metabolism of folic acid in cirrhosis. Ann. Int. Med. *45*:1027, 1956.

105. Jaques, W. E.: The incidence of portal cirrhosis and fatty metamorphosis in patients dying with diabetes mellitus, New Engl. J. Med. *249*:442, 1953.

106. Jarrold, T., and Vilter, R. W.: Hemolytic observations in patients with chronic hepatic insufficiency. Sternal bone marrow morphology and bone marrow plasmacytosis, J. Clin. Invest. *28*:286, 1949.

107. Johnson, J. B.: The pathogenesis of azotemia in hemorrhage from the upper gastro-intestinal tract, J. Clin. Invest. *20*:161, 1941.

108. Johnston, R. F., and Loo, R. V.: Hepatic hydrothorax; studies to determine the source of the fluid and report of 13 cases, Ann. Int. Med. *61*:385, 1964.

109. Jolliffe, N., and Jellinek, E. M.: Vitamin deficiencies and liver cirrhosis in alcoholism. VII. Cirrhosis of the liver, Quart. J. Stud. Alcohol *2*:544, 1941.

110. Jolliffe, N., Wortis, H., and Stein, M. H.: Vitamin deficiencies and liver cirrhosis in alcoholism, Quart. J. Stud. Alcohol *2*:73, 1941.

111. Jones, P. N., Weinstein, I. M., Ettinger, R. H., and Capps, R. B.: Decreased red cell survival associated with liver disease, Arch. Int. Med. *95*:93, 1955.

112. Kalk, H.: Die chronischen Verlaufsformen der Hepatitis epidemica in Beziehung zu ihren anatomischen Grundlagen, Dtsch. med. Wschr. *72*:308, 1947.

113. Kontos, H. A., Shapiro, W., Mauck, H. P., and Patterson, J. L., Jr.: General and regional circulatory alterations in cirrhosis of the liver, Am. J. Med. *37*:526, 1964.

114. Kark, R. M., Morey, G. R., and Paynter, C. R.: Refeeding (nutritional) gynecomastia in cirrhosis of the liver. I. Clinical observations, Am. J. Med. Sci. *222*:154, 1951.

115. Karsner, H. T.: Morphology and pathogenesis of hepatic cirrhosis, Am. J. Clin. Path. *13*:569, 1943.

116. Keefer, C. S., and Fries, E. D.: The fatty liver—its diagnosis and clinical course, Trans. Ass. Am. Physicians *57*:283, 1942.

117. Kelty, R. H., Baggenstoss, A. H., and Butt, H. R.: The relation of the regenerated liver nodule to the vascular bed in cirrhosis, Gastroenterology *15*:285, 1950.

118. Kerr, D. N. S., Pearson, D. T., and Read, A. E.: Infection of ascitic fluid in patients with hepatic cirrhosis, Gut *4*:394, 1963.

119. Kessler, B. J., Seife, M., and Lisa, J. R.: Use of choline supplements in fatty metamorphosis of the liver, Arch. Int. Med. *86*:671, 1950.

120. Kiessling, K. H., and Tobé, U.: Degeneration of liver mitochondria in rats after prolonged alcohol consumption, Exp. Cell Res. *33*:350, 1964.

121. Kimber, C., Deller, D. J., Ibbotson, R. N., and Lander, H.: The mechanism of anaemia in chronic liver disease, Quart. J. Med. *34*:33, 1965.

122. Kirschbaum, J. D., and Sure, N.: Alcoholic cirrhosis of the liver, J. Lab. Clin. Med. *28*:721, 1943.

123. Klatskin, G.: Effect of alcohol on the liver, J.A.M.A. *170*:1671, 1959.

124. ————: Newer concepts of cirrhosis, Arch. Int. Med. *104*:899, 1959.

125. Klatskin, G., and Rappaport, E. M.: Late residuals in presumably cured acute infectious hepatitis, Ann. Int. Med. *26*:13, 1947.

126. Klatskin, G., Salter, W. T., and Humm, F. D.: Gynecomastia due to malnutrition. I. Clinical studies, Am. J. Med. Sci. *213*:19, 1947.

127. Klatskin, G., and Yesner, R.: Factors in the treatment of Laennec's cirrhosis. I. Clinical and histological changes observed during a control period of bed-rest, alcohol withdrawal, and a minimal basic diet, J. Clin. Invest. *28*:723, 1949.

128. Klopstock, F.: Über Milztumor, Icterus und Ascites bei Lebercirrhose, Virchows Arch. path. Anat. *187*:111, 1907.

129. Koszalka, M. F., Lindert, M. C. F., Snodgrass, H. M., and Lerner, H. B.: Hepatitis and its sequelae, including the development of portal cirrhosis, Arch. Int. Med. *84*:782, 1949.

130. Krarup, N. B., and Roholm, K.: The development of cirrhosis of the liver after acute hepatitis, elucidated by aspiration biopsy, Acta med. scand. *108*:306, 1941.

131. Kunkel, H. G., Labby, D. H., Ahrens, E. H., Shank, R. E., and Hoagland, C. L.: The use of concentrated serum al-

bumin in the treatment of cirrhosis of the liver, J. Clin. Invest. 27:305, 1948.

132. Kunkel, H. G., Labby, D. H., and Hoagland, C. L.: Chronic liver disease following infectious hepatitis. I. Abnormal convalescence from initial attack, Ann. Int. Med. 27:202, 1947.

133. Leevy, C. M., Zinke, M., Baber, J., and Chey, W. Y.: Observations on the influence of medical therapy on portal hypertension in hepatic cirrhosis, Ann. Int. Med. 49:837, 1958.

134. Leevy, C. M., Zinke, M. R., White, T. J., and Gnassi, A. M.: Clinical observations on the fatty liver, Arch Int. Med. 92:527, 1953.

135. Lewis, J. H., Ferguson, J. H., Spaugh, E., Fresh, J. W., and Zucker, M. B.: Acquired hypoprothrombinemia, Blood 12:84, 1957.

136. Lieber, C. S.: Metabolic derangement induced by alcohol, Ann. Rev. Med. 18:35, 1967.

137. Lieber, C. S., Jones, D. P., and DeCarli, L. M.: Effects of prolonged ethanol intake: production of fatty liver despite adequate diets, J. Clin. Invest. 44:1009, 1965.

138. Lieberman, F. L., and Reynolds, T. B.: Renal failure with cirrhosis; observations on the role of diuretics, Ann. Int. Med. 64:1221, 1966.

139. Lipp, W. F., and Lipsitz, M. H.: The clinical significance of the co-existence of peptic ulcer and portal cirrhosis, with special reference to the problem of massive hemorrhage, Gastroenterology 22:181, 1952.

140. Lloyd, C. W., and Williams, R. H.: Endocrine changes associated with Laennec's cirrhosis of the liver, Am. J. Med. 4:315, 1948.

141. Loeper, M., Loewe-Lyon, S., and Netter, A.: Les télangiectasies éruptives des hépatiques, Sang 11:677, 1937.

142. Lowry, J. V., Ashburn, L. L., Daft, F. S., and Sebrell, W. H.: Effect of alcohol in experimental liver cirrhosis, Quart. J. Stud. Alcohol 3:168, 1942.

143. Lucké, B.: The pathology of fatal epidemic hepatitis, Am. J. Path. 20:471, 1944.

144. Maddrey, W. C., and Iber, F. L.: Familial cirrhosis: a clinical and pathological study, Ann. Int. Med. 61:667, 1964.

145. McCartney, J. S.: Latent cirrhosis of the liver, Arch. Path. 16:817, 1933.

146. McDermott, W. V., Jr., Palazzi, H., Nardi, G. L., and Mondet, A.: Elective portal systemic shunt: an analysis of 237 cases, New Engl. J. Med. 264:419, 1961.

147. McIndoe, A. H.: Vascular lesions of portal cirrhosis, Arch. Path. Lab. Med. 5:23,1928.

148. McNee, J. W.: Liver and spleen: their clinical and pathological association, Brit. Med. J. 1:111, 1932.

149. Mallory, F. B.: Cirrhosis of the liver, New Engl. J. Med. 206:1231, 1932.

150. Mann, J. D., Wakim, K. G., and Baggenstoss, A. H.: The vasculature of the human liver: a study by the injection-cast method, Proc. Mayo Clin. 28:227, 1953.

151. Meigs, J. V., Armstrong, S. H., and Hamilton, H. H.: A further contribution to the syndrome of fibroma of the ovary with fluid in the abdomen and chest; Meigs syndrome, Am. J. Obstet. Gynec. 46:19, 1943.

152. Moon, V. H.: Histogenesis of atrophic cirrhosis, Arch. Path. 13:691, 1932.

153. ———: Experimental cirrhosis in relation to human cirrhosis, Arch. Path. 18:381, 1934.

154. Morlock, C. G., and Hall, B. E.: Association of cirrhosis, thrombopenia, and hemorrhagic tendency, Arch. Int. Med. 72:69, 1943.

155. Morrione, T. G.: Effect of estrogens on the testis in hepatic insufficiency, Arch. Path. 37:39, 1944.

156. Moschcowitz, E.: The pathogenesis of splenomegaly in hypertension of the portal circulation: "congestive splenomegaly," Medicine 27:187, 1948.

157. Moser, R. H., Rosenak, B. D., Pickett, R. D., and McIntire, C. R.: The prognosis of portal cirrhosis, an analysis of 62 cases, Gastroenterology 18:86, 1951.

158. Murphy, T. L., Chalmers, T. C., Eckhardt, R. D., and Davidson, C. S.: Hepatic coma, New Engl. J. Med. 239:605, 1948.

159. Murray, J. F., Dawson, A. M., and Sherlock, S.: Circulatory changes in chronic liver disease, Am. J. Med. 24:358, 1958.

160. Naeye, R. L.: Hemophilioid factors: acquired deficiencies in several hemorrhagic states, Proc. Soc. Exp. Biol. Med. 94:623, 1957.

161. Nazari, B.: Dupuytren's contracture associated with liver disease, J. Mt. Sinai Hosp. 33:69, 1966.

162. Norkin, S. A., Weitzel, R., Campagna-Pinto, D., MacDonald, R. A., and Mallory, G. K.: "Alcoholic" hyalin in human cirrhosis; histochemical studies, Am. J. Path. 37:49, 1960.

163. Ophuls, W.: A Stastical Survey of Three Thousand Autopsies, Stanford, Calif., Stanford Univ. Press, 1926.

164. Orenstein, L. L., and Goldfarb, W.: Note on incidence of syphilis in alcoholics, Quart. J. Stud. Alcohol 1:413, 1940.

165. Palmer, E. D., and Brick, I. B.: Sources of upper gastrointestinal hemorrhage in cirrhotic patients with esophageal varices, New Engl. J. Med. 248:1057, 1953.

166. Palmer, E. D., Brick, I. B., and Jahnke, E. J., Jr.: Esophageal varices without hemorrhage in cirrhosis: a proper indication for shunting procedures, New Engl. J. Med. 250:863, 1954.

167. Papper, S., Belsky, J. L., and Bleifer, K. H.: Renal failure in Laennec's cirrhosis of the liver. I. Description of clinical and laboratory features, Ann. Int. Med. 51:759, 1959.

168. Patek, A. J., Jr.: Treatment of alcoholic cirrhosis of the liver with high vitamin therapy, Proc. Soc. Exp. Biol. Med. 37:329, 1937.

169. ———: An evaluation of dietary factors in the treatment of Laennec's cirrhosis of the liver, J. Mt. Sinai Hosp. 14:1, 1947.

170. Patek, A. J., Jr., and deFritsch, N. M.: Evidence for genetic factors in the resistance of the rat to dietary cirrhosis, Proc. Soc. Exp. Biol. Med. 113:820, 1963.

171. Patek, A. J., Jr., deFritsch, N. M., and Hirsch, R. L.: Strain differences in susceptibility of the rat to dietary cirrhosis, Proc. Soc. Exp. Biol. Med. 121:569, 1966.

172. Patek, A. J., Jr., deFritsch, N. M., Kendall, F. E., and Hirsch, R. L.: Corn and coconut oil effects in dietary cirrhosis of rats, A.M.A. Arch. Path. 75:264, 1963.

173. Patek, A. J., Jr., Kendall, F. E., deFritsch, N. M., and Hirsch, R. L.: Effects of unsaturated fats on dietary-induced cirrhosis in the rat, A.M.A. Arch. Path. 79:494, 1965.

174. Patek, A. J., Jr., Oken, D. E., Sakamoto, A., deFritsch, N., and Bevans, M.: Recovery from dietary cirrhosis of the liver in the rat. Changes in hepatic collagen and in microscopic appearance, A.M.A. Arch. Path. 69:168, 1960.

175. Patek, A. J., Jr., and Post, J.: Treatment of cirrhosis of the liver by a nutritious diet and supplements rich in vitamin B complex, J. Clin. Invest. 20:481, 1941.

176. Patek, A. J., Jr., Post, J., Ratnoff, O. D., Mankin, H., and Hillman, R. W.: The dietary treatment of cirrhosis of the liver. Results in 124 patients observed during a ten year period, J.A.M.A. 138:543, 1948.

177. Patek, A. J., Jr., Post, J., and Victor, J. C.: The vascular "spider" associated with cirrhosis of the liver, Am. J. Med. Sci. 200:41, 1940.

178. Patek, A. J., Jr., Seegal, D., and Bevans, M.: The coexistence of cirrhosis of the liver and glomerulonephritis. Report of 14 cases, Am. J. Med. Sci. 221:77, 1951.

179. Perera, G. A.: The plasma volume in Laennec's cirrhosis of the liver, Ann. Int. Med. 24:643, 1946.

180. Peterson, O. L., Deutsch, E., and Finland, M.: Therapy with sulfonamide compounds for patients with damage to the liver, Arch. Int. Med. 72:594, 1943.

181. Phillips, G. B., and Davidson, C. S.: Acute hepatic insufficiency of the chronic alcoholic: clinical and pathological study, A.M.A. Arch. Int. Med. 94:585, 1954.

182. Phillips, G. B., Schwartz, R., Gabuzda, G. J., Jr., and Davidson, C. S.: The syndrome of impending hepatic coma in patients with cirrhosis of the liver given certain nitrogenous substances, New Engl. J. Med. 247:239, 1952.

183. Plough, I. C., Patek, A. J., Jr., and Bevans, M.: The relative effects of protein, choline, and methionine in the treatment of experimental dietary cirrhosis in the rat, J. Exp. Med. 96:221, 1952.

184. Pollack, A. D., and Gerber, I. E.: Abdominal visceral lesions associated with primary disease of the liver, Arch. Path. 36:608, 1943.

185. Pollard, H. M., Gracie, W. A., Jr., and Sisson, J. C.: Extrahepatic complications associated with cirrhosis of the liver, J.A.M.A. 169:318, 1959.

186. Popper, H., and Schaffner, F. (eds.): Response of the liver to injury in Progress in Liver Disease, vol. 1, p. 86, New York, Grune and Stratton, 1961.

187. Popper, H., Steigmann, F., Meyer, K., Kozoll, D. D., and Franklin, M.: Correlation of liver function and liver structure: clinical applications, Am. J. Med. 6:278, 1949.

188. Popper, H., and Szanto, P. B.: Fatty

liver with hepatic failure in alcoholics, J. Mt. Sinai Hosp. 24:1121, 1957.

189. Popper, H., Szanto, P. B., and Parthasarathy, M.: Florid cirrhosis. A review of 35 cases, Am. J. Clin. Path. 25:889, 1955.

190. Porta, E. A., Hartroft, W. S., and de la Iglesia, F. A.: Hepatic changes associated with chronic alcoholism in rats, Lab. Invest. 14:1437, 1965.

191. Post, J., Benton, J. G., Breakstone, R., and Hoffman, J.: The effects of diet and choline on fatty infiltration of the human liver, Gastroenterology 20:403, 1952.

192. Post, J., Gellis, S., and Lindenauer, H. J.: Studies on the sequelae of acute infectious hepatitis, Ann. Int. Med. 33:1378, 1950.

193. Post, J., and Rose, J. V.: Clinical, functional and histological studies in Laennec's cirrhosis of the liver, Am. J. Med. 8:300, 1950.

194. Post, J., Rose, J. V., and Shore, S. M.: Intravenous use of salt-poor human albumin. Effects in thirty-four patients with decompensated hepatic cirrhosis, A.M.A. Arch. Int. Med. 87:775, 1951.

195. Rao, M. V. R.: An investigation into "decompensated portal cirrhosis," Indian J. Med. Res. 21:389, 1933.

196. Rappaport, A. M.: Acinar units and the pathophysiology of the liver in Rouiller, C. (ed.): The Liver —Morphology, Biochemistry, Physiology, vol. I, pp. 266-320, New York, Academic Press, 1963.

197. Ratnoff, O. D.: Bleeding Syndrome; A Clinical Manual, Springfield, Ill., Thomas, 1960.

198. Ratnoff, O. D., and Patek, A. J., Jr.: The natural history of Laennec's cirrhosis of the liver, Medicine 21:207, 1942.

199. Reinberg, M. H., and Lipson, M.: The association of Laennec's cirrhosis with diabetes mellitus, Ann. Int. Med. 33:1195, 1950.

200. Report of Pathologists on Cirrhosis Study: Tr. 6th Liver Injury Conf., New York, Macy, 1947.

201. Reynolds, T. B., Geller, H. M., Kuzma, O. T., and Redecker, A. G: Spontaneous decrease in portal pressure with clinical improvement in cirrhosis, New Engl. J. Med. 263:734, 1960.

202. Reynolds, T. B., Redeker, A. G., and Kuzma, O. T.: Role of alcohol in pathogenesis of alcoholic cirrhosis in McIntyre, N., and Sherlock, S. (eds.): Therapeutic Agents and the Liver, p. 131, Philadelphia, Davis, 1965.

203. Richardson, W.: A note on racial incidence in portal cirrhosis, New Engl. J. Med. 218:257, 1938.

204. Ricketts, W. E., Lushbaugh, C. C., Kirsner, J. B., and Palmer, W. L.: Pathologic observations in portal cirrhosis, Gastroenterology 14:491, 1950.

205. Rivera, A., Rojas, E., and Sepúlveda, B.: Correlación entre las alteraciones anatómicas y funcionales del hígado, Rev. invest. clin. 4:137, 1952.

206. Rodman, T., Sobel, M., and Close, H. P.: Arterial oxygen unsaturation and the ventilation-perfusion defect of Laennec's cirrhosis, New Engl. J. Med. 263:73, 1960.

207. Rolleston, H. D., and McNee, J. W.: Diseases of the Liver, Gall-Bladder, and Bile-Ducts, ed. 3, London, Macmillan, 1929.

208. Romano, J.: Deficiency syndromes associated with chronic alcoholism: clinical study, Am. J. Med. Sci. 194:645, 1937.

209. Rosenak, B. D., Moser, R. H., and Howell, J. D.: Chronic and recurrent infectious hepatitis; its relationship to cirrhosis of the liver, J. Indiana Med. A. 42:897, 1949.

210. Rosenberg, D. H., and Walters, A.: Macrocytic anemia in liver disease, particularly cirrhosis, Am. J. Med. Sci. 192:86, 1936.

211. Rössle, R.: Entzündung der Leber in Henke, F., and Lubarsch, O.: Handbuch der speziellen pathologischen Anatomie und Histologie, Berlin, Springer, 1930.

212. Rowntree, L. G.: Considerations in cirrhosis of the liver, J.A.M.A. 89:1590, 1927.

213. Rupp, J., Cantarow, A., Rakoff, A. E., and Paschkis, K. E.: Hormone excretion in liver disease and in gynecomastia, J. Clin. Endocr. 11:688, 1951.

214. Russakoff, A. H., and Blumberg, H.: Choline as an adjuvant to the dietary therapy of cirrhosis of the liver, Ann. Int. Med. 21:848, 1944.

215. Rydell, R., and Hoffbauer, F. W.: Multiple pulmonary arteriovenous fistulas in juvenile cirrhosis, Am. J. Med. 21:450, 1956.

216. Schiff, L.: The use of steroids in liver disease, Medicine 45:565, 1966.

217. Schiff, L., Rich, M. L., and Simon, S. D.: The "haematopoietic principle" in the

diseased human liver, Am. J. Med. Sci. *196*:313, 1938.

218. Schiff, L., and Stevens, R. J.: Elevation of urea nitrogen content of the blood following hematemesis or melena, Arch. Int. Med. *64*:1239, 1939.

219. Schmitker, M. A., and Hass, G. M.: Histologic study of liver in patients affected with peptic ulcer, Am. J. Dig. Dis. *1*:573, 1934.

220. Schultz, J. C., Adamson, J. S., Jr., Workman, W. W., and Norman, T. D.: Fatal liver disease after intravenous administration of tetracycline in high dosage, New Engl. J. Med. *269*:999, 1963.

221. Schumacher, G. A.: Causative factors in the production of Laennec's cirrhosis with special reference to syphilis, Am. J. Med. Sci. *194*:693, 1937.

222. Sears, G. G., and Lord, F. T.: The symptoms and treatment of hepatic cirrhosis in the light of seventy-eight autopsies, Trans. Ass. Am. Physicians *17*:598, 1902.

223. Semmola, M., and Gioffredi, C.: 20th Cent. Pract., Baltimore, Wood, *9*:573, 1897.

224. Sepúlveda, B., Rojas, E., and Landa, L.: La etiologia de la cirrosis del higado tipo Laennec, Rev. invest. clin. *4*:321, 1952.

225. Sheehy, T. W., and Berman, A.: Anemia of cirrhosis, J. Lab. Clin. Med. *56*:72, 1960.

226. Sherlock, S.: Diseases of the Liver and Biliary System, ed. 3, Philadelphia, Davis, 1963.

227. Sherlock, S.: Post-hepatitic cirrhosis, Lancet *1*:817, 1948.

228. Shils, M. E., and Stewart, W. B.: Preventive influence of certain amino acids on experimental fatty liver of portal type, Proc. Soc. Exp. Biol. Med. *87*:629, 1954.

229. Simpson, D. P.: Hepatic regeneration and hyperplasia, Med. Clin. N. Amer. *47*:765, 1963.

230. Spies, T. D., and DeWolf, H. F.: Observations on the etiological relationship of severe alcoholism to pellagra, Am. J. Med. Sci. *186*:521, 1933.

231. Stahl, J., Roger, S., and Witz, J.: Essai d'interprétation du mécanisme de l'épreuve d'hyperammonièmie provoquée chez les cirrhotiques, C. R. Soc. Biol. *146*:1787, 1952.

232. Statistical Bulletin, Metropolitan Life Insurance Co., *46*:6, 1965; *48*:7, 1967.

233. Strauss, M. B.: The etiology of "alcoholic" polyneuritis, Am. J. Med. Sci. *189*:378, 1935.

234. Summerskill, W. H. J., Wolfe, S. J., and Davidson, C. S.: Response to alcohol in chronic alcoholics with liver disease, Lancet *1*:335, 1957.

235. Takada, A., Porta, E. A., and Hartroft, W. S.: Regression of dietary cirrhosis in rats fed alcohol and a "super diet," Am. J. Clin. Nutr. *20*:213, 1967.

236. Tanyol, H.: Correlation of hernia with portal cirrhosis. A reevaluation of the role of ascites, Am. J. Dig. Dis. *3*:444, 1958.

237. Tenney, B., Jr., and King, R. B.: Pregnancy coincident with cirrhosis of the liver; report of case, New Engl. J. Med. *208*:1157, 1933.

238. Thayer, W. S.: On the presence of a venous hum in the epigastrium in cirrhosis of the liver, Am. J. Med. Sci. *141*:313, 1911.

239. Thompson, W. P.: The pathogenesis of Banti's disease, Ann. Int. Med. *14*:255, 1940.

240. Thorn, G. W., Armstrong, S. H., Jr., and Davenport, V. D.: Chemical, clinical, and immunological studies on the products of human plasma fractionation. XXXI. The use of salt-poor concentrated human serum albumin solution in the treatment of hepatic cirrhosis, J. Clin. Invest. *25*:304, 1946.

241. Tirimurti, T. S., and Rao, M. V. R.: The incidence of portal cirrhosis of the liver in Vizagapatam, based on a critical study of autopsy records and observations, Indian M. Gaz. *69*:74, 1934.

242. Tisdale, W. A., and Klatskin, G.: The fever of Laennec's cirrhosis, Yale J. Biol. Med. *33*:94, 1960.

243. Trowell, H. C.: Malignant malnutrition (Kwashiorkor), Trans. Roy. Soc. Trop. Med. Hyg. *42*:417, 1949.

244. Tucker, H. F., and Eckstein, H. C.: Effect of supplementary methionine and cystine on production of fatty livers by diet, J. Biol. Chem. *121*:479, 1937.

245. Tumen, H. J.: Cirrhosis of the liver *in* Bockus, H. L.: Gastro-enterology, vol. 3, pp. 293-332, Philadelphia, Saunders, 1947.

246. Tumen, H., and Bockus, H. L.: Clinical significance of serum proteins in hepatic diseases compared with other liver function tests, Am. J. Med. Sci. *193*:788, 1937.

247. Tyagaraja, S.: Early pathological changes in the liver in the tropics with special reference to cirrhosis, Ceylon J. Med. Sci. (Section D) 4:119, 1937.

248. Vachon, A., Tête, R., Paliard, P., and Malluret, J.: Les septicémies et bactériémies des cirrhoses alcooliques, Rev. Lyon. méd. 15:343, 1966.

249. Vedel, and Puech, A.: Considerations sur les épanchements pleuraux au cours de la cirrhose de Laënnec, Bull. Soc. sc. méd. et biol., Montpellier 8:120, 1927.

250. Victor, M., Adams, R. D., and Cole, M.: The acquired (non-Wilsonian) type of chronic hepatocerebral degeneration, Medicine 44:395, 1965.

251. Vint, F. W.: Cirrhosis of the liver in East African natives, Kenya E. Afr. med. J. 7:349, 1931.

252. Volwiler, W., Jones, C. M., and Mallory, T. B.: Criteria for the measurement of results of treatment in fatty cirrhosis, Gastroenterology 11:164, 1948.

253. Wakim, K. C., and Mann, F. C.: The intrahepatic circulation of blood, Anat. Rec. 82:233, 1942.

254. Waldstein, S. S., Popper, H., Szanto, P. B., and Steigmann, F.: Liver cirrhosis. Relation between function and structure based on biopsy studies, A.M.A. Arch. Int. Med. 87:844, 1951.

255. Wang, C. F.: Cirrhosis of the liver. I. Etiology, symptomatology, liver function tests and gastric juice findings, Chin. J. Med. 50:891, 1936.

256. Waterlow, J. C.: Fatty liver disease in infants in the British West Indies, Med. Res. Council Special Report Series, No. 263, p. 78, 1948.

256a. Watson, C. J.: The prognosis and treatment of hepatic insufficiency, Ann. Int. Med. 31:405, 1949.

257. Watson, C. J., and Hoffbauer, F. W.: The problem of prolonged hepatitis with particular reference to the cholangiolitic type and to the development of cholangiolitic cirrhosis of the liver, Ann. Int. Med. 25:195, 1946.

258. Wavburn, E., and Guerard, C. R.: Relation between multiple peripheral neuropathy and cirrhosis of the liver, Arch. Int. Med. 66:161, 1940.

259. Webster, G. T.: Cirrhosis of the liver among rats receiving diets poor in protein and rich in fat, J. Clin. Invest. 21:385, 1942.

260. Wertheimer, E., Shapiro, B., and Fodor-Salomonowicz, I.: Stability of fibrinogen in normal and pathological plasma, Brit. J. Exp. Path. 25:121, 1944.

261. Westerfeld, W. W.: The intermediary metabolism of alcohol, Am. J. Clin. Nutr. 9:426, 1961.

262. Westerfeld, W. W., and Schulman, M. P.: Metabolism and caloric value of alcohol, J.A.M.A. 170:197, 1959.

263. Whitesell, F. B., Jr., and Snell, A. M.: Thrombopenia and increased capillary fragility in hepatic disease, JA.M.A. 140:1071, 1949.

264. Wilbur, D. L., Wood, D. A., and Willett, F. M.: Primary carcinoma of the liver, Ann. Int. Med. 20:453, 1944.

265. Wilgram, G. F.: Experimental Laennec type of cirrhosis in monkeys, Ann. Int. Med. 51:1134, 1959.

266. Winje, M. E., Harper, A. E., Benton, D. A., Boldt, R. E., and Elvehjem, C. A.: Effect of dietary amino acid balance on fat deposition in livers of rats fed low protein diets, J. Nutr. 54:155, 1954.

267. Wolfe, S. J., Summerskill, W. H. J., and Davidson, C. S.: Thickening and contraction of palmar fascia (Dupuytren's contracture) associated with alcoholism and hepatic cirrhosis, New Engl. J. Med. 255:559, 1956.

268. Wollaeger, E. E., and Keith, N. M.: Epigastric thrill and murmur in a case of cirrhosis of the liver with general vascular signs of arteriovenous fistula, Proc. Staff Meet., Mayo Clin. 13:33, 1938.

269. Yang, C. S., Cirrhosis of the liver. Report of 84 cases, Nat. M. J. China 14:195, 1928.

270. Yenikomshian, H. A.: Non-alcoholic cirrhosis of the liver in Lebanon and Syria, J.A.M.A. 103:660, 1934.

271. Yonemoto, R. H., and Davidson, C. S.: Herniorrhaphy in cirrhosis of the liver with ascites, New Engl. J. Med. 255:733, 1956.

272. Zaki, F. G., Hoffbauer, F. W., and Grande, F.: Fatty cirrhosis in the rat. VIII. Effect of dietary fat, A.M.A. Arch. Path. 80:323, 1965.

273. Zieve, L.: Jaundice, hyperlipemia, and hemolytic anemia: a heretofore unrecognized syndrome associated with alcoholic fatty liver and cirrhosis, Ann. Int. Med. 48:471, 1958.

274. Zieve, L., and Hill, E.: Influence of alcohol consumption on hepatic function in healthy gainfully employed men, J. Lab. Clin. Med. *42*:705, 1953.

275. ————: Two varieties of hemolytic anemia in cirrhosis, S. Med. J. *54*:1347, 1961.

Texts:

276. Kleckner, M. S., Jr.: Cirrhosis of the Liver. Springfield, Ill., Thomas, 1960.
Popper, H. and Schaffner, F.: Liver: Structure and Function. New York, Blakiston, 1957.
Sherlock, S. See reference 226.

19

Postnecrotic Cirrhosis

ARTHUR J. PATEK, JR., M.D.

Postnecrotic cirrhosis of the liver has been variously named "healed or chronic yellow atrophy," "toxic cirrhosis,"[31] "posthepatitic cirrhosis," "multiple nodular hyperplasia"[32] and "coarsely nodular cirrhosis." Marchand was probably the first to delineate this type from Laennec's, or alcoholic, cirrhosis. Although many workers believe that clinical

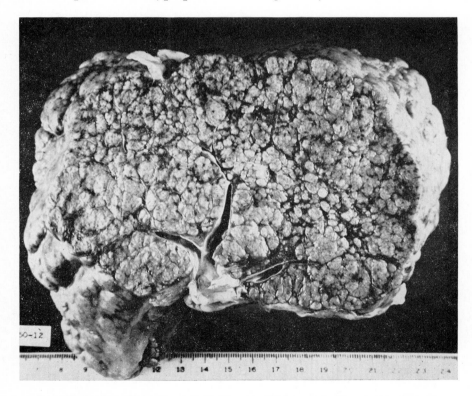

Fig. 19–1. (A) Coarsely nodular liver exhibits marked variation in pattern and character of nodulation. Of note are the broad trabecularlike bands of connective tissue which course irregularly. (B) Close-up macroscopic view, emphasizing the variable size of the large regenerated nodules and the irregular nature of the scarring. (C) Photomicrograph, revealing the characteristic broad septal scarring. The large parenchymal nodules reveal no pseudolobulation but contain multiple distorted lobules, many portal canals and asymmetrically located central veins.

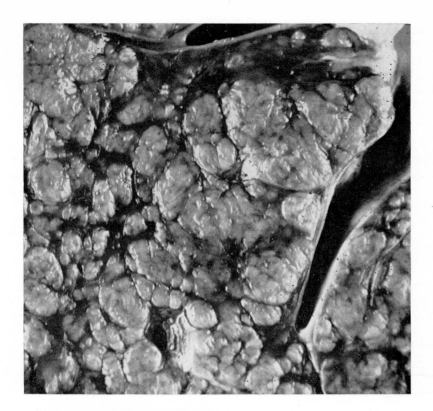

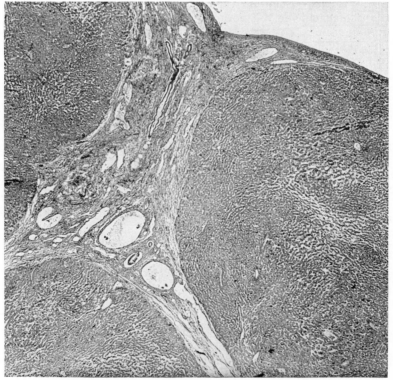

FIG. 19–1. (*Continued*). B (*Top*). C (*Bottom*).

and pathologic distinctions between these cirrhoses are not feasible on the basis of available data, the trend is to regard postnecrotic cirrhosis as an entity.

PATHOLOGY

The liver appears small and discolored. Its surface shows depressed areas and large nodules of varying size (Fig. 19–1). At times a large portion of a lobe, in particular the left lobe, is atrophied. The depressed areas, which are composed of broad and narrow bands of connective tissue containing few if any parenchymal cells, probably represent collapsed stroma.

One may find several portal triads bunched together in one area of scar tissue. Hyperplasia of cholangiole-like structures also is common in the septa, together with an inflammatory cellular reaction.[48] The nodules represent proliferating liver cells which lack the orderly arrangement of normal liver tissue. In some areas focal necroses are present. Fatty changes are slight or absent. Frequently, bizarre liver cells are seen. In other portions of the liver the normal lobular structure may be retained.

These findings may be contrasted with Laennec's cirrhosis, in which the liver typically shows finely diffuse and uniform changes. Small nodules of liver cells are surrounded by narrow bands of connective tissue, giving the effect of an orderly arrangement. Bizarre liver cells are uncommon, but fatty changes usually are pronounced.

Intermediate forms of cirrhosis occur which make the differentiation almost impossible, as pointed out by a group of pathologists conferring on this subject.[42] In order to show up the differences between these diseases, Baggenstoss and Stauffer compared 43 fatal cases each of "posthepatitic" cirrhosis and alcoholic cirrhosis.[2] In the first group the clinical data suggested viral hepatitis as the causative agent. Other causes for hepatitis were excluded. The alcoholic group presumably excluded other causes for hepatic damage except for 2 cases with history of viral hepatitis 3 and 9 years previously. In the alcoholic group jaundice occurred in 86 per cent, an unusu-

ally high incidence. In their detailed analysis, the authors point out the overlapping that occasionally occurs. In 7 cases of posthepatitic cirrhosis the pathology was similar to Laennec's, and in 4 cases of alcoholic cirrhosis the reverse was true.

There is little doubt that certain cases of chronic, progressive hepatitis lead to diffuse cirrhosis that closely resembles the alcoholic type. However, the reverse situation is less plausible. When the postnecrotic type of cirrhosis occurs in an alcoholic, it seems more likely that the patient had indeed postnecrotic cirrhosis, or a mixed lesion. In 13 of 45 cases[39] with classic pathologic features of postnecrotic cirrhosis there was associated alcoholism. In two larger and more recent series the incidence of alcoholism was 35[28] and 56 per cent[15] respectively.

INCIDENCE

Postnecrotic cirrhosis comprised 8.4 per cent of a series of 550 cases of cirrhosis reported by Mallory.[31] Karsner estimated that 10 per cent of his cases of cirrhosis were of this group.[23] In 124 cases of cirrhosis reported from our medical service,[36] 15 (11 per cent) were presumed to be postnecrotic. Of these, 7 were proved at autopsy. In England, where alcoholism is less frequent than in the past, postnecrotic cirrhosis is becoming relatively more frequent.[24, 46, 49]

AGE AND SEX

All ages are involved. The distribution in Baggenstoss and Stauffer's series was 4 to 77 years, with an average age of 36.[2] In another series the average age was 57, with 75 per cent of patients being 50 years or more.

The sex distribution appears to be about equal for males and females. In 4 reported series the per cent males were respectively 63,[31] 40,[2] 40[39] and 59.[28] In a series of 108 cases reported from Denmark over 95 per cent occurred in women, the large majority of whom were over 45 years of age.[6] This represented a special group of cases, etiology undetermined, and for the most part a subacute form of the disease.

Since postnecrotic cirrhosis apparently

can follow hepatic injury due to several different unrelated causes, the wide age distribution and relatively equal sex incidence (except for the Danish experience) is not surprising.

ETIOLOGY

In searching for factors that might bear on etiology, a series of 45 autopsied cases was analyzed.[39] The data are shown in Table 19–1. Similar findings have been reported by others.[15, 24, 27, 28, 46] In roughly a fourth to one-half the cases no etiology is apparent. On this account the disease has been described as cryptogenic. Fifteen to 45 per cent give a history of antecedent hepatitis, or an illness that resembles viral hepatitis. In some of these, hepatitis has occurred in the past, with a latent period of 5 or more years before signs of cirrhosis appeared. More often the disease seems to be initiated by acute hepatitis which then progresses to cirrhosis. On the basis of studies with serial needle biopsies of the liver[26, 43, 46] there is little doubt that postnecrotic cirrhosis can evolve from viral hepatitis, although proof of viral etiology is wanting.

The relation to viral hepatitis is special, for, of the total number of known cases of viral hepatitis, only a small percentage develop postnecrotic cirrhosis, estimated at 0.7 to 3.5 per cent in sporadic cases.[28, 38] In two large epidemics of hepatitis there were virtually no instances of postnecrotic cirrhosis.[11, 55] Presumably these were mild.

The incidence among anicteric cases has not been studied as extensively, but some evidence suggests that such patients are more prone to develop the disease. Klatskin has described 9 cases of nonicteric hepatitis which culminated in postnecrotic cirrhosis.[26] In a recent report from Taiwan, 5 of 36 patients (14 per cent) with anicteric hepatitis, proved by biopsy, developed postnecrotic cirrhosis.[10] It seems plausible that patients who develop postnecrotic cirrhosis without apparent cause have had anicteric viral hepatitis. A serious handicap is the lack of means to establish whether the antecedent hepatitis was viral in nature, or due to a particular strain of virus, or due to the same virus as that of infectious hepatitis.

TABLE 19–1.   ANTECEDENT FACTORS IN 45 CASES OF POSTNECROTIC CIRRHOSIS

	NUMBER OF PATIENTS
Past history (5 to 12 years) of jaundice or hepatitis	6
Present illness initiated by acute hepatitis	12
Hepatotoxic chemicals (CCl_4; arsenicals)	8
Chronic alcoholism	13
No apparent contributory factors	12
Malnutrition—data inadequate	

Other viruses, notably that of infectious mononucleosis, often produce anicteric hepatitis. In certain epidemics such as that in Denmark in the 1940's the viral strain was unusually virulent.[6]

Ordinarily infectious hepatitis is a benign disease followed by complete healing. The rare occurrence of postnecrotic cirrhosis suggests that other modifying conditions predispose to this disease. Differences in strain virulence, as suggested above, are probably involved. The susceptibility of the host may also be important. Infectious hepatitis may be particularly severe during pregnancy. The high incidence of postnecrotic cirrhosis in Denmark was predominantly in postmenopausal women.

Environmental factors may be important, in particular alcoholism. The incidence of alcoholism in several series in the United States is 30 to 50 per cent.[15, 28, 39] It is much less conspicuous in Europe.[24] The mechanism whereby alcoholism predisposes to this lesion is not known. It is possible that alcohol serves to lower resistance to the hepatitis virus or to interfere with an immune or protective response. A high incidence of alcoholism among carriers of hepatitis virus has been reported.[34] This may or may not bear on the problem.

PATHOGENESIS

The studies of Daft, Sebrell and Lillie,[12] Himsworth and Glynn[19a] and others[17, 44] show the importance of nutritional factors in experimental necrosis of the liver. Rats placed on low-protein diets deficient in tocopherol, cystine or selenium develop massive necrosis of the liver.[19, 44, 45] The lesions are prevented by appropriate supplements of tocopherol, cystine or methionine as a source of cystine. Whether there is a human counterpart to this experimental disease is unknown. It has been suggested that the atypical nodular cirrhosis seen in the African Rand and in the Punjab of India are analogous lesions.

Smetana believes that postnecrotic cirrhosis is the "result of healing and repair of destroyed parenchyma after a single, severe, near-fatal injury to the liver produced by viral hepatitis."[47] The nodules often appear to be of the same age. However, in other instances the lesions seem to be the end result of chronic viral hepatitis over a considerable period of time.

The basis for the progressive nature of the disease is not understood. Several possibilities have been suggested, such as continued active viral infection and anoxic necrosis of regenerating lobules. In the case of lupoid hepatitis, which is a form of postnecrotic cirrhosis in young persons, it has been suggested that activity of the disease is related to an autoimmune process.[14, 29, 30] Evidence for this is not sufficiently specific.[9]

SYMPTOMATOLOGY

The chief symptoms and signs of the disease, as observed in a series of 45 cases,[39]

are shown in Tables 19–2 and 19–3. Their incidence is compared with similar data obtained in a series of Laennec's cirrhosis.[40] Comparison with other reported series of cases reveals differences in the incidence of various symptoms and signs. However, the differences are not important, and they appear to reflect the selectivity of cases under study, as well as the stage of the disease at which hospitalization occurred.

The onset in 12 instances of postnecrotic cirrhosis resembled acute viral hepatitis with malaise, anorexia, nausea, vomiting, abdominal distress, jaundice, light-colored stools and dark urine. This syndrome is decidedly at variance with Laennec's cirrhosis, in which this stormy onset would be unusual. However, in other patients the illness began gradually, and the initial symptoms provided no clue to the type of cirrhosis present.

In tracing the history of cryptogenic cases, one finds that a considerable number of patients give the story of recovering from hepatitis 5 to 15 years before the onset of hepatic failure. This variability in onset was described long ago by Bloomfield.[8] Kelsall, Stewart and Witts noted that 17 of 35 patients developed the disease with an abrupt onset resembling acute hepatitis, whereas 18 developed symptoms gradually.[24] Sherlock[46] and Klatskin[26] have reported similar findings.

Abdominal pain was a common complaint,

TABLE 19–2. SYMPTOMS OF POSTNECROTIC CIRRHOSIS IN 45 PATIENTS[39] COMPARISON WITH LAENNEC'S CIRRHOSIS (386 PATIENTS)

SYMPTOMS	NUMBER OF CASES	PER CENT OF CASES	PER CENT OF CASES OF LAENNEC'S CIRRHOSIS[40]
Abdominal pain	35	78	31
Anorexia	26	58	35
Nausea	21	47	33
Weight loss	18	40	53
Hemorrhagic phenomena	18	40	26
Hematemesis	15	33	27
Vomiting	15	33	30
Weakness at or near onset	14	31	21
Diarrhea	13	29	20
Malaise at or near onset	10	22	3
Pruritus	7	16	3
Oligomenorrhea or amenorrhea	7 of 27 ♀	26	7

TABLE 19–3. PHYSICAL SIGNS OF POSTNECROTIC CIRRHOSIS IN 45 PATIENTS[39]
COMPARISON WITH LAENNEC'S CIRRHOSIS (386 PATIENTS)

PHYSICAL SIGNS	NUMBER OF CASES	PER CENT OF CASES	PER CENT OF CASES OF LAENNEC'S CIRRHOSIS[40]
Jaundice	40	89	65
Ascites	40	89	78
Palpable liver	34	76	75
Edema	32*	71	61
Palpable spleen	19	42	44
Fever without apparent cause	18	40	24
Hemorrhoids	15	33	27
Dilated veins	14	31	24
Hydrothorax	12	27	6
Liver breath	11	24	..
Vascular spiders	10	22	..
Acneiform rash	9	20	..
Palmar erythema	7	..	..

* Including 2 patients without ascites, 4 patients before ascites was noted, and 2 patients with nephritis.

being present in almost 80 per cent of patients. Except for one patient with peptic ulcer and one with portal vein thrombosis, the pain apparently was related to the hepatic disease. It usually is episodic and at times is associated with jaundice and fever. Occasionally, it is severe, crampy and colicky, and may simulate biliary colic.[54]

In addition to abdominal pain, 41 of 45 patients had one or more symptoms referable to the gastrointestinal tract, such as anorexia, nausea, vomiting, "heartburn" or diarrhea. These symptoms—abdominal pain and gastrointestinal distress—seemed to be more pronounced and frequent in postnecrotic than in Laennec's cirrhosis.

Bleeding tendencies in the form of epistaxis, gingival bleeding and purpura were frequent in this series as well as others.[2, 7, 15, 24]

The physical signs of postnecrotic cirrhosis are similar to those of Laennec's, the differences being qualitative or related to time. Malnutrition, for example, is less conspicuous in the postnecrotic type; one third of the patients were described as well nourished. Jaundice is an early and persistent sign, and it is apt to be fairly marked in degree. When it is accompanied by clay-colored stools the disease picture may be

mistaken for primary biliary cirrhosis.[21] In the latter, higher values for serum cholesterol, alkaline phosphatase and serum lipids are the rule.

Ascites, one of the first signs of hepatic failure in Laennec's cirrhosis, is a relatively late sign in postnecrotic cirrhosis and indicates far-advanced disease. Once it appears it tends to remain constant. In the series of MacDonald and Mallory only 30 per cent of 168 patients had ascites on admission to the hospital, whereas 70 per cent had ascites at the time of autopsy.[28]

LABORATORY FINDINGS

Laboratory findings in 45 cases are indicated in Table 19–4. Here, too, the changes are similar to those encountered in Laennec's cirrhosis but with some qualitative differences. Serum globulin, serum bilirubin and alkaline phosphatase tend to be somewhat higher in postnecrotic cirrhosis. According to Watson[51] and Baggenstoss and Stauffer[2] moderate leukocytosis is commonplace in Laennec's but unusual in postnecrotic cirrhosis. During periods of activity, characterized by fever and jaundice, serum transaminase values may be increased, particularly the SGOT.[43]

TABLE 19–4. LABORATORY FINDINGS IN 45 CASES OF POSTNECROTIC CIRRHOSIS[39]
CHARACTER CHANGES

Red blood count	3 to 4 million per cu. mm.
Hemoglobin	9 to 12 Gm. per 100 cc.
Mean corp. volume	100 to 113 cu. mm.
Reticulocytosis	Occasional
Fragility test	Normal
White blood count	Normal
Differential count	Normal (Eosinophils 7 to 14% in 4 patients)
Sedimentation rate	More than 20 mm./hr. in 70%
Serum albumin	Less than 3.0 Gm. in 80%
Serum globulin	More than 4.1 Gm. in 50% (chiefly gamma)
Cephalin flocculation	Positive in over 90%
Thymol turbidity	Positive in over 90%
Bromsulphalein retention	Positive in over 90%
Serum bilirubin	More than 5 mg./100 cc. in 50%
Urine urobilinogen	Increased in over 90%
Stool stercobilinogen	Occasional decrease (7 of 24 patients)
Alkaline phosphatase	Less than 10 B.U. in 10 ⎫
	Between 10 and 19 B.U. in 9 ⎬ (total, 22 patients)
	Between 22 and 28 B.U. in 3 ⎭

DIAGNOSIS

It is apparent from the foregoing discussion, that the criteria are not sharply defined. The chief difficulty arises when pathologic findings include features of both Laennec's and postnecrotic cirrhosis. It has been suggested that in these cases postnecrotic cirrhosis represents a final pathway of portal cirrhosis.[37] This is not entirely satisfactory as an explanation, since the majority of cases of Laennec's cirrhosis at autopsy do not reveal this progression. Moreover the majority of postnecrotic cirrhoses are seen in nonalcoholics. For the present it seems more reasonable to regard this intermediate group as "mixed" or unclassified.

Another subgroup of postnecrotic cirrhosis presents cholestatic features which suggest primary biliary cirrhosis.[50] In general these patients show more signs of hepatocellular injury than do those with primary biliary disease. In the latter, cholestasis and hepatosplenomegaly are common but with little functional derangement until late in the disease. Needle biopsy of the liver may be helpful in differentiating these cases.

COMPLICATIONS

The complications encountered relate chiefly to *infection* and *esophageal hemor-rhage*. In a series of 45 cases infections were frequent: 8 had peritonitis, 8 had pneumonia, and 5 had phlegmonous enteritis.[39] Chronic glomerulonephritis occurred in 3, and pyelonephritis in 4 patients. Hematemesis, presumably from esophageal varices, occurred in 33 per cent, as compared with 27 per cent of a series with Laennec's cirrhosis (cf. Table 19–2). Baggenstoss and Stauffer[2] reported hematemesis to be less frequent in the postnecrotic group.[2] It is possible that the differences are not significant but are related to the small number of cases involved.

In a series of 60 cases Kleckner recorded gastrointestinal hemorrhage in 30 per cent.[27] Garceau and associates reported upper gastrointestinal bleeding in 53 per cent of 154 cases—an unusually high incidence.[15] In the latter series there was also a high incidence of alcoholism (56 per cent).

Cholelithiasis is a fairly common complication. This was found in 23 per cent of the cases reported by MacDonald and Mallory.[28]

Hepatoma is more frequent in postnecrotic cirrhosis than in Laennec's cirrhosis. The usual incidence in Laennec's cirrhosis is about 4 per cent, whereas 10 to 15 per cent is not uncommon in postnecrotic cirrhosis. (See Chap. 24, Tumors of the Liver.)

18. Harvey, A. M., Shulman, L. E., Tumulty, P. A., Conley, C. L., and Schoenrich, E. H.: Systemic lupus erythematosus: review of the literature and clinical analyses of 138 cases, Medicine *33*:291, 1954.

19. Himsworth, H. P., and Glynn, L. E.: Massive hepatic necrosis and diffuse hepatic fibrosis (acute yellow atrophy and portal cirrhosis): their production by means of diet, Clin. Sci. *5*:93, 1945.

19a. ———: Toxipathic and trophopathic hepatitis, Lancet *1*:457, 1944.

20. Holman, H., and Tomasi, T.: "Lupoid" hepatitis, Med. Clin. N. Amer. *44*:633, No. 3, 1960.

21. Jones, W. A., and Tisdale, W. A.: Post-hepatitic cirrhosis clinically simulating extrahepatic biliary obstruction (so-called "primary biliary cirrhosis"), New Engl. J. Med. *268*:629, 1963.

22. Joske, R. A. and King, W. E.: The "L. E.-Cell" phenomenon in active chronic viral hepatitis, Lancet *2*:477, 1955.

23. Karsner, H. T.: Morphology and pathogenesis of hepatic cirrhosis, Am. J. Clin. Path. *13*:569, 1943.

24. Kelsall, A. R., Stewart, A., and Witts, L. G.: Subacute and chronic hepatitis, Lancet *2*:195, 1947.

25. Kern, F., Jr., Vinnik, I. E., Struthers, J. E., Jr., and Hill, R. B.: The treatment of chronic hepatitis with adrenal cortical hormones, Am. J. Med. *35*:310, 1963.

26. Klatskin, G.: Subacute hepatic necrosis and postnecrotic cirrhosis due to anicteric infections with hepatitis virus, Am. J. Med. *25*:333, 1958.

27. Kleckner, M. S.: Cirrhosis of the Liver, Springfield, Ill., Thomas, 1960.

28. MacDonald, R. A., and Mallory, G. K.: Natural history of postnecrotic cirrhosis. A study of 221 autopsy cases, Am. J. Med. *24*:334, 1958.

29. MacKay, I. R.: The problem of persisting destructive disease of the liver, Gastroenterology *40*:617, 1961.

30. Mackay, I. R., Taft, L. I., and Cowling, D. C.: Lupoid hepatitis, Lancet *2*:1323, 1956.

31. Mallory, F. B.: Cirrhosis of the liver, New Engl. J. Med. *206*:1231, 1932.

32. Marchand, F.: Ueber Ausgang der acuten Leberatrophie in multiple knotige Hyperplasie, Beitr. Path. Anat. *17*:206, 1895.

33. Mistilis, S. P., and Schiff, L.: Steroid therapy in chronic hepatitis, Arch. Int. Med. *113*:54, 1964.

34. Neefe, J. R., Norris, R. F., Reinhold, J. G., Mitchell, C. B., and Howell, D. S.: Carriers of hepatitis virus in the blood and viral hepatitis in whole blood recipients. I. Studies on donors suspected as carriers of hepatitis virus and as sources of post-transfusion viral hepatitis, J.A.M.A. *154*:1066, 1954.

35. Nefzger, M. D., and Chalmers, T. C.: The treatment of acute infectious hepatitis; ten year follow-up study of the effects of diet and rest, Am. J. Med. *35*: 299, 1963.

36. Patek, A. J., Jr., Post, J., Ratnoff, O. D., Mankin, H., and Hillman, R. W.: The dietary treatment of cirrhosis of the liver. Results in 124 patients observed during a ten year period, J.A.M.A. *138*:543, 1948.

37. Popper, H., Rubin, E., Krus, S., and Schaffner, F.: Postnecrotic cirrhosis in alcoholics, Gastroenterology *39*:669, 1960.

38. Post, J., Gellis, S., and Lindenauer, H. J.: Studies on sequelae of acute infectious hepatitis, Ann. Int. Med. *33*:1378, 1950.

39. Ratnoff, O. D., and Patek, A. J., Jr.: Postnecrotic cirrhosis of the liver, J. Chron. Dis. *1*:266, 1955.

40. ———: The natural history of Laennec's cirrhosis of the liver, Medicine *21*:207, **1942.**

41. Read, A. E., Sherlock, S., and Harrison, C. V.: Active "juvenile" cirrhosis as part of a systemic disease, and the effect of corticosteroid therapy, Gut *4*:378, 1963.

42. Report of Pathologists on Cirrhosis Study: Tr. 6th Liver Injury Conf., New York, Macy, 1947.

43. Schaefer, J. W., Schiff, L., Gall, E. A., and Oikawa, Y.: Progression of acute hepatitis to postnecrotic cirrhosis, Am. J. Med. *42*:348, 1967.

44. Schwartz, K.: Dietetic hepatic injuries and the mode of action of tocopherol, Ann. N. Y. Acad. Sci. *52*:225, 1949.

45. Schwartz, K., and Faltz, C. M.: Selenium as integral part of factor 3 against dietary necrotic liver degeneration, J. Am. Chem. Soc. *79*:3292, 1957.

46. Sherlock, S.: Post-hepatitis cirrhosis, Lancet *1*:817, 1948.

47. Smetana, H. F.: Histogenesis of coarse nodular cirrhosis, Lab. Invest. *5*:175, 1956.

48. Steiner, P. E.: Precision in the classification of cirrhosis of the liver, Am. J. Path. *37*:21, 1960.

49. Summerskill, W. H. J., Davidson, C. S.,

Dible, J. H., Mallory, G. K., Sherlock, S., Turner, M. D., and Wolfe, S. J.: Cirrhosis of the liver. A study of alcoholic and non-alcoholic patients in Boston and London, New Engl. J. Med. 262:1, 1960.

50. Tisdale, W. A.: Subacute hepatitis, N. Engl. J. Med. 268:85, 138, 1963.

51. Watson, C. J.: Some observations on recognition and treatment of the commoner forms of hepatic cirrhosis, Minnesota Med. 35:125, 1952.

52. Willcox, R. G., and Isselbacher, K. J.: Chronic liver disease in young people.

Clinical features and course in 33 patients, Am. J. Med. 30:185, 1961.

53. Williams, R.: The place of steroid therapy in the treatment of liver disease, Med. Clin. N. Amer. 47:801, 1963.

54. Yazigi, R., Armas-Cruz, R., Silva, S., and Ossandon, M.: Fibrosis and nodular hyperplasia of the liver (post-necrotic cirrhosis): clinical and pathological study of 9 cases, Gastroenterology 18:587, 1951.

55. Zieve, L., Hill, E., Nesbitt, S., and Zieve, B.: The incidence of residuals of viral hepatitis, Gastroenterology 25:495, 1953.

20

Biliary Cirrhosis

WILLIAM T. FOULK, M.D., AND ARCHIE H. BAGGENSTOSS, M.D.

Biliary cirrhosis is that hepatic cirrhosis which develops as a consequence of obstructive biliary tract disease. An obstructive lesion may be located in the extrahepatic biliary tree (obstructive or secondary biliary cirrhosis), or obstruction may be due to an inflammatory lesion, usually of obscure cause, of the interlobular bile ducts (primary biliary cirrhosis). Certain clinical features characterize the disease. Cirrhosis develops slowly over months or years. Robust health is frequently maintained for several years despite evidence of obstructive biliary disease, such as pruritus, jaundice, hepatomegaly, splenomegaly and increased serum levels of alkaline phosphatase, cholesterol and phospholipids. In some instances, very high serum lipid levels lead to the appearance of xanthomatous deposits in the skin. Hepatocellular function remains good for long periods with normal albumin and prothrombin levels in the serum.

In its broad clinical context the syndrome may be observed in the absence of histologic criteria for the diagnosis of cirrhosis. Classic clinical features may be observed when hepatic morphology is that of a chronic, nonsuppurative cholangitis with an inflammatory process of the portal ductules and periductules without cirrhosis. Needle biopsy may distinguish secondary from primary biliary cirrhosis but in some cases may be inadequate for a definitive differentiation between extrahepatic biliary obstruction and the intrahepatic lesion of primary biliary cirrhosis. When there has been no gallbladder or biliary tract surgery prior to the onset of symptoms and when abdominal pain or recurrent chills and fever are absent, it may be difficult to separate the secondary from the primary disease. Increase in serum levels of free cholesterol and phospholipids with xanthomatosis is a striking feature when present. Hyperlipemia may occur in both primary and secondary biliary cirrhosis; however, it is likely that severe hyperlipemia is more frequently absent than present. It may be that selection of cases of primary biliary cirrhosis has been inaccurate because of insistence on a particular level of serum cholesterol or lipids for confirmation of the diagnosis.

PRIMARY BILIARY CIRRHOSIS OF UNKNOWN CAUSE

In most cases of primary biliary cirrhosis the cause is obscure. The disease occurs most frequently in women in the fourth to sixth decades of life. Most series of cases reported a low incidence in males,[3, 29, 82] although others have not found this sex distribution.[21, 72] Perhaps the female preponderance has been due to some extent to a tendency to require the findings of extreme hyperlipemia and xanthomatosis for the diagnosis of primary biliary cirrhosis. Among patients with primary biliary cirrhosis, hyperlipemia may be more likely to develop in women than in men, but the clinical diagnosis now seems to be made more frequently in the absence of xanthomatosis. Nonxanthomatous primary biliary cirrhosis probably predominates, even in women. No familial, congenital or ethnic

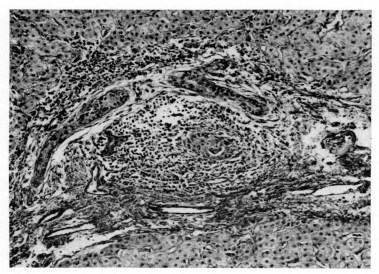

Fig. 20–1. Biopsy, after an illness of 10 months, interpreted as chronic nonsuppurative cholangitis of interlobular ducts, with focal necrosis of limiting plate with lymphocytic and Kupffer cell reaction. (Hematoxylin and eosin; × 155.)

predisposition to the disease has been reported.

ILLUSTRATIVE CASE

When this 38-year-old woman was seen in February, 1958, she had pruritus, jaundice and fatigue. The pruritus had begun the previous May, and the jaundice, 1 month later; in September of that year she had noted increased fatigue. She reported having dark urine and light-colored stools. There was no history of allergy, drug exposure, hepatitis or blood transfusions.

Examination revealed icterus of the skin and sclerae. The skin was dry, thickened and excoriated. The edge of the liver was rounded, smooth and not tender and was palpable 6 cm. below the costal margin; the spleen was not palpable.

Laboratory Findings. The pertinent laboratory data were: serum bilirubin, total 5.0 mg./100 ml. and direct 4.6 mg./100 ml.; alkaline phosphatase, 110.7 K-A units; thymol turbidity, 2 units; cephalin cholesterol flocculation, 3+; cholesterol, 612 mg./100 ml. plasma; phospholipids, 823 mg./100 ml. plasma; fatty acids, 744 mg./100 ml. plasma; total lipids, 1,356 mg./100 ml. plasma; albumin, 4.6 Gm./100 ml. serum; globulin, 3.25 Gm./100 ml. serum with slightly increased α_2 and β.

Surgical Findings. No gallstones or duct obstruction was found at operation or on a T-tube cholangiogram. Wedge biopsy of the liver revealed mild bile stasis and a chronic nonsuppurative cholangitis involving the interlobular

and septal ducts together with focal necrosis of the limiting plate with a lymphocytic and Kupffer cell reaction (Fig. 20–1).

Course. T-tube drainage relieved the pruritus completely. During 2 years of T-tube drainage, total lipids ranged from 700 to 1,000 mg./100 ml. plasma (Fig. 20–2); serum bilirubin, 2 to 6 mg./100 ml.; and alkaline phosphatase, 70 to 170 K-A units. Hepatomegaly persisted.

May 1960. The T-tube became plugged, drainage ceased and pruritus recurred.

June 1960. The patient was icteric and her skin was thick and excoriated. Total lipids were 3,218 mg./100 ml. plasma, with cholesterol 1,200 and phospholipids 2,000 mg./100 ml. Cholestyramine was given at a dosage of 10 Gm./day. The pruritus was relieved in 1 month, but total lipids remained at 2,000 mg./100 ml. (Fig. 20–2).

Nov. 1960. Xanthomata appeared on the palms and elbows.

Nov. 1961. The patient was tired but active. Jaundice persisted, pruritus was mild and the skin was dark and thickened. Xanthomata were on the palms, elbows, forearms, feet and gluteal folds. The liver was palpable 10 cm. below the costal margin and the spleen was palpable at 3 cm. Laboratory data were: total lipids, 2,074 mg./100 ml. plasma; alkaline phosphatase, 162 K-A units; serum bilirubin, 6.7 mg./100 ml.; fecal fat excretion, 30 Gm./24 hr.; albumin, 2.34 Gm./100 ml. serum, with normal globulin fractions. No varices were detectable roentgenographically. Needle biopsy of the liver revealed moderate bile stasis and a continuing necrosis of the limiting plate as well as focal necrosis with a polymorphonuclear and Kupffer cell reaction. Broadening and lengthening of portal tracts with septal formation was more advanced. Interlobular ducts were reduced in number.

April 1962. Mild pruritus and persistent jaundice were present. The skin was dark; the xanthomata were softer and smaller. Hepatosplenomegaly and moderate ascites were noted. Total lipids were 1,674 mg./100 ml. plasma.

Jan. and May 1962. Needle biopsies of the liver appeared similar to those seen in November, with a reduction in lobular parenchyma and many portal tracts without interlobular ducts (Fig. 20–3).

Sept. 1964. Gastrointestinal hemorrhage occurred.

July 1965. The patient died in hepatic coma. Bile ducts were patent at autopsy and the liver was nodular. Histologic examination revealed severe diffuse bile stasis and the presence of small regenerative nodules with broad internodular zones consisting of lymphocytes, fibroblasts and collagen. Lymphatic channels

were increased and interlobular ducts were reduced in number (Fig. 20–4).

This case illustrates the insidious onset, the slow but progressive course, the development of xanthomata and their subsidence with increasing cellular dysfunction, and the common terminal complications of gastrointestinal bleeding and hepatic coma, all of which are classic manifestations of primary biliary cirrhosis. Abdominal pain and symptoms of cholangitis are absent.

CLINICAL FINDINGS

The onset of primary biliary cirrhosis is most often insidious. A history of exposure to toxic agents, cholestatic drugs, jaundiced persons, blood transfusions or parenteral therapy is seldom obtained. In 10 per cent of 43 female patients with primary biliary cirrhosis the onset of symptoms occurred during pregnancy,[29] which may suggest some hormonal influence in the disease and

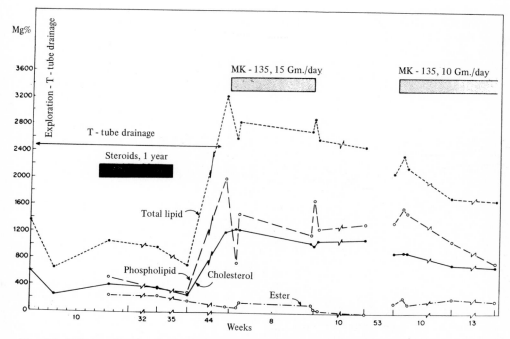

FIG. 20–2. Serum lipid values in patient with primary biliary cirrhosis. Note rapid decrease with drainage of the common bile duct and striking and rapid increase when external drainage terminated. Xanthomata appeared first after 8 weeks of cholestyramine (MK-135) therapy. Second trial of cholestyramine seemed more effective in lowering serum lipids; in this trial, xanthomata were beginning to resolve after 13 weeks.

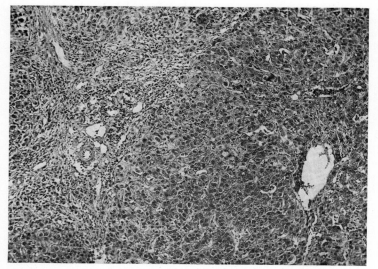

FIG. 20–3. Same case as Figure 20–1, biopsy 4 years later. Note continuing necrosis of limiting plate, broadening of portal tract, destruction of interlobular ducts and persistence of normal vascular relationships. (Hematoxylin and eosin; × 100.)

raises the question of a relationship in these patients to cholestatic jaundice of late pregnancy. An initial acute phase of illness is uncommon.

Pruritus is the commonest initial complaint and may be present for months or years before the onset of clinical jaundice. Pigmentation of the skin appears as the pruritus persists and is often darkest in areas accessible to scratching (Fig. 20–5). The skin becomes rough and thickened, probably due both to trauma and vitamin A deficiency. Later in the course of the disease

a growth of fine hair may develop on the face and extremities. Spider angiomata are less frequent and less prominent than in postnecrotic and alcoholic cirrhosis.

In those patients in whom persistently high serum levels of lipids develop, *xanthelasma* and plane and tuberous *xanthomata* are found (Fig. 20–6). In xanthelasma, yellowish plaques of lipid are deposited in the skin of the eyelids, commonly near the inner canthus. Xanthelasma occurs when the total serum lipid level is greater than 1,300 mg./100 ml. for several months. When the

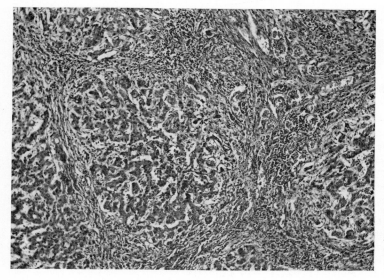

FIG. 20–4. Same case as represented in Figures 20–1 and 20–3, section taken at autopsy 8 years, 2 months after onset. Note regenerative nodules, bile stasis and atypical ductular proliferation. (Hematoxylin and eosin; × 75.)

FIG. 20–5. Pigmentation of skin in patient with primary biliary cirrhosis of 4 years' duration without hyperlipemia or xanthomata.

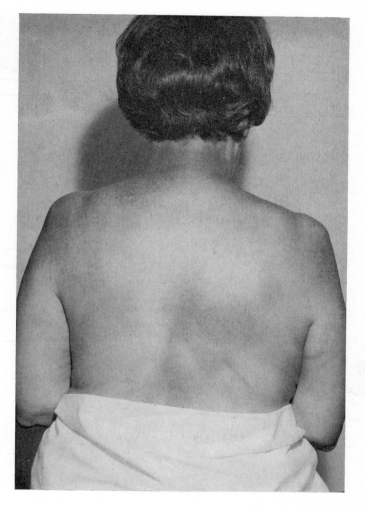

total serum lipid level persists above 2,000 mg./100 ml., plane and tuberous xanthomata develop.[1] Plane xanthomata are seen most often in the palmar creases, over the neck and trunk, and especially under the breasts. Tuberous xanthomata develop on extensor surfaces of the extremities, particularly on the elbows, knuckles, knees and Achilles tendon. On the hands and feet the deposits may be tender and sensitive to pressure. Xanthomata develop slowly and, as hepatic function deteriorates, they slowly resolve. The increase in serum lipid level must persist for several months before skin deposition is apparent. For this reason, xanthomata may be absent in the presence of

a high serum lipid level early in the disease and may persist for several months after the level has decreased later in the course of biliary cirrhosis.

Jaundice may be absent in the early stages of primary biliary cirrhosis and in some instances is not clinically evident for years. The absence of jaundice may imply that hepatocellular function remains good. We have followed a few patients for more than 10 years in whom clinical icterus has not appeared. In others, jaundice develops early in the course of the disease. With progression of the disease the jaundice usually becomes intense. Levels of serum lipids and alkaline phosphatase are increased but

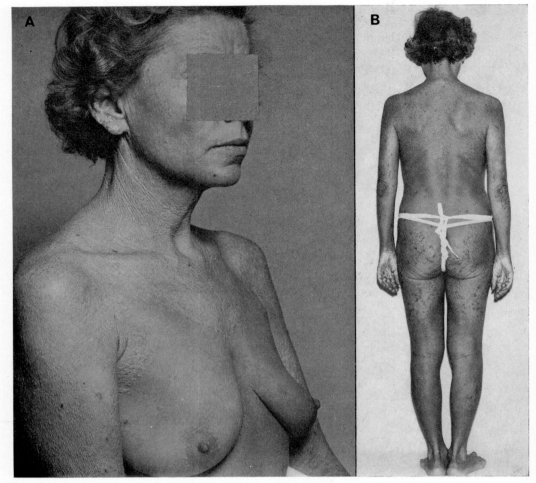

Fig. 20–6. Active, robust patient with xanthomatous primary biliary cirrhosis of 2 years' duration.

do not correlate with the level of serum bilirubin. The serum concentration of bile salts is usually increased. The characteristic increases in serum bile salts and alkaline phosphatase may reflect the primary ductal pathology and disturbed bile secretory physiology in the disease.

The *liver* is almost invariably enlarged and is usually palpable 4 to 10 cm. below the costal margin. Biliary cirrhosis, primary or secondary, is an unlikely diagnosis if the liver is not enlarged. The liver is firm, is sometimes irregularly nodular and is not tender. Splenomegaly is frequent and is observed more often in patients who have

histologic evidence of cirrhosis than of cholangiolitic hepatitis without cirrhosis. Splenomegaly does not necessarily indicate the presence of clinically significant portal hypertension, although the latter is an important complication of biliary cirrhosis. The spleen may enlarge several years prior to variceal bleeding or roentgenologic or esophagoscopic evidence of gastric or esophageal varices. Ascites and edema are late findings in primary biliary cirrhosis.

Diarrhea may be a complaint and, even in the absence of clinical jaundice, the description of the stool may suggest steatorrhea. Disturbances in bile flow and, perhaps, abnormalities in the chemical composition of the bile lead to impaired fat digestion and excess fat excretion in the stool. With this the fat-soluble vitamins A, D and K are malabsorbed. Because the liver cells function well until late in the disease process, the increased prothrombin time resulting from poor vitamin K absorption is readily corrected by parenteral vitamin K therapy or the oral administration of a water-soluble preparation of the vitamin. Failure of vitamin D and calcium absorption in the presence of steatorrhea results in osteomalacia. Later, as hepatocellular function and protein synthesis deteriorate, osteoporosis may complicate the osteomalacia.[83] Bone fractures related to minor trauma and collapse of vertebrae with pain and loss of height are common clinical findings.

Tests of hepatic function give results compatible with a diagnosis of obstructive jaundice. Serum cholesterol and alkaline phosphatase levels are increased early in the course of primary biliary cirrhosis, often when serum bilirubin levels are slightly increased or normal. The serum is clear rather than lactescent, even though lipid levels are high. This finding reflects the significant increase of serum phospholipid with lesser increase in neutral fat.[2] Serum triglycerides are normal or only mildly increased. Very high alkaline phosphatase levels are the rule: the average serum alkaline phosphatase value in 49 patients with primary biliary cirrhosis was 112 K-A units.[29] The source of the alkaline phosphatase appears to be the epithelium of bile ductules.[19] Transaminase levels in the serum are increased comparably to those in extrahepatic biliary obstruction. Cephalin cholesterol flocculation and thymol turbidity are variable and often normal. Protein synthesis is undisturbed early in the course of primary biliary cirrhosis, and serum albumin levels are normal until late in the disease when hepatocellular function begins to fail. An increase of the α_2- and β-globulins is frequently observed on electrophoresis; this probably reflects the hyperlipemic state because reportedly the serum lipids are associated with the β-globulin fraction in patients with biliary cirrhosis and hyperlipemia.[49] γ-Globulin levels in the serum may be normal or moderately increased.

Hematologic abnormalities include anemia, macrocytosis and the presence of target cells. As in all patients with cirrhosis, loss of blood is the most frequent cause of anemia and is usually due to bleeding esophageal varices. Anemia may occur in primary biliary cirrhosis before varices develop and may be the result of hemolysis. This has been confirmed by chromium-51 erythrocyte survival studies and by increases of fecal urobilinogen excretion to above normal levels during the period of hemolysis. The cause of the hemolytic episodes is not always clear. Hypersplenism plays a major role but deficiencies of vitamin B_{12}, folic acid and pyridoxine may be significant factors in the depressed erythrocyte survival.[41]

Primary biliary cirrhosis is usually fatal. The average duration of life from onset of symptoms is 5 years, with a range of 1 to 15 years. There are rare patients who, having run the gamut of symptoms—including deep jaundice, pruritus, hyperlipemia with xanthomatosis, osteoporosis and acute hemolytic episodes—are living a reasonably normal existence albeit with chronic but relatively inactive cirrhosis some 12 to 15 years after onset of symptoms (Figs. 20–16 and 20–17). One must assume that the processes that initiate and perpetuate the biliary cirrhosis become inactive. In the majority of cases, however, the disease pursues a relentless, if slow, course toward hepatocellular failure and portal hypertension with bleeding from esophageal varices.

The possibility of a silent extrahepatic biliary obstruction must not be overlooked. Unrelieved extrahepatic obstructive jaundice is also fatal and is discussed subsequently. For many years it has been advised that all patients in whom primary biliary cirrhosis is diagnosed have surgical exploration of the extrahepatic biliary tree. Surgery is well tolerated by patients with an intrahepatic obstructive process. Surgical exploration, if done, must include at least surgical cholangiography and wedge biopsy of the liver. Common duct exploration and tube drainage also should be considered. Prolonged surgical drainage of the common duct prevents pruritus and xanthomatosis.

Serum levels of bile acids and lipids tend to decrease rapidly after surgical biliary drainage (Fig. 20–2). Unfortunately, tubes in the common duct may become plugged. Stony debris forms in the tube and ducts, and the tube can erode the duct wall. For these reasons, surgical biliary drainage should not be continued for more than 6 to 9 months.

Recently, *percutaneous transhepatic cholangiography*[34] has been helpful in the exclusion of an extrahepatic biliary obstruction in patients with presumed primary biliary cirrhosis. Unfortunately, in this disease the intrahepatic ducts are small and few in number, and a good flow of contrast medium through the biliary ductal system is not achieved. Frequently, the biliary tree is not visualized. When this occurs, either the nonvisualization of an extrahepatic biliary block must be accepted as diagnostic of primary biliary cirrhosis or surgical exploration and cholangiography must be done as

a subsequent procedure to prove ductal patency.

TREATMENT

In primary biliary cirrhosis the symptoms are treated. To date, no agent can arrest the inflammatory ductular process which destroys the interlobular ducts, ductules and limiting plate with ultimate fibrosis and loss of lobular architecture. In view of some evidence suggesting that immune factors perpetuate primary biliary cirrhosis, immunosuppressive drugs might be useful therapeutic agents. Their use to date has been sporadic and no controlled study has been reported. Corticosteroids have not proved of therapeutic value.[83]

Pruritus may be relieved by surgical biliary drainage, as noted, but is usually equally well alleviated by the anion exchange resin, cholestyramine. This agent binds bile salts in the gut, preventing their enterohepatic circulation and usually induc-

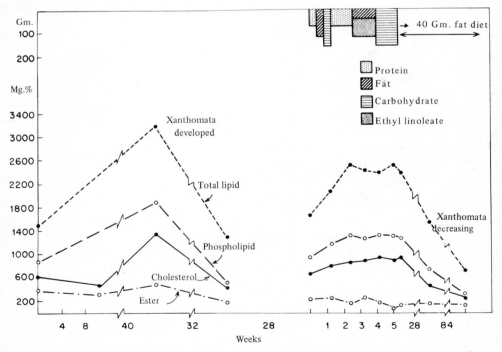

Fig. 20–7. Variability of serum lipids in patient with primary biliary cirrhosis, showing ineffectiveness of ethyl linoleate in reducing serum lipid levels in short-term trial and decrease of lipid levels as disease neared termination.

ing a decrease of serum bile acid levels.[17] Recently, bile acid concentrations on the skin have been reported to be higher in pruritic as opposed to nonpruritic hepatic disease.[79] Surgical drainage of the bile duct and cholestyramine both tend to decrease the serum lipid level and thus xanthomata may be absorbed or prevented (Fig. 20–2). Cholestyramine may increase the steatorrhea of primary biliary cirrhosis but its long-term use in these patients has had no apparent adverse effect.[78] If bile flow becomes completely obstructed, cholestyramine fails to relieve pruritus. Ten to 15 Gm. of cholestyramine given daily for more than 6 years in one patient has seemed to neither augment nor retard the progress of her disease. Cholestyramine given orally in dosages of 10 to 12 Gm. daily is indicated for the relief of pruritus and may prevent xanthomatosis in primary biliary cirrhosis. Methyl testosterone and norethandrolone have relieved pruritus, but both cause an increase in serum bilirubin levels; the mechanism by which these agents relieve pruritus is obscure.

Supplemental doses of vitamins A, D and K must be administered parenterally or water-soluble preparations must be given orally because the absorption of these vitamins is impaired in the presence of steatorrhea. A diet adequate in calories and protein should be provided. Protein intake may need to be restricted late in the disease when hepatocellular failure with evidence of encephalopathy ensues. Dietary restriction of fat or the provision of unsaturated or medium-chain triglycerides in the diet may diminish fatty diarrhea. Short-term trials of dietary supplementation of unsaturated fats have not significantly affected serum lipid levels (Fig. 20–7).

When bleeding from esophageal varices occurs, patients with primary biliary cirrhosis often tolerate surgical portal-systemic shunting well. Such an operation is definitely indicated in those patients who have variceal bleeding while hepatocellular function remains good. The procedure may be lifesaving and may permit several additional years of useful life. Construction of a portal-systemic shunt for hemorrhage occurring late in the disease, when hepatocellular failure is advanced, carries the same high risk and small chance of prolonging life as it does in advanced hepatocellular failure from any cause.

PRIMARY BILIARY CIRRHOSIS OF KNOWN CAUSE

Symptoms, clinical findings and abnormalities of hepatic function indistinguishable from those of primary or idiopathic biliary cirrhosis may be observed in association with viral hepatitis, after the administration of certain drugs or in some patients with chronic ulcerative colitis.

Clinicians have recognized for some time that tests of hepatocellular function may give relatively normal results in certain patients with viral hepatitis while signs and laboratory findings of obstructive jaundice predominate. Dubin and colleagues reported an epidemic of cholestatic viral hepatitis,[25] but with sporadic cases it is difficult to establish the viral etiology of a cholestatic episode. In most cases, the illness is brief and recovery is the rule. There is evidence that in rare instances cholangiolitic infectious hepatitis causes biliary cirrhosis.[44, 91] In these sporadic cases, the viral etiology of the syndrome cannot be proved because tests specific for detection of the virus have not been developed. Some clinical data strongly suggest that primary biliary cirrhosis occasionally occurs after infectious hepatitis.

It is more firmly established that drugs can cause chronic cholestatic jaundice and a clinical syndrome of primary biliary cirrhosis. In 1940, cholestatic jaundice was reported to be associated with arsphenamine therapy in 12 patients.[40] Biopsies of the liver showed inflammatory reaction around interlobular bile ductules and slight fibrosis. High plasma levels of cholesterol, alkaline phosphatase and bilirubin were observed. These patients all recovered, but chronic intrahepatic obstructive jaundice with xanthomatosis and histologic evidence of biliary cirrhosis occasionally has been reported.[18] We observed a young man in whom cholestasis developed after neoarsphenamine administration. He had pruritus, jaundice and xanthomatosis with a bilirubin level of 5.6 mg./100 ml. serum, alkaline phosphatase of 77 Bodansky units and cholesterol of 1,068 mg./100 ml. plasma. Three years later, clinical and laboratory findings were normal but liver biopsy showed cirrhosis. Fourteen years later he reported that his health was excellent.

Arsenicals are now less frequently used in therapy, but other drugs, particularly phenothiazines, currently are common etiologic agents in cholestatic jaundice which may be chronic and clinically may mimic primary biliary cirrhosis. Chlorpromazine is the most commonly incriminated etiologic agent but one can assume that any drug that causes cholestatic jaundice may produce severe and chronic symptoms and the complete clinical picture of primary biliary cirrhosis. Although it is generally assumed that chronic intrahepatic obstructive jaundice due to chlorpromazine ultimately resolves over a period of 2 to 3 years,[71] we have found that hepatic function abnormalities occasionally persist beyond 6 years. More recently, Walker and Combes described a case of biliary cirrhosis induced by chlorpromazine in which portal hypertension developed; death resulted from bleeding esophageal varices and hepatic failure.[89] Presumably, drug-induced biliary cirrhosis differs in no way from primary biliary cirrhosis, including the mode of death.

Some observations with respect to drug-induced chronic intrahepatic obstructive jaundice are of interest. Primary biliary cirrhosis is most often reported to occur preponderantly in females (85 to 90 per cent of cases) whereas the clinical picture of chronic arsphenamine jaundice is found predominantly in males. Of course, this may reflect only a higher incidence of arsphenamine therapy in men. Chlorpromazine jaundice affects males and females in equal numbers but those instances in which the clinical picture resembles primary biliary cirrhosis seem to be reported most often in women. Also it appears that pregnant women are more likely to develop cholestatic jaundice due to chlorpromazine. Extreme hyperlipemia leading to xanthomatosis is uncommon in males in reported series

of primary biliary cirrhosis,[29] but xanthomatosis has not been infrequent in males with drug-induced chronic intrahepatic obstructive jaundice. However, the selection of cases as examples of the so-called primary type of biliary cirrhosis may be somewhat biased.

Hepatic disease in association with chronic ulcerative colitis may present the clinical and laboratory profiles of obstructive jaundice (see also Chap. 8). Cirrhosis in chronic ulcerative colitis is usually of the postnecrotic type but portal zone inflammation[46] and pericholangitis[10, 88] as well as chronic cholestatic jaundice[43, 85] are found in some patients with chronic ulcerative colitis. Cases of biliary cirrhosis in association with chronic ulcerative colitis have been reported[43, 77, 88] and it has been suggested that the cirrhosis results from progression of the pericholangitis.[43] Holdsworth and coworkers found only one instance of biliary cirrhosis among 22 patients with ulcerative colitis and chronic liver disease.[43] They observed two patients with chronic cholestatic jaundice and a histologic picture of interlobular hepatitis or pericholangitis without cirrhosis. The question was raised whether biliary cirrhosis represents the final stage of a progression of chronic cholestatic jaundice. The effects of drugs and transfusions administered to patients with ulcerative colitis may tend to obscure the cause of chronic liver disease when it develops. That autoimmune hemolytic anemia is associated in some instances with biliary cirrhosis occurring with ulcerative colitis[77, 88] suggests the possibility of a common autoimmune basis for the hepatic and the colonic disease.

PATHOLOGY OF PRIMARY BILIARY CIRRHOSIS

In both types of biliary cirrhosis the pathologic disturbance is chronic and there is no general agreement as to what stage in the development of the lesion the term "cirrhosis" applies. This reflects the lack of agreement on a definition of hepatic cirrhosis in general. Gibson and Robertson defined hepatic cirrhosis as including parenchymal degeneration, fibrosis and nodular parenchymal repair.[35] We are in complete agreement

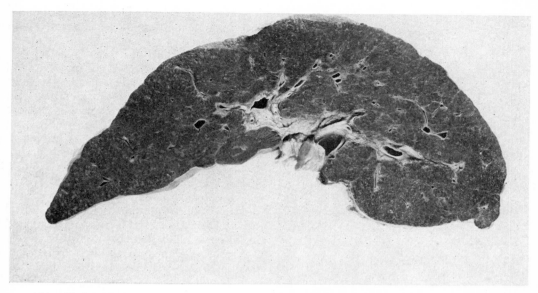

Fig. 20–8. Gross appearance of liver in primary biliary cirrhosis of 3 years' duration; weight at autopsy, 1,855 Gm.

with this concept. When a hepatic lesion reaches the stage of nodular parenchymal repair, the normal lobular and vascular pattern is distorted and central veins are either unidentifiable or markedly eccentric. For the purposes of this discussion, therefore, the term "biliary cirrhosis" refers to the hepatic lesion of the stage in which nodular regeneration is histologically identifiable.

Although the term "primary biliary cirrhosis" is widely used to designate the clinical syndrome described, only about half the cases so designated reveal cirrhosis as defined above morphologically. The precirrhotic stage of the syndrome is designated by various terms depending on the pathologist's conception of the initial injury, such as "cholestatic,"[23] "cholangiolitic or pericholangiolitic hepatitis,"[47, 91] "chronic intrahepatic obstructive jaundice,"[82] and, more recently, "chronic nonsuppurative cholangitis."[75] Although we are dealing with two phases of the same underlying pathologic process, the two stages will be described separately because they do have certain distinctive features.

Gross Appearance. *Precirrhotic Stage.* The liver is generally firm, larger than normal, dark green or brown (if jaundice is absent), and has a smooth surface. On section there are no definite lobular markings, but there may be a slight increase in connective tissue around the septal bile ducts. The grossly visible bile ducts are patent and appear normal.

Cirrhotic Stage. The liver is firm and usually dark green but granular or nodular (Fig. 20–8). The nodules are usually less than 0.5 cm. in diameter but are occasionally large and separated by broad scars indicative of postnecrotic cirrhosis.

Histologic   Appearance.   Precirrhotic Stage. Parenchymal injury is generally mild except in the area immediately adjacent to the portal tract, where it involves the limiting plate and adjacent hepatic laminae. Here, lytic necrosis of hepatic cells may be severe and is usually associated with a leukocytic and fibroblastic reaction which extends into the lobule (Fig. 20–9). Elsewhere in the lobule, individual cell necrosis of either lytic (hydropic) or acidophilic type and focal necrosis may occur but are not usually severe. The focal necrosis is generally associated with an increase in Kupffer cells, lymphocytes or polymorphonuclear leukocytes. Other alterations include increased Kupffer cells in the sinusoids, epithelioid cell granu-

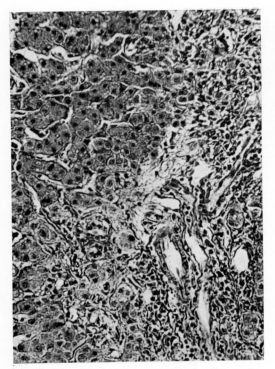

FIG. 20–9. Primary biliary cirrhosis of 1 year's duration. Precirrhotic stage, showing lytic necrosis of the limiting plate with leukocytic reaction. (Hematoxylin and eosin; × 200.) (Foulk, W. T., Baggenstoss, A. H., and Butt, H. R.: Gastroenterology 47:354. By permission of the publisher, Williams & Wilkins.)

lomas with giant cells and occasionally mild fatty changes. Granulomas, if one includes those observed in the portal tract, are present in about a third of cases.

Bile stasis, as indicated by pigmentation of liver and Kupffer cells and by bile plugs in the canaliculi, varies considerably from none to severe. The pigmentation is more often diffuse or periportal than centrolobular in distribution. The degree of bile stasis correlates roughly with the serum bilirubin level but exceptions are numerous in individual specimens.

The most consistent and pronounced evidence of hepatic injury is in the portal tracts, which are broadened and elongated in all cases. This increase in size is largely the result of increased numbers of lymphocytes, plasma cells, fibroblasts and neutrophilic leukocytes. Acidophilic leukocytes are observed in approximately a third of cases. The increase in lymphocytes is accompanied by formation of lymph follicles in about a third of cases. Fibroblastic proliferation and increase in collagen fibers is generally apparent and the portal venules often seem to be narrowed as a result of the fibrosis. Septal formation with linkage between portal tracts occurs occasionally and, more rarely, linkage with central veins is observed.

Inflammation around the interlobular and septal ducts is observed in all cases and this is often accompanied by varying degrees of

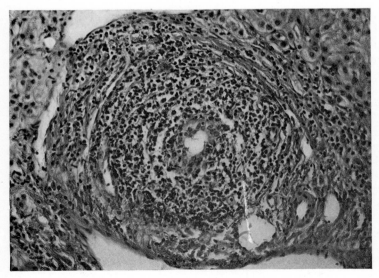

FIG. 20–10. Primary biliary cirrhosis of 3 years' duration. Precirrhotic stage, showing inflammation of interlobular duct (chronic nonsuppurative cholangitis). (Hematoxylin and eosin; × 200.) (Baggenstoss, A. H., Foulk, W. T., Butt, H. R., and Bahn, R. C.: Am. J. Clin. Path. 42:259. By permission of the publisher, Williams & Wilkins.)

FIG. 20–11. Primary biliary cirrhosis of 1½ years' duration. Precirrhotic stage, showing inflammation and necrosis of interlobular duct. (Hematoxylin and eosin; × 650.) (Baggenstoss, A. H., Foulk, W. T., Butt, H. R., and Bahn, R. C.: Am. J. Clin. Path. 42:259. By permission of the publisher, Williams & Wilkins.)

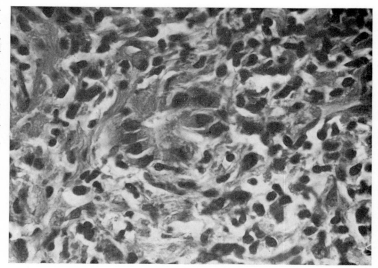

inflammation and degeneration of the ductal epithelium itself (Fig. 20–10). Vacuolar changes in the cytoplasm, leukocytes in the wall and lumen of the duct, nuclear pyknosis and karyorrhexis, and epithelial proliferation are frequently present. In some cases, necrosis of a portion of the circumference is observed with replacement by leukocytes or granulation or fibrous tissue (Fig. 20–11 and 20–12). In other instances the entire duct seems to be replaced by inflammatory or fibrous tissue and no trace of an interlobular duct can be found. In these cases with ductal injury, extraluminal periodic acid-Schiff (PAS)-positive, diastase-resistant material is sometimes demonstrated. Paraductal epithelioid cell granulomas with giant cells may also be present (Fig. 20–13), and these cells may contain a similar PAS-positive material which is considered to be a mucoprotein.

As a result of the inflammatory and destructive process, the visible interlobular ducts are reduced in number. In persons without hepatic disease and in portal, postnecrotic or obstructive biliary cirrhosis, the

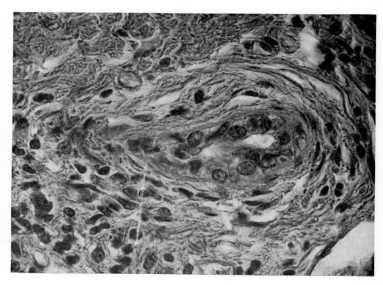

FIG. 20–12. Primary biliary cirrhosis of 4 years' duration. Precirrhotic stage, showing inflammation and fibrosis of interlobular duct. (Hematoxylin and eosin; × 650.) (Baggenstoss, A. H., Foulk, W. T., Butt, H. R., and Bahn, R. C.: Am. J. Clin. Path. 42:259. By permission of the publisher, Williams & Wilkins.)

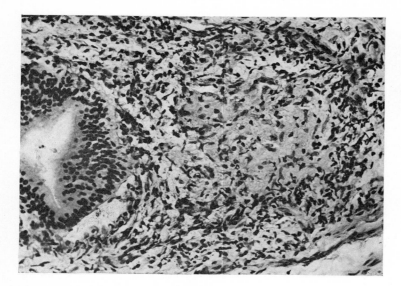

Fig. 20–13. Primary biliary cirrhosis of 9 months' duration. Precirrhotic stage, showing paraductal granuloma, inflammation and epithelial proliferation of interlobular duct. (Hematoxylin and eosin; × 300.)

mean number of interlobular biliary ducts per portal tract is greater than 1 and the mean proportion of portal tracts devoid of interlobular biliary ducts is less than 15 per cent.[6] In sharp contrast, in the syndrome of primary biliary cirrhosis, the mean number of interlobular ducts per portal tract is appreciably less than 1 and the mean proportion of portal tracts devoid of interlobular biliary ducts is greater than 60 per cent.[6]

In contrast to the reduction of interlobular ducts, a mild atypical ductular proliferation is often apparent. The origin of the resulting structures is disputed. Some in-

vestigators believe that they derive from interlobular ducts, whereas others believe that they derive from hepatic cell plates. They resemble small interlobular bile ducts but differ from them in having a tiny lumen or none at all, in their location at the peripheral zone of the portal tract, and in not being intimately associated with the hepatic arteriole and portal venule (Fig. 20–14). They almost always appear to be cut longitudinally, whereas the interlobular ducts are more frequently seen in transverse or tangential section. They are often surrounded by neutrophils, fibroblasts and col-

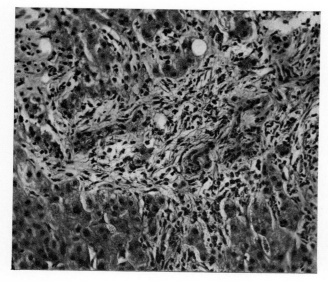

Fig. 20–14. Chronic cholangiolitic hepatitis of 8½ months' duration. Note atypical ductular proliferation at edge of portal tract. (Hematoxylin and eosin; × 200.)

FIG. 20–15. Primary biliary cirrhosis of 3½ years' duration. Cirrhotic stage, showing small regenerative nodule and absence of interlobular bile ducts. (Hematoxylin and eosin; × 100.)

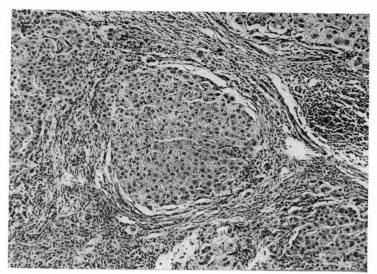

lagen fibers. Serial-section studies indicate that these structures are altered hepatic cell plates.[12]

These differences are emphasized because a count of the ducts in biopsy specimens may help to distinguish between primary biliary cirrhosis and obstruction of the extrahepatic bile ducts.[5] For an accurate count one must distinguish between true interlobular ducts and atypical ductular proliferation. In addition, counts are reliable only if at least 20 portal tracts are present in the biopsy specimen. When these conditions are met, primary biliary cirrhosis is strongly suspected if 60 per cent of the portal tracts are devoid of interlobular ducts. The occurrence of chronic nonsuppurative cholangitis is considered to be a reliable criterion for diagnosis, and frank necrosis of ducts (if present) is said to be pathognomonic of this stage of primary biliary cirrhosis.[75]

Cirrhotic Stage. Histologic examination reveals greater broadening and lengthening of the portal tracts by a mixed leukocytic reaction and fibrosis. Septal formation is more advanced, with linkage of portal tracts. The septa may demarcate individual lobules, end blindly or delineate large regions of parenchyma in which the vascular relationship and lobular architecture are still normal. Some of the septa join central veins with portal tracts, producing a seg-

mentation of the lobule and creating pseudolobules or regenerative nodules (Fig. 20–15). These are generally small (less than 0.5 cm. in diameter) and often are poorly delineated. The subdued character of the nodular regeneration is also indicated by the normal vascular relationships in large regions. At this stage active inflammation and degeneration of interlobular ducts are less evident, but the reduction in number is more obvious. Epithelioid cell granulomas with giant cells are rarely observed. The incidence of atypical ductular proliferation is no different than in specimens without cirrhosis. Bile stasis is generally more severe, especially in autopsy specimens.

Except for the absence of typical ductal proliferation, the cirrhosis resembles that observed after prolonged obstruction of the extrahepatic bile ducts and, if bile stasis is absent, may resemble portal (septal) cirrhosis. Occasionally at autopsy one observes postnecrotic cirrhosis.

Other Observations. At autopsy, jaundice, ascites and congestive splenomegaly are usually present. In our cases the spleen varied in weight between 320 and 1,600 Gm. (mean, 793 Gm.). Esophageal varices, hydrothorax, osteoporosis and cutaneous xanthomata are frequently observed. The lymph nodes at the hilus of the liver reveal hyperplasia of the reticuloendothelial cells of the sinuses and many of these cells con-

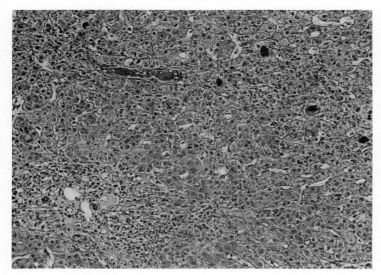

Fig. 20–16. Chronic cholangiolitic hepatitis of 11 months' duration. Note bile stasis and portal triaditis with necrosis of limiting plate. (Hematoxylin and eosin; × 150.) (Baggenstoss, A. H., Foulk, W. T., Butt, H. R., and Bahn, R. C.: Am. J. Clin. Path. 42:259. By permission of the publisher, Williams & Wilkins.)

tain brown pigment granules which do not stain for iron.

Histogenesis. The site of the initial injury and the earliest development of the lesion in primary biliary cirrhosis have been difficult to determine because investigators vary in their definitions of the syndrome and because biopsies are seldom obtained early in the course of illness. Because of the insidious onset of the disease, months and sometimes years elapse before a biopsy is obtained. Obviously, it is difficult or impossible to decipher the initial or early injury from the changes observed after these long intervals. Consequently, opinions regarding the initial or fundamental injury vary considerably and have led to a confusion of terms to designate the early or precirrhotic phase of the disorder.

Some investigators have held that the lesion is fundamentally a hepatitis of viral, toxic or unknown origin, which involves primarily the hepatic parenchymal cells.[24, 31, 44, 81, 92] Others have implicated the canals of Hering (cholangioles) as the main site of injury with the additional involvement of the adjacent parenchyma.[47, 51, 91] More recently the initial or primary lesion has been located in the interlobular and septal ducts,[74, 75, 93] whereas others have described involvement of both the interlobular ducts and the junction ducts or canals of Hering.[3, 6, 15, 42, 54, 56, 57, 60, 72] Lévy and associ-

ates followed the destruction of the ducts by reconstruction of serial sections and observed that the process began with the canals of Hering and included both interlobular and septal ducts.[54]

Our own observations[6] are in agreement with the findings of Lévy and co-workers who described involvement both of interlobular ducts and of the zone immediately adjacent to the portal tract, which includes the limiting plate and the canal of Hering. Whether the latter changes are the earliest or most significant in the development of the syndrome can be questioned, however, and it is our conviction that the ductal (not the ductular or cholangiolar) changes are the most significant in the progression of the lesion.

Although the site of the initial or primary injury to the liver may be in doubt, the later course of events has been followed by serial biopsies by a number of workers. These events include a continuing or recurrent necrosis of the limiting plate and adjacent laminae with an accompanying leukocytic and fibroblastic reaction here and in the adjacent portal tract, with inflammation and destruction of the interlobular ducts (Figs. 20–16 and 20–17). As a result of this process, both broadening and linear extension of the portal tracts occur with septal formation and linkage. The resulting loss of parenchymal elements leads to a pro-

FIG. 20–17. Primary biliary cirrhosis, same case as represented in Figure 20–16, of 10 years' duration. Note septal formation with nodular regeneration. (Hematoxylin and eosin; ×150.)

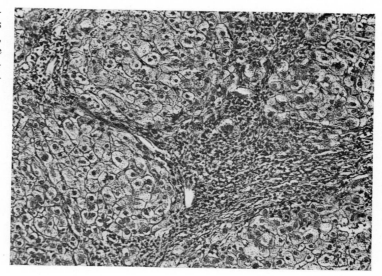

gressive diminution in the size of the lobule. A surprising feature of the process, even in patients who have been followed for years, is the preservation of a normal vascular relationship between portal and central veins. Gradually, however, in many instances the central vein comes to occupy an eccentric position and finally is incorporated in the broadening and lengthening mass of portal and periportal inflammatory tissue (Fig. 20–17). When this happens, any regeneration that occurs is no longer intralobular but eccentric and gives rise to regenerative nodules or pseudolobules which then fulfill the criteria for a diagnosis of cirrhosis.

Correlation of Histologic and Clinical Features. Several features of the histogenesis may be correlated with certain clinical features. It is conceivable that the early inflammatory process in the interlobular ducts allows the escape of certain constituents of the bile, such as the bile salts, without leakage of other elements, such as bilirubin, which continue to be excreted because hepatocellular function remains good. This might account for the long clinical history of pruritus prior to jaundice. When the inflammation and destruction become more severe, bile pigments may also escape, and this might account for the predominantly peripheral distribution of bile stasis in the lobule and the mild jaundice seen clinically. Still later, when the inflammatory process

leads to total destruction and fibrosis of the duct, obstruction occurs and may mimic extrahepatic obstruction clinically.

Other features of the histogenesis which deserve comment are the remarkable chronicity of the process and the superficial similarity of the cirrhosis (when present) to that of the secondary (obstructive) type. In our opinion, the ultimate fate of the interlobular ducts is probably the key to an understanding of these features. In addition to the early inflammatory and degenerative changes that have been observed, necrosis of part or all of the wall with fibrous obliteration of the duct also occurs.[6, 14, 15, 42, 47, 54, 60, 75, 93] Some investigators who have not observed the earlier changes nevertheless describe a marked reduction of the number of interlobular ducts.[39, 61, 82] This development offers an explanation for both the chronicity of the process and the histologic similarity to extrahepatic obstruction. Destruction of interlobular ducts deprives hepatic cells of normal excretory channels, and bile stasis as well as disruption of the canals of Hering could be expected as a consequence. If we assume that the interlobular ducts do not regenerate and that collateral drainage is insufficient to restore normal excretion, as is indicated by the studies of Buyssens,[12] then we have the basis for a continuing increase of biliary pressure in the ductules and cholangioles, with a continuing insult to the hepatic cells —especially to the "Achilles heel" of the hepatic lobule, the cholangioles (canals of Hering). This would in turn explain the chronicity and the inability of the liver to recover from an original insult which involved not only the ductules or cholangioles but also the interlobular ducts. If this concept is correct, then the changes observed in the interlobular ducts (whether they are the earliest lesion or not) are of the greatest importance to an understanding of the histogenesis of the lesion.

Etiology and Pathogenesis. If the inflammation, necrosis and destruction of the interlobular ducts are responsible for a permanent defect in biliary drainage, the immediate cause of these destructive changes remains to be elucidated. One may reasonably postulate that either a virus or a toxin produces the original injury. In most cases of either viral or drug-induced hepatitis, however, the clinical course is much shorter and complete recovery usually ensues. In such instances the zone including the limiting plate is also damaged or destroyed but hepatic cells and ductules regenerate completely and thus normal structure and function are restored. In the cases under study, however, we have evidence, even in the earliest biopsies, of inflammatory and destructive changes in the interlobular ducts in addition to the other changes. Whether this is the result of an affinity of the virus or toxin for the interlobular ducts (hepatosolenotropic agent) or of some weakness in the defensive reaction of the host remains unanswered. The fact that, in most cases, fewer ducts are found in later biopsies and at autopsy suggests that some ducts are continually being destroyed long after the original virus or toxin would be expected to be active. Thus possibly an autoimmune process is involved.

Immunologic Aspects of Primary Biliary Cirrhosis. Many bits of evidence suggest an immune basis for the development of primary biliary cirrhosis. A history of allergy has been observed by some investigators.[3] The clinical picture characteristic of chronic obstructive jaundice with hyperlipemia and xanthomatosis has occurred in some patients receiving chlorpromazine[71] or arsenicals.[18]

These drugs are considered to be hepatotoxic because of individual hypersensitivity. Eosinophilia is noted in some patients with cholestasis secondary to drug sensitivity. Instances have been reported of chronic obstructive liver disease associated with a histologic picture of biliary cirrhosis occurring after chlorpromazine therapy.[89] Although most patients with chronic chlorpromazine jaundice eventually recover completely, chronic drug jaundice due to chlorpromazine or arsenicals may be related to primary biliary cirrhosis.

Some patients with primary biliary cirrhosis have a positive lupus erythematosus (L.E.) clot test, but little reactivity has been observed with nuclear extracts, in contrast to the rule in systemic L.E. Reactivity in the serum in primary biliary cirrhosis has been with cytoplasmic antigens. Paronetto and associates have shown that macroglobulins accumulate in mesenchymal cells in the liver in early lesions of primary biliary cirrhosis.[66] Increased macroglobulin (IgM) levels in the serum have been reported by a number of investigators.[8, 27, 66, 84] Antibodies to bile ductular cells were found in the serum of 75 per cent of patients with primary biliary cirrhosis.[65] The antigen that binds these serum reactants is a mucoprotein that is present in the epithelium of proliferating bile ductules. A number of investigators[8, 23, 90] have found that the sera of virtually all patients with primary biliary cirrhosis contain non-organ-specific antibodies, probably directed against mitochondria and specifically against the crystae of the inner membrane.[7] The immunofluorescent test for mitochondrial antibodies has helped to differentiate primary biliary cirrhosis from prolonged obstructive jaundice and drug cholestasis.[8, 23, 38, 90] Sherlock and co-workers stated that the test may be positive in postnecrotic cirrhosis with cholestasis but not in extrahepatic obstruction, cholestatic drug jaundice or cholestatic jaundice occurring in chronic ulcerative colitis.[83] Hopefully, further application in larger series will confirm the usefulness of this test. An etiologic role in the perpetuation of liver disease could not be demonstrated for the tissue antibodies described.[23]

That primary biliary cirrhosis represents

the rare instance of an autoimmune process in the liver has been hypothesized.[48, 66] However, antiductular antibodies were present in the serum in 67 per cent of patients with viral hepatitis, 47 per cent of those with postnecrotic cirrhosis, 32 per cent of those with extrahepatic biliary obstruction and 10 per cent of normal subjects.[65] One must assume that, for unexplained reasons, in these patients the antigen-antibody complex does not form or is innocuous. The severity of the autoimmune process must vary among patients with primary biliary cirrhosis because a few patients seem to pass through all the typical clinical manifestations of the disease and yet remain active and reasonably well with quiescent cirrhosis for years. Although autoimmune phenomena may be of etiologic importance, such an explanation does not completely account for the clinical observations. It does seem likely, as suggested by Popper,[67] that primary biliary cirrhosis is characterized by a peculiar reactivity of the small bile ductules, which is initiated by a number of etiologic agents. That this reactivity is the result of immune processes is not proved.

Although cirrhosis has been produced experimentally by the repeated injection of various antigens,[9, 16, 28, 64] nothing in these models suggests autoimmunity, and the histologic appearance of the lesion does not remotely resemble that of primary biliary cirrhosis.

Steiner and associates concluded from their studies and a critical review of the literature in 1961 that up to that time there was no convincing human or experimental morphologic evidence that autoclasia initiates or self-perpetuates liver injury.[86] They could not, however, rule out autoimmunity as a possible contributory factor to the development of liver disease.

Milgrom and Witebsky proposed that the following criteria should be fulfilled in order to consider a disease as an autoimmune disorder: (1) direct demonstration of free circulating antibodies that are active at body temperature or the indirect demonstration of cell-bound antibodies; (2) identification of the specific antigen against which this antibody is directed; (3) production of antibodies against the same antigen in experimental animals; (4) appearance of pathologic changes in the corresponding tissues of an actively sensitized animal, basically similar to those of human disease; and (5) transfer of the disease by serum containing antibody or by immunologically stimulated lymphoid cells.[59] These criteria have not been met in regard to primary biliary cirrhosis.

OBSTRUCTIVE OR SECONDARY BILIARY CIRRHOSIS

Obstructive biliary cirrhosis may result from any pathologic process that blocks the extrahepatic biliary tree for a sufficiently prolonged period. Such processes include congenital atresia of bile ducts, choledocholithiasis, benign stricture of the common or hepatic bile ducts, various carcinomas arising within or involving the extrahepatic biliary channels, hydatid cysts and perhaps primary sclerosing cholangitis.

Here, as in primary biliary cirrhosis, is a lesion that usually progresses very slowly to cirrhosis. Cirrhosis may not be histologically evident for many months after onset of symptoms. A history of gallbladder or biliary tract surgery shortly preceding the onset of jaundice suggests surgical trauma to the biliary tree. Chills, fever and abdominal pain are valuable indicators of an extrahepatic obstructive lesion. (Rarely is abdominal pain a symptom in primary biliary cirrhosis. None of the patients with primary biliary cirrhosis described by Ahrens and co-workers had abdominal pain.[3] Vague abdominal distress was encountered in only 8 per cent of another series of 49 such patients.[29]) When the extrahepatic obstructing lesion is silent, as it is occasionally with common duct stone but especially with bile duct carcinoma, symptoms, clinical findings and laboratory studies may not help to differentiate secondary from primary biliary cirrhosis. Although most instances of obstructive biliary cirrhosis can be correctly diagnosed by clinical data, silent stones, strictures and tumors of the biliary tree may clinically mimic primary biliary cirrhosis. When this occurs, transhepatic or surgical cholangiography with wedge biopsy of the liver is required, as discussed under primary biliary cirrhosis.

The typical clinical picture in obstructive biliary cirrhosis is similar in major degree to that in primary biliary cirrhosis. Jaundice occurs earlier than in some patients with primary biliary cirrhosis, but in the few instances of choledocholithiasis without pain and in patients with carcinoma of the bile ducts, pruritus precedes clinical jaundice by several weeks. The skin darkens and thickens and, because the serum lipid disturbance is the same in both extrahepatic and intrahepatic obstructive processes, xanthelasma and xanthomata may appear if obstruction and hyperlipemia are persistent. Fatty diarrhea with attendant osteoporosis occurs. Bone thinning is less common when obstructive biliary cirrhosis is the result of a malignant obstruction because the course is usually short. Serum bilirubin levels may be low and jaundice intermittent in obstruction due to stone or stricture, but, as hepatocellular function fails late in the course, even an unrelieved, intermittent obstructing lesion may be associated with deep jaundice. Serum levels of alkaline phosphatase, cholesterol and phospholipids increase markedly with obstruction (Fig. 20–18). Increased levels of β-globulin may be equally as common in extrahepatic as in intrahepatic obstruction. An increase of IgM immunoglobulin in primary biliary cirrhosis is reportedly of value in differential diagnosis from chronic extrahepatic obstruction.[84] Tests of hepatocellular function show little deterioration over long periods. Serum albumin level and prothrombin times after vitamin K therapy are usually normal early in the course of secondary biliary cirrhosis. Portal hypertension with ascites and bleeding from esophageal varices are late manifestations.

Among adults, benign, often intermittent, obstructing lesions of the extrahepatic bile ducts lead most frequently to secondary biliary cirrhosis. Lindenauer and Child found biliary cirrhosis in 24 per cent of 50 patients operated on for common duct stricture and in 8 per cent of the 50 patients operated on for choledocholithiasis.[55] Even though cirrhosis may be present histologi-

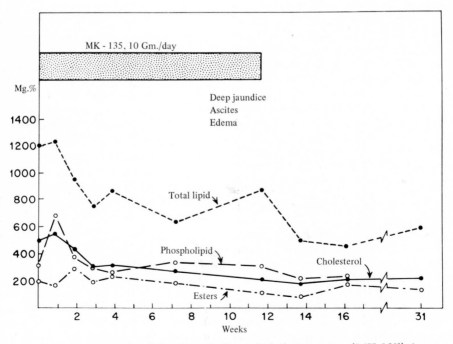

FIG. 20–18. Serum lipid levels and effect of cholestyramine (MK-135) in patient with obstructive biliary cirrhosis.

cally, probably in relatively few of these patients do late clinical manifestations of severe cirrhosis develop if the obstruction is relieved surgically.

Of 60 cases of obstructive biliary cirrhosis reported by Scobie and Summerskill[80], 50 per cent had ascites and gastrointestinal hemorrhage, which suggests that in this group cirrhosis was significant clinically as well as morphologically. Two thirds of the cases in this group were the result of postoperative stricture of the bile ducts, a lesion that is often not completely or permanently amenable to surgical repair. Malignant obstruction of the bile ducts is frequently relieved surgically, at least in a palliative manner, and the malignant disease terminates fatally before obstructive biliary cirrhosis develops. Malignant tumors of the papilla of Vater or of the common or hepatic bile ducts often progress slowly and may more likely lead to an obstructive biliary cirrhosis than does the usually more rapidly progressive carcinoma of the pancreas. Primary sclerosing cholangitis, a rare lesion of the biliary tree, may lead to biliary cirrhosis[36] and has been associated with unrecognized carcinoma of the biliary tree and chronic ulcerative colitis.[4, 37]

Progression of secondary biliary cirrhosis to significant hepatocellular failure is generally slow. Every effort must be made to diagnose and relieve the extrahepatic obstruction. Hemorrhage from esophageal varices may occur while hepatocellular function remains reasonably intact. In such instances, a portal-systemic shunt is indicated and well tolerated. Subsequent surgical attempts to relieve a demonstrable extrahepatic obstruction should then be considered. Medical treatment of established and clinically significant secondary biliary cirrhosis is no different from that of primary biliary cirrhosis.

ILLUSTRATIVE CASE

In May 1959, a 27-year-old married woman underwent cholecystectomy for cholelithiasis with recurrent biliary colic but no jaundice. Five days postoperatively jaundice with dark urine developed. Bile drainage from the wound persisted for 2 months. When the drainage ceased, chills, fever and jaundice increased. In August 1959 a common duct stricture was repaired, and the jaundice cleared. In January 1960 she had recurrent chills and fever at monthly intervals with reappearance of jaundice and development of pruritus. A second attempt to repair the stricture was made in July 1960 but symptoms of recurrent cholangitis persisted.

At that time she had icteric skin and sclerae and xanthelasma. The liver was firm, regular and smooth and was palpable 4 cm. below the right costal margin; there was no splenomegaly. Results of laboratory studies were: serum bilirubin, total 8.7 mg./100 ml., direct 7.2 mg./100 ml.; alkaline phosphatase, 115 K.-A. units; cholesterol, 504 mg./100 ml. plasma; cholesterol esters, 92 mg./100 ml. plasma; phospholipids, 486 mg./100 ml. plasma; total lipids, 1,408 mg./100 ml. plasma; prothrombin time, normal; albumin, 3.13 Gm./100 ml. serum; β-globulin, 1.22 Gm./100 ml. serum (slightly higher than normal).

In December 1960, exploration revealed a stricture 1 cm. below the bifurcation of the right and left hepatic ducts; Roux-en-Y hepaticojejunostomy was done. Liver biopsy was reported to show bile stasis and pericholangitis. Postoperatively, bile peritonitis developed. The patient recovered slowly and the jaundice faded but recurrent cholangitis continued.

Course. Aug. 1961. Laboratory data were: bilirubin, 3.0 mg./100 ml. serum; cholesterol, 672 mg./100 ml. plasma; alkaline phosphatase, 116 K.-A. units. Hepaticojejunostomy was performed with insertion of a Vitallium tube. She continued to have low-grade clinical icterus and recurrent cholangitis.

March 1963. The jaundice was deeper, the skin was darker, and the xanthelasma persisted. The liver was palpable 6 cm. below the costal margin.

Jan. 1964. Deep jaundice, edema and splenomegaly were noted. The liver still was 6 cm. below the costal margin. Laboratory data were: bilirubin, 8 mg./100 ml. serum; cholesterol, 354 mg./100 ml. plasma; albumin, 2.4 Gm./100 ml. serum.

Oct. 1965. The patient died in hepatic coma, 6 years after cholecystectomy and 4 unsuccessful attempts to repair a common duct stricture.

At autopsy the following anatomic diagnoses were made: multiple previous operations for postcholecystectomy stricture of the common bile duct; partial stricture of the left hepatic duct and complete stricture of the right hepatic duct; acute and chronic cholangitis with intrahepatic abscesses in the right lobe of the liver; early obstructive (secondary) biliary cirrhosis; splenomegaly (1,100 Gm.); ascites (3,000 ml.); bilateral suppurative pyelonephritis; edema of the lower extremities; xanthelasma; and moderate coronary and aortic atherosclerosis. Histologic sections of the liver revealed an organizing abscess, chronic cholangitis with periportal and periductal fibrosis, septal formation, bile stasis and a few regenerative nodules.

The patient's problem is obvious from her history of jaundice with recurrent chills and fever which occurred shortly after a cholecystectomy for cholelithiasis. The physical findings and laboratory data differ in no way from those of primary biliary cirrhosis. Preoperative transhepatic cholangiography might have permitted better evaluation of the problem and careful preoperative planning for successful surgical repair of the stricture.

Pathology. The stages preceding the development of true cirrhosis in extrahepatic obstruction of the bile ducts perhaps can best be designated as extrahepatic obstructive jaundice in the early stages and as biliary fibrosis in the more advanced stages. The stage of biliary fibrosis in which bands of collagen radiate out into the lobule from portal tracts and sometimes join adjacent portal tracts (linkage) while normal vascular relationships are retained is not infrequently called "biliary cirrhosis" but is not considered as such in the following discussion.

The exact cause of the cirrhosis that follows prolonged extrahepatic biliary obstruction is not clear even though it has been recognized since the latter half of the nineteenth century.[53, 62, 69] Controversy exists regarding the role, in the pathogenesis of secondary biliary cirrhosis, of obstruction *per se* and of the infection in the biliary channels which frequently complicates obstruction, particularly when the latter is incomplete as is common in choledocholithiasis and benign stricture of extrahepatic ducts. The development of cirrhosis after aseptic common bile duct ligation in animals and its occurrence in infants with congenital atresia of bile ducts support the concept that the lesion can result from obstruction alone.

The inflammatory process that develops around intrahepatic ducts and ductules in unrelieved extrahepatic obstruction seems to be of significance in the pathogenesis of secondary biliary cirrhosis. The cause of this secondary inflammation is not clearly established but appears to be related to the escape of biliary constituents from injured bile ducts.

The time required for cirrhosis of the liver to develop in unrelieved extrahepatic obstruction is variable. In infants with congenital atresia of bile ducts, irreversible biliary cirrhosis develops after 5 to 6 months. However, Gellis states that during the first 4 months of life there is no correlation between duration of obstruction and severity of cirrhosis.[33] Scobie and Summerskill found a wide range of time intervals between the onset of biliary obstruction in adults and the confirmation of obstructive biliary cirrhosis.[80] The mean interval was longest in patients with common duct stricture (7 years), shorter in patients with choledocholithiasis, and only 9 to 10 months in seven patients with biliary cirrhosis secondary to malignant obstruction of the bile ducts. It was also noted in this group of 60 patients with cirrhosis secondary to bile duct obstruction that, in those patients who had fever, chills and intermittent jaundice suggestive of cholangitis, cirrhosis developed much more slowly than it did in those without such symptoms. Cholangitis is likely to occur when bile duct obstruction is incomplete; the more complete the bile duct obstruction, the more rapidly obstructive biliary cirrhosis develops.

Biliary cirrhosis secondary to chronic obstructive lesions in the extrahepatic bile ducts is best discussed separately for adults and for children. In children, secondary biliary cirrhosis occurs predominantly as a result of congenital atresia or absence of bile ducts; in adults the obstruction of the extrahepatic bile ducts is usually due to strictures, gallstones or neoplasms.

Biliary Cirrhosis Secondary to Congenital Atresia or Agenesis of Extrahepatic Bile Ducts. These cases are of special interest because: (1) they afford an opportunity to observe the development of cirrhosis from a purely obstructive lesion uncomplicated in the early stages at least by an infective process; (2) compared with obstructive lesions in the adult the incidence of cirrhosis is extremely high; and (3) the development of cirrhosis is unusually rapid.[58, 63]

Gross Appearance. The liver is dark green, enlarged and smooth in the precirrhotic stage but granular in the cirrhotic stage (Fig. 20–19). The liver may be enlarged up to four times normal size.[20] The cut surface reveals broad scars along the vessels and bile ducts and small regenerative nodules separated by relatively broad internodular scars. Dilatation of the large interhepatic bile ducts can sometimes be recognized (Fig. 20–19).

Histologic Appearance. In the precirrhotic phase, centrilobular cholestasis with feathery degeneration of liver cells, periportal inflammation and fibroblastic proliferation, and an apparent increase in interlobular ducts are the predominant changes. When acidophilic and lytic degeneration of individual cells, acidophilic bodies, pseudoductular proliferation and multinucleated

parenchymal giant cells are present, the condition is difficult to distinguish from neonatal hepatitis.[76] The giant cell reaction is said to appear in 15 to 66 per cent of cases.[45, 87]

In the cirrhotic stage vascular relationships become abnormal and regenerative nodules of variable size and shape are observed (Fig. 20–20). Cholestasis is severe and bile plugs may be observed in the canaliculi and microcalculi, in the interlobular ducts (Fig. 20–20).

The nodular parenchyma frequently reveals focal eosinophilic and lytic necrosis and feathery degeneration of scattered cells. Pseudoductular proliferation is prominent, but multinucleated parenchymal giant cells are not seen as frequently as in the precirrhotic stage. The internodular bands of connective tissue are of variable width and contain numerous ducts, both typical and atypical. The inflammatory reaction is usually mild and consists largely of lymphocytes, mononuclear cells and, rarely neutrophilic leukocytes.

In all but 3 of 40 cases of congenital bili-

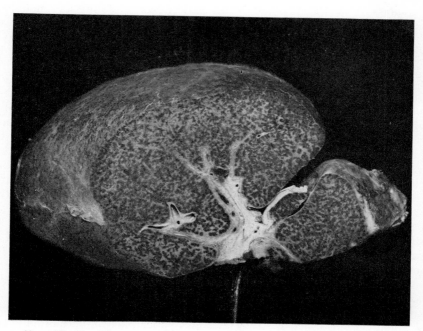

Fig. 20–19. Obstructive biliary cirrhosis in 3-month-old infant with congenital atresia of extrahepatic bile ducts. The liver weighed 92 Gm. (normal, 140 Gm.). Note dilated ducts and scarring of portal tracts.

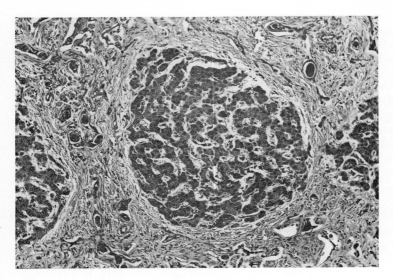

Fig. 20–20. Liver section from 8-month-old infant with obstructive biliary cirrhosis due to congenital atresia of extrahepatic bile ducts. The liver weighed 314 Gm. (normal, 254 Gm.). Note the regenerative nodule and dilated interlobular ducts containing bile. (Hematoxylin and eosin; × 100.) (Myers, R. L., Baggenstoss, A. H., Logan, G. B., and Hallenbeck, G. A.: Pediatrics 18:767. By permission of the publisher, American Academy of Pediatrics.)

ary atresia that we studied there was evidence of cirrhosis; in the 3 exceptions the patients were less than 5 months old.[63] However, in seven other patients who were under 5 months of age histologic signs of cirrhosis were already evident, which emphasizes the observation of Gellis[33] that the age of the infant does not correlate with the degree of histologic change. These cases also emphasize the fact that cirrhosis may develop rapidly and is invariable if the obstruction is not relieved. If the obstruction is relieved in time, reparative processes restore a functionally and morphologically normal liver. Data indicate that this is true even if histologic evidence of cirrhosis is present.[11]

Secondary (Obstructive) Biliary Cirrhosis in Adults. True cirrhosis as defined here rarely occurs as a result of obstruction of the extrahepatic bile ducts. The histologic and diagnostic features of the precirrhotic stages (extrahepatic obstructive jaundice and biliary fibrosis) have been adequately covered in numerous publications and are not reviewed here.[32, 57, 68] Gibson and Robertson found only 21 instances (8.6 per cent) of true cirrhosis at autopsy in 244 cases of extrahepatic obstruction of the bile ducts.[35] In general, benign lesions (such as strictures and gallstones) which lead to prolonged and intermittent obstruction are more likely to cause cirrhosis. Thus, only 4 per cent of

neoplastic lesions, in contrast to 18 per cent of benign lesions, resulted in cirrhosis.[35] Patients with neoplastic obstruction probably die of neoplastic disease before nodular regeneration can develop.

Gross Appearance. The liver is usually enlarged and dark green or greenish brown, and it has a granular or nodular surface (Fig. 20–21). It cuts with increased resistance and the large ducts near the hilus are dilated and accompanied by an increased amount of connective tissue.

Histologic Appearance. In early obstructive biliary cirrhosis, regenerative nodules are few in number and poorly delineated.[22] A large portion of the parenchyma may still show a fairly normal lobular pattern with normal vascular relationships. In these areas the portal tracts are stellate and broadened with septa extending into the parenchyma or linking with adjacent portal tracts and occasionally with central veins. The widening of the portal tracts is largely the result of fibroblastic proliferation and collagen formation; to a lesser extent it is due to lymphocytes, mononuclear and neutrophilic leukocytes and typical ductal and atypical ductular proliferation (Fig. 20–22). The connective tissue fibers have a loose edematous appearance and are often in concentric configuration around the bile ducts (Fig. 20–22). Bile stasis may be moderate or severe with pigmentation of parenchymal and

FIG. 20–21. Early obstructive biliary cirrhosis due to stricture of common bile duct of 2 years' duration. The liver weighed 1,900 Gm. (normal 1,600 Gm.).

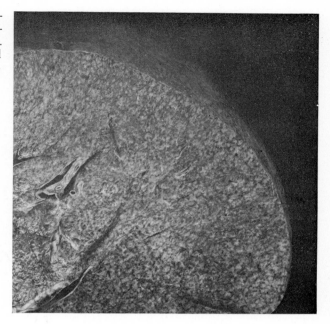

Kupffer cells, bile thrombi in the canaliculi and ductules, and, more rarely, microcalculi in the interlobular ducts. Foci of the liver cells, usually adjacent to portal tracts, which present lytic necrosis with bile stasis, are often observed and are known as "bile infarcts." Occasionally, large masses of pigment known as "bile lakes" are seen in or adjacent to portal tracts. They are surrounded by necrotic liver cells or a mild mesenchymal reaction. They have been in-

terpreted as extravasates of bile from destroyed bile ducts or as evidence of necrosis of liver cells at the periphery of the lobule (Fig. 20–23).

Focal and individual cell necrosis of either eosinophilic or lytic type is frequently observed. The latter type involves cells which have a rarefied cytoplasm in which a fine, brown pigmented, protoplasmic network is found. The nucleus may be pyknotic or absent and the condition is also desig-

FIG. 20–22. Early obstructive biliary cirrhosis; patient had jaundice for 2½ years. Note regenerative nodules, other areas with perilobular fibrosis but normal vascular relationships, and paraductal concentric fibrosis. (Hematoxylin and eosin; × 30.)

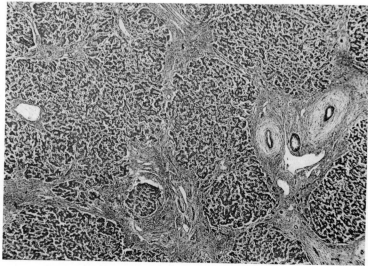

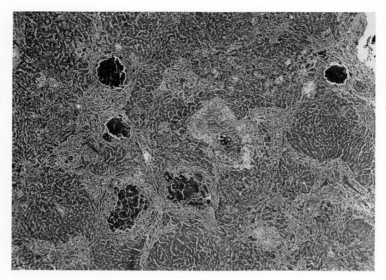

FIG. 20–23. Early obstructive biliary cirrhosis; patient had jaundice for 9 months. Note irregular, poorly delineated, regenerative nodules and "bile lakes." (Hematoxylin and eosin; × 30.)

nated as "feathery degeneration." It involves scattered cells as well as those constituting the bile infarcts.

In advanced biliary cirrhosis the same changes are present but nodular regeneration is more advanced and the fibrous tissue is more condensed. The pattern may resemble septal (portal) cirrhosis except for the severe bile stasis and the greater apparent increase in typical interlobular ducts (Fig. 20–24). Occasionally, however, the regenerative nodules assume garland and other bizarre shapes[22] (Fig. 20–25). Also, occa-

sionally, the areas of collapse and scarring are so broad that remnants of three or more portal tracts can be discerned in the scar. These cases, therefore, may qualify as examples of postnecrotic cirrhosis resulting from biliary tract obstruction. In some of these instances, interlobular ducts are reduced in number and atypical ductular proliferation is absent.

Secondary (obstructive) biliary cirrhosis is frequently complicated by bacterial infection. This occurs more often when the obstruction is due to stricture or choledo-

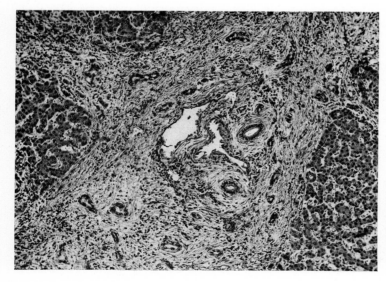

FIG. 20–24. Obstructive biliary cirrhosis due to stricture of common bile duct of 2½ years' duration, showing apparent increase in interlobular ducts. (Hematoxylin and eosin; × 90.)

FIG. 20–25. Obstructive biliary cirrhosis due to stricture of common bile duct of 14 years' duration, showing garland-shaped regenerative nodules and reduction in interlobular ducts. (Hematoxylin and eosin; × 30.)

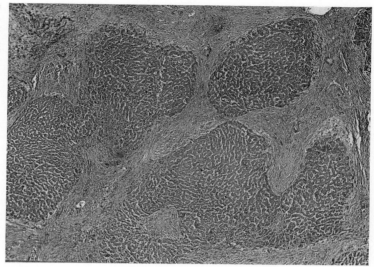

cholithiasis than when it is neoplastic. The most common bacteria are *Escherichia coli, Aerobacter aerogenes, Streptococcus faecalis* and *Proteus* species. The infection may be manifested as suppurative cholecystitis, cholangitis or pylephlebitis. The liver is invaded by pyogenic bacteria through the portal vein branches or, less often, through the bile ducts. The hematogenous and lymphatic routes are considered more important than is ascending infection through the bile ducts.[68] When the infection is severe, pylephlebitis or cholangitic abscesses may result.

Complications of the cirrhotic process occur, such as portal hypertension with splenomegaly and esophageal varices and ascites, but the incidence is not as high as in portal cirrhosis.[22] These complications are most frequent in cases of advanced biliary cirrhosis in which the greater part of the parenchyma has been converted into regenerative nodules.[22, 73] The principal causes of death are hepatic insufficiency, hemorrhage from varices, renal insufficiency and intercurrent infection.

LIPID ALTERATIONS IN BILIARY CIRRHOSIS

Hepatic disease with biliary obstruction is associated with a unique disturbance of serum lipids. The characteristics of the serum lipid pattern are an increase of free cholesterol and phospholipid with low cholesterol ester and normal neutral fat levels. Typically the serum is clear; despite high lipid levels, lactescence is rarely observed in fasting serum. A correlation exists between free cholesterol level and phospholipid level in extrahepatic bile duct obstruction, primary and secondary biliary cirrhosis, and the acute phase of infectious hepatitis.[26] In certain patients this characteristic alteration of lipids is more striking than in others. The reason for individual variation in the degree of lipid alteration in patients with apparently identical obstructive hepatic processes is unknown but may be related to the degree of secretory failure for bile acid salts. Serum lipid levels do not correlate with fatty change of the liver.[52]

Cholesterol and phospholipid fractions of serum are bound mainly to proteins and, on zone electrophoresis, migrate with a mobility similar to that of beta-lipoproteins.[50] Alpha-lipoproteins (high density lipoproteins) in the sera are diminished or absent in obstructive hepatic disease in analyses made by preparative or analytical ultracentrifugation, but, on electrophoretic and immunochemical analyses, are markedly increased in biliary cirrhosis. These alpha-lipoproteins are antigenically identical to but contain more phospholipid than the normal form, float in the density region

1.006 to 1.063, and swell the concentration of low-density lipoprotein.[30] Some patients with biliary obstruction may have an increase in true beta-lipoprotein that also contains greater than usual amounts of phospholipid. Release of lipid into the plasma from the liver may be increased because normal flow of phospholipids and cholesterol is obstructed and because the enterohepatic cycle of cholesterol is interrupted, which alters lipoprotein synthesis.

Serum lipoproteins are of very high molecular weight, with free cholesterol and phospholipid constituting the major fraction of the molecule. The lipids in the serum are bound to protein in such a way that they are very soluble in aqueous solution.[48] A high concentration of the hydrophilic lipid, lecithin, in the phospholipids is important in producing these soluble lipoproteins. Bile acids are factors in the increase in serum lipid levels in obstructive jaundice.[13] A direct correlation has been observed between serum bile salt levels and cholesterol levels.[70] The degree of excretory failure for bile salts may be of importance in the development of hyperlipemia in hepatic obstructive disease.

REFERENCES

1. Ahrens, E. H., Jr., and Kunkel, H. G.: The relationship between serum lipids and skin xanthomata in eighteen patients with primary biliary cirrhosis, J. Clin. Invest. 28:1565, 1949.
2. ———: The stabilization of serum lipid emulsions by serum phospholipids, J. Exp. Med. 90:409, 1949.
3. Ahrens, E. H., Jr., Payne, M. A., Kunkel, H. G., Eisenmenger, W. J., and Blondheim, S. H.: Primary biliary cirrhosis, Medicine. 29:299, 1950.
4. Altemeier, W. A., Gall, E. A., Zinninger, M. M., and Hoxworth, P. I.: Sclerosing carcinoma of the major intrahepatic bile ducts, A.M.A. Arch. Surg. 75:450, 1957.
5. Baggenstoss, A. H.: Morphologic and etiologic diagnoses from hepatic biopsies without clinical data, Medicine. 45:435, 1966.
6. Baggenstoss, A. H., Foulk, W. T., Butt, H. R., and Bahn, R. C.: The pathology of primary biliary cirrhosis with emphasis

7. on histogenesis, Am. J. Clin. Path. 42: 259, 1964.
7. Berg, P. A., Doniach, D., and Roitt, I. M.: Mitochondrial antibodies in primary biliary cirrhosis. I. Localization of the antigen to mitochondrial membranes, J. Exp. Med. 126:277, 1967.
8. Bevan, G.: Primary biliary cirrhosis—positive antibody tests associated with increased immunoglobulin (IgM), Proc. Roy. Soc. Med. 59:567, 1966.
9. Blackwell, J. B.: Cirrhosis resulting from repeated injections of antigen, J. Path. Bact. 90:245, 1965.
10. Boden, R. W., Rankin, J. G., Goulston, S. J. M., and Morrow, W.: The liver in ulcerative colitis: the significance of raised serum-alkaline-phosphatase levels, Lancet 2:245, 1959.
11. Bunton, G. L., and Cameron, R.: Regeneration of liver after biliary cirrhosis, Ann. N. Y. Acad. Sci. 111:412, 1963.
12. Buyssens, N.: La prolifération des canaux biliaires et la formation de structures tubulaires au cours des affections hépatiques en pathologie humaine et expérimentale, Rev. Belg. Path. 29:5, 1962.
13. Byers, S. O., Friedman, M., Biggs, M. W., and Gunning, B.: Observations concerning the production and excretion of cholesterol in mammals. IX. The mechanism of the hypercholesteremic effect of cholic acid, J. Exp. Med. 97:511, 1953.
14. Cameron, G. R., and Hou, P. C.: Biliary Cirrhosis (Pathological Monographs No. 1), Springfield, Ill., Thomas, 1962, 214 pp.
15. Cameron, R.: Some problems of biliary cirrhosis, Brit. Med. J. 1:535, 1958.
16. Campbell, J. A. H.: Experimental nondietary cirrhosis in rats, Brit. J. Exp. Path. 42:290, 1961.
17. Carey, J. B., Jr.: Lowering of serum bile acid concentrations and relief of pruritus in jaundiced patients fed a bile acid sequestering resin (Abstr.), J. Lab. Clin. Med. 56:797, 1960.
18. Chanutin, A., and Ludewig, S.: Blood lipid studies in a case of xanthomatosis associated with hepatic damage, J. Lab. Clin. Med. 22:903, 1937.
19. Clubb, J. S., Neale, F. C., and Posen, S.: The behavior of infused human placental alkaline phosphatase in human subjects, J. Lab. Clin. Med. 66:493, 1965.
20. Craig, J. M., Gellis, S. S., and Hsia, D. Y. Y.: Cirrhosis of the liver in infants

and children, Am. J. Dis. Child. *90*:299, 1955.

21. Dauphinee, J. A., and Sinclair, J. C.: Primary biliary cirrhosis, Canad. Med. Ass. J. *61*:1, 1949.

22. Doehlert, C. A., Jr., Baggenstoss, A. H., and Cain, J. C.: Obstructive biliary cirrhosis and alcoholic cirrhosis: comparison of clinical and pathologic features, Am. J. Clin. Path. *25*:902, 1955.

23. Doniach, D., Roitt, I. M., Walker, J. G., and Sherlock, S.: Tissue antibodies in primary biliary cirrhosis, active chronic (lupoid) hepatitis, cryptogenic cirrhosis and other liver diseases and their clinical implications, Clin. Exp. Immun. *1*:237, 1966.

24. Dubin, I. N.: Cholestatic hepatitis (primary pericholangitis; cholangiolitic hepatitis), Bull N. Y. Acad. Med. *32*:396, 1956.

25. Dubin, I. N., Sullivan, B. H., Jr., LeGolvan, P. C., and Murphy, L. C.: The cholestatic form of viral hepatitis: experiences with viral hepatitis at Brooke Army Hospital during the years 1951 to 1953, Am. J. Med. *29*:55, 1960.

26. Eder, H. A., Russ, E. M., Pritchett, R. A. R., Wilber, M. M., and Barr, D. P.: Protein-lipid relationships in human plasma: in biliary cirrhosis, obstructive jaundice, and acute hepatitis, J. Clin. Invest. *34*: 1147, 1955.

27. Fahey, J. L.: Antibodies and immunoglobulins. II. Normal development and changes in disease, J.A.M.A. *194*:255, 1965.

28. Fennell, R. H., Jr.: Chronic liver disease induced in rats by repeated anaphylactic shock, Am. J. Path. *47*:173, 1965.

29. Foulk, W. T., Baggenstoss, A. H., and Butt, H. R.: Primary biliary cirrhosis: re-evaluation by clinical and histologic study of 49 cases, Gastroenterology *47*:354, 1964.

30. Fredrickson, D. S., Levy, R. I., and Lees, R. S.: Fat transport in lipoproteins: an integrated approach to mechanisms and disorders, New Engl. J. Med. *276*: 273, 1967.

31. Gall, E. A., and Braunstein, H.: Hepatitis with manifestations simulating bile duct obstruction (so-called "cholangiolitic hepatitis"), Am. J. Clin. Path. *25*:1113, 1955.

32. Gall, E. A., and Dobrogorski, O.: Hepatic alterations in obstructive jaundice, Am. J. Clin. Path. *41*:126, 1964.

33. Gellis, S. S.: Jaundice and liver disease in infancy and childhood, Postgrad. Med. *41*:48, 1967.

34. George, P.: Percutaneous transhepatic cholangiography, *in* Thomson, T. J., and Gillespie, I. E. (eds.): Postgraduate Gastroenterology, London, Baillière, Tindall & Cassell, 1966, p. 309.

35. Gibson, W. R., and Robertson, H. E.: So-called biliary cirrhosis, Arch. Path. *28*: 37, 1939.

36. Glenn, F., and Whitsell, J. C., II: Primary sclerosing cholangitis, Surg. Gynec. Obstet. *123*:1037, 1966.

37. Goldgraber, M. B., and Kirsner, J. B.: Chronic granulomatous cholecystitis and chronic fibrosing choledochitis associated with chronic ulcerative colitis: a case report, Gastroenterology *38*:821, 1960.

38. Goudie, R. B., Macsween, R. N. M., and Goldberg, D. M.: Serological and histological diagnosis of primary biliary cirrhosis, J. Clin. Path. *19*:527, 1966.

39. Hamilton, J. D.: The pathology of primary biliary cirrhosis, Lab. Invest. 8:701, 1959.

40. Hanger, F. M., Jr., and Gutman, A. B.: Postarsphenamine jaundice apparently due to obstruction of intrahepatic biliary tract, J.A.M.A. *115*:263, 1940.

41. Herbert, V.: Hematopoietic factors in liver diseases, *in* Popper, H., and Schaffner, F. (eds.): Progress in Liver Diseases, vol. 2, New York, Grune & Stratton, 1965, p. 57.

42. Hoffbauer, F. W.: Primary biliary cirrhosis: observations on the natural course of the disease in 25 women, Am. J. Dig. Dis. n.s. 5:348, 1960.

43. Holdsworth, C. D., Hall, E. W., Dawson, A. M., and Sherlock, S.: Ulcerative colitis in chronic liver disease, Quart. J. Med. *34*:211, 1965.

44. Jones, W. A., and Tisdale, W. A.: Posthepatitic cirrhosis clinically simulating extrahepatic biliary obstruction (so-called "primary biliary cirrhosis"), New Engl. J. Med. *268*:629, 1963.

45. Kasai, M., Yakovac, W. C., and Koop, C. E.: Liver in congenital biliary atresia and neonatal hepatitis: a histopathologic study, Arch. Path. *74*:152, 1962.

46. Kimmelstiel, P., Large, H. L., Jr., and Verner, H. D.: Liver damage in ulcerative colitis, Am. J. Path. *28*:259, 1952.

47. Kühn, H. A., Müller, W., and Pfister, R.: Über chronische Cholangiolitis und ihre

Beziehung zur primären biliären Cirrhose, Z. klin. Med. *154*:462, 1957.

48. Kunkel, H. G.: Biliary cirrhosis, *in* Schiff, L. (ed.): Diseases of the Liver, Philadelphia, Lippincott, 1956, p. 467.

49. Kunkel, H. G., and Ahrens, E. H., Jr.: The relationship between serum lipids and the electrophoretic pattern, with particular reference to patients with primary biliary cirrhosis, J. Clin. Invest. *28*:1575, 1949.

50. Kunkel, H. G., and Slater, R. J.: Lipoprotein patterns of serum obtained by zone electrophoresis, J. Clin. Invest. *31*: 677, 1952.

51. Lauda, E.: Die hypertrophische Lebercirrhose, M'ed. Klin. *51*:557, 1956.

52. Leevy, C. M.: Fatty liver: a study of 270 patients with biopsy proven fatty liver and a review of the literature, Medicine *41*:249, 1962.

53. Legg, J. W.: Article XII. On the changes in the liver which follow ligature of the bile ducts, St. Barth. Hosp. Rep. *9*:161, 1873.

54. Lévy, V. G., Opolon, P., and Caroli, J.: Cirrhoses biliaires primitives: contribution au diagnostic. Etude anatomopathologique par la méthode de reconstruction, Sem. Hôp. Paris *40*:1749, 1964.

55. Lindenauer, S. M., and Child, C. G., III: Disturbances of liver function in biliary tract disease, Surg. Gynec. Obstet. *123*: 1205, 1966.

56. MacMahon, H. E.: Biliary xanthomatosis (xanthomatous biliary cirrhosis), Am. J. Path. *24*:527, 1948.

57. ———: Biliary cirrhosis: differential features of the five types, Lab. Invest. *4*:243, 1955.

58. MacMahon, H. E., and Mallory, F. B.: Obstructive cirrhosis, Am. J. Path. *5*:645, 1929.

59. Milgrom, F., and Witebsky, E.: Autoantibodies and autoimmune diseases, J.A.M.A. *181*:706, 1962.

60. Moschcowitz, E.: Morphology and pathogenesis of biliary cirrhosis, A.M.A. Arch. Path. *54*:259, 1952.

61. Movitt, E. R.: Biliary cirrhosis in adults: a study based on needle biopsy of the liver, Ann. Int. Med. *45*:242, 1956.

62. Moxon, W.: Simple stricture of hepatic duct, causing chronic jaundice and xanthelasma, Tr. Path. Soc. London *24*:129, 1873.

63. Myers, R. L., Baggenstoss, A. H., Logan, G. B., and Hallenbeck, G. A.: Congenital atresia of the extrahepatic biliary tract: a clinical and pathologic study, Pediatrics *18*:767, 1956.

64. Paronetto, F., and Popper, H.: Chronic liver injury induced by immunologic reactions: cirrhosis following immunization with heterologous sera, Am. J. Path. *49*: 1087, 1966.

65. Paronetto, F., Schaffner, F., Mutter, R. D., Kniffen, J. C., and Popper, H.: Circulating antibodies to bile ductular cells in various liver diseases, J.A.M.A. *187*:503, 1964.

66. Paronetto, F., Schaffner, F., and Popper, H.: Immunocytochemical and serologic observations in primary biliary cirrhosis, New Engl. J. Med. *271*:1123, 1964.

67. Popper, H.: Primary biliary cirrhosis, Rev. int. Hépat. *16*:239, 1966.

68. Popper, H., and Schaffner, F.: Liver: Structure and Function, New York, McGraw-Hill, 1957, 777 pp.

69. Pye Smith, P. H.: Xanthelasma (vitiligoidea plana) of skin, peritoneum and mucous membrane, associated with jaundice: autopsy, Tr. Path. Soc. London *24*: 250, 1873.

70. Rautureau, M., Lemonnier, F., and Chevrel, B.: Les acides biliaires dans les cirrhoses biliaires primitives, Rev. int. Hépat. *16*:193, 1966.

71. Read, A. E., Harrison, C. V., and Sherlock, S.: Chronic chlorpromazine jaundice: with particular reference to its relationship to primary biliary cirrhosis, Am. J. Med. *31*:249, 1961.

72. Ricketts, W. E., and Wissler, R. W.: Cholangiolitic biliary cirrhosis (primary biliary cirrhosis), Ann. Int. Med. *36*:1241, 1952.

73. Roth, D.: Pathologic anatomy of the cirrhotic liver with portal hypertension, Am. J. Dig. Dis. *4*:721, 1959.

74. Rubin, E., Schaffner, F., and Popper, H.: Localization of the basic injury in primary biliary cirrhosis, J.A.M.A. *183*:331, 1963.

75. ———: Primary biliary cirrhosis: chronic non-suppurative destructive cholangitis, Am. J. Path. *46*:387, 1965.

76. Ruebner, B. H., and Miyai, K.: The pathology of neonatal hepatitis and biliary atresia with particular reference to hemopoiesis and hemosiderin deposition, Ann. N. Y. Acad. Sci. *111*:375, 1963.

77. Schaffner, F. (ed.): Clinico-pathological Conference: Diarrhea, anemia and severe

cholestatic jaundice, J. Mt Sinai Hosp. *29*: 239, 1962.

78. Schaffner, F., Klion, F. M., and Latuff, J.: The long term use of cholestyramine in the treatment of primary biliary cirrhosis, Gastroenterology *48*:293, 1965.

79. Schoenfield, L. J., Sjövall, J., and Perman, E.: Bile acids on the skin of patients with pruritic hepatobiliary disease, Nature *213*:93, 1967.

80. Scobie, B. A., and Summerskill, W. H. J.: Hepatic cirrhosis secondary to obstruction of the biliary system, Am. J. Dig. Dis. *10*:135, 1965.

81. Shay, H., and Harris, C.: Changing concepts of "xanthomatous biliary cirrhosis," Am. J. Med. Sci. *223*:286, 1952.

82. Sherlock, S.: Primary biliary cirrhosis (chronic intrahepatic obstructive jaundice), Gastroenterology *37*:574, 1959.

83. Sherlock, S., Datta, D. V., and Walker, J. G.: Prognosis and treatment of primary biliary cirrhosis, Rev. int. Hépat. *16*:217, 1966.

84. Sotgiu, G., Pisi, E., and Cavalli, G.: Hepatite et cirrhose biliaires primitives: aspects étiopathogénétiques, cliniques, histologiques et immunologiques, Rev. int. Hépat. *16*:251, 1966.

85. Stauffer, M. H., Sauer, W. G., and Baggenstoss, A. H.: Cholestatic jaundice with ulcerative colitis, *in* Demling, L., Demole, M., and Popper, H. (eds.): Topical Problems in Diseases of the Liver (2nd World Congress of Gastroenterology), vol. 3, New York, Karger, 1963, p. 220.

86. Steiner, J. W., Carruthers, J. S., Baumal, R., and Kalifat, S. R.: Experimental immunologic liver injury and the concept of autodestruction, Canad. Med. Ass. J. *85*: 1369; 1425, 1961.

87. Stowens, D.: Congenital biliary atresia, Ann. N. Y. Acad. Sci. *111* (Pt. V):337, 1963.

88. Vinnik, I. E., and Kern, F., Jr.: Liver diseases in ulcerative colitis: a review, Arch. Int. Med. *112*:41, 1963.

89. Walker, C. O., and Combes, B.: Biliary cirrhosis induced by chlorpromazine, Gastroenterology *51*:631, 1966.

90. Walker, J. G., Doniach, D., Roitt, I. M., and Sherlock, S.: Serological tests in diagnosis of primary biliary cirrhosis, Lancet *1*:827, 1965.

91. Watson, C. J., and Hoffbauer, F. W.: The problem of prolonged hepatitis with particular reference to the cholangiolitic type and to the development of cholangiolitic cirrhosis of the liver, Ann. Int. Med. *25*: 195, 1946.

92. Wepler, W.: Zur Atiologie und Pathogenese der primaren biliaren Cirrhose, Rev. int. Hépat. *16*:151, 1966.

93. Williams, G. E. G.: Pericholangiolitic biliary cirrhosis, J. Path. Bact. *89*:23, 1965.

21

Hemochromatosis

THEODORE L. ALTHAUSEN, M.D., AND *VICTOR M. SBOROV*, M.D.

Hemochromatosis was first described by Trousseau in 1865.[84] Since that time more than 1,100 cases of this disease have been reported in the literature.[59] Despite its relative rarity, hemochromatosis has intrigued clinicians and investigators far out of proportion to its statistical importance. Numerous publications have recorded case histories, physical findings, histologic changes, laboratory data, studies of metabolism and other aspects of this disease. Even single case reports, whose only purpose is to call attention to some hitherto undescribed feature of hemochromatosis, are not uncommon in the literature.

There are two principal reasons for the great interest in this condition: First, a gross perversion of iron metabolism is involved, the study of which has shed considerable light on normal iron metabolism and promises further advances. Second, hemochromatosis often manifests both diabetes mellitus and hepatic cirrhosis, a rare combination which offers unusual opportunities for studying the activities of both the pancreas and the liver, especially in regard to carbohydrate metabolism.

The early detailed descriptions of its clinical manifestations, the many speculations regarding its etiology and the gradual improvement in diagnostic methods make up one important part of the history of hemochromatosis. Overshadowing these in practical importance are the various therapeutic regimens which have been tried and their success in prolonging the lives of the patients and in altering the clinical manifestations of this disease.

Three milestones mark the outstanding advances in the therapy of hemochromatosis. The first, undoubtedly, was the introduction of insulin and its use in the control of diabetes mellitus, a member of the classic triad formerly needed for the diagnosis of hemochromatosis.[3] Early enthusiasm regarding the efficacy of insulin in ameliorating the course of the disease and lightening the skin pigmentation in hemochromatosis was dimmed when it was found that despite such therapy the disease progressed and death resulted from other complications.

The importance of insulin in the management of these patients is undeniable, but the hypothesis that it alters the fundamental mechanisms of hemochromatosis and halts its progress is no longer tenable. In the late 1930's and early 1940's, when the introduction of dietary measures proved to be successful in the management of chronic liver disease, it was hoped that similar measures would further improve the prognosis in hemochromatosis. Unfortunately, this approach has made only a modest contribution toward improving the outlook in this disease.

The application of modern research technics to the problem of iron metabolism in past years has resulted in a fundamental understanding of the absorption, utilization, storage and excretion of iron by the human body.[39, 40] The natural extension of this knowledge to therapy has resulted in procedures by which, under favorable circumstances, large amounts of iron can be removed from the tissues of patients suffering from hemochromatosis.[21, 31] This treatment improves general well-being, strength, ability to work and clinical as well as laboratory manifestations of pancreatic and hepatic function. Thus, with modern methods of diagnosis, both histologic and biochemical, and with current means of therapy, the outlook for the patient with early manifestations of hemochromatosis is relatively hopeful.

INCIDENCE

Because of the widespread interest in this disease, it is probable that an unusually large proportion of recognized cases has been reported. However, the incidence of this disease varies considerably. Of 335,765 patients admitted to the University of California Hospital through 1960, 48 were diagnosed as having hemochromatosis, or a ratio of 1 case to about 7,000 hospital admissions. On the other hand, Finch and Finch, from an extensive compilation of cases from the literature, arrived at the incidence of 1 case in 20,000 hospital admissions.[32] The same authors concluded that this disease is usually recognized once in 7,000 hospital deaths, while MacDonald and Mallory reported the incidence at the Boston City Hospital to be 1 in 800 hospital deaths.[59]

In a geographic review of hemochromatosis by questionnaire, MacDonald determined that the average rate of occurrence of hemochromatosis in the United States is 178 per 100,000 necropsies and in other countries 180 per 100,000 necropsies.[58] The clinical occurrence in his survey was 9.5 cases per 100,000 hospital admissions in the United States and 70 per 100,000 admissions in other countries.

The diagnosis is more common in the morgue than in the clinic probably because the disease is more difficult to recognize during life. However, Butt and Wilder,[16] in a study covering a 15-year period at the Mayo Clinic, reported 30 cases in which the diagnosis was made during life, and one of us (T.L.A.) studied 15 patients with this disease during a sabbatical leave in Melbourne, Australia.[2]

Statistics show by far the greatest incidence of hemochromatosis in males. It usually occurs between the ages of 35 and 60 years, reaching a peak between 45 and 50 years. Well-authenticated cases of hemo-

chromatosis in females have been described.[78] Of the total 1,100 cases reported in the literature, only just under 60 occurred in women, making a ratio of 17:1. As a rule women develop the disease later in life than men. That the disease in women is diagnosed most often past the menopause is of some importance in view of current concepts of the excretion of iron by the human body.

Familial cases of hemochromatosis have been described and in recent years studied extensively because of the assumption by Sheldon[78] and others that an "inborn error" of iron metabolism is the cause of this disease and because of the growing interest in genetic causation of diseases. In a considerable number of such studies asymptomatic relatives of patients with hemochromatosis were also examined and subjected to biochemical tests concerned with iron metabolism. As a result of these studies almost as many instances of clinical hemochromatosis in siblings, usually male, were described in the last 6 years as in the entire medical literature up to 1955. For example, Boulin and Bamberger collected over 60 familial cases.[14]

Among these families is one reported by Kappeler in which 3 siblings were affected by clinical hemochromatosis, while 4 out of 6 of their children had abnormally high concentrations of iron in the serum.[49] Pirart and Gatez described a family in which a brother, a sister and a sister's daughter had clinical hemochromatosis.[69] Dillingham published the clinical data on a family in which 4 siblings suffered from typical hemochromatosis proved by either skin or liver biopsy.[23] The last family is of particular significance from the point of view of a genetic tendency to this disease because 3 of the affected siblings were females and therefore were partially protected from iron overload of the body by loss of iron in the menstrual blood.

Studies of large numbers of asymptomatic relatives of patients with hemochromatosis have shown that approximately half of the adult male siblings and of the male offspring over the age of 15 years had abnormally high serum iron levels and coefficients of iron saturation.[22] Against these findings has been cited the rarity of clinical hemochromatosis in consecutive generations. On the basis of newer findings, this observation has been explained by transmission of the disease by a dominant mendelian autosomal genetic defect of incomplete penetrance or of variable expressivity in different generations. On the other hand, a recent study of a family survey reporting hemochromatosis in two sisters aged 21 and 23 suggests that there is also a classic autosomal recessive form of the disease where heterozygous relatives cannot be detected with the usual methods.[29]

Family surveys have resulted in the early detection of cases of hemochromatosis in young persons and have provided means by which the disease in such cases can be aborted. Perkins and co-workers have reported a case of a boy aged 13 years found to have classic hemochromatosis.[66] Over a 3 year period, 38 liters of blood were removed, resulting in considerable clinical improvement. Reports of this type also illuminate the effects of this condition in the puberty period in contrast to that in the more adult subject.

ETIOLOGY AND PATHOGENESIS

Through the years a number of hypotheses have been proposed to explain the abnormal accumulation of iron in the tissues of various organs and the pathophysiology of the clinical manifestations in hemochromatosis. Whatever hypothesis one entertains, it must be consistent with the concept that the disease develops over a period of many years. In hemochromatosis the amount of iron in the tissues varies from 10 to 50 Gm.[20] Even if the entire 5 to 15 mg. of iron contained in the average daily diet were absorbed, it would take 6 to 30 years to accumulate the large deposits in the tissues of patients with hemochromatosis. This is all the more true since it is highly unlikely that intestinal absorption of iron is ever complete.[77]

One of the earliest and most attractive theories, even today, is that excessive hemolysis of red blood cells in hemochromatosis liberates iron, which is deposited in the tissues of the body.[34, 78] For example, in untreated pernicious anemia,

hemolytic anemias and refractory anemias, increased amounts of iron often are found in the liver and other tissues of the body, even when no blood transfusions have been given. A number of possible explanations for such hemolysis have been advanced; however, despite careful studies of pigment metabolism and red cell turnover, excessive destruction of red blood cells in hemochromatosis has not been proved.

In spite of the negative outcome of these studies, the red blood cell is undoubtedly one of the most logical sources of iron. Indeed, several reports describe a form of hemochromatosis of exogenous origin following multiple blood transfusions to anemic patients.[77, 87] As demonstrated by radioactive studies in anemias of various types the uptake of iron from the gastrointestinal tract is increased.[25] Thus, the excessive deposition of iron in anemic individuals may result from a combination of factors, rather than from a single factor.

The frequent occurrence in South African natives of another exogenous form of hemochromatosis of dietary origin has been described by Gillman and Gillman.[35] These authors also observed features of this disease in pellagra and other forms of malnutrition due chiefly to a staple diet of corn. They concluded that this form of hemochromatosis is caused by a derangement of metabolism which finally results in widespread dissemination and deposition of iron pigment in the tissues. They stated that the concomitant hepatic cirrhosis is not necessarily the result of the deposition of iron in the liver but may have been preexistent or due to other causes.

Bothwell et al. have reviewed the evidence comparing idiopathic hemochromatosis and Bantu hemochromatosis.[12] They found distinct differences in these entities: Iron was more concentrated in the spleen in Bantu hemochromatosis than in idiopathic hemochromatosis and the distribution of iron deposits within the liver in the two forms differed. These differences tend to show that idiopathic hemochromatosis is a separate entity rather than a variation of nutritional cirrhosis resulting from a high dietary intake of iron. That the coincident occurrence of cirrhosis and heavy iron deposits in the liver is a matter of association or common etiology rather than a cause-and-effect relationship is considered by some authors.[56]

The nutritional hemochromatosis described by the Gillmans is now thought to be related to a disturbance of the iron-phosphorus ratio in the diet, whereas the fatty and fibrous tissue changes seen in the livers of the South African natives with this condition may be the manifestation of an independent nutritional liver disease.[35] Hegsted and co-workers demonstrated that rats fed a diet low in phosphorus with liberal additions of iron develop an increase in iron absorption and storage.[42] A similar situation exists in South Africa, where a high dietary intake of iron with a very low proportion of phosphorus favors excessive absorption of iron. A detailed survey of a group of patients by Althausen and co-workers showed no deficiency in the phosphate intake and only slightly increased iron content of the diet[2] (Fig. 21–1).

Knutsen suggested that hemochromatosis results from a primary cirrhosis of the liver and the pancreas which leads to an abnormality of iron metabolism and a progressive deposition of iron in the tissues.[52] He also postulated that the formation of the related iron-free pigment, hemofuscin, also present in the tissues in hemochromatosis, stems from an abnormality of sulfur-protein metabolism caused by hepatic dysfunction. This hypothesis is partially supported by the fact that markedly elevated serum iron levels are known to occur in acute viral hepatitis and in some cases of chronic liver disease.[67]

Sheldon concluded that hemochromatosis results from a congenital endogenous disturbance of the intermediary metabolism of iron which manifests itself partly by the formation of iron-containing hemosiderin in the tissues and partly by the formation of iron-free melanin in smooth muscle, connective tissue and skin.[78] At one time Mallory advanced the hypothesis that copper poisoning causes hemochromatosis. He and his co-workers produced cirrhosis of the liver with pigmentation of several parenchymatous organs resembling that of hemochromatosis by feeding large amounts of copper acetate to animals.[60] In addition, they elicited a history of industrial exposure to copper from several patients with hemochromatosis. Herkel found that the livers of patients dying from hemochromatosis contained greatly increased amounts of copper, although the same was true of patients with hepatic cirrhosis and normal infants.[44]

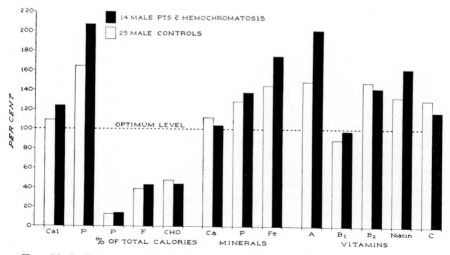

F IG. 21–1. Dietary intake in per cent of optimum amount recommended by National Research Council compared in 14 male patients with hemochromatosis and 25 male controls. (Althausen, T. L., et al.: Tr. Ass. Am. Physicians 63:209)

Although one group of investigators confirmed the animal experiments of Mallory et al., several other workers were unable to do so.[4] Mallory's theory was widely accepted for a time but was gradually abandoned when it became apparent that few patients with hemochromatosis had been exposed to copper, and that relatively enormous amounts of copper were required to produce hepatic lesions in experimental animals.

Once alcoholism was considered as an important contributing cause of hemochromatosis, particularly since a large proportion of reported cases occurred in chronic alcoholics. For instance, MacDonald has pointed out that alcoholism is found in 29 to 85 per cent of cases of hemochromatosis.[56] Yet hemochromatosis occurs in total abstainers as well and therefore alcoholism cannot be the only cause of the disease. Dubin suggests that excessive intake of alcohol accelerates the development of hemochromatosis.[26]

MacDonald has challenged the prevailing concepts of the pathogenesis of hemochromatosis and concluded that in most cases endogenous hemochromatosis is a variant of portal cirrhosis and of endogenous hemosiderosis.[56] In a few cases, in his opinion, the disease results from two coexisting conditions, such as nutritional deficiency or hepatic disease plus a hematologic disease or environmental condition leading to increased iron absorption. This concept of the pathogenesis of hemochromatosis is supported by the results of recently reported animal experiments.[38] In one study, rats loaded with iron and fed ethionine and a low protein diet developed cirrhosis of the liver in a much shorter time than their controls in which the iron-loading was omitted. This study suggests that a combination of hepatic damage plus an iron overload produces hemochromatosis.

Information concerning iron metabolism in the normal state, in hematologic disorders and in hemochromatosis indicates that a fundamental defect underlies the increased absorption of iron from the gastrointestinal tract in hemochromatosis.[1, 25, 68] The cause of this increase and the exact mechanism involved are undetermined. The increased absorption of iron, plus the lack of a natural mechanism for excreting excesses of iron from the body, accounts for the widespread deposition and storage of iron pigment in the tissues and the resultant secondary changes in their structure and function.

Considerable controversy has stemmed from attempts to differentiate between hemochromatosis and hemosiderosis.[5, 51] Some investigators regard them as two distinct entities with different clinical and prognostic implications.[41, 51, 64] Excessive deposition of iron in the tissues after numerous transfusions and administration of large amounts of iron by mouth or by vein to patients with refractory anemia has been termed hemosiderosis to distinguish this condition from hemochromatosis in the asymptomatic stage. Animal experiments with iron overloading for varying periods of time have led to the conclusion that chronic iron toxicity does not result in experimental hemochromatosis.[73]

On the contrary, in humans, cases of so-called hemosiderosis of exogenous origin indistinguishable from classic hemochromatosis have been reported in considerable numbers.[10, 77, 87] Further evidence is reported by Richter based on the results of chemical analyses, serologic tests and electron microscopy.[74] He found that hemosiderin granules from patients with endogenous and exogenous hemochromatosis were qualitatively similar in composition of inorganic iron, ferritin and apoferritin. He tentatively concluded that a similar abnormal pathway in the cellular metabolism of ferritin is responsible for both conditions.

A patient with exogenous hemochromatosis, a 59-year-old white male, was first studied in New Zealand 9 years before being studied by us at the University of California Hospital. He had sought medical help for an anemia, having enjoyed good health until then. After careful studies, including the finding of a hypoplastic bone marrow, the diagnosis of aplastic anemia was made. In the following 9-year period he required over 300 units of whole blood to maintain a satisfactory hemoglobin level. Supportive therapy included 0.9 Gm. of ferrous sulfate daily during this entire period.

In the last 2 or 3 years of medical observation in New Zealand, the liver and spleen had

IRON METABOLISM - NORMAL

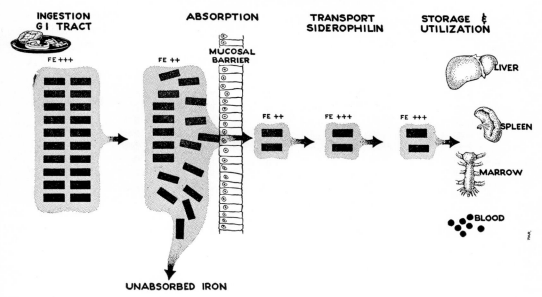

FIGURE 21-2

enlarged gradually. Shortly before admission at the University of California Hospital he noticed that his skin had become slate gray. There was no history of jaundice, ascites, weakness or symptoms suggestive of diabetes mellitus. A liver biopsy 6 months prior to the present hospitalization was reported to show "cirrhosis and hemosiderosis."

Our physical examination revealed moderate obesity and no distress. No jaundice was present. A slate gray and brownish pigmentation was noted over the dorsum of the hands, the face and the exposed portion of the neck. The distribution of the body hair was normal. Blood pressure was 158/82. The heart was not enlarged. The heart rate was normal, and no cardiac arrhythmia was present. The liver was enlarged to 8 cm. above and 10 cm. below the right costal margin in the mid-clavicular line. The spleen was palpated 6 cm. below the costal margin. The liver and spleen were firm and not tender. The testicles were small and atrophic.

Laboratory studies for hemosiderin in urinary sediment were negative. A urinalysis was normal except for 2+ albuminuria. A sternal bone marrow aspiration showed a hypoplastic marrow with abundant deposits of hemosiderin. Results of the following tests were within normal limits: prothrombin time, thymol turbidity, zinc turbidity, serum bilirubin, serum albumin and globulin, alkaline phosphatase, total cholesterol, per cent cholesterol esters, cephalin cholesterol flocculation and intravenous hippuric acid. An oral glucose tolerance test showed a diabetic curve, with a fasting blood sugar of 128 mg./100 cc. and a peak of 196 mg./100 cc., which was reached at 1 hour.

An electrocardiogram showed borderline ST and T wave changes. A skin biopsy was negative for hemosiderin. A liver biopsy demonstrated marked portal and periportal fibrosis with bile duct proliferation. Portal areas were filled with macrophages containing large amounts of iron. A gastrointestinal x-ray study was negative for esophageal varices. Further clarifying studies of the basic hematologic disease demonstrated a factor of hypersplenism. Splenectomy resulted in maintenance of a stable hemoglobin level.

The difference between hemochromatosis and hemosiderosis, in our opinion, consists of the presence or the absence of clinical disease. In endogenous hemosiderosis the mucosa of the gut absorbs excessive amounts of iron from food, which is the sole source of iron in this condition (Figs. 21-2, 3). The dietary iron is deposited primarily in the parenchymatous organs,

IRON METABOLISM - ENDOGENOUS HEMOCHROMATOSIS

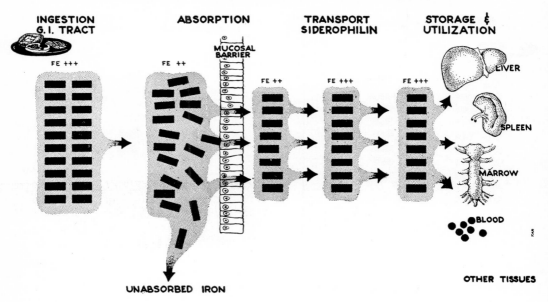

FIGURE 21–3

notably the liver, pancreas and heart. If present in large amounts for a sufficiently long time these deposits lead to the clinical picture of endogenous hemochromatosis. Exogenous hemosiderosis results when iron is administered for refractory anemias by multiple blood transfusions or parenteral injections of medicinal iron and is deposited primarily in the reticuloendothelial system, where it is relatively innocuous.

In such cases increased amounts of iron are also absorbed by the intestine from food and medicinal preparations of iron (Fig. 21–4) and are deposited in parenchymatous organs. A classic example of this is iron-loading, pyridoxine-deficient anemia. Increased absorption of iron, plus lack of utilization, results in large accumulations of iron in the tissues and secondary organ fibrosis with clinical cardiac, hepatic and pancreatic decompensation.[89] In some patients part of the injected iron apparently also finds its way into the parenchymatous organs and in combination with iron entering from the gut produces typical exogenous hemochromatosis. Admittedly, in many cases of refractory anemia, energetic parenteral therapy may result in asymptomatic

accumulation of total body iron in amounts equal to those found in full-blown endogenous hemochromatosis. This is explained by the accumulation of iron over a shorter period and the relatively harmless localization of a portion of the iron without altering the concept that the essential differences between hemosiderosis and hemochromatosis, whether endogenous or exogenous, are quantitative and chronologic rather than qualitative.[5, 6] Some investigators have attached significance to the fact that hemofuscin is present in hemochromatosis and absent in hemosiderosis.[41] This also is not a fundamental distinction, since hemofuscin may form in other diseases.[26]

Certain structures in the body, when infiltrated with iron, undergo fibrosis and suffer a marked disturbance of function (e.g., pancreatic islets), whereas others show no anatomic or functional abnormalities (e.g., chief cells of the gastric mucosa).[2] It is possible that the former structures are more susceptible than the latter to iron and that therefore their architecture and metabolism are interfered with more readily. The duration of involvement of various organs also may be of impor-

IRON METABOLISM – EXOGENOUS HEMOCHROMATOSIS

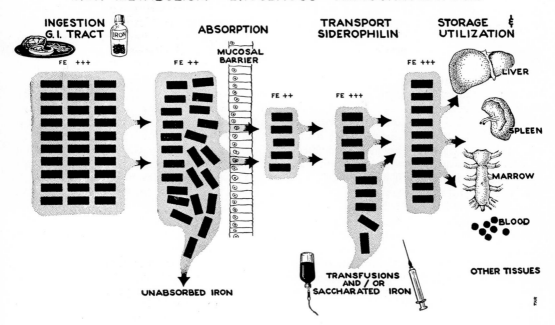

FIGURE 21–4

tance. Certain organs that store iron readily, such as the liver and pancreas, become involved at a much earlier stage of the disease, and thus show structural and functional changes before other organs that store iron less readily.

Since hemochromatosis is so rare in females, particularly during the child-bearing age, loss of iron through menstrual bleeding is thought to prevent clinical manifestations of the disease. It has been estimated that during the reproductive life 15 Gm. of iron is lost in this manner. Each childbirth accounts for a further loss of approximately 500 mg. of iron.[40] Consistent with this concept is the observation that hemochromatosis occurs only in middle-aged women or in women who have disturbances associated with a grossly diminished menstrual flow and are usually childless.[2, 46]

CLINICAL FEATURES

HISTORY

Since hemochromatosis is a multiple system disease, it is manifested by a wide variety of symptoms. These symptoms can be divided into those that are nonspecific or general and those that relate to some organ system of the body. The outstanding general symptoms are weakness, fatigability, loss of weight and lack of energy and initiative. These symptoms, which are found in varying degrees in most patients with proved hemochromatosis, are gradual in onset, but progressive; in many instances they are noted to persist despite therapy for the coexistent diabetes and hepatic disease. Frequently, these general complaints antedate the diagnosis of the disease by many years.

The major manifestations of the disease consist of the classic triad of pigmentation of the skin, diabetes mellitus and cirrhosis of the liver. This triad was noted at the time of diagnosis in over 80 per cent of the cases described in the literature.[32, 78] The fact that more specific diagnostic procedures were lacking until recently makes it easy to understand why these three manifestations were seen in such a large proportion of the reported cases, since by definition they comprise the clinical syndrome of hemochromatosis. Use of current diagnostic technics, the greater awareness of the many expressions of the disease and the widespread testing and examining of relatives of patients with clinical hemochromatosis undoubtedly will lead to recognition of the disease at an earlier stage, and many patients will lack the classic triad when they first come under medical observation. A recent survey has justifiably called attention to the wide variety of diagnostic criteria for hemochromatosis used by pathologists and clinicians.[59] Earlier diagnosis poses the problem of a more precise definition of hemochromatosis, and specific minimum criteria for such a diagnosis must be established.

Skin pigmentation, although probably present in 90 per cent of patients at the time of diagnosis when looked for, has been reported as a prominent feature in only 30 per cent of cases.[32] Its presence and the details concerning its development must be established by careful interrogation. The time at which the increase in pigmentation began can rarely be fixed exactly. As a rule, the patient is aware only that his skin has been dark for a number of years, sometimes for decades, and has become darker in the period immediately preceding medical observation. Only 10 to 15 per cent show pigmentation of the mucous membranes.

In contrast, the onset of the symptoms of diabetes mellitus, particularly polydipsia and polyuria, can be established with relative exactness. These symptoms, along with weight loss which usually is also related to the diabetes, generally can be controlled without difficulty by means of diet and insulin.[4, 16] About three fourths of the 82 per cent of patients who have diabetes mellitus require insulin.

In hemochromatosis, the principal symptoms related to the liver are hepatic enlargement and tenderness; ascites and jaundice are much less frequent. Anorexia, diarrhea and other gastrointestinal symptoms which may also reflect involvement of the liver are often present. In general, surprisingly few symptoms specifically referable to the liver are noted in hemochromatosis despite the long standing and extensive hepatic involvement in all reported cases.

Symptoms referable to the cardiovascular system, such as arrhythmias, palpitation, exertional dyspnea, orthopnea, ankle edema and angina pectoris, have been recorded at the time of diagnosis in about 15 per cent of patients with this disease.[45] However, Finch and Finch state that about one third of all patients subsequently develop symptoms referable to the heart.[32] The type and severity of the cardiovascular manifestations have not been found to correlate with the presence and extent of hemosiderin deposits in the myocardium. For this reason, it is often difficult to determine whether these symptoms result from the hemochromatosis or from a coexistent cardiovascular disease. However, age may provide a clue, since patients in whom cardiovascular manifestations are related to excessive deposits of iron in the myocardium develop such manifestations at an earlier age than patients with degenerative cardiovascular disease. The rate at which iron is deposited in the myocardium may be of far greater significance in the development of cardiac symptoms than the amount of hemosiderin present.[66]

Impotence and lack of libido are frequent complaints of patients with hemochromatosis.[4] Whether these, along with spider nevi and palmar erythema, are evidence of hepatic insufficiency or of a primary endocrine abnormality of the hypophysis, adrenal glands or gonads is not known.

PHYSICAL EXAMINATION

Pigmentation of the skin and mucous membranes—one of the classic triad of symptoms in hemochromatosis—should alert the physician immediately to a possible diagnosis of this disease. The pigmentation usually considered characteristic is "bluish gray" or "slaty" in color, as distinguished from a more extensive generalized brown pigmentation due to simple melanin deposition in the skin (Plate 1). In our experience, both types of pigmentation appear prominently on the forearms, and somewhat less so on the face, neck, upper arms, hands, legs and feet.[2] Sometimes the distribution of the bluish-gray pigmentation is generalized, but even then it is more prominent on the parts mentioned. However, Sheldon found the pigmentation more abundant in the axillary and the inguinal folds and around the genitalia.[78] The nature and the distribution of the pigmentation seem to be too variable to constitute a pathognomonic sign, especially if the slaty tint is missing.

Pigmentation of the mucous membrane is also fairly common, as evidenced by Sheldon's report of this finding in 16.7 per cent of 197 collected patients with hemochromatosis.[78] The mucous membranes of the mouth, particularly the inside of the cheeks, are the most frequent site of this type of pigmentation. The pigment usually occurs in localized plaques or areas, rather than as generalized deposits. Pigmentation has been found also in the conjunctiva and, at autopsy, in the trachea, esophagus and stomach. The depth of pigmentation is variable, even in untreated patients. A deepening of the pigmentation has been noted after bouts of alcoholism, incident to aggravation of diabetes, and in the terminal stages of the disease.[78] Conversely, diminution in pigmentation has been observed repeatedly following the use of insulin in patients with previously uncontrolled diabetes.[3, 16] The reason for this decrease is not clear.

The skin of patients with hemochromatosis usually is shiny and dry or scaly. On palpation it is found to be of fine texture and considerably atrophied.

The liver is involved in all cases of hemochromatosis; in fact, enlargement of the liver is the most consistent clinical feature of this disease. It has been found to be palpably enlarged in as many as 93 per cent of cases.[32] Characteristically, the liver is hard, smooth and in some instances tender. Usually, the enlargement is massive and diffuse, affecting both the right and the left lobes, although cases have been noted in which the left lobe was not palpable. It has also been described as coarsely nodular on palpation.

The spleen is palpable in about 50 per cent of cases. Clinical jaundice has been reported in only 10 per cent of cases.[16] Ascites is noted in about 35 per cent of all reported cases and is usually present only in the later stages of the disease. Spider nevi are found in about 60 per cent of diagnosed cases. Bleeding from ruptured esophageal varices has resulted in death in some cases. Use of modern roentgenologic methods and esophagoscopy can be expected to demonstrate esophageal varices in a fairly large number of patients.[15]

Myocardial involvement, evidenced by arrhythmias and symptoms of congestive heart failure, also occurs. Among their collected patients with hemochromatosis, Bothwell and Alper noted 33 cases with clinical heart failure[11] and Horns, in a review of English and American literature, noted 9 cases in which cardiac symptoms and signs were prominent[45]; Finch noted that in 15 per cent of cases the initial complaints included cardiac symptoms. About one third of all patients later develop symptoms referable to the heart, and approximately the same number ultimately die of cardiac complications. Cardiac involvement is thus the most important cause of death in hemochromatosis.[32]

According to Horns, the most common electrocardiographic change noted among patients with myocardial damage was low voltage. He also found complete heart block and auricular fibrillation in each of two cases respectively. Finch pointed out that symptoms of heart failure may develop rapidly, sometimes within only a few days. Cyanosis of the skin is a prominent feature in some of these patients; and when heart failure develops, both ventricles usually become dilated so that the cardiac silhouette assumes a globular shape resembling that seen in beriberi or with a pericardial effusion. The relatively infrequent incidence of symptoms and objective findings indicative of myocardial involvement is surprising in view of the extensive deposits of hemosiderin found in the myocardium of almost all patients examined postmortem.

In hemochromatosis the body hair is characteristically sparse, soft and thin.[2] In men, the pattern of distribution may be feminine. Whether the hair changes are caused by the disease or whether hemochromatosis is more common in individuals with hair of this type and distribution is not known. Endocrine changes with lack of development of secondary sexual characteristics are more common when the disease appears early in life.[66]

In one group of 20 male patients more

than half had atrophic or soft testicles and some had a small penis.[78]

IRON METABOLISM

In the past several years much investigative effort has been directed toward accumulation of fundamental information about how the human body metabolizes iron. Certain concepts have been developed which, although not finally established, serve to clarify our understanding of iron metabolism.[63]

Granick demonstrated that normally iron is absorbed from the gastrointestinal tract in the region of the duodenum and, more specifically, in the area just distal to the pyloric sphincter.[39] When large amounts of iron are ingested, the more distal portions of the small intestine probably also participate in its absorption. The limitation of the absorptive area in the gastrointestinal tract is probably related more closely to the chemical availability of the iron than to the selective character of the intestinal site.

Iron is absorbed most readily when in the ferrous rather than the ferric form, and its absorption is influenced by conditions in the intestinal lumen. For example, achlorhydria, alkaline medications and diets high in phosphorus content decrease the absorption of iron from ingested food.[87]

According to Granick, the ingested iron becomes bound in the intestinal tract to a protein acceptor called apoferritin, which is present in limited amounts.[40] The combined form, known as ferritin, releases the iron to the plasma; then apoferritin combines again with ferrous iron. Granick postulated that the apoferritin-ferritin system regulates the absorption of iron from the gastrointestinal tract by blocking further uptake when the available apoferritin is combined with iron. In experiments performed subsequently, Heilmeyer found no evidence to indicate that an increased amount of ferritin in the intestinal mucosa reduces iron absorption.[43] He concluded that the ferritin system in the gastrointestinal tract merely mediates the absorption of iron, so that when much iron is absorbed, much ferritin is present, and when less iron is absorbed, less ferritin is present.

Detailed studies have recently clarified certain features of iron kinetics in the intestine.[91] Following parenteral injection of iron-59, it was noted that the injected iron is concentrated in newly formed cells of the crypts of Lieberkühn. The iron remains in these cells for their entire life span. Thus it is presumed that the subsequent absorptive potential for each mucosal cell for iron was determined at the time of its formation. The amount of the iron incorporated into the cell is dependent on the plasma iron clearance, which in turn is related to the then current requirements. Thus when the marrow requires iron for increased erythropoiesis, less iron is available for incorporation into the developing mucosal cell. The absorptive capacity of these cells for iron from the intestinal lumen is then increased. This provides a baseline regulation of iron absorption which changes according to the changing requirements for iron. The mucosal regulation or "self inhibition" of iron absorption is postulated to be operative within the limits of the usual levels of dietary iron. With the oral administration of large amounts of iron, this regulatory mechanism can be overcome and large, even toxic, amounts of iron can be absorbed. Despite evidence such as this, there is continued debate as to the existence of a mucosal regulatory mechanism and its precise function.

In the plasma, the nonheme iron is bound to a protein called transferrin (siderophilin).[72] Transferrin is a beta-1 globulin which binds not only iron but copper and zinc as well.[81] This protein makes up about 3 per cent of the total serum protein and migrates electrophoretically with the beta-1 globulin. Quantitative determinations of transferrin can be made directly only by means of immunochemical technics with antitransferrin serum. The iron-binding protein content of the blood is determined indirectly by measurement of the total iron-binding capacity of the serum (TIBC).[55] This indicates the total amount of iron that can be bound by transferrin in the serum. Transferrin values are high in chronic iron deficiency (TIBC over 400 μg./100 ml. serum). Transferrin values are low in all conditions that interfere with the synthesis of plasma proteins

(TIBC under 260 μg./100 ml.). Normally, the TIBC is approximately 300 μg./100 ml. of serum; usually only approximately half of this capacity is utilized.[37, 47] In hemochromatosis, serum iron levels as high as 480 μg. have been reported.[2] The level of serum iron usually reflects the amount of iron available for the synthesis of hemoglobin.[39, 48] This level does not regulate the movement of iron from the intestinal mucosa into the blood.[80]

Iron does not circulate in the blood in the free state except in patients in the terminal stages of hemochromatosis or in persons given massive amounts of iron intravenously.[39] If an excessive amount (greater than 10 mg. of iron) is given intravenously, the subject reacts with flushing, nausea and vomiting.[53] The complete binding of iron to protein, both in the blood and in the tissues, is believed to account for the exceedingly small amounts of iron normally lost from the human body. The daily loss of iron in the urine is 0.1 to 1.3 mg., according to different investigators[86]; in addition, minute amounts are lost in desquamated cells of the skin. Small amounts of iron in the bile and other digestive secretions also reach the gastrointestinal tract but are subject to reabsorption. Much of the iron incorporated into the developing intestinal mucosal cells, as noted above, is lost when the cells are sloughed at the villus tip.[18]

In the normal person, 75 to 85 per cent of the total body iron is contained in the hemoglobin of the red blood cells and muscle, 15 per cent (in the form of ferritin) is stored in the gastrointestinal tract, the liver and the spleen, and approximately 1 per cent is contained in the heme enzymes of the cells.[39] The average diet provides 5 to 15 mg. of iron daily, of which approximately 0.5 mg. is absorbed.

In idiopathic hemochromatosis, excessive amounts of iron are absorbed. This has been demonstrated by the use of iron balance technics. In normal subjects, after oral administration of small amounts of radioactive iron in the ferric form, Peterson and Ettinger found the absorption of iron from the gastrointestinal tract to be 1.5 to 4.4 per cent of the ingested amount.[68] In patients with hemochromatosis 20 to 45 per cent of the ingested iron was absorbed. It was shown further that in patients with increased iron stores, the uptake of radioactive iron in the red blood cells cannot be used as an index of iron absorption. The authors concluded that the only reliable way to measure iron absorption is by the balance technic.

Other studies using this method indicate that iron absorption in patients with fully developed but untreated hemochromatosis is similar to that of normal individuals, whereas after repeated venesection, as much as 88.5 per cent of iron ingested in the form of ferrous chloride is again absorbed.[17]

As data continue to accumulate with the use of balance technics and radioiron absorption, inconsistencies become apparent. The amount of iron absorbed normally at different times by the same individual may vary. Variations have also been noted in hemochromatosis from cases to case. Different stages of the disease and different physiologic conditions undoubtedly account for many of the discrepancies noted.[57]

Studies by Gitlow and Beyers have indicated that in hemochromatosis not only the intestinal mucosa but other tissues as well develop a greater affinity for iron.[36] The consequent gross overloading of the iron depots of the body over a period of many years eventually results in the clinical manifestations of this disease. Whereas the total body iron normally is about 4.5 Gm., in hemochromatosis it may be more than 50 Gm. This iron, in the form of hemosiderin, a ferric hydroxide polymer which microscopically has the appearance of granular brown particles, is deposited in most of the tissues of the body in hemochromatosis.

The available facts indicate that a greater than normal absorption of iron over a period of years is responsible for the final picture of massive iron deposition in the tissues in hemochromatosis.[4, 5] Since only small amounts of iron are lost normally, except during menstruation and as a result of parturition, this disease can be controlled only by (1) blocking absorption of iron and (2) removing excess storage iron by repeated withdrawal of red blood cells or by increasing the elimination of iron through normal channels.[21, 62]

LABORATORY FEATURES

SERUM IRON

Quantitative determinations of serum iron are a valuable aid in the diagnosis of hemochromatosis. An increase in the serum iron level is one of the earliest abnormalities of iron metabolism which can be measured, and was found by Finch in 31 of 32 cases in the symptomatic stage of hemochromatosis.[30] Althausen and co-workers found initial abnormal serum iron levels in 12 of 18 cases of proved hemochromatosis (Fig. 21–5).[2] Serial determinations in 5 of the 18 cases after an average interval of 15 months showed a significant increase in each case, including 3 cases in which the serum iron rose from a normal or high normal to a definitely abnormal level. Furthermore, iron levels above 150 μg./100 ml. of serum have been noted in about 20 per cent of asymptomatic relatives of patients with hemochromatosis.[13]

According to Houston and Thompson, serum iron levels rose considerably after oral administration of 1 Gm. of ferrous sulfate to normal subjects.[47] However, the same amount of ferrous sulfate administered to 7 patients with hemochromatosis in whom fasting serum iron levels were high resulted in little or no rise in iron levels.

Although the concentration of iron-binding protein in the blood is not changed in hemochromatosis, the percentage of this protein saturated with iron is high. Houston and Thompson found it to be approximately twice as high in patients with hemochromatosis as in normal controls.

A test for determining the iron-binding capacity of the blood has been described by Rath and Finch.[72] The method is based on the observation of Schade that transferrin, which is colorless, assumes a salmon color when it combines with iron. When the transferrin becomes saturated with iron, the color curve (absorption maximum 470 to 480 mμ) shows a sharp break at the exact point where free iron can be demonstrated by bio-assay. As noted, no significant increase in serum iron concentration follows oral or intravenous administration of iron to patients with saturated iron-binding capacity, such as occurs in hemochromatosis.[47]

HEPATIC FUNCTION

In hemochromatosis impairment of liver function shows a surprising lack of correlation with either hemosiderin deposits or structural changes in the liver. Butt and Wilder reported that liver function was often within normal limits in their patients.[16] In another comprehensive study, hippuric acid synthesis was found to be depressed in

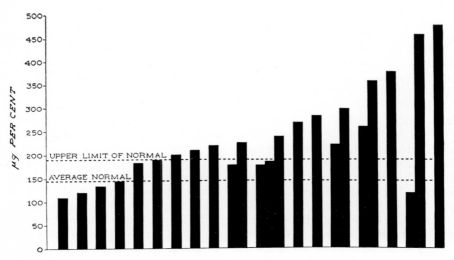

FIG. 21–5. Serum iron levels in 18 patients with hemochromatosis. (Althausen, T. L., et al.: Ass. Am. Physicians 63:209.)

TABLE 21–1.   RESULTS OF LIVER FUNCTION TESTS IN 15 PATIENTS WITH HEMOCHROMATOSIS

Case No.	Cephalin Floccu- lation	Thymol Floc- cula- tion	Thymol Tur- bidity, Units	Gamma Globulin, Gm./100 cc.	Serum Albumin, Gm./100 cc.	Hippuric Acid Synthesis, Gm.	Bromsulph- alein Retention, 45 Min., %	Liver Biopsy Specimen
1	0	0	6	1.03	5.5	0.42	10	Hemosiderin only
2	0	0	4.6	1.05	4.8	0.82	5	Hemosiderin only
3	0	0	5	1.30	5.2	0.72	5	Multinodular cirrhosis
4	0	0	3.5	1.03	4.7	0.22	5	Multinodular cirrhosis
5	0	0	5.5	1.26	4.0	0.59	5	Hemosiderin only
6	++	0	12.5	1.32	3.9	0.42	20	Multinodular cirrhosis
7	+	0	8	1.43	4.3	0.23	10	Multinodular cirrhosis
8	0	0	7	1.35	6.4	0.20	10	Multinodular cirrhosis
9	0	0	7	1.30	3.9	0.79	20	Multinodular cirrhosis
10	0	0	5.2	. . .	4.0	0.80	7	No Biopsy
11	+	0	8.6	1.12	6.2	0.97	. .	Multinodular cirrhosis
12	0	0	7.3	1.21	6.2	0.22	5	Laennec cirrhosis
13	0	0	9.5	1.49	4.8	0.33	15	Laennec cirrhosis
14	0	0	6.5	1.13	5.2	0.39	5	Multinodular cirrhosis
15	+	0	9.6	1.52	4.3	0.29	5	Multinodular cirrhosis
Normal	0 to +	0	< 5	< 1.24	> 4	> 0.7	< 5	

(Althausen et al.: Arch. Int. Med. 88:553.)

two thirds of the 15 patients studied, while Bromsulphalein retention and gamma globulin levels were abnormally high in half the cases.[2] An even smaller proportion of patients showed other manifestations of hepatic involvement (Table 21–1). Rigas reported a study of serum proteins in hemochromatosis.[75] In this study electrophoretic measurements showed the predominant abnormality to be a lowering of *alpha*-globulin. The *beta*-globulin did not appear to be affected. It was concluded that this change was not specific and might be attributable to the presence of liver disease or diabetes mellitus.

These data seem to indicate a lesser degree of hepatic insufficiency in hemochromatosis than in other forms of cirrhosis with a comparable degree of fibrosis. A slower progression of the disease may account for this difference.

PANCREATIC FUNCTION

The exocrine function of the pancreas was studied in 13 patients with hemochromatosis[2] (Table 21–2). In 5 of these patients the ability to break down gelatin apparently was impaired, probably due to insufficient secretion of trypsin. A secretin response test was performed in 7 patients in this group; in only one case was the total amount of bicarbonate secreted lower than that secreted by control subjects, while 4 of the patients showed hypersecretion of a dilute pancreatic juice.*

The laboratory features of diabetes in hemochromatosis are variable. In many cases diabetes mellitus is detected only by the glucose tolerance test;[16] in others, diabetes is frank. Both insulin-sensitive and insulin-resistant types of diabetes have been noted[4]; this variation may result from involvement of other organs which influence carbohydrate metabolism, such as the liver, pituitary and adrenals.

Of considerable interest in the consideration of the etiology of hemochromatosis and the physiology of iron absorption are reports that pancreatic enzymes normally inhibit absorption of iron.[65] The relationship between the pancreatic fibrosis com-

* Dreiling, in a study of 71 patients with chronic inflammatory disease of the pancreas, reported this same finding in the only patient with hemochromatosis.[24] The only other patient in this series in whom the volume of pancreatic juice secreted was unusually large had "pancreatic fibrosis and hepatic cirrhosis" shown by biopsy.

TABLE 21-2.   RESULTS OF PANCREATIC FUNCTION TESTS IN 13 PATIENTS
WITH HEMOCHROMATOSIS

CASE No.	RISE IN AMINO NITROGEN OF BLOOD, MG./100 CC.		DUODENAL CONTENTS AFTER SECRETIN		
	After Gelatin	After Glycine	Volume, cc.	Bicarbonate Concentration, mM./cc.	Total Bicarbonate, mM.
1	3.6	3.8	107	0.110	11.7
3	2.7	..	350	0.060	21.1
4	2.2	6.4	187	0.038	6.4
5	6.3	..	...	....	...
6	1.7	3.4	...	....	...
7	3.7	..	...	....	...
8	4.1	..	223	0.064	14.4
9	3.5	..	...	....	...
11	2.0	..	...	....	...
12	0.5	3.2	333	0.072	24.8
13	0.9	4.1	166	0.093	15.4
14	1.6	3.0	480	0.052	25.4
15	1.8	4.6	...	....	...
Normal	2.0	2.5	90–192	72–128	10.7–17.75

(Althausen et al.: Arch. Int. Med. 88:553.)

monly associated with hemochromatosis and the contribution of increased iron absorption due to this factor must be evaluated in some of the cases encountered. Certain of the reports indicate that administration of pancreatin suppresses excessive iron absorption, but this effect has been found to date to be far from consistent.

THE BLOOD

Anemia was reported by earlier observers to be a prominent feature of endogenous hemochromatosis[78]; later investigators were unable to confirm this finding,[77] and recently it was shown that both the formation of hemoglobin and the life span of the erythrocytes are normal in this disease.[70] Thus, the very absence of hematologic abnormalities helps to distinguish between the endogenous and exogenous types of hemochromatosis. Studies of the other formed blood elements have shown only inconstant deviations from normal.

PATHOLOGY

In hemochromatosis practically all tissues of the body show the characteristic deposits of hemosiderin, although certain tissues are involved more extensively than others. Of special importance are abnormalities of the skin, liver, pancreas, heart, stomach and endocrine organs.

Skin. Grossly, the skin appears thin and dry, with a notable sparseness of hair. Microscopic study shows atrophy of the epidermis, hair follicles and sebaceous glands. Sometimes the epidermis is reduced to a sheet only 4 or 5 cells deep; the interpapillary processes are flattened. Areas of pigmentation show a marked increase in melanin, particularly in the basal layers of the epidermis. Hemosiderin, if present, occurs as small granules diffusely distributed through the corium and about the acini of the sweat glands. Occasional clumps of hemofuscin, a sulfur-containing iron-free pigment, are found just under the epidermis and sometimes in the walls of blood vessels.

It is believed that the deposits of hemosiderin in the skin are too scanty to show any detectable color and that the increase of melanin is responsible for the brown pigmentation. The "slaty" bluish-gray appearance of certain areas is thought to be produced by viewing an increased amount of melanin through a greatly reduced number of superficial epidermal cells.[2]

Liver. The liver in hemochromatosis is usually greatly enlarged and weighs about

2,200 Gm. At autopsy the liver is reddish brown and has a hobnail appearance. It is firm in consistency and feels gritty on sectioning. Microscopic examination reveals two outstanding features: extensive pigmentation and pronounced fibrosis. Two types of pigment are present: hemosiderin and hemofuscin. In the hepatic cells the hemosiderin appears as fine, dustlike particles, either scattered or in clumps. Eventually, these conglomerates fill up the entire cell and apparently destroy it.

Examination of liver sections by electron microscopy has shown that the iron deposits consist of isolated ferritin molecules scattered throughout the protoplasm, of paracrystalline accumulations of ferritin molecules and of clumps of hemosiderin composed of ferritin in association with lipids, carbohydrates and other unknown substances. With rare exceptions, no ferritin is found in the nuclei or the mitochondria of the hepatic cells.[9] The observation that in all types of hemochromatosis the electron-microscopic picture was similar supports the view that the pathogenesis is identical, regardless of type.

Although it is often difficult to determine what portion of the lobule is involved most, the periphery appears to contain the most hemosiderin. Hemosiderin is also found in the broad bands of fibrous tissue usually present, in the connective tissue cells and in the extracellular areas. The Kupffer cells are distended with hemosiderin and are easily recognized. Hemosiderin is found also in the walls of the capillaries of the liver capsule and in the cells of the bile ducts. Hemofuscin is present in much smaller amounts in the walls of the large arteries and veins in the liver capsule, in the connective tissue and, to a lesser extent, in the hepatic polygonal cells.

In addition to the enormous amounts of hemosiderin, the liver shows the structural alterations of portal cirrhosis, with varying amounts of intralobular fibrosis. Indeed, in patients treated by repeated phlebotomy which succeeded in removing virtually all iron deposits from the liver, serial liver biopsies have shown a picture indistinguishable from that of simple portal cirrhosis.[20]

Furthermore, no lessening of fibrosis was apparent after venesections.

Pancreas. The pancreas may or may not be enlarged. In most cases it is deeply pigmented and exhibits a reddish-brown color similar to that of the liver; it is more firm in consistency than the normal pancreas.

Microscopic examination of the pancreatic tissue always shows heavy deposits of hemosiderin, especially in the acinar cells and in the islets of Langerhans. The degree of pigmentation of the islets has no consistent relation to the degree of diabetes mellitus. In most of the reported cases the number of islets of Langerhans was diminished, and in some they could not be identified. Hemofuscin granules also can be detected in the pancreatic tissue. Other pathologic changes consist of fibrosis found in about 90 per cent of cases and a marked relative increase in the number of acinar cells, many of which show degenerative changes. At times a fatty metamorphosis is evident.

Heart. Upon gross examination the heart is usually enlarged and often deep brown. Hemosiderin is found in the heart muscle fibers in nearly all cases of hemochromatosis. Characteristically, the hemosiderin is arranged at the poles of the nuclei. These deposits have resulted in degenerative changes in a few instances but rarely cause fibrosis.

The deposits of hemosiderin in the myocardium are not always related quantitatively to the degree of heart involvement as manifested clinically. As explanation, it has been postulated that the rate of disposition of hemosiderin plays an important part in determining the degree of damage to the heart muscle.

Stomach. In rare cases of hemochromatosis the gastric mucosa shows a brown pigmentation to the naked eye. Considerable amounts of hemosiderin were found in the chief cells of the gastric mucosa in 11 cases studied with biopsy by Althausen and co-workers[2] (Plate 1). The intensity of pigmentation in the liver correlated roughly with that in the gastric mucosa. A gastric analysis after histamine administration revealed normal values for hydrochloric acid and normal or slightly low values for pepsin in 9 patients in whom the gastric mucosa, apart from the deposits of hemosiderin, appeared normal histologically.

These findings indicate that hemosiderin in the chief cells, even in large amounts, had little or no effect on their secretory activity. In two cases in which some atrophy of the chief and the parietal cells was noted, the secretion of hydrochloric acid and of pepsin was lowered. The atrophy probably was not due to the presence of iron, since the parietal cells of the gastric glands, which contained little or no iron, atrophied to the same degree as the chief cells, which contained large amounts of iron.

Endocrine Glands. Hemosiderin deposits are found in the hypophysis, adrenals, testes, and thyroid and parathyroid glands.[69] These are of interest in view of the endocrinopathies which may be present in hemochromatosis. No specific abnormalities of thyroid or parathyroid function have been reported. Clinical manifestations of "feminization," such as hypoplasia of the male genitalia and sparsity of body hair, are frequent. The testes may be atrophic but usually contain little hemosiderin. These changes have not been correlated with morphologic changes in the pituitary or the adrenals, and no other acceptable explanation has been advanced.[4]

Melanin pigmentation and physical weakness so often found in hemochromatosis have been ascribed to adrenal insufficiency. However, this relationship has not been clearly demonstrated, and the water and electrolyte metabolism in hemochromatosis is found to be normal in almost all cases. Two of our cases were first misdiagnosed as Addison's disease; in these patients blood electrolytes and blood pressure were normal. Blood pressure was normal or high in all but one of the remaining 21 cases in this series.[2]

DIAGNOSIS

The principal physiologic abnormality in hemochromatosis is increase in storage iron, regardless of its source. It is believed that if sufficient iron is in the tissues over long enough periods of time, changes will take place leading to the classic manifestations of this disease, namely, hepatic cirrhosis,

diabetes mellitus and skin pigmentation.[5] The diagnosis of hemochromatosis depends, therefore, upon the demonstration of increased stores of iron, plus an empiric delineation of certain additional clinical features. Thus, the term "hemosiderosis" or "prehemochromatosis" might be used to signify increased amounts of tissue iron alone, and the term "hemochromatosis" to indicate a characteristic combination of abnormal accumulations of iron plus clinical evidence pointing to involvement of the liver, pancreas and skin. Some physicians prefer the term "iron storage disease" to describe the basic abnormality.[27] Additional terms delineating etiology, the site of iron deposition or the resulting diseases or complications have been proposed to describe the complete entity.

The diagnosis of hemochromatosis should be considered by the examining physician in all patients with increased pigmentation of the skin who evidence symptoms of weakness, fatigability and liver enlargement or pain. Polyphagia, polyuria, polydipsia and other symptoms of diabetes in a patient with increased pigment likewise is suggestive of hemochromatosis, as is the combination of diabetes mellitus and hepatic cirrhosis, even in the absence of increased pigmentation of the skin. Diabetes and evidence of hepatic disease in a pigmented patient justify a tentative diagnosis of hemochromatosis, subject to confirmation by laboratory procedures. When suspicion is aroused, other abnormalities commonly encountered in the history and the physical examination of patients with hemochromatosis should be looked for, particularly in regard to the texture of the skin, distribution of hair, and condition of the testicles or menstrual history.

The results of liver and pancreatic function tests may be entirely within normal limits. Demonstration of abnormal liver and pancreatic function does not constitute proof that hemochromatosis is present. However, the finding of a "diabetic" glucose tolerance curve or of impaired liver function in suspected cases, greatly strengthens other evidence.

The most useful diagnostic tests are based on demonstration of abnormal iron metabolism. The laboratory findings of elevated serum iron and decreased iron-binding capacity of the serum are strongly suggestive in establishing the diagnosis; they are not decisive, however, since relatives of patients with hemochromatosis may exhibit similar abnormalities without showing other overt evidence of the disease.[13, 61] Markedly elevated serum iron levels also may be found in patients with hepatitis or cirrhosis of the liver due to other causes, although the extremely high levels which may occur in hemochromatosis have not been described in patients with chronic liver disease[67] (Fig. 21-6).

The sine qua non in this disease is the demonstration of abnormal amounts of iron in the tissues. However, the presence of hemosiderin granules in epithelial cells desquamated into the urine is strongly suggestive of the diagnosis.[76] Since only a minority of patients with hemochromatosis show this finding, the disease cannot be ruled out by its absence.

Biopsies of certain tissues are useful in the diagnosis.

Skin. If positive, the skin biopsy clinches a diagnosis of hemochromatosis, provided that local sources of hemosiderin, such as varicose veins and "vagabond's disease," can be excluded.[2] If the skin biopsy is negative, the disease cannot be ruled out. In 13 cases of hemochromatosis with pigmentation in which a biopsy was done, Althausen found that only 7 had detectable amounts of hemosiderin in the skin.[2] Blue discoloration of the skin following intradermal injection of acidified potassium ferrocyanide (Fishback test[33]) had been proposed as a diagnostic aid in hemochromatosis, but this test is even less reliable than the presence of hemosiderin in the cells of the urinary sediment or in the skin.

Stomach. In Althausen's experience, gastric biopsy showed considerable deposits of hemosiderin in the chief cells of the gastric glands in all of 11 patients subjected to this procedure.[2] These results suggest that gastric biopsy is a far more reliable means of diagnosis in hemochromatosis than biopsy of the skin.

Liver. Of all measures for diagnosing hemochromatosis, liver biopsy is the most

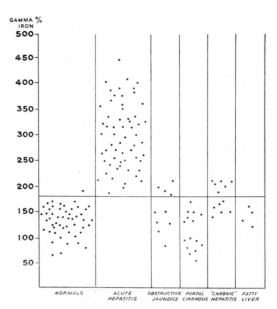

FIG. 21-6. Serum iron levels compared in normal subjects and in patients with various liver and biliary tract diseases. (Peterson, R. E.: J. Lab. Clin. Med. 39: 225.)

satisfactory.[21, 50, 83] Since the liver is the main storehouse for iron in the body, the absence of increased amounts of iron in this organ rules out this disease decisively. By the same token, the increased amounts of iron in the liver, even if the other characteristic findings of hemochromatosis are lacking, probably means that the disease is in an early stage, provided that other forms of siderosis caused by repeated blood transfusions, administration of iron or nutritional imbalance can be ruled out. Admittedly, as pointed out by Davis, liver biopsy is less satisfactory in hemochromatosis than in other hepatic diseases, since there is more pain, greater risk of hemorrhage and less certainty of obtaining an adequate specimen.[21] Despite certain dangers attendant to its use, even with proper precautions, the liver biopsy stands *alone* in its value in the diagnosis of hemochromatosis and should be used in all suspected cases, provided that no contra-indications are present.

Sosman and associates (as cited by Marble and Bailey[61]) have called attention to the diagnostic use of x-ray examination of the liver. They demonstrated an increase in liver density and a double contour line along the diaphragmatic border in 9 of 10 patients with hemochromatosis studied by means of x-ray films of the abdomen. Although other investigators have searched for this sign,[79] it has not been found with any consistency to date.

Bone Marrow. Examination of the aspirated sternal marrow for increased amounts of hemosiderin is a highly accurate means of diagnosis, according to Rath and Finch, who stated that hemochromatosis can be positively excluded when increased amounts of hemosiderin are *not* demonstrated.[71]

TREATMENT

Treatment of the patient with hemochromatosis is concerned with the specific metabolic anomalies of excessive absorption and deposition of iron and with the organs directly affected by the disease, such as the liver, pancreas and heart.

Phlebotomy. Effective treatment of excessive accumulation of iron in the body was first tried by Balfour in 1942 and reintroduced almost simultaneously by Finch in 1947[30] and by Davis and Arrowsmith in 1948.[21] It consists in removal of 500 ml. of blood from the patient, first at intervals of 2 to 7 days, and later at longer intervals as indicated by the circumstances of the individual case. This regimen usually results in an initial fall in the hemoglobin and the hematocrit until bone marrow responds to bleeding by increasing the rate of red blood cell production, after which these indicators are maintained within 10 per cent of their pretreatment levels. During this time the serum iron level remains high until the available stores of iron are near exhaustion. After this point is reached, blood loss anemia develops.[31]

Some clinicians have claimed that mobilization of iron from the body is more rapid during the initial stages than later in the course of phlebotomies. In one patient the initial rate was calculated to be 130 mg./day, which gradually fell to 20 mg./day, possibly due to fixation of a portion of hemosiderin in the iron stores in larger aggre-

gates.[19] Since the total stores of iron in hemochromatosis are 25 to 60 Gm. and each phlebotomy removes 200 to 250 mg. of iron, the exhaustion of stored iron usually takes 1 to 3 years. However, the length of this period also depends to some extent on the amount of iron in the diet, the degree of increased absorption and the rate at which iron is lost from the body through natural channels. The last factor is especially important in women during the reproductive period when losses of iron incident to each menstrual period and to parturition average 25 mg. and 0.5 Gm., respectively.

During treatment, serum iron or hematocrit should be determined before each phlebotomy, and when the values become subnormal, bleeding should be continued at a reduced rate to maintain these indicators at a slightly subnormal level. In most reported cases the amount of blood removed before the maintenance period is 12 to 20 liters. However, in some instances 50 to 60 liters was taken during periods up to 2 years, and in one case 96.4 liters was taken in less than 4 years (Table 21–3).

During the maintenance period the removal of 250 to 500 ml. of blood every 2 to 3 months, amounting to 1 to 2 liters of blood a year, is usually sufficient. The rate of removal is determined chiefly by the rate at which new iron is absorbed from the diet, which can be predicted roughly by the age of the patient at the onset of symptomatic hemochromatosis and the amount of iron that must be removed to deplete the amount stored.

When phlebotomy as treatment for hemochromatosis was in the experimental stage, it was considered necessary to separate the plasma from the blood cells by centrifugation and to reinject it. Further experience showed this precaution to be unnecessary except in alcoholics, provided that the patients were maintained on a diet adequate in calories and moderately high in proteins. However, alcoholic patients, especially if their diet was poor, tended to develop hypoproteinemia with edema and ascites, which requires return of the removed plasma.

This safe and relatively simple treatment has proved to be effective. Subjectively, a few weeks after venesection is initiated, the patient usually begins to feel stronger and to eat better, and the abdominal pain and aches in the extremities disappear. After several months many patients can resume a full work schedule. In a few cases even libido returns. Objectively, pigmentation of the skin fades, and body weight increases. The liver diminishes in size, and tenderness subsides. Spider angiomata disappear, and the function of the heart, if affected, may improve. However, the lack of hair persists.

On the laboratory side, the serum iron level almost always drops, and the saturation of the iron-carrying globulin is decreased to about one third of total capacity without production of anemia. In one case, pre-existing anemia and leukopenia due to "hypersplenism" were corrected by phlebotomies.[85] Liver function tests almost always show improvement, and the glucose tolerance curve usually becomes more normal. In many cases the insulin requirement is also reduced. Abnormalities in the electrocardiogram, if originally present, are often lessened. Tests of thyroid and of pituitary function have been reported to return toward normal.[55]

Anatomically, serial liver biopsies show a remarkable reduction in hemosiderin deposits, amounting to virtual disappearance of the iron pigment. However, no decrease in the degree of hepatic fibrosis has been reported, even after several years of continued treatment by phlebotomy, and malignant hepatomas can still arise.[54] Pancreatic fibrosis is apparently also not resolved by this treatment, since one patient developed diabetes and another became jaundiced due to fibrosis of the pancreas, 9 and 15 months, respectively, after phlebotomies were started.[54]

Occasionally, the bone marrow of a patient who is being bled fails to respond. In one variant the initial reduction in hemoglobin and hematocrit continues to drop below the usual level, and if the decrease amounts to 25 per cent, either an incorrect diagnosis or the presence of a malignant hepatoma should be considered. In another variant, the serum iron concentration may fall, and an iron-deficiency anemia may develop later in the course of treatment even

TABLE 21–3. QUANTITIES OF BLOOD AND IRON REMOVED BY REPEATED PHLEBOTOMIES FROM 5 PATIENTS WITH HEMOCHROMATOSIS

PATIENT	BLEEDING (liters)	TIME (months)	IRON (Gm.)
P. S.	40	22	20
A. W.	40	16	20
G. P.	51	21	26
R. B.	8	4	?
B. M. U.	103	54	52

Modified from Davis, W. D., Jr., and Arrowsmith, W. R.: Ann. Int. Med. 39:723.

though the iron stores are still excessive. This happens when, for some unknown reason, the iron stores are less available than usual. In such cases phlebotomy should be discontinued temporarily and resumed at a later date when the iron stores again become available.[31] Weintraub points out that energetic phlebotomy should be considered in the pyridoxine-responsive iron-loading anemias not only to remove excess iron but also to prevent excess iron from re-accumulating.[90] In such cases, it has been possible to remove large amounts of iron despite the moderately severe anemia.

A patient studied by one of us (V.M.S.) illustrates improvement from repeated phlebotomies.

A 50-year-old army officer gave a history of fatigue and anorexia, which had developed gradually over an 8-month period. One month after these symptoms first occurred, he noted moderate jaundice and dark urine, which lasted for 3 months and then gradually diminished. At the time of admission to the hospital he complained of fatigue, weakness, anorexia, abdominal distention and a gradual loss of 15 pounds in weight. The patient used only small amounts of alcohol and had been exposed to no other hepatotoxic materials.

Physical examination showed a normally developed and nourished man with no evidence of pigmentation in the skin or the mucous membranes. Body hair was sparse. Palmar erythema and a few spider nevi over the face, neck and shoulders were noted. The liver was enlarged to 7 cm. below the right costal margin and was tender on palpation and percussion. The spleen was not palpable. A small amount of ascites was found. The penis was normal, but the testes were soft.

The hemoglobin, the red and the white blood cell and differential counts were normal; results of tests for serum bilirubin, alkaline phosphatase, serum proteins and thymol turbidity were all within normal limits. Bromsulphalein retention was 20 per cent in 45 minutes (5 mg./kilo). The serum iron was 275 μg% and the serum iron-binding capacity was fully saturated. The glucose-tolerance test showed a diabetic curve although a number of urine specimens were negative for sugar. Hemosiderin could not be demonstrated in the urine.

A biopsy of the skin and gastric mucosa showed no hemosiderin deposition. A sternal bone marrow aspiration was strongly positive for hemosiderin. A liver biopsy specimen taken prior to treatment is illustrated in Plate 1. Treatment consisting of bed rest and a high-protein, high-caloric diet with multiple vitamin supplements was only partially successful; the patient continued to complain of fatigue and lack of initiative, but to a lesser degree than previously.

Six months after admission a program of frequent phlebotomies was begun, and the patient was given added dietary phosphate to help lessen absorption of ingested iron. At this time the red blood count was 5.3 million cells, hemoglobin 15 Gm. and hematocrit 45 per cent. The liver was 14 cm. and the spleen 2 cm. below the costal margin. During the next 10-month period, 24,000 cc. of blood was removed by means of 39 phlebotomies. At the end of this time the red blood count was 4.1 million cells, hemoglobin 13.2 Gm., hematocrit 44 per cent and reticulocyte count 4.5 per cent. Bromsulphalein retention was lowered to 5 per cent; results of other liver function tests remained normal. The serum iron measured 220 μg.%. During the next 4 months it became necessary to reduce the phlebotomies to one every 2 to 4 weeks.

After 14 months of therapy a total of 37,000 cc. of blood had been removed, which accounted for approximately 15 Gm. of iron. The red blood count was 3.0 million cells, hemoglobin 8.5 Gm., and hematocrit 34 per cent; the serum iron was 40 μg.%. Examination of the sternal marrow revealed changes consistent with iron deficiency anemia. A liver biopsy specimen obtained at this time is illustrated in Plate 1. A glucose-tolerance test showed some improvement but was still abnormal.

Since the beginning of treatment with phlebotomy, the patient tolerated more physical activity, and his sense of well-being increased.

In spite of slight anemia the patient complained of a fullness in the head and dizziness, which heretofore had always been relieved by venesection. However, results of a blood-volume determination were within normal limits. Enlargement and tenderness of the liver persisted, but the spleen was no longer palpable. During the following 12 months the patient was bled on 6 more occasions to maintain a moderate anemia and to perpetuate the marked clinical improvement.

Biochemical Approach. *Desferrioxamine-B.* An alternative method is available for the removal of tissue iron in hemosiderosis and hemochromatosis.[62, 82] Although earlier attempts at treatment of these conditions with chelating agents such as EDTA, BAL and penicillamine removed only small amounts of iron through the kidney, they gave promise of a biochemical approach to this problem. In 1960, desferrioxamine-B, or Desferal, a new, potent, iron-eliminating agent, was developed by Ciba Laboratories. A series of reports confirm that this compound removes significant amounts of iron from patients with endogenous hemochromatosis and iron-overloading anemias. Results are most satisfactory with continuous intravenous infusions of 25 mg./body weight, although the drug is also effective when injected intramuscularly in a dose of 600 mg. twice daily. Oral administration of Desferal is ineffective because it fails to be absorbed from the gastrointestinal tract. Its use by this route, however, is recommended in acute iron poisoning for the purpose of combining with the ingested iron in the stomach and upper intestine.

Urinary excretion of iron is greatest when the iron-binding capacity is over 75 per cent saturated. Although Desferal has a strong affinity for ferritin, hemosiderin and transferrin iron, it does not chelate hemoglobin iron. In a normal subject, therefore, it is difficult to cause an increase in urinary iron excretion greater than 5 times normal, whereas in conditions with excessive iron deposition, regardless of cause, iron excretion is 10 to 15 times normal. Reportedly with use of Desferal 25 to 54 mg. of iron has been excreted per day. In one case of hemochromatosis, 7.2 Gm. of iron was removed in less than 2 years.

Few significant side effects from Desferal administration have been noted in humans, although possible cataract formation in dogs has been reported. It can be used either as adjunctive therapy with phlebotomy or alone when severe anemia precludes the use of phlebotomy.

Diet and Other Drugs. Diets low in iron are by necessity also very low in the protein needed to replace the drain on plasma proteins during active treatment by phlebotomy. Such diets are unpalatable and ineffective. The same is true of diets with a high phosphate content or medicinal administration of phosphates in an effort to decrease intestinal absorption of iron. Attempts to achieve the same objective by raising the pH of the duodenal contents with aluminum hydroxide gel or other neutralizing preparations which maintain the ingested iron in the less absorbable ferric form have also failed.[21]

Topical Therapy. Treatment of the organs directly affected by hemochromatosis is largely symptomatic. With the use of insulin, the management of the associated diabetes mellitus has presented no particular problem, except under unusual circumstances. Both insulin-hypersensitive and insulin-resistant types of diabetes occur in hemochromatosis. In this condition the diet must be moderately high in protein and adequate in calories and vitamins. This is particularly important because of the coexistence of hepatic disease. Sufficient insulin prevents hyperglycemia and glycosuria. In patients in whom treatment by phlebotomy is contraindicated, administration of large doses of pancreatin may be prescribed as an adjunct to desferrioxamine-B therapy in an attempt to limit absorption of iron.[65] Usually, no medication is required as a substitute for digestive enzymes of the pancreas in hemochromatosis. As a remedy for indigestion or to improve nutrition, pancreatic extracts may be tried, especially if enzyme secretion by the pancreas is known to be deficient.

Therapy of the associated liver disease is mainly dietary; large amounts of protein and carbohydrate and moderate amounts of fat, as well as abstinence from alcohol, are prescribed. If liver function is stable, as is usually the case, physical activity may be advised as tolerated. However, activities are restricted whenever deterioration or lack of improvement in hepatic function is observed.

Heart failure and cardiac arrhythmias are managed in the usual way with digitalis preparations, quinidine, diuretic agents and restriction of salt intake. The success of these measures apparently depends to a large degree on whether the cardiac involvement in a given patient is part of hemochromatosis or is unrelated to it. In the former case, the cardiac manifestations occur mostly in younger patients, and the results of treatment are poor; in the latter case, the manifestations usually are seen in older individuals, and the results of therapy are more favorable.

In some patients testosterone, given parenterally in moderate doses improves nitrogen balance and general well-being; in others, it improves libido and secondary sex characteristics.

PROGNOSIS

Before the discovery of insulin, survival of patients after the diagnosis of hemochromatosis was only several weeks to a few months. The use of insulin and modern therapy for cirrhosis of the liver extended this average life expectancy to 4.4 years. A few patients survived for 20 to 30 years. However, despite such treatment, the disease usually progressed steadily, and death resulted from complications of cirrhosis of the liver, from cardiac failure, diabetes or intercurrent infections, especially pneumonia.

Repeated phlebotomies and use of iron chelating materials can further prolong life and often restore the patient's ability to earn a living as well as to enjoy life. However, more time is required to establish whether freeing the body from excessive stores of iron reverses the disease process and, if so, at what stage of the disease venesection must be started.

INCREASED IRON STORES IN RELATIVES OF PATIENTS WITH CLINICAL HEMOCHROMATOSIS

The interesting and pertinent question arises as to whether asymptomatic close relatives of patients with clinical hemochromatosis who have increased iron stores should be treated prophylactically by venesection. Several reports have been published by investigators who examined such persons. One result of such studies was the finding of new clinical cases of this disease, particularly among siblings of patients who sought medical assistance. Another result was the discovery that approximately one half of asymptomatic adult siblings of patients suffering from hemochromatosis, and a like proportion of asymptomatic male offspring over the age of 15 years, had abnormally high plasma iron values and an increase in the iron-saturation coefficient of the iron-binding protein.[22] Such findings almost always point to early hemochromatosis, provided that other causes, chiefly acute viral hepatitis, increased hemolysis and reduced bone marrow activity can be ruled out.

Some close relatives of patients with hemochromatosis, even those who do not have elevated serum iron levels, may have increased iron stores and fibrosis and fatty infiltration of the liver as shown by needle biopsy. Finally, increased deposits of hemosiderin in bone marrow obtained by puncture were found in all 22 cases of hemochromatosis examined by Finch and Finch, who consider this test to be one of the most reliable for the diagnosis of iron-storage disorders.[32]

These reasons indicate a need for a screening examination of all adult siblings and sons over 15 years of age of patients with hemochromatosis for elevated serum iron levels, associated with increased iron saturation of ferritin and excessive deposits of hemosiderin in the bone marrow. The finding of any of these abnormalities should lead to liver biopsy or, in case of refusal to undergo this operation, to a therapeutic test with repeated phlebotomies in order to ascertain the amount of available storage iron. In negative or doubtful cases the screening examinations should be repeated periodically. If the results are positive, a preventive course of phlebotomies should be seriously considered,[22] at least until further investigations definitely establish the etiology of hemochromatosis. Whether cirrhosis of the liver, diabetes, pigmentation and other features of clinical hemochromatosis will develop in these presumably predisposed individuals if accumulation of excessive deposits of iron is prevented should prove to be of great interest.

REFERENCES

1. Alper, T., Savage, D. V., and Bothwell, T. H.: Radioiron studies in a case of hemochromatosis, J. Lab. Clin. Med. 37: 665, 1951.
2. Althausen, T. L., Doig, R. K., Weiden, S., Motteram, R., Turner, C. N., and Moore, A.: Hemochromatosis. Investigation of twenty-three cases with special reference to etiology, nutrition, iron metabolism and studies of hepatic and pancreatic function, Arch. Int. Med 88:553, 1951.
3. Althausen, T. L., and Kerr, W. J.: Hemochromatosis. A report of three cases with results of insulin therapy in one case, Endocrinology 11:377, 1927.
4. ————: Hemochromatosis. II. A report of three cases with endocrine disturbances and notes on a previously reported case Discussion of etiology, Endocrinology 17: 621, 1933.
5. Aufderheide, A. C., Horns, H. L., and Goldish, R. J.: Secondary hemochromatosis. I. Transfusion (exogenous) hemochromatosis, Blood 8:824, 1953.
6. ————: Secondary hemochromatosis. II. Report of case not attributable to blood transfusion, Blood 8:837, 1953.
7. Balfour, W. M., Hahn, P. F., Bale, W. F., Pommerenke, W. T., and Whipple, G. H.: Radioactive iron absorption in clinical conditions: normal, pregnancy, anemia, and hemochromatosis, J. Exp. Med. 76: 15, 1942.
8. Berk, J. E., and Lieber, M. M.: Primary carcinoma of the liver in hemochromatosis, Am. J. Med. Sci. 202:708, 1941.
9. Bessis, M., and Caroli, J.: A comparative study of hemochromatosis by electron microscopy, Gastroenterology 37:538, 1959.
10. Block, M., Bethard, W., and Jacobson, L.: Secondary hemochromatosis, J. Lab. Clin. Med. 40:781, 1952.
11. Bothwell, T. H., and Alper, T.: The cardiac complications of hemochromatosis; report of a case with a review of the literature, S. Afr. J. Clin. Sci. 2:226, 1951.
12. Bothwell, T. H., Abrahams, C., Bradlow,

PLATE 1

Hemochromatosis

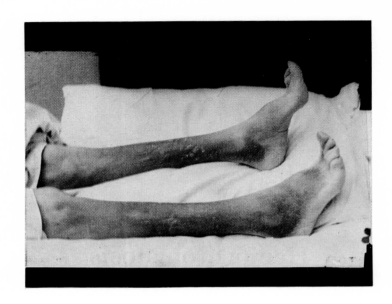

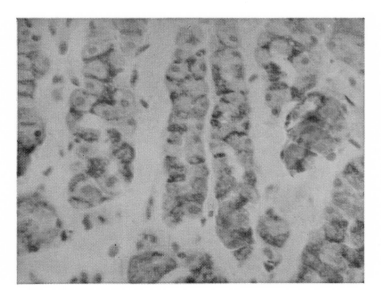

(A, *Top*). Characteristic melanosis of the skin in hemochromatosis. (Althausen, T. L., and Kerr, W. J.: Endocrinology 11:377-422.)

(B, *Bottom*). Biopsy specimen of gastric mucosa from a patient with hemochromatosis. Chief cells of tubular glands are laden with hemosiderin, while the parietal cells are practically free of this pigment (ferric ferrocyanide and hematoxylin. × 450). (Althausen, T. L., et al.: A. M. A. Arch. Int. Med. 88:553-570)

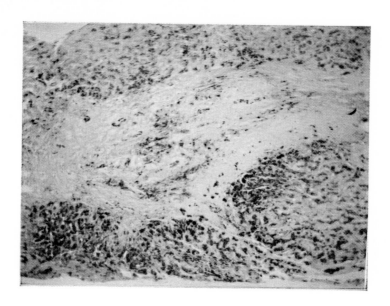

(C, *Top*). Biopsy specimen of liver from a patient with hemochromatosis before treatment with multiple phlebotomies. Extensive portal cirrhosis is present, with massive deposition of hemosiderin in the polygonal and reticuloendothelial cells (ferric ferrocyanide and hematoxylin. × 200).

(D, *Bottom*). Biopsy specimen of liver from the same patient as in C, taken after removal of 37,000 cc. of blood in a 14-month period. Portal fibrosis persists unchanged despite the almost complete removal of iron from the liver (ferric ferrocyanide and hematoxylin. × 200).

B. A., and Charlton, R. W.: Idiopathic and Bantu hemochromatosis. Comparative histological study, Arch. Path. 79:163, 1965.

13. Bothwell, T. H., Cohn, I., Abrahams, O. L., and Perold, S. M.: A familial study in idiopathic hemochromatosis, Am. J. Med. 27:730, 1959.

14. Boulin, R., and Bamberger, J.: L'hémochromatose familiale, Sem. Hôp. Paris 29: 3153, 1953.

15. Brick, I. B., and Palmer, E. D.: Esophageal varices and vascular spiders (nevi araneosi) in cirrhosis of the liver, J.A.M.A. 155:8, 1954.

16. Butt, H. R., and Wilder, R. M.: Hemochromatosis; report of 30 cases in which the diagnosis was made during life, Arch. Path. 26:262, 1938.

17. Chodos, R. B., Ross, J. F., Apt, L., Pollycove, M., and Halkett, J. A. E.: The absorption of radioiron-labeled foods and iron salts in normal and in iron-deficient subjects and in idiopathic hemochromatosis, J. Clin. Invest. 36:314, 1957.

18. Conrad, N. E., Jr., and Crosby, W. H.: Intestinal mucosal mechanisms controlling iron absorption, Blood 22:406, 1963.

19. Crosby, W. H.: Treatment of hemochromatosis by energetic phlebotomy; one patient's response to the letting of 55 litres of blood in 11 months, Brit. J. Haemat. 4:82, 1958.

20. Davis, W. D., and Arrowsmith, W. R.: The effect of repeated phlebotomies in hemochromatosis, J. Lab. Clin. Med. 39: 526, 1952.

21. ———: The treatment of hemochromatosis by massive venesection, Ann. Int. Med. 39:723, 1952.

22. Debré, R., Dreyfus, J. C., Frézal, J., Labie, D., Lamy, M., Maroteaux, P., Schapira, F., and Schapira, G.: Genetics of haemochromatosis, Ann. Human Genet. 23:16, 1958.

23. Dillingham, C. H.: Familial occurrence of hemochromatosis; report of 4 cases in siblings, New Engl. J. Med. 262:1128, 1960.

24. Dreiling, D. A., Sr.: Studies in pancreatic function. V. The use of the secretin test in the diagnosis of pancreatitis and in the demonstration of pancreatic insufficiencies in gastrointestinal disorders, Gastroenterology 24:540, 1953.

25. Dubach, R., Callender, S. T., and Moore, C. V.: Studies in iron transportation and metabolism. VI. Absorption of radioactive iron in patients with fever and with anemias of varied etiology, Blood 3:526, 1948.

26. Dubin, I. N.: Idiopathic hemochromatosis and transfusion siderosis, Am. J. Clin. Path. 25:514, 1955.

27. Duncan, T. G.: Iron storage disease, Med. Clin. N. Amer. 49:1361, 1965.

28. Evans, J.: Treatment of heart failure in haemochromatosis, Brit. Med. J. 1:1075, 1959.

29. Felts, J. H., Nelson, J. R., Herndon, C. N., and Spurr, C. L.: Hemochromatosis in two young sisters, Ann. Int. Med. 67:117, 1967.

30. Finch, C. A.: Iron metabolism in hemochromatosis, International Society of Hematology, 1948.

31. ———: Pathological and clinical aspects of iron overload in Bothwell, T., and Finch, C. A. (eds.): Iron Metabolism, Boston, Little, 1962.

32. Finch, S. C., and Finch, C. A.: Idiopathic hemochromatosis, an iron storage disease. A. Iron metabolism in hemochromatosis, Medicine 34:381, 1955.

33. Fishback, H. R.: Clinical demonstration of iron in the skin in hemochromatosis, J. Lab. Clin. Med. 25:98, 1939.

34. Frandsen, S.: On the metabolism of iron in hemochromatosis, Acta med. scand. 128:186, 1947.

35. Gillman, J., and Gillman, T.: The pathogenesis of cytosiderosis (hemochromatosis) as evidenced in malnourished Africans, Gastroenterology 8:19, 1947.

36. Gitlow, S. E., and Beyers, M. R.: Metabolism of iron. I. Intravenous iron tolerance tests in normal subjects and patients with hemochromatosis, J. Lab. Clin. Med. 39:337, 1952.

37. Gitlow, S. E., Beyers, M. R., and Colmore, J. P.: Metabolism of iron. II. Intravenous iron tolerance tests in Laennec's cirrhosis, J. Lab. Clin. Med. 40:541, 1952.

38. Goldberg, L., and Smith, J. P.: Iron overloading and hepatic vulnerability, Am. J. Path. 36:125, 1960.

39. Granick, S.: Iron metabolism and hemochromatosis, Bull. N. Y. Acad. Med. 25: 403, 1949.

40. ———: Iron metabolism, Bull. N. Y. Acad. Med. 30:81, 1954.

41. Hedinger, C.: Zur Pathologie der Hämochromatose; Hämochromatose als Syndrom, Helvet. med. acta, Supp. 32, pp. 1-109, 1953.

42. Hegsted, D. M., Finch, C. A., and Kinney, T. D.: The influence of diet on iron absorption: The interrelationship of iron and phosphorus, J. Exp. Med. 90:147, 1949.

43. Heilmeyer, L.: Ferritin in Wallerstein, R. O., and Mettier, S. R. (eds.): Iron in Clinical Medicine, pp. 24-42, Berkeley, Univ. California Press, 1958.

44. Herkel, W.: Über die Bedeutung des Kupfers (Zinks und Mangans) in der Biologie und Pathologie, Beitr. path. Anat. 85:513, 1930.

45. Horns, H. L.: Hemochromatosis, Am. J. Med. 6:272, 1949.

46. Houston, J. C.: Phlebotomy for haemochromatosis; effect of removing 52 pints of blood in 16 months, Lancet 1:766, 1953.

47. Houston, J. C., and Thompson, R. H. S.: The diagnostic value of serum iron studies in haemochromatosis: Observations on seven patients, Quart. J. Med. 21:215, 1952.

48. Huff, R. L., Hennessy, T. G., Austin, R. E., Garcia, J. F., Roberts, B. M., and Lawrence, J. H.: Plasma and red cell iron turnover in normal subjects and in patients having various hematopoietic disorders, J. Clin. Invest. 29:1041, 1950.

49. Kappeler, R.: Familiäre Hämatochromatose, Schweiz. med. Wschr. 86:477, 1956.

50. King, W. E., and Downie, E.: Haemochromatosis: Observations on the incidence and on the value of liver biopsy in diagnosis, Quart. J. Med. 17:247, 1948.

51. Kleckner, M. S., Baggenstoss, A. H., and Weir, J. F.: Hemochromatosis and transfusional hemosiderosis, Am. J. Med. 16:382, 1954.

52. Knutsen, B.: Hemochromatosis; case report with special reference to symptomatology and pathogenesis, Acta med. scand. 114:280, 1943.

53. Laurell, C. B.: Iron transportation in Wallerstein, R. O., and Mettier, S. R. (eds.): Iron in Clinical Medicine, pp. 8-23, Berkeley, Univ. California Press, 1958.

54. Ley, A. B.: The management of hemochromatosis, Med. Clin. N. Amer. 44:789, 1960.

55. McAllen, P. M., Coghill, N. F., and Lubran, M.: The treatment of haemochromatosis, Quart. J. Med. 26:251, 1957.

56. MacDonald, R. A.: Idiopathic hemochromatosis, A.M.A. Arch. Int. Med. 107:606, 1961.

57. ———: Idiopathic hemochromatosis. Genetic or acquired? Arch. Int. Med. 112:184, 1963.

58. ———: Hemochromatosis and cirrhosis in different geographic areas, Am. J. Med. Sci. 249:36, 1965.

59. MacDonald, R. A., and Mallory, G. K.: Hemochromatosis and hemosiderosis; study of 211 autopsied cases, A.M.A. Arch. Int. Med. 105:686, 1960.

60. Mallory, F. B., Parker, F., and Nye, R. N.: Experimental pigment cirrhosis due to copper and its relation to hemochromatosis, J. Med. Res. 42:461, 1921.

61. Marble, A., and Bailey, C. C.: Hemochromatosis, Am. J. Med. 11:590, 1951.

62. Moeschlin, S., and Schnider, U.: Treatment of primary and secondary hemochromatosis and acute iron poisoning with a new, potent iron-eliminating agent (desferrioxamine-B), New Engl. J. Med. 269:57, 1963.

63. Moore, C. V., and Dubach, R.: Metabolism and requirements of iron in the human, J.A.M.A. 162:197, 1956.

64. Motteram, R.: Observations on Haemosiderosis; Studies in Pathology, p. 191, Melbourne, Melbourne Univ. Press, 1950.

65. Murray, M. J., and Stein, N.: Does the pancreas influence iron absorption? A critical review of information to date, Gastroenterology 51:694, 1966.

66. Perkins, K. W., McInnes, I. W. S., Blackburn, C. R. B., and Beal, R. W.: Idiopathic hemochromatosis in children, Am. J. Med. 39:118, 1965.

67. Peterson, R. E.: The serum iron in acute hepatitis, J. Lab. Clin. Med. 39:225, 1952.

68. Peterson, R. E., and Ettinger, R. H.: Radioactive iron absorption in siderosis (hemochromatosis) of the liver, Am. J. Med. 15:518, 1953.

69. Pirart, J., and Gatez, P.: L'étiologie de l'hémochromatose non transfusionelle: revue de la question; étude de l'hérédité dans 21 familles, Sem. hôp. Paris 34:1044, 1958.

70. Pollycove, M.: Verbal communication.

71. Rath, C. E., and Finch, C. A.: Sternal marrow hemosiderin; method for determination of available iron stores in man, J. Lab. Clin. Med. 33:81, 1948.

72. ———: Chemical, clinical and immunological studies on the products of human plasma fractionation. XXXVIII. Serum iron transport. Measurement of iron-bind-

ing capacity of serum in man, J. Clin. Invest. 28:79, 1949.

73. Rather, L. J.: Hemochromatosis and hemosiderosis: Does iron overload cause diffuse fibrosis of the liver? Am. J. Med. 21:857, 1956.

74. Richter, G. W.: The nature of storage iron in idiopathic hemochromatosis and in hemosiderosis: electron, optical, chemical, and serologic studies on isolated hemosiderin granules, J. Exp. Med. 112:551, 1960.

75. Rigas, D. A., and Finch, S. C.: Electrophoretic studies of serum proteins in hemochromatosis, Am. J. Med. Sci. 237:566, 1959.

76. Rous, P.: Urinary siderosis, J. Exp. Med. 28:645, 1918.

77. Schwartz, S. R., and Blumenthal, S. A.: Exogenous hemochromatosis resulting from blood transfusions, Blood 3:617, 1948.

78. Sheldon, J. H.: Haemochromatosis, London, Oxford, 1935.

79. Steinback, H.: Personal communication.

80. Stewart, W. B.: Some aspects of the metabolism of iron (Abstract), Bull. N. Y. Acad. Med. 29:818, 1953.

81. Surgenor, D. M., Koechlin, B. A., and Strong, L. E.: Chemical, clinical and immunological studies on the products of human plasma fractionation. XXXVII. The metal combining globulin of human plasma, J. Clin. Invest. 28:73, 1949.

82. Thompson, R. B., Owen, D. M., and Bell, W. N.: Desferal therapy in iron storage disease, Am. J. Med. Sci. 253:453, 1967.

83. Topp, J. H., and Lindert, M. C. F.: The diagnosis of hemochromatosis by means of needle biopsy of the liver, Gastroenterology 10:813, 1948.

84. Trousseau, A.: Clinique médicale de l'Hôtel-Dieu de Paris, ed. 2, p. 672, Paris, Baillière, 1865.

85. Vaisrub, S., and Karlinsky, W.: Iron deficiency anemia in case of hemochromatosis treated by repeated phlebotomy, Canad. Serv. M. J. 12:81,1956.

86. Vannoti, A., and Delachaux, A.: Iron Metabolism and Its Clinical Significance, London, Muller, 1949.

87. Wallerstein, R. O., and Robbins, S. L.: Hemochromatosis after prolonged oral iron therapy in a patient with chronic hemolytic anemia, Am. J. Med. 14:256, 1953.

88. Warren, S., and Drake, E. I., Jr.: Primary carcinoma of the liver in hemochromatosis, Am. J. Path. 27:573, 1951.

89. Weintraub, L. R.: The iron storage diseases. Seminars in hematology, Vol. 3, No. 4, 340, 1966.

90. Weintraub, L. R., Conrad, M. E., and Crosby, W. H.: Iron loading anemia: treatment with repeated phlebotomies and pyridoxine, New Engl. J. Med. 275:169, 1966.

91. Wheby, M. S.: Regulation of iron absorption, Gastroenterology 50:888, 1966.

22

The Liver in Hepatolenticular Degeneration

J. M. WALSHE, SC.D., F.R.C.P.

Since the first edition of this book was published more than 10 years ago much has been learned about the pathogenesis and treatment of Wilson's disease (hepatolenticular degeneration) so that many of the questions asked in Matthews' admirable chapter[30] can now be answered. As a result of recent advances Wilson's disease is one of the very few chronic diseases of not only the liver but also of the nervous system for which treatment is specific and highly effective.[56, 60] Until now hepatolenticular degeneration fell largely within the province of the neurologist; this perhaps is hardly surprising following Wilson's justly famous original description in Brain.[61] Nevertheless the occasional publication of well-documented accounts of cases of "hepatic" or "abdominal" Wilson's disease[8, 13, 28] should have awakened hepatologists to the possibility of recognizing this disease before the march of events led the patient to the neurologic clinic.

Hepatolenticular degeneration is not a disease of either the liver or the nervous system but an inborn error of metabolism in the exact sense intended by Garrod[19] in 1908; it is inherited in an autosomal recessive fashion[2, 4, 5] and involves not the metabolism but the transport and storage of copper in the body. Although it is now widely held that Wilson's disease is an error of copper metabolism, this is a misconception, for copper, in its role as a four electron transfer oxidase, is the only pathway for the biological reduction of molecular oxygen to water,[51] and a breakdown of this metabolic process is incompatible with life.

GENETICS

Wilson's disease is probably one of the less common inborn errors of metabolism. Bearn has calculated that the general gene frequency is of the order of 1 in 500 in the population, giving a disease incidence of about 1 in 1,000,000. This may well be an underestimate, at least as far as Great Britain is concerned, where, with a birth rate of approximately 1,000,000 per annum, only one new case should be seen each year whereas, on the average, I see three new cases each year and surely others are seen at different centers or remain undiagnosed. The disease has been reported not only in Europeans but also in Middle Eastern, African and Asian races. The frequency appears to be high in Japan, where Arima and Sano recently reported data on almost 200 cases[3]; however, the consanguinity rate among parents was so high that the gene frequency may not be significantly greater than in other countries.

Wilson originally suspected that an environmental rather than a genetic factor was responsible, but it is now accepted, largely following the work of André and van Bogaert[2] and Bearn,[4, 5] that the disease is genetically determined and is inherited in a recessive fashion. In Bearn's series of patients seen in New York the consanguinity rate was 46 per cent,[5] and reportedly in Japan it reached 68 per cent in small cities although it was lower in the large centers of population.[3] Among my own cases seen in the United Kingdom (which include a few from Western Europe), in 51 families

796

there were 4 cases of first-cousin marriage and one of incest. Linkage studies for blood group antigens from these families has produced no significant findings.[42] Among 78 siblings of the propositi no less than 17 (22 per cent) were proved or highly probable cases of Wilson's disease, a close approximation to the expected 25 per cent for a recessive mode of inheritance.

CLINICAL FEATURES

Among cases seen in the United Kingdom the age of onset of symptoms has varied from 6 to 39 years. Although it is generally held that the disease is more common in boys than in girls,[15, 30] this has not been my own experience; in 65 cases there were 34 males and 31 females, but among all the siblings of these families there were 66 male and 57 female offspring, which shows, in fact, that the incidence among males has been slightly less than among females. The average age of onset among males has been 14.6 years, compared to 12.9 years for females. The youngest patient, a girl, presented at 6 years of age with jaundice, whereas the oldest, a man of 39 years, complained of tremor (see Fig. 22–1).

Manifestations of liver involvement in Wilson's disease are by no means as rare as has previously been believed, and in many cases these are the earliest symptoms. No less than 30 of 65 patients studied first sought medical advice because of symptoms of liver disease such as jaundice, ascites, edema, a hemorrhagic tendency or acne and amenorrhea. In 8 of these cases hemolysis was also present, and the combination of hepatic and hemolytic jaundice should always alert the physician to the likelihood of Wilson's disease as the correct diagnosis.

Of the 65 patients, 26 first complained of neurologic disease; symptoms were again protean, consisting of tremor, rigidity, awkwardness of gait, clumsiness with the hands, deteriorating performance at school, childish behavior, slurring of speech, cramps and personality changes; single examples have also been seen of a schizophrenic-like psychosis and of seizures (Fig. 22–2). Such cases are, however, unlikely to present at the hepatic or gastroenterological clinic.

A rare cause of complaint is high, swinging fever which may last several weeks before localizing signs draw attention to either the liver or the central nervous system. Spontaneous fractures or bone pains are occasionally seen,[32] and in fact boney changes are not uncommon in this disease[17] (see Fig. 22–3). When the disease has been diagnosed by genetic screening in individuals who have not yet developed symptoms, it has been common to find disturbed tests of liver function and careful clinical examination may also detect enlargement of the liver or spleen and vascular spider angiomata.

In the past, hepatic manifestations of Wilson's disease have received little atten-

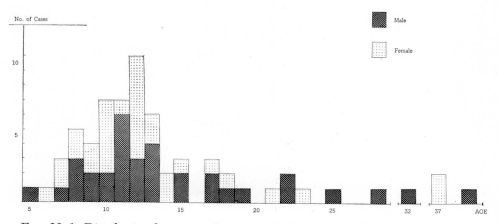

FIG. 22–1. Distribution by age and sex of 65 patients with Wilson's disease at the time of first symptoms.

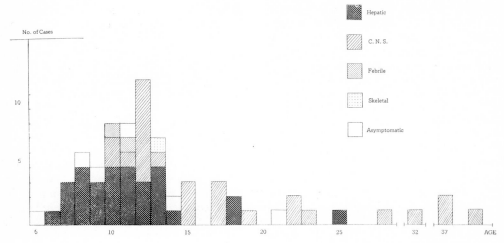

Fɪɢ. 22–2. Distribution by age and first symptoms of 65 patients with Wilson's disease at the time of onset.

tion except as subsidiary phenomena in a predominantly neurologic disorder, and, until recent years, much of the literature on this disease has appeared in the neurologic journals, although some writers have stressed the hepatic aspects.[13, 18, 49, 57, 58] Osborn and Walshe demonstrated recently the pri- mary role of the liver in the metabolic sequence that leads to the clinical manifestations of Wilson's disease,[37] so that it is logical to consider first the hepatic aspects of the disease and only later to refer more briefly to those cases in which the presenting symptoms involve the central nervous

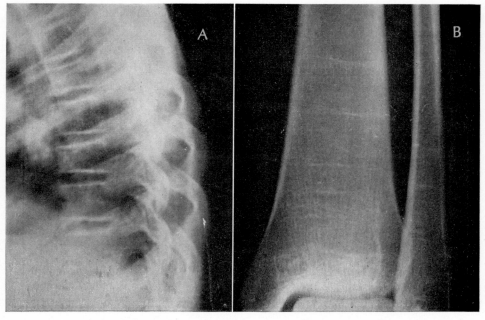

Fɪɢ. 22–3. Skeletal changes in Wilson's disease; (A) Porotic vertebrae and wedging of mid-dorsal vertebral bodies. (B) Multiple Harris' lines at the lower end of the tibia and fibula.

system, in which cases liver dysfunction is apt to be only a late or minor component of the illness.

EARLY, HEPATIC, WILSON'S DISEASE

While, apart from the Kayser-Fleischer ring, there is no single diagnostic sign of Wilson's disease, the possibility should be borne in mind in all children or adolescents with liver disease, particularly when accompanied by hemolysis or a history that an elder sibling, or siblings, have died of chronic, subacute or even acute liver failure. The hepatic signs and symptoms of Wilson's disease are as varied as are the signs of brain damage, and particularly in young children the illness may be acute so that death may occur within a week of onset,

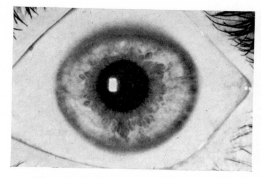

FIG. 22–5. Kayser-Fleischer ring showing decreased density of the pigment in the lateral crescents. Because the rings are brown they are much more easily seen on a blue than on a brown iris.

and in untreated patients the mortality is high. Since among families with proved cases of Wilson's disease the incidence of death from acute or subacute liver failure is high among elder siblings, there is little doubt that these are examples of the same illness.

No less than half of the 30 patients presenting with liver damage and comprising the present series died of liver failure or portal hypertension and hemorrhage; the most acute illness lasted only 5 days and eight of these patients died in less than 10 weeks. Only two cases were diagnosed during life. Wilson's disease is usually much more chronic and may last for several years, being punctuated by episodes of increasing jaundice, variceal hemorrhage or hemolytic crises intermixed with periods of relative good health before liver failure or an exsanguinating hemorrhage brings this sorry story to a close. Sometimes hepatic signs disappear completely to be replaced months or years later by tremor or other evidence of central nervous system involvement, but the mechanism of this apparent spontaneous improvement is obscure. Eight such patients were correctly diagnosed only after nervous system disease had developed; all had Kayser-Fleischer rings and splenic or hepatic enlargement as a permanent legacy of the earlier stage of their illness.

Routine laboratory tests of liver function are seldom severely disturbed once

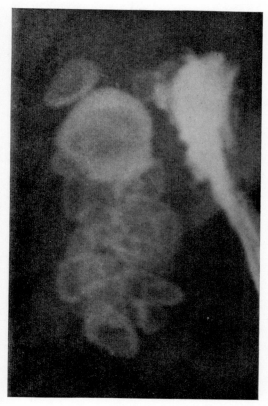

FIG. 22–4. Symptomless gallstones found during the course of a barium swallow examination. The patient had had a series of hemolytic episodes 15 years previously.

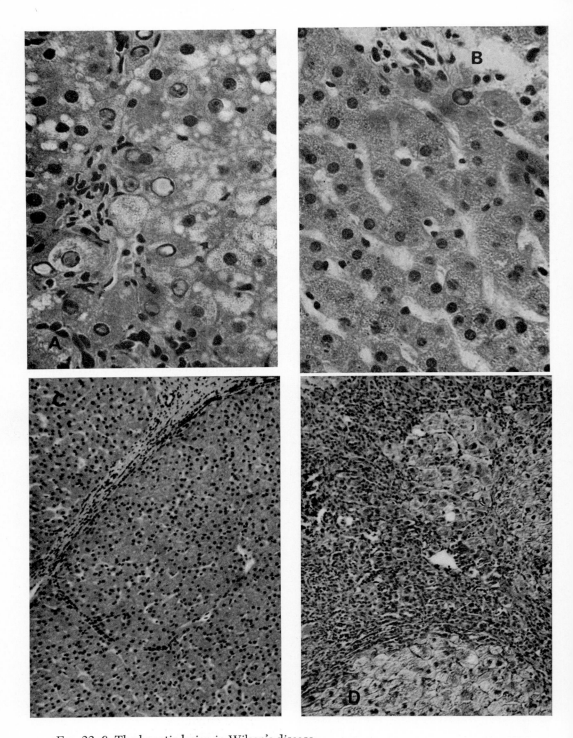

FIG. 22–6. The hepatic lesion in Wilson's disease.
(A) Needle biopsy, presymptomatic stage; cytoplasmic fat droplets, glycogen nuclei and periportal infiltration. (B) Needle biopsy, early symptomatic stage; pigment deposits in the cells giving a positive stain for copper rubeanic acid. (C) Operation biopsy, early neurologic stage with abnormal liver function tests; early fibrosis. (D) Needle biopsy, clinical liver disease; active cirrhosis. *(Fig. 22–6. E and F on facing page.)*

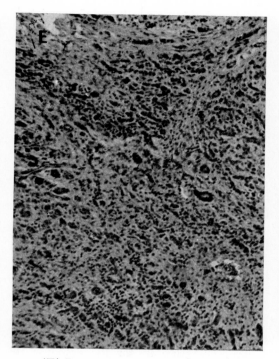
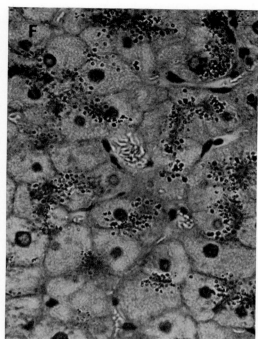

(E) Postmortem section, subacute liver atrophy.

(F) Needle biopsy, heavy hemosiderin deposits; active chronic hepatitis with edema and ascites.

the acute episode of the illness is passed. This self-limiting type of liver damage may present either as a transient illness lasting only a few weeks and called, at the time, acute hepatitis or it may smoulder for several years punctuated by severe hemolytic crises requiring transfusion and reactivated by any and every intercurrent infection. Symptomless gallstones are not uncommon in such patients (see Fig. 22–4) and splenic infarcts or even thrombosis of the splenic vein are a rare cause of obscure abdominal pain. Finally the onset of neurologic disease has led to the correct diagnosis and institution of effective therapy. Among those patients first seen in the hepatic stage of Wilson's disease the diagnosis was established relatively early in eight and all these have had a most satisfactory response to treatment with no recurrence of signs or symptoms of liver damage.

It is not possible to say at what stage the Kayser-Fleischer ring develops, but in patients with hepatic disease only two un- doubted cases have been seen in whom it was not possible to detect the rings under slit lamp examination. In two presymptomatic patients the rings developed about 1 year after prophylactic treatment was temporarily interrupted. These rings are so easily sought and are such a characteristic physical sign of the disease (see Fig. 22–5) that they should always be looked for in children or young adults with liver disease. The ring appears first as a thin top crescent at the outer margin of the cornea and can usually be seen with a hand lens if viewed obliquely from above in a good light. It is next seen in the lower corneal crescent before it extends from above and below to meet laterally and complete the ring. Under treatment it disappears in the reverse order so that the top crescent is the last place in which the ring can be seen.

Thus, apart from the corneal rings, the hepatic manifestations of Wilson's disease have no specifically characteristic features and any or all signs or symptoms of acute or chronic liver damage can be found. Fluid retention is a common presenting sign, but jaundice, abdominal pain, vomiting and nose bleeds have all been seen, as also have acne and amenorrhea.

The pathologic changes in the liver (Fig. 22–6), like the clinical features, are not diagnostic of Wilson's disease except in those cases in which it is possible to demonstrate copper in the tissues by special staining technics. The illustrations in Wilson's original description suggest that both diffuse hepatic fibrosis and postnecrotic scarring might be expected.[61] Franklin and Baumann[18] found typical multilobular cirrhosis in six patients at postmortem examination and Anderson and Popper[1] concluded from a histologic study of 20 cases that the changes were postnecrotic, but they also noted a great variation in the activity of the disease process; characteristic, though not diagnostic, were fatty changes in degenerating liver cells, glycogen nuclei and excessively large Kupffer cells. Electron microscopic studies also showed increased density of the lysozymes,[46] and enzyme studies showed an associated reduction of the acid phosphatase in these cells. Iron pigment is sometimes seen in the hepatic parenchymal cells in Wilson's disease and is, presumably, the legacy of an earlier episode of hemolysis.

HEPATIC MANIFESTATIONS IN ADVANCED WILSON'S DISEASE

Clinical evidence of liver damage is not, apparently, an inevitable sequelae of increased copper storage in Wilson's disease, whatever may be the pathologic changes in the liver. One patient has been studied who, after 20 years of disabling ataxia, has no enlargement of the liver or spleen, no vascular spiders and no abnormality in laboratory tests of liver function. Twenty-six of the patients seen in the present series gave no history of liver disease, but the majority of these have been protected by early diagnosis and treatment. However, about half of these patients, when first seen, had palpable livers and spleens; sometimes the spleen alone has been enlarged and this was apt to be associated with hypersplenism and thrombocytopenia. The serum proteins and liver function tests are seldom significantly disturbed, but the serum transaminases may be moderately elevated. Fluid retention is sometimes seen as a late sign in untreated or neglected cases and these may also develop esophageal varices leading to severe hemorrhage. Fortunately the infinitely distressing picture of long-standing untreated Wilson's disease is now rare so that it is difficult to draw any conclusions on its natural history from cases seen today, but death from liver failure or exsanguinating hemorrhage is occasionally encountered which suggests that late hepatic involvement may have played a more prominent part in the past than at present.

DIAGNOSIS

Once the diagnosis of Wilson's disease is suspected every effort should be made to confirm or refute it, for the response to treatment with penicillamine has revolutionized the prognosis. Moreover, the high mortality and often rapid course of the untreated illness make this a matter of some urgency. The simplest and most reliable of all diagnostic procedures is identification of the *Kayser-Fleischer corneal ring;* if it can not be seen with the naked eye or with a hand lens then a slit lamp or gonioscopy should be employed. A positive finding is diagnostic of Wilson's disease but on occasions the early hepatic stages of the illness develop before pigment becomes visible in the cornea. However, probably once signs of central nervous system involvement occur the ring is always present.

In most cases it is desirable to confirm the diagnosis by biochemical tests. Probably the most valuable screening test is determination of the serum oxidase activity against paraphenylenediamine (or its dimethyl derivative) as an estimate of the *serum ceruloplasmin concentration.* This is low or even absent in most cases of Wilson's disease[47] but may approach normal values in the early hepatic stages of the illness.[36] Alternatively, it is possible that when ceruloplasmin synthesis is only partially inhibited the illness tends to follow a predominantly hepatic rather than a neurologic course. If estimation of the serum ceruloplasmin gives an equivocal answer, determination of the serum copper is unlikely to be of help, for ceruloplasmin is the copper-carrying protein in the serum. Rarely is the normal concentration of ceruloplasmin less than 25 mg./100 ml. or the copper below 90 μg./100 ml. The excretion of copper in the urine is almost always increased except in the very early stages of the illness. For a normal adult the 24 hour excretion is less than 50 μg., but in biliary obstruction this figure may be exceeded three- or fourfold.[25] In Wilson's disease the amount of copper excreted in the urine varies with the size of the excess body pool of the metal, but may reach 1,000 μg. daily in those patients whose tissue proteins are saturated with copper. While the results of these determinations may confirm the diagnosis beyond reasonable doubt, it must be remembered that not only in hepatic Wilson's disease are there relatively high serum ceruloplasmin and copper concentrations but in severe liver damage from other causes there may be, as a temporary phenomenon, depressed levels of ceruloplasmin in the blood, presumably resulting from failure of protein synthesis in the liver.[9]

Recourse to estimation of uric acid excretion or amino acid patterns in the urine are unlikely to be of value in deciding a difficult case, and it may be necessary to estimate the *copper content of liver biopsy* tissue or to revert to studies with *radioactive copper*. The copper concentration in normal liver tissue is 4 to 8 μg./Gm. wet weight, whereas in Wilson's disease, once symptoms develop, it is usually greater than 50 μg./Gm. wet weight and may be much higher. If radiocopper is used, the simplest estimation is the ratio of radioactivity in the plasma at 24 hours to that at 2 hours (a dose of at least 100 μc, given intravenously, is necessary for this determination). In normal individuals the ratio is greater than 0.8, whereas in patients it is almost invariably less than 0.3, even if the concentration of ceruloplasmin is relatively high.[53] If, however, neither technic is available, it may help to estimate the *urine copper excretion* after a test dose of penicillamine. A normal person usually excretes less than 300 μg. in 6 hours after taking 500 mg. of the drug, whereas, under the same conditions, it is extremely rare for an untreated patient to excrete less than 700 μg. copper.

PATHOGENESIS

The literature on this subject has of recent years become a veritable battlefield, but it is not intended to fight yet again the wars of far away and long ago as has, of late, been the wont of so many retired generals: better to tabulate the established facts and let these point the way ahead. It has long been suspected[45] and is now established[12, 14, 15] that copper is deposited in excess in most tissues of the body in symptomatic Wilson's disease, particularly in those tissues which bear the brunt of the illness, namely the liver, brain and kidneys.[12] Copper inhibits many enzyme systems,[43] particularly those dependent upon the presence of an —SH radical at the active center.[29] Recently it has been shown that ionic copper (Cu^{2+}) inhibits pyruvate oxidase in brain and also the cerebral membrane ATPase,[39, 40] leading, in turn, to a diminution of the adenosine triphosphate, phosphocreatine and potassium content of the tissue.[16] Finally there is overwhelming evidence that patients with Wilson's disease who are kept in a prolonged state of negative copper balance will undergo considerable improvement if not complete remission of symptoms.[60] Thus deposition of copper in the tissues is responsible for the pathologic and functional changes that are characteristic of Wilson's disease.

If it is accepted, and the evidence available leaves little room for doubt, that copper is the pathogenic agent in this disease, then it is necessary to consider first the normal fate of copper in the body and afterward by what means and in what way abnormalities of copper transport and storage occur in Wilson's disease.

The normal physiology of copper is the subject of recent review articles[50, 60] and is summarized only briefly here. It has

PLASMA RADIOACTIVITY

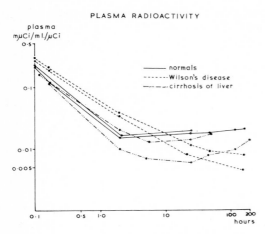

FIG. 22–7. Plasma radioactivity. Concentration of radiocopper in the serum $(m\mu c/ml./\mu c$ injected) in 2 control subjects, 2 patients with chronic hepatic disease and 2 patients with Wilson's disease, 1 presymptomatic and 1 with advanced neurologic disease. (Reproduced from Brain.[60])

been calculated that between 100 and 150 mg. of copper are present in a normal adult man and that 2 to 4 mg. is consumed daily in the diet. Most of this copper is probably in organic combination, but drinking water, particularly that supplied in copper pipes, may contain appreciable amounts of Cu^{2+}. Copper is absorbed from the stomach or upper small intestine and studies with radiocopper chloride show that absorption begins within 15 minutes of oral ingestion so that radioactivity can be detected in the liver, plasma and red cells.[38] Thirty to 70 per cent of a dose of labeled copper so administered is eventually absorbed and the remainder is excreted via the stools. Once absorbed, copper must pass via the portal vein into the liver where much is retained[37] and incorporated into hepatic copper proteins.[31] Copper that passes through the liver appears in the plasma mostly attached to serum albumin,[6] while a small amount is present in a form that can pass through a semipermeable membrane,[35,59] and this fraction may be bound to amino acids.[33] It is probably this amino acid–copper complex that is excreted

in the urine where it can be detected soon after the labeled metal is administered and probably also corresponds to the fraction that produces the normal urinary copper. This early plasma radioactivity rapidly disappears as the metal is taken up by the liver,[34,37] where it is incorporated into liver copper proteins and into the blue copper protein ceruloplasmin. This alpha-globulin of M.W. 160,000 contains 8 atoms of copper in cuprous-cupric pairs[26,27]; this protein with its radioactive label is then returned to the plasma, leading to a secondary rise in plasma radioactivity (see Fig. 22–7).

Ceruloplasmin is a protein of unknown function or fate,[23] though it is a weak oxidase for certain aromatic amines but has a pH and activity that hardly suggest any physiological significance. Since the copper atoms in the ceruloplasmin molecule are not exchangeable *in vivo*,[48,54] it hardly seems likely that this is a transport protein for copper. The concentration of ceruloplasmin in blood does vary in certain disease states; it is high in many chronic infections and pregnancy and low in the nephrotic syndrome (due to loss of protein in the urine),[11] in protein-losing gastroenteropathy[50] and in severe liver failure.[9] Some of the absorbed copper is excreted in the bile and as much as 10 per cent has been recovered within 24 hours of injection in patients with external biliary drainage.[38] Isotope studies have, as yet, revealed nothing of the long-term fate of absorbed copper but the metal is present in all tissues with particularly high concentrations in some of the pigmented nuclei of the brain. In the brain, as in the liver, it is present in specific copper-protein combinations[41]; it is present in hair [20] and in the enzyme tyrosinase mostly localized in the skin. But the most vital role of the metal is in the final pathway for the biologic reduction of oxygen to water by cytochrome C oxidase as the terminal step in the electron transfer chain. Life as we know it on this planet appears to be largely dependent on copper for the final supply of energy at the cellular level.[51]

At many points the transport, storage or

functional activity of copper could be disorganized, but there is no general disruption in Wilson's disease. If one accepts the theory "one gene one enzyme or polypeptide chain," then it is probable that only at a single point in its normal pathway of utilization is the handling of the metal disturbed. Due to this single abnormality, excess copper accumulates in the body, thereby giving rise to multiple enzyme defects in various systems or organs and producing the pleomorphic clinical picture known as Wilson's disease. Pigment is formed normally and a breakdown in the function of cytochrome C oxidase would surely be incompatible with life.

Orally administered radiocopper is readily absorbed at a rate which does not appear to differ from normal to any significant extent, but the radioactivity in plasma does show a characteristic pattern. Shortly after radiocopper is administered, there tends to be a greater amount of labeled metal able to pass from plasma through a semipermeable membrane[35] and larger amounts are correspondingly found in the urine; at this early stage too the plasma levels are rather higher than in normal individuals. However, most of the radiocopper is attached to the albumin, but it is not removed from this by the liver and it remains albumin-bound for as long as the half-life of the isotope permits study; thus there is no secondary rise in plasma radioactivity, as occurs in the normal individual, but a steady fall which has been shown to continue for as long as 200 hours (Fig. 22–7). There are at present no published figures for the rate at which radiocopper is excreted in the bile in Wilson's disease, but less radioactivity is detected in the stools[10] though whether this is due to greater absorption or lesser excretion than normal is one of the major unanswered questions in regard to this disease. Meantime abnormal amounts of copper accumulate, first in the liver and, after this has become saturated, in other tissues.[37] Evidence suggests that the protein-copper combinations differ from normal quantitatively in their degree of saturation with the metal rather than qualitatively in the nature of the protein.[31, 41] The excess copper so deposited leads sooner or later to necrosis of liver parenchymal cells, as illustrated by a rise in the serum transaminases, and this is eventually followed by the development of fibrosis and scarring. When the liver is finally saturated with copper it can no longer clear the metal from the plasma so that it comes to be deposited in other sites (See Fig. 22–8), principally the kidneys leading to tubular defects and in the brain where it produces the motor and occasionally psychiatric disturbances that characterize the disease.

Quantitative studies of the fate of injected radiocopper[37] clearly show how the pattern of uptake by the liver and clearance of the isotope from the plasma change as the disease progresses but revert to the original state following prolonged decoppering with penicillamine (Fig. 22–9). Thus early in the illness, before the onset of symptoms, uptake of copper by the liver and excretion in the urine cannot necessarily be distinguished from the normal, but even in these cases there is no secondary rise in plasma radioactivity due to incorporation of the metal into ceruloplasmin; detection of this defect probably remains the single most reliable test for the diagnosis of Wilson's disease.[53] While the mechanism of the positive copper balance in these patients remains obscure,[10] it could be due to either increased intestinal absorption or decreased biliary excretion of the metal; furthermore, the relationship of the mechanism of biliary excretion to the failure to incorporate copper into ceruloplasmin cannot be determined until there is some clue as to the physiological role of the protein. In this connection, some indirect evidence is available; in those patients with Wilson's disease who have been successfully treated with penicillamine a stage is commonly reached when there are no symptoms of the disease and no detectable oxidase activity in the serum. This suggests that ceruloplasmin is not essential for normal health provided some other mechanism is found to control the excretion of copper from the body and hence to establish a normal copper balance.

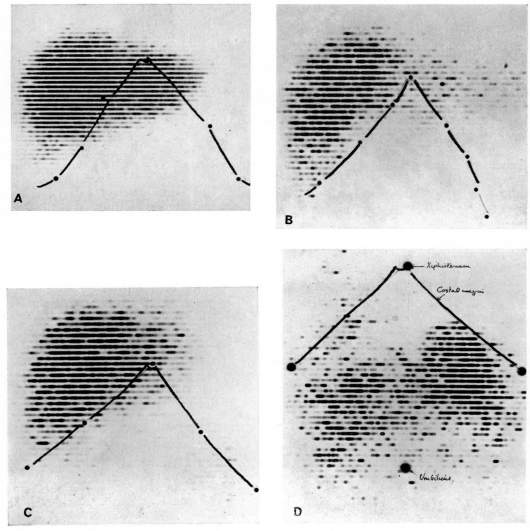

Fig. 22–8. Scintiscans of the abdomen approximately 4 hours after intravenous injection of radiocopper:

(A) Normal individual showing liver only outlined.

(B) Presymptomatic Wilson's disease showing the liver slightly less well outlined than in the control.

(C) Early hepatic Wilson's disease; the liver is still well outlined but faint renal shadows can also be seen.

(D) Neurologic Wilson's disease; little radiocopper is in the liver but the kidneys have taken up much of the isotope. (*Fig. 22–8. E and F on facing page.*)

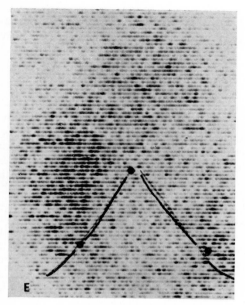

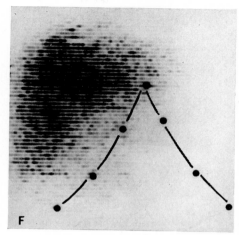

(E) Advanced, neglected Wilson's disease. Radioactivity is widely distributed over the thoracic and abdominal regions; density in the hepatic area is slightly increased.

(F) Treated Wilson's disease; in this patient liver function had been restored by 6 years' treatment with penicillamine.

TREATMENT

It would be arguing in a circle to say that the object of treatment must be the removal of copper because this is the pathogenic agent; nevertheless, this must indeed be the aim—to establish and maintain a negative copper balance—for only by doing this can the disease process be arrested and reversed. Treatment directed to the management of signs or symptoms of liver damage is purely supportive and is not an end in itself; this aspect of the problem is not referred to here, for it is more than adequately dealt with in other chapters of this book. However, I cannot stress too strongly that no patient should be subjected to hepatic or portal surgery unless as an urgent lifesaving measure; the end results are often disastrous, leading to either rapid progression of Wilson's disease or hepatic failure, or, if the patient survives the operation, he may be a psychiatric casualty. Possibly the combination of a raised blood concentration of the ammonium ion and of copper are synergistic in their toxic action.

Various procedures were suggested in the past to deplete the body stores of copper. Cumings was the first to realize the possibility of this when he suggested that the dithiol "BAL" (dimercaptopropanol) deserved a trial in the treatment of Wilson's disease.[14] However, the results with this drug were unpredictable and on the whole did not live up to expectations, but its use has died hard despite the frequency of relapse following a good initial response and despite the painful nature of the injection and the frequent occurrence of toxic reactions.

Another powerful chelating agent, though not structurally related to BAL, is ethylenediamine tetraacetic acid (Versene); it is inconstantly absorbed when given by mouth and, like BAL, calls for an act of endurance by the patient, for it must be given by either intravenous infusion or bulky intramuscular injection.[7] Its use has not alleviated the symptoms of Wilson's disease. The use of the even more powerful analogue diethylenetriamine pentaacetic acid is probably subject to the same limitations.

Ion exchange resins and potassium sulfide have been given by mouth in an attempt to

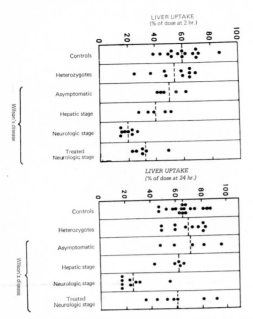

FIG. 22–9. Percentage uptake of intravenously injected radiocopper by the liver. As Wilson's disease progresses this function becomes increasingly impaired by comparison with that of control subjects. Once treatment with penicillamine is instituted this progress of events is reversed so that concentrating ability returns toward normal.

(*Top*) Liver uptake 2 hours after injection of radiocopper. (*Bottom*) Liver uptake 24 hours after injection of radiocopper.

reduce the absorption of dietary copper[12] but are probably an unnecessary adjunct to chelation therapy. Cortisone, high protein diets and single amino acids in high dosage[30] can be similarly dismissed from the list of useful therapeutic agents. This leaves two further thiol compounds for consideration, namely, diethyldithiocarbamate[55] and β,β-dimethylcysteine, penicillamine.[56] Sunderman, White and Sunderman reported the successful use of dithiocarbamate in a single case and claimed that it produced a strongly negative copper balance when given either by vein to promote urinary excretion or by mouth to increase the fecal excretion of copper.[55] Attempts to confirm the fecal excretion of copper following oral administration of dithiocarbamate using

both chemical[24] and radiochemical methods[60] have failed to demonstrate any increase in the loss of metal via this route.

This leaves penicillamine,

$$\begin{matrix} CH_3 \\ CH_3 \end{matrix} \!\!\Big\rangle\! C \cdot SH \cdot CH \cdot NH_2 \cdot COOH,$$

as the only remaining therapy for the treatment of Wilson's disease. The high mortality in the hepatic stage of the illness, as described, might well lead to the conclusion that no form of treatment is likely to be of benefit. This, however, is not the case, for in only a minority of these patients was the diagnosis made during life. All patients in whom the diagnosis was made prior to the terminal phase of the illness and who received a dose of penicillamine adequate to establish and maintain a negative copper balance have recovered so that their liver function tests have become normal (see Fig. 22–10) and clinical signs of active liver disease have disappeared even though the liver or spleen may remain palpable for a considerable period. Similarly, hemolysis has not recurred in any patient once treatment has been started. Four of six patients diagnosed before the onset of clinical symptoms had marked elevation of the serum transaminases and a fifth had positive floccula-

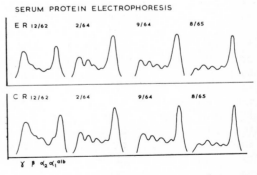

FIG. 22–10. Changes in the electrophoretic pattern of serum proteins of two sisters with hepatic Wilson's disease. The elder girl, E. R., was in hepatic precoma when first seen; her sibling, C. R., had no symptoms but was found to have an enlarged spleen and vascular spiders. Both children were started on penicillamine in December 1962 and have taken it continuously since that date.

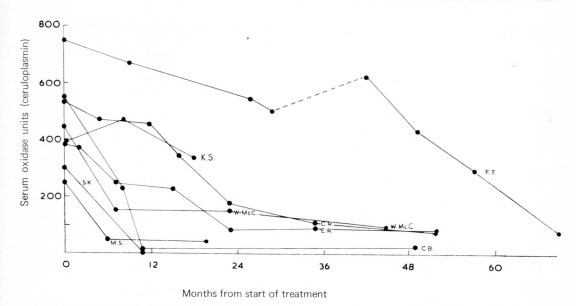

FIG. 22–11. Effect of penicillamine treatment on oxidase activity of serum in 8 patients with Wilson's disease in whom the ceruloplasmin concentration was significantly above average (800 oxidase units is approximately equivalent to 30 mg./100 ml. of ceruloplasmin). Note the rise in oxidase activity of the serum of F. T. when prophylactic treatment was temporarily interrupted; during this time Kayser-Fleischer rings became visible.

tion tests; these tests all returned to normal once therapy was instituted.

Since hepatic Wilson's disease can run a rapidly fatal course, treatment should be started as soon as possible and should not be delayed in the interest of purely esoteric investigations. However, it is desirable to know basal figures for serum copper and ceruloplasmin and for the excretion of copper in the urine. Once these are known D-penicillamine should be started. A dose of 500 mg. free base (or 600 mg. of the hydrochloride) given before meals three times daily is adequate for most cases but occasionally more is needed, particularly if the clinical condition is desperate. A dose of this size should promote a cupriuresis of at least 2,000 μg. copper daily, but if necessary the dose must be stepped up until this is achieved. The actual amount of copper mobilized will depend, to some extent, on the degree of saturation of the tissues with the metal, and patients with a great excess load may excrete as much as 8,000 or 9,000 μg. every 24 hours for the first few days of treatment. As time goes on and the excess body load of copper is depleted, the amount

recovered in the urine will diminish but this does not mean that the patient is becoming resistant to the drug[60] and it is not necessarily an indication for increasing the dose. When, and only when, the body

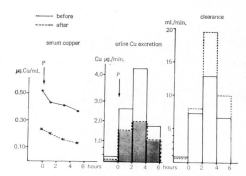

FIG. 22–12. Mean results of endogenous copper clearance studies on 22 patients with Wilson's disease when first seen and again after an average period of 33 months' treatment with D-penicillamine HCl. All treatment was stopped for 48 hours before the test and 600 mg. of D-penicillamine HCl (arrow P on chart) was given at zero time. (Reproduced from Brain.[60])

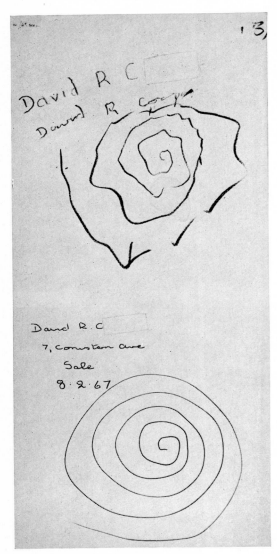

FIG. 22–13. Handwriting of a patient with Wilson's disease shortly after the start of treatment, February 1966, and 1 year later in February 1967. During this time he had taken 1,500 mg. of D-penicillamine HCl daily.

stores of excess copper are becoming significantly depleted the concentration of copper in the serum will fall as also will that of ceruloplasmin, though it may be many months before this happens (see Fig. 22–11). Similarly the basal urine copper excretion eventually returns to normal, as

also does the amount of copper excreted in response to a test dose of penicillamine (Fig. 22–12). As these parameters improve there will be a corresponding clinical improvement (Fig. 22–13). Failure to achieve these results can be ascribed only to inadequate dosage of penicillamine or to drug intolerance. Remember that a patient does not necessarily take or continue to take the medicine prescribed, and this should be considered if there is an unsatisfactory response to a theoretically adequate dose of penicillamine.

In my own experience penicillamine alone has proved to be a highly effective treatment for both the hepatic and neurologic signs of Wilson's disease. The addition of potassium sulfide or Carbo-Resin to prevent copper absorption has not been necessary, but it is probably sensible to advise the patient to avoid those foods with the highest copper contents, such as shellfish, dried fruit, nuts, chocolate, mushrooms and liver,[50] but so many foods have measurable amounts of copper that it would be easy to induce a state of malnutrition by overzealous attempts to design a copper-free diet. Whisky is made in copper stills and in most modern homes water is delivered through copper pipes which may cause something of a problem though once the disease is under control it should not give rise to undue worry. Whether or not the dose of penicillamine should be reduced once clinical remission has been achieved depends partly on the size of the initial dose and partly on the degree of supervision which can be maintained during the follow-up period. Few patients are likely to remain in negative copper balance on less than 900 mg. of penicillamine hydrochloride daily (or correspondingly less for children), and to reduce the dose below this level, one would risk reaccumulation of copper stores and return of symptoms. If it is necessary for any reason to give a smaller dose, the serum copper concentration and basal urine copper excretion should be estimated at not less than 3 monthly intervals and the dose again increased if they show any tendency to rise.

Unfortunately penicillamine, like all powerful drugs, produces toxic reactions in a small proportion of patients. Nausea and gastric irritation can be overcome by giving enteric-coated tablets and, if necessary, pressure must be brought to bear on the manufacturers to provide these.* Weight loss has been observed in some patients without any apparent cause and a positive L.E. cell phenomenon has been found in the serum of two patients though it has not as yet necessitated stopping treatment. Purpura have also been seen, commonly associated with hypersplenism and can usually be controlled with a short course of steroids. Thrombocytopenia and leukopenia have also been reported but have not proved troublesome in the present series. One should know the platelet count before starting treatment, for it is often low in untreated cases. The nephrotic syndrome has been recorded; Sternlieb recently reviewed this, concluding that DL-penicillamine had been used in all cases reported so far.[52] Unfortunately D-penicillamine also induces this serious complication.[44] In some cases it has been possible to restart treatment under steroid cover once proteinuria has subsided. I have seen this toxic reaction to the D-isomer develop no less than 6 years after the start of treatment and it has been shown to be due, almost certainly, to an immune response.[28a] Urticarial reactions also occur occasionally, soon after treatment is started, and can usually be controlled easily by temporarily reducing the dose of penicillamine and giving an antihistaminic. Penicillamine also induces changes in collagen[22] and this may give rise to hemorrhages into the skin over pressure points, but this has been reported only in patients who take more than 2 Gm. daily for more than a year. Finally, L-penicillamine and to a lesser extent the D-isomer, are pyridoxine (vitamin B_6) antimetabolites and although severe pyridoxine deficiency has not been recorded for patients taking D-penicillamine,[21] it is a wise precaution to give them at least 50 mg. of the vitamin weekly.

Recently the whole subject of toxic reactions to penicillamine has been reviewed at a symposium and the proceedings have been published in the Postgraduate Medical Journal for October, 1968.

GENETIC COUNSELING

Now that there is a highly effective treatment for Wilson's disease many young people are going to grow up who would otherwise have died. They will be to all intents and purposes normal except that they need a daily dose of penicillamine for the rest of their lives or until some alternative therapy becomes available. They will be fertile and many will have the foresight to ask about the possible effect on their children. We all carry one or more abnormal genes in our makeup, but this does not stop us from breeding if we so desire; indeed, the human race would have no future if carriers of abnormal genes were forbidden to procreate.† Prior knowledge of what the abnormal gene may be is therefore no bar to having children, provided that it is realized that to marry a close relative brings a grave risk of having children with Wilson's disease. The risk of marrying a carrier on random mating is probably not greater than 1 chance in 200 and may be as low as 1 in 500. Should such a mischance occur the risk to the child is 1 in 2 of developing Wilson's disease and if this does not occur he is certainly a carrier of the genetic defect. These facts should be explained to the patient who can then make up his own mind and reach an informed decision. To forbid the patient the normal hopes and expectations of a married life is unjust and unreasonable, provided that both patient and consort are conversant with the facts.

REFERENCES

1. Anderson, P. J., and Popper, H.: Changes in hepatic structure in Wilson's disease, Am. J. Path. 36:483, 1960.
2. André, J., and van Bogaert, L.: Études génétiques et anatomiques sur la dégénérescences hépato-lenticulaire, Bull. Ass. d'Études physiopathol. du foie 5:3, 1948.
3. Arima, M., and Sano, I.: Genetical studies

* In England these are provided by Dista Products Ltd. of Speke, Liverpool, and are most satisfactory.

† There may well be those who do not consider this to be such an undesirable state of affairs.

of Wilson's Disease, in Japan, *in* The International Symposium on Wilson's Disease, Toyko, 1966, Birth Defects: Original Article Series, 4:54, 1968.

4. Bearn, A. G.: Genetic and biochemical aspects of Wilson's disease, Am. J. Med. 15:442, 1953.

5. ———: A genetical analysis of thirty families with Wilson's disease (hepatolenticular degeneration), Ann. Hum. Genet. 24:33, 1960.

6. Bearn, A. G., and Kunkel, H. G.: Localization of Cu^{64} in serum fractions following oral administration: an alteration in Wilson's disease, Proc. Soc. Exp. Biol. Med. 85:44, 1954.

7. Bickel, H., Neale, F. C., and Hall, G.: A clinical and biochemical study of hepatolenticular degeneration (Wilson's disease), Quart. J. Med. 26:527, 1957.

8. Bramwell, B.: Familial cirrhosis of the liver: four cases of acute fatal cirrhosis of the liver in the same family, the patients being respectively nine, ten, fourteen and fourteen years of age; suggested relationship to Wilson's progressive degeneration of the lenticular nucleus, Edinb. Med. J. 17:90, 1916.

9. Briggs, J., and Walshe, J. M.: Caeruloplasmin in liver disease: a diagnostic pitfall, Lancet 2:263, 1962.

10. Bush, J. A., Mahoney, J. P., Markowitz, H., Gubler, C. J., Cartwright, G. E., and Wintrobe, M. M.: Studies on copper metabolism. XVI. Radioactive copper studies in normal subjects and in patients with hepatolenticular degeneration, J. Clin. Invest. 34:1766, 1955.

11. Cartwright, G. E., Gubler, C. J., and Wintrobe, M. M.: Studies on copper metabolism. XI. Copper and iron metabolism in the nephrotic syndrome, J. Clin. Invest. 33:685, 1954.

12. Cartwright, G. E., Hodges, R. E., Gubler, C. J., Mahoney, J. P., Daum, K., Wintrobe, M. M., and Bean, W. B.: Studies on copper metabolism. XIII. Hepatolenticular degeneration, J. Clin. Invest. 33:1487, 1954.

13. Chalmers, T. C., Iber, F. L., and Uzman, L. L.: Hepatolenticular degeneration (Wilson's disease) as a form of idiopathic cirrhosis, New Engl. J. Med. 256:235, 1957.

14. Cumings, J. N.: The copper and iron content of brain and liver in the normal and in hepatolenticular degeneration, Brain 71:410, 1948.

15. ———: Heavy Metals and the Brain. Oxford, Blackwell's Scientific Publications, Springfield, Ill., Thomas, 1959.

16. Epstein, P. S., and McIlwain, H.: Actions of cupric salts on isolated cerebral tissue, Proc. Roy. Soc. B 166:295, 1966.

17. Finby, N., and Bearn, A. G.: Roentgenographic abnormalities of the skeletal system in Wilson's disease (hepatolenticular degeneration), Am. J. Roentgenol. 79:603, 1958.

18. Franklin, E. C., and Baumann, A.: Liver dysfunction in hepatolenticular degeneration, Am. J. Med. 15:450, 1953.

19. Garrod, A. E.: Inborn errors of metabolism (Croonian Lectures), Lancet 2:1, 73, 142, 214, 1908.

20. Gibbs, K., and Walshe, J. M.: A study of copper content of hair in normal families and those with Wilson's disease, J. med. Genet. 2:181, 1965.

21. ———: Penicillamine and pyridoxine requirements in man, Lancet 1:175, 1966.

22. Harris, E. D., Jr., and Sjoerdsma, A.: Effect of penicillamine on human collagen and its possible application to treatment of scleroderma, Lancet 2:996, 1966.

23. Holmberg, C. G.: Development of knowledge of caeruloplasmin *in* Walshe, J. M., and Cumings, J. N. (eds.): Wilson's Disease: Some Current Concepts, Oxford, Blackwell's Scientific Publications, 1961.

24. Hsia, Y. E., Combs, J. T., Hook, L., and Brandt, I. K.: Hepatolenticular degeneration: the comparative effectiveness of D-penicillamine, potassium sulphide and diethyldithiocarbamate as decoppering agents, J. Pediat. 68:921, 1966.

25. Hunt, A. H., Parr, R. M., Taylor, D. M., and Trott, N. G.: Relation between cirrhosis and trace metal content of liver with special reference to primary biliary cirrhosis and copper, Brit. Med. J. 2:1498, 1963.

26. Kasper, C. B., and Deutsch, H. F.: Physicochemical studies of human ceruloplasmin, J. Biol. Chem. 238:2325, 1963.

27. Kasper, C. B., Deutsch, H. F., and Beinert, H.: Studies on the state of copper in native and a modified ceruloplasmin, J. Biol. Chem. 238:2338, 1963.

28. Kehrer, F.: Der Ursachenkreis des Parkinsonismus (Erblichkeit, Trauma, Syphilis), Arch. Psychiat. Nervenkr. 91:187, 1930.

28a. Lachmann, P. J., and Walshe, J. M.: Unpublished observations.

29. Massey, V., and Veeger, C.: Studies on the reaction mechanism of lipoyl dehydrogenase, Biochim. Biophys. Acta 48: 33, 1961.

30. Matthews, W. B.: Hepatolenticular degeneration in Schiff, L. (ed.): Diseases of the Liver, Philadelphia, Lippincott, 1956.

31. Morell, A. G., Shapiro, J. R., and Scheinberg, I. H.: Copper-binding protein from human liver in Walshe, J. M., and Cumings, J. N. (eds.): Wilson's Disease: Some Current Concepts, Oxford, Blackwell's Scientific Publications, 1961.

32. Morgan, H. G., Stewart, W. K., Lowe, K. G., Stowers, J. M., and Johnstone, J. H.: Wilson's disease and the Fanconi syndrome, Quart. J. Med. 31:361, 1962.

33. Neumann, P. Z., and Sass-Kortsak, A.: The state of copper in human serum: evidence for an amino acid–bound fraction, J. Clin. Invest. 46:646, 1967.

34. Osborn, S. B., and Walshe, J. M.: The effect of penicillamine and dimercaprol on turnover of copper in patients with Wilson's disease, Lancet 1:70, 1958.

35. ———: Filterable and non-filterable serum copper. (2) Studies with ^{64}Cu, Clin. Sci. 26:213, 1964.

36. ———: Studies with radiocopper (^{64}Cu, ^{67}Cu). A distinction between the hepatic and neurological forms of Wilson's disease in The International Symposium on Wilson's Disease, Toyko, 1966, Birth Defects: Original Article Series, 4:41, 1968.

37. ———: Studies with radioactive copper (^{64}Cu and ^{67}Cu) in relation to the natural history of Wilson's disease, Lancet 1:346, 1967.

38. ———: Studies with radioactive copper (^{64}Cu); the fate of orally ingested copper. Unpublished.

39. Peters, R. A., and Walshe, J. M.: Studies on the toxicity of copper. (1) The toxic action of copper in vivo and in vitro, Proc. Roy. Soc. B 166:273, 1966.

40. Peters, R. A., Shorthouse, M., and Walshe, J. M.: Studies on the toxicity of copper. (2) The behaviour of microsomal membrane ATPase of the pigeon's brain tissue to copper and some metallic substances, Proc. Roy. Soc. B 166:285, 1966.

41. Porter, H.: Copper proteins in brain and liver in the normal and in Wilson's disease, in The International Symposium on Wilson's Disease, Toyko, 1966, Birth Defects: Original Article Series, 41:23, 1968.

42. Race, R. R., Sanger, R., and Walshe, J. M.: Unpublished observations.

43. Rees, K.: Copper as an enzyme poison in Walshe, J. M., and Cumings, J. N. (eds.): Wilson's Disease: Some Current Concepts, Oxford, Blackwell's Scientific Publications, 1961.

44. Rosenberg, L. E., and Hayslett, J. P.: Nephrotoxic effects of penicillamine in cystinuria, J.A.M.A. 201:698, 1967.

45. Rumpel, A.: Über das Wesen und die Bedeutung der Leberveränderungen und der Pigmentierungen bei den damit verbundenen Fällen von Pseudosklerose, Dtsch. Z. Nervenheilk. 49:54, 1913.

46. Schaffner, F., Sternlieb, I., Barka, T., and Popper, H.: Hepatocellular changes in Wilson's disease, Am. J. Path. 41:315, 1962.

47. Scheinberg, I. H., and Gitlin, D.: Deficiency of ceruloplasmin in patients with hepatolenticular degeneration (Wilson's disease), Science 116:484, 1952.

48. Scheinberg, I. H., and Morell, A. G.: Exchange of ceruloplasmin copper with ionic Cu^{64} with reference to Wilson's disease, J. Clin. Invest. 36:1193, 1957.

49. Scheinberg, I. H., and Sternlieb, I.: The liver in Wilson's disease, Gastroenterology 37:550, 1959.

50. ———: Copper metabolism, Pharmacol. Rev. 12:355, 1960.

51. Schubert, J.: Copper and Peroxides in Radiobiology and Medicine, Springfield, Ill., Thomas, 1964.

52. Sternlieb, I.: Penicillamine and the nephrotic syndrome. J.A.M.A. 198:1311, 1966.

53. Sternlieb, I., Morell, A. G., Bauer, C. D., Combes, B., De Bobes-Sternberg, S., and Scheinberg, I. H.: Detection of the heterozygous carrier of the Wilson's disease gene, J. Clin. Invest. 40:707, 1961.

54. Sternlieb, I., Morell, A. G., Tucker, W. D., Greene, M. W., and Scheinberg, I. H.: Incorporation of copper into ceruloplasmin in vivo: Studies with copper^{64} and copper^{67}, J. Clin. Invest. 40:1834, 1961.

55. Sunderman, F. W., Jr., White, J. C., and Sunderman, F. W.: Metabolic balance studies in hepatolenticular degeneration treated with diethyldithiocarbamate, Am. J. Med. 34:875, 1963.

56. Walshe, J. M.: Penicillamine, a new oral therapy for Wilson's disease, Am. J. Med. 21:487, 1956.

57. ———: Wilson's disease, the presenting symptoms, Arch. Dis. Childh. 37:253, 1962.

58. ———: Copper metabolism and the liver, Postgrad. Med. J. 39:188, 1963.

59. ———: Filterable and non-filterable serum copper. (1) The action of penicillamine, Clin. Sci. 25:405, 1963.

60. ———: The physiology of copper in man and its relation to Wilson's disease, Brain 90:149, 1967.

61. Wilson, S. A. K.: Progressive lenticular degeneration; a familial nervous disease associated with cirrhosis of the liver, Brain 34:295, 1912.

23

The Liver in Circulatory Failure

SHEILA SHERLOCK, M.D.

The hepatic veins enter the inferior vena cava very close to its entrance into the right auricle, and a rise in pressure in the right auricle is transmitted readily to the hepatic veins. Liver cells are particularly vulnerable to oxygen deprivation; therefore, diminished hepatic oxygen supply consequent upon a failing heart, lowered blood pressure or any cause of a reduced hepatic blood flow is reflected in impaired function of liver cells. Hepatic dysfunction is to be expected in both peripheral circulatory failure with a lowered blood pressure and in right-sided congestive heart failure, with a rise in right auricular pressure or lowered cardiac output.

HEPATIC CHANGES IN ACUTE HEART FAILURE AND SHOCK

Hepatic changes occur in shock and are particularly common with myocardial infarction,[13] with acute heart failure of all types and in many other conditions, including crushing and severe trauma, burns, hemorrhage, sepsis, pulmonary embolism, peritonitis and blackwater fever.[10, 16, 74]

Histologic features are:

1. Congestion of the central hepatic vein with local hemorrhage from it (Fig. 23-1).

2. Focal necrosis of liver cells which is usually centrilobular but occasionally appears to be mid-zonal, perhaps due to the section being cut in a plane that missed the adjacent central vein.

3. The necrotizing liver cells take eosin stains in contrast with the basophilia of normal liver cells. The cytoplasm may show hydropic change, reminiscent of that observed in carbon tetrachloride poisoning, but fatty change is not seen.

4. Nuclear changes in the necrotic zone are prominent, with pyknosis and disintegration and fading of the nuclei (Fig. 23-2).

5. There may be polymorphonuclear infiltration around the focal necrosis.

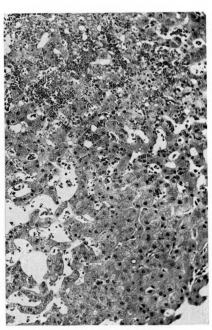

FIG. 23-1. Ischemic heart failure. Serum bilirubin 2.1 mg./100 ml. Liver cells have disappeared from the center of the lobule and are replaced by frank hemorrhage. (Hematoxylin and eosin; × 120.) (Sherlock, S.: Brit. Heart J. 13:273.)

6. The essential reticulin structure of the liver is preserved within the necrotic zone.[13]

7. With recovery from the shock, particularly in traumatic cases, mitoses may be prominent in the hepatic cell nuclei.[10] This may represent part of the reparative process.

8. Sometimes, and for no obvious reason, the left lobe of the liver suffers more than the right. This is similar to that seen in acute viral hepatitis where the left lobe also may be more necrotic than the right.[40]

Electron microscopy shows cytoplasmic edema, swollen and disorganized mitochondria and increase in number and size of lysosomes.[24]

TOXIC AND CONGESTIVE CENTRAL HEPATIC NECROSIS

Wallach and Popper analyzed the clinical and the gross anatomic findings in 100 patients in whom autopsy revealed central hepatic necrosis (not including primary hepatic disease).[74] Two main groups could be recognized, depending on whether or not congestive heart failure was present. Histologic changes in the heart failure or "congestive" cases included large central veins with wide branches piercing through the walls of the larger vessels, marked disappearance and atrophy of the liver cells, but no fragments or remnants of cells and, usually, dilatation of sinusoids. The "toxic" cases were distinguished by fragmentation of the nucleus, exudative cells encircling the affected cells, and, despite occasionally wide sinusoids, small central veins with narrow piercing branches and dissociation of liver cell cords. These differences might be related to the increased venous pressure in the congestive cases and the presence of a circulating injurious substance in the toxic instances.

PATHOGENESIS OF HEPATIC CHANGES

The extent of the changes can be related to the duration of the shock state; if it exists longer than 24 hours, hepatic necrosis is almost constant; if less than 10 hours, it is unusual.

The fall in systemic blood pressure is most important. This leads to a fall in the blood flow through the portal vein on which the liver mainly depends for its oxygen supply. In addition, the falling blood pressure proportionately lowers the oxygen content of the portal venous blood.[42] Therefore, the hepatic cells are more dependent for oxygen on the hepatic arterial blood flow. However, this is reduced also as

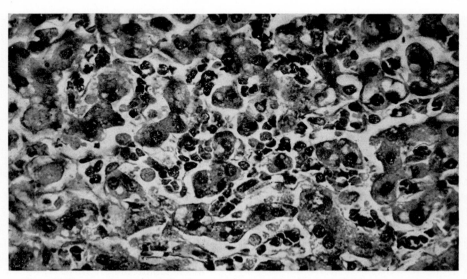

FIG. 23–2. Crush injury. Shrinkage of liver cells with nonfatty vacuoles appearing in cytoplasm and nonfatty globules lying free between cells and sinusoids. (Hematoxylin and eosin; × 430.) (Bywaters, E. G. L.: Clin. Sci. 6:19.)

a result of vasoconstriction consequent on the fall in systemic blood pressure. Therefore, the hepatic cells are anoxic, and the cells at the center of the lobules, which receive blood at a lower oxygen tension than at the periphery[6] and are more susceptible to a fall in the oxygen supply to the liver, become necrotic.

In the dog the outflow of blood from the liver is controlled by a sluice mechanism located near the caval orifices of the main hepatic vein.[3] Contraction of muscles in the walls of hepatic veins in this area causes diminution of outflow of blood from the liver, which swells. Active constriction of hepatic venous radicles in man has been postulated so that the intralobular blood flow is impeded. This is put forward as a significant factor in the pathogenesis of the centrilobular lesions occurring in anaphylactic shock, in blackwater fever (malignant malaria) and in congestive heart failure.[44, 45] However, this mechanism never has been demonstrated in man and seems to be unlikely, for in man the hepatic veins have little plain muscle in their walls.[52]

The Liver and the Metabolic Changes That Occur in Peripheral Circulatory Failure

Results have been based largely on observations of experimental animals, and it has been shown clearly that the liver in shock functions abnormally.

1. It is unable to store glycogen normally and to convert lactate and pyruvate to glycogen.[20]

2. The oxygen consumption of liver slices from shocked animals is diminished.[60]

3. There is a failure to deaminate amino acids with a rise in the blood amino-acid nitrogen content.[76]

There are a few observations along similar lines in shock in man. Davidson and co-workers noticed a rise in the level of the blood lactic acid and alpha-amino nitrogen in medical shock, and some of their patients also showed mild icterus and an increase in the prothrombin time.[14] All these suggested hepatic involvement. Bywaters also observed jaundice in some of the severely traumatized patients whom he studied.[10]

POSTOPERATIVE JAUNDICE

Jaundice that develops soon after a surgical procedure may have multiple causes.[26] Increased pigment load follows blood transfusion, particularly if the blood has been stored for some days. The hemoglobin in 500 ml. of stored blood contains about 250 ml. of bilirubin, the normal daily production. Extravasated blood in the tissues gives an additional bilirubin load.

Hepatocellular function is impaired following an operation, administration of anesthetics or shock. Hepatic perfusion is reduced. This is particularly evident if the patient is in incipient circulatory failure and the cardiac output is already reduced. Simultaneously the kidney suffers from reduced renal blood flow.

Administration of halothane anesthetics, especially if multiple, may be followed within a few days of the operation by a hepatitis-like picture. Other drugs used in the operative period, such as promazines or hydrazine oxidase inhibitors must also be considered as the cause of the icterus. Sepsis *per se* can produce deep jaundice which may be cholestatic.

In addition a *cholestatic jaundice* may appear postoperatively. It is noted on the first or second postoperative day, reaches its height between the fourth and tenth day, and disappears by 14 to 18 days. Serum biochemical changes are variable. Sometimes alkaline phosphatase and transaminase levels are increased.[65] Serum bilirubin may rise to levels of 23 to 39 mg./100 ml. The picture simulates extrahepatic biliary obstruction. These patients have all had an episode of shock, been transfused and suffered heart failure of recent onset. Centrizonal hepatic necrosis, however, is not conspicuous and hepatic histology shows only minor abnormalities. The mechanism of the cholestasis is uncertain. This picture must be recognized, and if necessary needle biopsy of the liver performed. In these patients, surgical intervention to relieve a nonexistent obstruction would be disastrous.

Jaundice After Cardiac Surgery

Jaundice is particularly liable to follow major heart surgery.[58] In one series of 232 patients the overall incidence was 13 per cent, 55 per cent with mitral valve disease and 5 per cent when the aortic valve was involved. Postoperative jaundice (serum bilirubin greater than 3 mg.) was seen in 63 (8.6 per cent) of 736 patients having open heart operations. Fifty-eight of the 63 had acquired heart disease.[62] Jaundice was greater the more severe the valvular pathology, being particularly marked in cases of double or triple valve replacements.

The patient may have preoperative disturbance of hepatic function with centrizonal necrosis, consequent upon prolonged heart failure. Patients over 50 years of age are very liable. Hypotension and shock are frequent in the operative period, further reducing hepatic blood flow.[48] Hypothermia may contribute.[32]

Large quantities of stored blood are used. The life-span of this blood may be further reduced by passage through the heart-lung machine.[1] Plasma hemoglobin (indicating hemolysis) can be raised after heart surgery.[39] Mechanical prostheses may decrease the survival time of red cells.[1, 39] The bilirubin load on the liver cell is therefore increased.

The cholestatic picture following operations may also be seen. In these patients hepatic necrosis is minimal. Surprisingly, alkaline phosphatase may be normal or only slightly increased. Serum transaminases are raised.[39]

Infections, drugs (including anticoagulants) and anesthetics must also be considered.

Virus (transfusion) hepatitis is also likely to develop after cardiac surgery. This is not usual less than 2 weeks postoperatively.

EXPERIMENTAL CHRONIC HEPATIC VENOUS CONGESTION

In the experimental animal, individual ligation of all the hepatic veins is impossible, and the usual method is to constrict the inferior vena cava by a cellophane band placed above the entry of the hepatic veins, thus obstructing the venous return from the liver.

STRUCTURAL CHANGES

Structural changes in the liver[8, 9, 29, 70, 78]

are essentially similar to those seen in congestive heart failure. The whole liver swells, and the hepatic veins dilate with congestion of the sinusoids. Centrilobular hemorrhage and necrosis of liver cells follow, and the extent is proportional to the amount of hepatic venous obstruction. Connective tissue proliferates round the central vein, giving a picture analogous to cardiac cirrhosis. The liver cells adjoining the portal tracts are well preserved, and the tracts themselves show little change. In acute hepatic venous occlusion the lymphatics are greatly dilated but this later subsides.

FUNCTIONAL CHANGES

Functional changes in the liver include the accumulation of ascites. It has been suggested that this ascites forms by outpouring of hepatic lymph into the peritoneum. Increased liver lymph flow is the first sign of venous congestion of the liver,[9] and in the dog occlusion of the hepatic venous return results in a 10- to 20-fold increase of liver lymph flow having a high protein content.[73] The hepatic sinusoids are related intimately to the hepatic lymphatics, and the increase in sinusoidal pressure may be related to the overproduction of lymph. Although there is an undoubted increase in hepatic lymph flow, there are no obvious anatomic connections between the liver lymphatics and the peritoneal cavity.

Hepatic venous congestion in the dog results in sodium retention in the ascitic fluid.[64] Two explanations have been offered. The low tissue pressure in the peritoneal cavity may trap sodium and chloride; alternatively, the retention may be a renal compensatory mechanism to offset the loss of body fluids, plasma proteins and electrolytes into the peritoneal cavity. It has even been postulated that the sodium retention of congestive heart failure may be related in part to the hepatic venous congestion occurring in that condition.

LIVER FUNCTION TESTS

Liver function tests are little affected. The plasma nonprotein nitrogen, glucose or prothrombin time show little change; although the serum protein concentration may fall, this may be related to loss of protein into the ascites rather than hepatic cellular dysfunction. It seems unlikely that the disturbed hepatic function tests in congestive heart failure are due to hepatic venous congestion alone. Some other factor must be playing a part, and this may well be the concomitant anoxia of the liver.[29]

THE LIVER IN CONGESTIVE (RIGHT-SIDED) HEART FAILURE

Postmortem hepatic autolysis is particularly rapid in the patient dying in heart failure.[53, 67] In the agonal period and in the 12 hours after death, the liver cells shrink and disappear, and the remaining cells become dissociated from each other. Glycogen is lost from the liver cells, the parasinusoidal spaces are opened up, and the liver cell columns are shrunken. The sinusoids contain less blood than in life. The appearance of fat in the liver cells in heart failure is also a postmortem phenomenon. Autopsy material is therefore unreliable for the assessment of the effects of cardiac failure on the liver in life. Accurate histologic data can be obtained only by aspiration liver biopsy. Hemorrhage might be anticipated from puncture of the "congested" liver of heart failure, but 41 biopsies performed in one series and 75 in another were uncomplicated and well tolerated.[67, 75]

MACROSCOPIC CHANGES

At autopsy the liver usually is enlarged, but liver weights are variable and bear no relation to the clinical assessment of hepatic size. This may be due to drainage of blood, postmortem, from an overdistended liver into other organs. The liver is purplish, with rounded edges. If there is gross fibrosis and a cardiac cirrhosis, the liver may be small, but it is never so irregular and never has the same degree of nodular regeneration of liver cells as is seen in a classic Laennec's cirrhosis.

The cut surface (Fig. 23–3) shows prominence of the hepatic veins, which may be thickened in a chronic case. The organ drips blood. If a cardiac cirrhosis is present, the liver cuts with difficulty. The lobules are prominent, with yellow and red areas alternating; the red represents the hemor-

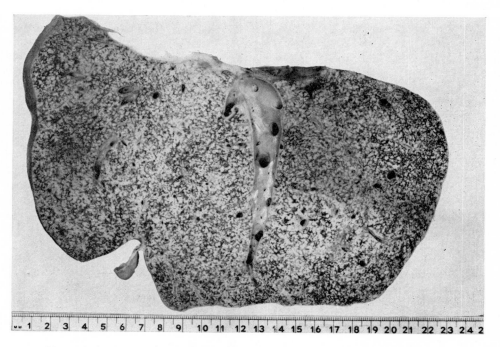

FIG. 23–3. Cut surface of liver from patient dying from congestive heart failure. Note dilated hepatic veins. Light areas corresponding to peripheral fatty zones alternate with dark areas corresponding to central zonal congestion and hemorrhage.

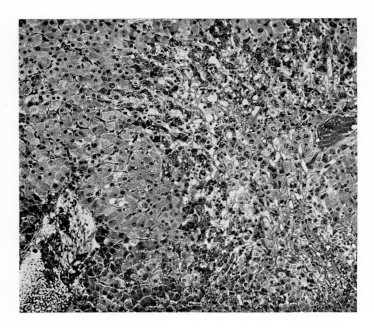

FIG. 23–4. Cor pulmonale. Serum bilirubin 3.4 mg./100 ml. Gross centrilobular congestion and liver cell necrosis. Pigment increase is seen in the degenerating liver cells. Liver cells at the periphery of the lobule are relatively normal. (Hematoxylin and eosin; × 120.) Sherlock, S.: Brit. Heart J. *13*:273.)

rhagic centers of the lobules, and the yellow the fatty periphery. This appearance has been likened to a nutmeg.[30] In a longstanding case of heart failure, the red and yellow areas may coalesce, giving the cut surface the appearance of a fern leaf.

HISTOLOGIC CHANGES

The general anatomy of the lobule is usually intact, the portal tracts bearing their normal relationship to the central hepatic vein. Sometimes the lobular pattern is reversed, the portal tract apparently lying centrally with a ring of surrounding fibrous tissue passing from central vein to central vein. This is characteristic of cardiac cirrhosis (Fig. 23–6).

The central vein always is dilated, and the sinusoids entering it are engorged for a variable distance toward the periphery of the lobule (Fig. 23–4). In severe cases there is frank hemorrhage from the sinusoids, with focal necrosis of the liver cells. This may be attributed to the lowered blood pressure and shock state. The liver cell columns are usually atrophic, particularly toward the centers of the lobule, and appear to be attenuated. The liver cells show a variety of degenerative changes in the central area. The cytoplasm is shrunken with excessive granularity, and the nuclei show fragmentation and pyknosis, diminishing in intensity as the portal zones are reached. Apart from cardiac cirrhosis the portal tracts are usually normal. Each portal tract is surrounded by relatively normal cells to a depth that varies inversely with the extent of the centrilobular necrosis.

Diffuse loss of glycogen is noted only agonally. Surviving cells usually contain their normal complement of glycogen, and this is true not only of the relatively normal portal zones but also of the surviving liver cells lying amid debris at the center of the lobule. Biopsy sections show significant fatty change in only about one third of sections and then only a few scattered globules, usually at the periphery of the lobule. This absence of fat in material obtained in life contrasts with the usual postmortem picture described in textbooks of pathology.

The liver cells at the center of a lobule are packed with pigment granules, and as the cell disintegrates completely the pigment lies free amid cellular debris. The brown pigment is probably a lipochrome.

Methylene blue stains sometimes show an excess of bile pigment in the minute bile channels (bile thrombi), especially in the periportal zones. These are most conspicuous in the deeply jaundiced patients.

If the heart condition does not respond to

therapy, the necrosis spreads toward the periphery of the hepatic lobule. If the cardiac failure responds to treatment, the centrilobular necrosis may heal and, even if there is a definite cardiac cirrhosis, hepatic function may be adequate.

Electron microscopy shows that the centrizonal cells disappear because of atrophy rather than necrosis.[61] This atrophy may be related to extensive fibrosis, especially in the space of Disse, where blood-liver cell exchange is impaired. This fibrosis follows formation of new fibers rather than condensation of pre-existing stroma. Canalicular dilation and rupture may also be seen.

FIBROUS TISSUE CHANGES AND CARDIAC CIRRHOSIS

In the mildest cases the reticulin pattern of the liver is normal. The occasional asso-

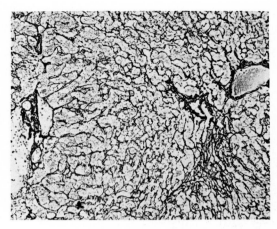

FIG. 23–5. Same section as in Fig. 23–4. Reticulin stains show condensation at the lobular center. (Hematoxylin and eosin; × 120.) (Sherlock, S.: Brit. Heart J. *13*:273)

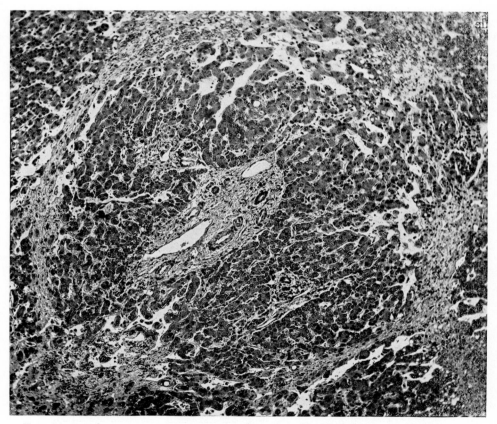

FIG. 23–6. Fibrous tissue bands pass from central vein to central vein. There is "reversed lobulation" and a fully developed cardiac cirrhosis. Portal tracts show only slight fibrosis. (Hematoxylin and eosin; × 90.)

ciation of much liver damage with an intact reticulin framework in the lobule usually is seen in acute heart failure. The next stage is centrizonal reticulin condensation. Hepatic cells have been lost from the centers of the lobule, and this has resulted in collapse of the reticulin stroma—a very common finding in heart failure.

Then follows centrizonal reticulin proliferation. Not only are the reticulin fibers more closely packed together but also there is actual production of new reticulin at the center of the lobule. This is seen as golden yellow fibers in the silver-impregnated sections (Fig. 23–5). A centrizonal increase in collagen is found also. The central vein shows fibrous thickening of its wall, and intimal proliferations with loose connective tissue fibers may be seen[12] (phlebosclerosis). The connective tissue extends outward for a variable distance but does not reach the periphery of the lobule.

If heart failure continues or relapses, the connective tissue from one hepatic vein joins the connective tissue from the central areas of adjoining lobules. The portal areas become surrounded by a ring of fibrous tissue, passing from central vein to central vein. This gives the appearance of reversed lobulation. This lesion is a frank cardiac cirrhosis (Fig. 23–6). The portal tracts may remain unaffected, but in long-standing cases often they are involved also. The bile ducts proliferate, fibroblasts are seen, and sometimes there is also a little round-celled proliferation. When there are changes in both central areas and portal tracts a complex "mixed" picture results (Fig. 23–7). This may be difficult to distinguish from the usual type of portal cirrhosis. However, careful study usually demonstrates that the maximal fibrosis is centrizonal. In some instances, nodular regeneration of liver cells may be seen, but this is never as conspicuous as that of ordinary Laennec's or portal cirrhosis.

If the heart failure continues, the fibrosis progresses so that terminally a "mixed" picture of central cardiac and portal cirrhosis is seen. However, if the failure responds to therapy not only does the centrizonal necrosis heal but the cirrhosis regresses, the fibrous tissue bands becoming narrower and acellular. This type of (latent) cardiac cirrhosis may cause no functional hepatic

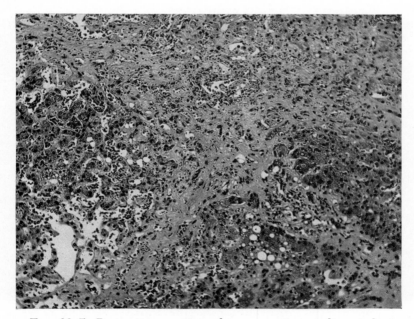

Fig. 23–7. Postmortem sections show an active cardiac cirrhosis. Portal tracts are also involved, giving a mixed portal and cardiac cirrhosis. (Hematoxylin and eosin; × 120.)

TABLE 23–1. HEPATIC RETICULIN CHANGES RELATED TO THE EXTENT OF HEPATIC
CELL NECROSIS AND TO THE TYPE OF HEART FAILURE

	RETICULIN PATTERN CHANGES (NO. OF PATIENTS)			
	Normal	Centrizonal Condensation	Centrizonal Proliferation	Cardiac Cirrhosis
Extent of hepatic necrosis:				
Grade 1	16	1	1	0
2	3	2	3	7
3	4	5	2	6
Type of heart failure:				
Primary valvular mitral	3	2	2	11
Primary valvular aortic	4	2	0	0
Cor pulmonale	7	1	2	2
Hypertensive	6	1	1	0
Ischemic	3	2	1	0

(Sherlock, S.: The liver in heart failure; relation of anatomical, functional and circulatory changes, Brit. Heart J. 13:273)

disturbance. If heart failure again supervenes the acute changes again appear.

CLINICAL ASSOCIATIONS (TABLE 23–1)

Centrizonal hepatic cell necrosis occurs in all forms of heart failure, but the severer grades usually are associated with mitral stenosis or constrictive pericarditis. In general, the longer the patient has been in failure the greater is the extent of the underlying damage to the liver. If failure exists for longer than 60 days, a severe hepatic lesion can be expected.

Cardiac cirrhosis is most often associated with mitral stenosis complicated by tricuspid valvular incompetence. It is an almost constant complication of constrictive pericarditis. However, cardiac cirrhosis can occur with all forms of heart failure, provided that they continue for a sufficient length of time or that there are repeated episodes of failure. The incidence depends on the strictness of the histologic criteria adopted for diagnosis. The term "cardiac cirrhosis" should be used only if there is an alteration in the architectural pattern of the liver as well as fibrosis. With these criteria an incidence of 0.4 per cent of all autopsies seems reasonable.[34]

Centrizonal Hepatic Necrosis. The liver cells at the center of the lobule receive blood at a lower oxygen tension than at the periphery[6] and therefore are more sus-

ceptible to any fall in the oxygen supply to the liver. Anoxia is known to cause both degeneration of central liver cells[46] and dilatation of sinusoids.[66] Intravital fluorescence microscopy studies have shown that hypoxia slows down the rate of secretion of liver cells.[55] This is especially so in the centrizonal cells which finally become necrotic. Catheterization studies in man have shown that as the cardiac output diminishes, the hepatic blood flow diminishes in proportion.[49] The oxygen supply to the liver decreases with diminishing cardiac output, and the centrizonal hepatic necrosis in heart failure can be related to the degree of depression in cardiac output.

The oxygen supply to the liver depends on not only the hepatic blood flow but also the oxygen content of the portal venous and hepatic arterial blood. The arterial oxygen saturation in most types of congestive heart failure is reduced only a little, and this factor is of importance only in patients with pulmonary or congenital heart disease having a lowered arterial oxygen content. The portal venous oxygen level may be reduced in congestive heart failure, and certainly the hepatic vein catheterization studies have shown that the hepatic venous oxygen content is lower than normal.[18, 50] The liver cells are perfused slowly with poorly oxygenated blood, and this must play a part in the genesis of the centrizonal necrosis.

The hepatic venous pressure is raised in heart failure, reflecting the rise in pressure in the right side of the heart, and this might conduce to the centrizonal necrosis.[50] Severe hepatic necrosis usually is associated with a high hepatic venous pressure, and patients with constrictive pericarditis with greatly elevated hepatic venous pressures also have severe centrizonal necrosis. However, as Bolton[8] pointed out, it is doubtful whether the centrizonal changes produced by passive venous congestion are purely mechanical, since the rise in pressure must extend from the hepatic vein through the lobule to the portal veins.

In summary, it seems likely that the centrizonal changes in heart failure result from a combination of hepatic anoxia and hemorrhage from distended sinusoids, due to the increase in the venous pressure.

Cardiac Cirrhosis. The fibrotic changes in the liver occur secondary to the anoxic, centrizonal necrosis and are probably reparative. This central fibrosis then proceeds to a centrizonal cirrhosis. The relative rarity of this condition probably is related to the infrequency of prolonged heart failure. Most patients die in the stage of centrizonal reticulin condensation and never pass to the proliferative, regenerative phase. Repeated episodes of failure are necessary for the development of a full cardiac cirrhosis.[35] Patients with rheumatic mitral stenosis, especially with tricuspid valve incompetence, responding intermittently to treatment, are therefore particularly prone to develop cardiac cirrhosis. If patients with other forms of heart failure survive for a sufficient length of time, they too can develop the same lesion.

Although the connective tissue in heart failure is primarily centrizonal, in the later stages the portal tracts become involved. Fibrous bands link not only central areas but also portal tracts. This may account for the reported frequency of portal cirrhosis in heart failure.[27] However, if serial hepatic biopsies are taken, it is shown that the essential cirrhosis of heart failure is centrizonal and that involvement of the portal tracts is merely a later, confusing feature.[67]

Cardiac cirrhosis *per se* does not seem to have any deleterious effect on the patient. It must be distinguished from the symptom of cardiac jaundice, for patients with cardiac cirrhosis are not more jaundiced than those in heart failure but without hepatic fibrosis. Cardiac cirrhosis does not seem to cause any specific alteration in the serum protein values. The centrizonal fibrosis of heart failure does not seem to cause obstruction to the portal venous blood flow. Superficial abdominal veins are not distended, hematemesis does not occur, and esophageal varicosities are not seen at autopsy. The spleen is not larger in cardiac cirrhosis than in heart failure without cirrhosis. It is only in severe cardiac cirrhosis associated with constrictive pericarditis that symptomatic portal hypertension might be considered.

Clinical recognition of cardiac cirrhosis usually is impossible.[65, 67] It should be suspected in mitral disease with repeated episodes of heart failure, especially if there is associated tricuspid valve incompetence, or in constrictive pericarditis. Most patients with heart failure and deep jaundice have also cardiac cirrhosis, but most patients in whom cirrhosis is present will give no clinical indications of this lesion, and the diagnosis is purely academic, confirmed at autopsy.

If the heart failure is controlled, acute hepatic changes disappear, and the liver shows only avascular fibrous bands passing between central veins. The hepatic cirrhosis is quiescent or latent. This type of cirrhosis is of no clinical significance.

CLINICAL EXAMINATION IN CONGESTIVE HEART FAILURE

Edematous areas may not be jaundiced. Bile pigment is attached to protein and does not enter the edema fluid because of its low protein content.[47] However, this may not be true, as no correlation has been found between the bilirubin and the protein content of edema fluid.[37] The jaundice is not associated with pruritus.

The urine is dark and concentrated and shows excess of urobilinogen. If the jaundice is deep, bile pigment may be detected in the urine.[67] The stools are usually darker in color than normal, and fecal stercobilinogen is increased. Occasionally, however, if the jaundice is very deep, the stools may be gray in color.[21]

Liver. The patient may complain of spontaneous right abdominal pain, similar to that experienced in the early stages of acute infective hepatitis. In both conditions the pain probably is due to stretching of nerve endings in the capsule of the liver.

The liver usually is enlarged, the lower edge often extending to the umbilicus. The edge is firm, smooth and tender on palpation. Tender enlargement of the liver is an early sign of congestive heart failure, often preceding peripheral edema.

Hepatic Pulsation. A rise in pressure in the right auricle is transmitted readily not only to the neck veins but also to the inferior vena cava and the hepatic veins. This transmission of pressure from the right auricle to the hepatic veins is particularly conspicuous in tricuspid valve incompetence when pressure tracings taken from the hepatic veins show a contour similar to those obtained from the right auricle. In both the normal interval between the "c" and the "v" waves of the phlebogram is obliterated. Correct timing of the pulsation is important, and if necessary hepatic pulse tracings are recorded. These are compared with those from the jugular vein and with simultaneous phonocardiograms.[11] These procedures may be especially valuable if surgery of the tricuspid valve is contemplated. Terry described coupled hepatic pulsation in tricuspid incompetence.[71] This can be distinguished from extrasystoles in which the pulse is felt over the liver but never reaches the peripheral artery.

The pulsation is palpable and occurs during ventricular systole. Its expansile nature may be felt bimanually with one hand over the liver in the right upper quadrant of the abdomen and the other over the right lower ribs posteriorly. This expansibility distinguishes it from the palpable epigastric pulsation due to the aorta or to a hypertrophied right ventricle. Highly vascular tumors sometimes cause the liver to pulsate, but they are very rare. If a cardiac cirrhosis develops, the pulsation is lost.

Hepatojugular Reflux. In heart failure, if pressure is applied over the liver in the epi-

gastrium, the large veins of the neck are seen to fill. The hepatic compression increases the venous return and intensifies the distention in the neck veins due to the inability of the failing right heart to handle the increased blood flow. Increased tone in the jugular veins in heart failure may augment this effect.[15] Therefore, the reflux is seen particularly well in heart failure. It is of value: (1) to better identify the upper levels of venous pulsation in the neck; (2) to establish the patency of venous channels between the hepatic and jugular veins. Therefore, reflux is negative in Budd-Chiari's disease (hepatic venous occlusion) or with blockage of the main mediastinal or jugular veins.

Spleen. The spleen may be enlarged and palpable. This may have various explanations and does not necessarily indicate cardiac cirrhosis.

Ascites. The ascites of heart failure may be related to three factors: rise in hepatic venous pressure; change in the plasma protein concentration; sodium retention.

Rise in Venous Pressure. In animals, experimental obstruction to the venous return from the liver is a common way of producing ascites. The rise in the hepatic venous pressure in congestive heart failure is probably of similar importance. The "hepatic venous outflow block" is analogous to that found in all forms of cirrhosis and is believed to be of importance in the genesis of ascites.

Plasma Protein Changes. The plasma proteins tend to be lowered in congestive heart failure due to malnutrition, to the patient's being on a restricted diet and having no appetite, to liver cell destruction with impaired protein synthesis, and to loss of protein into edema and ascites.

Sodium Retention. In congestive heart failure excretion of sodium is difficult, for sodium is retained in the tissues and holds water with it. Although this may not initiate the fluid retention of heart failure, it is probably of importance in its perpetuation.

Therefore, the patient who develops ascites has a particularly high venous pressure, a low cardiac output and associated, severe, centrizonal liver cell damage. This description can be applied to mitral stenosis with tricuspid incompetence and constrictive pericarditis, and it is with these two conditions that ascites is closely associated. Occasionally, ascites is out of all proportion to the edema and to the other symptoms of congestive heart failure.

Impending Hepatic Coma. Confusion, lethargy and coma occasionally accompany heart failure and are usually related to cerebral anoxia. Occasionally, the whole picture of impending hepatic coma is seen. This may follow severe, acute, centrizonal hepatic necrosis, for instance after myocardial infarction, or in patients with chronic congestive failure given ammonium chloride[72]; and increased arterial ammonium level has been noted in heart failure.[5]

PROGNOSIS AND TREATMENT

The prognosis of the liver changes in heart failure is that of the heart disease which caused them. Cardiac jaundice, particularly if deep, is always a bad omen un-less associated with a sudden, frank pulmonary infarct.

Cardiac cirrhosis *per se* does not carry a bad prognosis, and if the heart failure responds to treatment, the cirrhosis can be expected to become latent.

Treatment is that of the heart failure. Diet should be adequate in protein, and it must be remembered that the salt-free diet used for the treatment of congestive heart failure may be inadequate in other respects and may need supplementing.

LIVER FUNCTION TESTS
(TABLE 23–2)

Serum Bilirubin Concentration. The serum bilirubin is raised with congestive heart failure, but very high values are unusual.

The level of the serum bilirubin corresponds closely to the degree of clinical heart failure. It has been suggested that when cardiac compensation is attained and the

TABLE 23–2. BIOCHEMICAL RESULTS IN 50 PATIENTS WITH HEART FAILURE

EXTENT OF HEPATIC NECROSIS	SERUM BILIRUBIN MG./100 ML.		SERUM ALK. PHOSPHATASE UNITS/100 ML.		SERUM ALBUMIN GM./100 ML.		SERUM GLOBULIN GM./100 ML.		BROMSULPHALEIN PERCENTAGE RETENTION AT 30 MINUTES	
	No. of Cases	Mean	No. of Cases	Mean	No. of Cases	Mean	No. of Cases	Mean	No. of Cases	Mean
Normal	—	(0.5–1)	—	(4–13)	—	(3.4–5.0)	—	(1.5–3.0)	—	(0–10)
Grade 1	18	1.1 0.24* (0.5–4.7) †	17	9.3 1.07 (6.0–25.0)	16	4.1 0.10 (3.4–4.7)	16	2.5 0.15 (1.4–3.6)	6	11.3 (2–30)
Grade 2	15	2.0 0.33 (0.5–5.0)	15	10.3 1.21 (6.0–20.0)	15	3.5 0.18 (2.2–4.7)	15	2.9 0.17 (1.4–4.2)	7	18.0 (1–48)
Grade 3	17	3.3 0.13 (0.9–7.4)	13	12.3 1.03 (4.7–26.0)	12	3.5 0.21 (2.4–5.1)	12	2.9 0.13 (1.6–3.7)	8	24.6 (7–53)
Total	50	2.1 0.19 (0.5–7.4)	45	10.5 0.73 (4.7–26.0)	43	3.7 0.11 (2.2–5.1)	43	2.8 0.12 (1.4–4.2)	21	19.0 2.53 (1–53)

* = standard error of mean.   † = range.
(Sherlock, S.: The liver in heart failure; relation of anatomical, functional and circulatory changes, Brit. Heart J. *13*:273)

total serum bilirubin remains raised, permanent hepatic damage is present.[63] However, the serum bilirubin may be normal in the presence of cardiac cirrhosis if this is compensated.

Bromsulphalein Test. This is the most sensitive method of detecting hepatic involvement in congestive heart failure.[4, 25] Results parallel both the clinical severity of failure[18] and the hepatic cell necrosis as shown by biopsy.[67] The lowered hepatic blood flow in heart failure may contribute to the abnormal Bromsulphalein test.[7]

If the Bromsulphalein test remains ab-

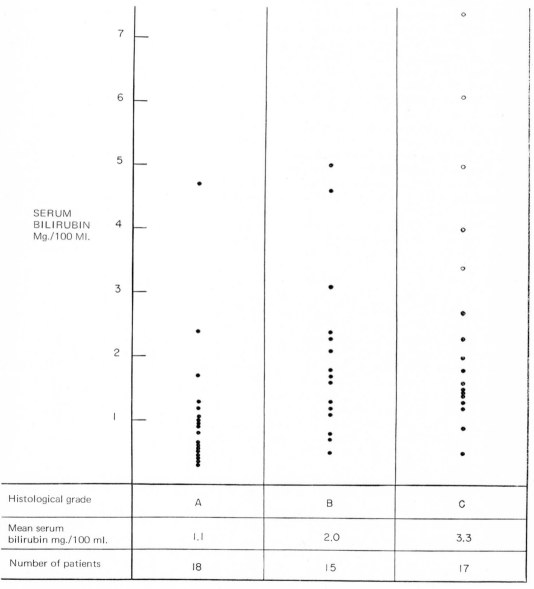

Histological grade	A	B	C
Mean serum bilirubin mg./100 ml.	1.1	2.0	3.3
Number of patients	18	15	17

Fig. 23–8. Relationship of extent of hepatic necrosis to serum bilirubin concentration. (Sherlock, S.: Brit. Heart J. *13*:273.)

normal after clinical recovery from the heart failure, there may be cardiac cirrhosis.[18]

The *serum alkaline phosphatase* concentration is usually normal.

The *serum total cholesterol* level is usually normal. If the failure is of rheumatic etiology, it may be depressed, perhaps because the illness has been of long duration and is associated with much malnutrition.[51]

Serum Protein Levels. Although the mean values for total serum protein, serum albumin and serum globulin may be normal, there is much variation in the individual patient. In one series of 43 patients with congestive heart failure, 12 had a serum albumin value less than the normal lower limit of 3.4 Gm./100 ml., and 18 patients had a serum globulin level above the upper normal limit of 3 Gm./100 ml. In another series, 29 per cent of patients had a depressed serum albumin. Low serum albumin values occur in severe hepatic necrosis and must be due in part to defective hepatic synthesis of protein. They also occur in the patients with the most edema in whom protein, particularly albumin, is lost into edema fluid. With recovery from the heart failure plasma proteins return to normal.

Serum Transaminase Values. A rise in serum glutamic oxaloacetic transaminase and to a lesser extent in serum glutamic pyruvic transaminase occurs in heart failure irrespective of pulmonary or myocardial infarction.[2] It is higher in acute than chronic failure[57] and is proportional to the degree of shock and the extent of centrizonal necrosis.[57] In a patient with myocardial infarction SGOT levels rise higher, and values over 400 units suggest that hepatic congestion is also present.[69] Serum transaminases may increase in patients with congestive heart failure given phenindione or other coumarol anticoagulants.[68, 77]

Summary. Abnormal hepatic function tests in patients with congestive heart failure are an index of the centrizonal hepatic necrosis and atrophy of liver cells.

CARDIAC JAUNDICE

Incidence. Although overt jaundice is rare, biochemical jaundice, as evidenced by a raised serum bilirubin concentration, is a common finding in congestive heart failure.[29, 36, 59] In one series of 50 patients in congestive heart failure, 34 had serum bilirubin levels greater than 1 mg./100 ml., and in 16 of these the value exceeded 2 mg./100 ml. Moreover, in 8 of the subjects jaundice was deep with a serum bilirubin greater than 4.5 mg./100 ml. The three highest values were 18.0, 21.5 and 22.0 mg./100 ml. and compare with the levels found in mechanical obstruction of the common bile duct. Heart disease with or without congestive failure was the commonest association in a large series of patients with unconjugated hyperbilirubinemia but without evidence of hemolysis.[38]

Jaundice and the Cause of the Heart Failure. Mild degrees of jaundice may occur with all the common varieties of heart failure—valvular, hypertensive, ischemic or pulmonary. Deeper icterus has a closer association with valvular heart disease and in particular with mitral stenosis, especially if there is an associated tricuspid valve incompetence. The incidence increases with prolonged congestive heart failure, and repeated bouts also contribute to the incidence.

Etiology. *Hepatogenous Jaundice.* This implies that in heart failure the liver cells are inadequate to excrete all the bile pigment. The impaired liver function tests are in keeping with this concept, and in general the greater the extent of liver cell necrosis the deeper the icterus (Fig. 23–8). However, there are many exceptions to this rule, and in particular the occurrence of tricuspid incompetence with severe liver damage but without clinical icterus. Liver cell damage cannot entirely explain cardiac jaundice.

Cholestatic Mechanical Jaundice. Eppinger believed that cardiac jaundice was due to obstruction of bile capillaries, both by pressure on the outside by distended veins and by inspissated bile thrombi within.[17] The obstruction may be related to the height of the venous pressure within the hepatic lobule. The normal biliary secretory pressure is 20 to 30 cm. water.[41] Many patients with heart failure have right auricular pressures of 20 cm. water. The hepatic venous pressure has been shown to be higher than this and may be greater than the pressure at which bile can be secreted.[18, 50] A mechanical obstruction to the intralobular bile canaliculi might exist. Moreover, patients with deep jaundice often have very high right auricular pressures, and a statistical correlation may be established between the depth of jaundice and the venous filling pressure of the right heart.[67] The usually close association of tricuspid valve incompetence (with presumably high hepatic venous pressures) and deep jaundice has been noted. In dogs, reduction of hepatic blood flow with an increase in hepatic venous pressure produced a fall in bile flow.[54] Hepatic oxygen uptake and relative storage capacity of Bromsulphalein remained unchanged. The biliary excretory blockade was postulated due to encroachment of engorged blood vessels in biliary channels. A similar mechanism might be important in congestive heart failure.

Inspissation of bile in the minute canaliculi to form "bile thrombi" is commonly evidence of biliary obstruction. Bile thrombi are conspicuous in the liver in deep cardiac jaundice but are seen in every condition where jaundice is deep, and particularly when the bile is viscid, as in hemolytic crises. Therefore, their presence is not necessarily indicative of biliary obstruction.

Other evidence against the hepatic venous-obstructive theory of cardiac jaundice may be given. The relationship between high venous pressure and jaundice is not constant, and some patients with tricuspid incompetence and very high hepatic venous pressures are not jaundiced. At autopsy the gallbladder and the bile passages, in even those most deeply jaundiced, are full of dark bile, and with rare exceptions the feces are darker than normal and not suggestive of cholestasis. Further, the biochemical data are unlike those of biliary obstruction. Serum alkaline phosphatase is normal, as are the blood cholates. Urobilinogen is present in excess in the urine. Intrahepatic biliary obstruction related to high venous pressure is therefore unlikely to be an important cause of cardiac jaundice.

It is doubtful whether bile thrombi alone can ever result in clinical jaundice, for they never are present in sufficient amounts so that significant numbers of bile channels are blocked.

Hemolytic Jaundice. The icterus of heart failure is often related to hemorrhages into the tissue, particularly pulmonary infarctions. The sudden appearance of jaundice following the clinical features of an infarct, whether pulmonary, splenic or renal, in a patient with congestive heart failure is well recognized.[28] Similar infarcts in patients without heart failure do not result in jaundice.[36] It is postulated that the excess of bilirubin produced in the infarcted tissues cannot be excreted by a liver damaged by heart failure; therefore, jaundice results.

Many points favor this hypothesis. Excess iron pigment present in the tissues in heart failure; and congestion, particularly in the lungs, may be even more important than frank infarction. Even without frank infarcts the pulmonary alveoli usually contain "heart failure" cells. These macrophages show iron pigment, presumably derived from red blood corpuscles. Bilirubin also must have been formed, constituting an additional excretory load on the liver. Although there are exceptions, patients with pulmonary infarction show a higher serum bilirubin level than those without (Table 23–3). In one reported series of 424 autopsies on patients who had heart failure, jaundice was noted in 4 per cent of the whole series, but in 10.5 per cent of those with infarcts.[36] In some patients jaundice develops after infarction, although the right auricular pressure and the cardiac output are not changed, and liver biopsy shows only minimal histologic changes. In these patients jaundice can be associated only with infarction. Patients with minimal liver cell damage in heart failure who become jaundiced usually have clear evidence of pulmonary infarcts.[67] Biochemical results support a hemolytic etiology. The stools are dark,[19] the urine contains excess urobilin, and serum biochemical findings are compatible.

At the same time, pigment overload cannot be the only cause of cardiac jaundice. Rich and Resnik introduced into the tissues of patients with heart failure a volume of blood equal to that found in pulmonary infarctions and failed to increase the serum

TABLE 23–3. THE RELATION OF SERUM BILIRUBIN CONCENTRATION AND
PULMONARY INFARCTION

		HISTOLOGY OF LIVER GRADE						TYPE OF HEART FAILURE (NO. OF CASES)				
		1		2		3						
No. OF PA-TIENTS	MEAN SERUM BILI-RUBIN	No.	Serum bili-rubin (mean)	No.	Serum bili-rubin (mean)	No.	Serum bili-rubin (mean)	Mitral val-vular	Aor-tic val-vular	Cor pul-mo-nale	Hy-per-ten-sive	Ische-mic
Without pulmonary infarction												
28	1.4	11	0.9	10	1.6	7	2.1	7	2	11	4	4
With pulmonary infarction												
14	3.2	3	2.6	4	3.1	7	3.5	9	2	1	2	0

(Sherlock, S.: The liver in heart failure; relation of anatomical, functional and circulatory changes, Brit. Heart J. *13*:273)

bilirubin level.[56] Although bilirubinuria is not found in hemolytic icterus, it is often found in cardiac jaundice, and occasionally the stools are pale. Finally, jaundice may occur without pulmonary infarction and may be particularly conspicuous in association with tricuspid incompetence in which pulmonary vascular congestion is minimal.

Summary. Cardiac jaundice is very complex. Support can be found for hepatocellular, cholestatic and hemolytic theories. In most patients multiple factors are present, the most important being hepatocellular anoxia and increased pigment overload of the liver cells, resulting from the liberation of blood into the tissues.

THE LIVER IN CONSTRICTIVE PERICARDITIS

Hepatic changes are particularly severe but are essentially similar to those described in right-sided heart failure.

Macroscopically, if the constriction has been prolonged there is usually a cardiac cirrhosis. The capsule of the liver is greatly thickened and has been likened to one of sugar icing (*Zuckergussleber*).

Microscopically, the picture is of centrilobular cardiac congestion and necrosis, progressing to a mixed portal and cardiac type of cirrhosis. Portal zone connective tissue and new bile duct formation may be particularly prominent.[34]

Clinical Features. The patient is not jaundiced. The liver is enlarged, and the edge is hard; it does not pulsate. The spleen is usually palpable. Ascites is prominent, and the resultant dyspnea and abdominal swelling may be the main complaints. Peripheral edema may or may not accompany the ascites. The most important factor in the ascites formation is venous obstruction.

There may be considerable difficulty in distinguishing constrictive pericarditis from chronic hepatocellular failure with ascites. In both, the jugular venous pressure in the neck is raised, although it is usually higher with constrictive pericarditis. The diagnosis is made by the paradoxical pulse, the radiologic demonstration of calcium in the pericardium, the characteristic electrocardiogram and cardiac catheterization.

Biochemical Findings. The serum bilirubin level is rarely higher than 2 mg./100 ml., the Bromsulphalein retention test is positive and serum proteins are altered with a level albumin and a high globulin value.

Treatment. Treatment is that of the cardiac condition. If pericardectomy is possible, prognosis as regards the liver is good, although recovery may be slow. Within 6 months of a successful operation, liver function tests improve, and the liver shrinks.[43] The cardiac cirrhosis cannot be expected to resolve completely, but the fibrous bands in the liver become narrower and avascular, and it is doubtful if they can cause clinical symptoms.

If the pericardial lesion is inoperable, treatment is that of any cirrhosis with ascites, namely, dietary sodium restriction and diuretics with salt-free protein supplements.

THE LIVER IN BACTERIAL ENDOCARDITIS

The liver may show focal necrosis of liver cells with surrounding polymorphonuclear infiltration, presumably embolic in nature. Congestive changes may occur if the patient is in heart failure but are unusual, and cardiac cirrhosis is rare.

ANTICOAGULANT THERAPY AND THE LIVER

Anticoagulants such as the coumarins or phenindione cause a reduction in factor VII (proconvertin) and prothrombin and also factor X (Stuart factor) early in therapy and Christmas (PTC) factor later.[23] These factors may be lowered spontaneously in hepatobiliary disease. Patients with hepatic disease or those who develop it while receiving anticoagulant therapy, show a particularly profound depression of the clotting mechanism.[68, 77] This may account for the increased sensitivity to anticoagulants of patients with heart failure when hepatic congestion develops,[31] or if they have an intercurrent acute virus hepatitis.[33]

Phenindione (phenylindanedione) rarely causes a sensitivity type reaction, and 15 cases of jaundice of cholestatic or hepatocellular type have been recorded following its use.[22]

REFERENCES

1. Anderson, M. N., Gabrieli, E., and Zizzi, J. A.: Chronic hemolysis in patients with ball-valve prostheses, J. Thorac. Cardiovasc. Surg. *50*:501, 1965.
2. Bang, N. U., Iversen, K., Jagtt, T., and Tobiassen, G.: Serum glutamic-oxaloacetic transaminase activity as an index of centrilobular liver cell necrosis in cardiac and circulatory failure, Acta med. scand. *164*: 385, 1959.
3. Bauer, W., Dale, H. H., Poulsson, L. T., and Richards, D. W.: The control of circulation through the liver, J. Physiol. *74*: 343, 1932.
4. Bernstein, M., Le Winn, E. B., and Simkins, S. J.: Heart disease and liver function, J. Lab. Clin. Med. *28*:1, 1942.
5. Bessman, A. N., and Evans, J. M.: The blood ammonia in congestive heart failure, Am. Heart J. *50*:715, 1955.
6. Blalock, A., and Mason, M. F.: Observations on blood flow and gaseous metabolism of liver of unanesthetized dogs, Am. J. Physiol. *117*:328, 1936.
7. Blumberg, N., and Schloss, E. M.: The effect of circulatory factors on the Bromsulphalein test in liver disease, Am. J. Med. Sci. *213*:470, 1947.
8. Bolton, C.: The pathological changes in the liver resulting from passive venous congestion experimentally produced, J. Path. Bact. *19*:258, 1914.
9. Bolton, C., and Barnard, W. G.: The pathological occurrences in the liver in experimental venous stagnation, J. Path. Bact. *34*:701, 1931.
10. Bywaters, E. G. L.: Anatomical changes in the liver after trauma, Clin. Sci. *6*:19, 1946.
11. Calleja, H. B., Rosenow, O. F., and Clark, T. E.: Pulsations of the liver in heart disease, Am. J. Med. *30*:202, 1961.
12. Castberg, T.: Vascular changes in chronic passive congestion of the liver, Acta path. microbiol. scand. *30*:358, 1952.
13. Clarke, W. T. W.: Centrilobular hepatic necrosis following cardiac infarction, Am. J. Path. *26*:249, 1950.
14. Davidson, C. S., Lewis, J. H., Tagnon, H. J., Adams, M. A., and Taylor, F. H. L.: Medical shock: abnormal biochemical changes in patients with severe acute medical illnesses, with and without peripheral vascular failure, New Engl. J. Med. *234*: 279, 1946.
15. de Pasquale, N., and Burch, G. E.: The hepatojugular reflux, Arch. Int. Med. *102*: 426, 1958.
16. Ellenberg, M., and Osserman, K. E.: Role of shock in the production of central liver cell necrosis, Am. J. Med. *11*:170, 1951.
17. Eppinger, H.: Die Leberkrankheiten, Vienna, Springer, 1937.
18. Evans, J. M., Zimmerman, H. J., Wilmer, J. G., Thomas, J. L., and Ethridge, C. B.: Altered liver function of chronic

congestive heart failure, Am. J. Med. *13*: 704, 1952.

19. Fishberg, A. M.: Jaundice in myocardial insufficiency, J.A.M.A. *80*:1516, 1923.

20. Haist, R. E., and Hamilton, J. I.: Reversibility of carbohydrate and other changes in rats shocked by a clamping technique, J. Physiol. *102*:471, 1944.

21. Halbersleben, D.: Jaundice with gray stools during congestive heart failure, Medical Papers Dedicated to Henry Asbury Christian, p. 115, Baltimore, Waverly Press, 1936.

22. Hargreaves, T., and Howell, M.: Phenindione jaundice, Brit. Heart J. *27*:932, 1965.

23. Hicks, N. D., and Bonnin, J. A.: The behavior of coagulation factors during anticoagulant therapy with especial reference to the one-stage test as an index of therapy, Brit. J. Haemat. *5*:194, 1959.

24. Holden, W. D., de Palma, R. G., Drucker, W. R., and McKalen, A.: Ultrastructural changes in hemorrhagic shock: electron microscopic study of liver, kidney and striated muscle cells in rats, Ann. Surg. *162*:517, 1965.

25. Jolliffe, N.: Liver function in congestive heart failure, J. Clin. Invest. *8*:419, 1939.

26. Kantrowitz, P. A., Jones, W. A., Greenberger, N. J., and Isselbacher, K. J.: Postoperative hyperbilirubinemia simulating obstructive jaundice, New Engl. J. Med. *276*:591, 1967.

27. Katzin, H. M., Waller, J. V., and Blumgart, H. L.: "Cardiac cirrhosis" of the liver. A clinical and pathological study, Arch. Int. Med. *64*:457, 1939.

28. Keefer, C. S., and Resnik, W. H.: Jaundice following pulmonary infarction in patients with myocardial insufficiency. I. A clinical study, J. Clin. Invest. *2*:375, 1926.

29. Kershner, D., Hooton, T. C., and Feinberg, W. G.: Chemical studies on experimental hepatic congestion in the dog, Arch. Surg. *57*:24, 1948.

30. Kiernan, F.: The anatomy and physiology of the liver, Phil. Trans. Roy. Soc., London *123*:711, 1833.

31. Killip, T., III, and Payne, M. A.: High serum transaminase activity in heart disease, circulatory failure and hepatic necrosis, Circulation *21*:646, 1960.

32. Kingsley, D. P. E.: Hepatic damage following profound hypothermia and extracorporeal circulation in man, Thorax *21*: 91, 1966.

33. Kliesch, W. F., Young, P. C., and Davis, W. D., Jr.: Dangers of prolonged anticoagulant therapy in hepatic disease, J.A.M.A. *172*:223, 1960.

34. Koletsky, S., and Barnebee, J. H.: "Cardiac" or congestive cirrhosis. Pathologic and clinical aspects, Am. J. Med. Sci. *207*: 421, 1944.

35. Kotin, P., and Hall, E. M.: "Cardiac" or congestive cirrhosis of liver, Am. J. Path. *27*:561, 1951.

36. Kugel, M. A., and Lichtman, S. S.: Factors causing clinical jaundice in heart disease, Arch. Int. Med. *52*:16, 1933.

37. Layne, J. A., Schemm, F. R., and Hurst, W. W.: Further comparative studies on ascites in liver and heart disease, Gastroenterology *16*:91, 1950.

38. Levine, R. A., and Klatskin, G.: Unconjugated hyperbilirubinemia in the absence of overt hemolysis, Am. J. Med. *36*:541, 1964.

39. Lockey, E., McIntyre, N., Ross, D. N., Brookes, E., and Sturridge, M. F.: Early jaundice after open-heart surgery, Thorax *22*:165, 1967.

40. Lucké, B.: The pathology of fatal epidemic hepatitis, Am. J. Path. *20*:471, 1944.

41. McMaster, P. D., Broun, G. O., and Rous, P.: Studies on the total bile. III. On the bile changes caused by a pressure obstacle to secretion, and on hydrohepatosis, J. Exp. Med. *37*:685, 1923.

42. McMichael, J.: The oxygen supply of the liver, Quart. J. Exp. Physiol. *27*:73, 1937.

43. McMurray, C. M., Cayer, D., and Cornatzer, W. E.: Chronic adhesive pericarditis due to the rheumatic state, associated with liver damage, serous effusions and pigmentation, Gastroenterology *17*:294, 1951.

44. Maegraith, B. G.: Micro-anatomy of the hepatic vascular system, p. 181, Tr. 10th Liver Injury Conf., New York, Macy, 1951.

45. Maegraith, B. G., Andrews, W. H. H., and Wenyon, C. E. M.: Studies on the liver circulation. I. Active constriction of the hepatic venous tree in anaphylactic shock, Ann. Trop. Med. *43*:225, 1949.

46. Martin, G. H., Bunting, C. H., and Loevenhart, A. S.: The morphological changes in the tissues of the rabbit as a result of reduced oxidations, J. Pharmacol. *8*:112, 1916.

47. Meakins, J.: Distribution of jaundice in circulatory failure, J. Clin. Invest. *4*:135, 1927.

sOK

48. Mundth, E. D., Keller, A. R., and Austen, W. G.: Progressive hepatic and renal failure associated with low cardiac output following open heart surgery, J. Thorac. Cardiovasc. Surg. 53:275, 1967.

49. Myers, J. D., and Hickman, J. B.: An estimation of the hepatic blood flow and splanchnic oxygen consumption in heart failure, J. Clin. Invest. 27:620, 1948.

50. Paton, A., Reynolds, T. B., and Sherlock, S.: Assessment of portal venous hypertension by catheterisation of hepatic vein, Lancet 1:918, 1953.

51. Poindexter, C. A., and Bruger, M.: Cholesterol content of the blood in heart disease, Arch. Int. Med. 61:714, 1938.

52. Popper, H.: Über Drosselvorrichtungen an Lebervenen, Klin. Wschr. 10:2129, 1931.

53. ———: Significance of agonal changes in human liver, Arch. Path. 46:132, 1948.

54. Preisig, R., Another, A. B. C., and Bradley, S. E.: Bile formation during hepatic ischemia in the dog, in preparation, 1968.

55. Reese, A. J. M.: The effect of hypoxia on liver secretion studied by intravital fluorescence microscopy, Brit. J. Exp. Path. 41:527, 1960.

56. Rich, A. R., and Resnik, W. H.: On the mechanism of the jaundice following pulmonary infarction in patients with heart failure, Bull. Johns Hopkins Hosp. 38:75, 1926.

57. Richman, S. M., Delman, A. J., and Grob, D.: Alterations in indices of liver function in congestive heart failure with particular reference to serum enzymes, Am. J. Med. 30:211, 1961.

58. Robinson, J. S., Cole, F. R., Gibson, P., and Simpson, J. A.: Jaundice following cardiopulmonary bypass, Thorax 22:232, 1967.

59. Routier, D., Cottet, J., and Molinghen, P.: Contribution à l'étude des fonctions hépatiques au cours de l'asystolie, Arch. Mal. Appar. dig. 25:801, 1935.

60. Russell, J. A., Long, C. N. H., and Wilhelmi, A. E.: Biochemical studies on shock. IV. Oxygen consumption of liver and kidney tissue from rats in hemorrhagic shock, J. Exp. Med. 79:23, 1944.

61. Safran, A. P., and Schaffner, F.: Chronic passive congestion of the liver in man. Electron microscopic study of cell atrophy and intralobular fibrosis, Am. J. Path. 50: 447, 1967.

62. Sanderson, R. G., Ellison, J. H., Benson, J. A., Jr., and Starr, A.: Jaundice following open-heart surgery, Ann. Surg. 165:217, 1967.

63. Schalm, L., and Hoogenboom, W. A. H.: Blood bilirubin in congestive heart failure, Am. Heart J. 44:571, 1952.

64. Schilling, J. A., McCoord, A. B., Clausen, S. W., Troup, S. B., and McKee, F. W.: Experimental ascites. Studies of electrolyte balance in dogs with partial and complete occlusion of the portal vein and of the vena cava above and below the liver, J. Clin. Invest. 31:702, 1952.

65. Schmid, M., Hefti, M. L., Gattiker, R., Kistler, H. J., and Senning, A.: Benign postoperative intrahepatic cholestasis, New Engl. J. Med. 272:545, 1965.

66. Seneviratne, R. D.: Physiological and pathological responses in the blood vessels of the liver, Quart. J. Exp. Physiol. 35:77, 1949.

67. Sherlock, S.: The liver in heart failure; relation of anatomical, functional and circulatory changes, Brit. Heart J. 13:273, 1951.

68. Sherlock, S., Barber, K. M., Bell, J. L., and Watt, P. J.: Anticoagulants and the liver, in Pickering, G. W. (ed.): Symposium on Anticoagulant Therapy, p. 14, London, Harvey and Blythe, 1961.

69. Shields, L. H., and Shannon, R. E.: Acute hepatic congestion as a factor in elevated serum oxaloacetic transaminase titres above 400 units, Am. J. Med. Sci. 236:438, 1958.

70. Simonds, J. P., and Jergesen, F. H.: Late changes in the liver induced by mechanical obstruction of the hepatic veins, Arch. Path. 20:571, 1935.

71. Terry, R. B.: Coupled hepatic pulsations in tricuspid incompetence (a new physical sign), Am. Heart J. 57:158, 1959.

72. Ticktin, H. E., Fazekas, J. F., and Evans, J. M.: Ammonia intoxication in a patient with congestive heart failure receiving ammonium chloride orally, New Engl. J. Med. 255:905, 1956.

73. Volwiler, W., Grindlay, J. H., and Bollman, J. L.: The relation of portal vein pressure to the formation of ascites—an experimental study, Gastroenterology 14: 40, 1950.

74. Wallach, H. F., and Popper, H.: Central necrosis of the liver, Arch. Path. 49:33, 1950.

75. White, T. J., Wallace, R. B., Gnassi, A. M., Kemp., N. F, Price, H. P., and Leevy, C. M.: Hepatic abnormalities in congestive

heart failure. Needle biopsy studies, Circulation 3:501, 1951.

76. Wilhelmi, A. E., Russell, J. A., Engel, M. G., and Long, C. N. H.: Some aspects of the nitrogen metabolism of liver tissue from rats in hemorrhagic shock, Am. J. Physiol. *144*:674, 1945.

77. Wróblewski, F., and Manso, C.: Effects of certain anticoagulants on serum enzyme activity, J.A.M.A. *167*:2163, 1958.

78. Zimmerman, H. M., and Hillsman, J. A.: Chronic passive congestion of the liver: an experimental study, Arch. Path. 9:1154, 1930.

24

Tumors of the Liver

EDWARD A. GALL, M.D.

Hepatic neoplasms, once considered insusceptible to therapeutic attack, can now be managed medically and surgically. Appreciation of the details of vascular patterns, the availability of innumerable "anticancer" agents, and greatly improved radiographic and surgical technics have served to bring liver tumors from the limbo of the academic into the realm of the pragmatic.[148, 157, 179, 181] Tumors of the liver are now more readily recognized and more readily and effectively treated. Their diagnosis, identity and biologic potential have come to have salient importance in determining methods of management and prognostic outlook.

The need for a clearer distinction clinically between lesions of primary and secondary nature requires no elaboration; examination of vital statistics pertaining to causes of death reveals an obviously impossible recorded frequency of "carcinoma of the liver." However, clinical recognition is not a simple matter, and tumors of the liver often represent unexpected observations at necropsy.[141] In the case of the benign lesion this is attributable to the relatively small size of the tumor or to the slow rate of growth which evokes few or no symptoms. On the other hand, malignant lesions often escape detection by reason of the obscuring manifestations of such underlying disorders as cirrhosis or primary extrahepatic carcinoma. Moreover, the enormous reserve capacity of the liver permits wide replacement with little perceptible interference with function. Obviously, any improvement in clinical recognition would require an increased awareness and anticipation of liver neoplasm, an understanding

of the miscellaneous clinical and laboratory phenomena which may herald these lesions and the development of newer diagnostic methods.[90, 194]

As a basis for discussion the following listing represents a working classification which serves as an outline for the subject matter of this chapter. It has the doubtful advantage of avoiding controversial terminology.

1. Primary epithelial neoplasm
   A. Parenchymal
   B. Ductal
   C. Combined (parenchymal and ductal)
2. Endothelial neoplasm
3. Hematopoietic neoplasm
4. Supporting-tissue neoplasm
5. Teratoid and embryonal neoplasm
6. Miscellaneous and uncertain neoplasm
7. Metastatic neoplasm
8. Pseudoneoplasm (including hamartoma)

PRIMARY EPITHELIAL NEOPLASM

TERMINOLOGY

A distinction between primary and secondary carcinoma of the liver has been recognized for at least a century.[237] Kelsch and Kiener[121] in 1876 delineated a tumor of hepatic-cell origin, but the two types of derivation—parenchymal and ductal—were not recognized until 1911, by Yamagiwa.[246] The term "hepatoma" was proposed initially by Monier-Vinard in 1910.[156] It was intended to designate a benign tumor of hepatic-cell origin in contradistinction to the then nondescript "adenoma" and multi-nodular hyperplasia.[209] In due course, the term "cholangioma" was introduced to represent the tumor arising from biliary ductal epithelium, thus distinguishing it from the parenchymal-cell lesion.[87] In 1888 Hanot and Gilbert devised a descriptive gross classification (massive, nodular and diffuse) which continues to have wide usage.[28, 60, 98]

INCIDENCE

Primary liver carcinoma has an infrequent, but seemingly growing, incidence. It is said to appear in 1 in 400 (0.25%) autopsy examinations with a recorded incidence range of 0.02 to 1.05 per cent.[24, 91, 96, 110, 134, 136, 195, 212, 241, 243] The latter figure (1:100) reflects a greater frequency in certain portions of Africa and the Orient (0.74 to 1.05%).[24, 91, 96] It is claimed that the rate is considerably higher in the colored races, but this apparently holds only in their native habitat. The Negro in Africa suffers a much higher incidence of liver cancer than the American Negro, whose rate parallels that of the Caucasian in the same area.[55, 104, 165, 243] In certain portions of Africa the incidence is 10 to 15 times that in the United States.[228]

In the selected population of individuals with malignant neoplasm, cancer of the liver comprises 1.5 per cent of the tumors encountered.[24, 44, 168, 212, 241, 243] Among patients with cirrhosis of the liver, a condition considered to be an important precursor of liver neoplasm, the rate of incidence in fatal cases is 1:25 (3.5 to 4.5%).[25, 96, 206] It is said to occur with at least twice this frequency in hemochromatosis[25, 195, 206, 241] although this experience has not been universal.[81]

Those who have considered primary hepatic cancer to be on the increase have attributed this to a heightened incidence of cirrhosis. A rising frequency of cirrhosis in the United States has been attributed to the repeal of Prohibition[61, 141, 143]; elsewhere, dietary deficiency and epidemics of hepatitis have been considered as contributory circumstances. A close, even cause and effect, relationship with viral hepatitis has been suggested.[122, 207]

Carcinoma of the liver is of more frequent occurrence in males.[91, 110, 241] The ratio is said to be 6:1 in hepatoma[134] and 2:1 in cholangioma.[91] As Gustafson has indicated, these ratios require adjustment in view of the disproportionately higher number of autopsies carried out in males.[96] This has proved to be a salient point in interpreting rates reported from Africa where women are rarely examined at necropsy.[55] It is his contention that the preponderance of men with hepatoma is more properly 2:1, and that with cholangioma the incidence is actually greater in women. In the Cincinnati General Hospital, where the usual male-female postmortem rate obtains, the corrected incidence of cholangioma is 1:1; with hepatoma, males predominate 4:1.[81]

Onset is usually in the 6th decade, the average age given being 55 years.[134] In our own series of 76 cases the average age was 63 years, with negligible difference between the two major types. However, it is claimed by some that cholangioma appears at a somewhat older age.[71] Despite a prevalence in middle and old age, many recorded cases are in children, infants and even the newborn.[54, 59, 123, 163, 171, 173, 208, 217] Hepatoma has been recorded in siblings.[117]

In Africa and Java hepatoma is a disease of youth and appears as one of the most common neoplasms among young men.[55, 104, 164]

ETIOLOGY

The essential cause of hepatic neoplasm is not known. Many possible precipitating causes have been suggested, but the most common underlying state is that resulting from tissue injury, necrosis and repair. This is certainly the case with hepatoma, in which cirrhosis so often precedes the inception of neoplasm.[40, 51] Such factors as the reactivation of growth potential in congenital rests[187] and the disturbance of growth characteristics as the result of anomalies of vascular supply[225] are proposed repeatedly but probably have little importance. The contributory influence attributed to parasitic disease,[24, 26, 100, 108, 110, 175] syphilis,[96, 197] nutritional deficiency,[241] alcoholism and hepatotoxic substances,[24, 96, 166, 241] all of which are included also among the causes of cirrhosis, lend some credence to the concept that many neoplasms of this variety reflect cytologic aberration supervening upon repair and regeneration. In the Cincinnati General Hospital series, evaluation of the types of cirrhosis accompanying liver cancer indicates that the postnecrotic and posthepatitic varieties predominate.[81] There appears to be no relationship between Laennec or alcoholic cirrhosis and liver neoplasm unless an end-stage postnecrotic scarring has supervened.[159]

Some 75 per cent of cases of hepatoma appear in association with pre-existing cirrhosis.[25, 71, 243] The range given in the literature is 39 to 87 per cent.[134, 243] Nor does the fact that the bulk of the liver appeared to be normal necessarily indicate that a given hepatoma arose *de novo* in a completely normal nidus.[18, 42, 56, 129] In our own material there were 27 cases in which hepatoma was unaccompanied by cirrhosis, but in at least 4 of these the tumor appeared to arise in a sharply localized area of scarring, simulating postnecrotic cirrhosis. Diffuse cirrhosis need not be the only stigma of prior cellular damage in the liver. In recent years a growing number of hepatic tumors have been encountered in otherwise unscarred livers; this has been particularly the case in childhood.[112, 211]

COINCIDENTAL DISEASE

The coincidence of cirrhosis with cholangioma is considerably less and generally is given as 50 per cent, with a reported range of 18 to 57 per cent.[78, 110, 134, 241] An uncritical assumption that the type of cirrhosis here is similar to that observed in hepatoma and thus precedes the neoplasm has led to a misconception of cause-and-effect relationship.

In 9 of our 20 cases with cholangioma, cirrhosis was also present.[81] However, in 7 of these the cirrhosis proved to be of biliary (obstructive) type and did not antecede the tumor but followed as a direct result of the obstruction produced by it. Hence, in this particular series, although tumor and cirrhosis co-existed in 45 per cent, the cirrhosis appeared to antedate the neoplasm in only

2 instances (actually, in 10 per cent of the 20 cases in the group).

On the other hand, there is indeed a background of obstruction or chronic bile duct inflammatory disease with some degree of frequency in cases of cholangioma.[71, 197, 246] The potentiality of this mechanism has support in the experiments of Stewart, Cantarow and Morgan, who observed the appearance of intraductal tumor-like overgrowth following the ligation of single, major bile ducts in the cat.[220] Clinical experience has provided a parallel to this in the significant number of cases in which extrahepatic bile duct carcinoma has been noted in individuals with long-standing biliary tract disease (calculus, stricture[197] and hepatic duct parasites[108]). In point also is the high degree of coincidence of gallbladder carcinoma and cholelithiasis. The mucosal epithelium of the bile ducts, both intrahepatic and extrahepatic, and of the gallbladder is histologically indistinguishable.

A large body of literature is devoted to the induction of hepatic tumors in experimental animals. Spontaneous hepatomas have been observed in the cat, the dog and the frog.[158, 243] They occur but are said to be rare in cattle and sheep.[73] Older mice and rats develop them not infrequently.[36, 90] It has been the latter animals in which experimental methods have resulted in a striking yield. Here, even more than in the human subject, cell injury and regeneration appear to provide the basis for abnormal growth release. Cytologic alterations in livers so treated have been considered by some to presage the development of neoplasm.[229] Although dietary deficiency alone may be effective, the incidence of liver carcinoma following the use of a variety of hepatotoxic substances is of very high order indeed. Among the toxic agents used are *p*-dimethylaminoazobenzene (butter yellow),[64, 166, 240, 241] *o*-aminoazotoluene (a scarlet-red derivative),[8, 9, 245, 248] 2-amino-5-azotoluene (another aniline dye)[66] and carbon tetrachloride.[62, 63] Some of the rat tumors produced in this fashion have proved to be transplantable, but this has not been accomplished with their human counterparts.

Investigation of deaths in domestic poul-

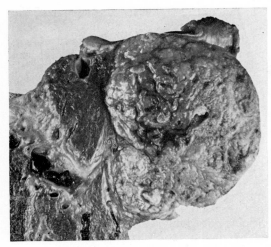

Fig. 24–1. Hepatoma, massive form. The entire left lobe of a cirrhotic liver has been replaced by a single neoplasm.

try has brought to light the existence of a hepatotoxic contaminant in the food utilized (groundnut meal). Identified as a product of *Aspergillus flavus*, extracts of this fungus have proved to be not only injurious to the liver parenchyma, but carcinogenic as well. [39, 57, 135, 138] Substances of this nature, designated aflatoxins, have world wide distribution and are in course of intensive investigation since they represent one of many toxic food sources in the diet staples of domesticated animals and man as well.

Gross Pathology

Parenchymal Neoplasm (Hepatoma). It has become customary to subclassify this tumor into the gross categories proposed by Hanot and Gilbert.[96, 98] Such a division does not imply any biologic distinction, and there is much overlapping in actual fact.

A *massive* form is characterized by a single large tumor with smaller nodules often distributed at its periphery (Fig. 24–1). The lesion may attain such proportions as to replace much or all of a major lobe and displace adjacent structures (stomach, kidney, spleen, diaphragm).

A *nodular* form is manifested by multiple discrete nodules, one or more of which are larger than the remainder but never reach the bulk attained in the massive type (Fig.

24–2). The lesser nodules may appear in satellite fashion or they may be distributed widely throughout the liver. The arrangement has given rise to debate as to whether or not this was the result of intrahepatic dissemination from a single source or a manifestation of multiple sites of origin.

The third manner of growth, a *diffuse* form, exhibits no discrete tumor formation (Fig. 24–3). There is wide and noncircumscribed extension throughout the liver with replacement of much of the parenchyma. The process has been referred to as "carcinomatous cirrhosis," a term considered unsuitable, since the prerequisites to cirrhosis do not obtain.[65] However, there are examples of diffusely distributed intrahepatic neoplasm in which the clinical features of biliary cirrhosis are mimicked.[41] This nomenclature should be utilized simply as a convenient means of description; there is no connotation of specificity of action.

The size attained by these tumors is a reflection of the reserve capacity of the liver and the malleability of contiguous viscera. Accordingly, early recognition is rare, and large tumors are the rule.[61, 92, 142] A dearth of stroma is a characteristic of hepatoma; hence, this tumor is considerably softer than other forms of carcinoma. Bile formation is a common feature, but it is rarely of a degree to impart a characteristic hue to the neoplasm. Color, though nondescript, is usually tan. A rich vascular component may result in a relatively soft, occasionally pulsatile, purplish red mass which has been mistaken for a hemangioma.[50, 86] Seepage of blood and even massive intraperitoneal hemorrhage occur with a fair degree of frequency.[30, 176, 204] Contiguity with the peritoneal surface may result in a friction rub.[79]

Venous intrusion is a prominent feature in hepatoma; either the portal or the hepatic vein may contain tumor thrombus.[71] This phenomenon serves as the basis for intrahepatic metastasis.[136] It may lead also to progression into the vena cava[93] or into the main trunk of the portal vein or its tributaries (Fig. 24–4). As with renal-cell carcinoma, caval propagation of hepatoma may proceed into the right atrial cavity[71] or result in pulmonary embolization.[221] Spontaneous non-neoplastic portal vein

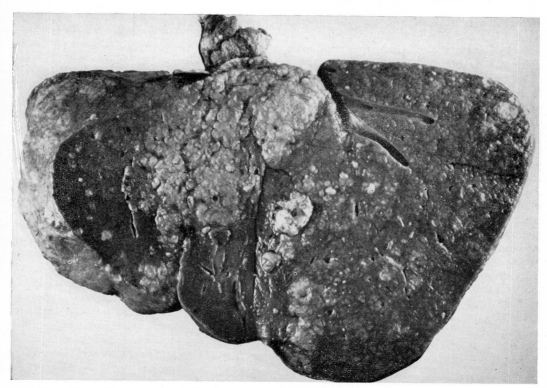

FIG. 24–2. Hepatoma, nodular form. A major mass abuts upon the upper border of a cirrhotic liver. Clusters of smaller nodules are distributed throughout the remainder of the organ. The tongue of neoplasm projecting above represents an extension into the vena cava via the hepatic vein.

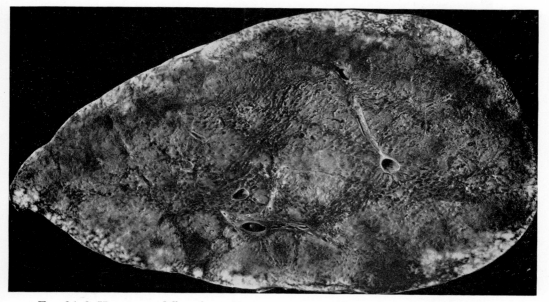

FIG. 24–3. Hepatoma, diffuse form. Transverse section of the liver, exhibiting diffuse neoplastic replacement of the parenchyma. Circumscribed nodulation is not apparent.

thrombosis is also an important complication.[241] This may result from venous stasis due to concomitant cirrhosis, neoplastic obtrusion or both. With these possibilities in mind, the sudden exacerbation of symptoms related to portal hypertension[71] or the appearance of evidence of inferior caval obstruction[241] should occasion prompt suspicion of hepatoma in the case of the patient with cirrhosis. Exceptionally, direct growth into the common bile duct has been recorded.[60]

Ductal Neoplasm (Cholangioma). The cholangioma lacks a characteristic gross appearance; on occasion, located in the hilar region, it fans out widely into the hepatic substance.[5, 6, 124, 204] It frequently appears as a single large, rather homogeneous, grayish-yellow mass which simulates metastatic carcinoma. Umbilication is seldom present, and a heavy stromal component gives it a more scirrhous quality than hepatoma. A variant of cholangioma believed to be of cholangiolar derivation has a diffusely distributed pattern.[137, 219] Seed-

ling metastases often occur throughout the liver, but the primary tumor is dominant.

The surrounding liver is smooth and noncirrhotic but may be deeply stained with bile, a feature contrasting with the tumor itself, which is not pigmented. Bile stasis of this order occurs only when the tumor, by reason of its location, obstructs major ducts. Said to constitute a special category in this location,[60] a number of these have had unusually prolonged courses; so long, indeed, that they have been mistaken clinically for non-neoplastic "sclerosing cholangitis."[5, 6, 124] Venous obstruction is not common, and portal thrombosis, when it does appear, is usually a result of secondary cholangitis and not tumor thrombosis. This form of tumor is not highly vascularized, and hemorrhage from it is not a common event.

Combined Form (Hepatocholangioma). This lesion resembles hepatoma in its gross characteristics and has no peculiar features which permit ready distinction.[3] It is probable that it is closely related to tumors of parenchymal origin and may well be a vari-

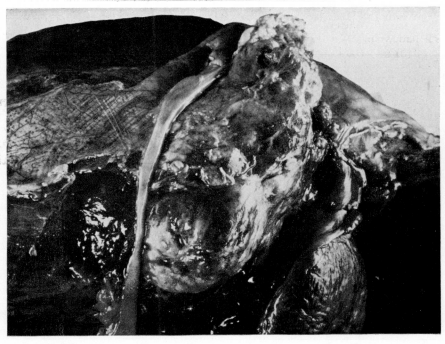

Fig. 24–4. Hepatoma. Tumor thrombus projecting into the inferior vena cava as a polypoid mass emerging from the hepatic vein.

ant of that group.[71] Certainly in the mechanism of action it resembles hepatoma more closely than it does primary duct cell tumor.

MICROSCOPIC PATHOLOGY

Hepatoma. The hepatoma exhibits a considerable range of cytologic structure and functional capacity. In larger tumors the histologic pattern often varies markedly from one portion to another. In the differentiated neoplasm, function is manifested by the secretion of bile.[110] Droplets appear within tumor cells, between them or within acini (Fig. 24–5). Though not manifested uniformly in all hepatomas, bile formation is of diagnostic aid when demonstrable.[136] Distinction of this pigment from hemosiderin, which may be abundant in hemorrhagic foci, usually is made with ease, although it may be necessary to have recourse to iron stains. It is of interest that hepatomas occurring in cases of hemochromatosis rarely contain significant amounts of the iron pigment so abundant elsewhere in the liver.[241] An exception to this is the case reported by Binford and co-workers. [29, 206]

Glycogen is also disproportionately scanty in hepatoma cells, although present in large

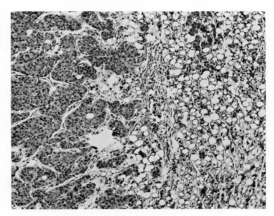

FIG. 24–6. Hepatoma. Alveolar pattern in which contrast between the neoplastic cells devoid of lipid and the markedly vacuolated surrounding parenchyma is well shown. × 80.

amounts in the parenchyma.[139] Here, too, exceptions occur, and the clarity of cytoplasmic staining under such circumstances may permit simulation of new growths of renal or adrenal origin. This may well be an explanation for the disputed primary intrahepatic hypernephroma. Glycogen deposition, as noted above, may be of such order as to deprive the affected individual of circulating glucose and to provoke manifestations of hypoglycemia.[7, 109, 125, 149, 231] Vacuolization due to intracellular lipid is uncommon in the hepatoma cell, and its sparsity may contrast the neoplasm very sharply with the surrounding fat-filled parenchyma (Fig. 24–6). It is claimed that hepatomas rich in lipid content are characterized by long survival and limited metastatic proclivity.[60]

On occasion it is difficult to distinguish the nodule of hepatoma from the actively regenerating nodule of cirrhosis.[241] When this does occur, contrast with the component elements in adjacent liver substance usually suffices (Fig. 24–7). Bizarre nuclei and cytoplasmic atypism are helpful distinguishing features. The presence of non-neoplastic biliary radicles and of regularly distributed Kupffer cells are important features indicating regenerative rather than neoplastic growth.

The most common growth pattern encountered is of a papillary or trabecular

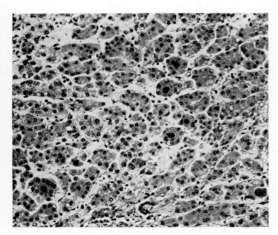

FIG. 24–5. Hepatoma. Photomicrograph demonstrating a papillary and trabecular pattern. The narrow fronds extend among sinusoid-like channels and there is relatively little stromal component. In the center of pseudoacini may be seen small droplets of inspissated bile. × 160.

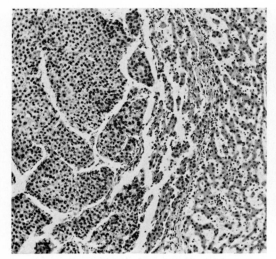

FIG. 24–7. Hepatoma. Solid masses of neoplastic elements do not resemble adjacent parenchymal cells. × 80.

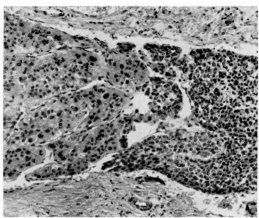

FIG. 24–8. Hepatoma. (*Top*) Undifferentiated form with large syncytial masses and bizarre nuclei to the left and a patternless small-cell component to the right. A resemblance to chorioepithelioma is apparent. × 160. (*Bottom*) Closely packed syncytial hepatoma elements with bizarre multinucleated forms. × 160.

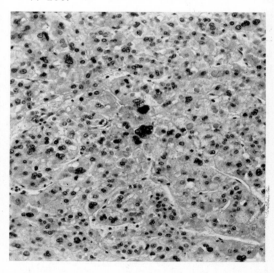

variety (Fig. 24–5). In this form there are cords of large polyhedral oxyphilic cells coursing as narrow fronds one or more cells thick. These are embraced by a delicate layer of flattened endothelium which in turn faces upon a sinusoidal network containing greater or lesser amounts of blood.[110] Stroma is scanty in relation to these channels but may be present as occasional coarse trabeculation, causing lobulation of the tumor. Less frequently encountered is an alveolar structure characterized by thick, rather solid masses of epithelium in some of which frank acini appear[136] (Fig. 24–7). In the instances in which acinus formation predominates, the structure of cholangioma is simulated and may lead to a mistaken classification as hepatocholangioma. Acinar cells are usually polyhedral, but they may be tall and columnar; on occasion they have been observed to be ciliated. Secretion is either bile or a brightly eosinophilic hyaline substance of unknown nature. It does not have the filmy basophilia of the mucoid substance secreted by ductal epithelium. A third variant exhibits little organoid pattern and consists of irregularly arranged large anaplastic cells containing one or more hyperchromatic or vesicular nuclei[136] (Fig. 24–8). The latter have bizarre configuration and may be observed in process of division.

The large pleomorphic cells with multiple nuclei bear some resemblance to abnormal placental trophoblast and probably represent the elements which have comprised so-called primary chorioepithelioma of the liver.

Cholangioma. Usually much more scirrhous than the hepatoma, the epithelium here is embedded in a relatively densely collagenized stroma which is not strikingly

rhagic. Abortive efforts at vessel formation result in poor lumen development and the appearance of solid cords of pleomorphic endothelium, exhibiting nuclear variations and mitotic figures in relative abundance (Fig. 24–11). Resemblance to the more vascular and anaplastic forms of hepatoma is apparent. One should avoid such errors of interpretation.[71, 133]

Tumor elements may line sinusoids and simulate lesions of Kupffer cell origin, a resemblance heightened by phagocytic activity and even extramedullary hematopoiesis. A spindle cell component with heavy hemosiderin pigmentation may suggest primary or metastatic melanoma to the unwary. Occasionally, the entire gamut of variations may appear in a single lesion.

Metastasis can proceed widely by way of the blood stream, but this is not common. Death is more often the result of hemorrhage.

Since most angiomas are small and innocuous, there are no related clinical symptoms.[13] They almost invariably represent incidental observations at exploration or necropsy. In infancy, however, both cutaneous and lymph node angiomatosis may also exist.[59] In the adult this is rarely the case, and no indication of the hepatic lesion may exist unless significant bulk is attained. Symptoms at this time are essentially those of hepatomegaly from any cause, although intra-abdominal hemorrhage is a common complication. Indeed, as in hepatoma, this may be both the initial and the fatal presenting manifestation.[71] A murmur or a venous hum may be audible through the abdominal wall in more extensive lesions, and a thrill may be palpable.[134] However, these are unusual phenomena and are not at all pathognomonic, since they have been encountered with vascular hepatomas and in relation to other masses in this portion of the abdomen.

In young children hepatic angiomas with arteriovenous communication have been known to cause cardiac hypertrophy,[49] cyanosis, cardiac murmurs and heart failure, a pattern easily mistaken for congenital heart disease.[52, 244] Indeed, these signs have been known to subside following roentgen therapy to or extirpation of the lesion.

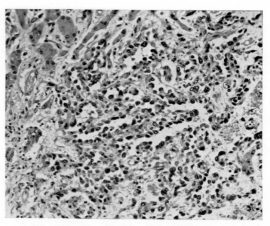

Fig. 24–11. Malignant angioma. Liver diffusely infiltrated by narrow channels resembling capillaries lined by bizarre endothelial cells. × 160. (Armed Forces Institute of Pathology, Accession 607019.)

Calcification in hemorrhagic extravasates may be visible in roentgenograms, but the degree of mineralization is generally very slight. Similarly located opaque deposits occur with tuberculosis, echinococcus disease, hepatolithiasis and subphrenic or liver abscess. A growing number of cases with hepatic neoplasm are being encountered in individuals to whom Thorotrast was administered 12 to 25 years earlier.[144, 223, 230] The livers containing persistently radioactive thorium dioxide are readily visible roentgenographically and are the seat of a curious form of granulomatous cirrhosis[107] and bizarre hematopoiesis.[14] The tumors encountered have been of varied types. Although many have been said to be of vascular nature ("endothelial sarcoma," "hemangioendotheliosarcoma") most of them are composed of phagocytic Kupffer cell-like elements.[161, 224] Similar hepatic neoplasms arise spontaneously in individuals who have not been exposed to Thorotrast.[14, 37]

Angiomas in the liver ordinarily neither require nor benefit from therapy. In the rare instance of a pedunculated lesion of sufficient size to require removal, resection is relatively simple, provided that due regard is given to the prevention of hemorrhage from the liver bed.[119, 202] The large tumors that are inaccessible to surgery are bene-

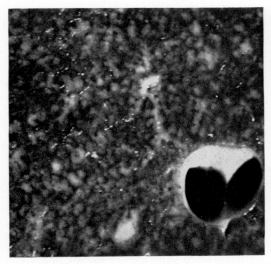
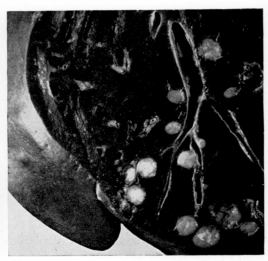

Fig. 24–12. (*Left*) Myeloid leukemia. Close-up view of a sectioned liver, demonstrating prominent though irregular streaking indicative of leukemic infiltration. (*Right*) Hodgkin's disease. Transverse section of the liver exhibiting nodular aggregates in malignant lymphoma.

fited by roentgen therapy in some instances. Ray has reported a large deep-seated cavernous process in which x-ray treatment was remarkably effective.[183]

Prognosis is affected by the extent and more particularly by the histologic nature of the angioma. It is rare, even with the large benign lesions, that serious implications exist, although there is danger that trauma to the liver in the presence of a bulky angioma may result in intractable hemorrhage.[13] On the other hand, the malignant angioma pursues a rapidly fatal course once its presence becomes manifest.[78, 210, 226]

HEMATOPOIETIC NEOPLASM

This group does not properly represent primary hepatic neoplasm. It is essentially indicative of liver involvement as part of systemic disease. Only in the exceptional case is the liver the sole or predominant site of the disease. Infiltration is common in myeloid leukemia but it is seldom seen in the monocytic form. On the other hand, the liver is often the seat of diffuse or nodular lesions in malignant lymphoma with or without lymphatic leukemia, the degree and the nature varying with the type of lymphoma.[82]

The enlarged organ is generally smooth and pallid and exhibits little else to gross inspection. Fine streak-like infiltrations are observed occasionally (Fig. 24–12, *left*) and in rare instances discrete nodules simulating metastatic carcinoma have been noted (Fig. 24–12, *right*). The latter circumstance is encountered more often in Hodgkin's disease and reticulum-cell sarcoma; it is exceptional in other blood dyscrasias.

The microscopic picture is identical with that observed in leukemia and lymphoma elsewhere in the body. There is a monotonous repetition (save in Hodgkin's disease) of whatever cell or pattern of growth characterizes the disease in a given patient. Frequently, portal areas are enlarged uniformly by the cellular infiltrate and this imparts the streaking observed with the unaided eye. Unusual focal growth leads to coarse nodularity. In certain forms, notably in myeloid leukemia, the sinusoids are made unduly prominent by heavy aggregations of leukemic myelocytes.

Smooth enlargement of the liver, frequently accompanied by splenomegaly, with a dragging sensation in the upper abdomen, are the nonspecific features directing clinical attention to this condition. As a rule the clinical syndrome is dominated by the usual systemic manifestations of leukemia. Jaundice is rare in the absence of complicating sepsis, and abnormality of liver function is variable and nonspecific. Despite the absence of symptoms pertinent to hepatic involvement, patients with the malaise attendant upon leukemia have a surprising degree of relief and even euphoria following roentgen therapy to the enlarged liver.

Needle biopsy of the liver is a valuable diagnostic adjunct in the hematopoietic disorders. A correct diagnosis has been established on several occasions in cases in which the peripheral blood picture has been equivocal and conventional marrow puncture has been unsuccessful.[19ᶜ]

SUPPORTING-TISSUE NEOPLASM

This group consists of fibromas, lipomas, leiomyomas and myxomas and their malignant counterparts. They are probably rare, although their incidence cannot be determined with certainty, since they constitute only minor incidental lesions at necropsy and seldom attain proportions which permit clinical recognition. Consequently, unless attended by extraordinary features they do not reach the medical literature. The few which do would seem to indicate a predominance of malignant forms, a situation which is undoubtedly more apparent than real. Shallow and Wagner believed that fewer than 100 cases of sarcoma of the liver had been recorded.[203] Herxheimer referred to 149 cases, but admittedly these were selected uncritically and probably included, among others, cases of lymphoma and metastatic lesions.[103]

Sarcomas of the liver have no special qualities that distinguish them clinically. The incidence in childhood appears to be disproportionately high, but the process is by no means limited to youth.[70, 134, 203, 210] They are prone to be bulky tumors, comparatively soft, hemorrhagic and are often cystic (Fig. 24–13). A translucent viscid quality is noted on sectioning.

The histologic structure is often bizarre

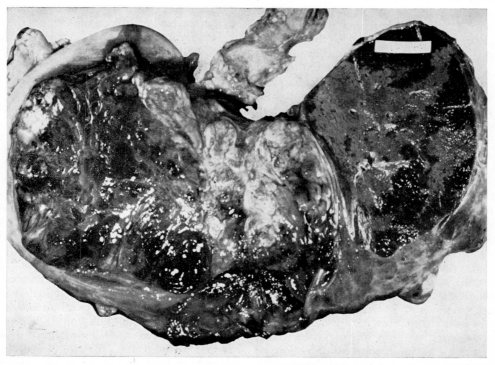

Fig. 24–13. Sarcoma of the liver. Huge sarcoma of the liver in the adult, replacing all of the right lobe. The tumor is cystic and necrotic.

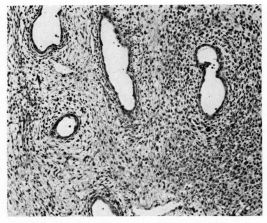

FIG. 24–14. Sarcoma of the liver. The lesion is obviously stromal, although dilated ductal elements may justify a diagnosis of carcinosarcoma (or adenosarcoma). However, the lining epithelium does not appear to be neoplastic. The photograph indicates the marked variation of cellularity observed in these lesions. × 80.

and is unlike that in sarcomas encountered elsewhere in the body.[19] Ewing stated that a pure spindle cell sarcoma with uniform structure had yet to be described in the liver.[71] The nomenclature for these tumors is representative of their unusual structure; i.e., myxosarcoma, rhabdomyosarcoma and alveolar, spindle cell, round cell, giant cell, angioplastic or angioreticular perithelial, syncytial and anaplastic sarcomas.[153, 154, 205, 242] They are often so pleomorphic that it is impossible to classify them definitively. A lesion that appears to be a sparsely nucleated myxoma in one area may have spindle cell or striated myoblast aggregates elsewhere and also may contain islands of bone or cartilage (Fig. 24–14). Epithelial components are encountered, but these may represent the residua of normal ducts included within the neoplasm. This should be distinguished from the mixed epithelial and mesenchymal variant of hepatoblastoma noted previously.[112] Despite evidence of rapid growth, metastasis is unusual.[113] Death occurs as the result of hemorrhage, necrosis, cachexia, secondary infection or widespread infiltration of the abdomen with displacement of vital viscera. A consider-able number succumb postoperatively following unsuccessful efforts at removal.

TERATOID AND EMBRYONAL NEOPLASMS

These exceptional lesions constitute an interesting group with curious morphologic variations. The adult teratoma and dermoid cyst are identical with like lesions encountered more commonly elsewhere.[101, 162] The appearance of islands of bone or cartilage in adenomas or cholangiomas in childhood[60, 84, 201, 243] is an occasional oddity. Some have contended that lesions with this pattern are actually mixed tumors.[208] They are observed infrequently and are somewhat more common in children.[2, 47, 48] In this age group the radiographic demonstration of a fine, irregular, calcific stippling in an enlarged liver may well suggest an embryonal or mixed tumor.[4] Dermoid cysts also have been described in the falciform ligament and the umbilical cord.[101, 201]

Milman and Grayzel found reports of only 27 cases of poorly differentiated mixed or embryonal tumors of the liver.[154] Termed "carcinosarcoma," "mixed embryonal tumor" or "embryonal hepatoma," some of these resemble the embryoma. (Wilms's tumor) of the kidney. They are composed of loose, edematous myxoid stroma, occasionally with islands of poorly developed cartilage or osteoid and isolated strands of primitive striated muscle. Anaplastic epithelium appears to emerge from stromal cells. It remains in an undifferentiated state or, as in the Wilms's tumor, proceeds to the development of bizarre ductal and acinar organoid structures (Fig. 24–15). In a few examples well-differentiated foci of fetal parenchyma appear. In one unusual case there was unilateral overgrowth of the torso and extremities.[4]

It is probable that included among the embryonal mixed tumors are instances of the bizarre sarcomas described in the preceding section. A clear separation is not always possible, although it would seem to be wiser to reserve the designation of embryonal mixed tumor for those with both stromal and epithelial neoplastic components.

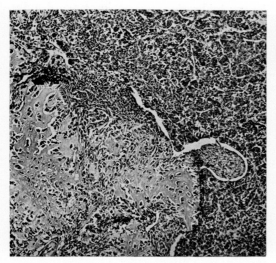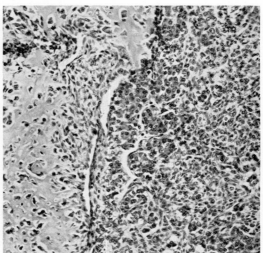

Fig. 24–15. (*Left*) Malignant embryonal tumor. Large island of osteoid surrounded by a highly cellular neoplasm in which epithelium-like clusters appear to emerge from an embryonal stromal background. × 160. (Armed Forces Institute of Pathology, Accession 497787.)

(*Right*) High-power view of the lesion shown in the figure at left. The cellular stromal lesion exhibits abortive duct formation. Note the primitive character of the osteoid. × 160.

Therapy would appear to be fruitless in the malignant lesions; almost all of the recorded cases have been fatal.[154, 247] There is no information available as to radiosensitivity. In view of the encouraging results with roentgen therapy in the Wilms's tumor and its similarity of structure to the embryonal tumor of the liver, this would appear to be an avenue of attack worthy of exploration.[128]

MISCELLANEOUS NEOPLASMS

In this group have been placed several rare neoplasms concerning which there has been controversy. It seems unlikely that such lesions as "hypernephroma," "melanoma" and "chorioepithelioma" have valid claims to hepatic origin.

The normal anatomic contiguity of the right adrenal to the posterior aspect of the liver is well known, and there is some indication that aberrant adrenal substance embedded within the substance of the right lobe is more common than has been recognized.[17, 103, 200] The assumption that this may be a nidus for the origin of intrahepatic adrenal cell neoplasm is reminiscent of the weary controversy relating to the cellular origin of the so-called "hypernephroma" of the kidney. Most of the cases cited have been in the right lobe. There is no doubt that neoplasm arising in an aberrant adrenal focus is a possibility, but with few exceptions[1, 61, 180] the cases cited in the literature are poorly documented and not convincing.[1, 180] Cases with sexual precocity and Cushing's disease have been reported; one patient exhibited ulcerations simulating those of the Zollinger-Ellison syndrome.[111] In many, the possibility of metastasis from an unrecognized extrahepatic source or the direct invasion from a primary neoplasm of the adjacent kidney or adrenal has not been adequately excluded. Hepatomas may be composed of clear cells arranged in trabecular fashion and conceivably may be mistaken for adrenal cortical or renal tubular neoplastic epithelium.

Few of the cases classified as primary melanoma of the liver withstand critical study. The liver is a well-known site of metastasis from melanoma of the skin and the ocular choroid. In each of these areas it is a common experience for an obscure, minute primary tumor to remain unnoticed in the presence of massive visceral dissemination. Excision of lesions of this nature may be followed by an unusually prolonged latent period before systemic distribution becomes manifest. Often physicians are confronted with metastatic melanoma in patients who deny or have forgotten the removal of a cutaneous lesion of innocuous appearance months or years earlier. Adherence to the dictum that a diagnosis of primary melanoma of the liver is permissible only after careful scrutiny of the eye and the skin probably would eliminate all of the cases cited.[103]

Primary hepatic chorioepithelioma seems to be an even less likely entity than melanoma. A curious aberrance of genital epithelium or an origin in a teratoma appear to be necessary prerequisites. Undoubtedly, a significant number of the cases recorded represent anaplastic and syncitial-cell variants of hepatoma which have much cytologic resemblance to chorioepithelioma. Undifferentiated bronchogenic carcinoma or obscure neoplasms of the ovary or the uterus are conceivable sources of hepatic metastases which also may simulate this condition.

METASTATIC NEOPLASM

Hepatic metastasis is anticipated in 35 to 50 per cent of all cases of neoplasm whatever the primary site.[25, 110, 134, 169] Indeed, secondary carcinoma is the most common malignant tumor encountered in the liver. It is estimated that the relative proportion of primary to secondary neoplasm in the liver is 1:20 with a range of 1:13 to 1:65.[25, 113, 243] The usual sites from which metastasis proceeds are the alimentary tract, pancreas, gallbladder, lung, breast, genitourinary system, eye and adrenal.[38] Most of these enter the liver via the vascular system, the portal vein being a favored route. The hepatic artery serves as the avenue of entry in those cases in which pulmonary lesions of either primary or secondary nature exist. Retrograde lymphatic progression is a less common route.

Multiplicity is the rule in secondary neoplasm in the liver, the individual lesions being circumscribed and spherical in nature.

Heavy infiltration and coalescence of adjacent nodules result in an irregular lobulated configuration. Enormous enlargement with weights up to 8,000 Gm. may result from massive seeding. Several investigators have noted cellular and nuclear enlargement and other curious alterations in hepatic parenchymal cells adjacent to and at a distance from the neoplastic nodules.[168, 170] Despite a high degree of parenchymal replacement, detectable jaundice usually is absent or relatively slight.[193, 235] Widely dispersed miliary metastatic carcinoma, stemming in particular from breast, prostate or colon cancers, may be associated with deep jaundice.[60] A somewhat related diffuse form of metastasis insinuates itself within sinusoids and causes hepatic enlargement but with retention of normal external contours and even lobular architecture.[214] This variant, too, is accompanied by severe icterus and, unless a primary site is detected, may be mistaken clinically for cirrhosis with liver failure.[41, 238] Calcification has been described as a feature of metastatic carcinoma in the liver, notably that stemming from intestinal neoplasms.[152]

The distribution of metastasis, at least in its early stage, appears to follow the flow of portal vein currents with predominant right-lobe or left-lobe involvement, depending upon the venous drainage of the viscus containing the primary neoplasm.[16] This predilection is soon lost, however, as the degree of liver infiltration increases.

An enlarged, coarsely nodular liver or one that is relatively smooth but contains several discrete nodules palpable through the abdominal wall should arouse suspicion of metastatic tumor.

The observation that the cirrhotic liver is an infrequent site of metastatic neoplasm[45, 192] has been disputed.[187, 208] There is certainly no lessened incidence of primary extrahepatic carcinoma in the necropsy population with cirrhosis.[81, 192] Nonetheless, a continuing and retrospective survey of well over 1,300 necropsy examples of cirrhosis lends much support to the contention that metastasis is relatively uncommon in this condition.[80] However, this is neither absolute nor indicative of a specific immunity.[192]

The needle biopsy method is unusually

effective in detecting metastatic tumors in the liver. Despite a seemingly blind approach, a number of individuals have demonstrated neoplasm in the liver in 70 to 80 per cent of cases in which it ultimately was proved to be present.[34, 74, 92, 195] This is a particularly noteworthy yield, since the degree of involvement in many was relatively sparse.

Yuhl and co-workers have proposed the use of radioactive albumin as a tracer substance with disproportionately higher predilective localization in hepatic than in extrahepatic metastasis.[249] Other radioactive substances conjugated with rose bengal,[10] Cholografin,[32] and vitamin B_{12}[216] have proved to be useful in mapping the distribution of metastatic tumor in the liver. Used separately or in combination with splenoportography,[160, 196] the detection of intrahepatic neoplasm has reached a high state of accuracy.

Overt derangement of liver function is not ordinarily apparent, although one or more commonly utilized liver function tests exhibit abnormality in the presence of hepatic metastasis. Many investigators have called attention to a disproportionate rise in the serum alkaline phosphatase under these circumstances and have emphasized the usefulness of this test in anticipating otherwise obscure liver metastases.[35, 43, 86, 92, 134, 151]

Bullard indicated that if cirrhosis, obstructive jaundice and bone disease were eliminated, the serum alkaline phosphatase, although by no means infallible, was a helpful indication of neoplastic disease of the liver.[34] It is thought to be particularly helpful in the recognition of metastasis developing after abdominal operations for extrahepatic carcinoma (colon) when the liver was found to be free at the time of laparotomy.

Mendelsohn and Bodansky observed considerable retention of Bromsulphalein and other dyes but noted that similar abnormalities occurred frequently in the absence of metastasis.[150] They found that 78 per cent of cases with liver metastases exhibited elevation of the serum alkaline phosphatase, a rise which occurred in only 10 per cent of cases in which metastasis was not present. Klotz stated that 64 per cent of nonicteric patients with hepatic neoplasm exhibited an abnormal rise of the serum alkaline phosphatase.[126] Ariel and Shahon, on the other hand, were unconvinced that any liver function test was of value as a search method for neoplasm.[12]

There appears to be no test that detects minimal metastasis.[172] This is obviously an essential need when radical surgical procedures are being contemplated.

Refinements of roentgen technic have permitted the detection of otherwise obscure intrahepatic tumors, both primary and secondary.[67, 69, 194] Certain types of mucin-secreting colon carcinomas undergo fine feathery calcification; the roentgen demonstration of this in the liver of a patient known to have had such a neoplasm has served to detect metastasis.[239] Esophageal varices, with or without bleeding, have been demonstrated in association with liver neoplasm in the absence of cirrhosis or other causes of portal hypertension.[83, 193]

Lembeck and others[130, 232] have called attention to the unique features of the serotonin syndrome (cutaneous cyanosis, facial flushing, abdominal cramps, diarrhea, sclerosis of right heart endocardium, etc.) appearing with carcinoid tumors metastatic to the liver.[130, 232] The liver is considered to be a prime site in the "detoxification" of the enterochromaffin cell product (serotonin) and thus a barrier to its systemic dispersion. In the instance of carcinoid this substance is produced in excess and having breached hepatic restraint by metastasis may result in the characteristic clinical phenomena as well as excessive urinary excretion of a serotonin product (5 hydroxyindole acetic acid). Edmondson[60] has cited two cases of carcinoid tumor of the liver without demonstrable extrahepatic site; in one of these the carcinoid syndrome was manifest.

PSEUDONEOPLASM

This is an unsatisfactory term, and there is no general agreement as to its meaning. It has been customary to consider as a pseudotumor or a pseudoneoplasm any clinically detectable mass simulating a tumor that proves to be non-neoplastic. Such lesions may be malformations of which the

Riedel beaver-tail lobe is a prime example or an exuberant reaction to injury of infectious or noninfectious nature.

Anomalous enlargement of one or another of the minor hepatic lobes is not as frequent as the Riedel lobe but may create some concern at abdominal exploration.[53] A peculiar knoblike projection is observed protruding from the superior surface of the liver in infants in which central defects of the diaphragm exist.[177] Aberrant hepatic substance may appear in the falciform ligament in contiguity with or separated from the main liver mass.[201] In each of these the histologic structure is essentially that of normal liver.

Localized non-neoplastic growth disturbances (hamartoma) appear as curious disarrangements of intrinsically normal hepatic components.[46, 95, 145, 185]

Infectious lesions, such as tuberculoma, gumma, helminthic disorders and other granulomatous processes, may mimic neoplasm but are distinguished readily by pathologic study. Since the concept of neoplasm first emerged, regenerating foci appearing in the damaged liver have been mistaken for neoplasm. As mentioned in the early portion of this chapter, clear distinction between the coarsely nodular cirrhotic liver and hepatoma still may create some confusion. This is not only the case with diffuse hepatic disease but also obtains in relation to isolated and discrete areas of repair as well. In the latter instance the appearance of one or more sharply circumscribed pallid nodules within an otherwise normal liver creates a situation in which it is virtually impossible to distinguish the lesion from metastatic carcinoma by gross inspection alone. The resemblance is so convincing that many have chosen to ignore the connotations of the microscopic examination and have designated this lesion as benign hepatoma, adenoma or hamartoma.[15, 23] Claims of successful excision of hepatoma may well reflect the removal of nodules of this nature.

The lesions present as single or multiple[3, 8, 9] sharply outlined nodules, gray or grayish brown in color, with seeming encapsulation.[18, 23] Usually embedded well within the substance of the liver, they may be in subcapsular location or project from the free surface. Microscopic examination should dispel the suspicion of neoplasm, for the structure is obviously that common to cirrhosis, albeit in localized form. The lobular pattern is distorted, and fibrous trabeculae course through the lesion in irregular fashion. The persistence of inflammation and the presence of disarranged biliary ductules within the mass of functioning parenchymal elements clearly exclude the possibility of hepatoma or other form of neoplasm. Warvi has emphasized the presence of ductules as a feature of prime differential diagnostic value.[237] As in hepatoma, occasional lesions of this type have been associated with polycythemia.[115]

To those who have differentiated this lesion sharply there has arisen the all too frequent controversy of nomenclature. Such names as solitary hyperplastic nodule, focal cirrhosis, localized cirrhosis and benign regenerative nodule have been proposed. It is not within the scope of this discussion to defend one or another term. The lesion is not common, and it suffices that the possibility of its existence be recognized when it is encountered at laparotomy. Although of little prognostic import, the possibility exists that in certain instances of hepatoma arising in a noncirrhotic liver, foci of this nature may represent the points of origin.

REFERENCES

1. Abell, I.: Primary hypernephroma of the liver, Ann. Surg. 87:829, 1928.
2. Alexander, M. K.: A mixed tumour of the liver in an adult, J. Path. Bact. 82:217, 1961.
3. Allen, R. A., and Lisa, J. R.: Combined liver cell and bile duct carcinoma, Am. J. Path. 25:647, 1949.
4. Allison, R. M., and Willis, R. A.: An ossifying embryonic mixed tumor of an infant's liver, J. Path. Bact. 72:155, 1956.
5. Altemeier, W. A., Gall, E. A., Culbertson, W. R., and Inge, W. W.: Sclerosing carcinoma of the intrahepatic (hilar) bile ducts, Surgery 60:191, 1966.
6. Altemeier, W. A., Gall, E. A., Zinninger, M. M., and Hoxworth, P. I.: Sclerosing carcinoma of the major intrahepatic bile ducts, A.M.A. Arch. Surg., 75:459, 1957.

7. Amromin, G. D.: Suggested mechanisms of extrapancreatic neoplasms and hypoglycemia (Correspondence), New Engl. J. Med. 268:682, 1963.

8. Andervont, H. B.: Studies on the occurrence of spontaneous hepatomas in mice of strains C3H and CBA, J. Nat. Cancer Inst. 11:581, 1950.

9. Andervont, H. B., Grady, H. G., and Edwards, J. E.: Induction of hepatic lesions, hepatomas, pulmonary tumors and hemangioendotheliomas in mice with o-aminoazotoluene, J. Nat. Cancer Inst. 3:131, 1942,

10. Ariel, I. M.: An aid for determining treatment of liver cancer by combined hepatic gammascanning, Surg. Gynec. Obstet. 121:267, 1965.

11. Ariel, I. M., and Pack, G. T.: Treatment of inoperable cancer of the liver by intraarterial radioactive isotopes and chemotherapy, Cancer 20:793, 1967.

12. Ariel, I. M., and Shahon, D. B.: Hepatic dysfunction in candidates for abdominal surgery, especially in patients with cancer, Cancer 3:608, 1950.

13. Aspray, M.: Calcified hemangiomas of the liver, Am. J. Roentgenol. 53:446, 1945.

14. Baker, H. de C., Paget, G. E., and Davson, J.: Haemangio-endothelioma (Kupffer-cell sarcoma) of the liver, J. Path. Bact. 72:173, 1956.

15. Bartlett, W. I., and Shellito, J. G.: Hamartoma of the liver, Surgery 29:593, 1951.

16. Bauer, W., Dale, H. H., Poulsson, L. T., and Richards, D. W.: The control of circulation through the liver, J. Physiol. 74:343, 1932.

17. Beer, E.: Über Nebennierenkeime in der Leber, Z. Heilk. 25:381, 1904.

18. Begg, C. F., and Berry, W. H.: Isolated nodular regenerative hyperplasia of the liver. The problem of their differentiation from neoplasm, Am. J. Clin. Path. 23:447, 1953.

19. Beggiato, U.: Un caso di mixosarcoma primitive del fegato a sintomatologia di ascesso epatico, Policlinico 34:885, 1927.

20. Behar, A., Moran, E., and Izak, G.: Acquired hypofibrinogenemia associated with a giant cavernous hemangioma of the liver, Am. J. Clin. Path. 40:78, 1963.

21. Behrle, F. C., Mantz, F. A., Jr., Olson, R. L., and Trombold, J. C.: Virilization

accompanying hepatoblastoma, Pediatrics 32:265, 1963.

22. Benson, C. D., and Penberthy, G. C.: Surgical excision of primary tumor of liver (hamartoma) in infant 7 months old with recovery, Surgery 12:881, 1942.

23. Benz, E. J., and Baggenstoss, A. H.: Focal cirrhosis of the liver: its relation to the so-called hamartoma (adenoma, benign hepatoma), Cancer 6:743, 1953.

24. Berk, J. E.: Primary tumors and cysts of the liver in Bockus, H. L.: Gastroenterology, vol. 3, pp. 353-379, Philadelphia, Saunders, 1946.

25. Berk, J. E., and Lieber, M. M.: Primary carcinoma of the liver in hemochromatosis, Am. J. Med. Sci. 202:708, 1941.

26. Berkheiser, S. W.: Recurrent liver cell adenoma, Gastroenterology 37:760, 1959.

27. Berman, C.: An analysis of the incidence of primary carcinoma of the liver amongst the Bantu in the Witersrand gold mines and in Johannesburg with special reference to the incidence of the disease amongst other races, S. Afr. J. Med. Sci. 5:54, 1940.

28. ———: Primary Carcinoma of the Liver: A Study in Incidence, Clinical Manifestation, Pathology and Aetiology, London, H. K. Lewis, 1951.

29. Binford, C. H., Lawrence, R. L., and Wollenweber, H. L.: Hemochromatosis with primary carcinoma of the liver, Arch. Path. 25:527, 1938.

30. Bloch, H., and Chazan, S.: Primary carcinoma of the liver with cirrhosis; report of a case, Arch. Pediat. 73:89, 1956.

31. Bolke, H., Jacobi, M., and Koven, M. T.: Primary carcinoma of the liver with bone metastasis, Ann. Int. Med. 1:1212, 1937.

32. Bonte, F. J., Krohmer, J. S., Elmendorf, E., Presley, N. L., and Andrews, G. J.: Scintillation scanning of the liver. II. Clinical applications, Am. J. Roentgenol. 88:275, 1962.

33. Bowden, L., and Kravitz, S.: Needle biopsy of the liver. A diagnostic aid in the treatment of cancer, Cancer 6:1010, 1953.

34. Bullard, R. W.: Alkaline phosphatase and metastatic liver disease, Surgery 19:379, 1946.

35. Bunce, J. O.: Serum alkaline phosphatase in liver disease. A concept of its significance, Gastroenterology 16:660, 1950.

36. Burns, E. L., and Schenken, J. R.: Spontaneous primary hepatoma in mice of

strain C3H. A study of incidence, sex distribution and morbid anatomy, Am. J. Cancer 39:25, 1940.

37. Burston, J.: Kupffer cell sarcoma, Cancer 2:798, 1958.

38. Butler, D. B., and Bargen, J. A.: Abdominal masses. III. Diseases of the liver, pancreas and spleen: metastatic tumors of the liver, acute cholecystitis, obstruction of the common bile duct, hepatic cirrhosis, tumors of the pancreas, and Banti's disease, Gastroenterology 19:32, 1951.

39. Butler, W. H., and Barnes, J. M.: Toxic effects of groundnut meal containing aflatoxin to rats and guinea pigs, Brit. J. Cancer 17:699, 1963.

40. Caminiti, R.: Über das solitäre Adenom der Leber mit Cirrhose, Arch. klin. Chir. 69:630, 1903.

41. Case records of the Massachusetts General Hospital; Case 43302, New Engl. J. Med. 257:187, 1957.

42. Castle, O. L.: Primary carcinoma of the liver in childhood, Surg., Gynec. Obstet. 18:477, 1914.

43. Cayer, D., and Sohmer, M. F.: The duration of life without operation in patients with tumors metastatic to the liver demonstrated by needle aspiration biopsy, Cancer 9:141, 1956.

44. Charache, H.: Primary carcinoma of the liver. Report of a case and review of the literature, Am. J. Surg. 43:96, 1939.

45. Chomet, B., Valaitis, J., and Pearah, G.: Metastatic carcinoma in the cirrhotic liver, Am. J. Med. Sci. 238:753, 1959.

46. Christopherson, W. M., and Collier, H. S.: Primary benign liver-cell tumors in infancy and childhood, Cancer, 6:583, 1953.

47. Clatworthy, H. W., Jr., Boles, E. T., Jr., and Kottmeier, P. K.: Liver tumors in infancy and childhood, Ann Surg. 154:475, 1961.

48. Clatworthy, H. W., Jr., Boles, E. T., Jr., and Newton, W. A.: Primary tumors of the liver in infants and children, Arch. Dis. Child. 35:22, 1960.

49. Cooper, A. G., and Bolande, R. P.: Multiple hemangiomas in an infant with cardiac hypertrophy; postmortem angiographic demonstration of the arteriovenous fistulae, Pediatrics 35:27, 1965.

50. Copeland, D. H., and Salmon, W. D.: The occurrence of neoplasm in the liver, lungs and other tissues of rats as a result of prolonged choline deficiency, Am. J. Path. 22:1059, 1946.

51. Counsellor, V. S., and McIndoe, A. H.: Primary carcinoma of the liver, Arch. Int. Med. 37:363, 1926.

52. Crocker, D. W., and Cleland, R. S.: Infantile hemangioendothelioma of the liver; report of three cases, Pediatrics 19:596, 1957.

53. Cullen, T. S.: Accessory lobes of the liver. An accessory hepatic lobe springing from the surface of the gallbladder, Arch. Surg. 11:718, 1925.

54. Dansie, C. B.: Primary growth of liver in infants, Lancet 2:228, 1922.

55. Davies, J. N. P.: Human implications; primary carcinoma of the liver in Africa, J. Nat. Cancer Inst. (Supp.) 15:1637, 1955.

56. Dhayagude, R. G.: An unusually large adenoma of the liver, J. Path. Bact. 33:215, 1930.

57. Dickens, F., and Jones, H. E. H.: The carcinogenic action of aflatoxin after its subcutaneous injection in the rat, Brit. J. Cancer 17:691, 1963.

58. Duckett, J. W., and Montgomery, H. G.: Resection of primary liver tumors, Surgery 21:455, 1947.

59. Edmondson, H. A.: Differential diagnosis of tumors and tumor-like lesions of liver in infancy and childhood, Am. J. Dis. Child. 91:168, 1956.

60. ———: Tumors of the liver and intrahepatic bile ducts. Atlas of Tumor Pathology, p. 216, Sect. VII, Fascicle 25, A.F.I.P., Washington, D.C., 1958.

61. Edmondson, H. A., and Steiner, P. E.: Primary carcinoma of the liver; a study of 100 cases among 48,900 necropsies, Cancer 7:462, 1954.

62. Edwards, J. E.: Hepatomas in mice induced with carbon tetrachloride, J. Nat. Cancer Inst. 2:197, 1941-2.

63. Edwards, J. E., and Dalton, A. J.: Induction of cirrhosis of the liver and of hepatomas in mice with carbon tetrachloride, J. Nat. Cancer Inst. 3:19, 1942.

64. Edwards, J. E., and White, J.: Pathologic changes, with special reference to pigmentation and classification of hepatic tumors in rats fed p-dimethyl-aminoazobenzene (butter-yellow), J. Nat. Cancer Inst. 2:157, 1941.

65. Eggel, H.: Über das primäre Carcinom der Leber, Beitr. path. Anat. 30:506, 1901.

66. Emmart, E. W.: The action of 2-amino-5-azotoluene in the production of liver tumors of rats and the behavior of these tumors in vitro, J. Nat. Cancer Inst. *1*: 255, 1940-1.

67. Epstein, B. S.: Diaphragmatic changes incident to hepatic neoplasms, Am. J. Roentgenol. *82*:114, 1959.

68. Escobar, M. A., and Trobaugh, F. E., Jr.: Erythrocythemia in primary carcinoma of the liver; a case report, Arch. Int. Med. *110*:339, 1962.

69. Evans, J. A., and Mujahed, Z.: Roentgenographic aids in diagnosis of neoplasms of liver and extrahepatic ducts, J.A.M.A. *171*:7, 1959.

70. Evans, N., and Hoxie, H. J.: Primary myxosarcoma of liver, Am. J. Cancer *31*:290, 1937.

71. Ewing, J.: Epithelial hyperplasia and tumors of the liver *in* Neoplastic Diseases, ed. 4, pp. 735-761, Philadelphia, Saunders, 1940.

72. Feasby, W. R.: Primary carcinoma of the liver, Canad. Med. Ass. J. *53*:486, 1945.

73. Feldman, W. H.: Neoplasms of Domesticated Animals, pp. 299, 311, Philadelphia, Saunders, 1932.

74. Fenster, L. F., and Klatskin, G.: Manifestations of metastatic tumors of the liver; a study of 81 patients subjected to needle biopsy, Am. J. Med. *31*:238, 1961.

75. Fisher, E. R., Hellstrom, H. R., and Fisher, B.: Rarity of hepatic metastases in cirrhosis— a misconception, J.A.M.A. *174*:366, 1960.

76. Fiske, F. A., and Aegeter, E. E.: Primary carcinoma of liver cells with peritoneal metastasis, Arch. Path. *24*:58, 1937.

77. Flood, C. A., Gutman, E. B., and Gutman, A. B.: Phosphate activity, inorganic phosphorus, and calcium of serum in disease of the liver and biliary tract. A study of 123 cases, Arch. Int. Med. *59*:981, 1937.

78. Foote, J.: Congenital hemangioendothelioma. A disease of early life, J.A.M.A. *73*:1042, 1919.

79. Fred, H. L., and Brown, G. R.: The hepatic friction rub, New Engl. J. Med. *266*:554, 1962.

80. Gall, E. A.: Unpublished data, Department of Pathology, Cincinnati General Hospital.

81. ———: Primary and metastatic carcinoma of the liver. Relationships to hepatic cirrhosis, Arch. Path. *70*:226, 1960.

82. Gall, E. A., and Mallory, T. B.: Malignant lymphoma: a clinical and pathological survey of 618 cases, Am. J. Path. *18*: 381, 1942.

83. Garrett, N., Jr., and Gall, E. A.: Esophageal varices without hepatic cirrhosis, A.M.A. Arch. Path. *55*:196, 1953.

84. Gasparian, G. I.: Über die primären Lebergeschwülste, Arch. klin. Chir. *153*: 435, 1928.

85. Geschickter, C. F., and Keasberg, L. E.: Tumors of blood vessels, Am. J. Cancer *23*:568, 1935.

86. Gibbons, T. B.: Hyperphosphatasemia in patients without jaundice with hepatobiliary disease, J.A.M.A. *164*:22, 1957.

87. Goldzieher, M., and von Bókay, Z.: Der primäre Leberkrebs, Virchows Arch. path. Anat. *203*:75, 1911.

88. Goodale, R. H.: Hemangioendothelioma of the liver, Arch. Path. *9*:528, 1930.

89. Gordon, B. S., Wolf, J., Krause, T., and Shai, F.: Peliosis hepatis and cholestasis following administration of norethandrolone, Am. J. Clin. Path. *33*:156, 1960.

90. Gover, P. A.: The incidence of tumours of the liver and other organs in a pure line of mice (Strong's CBA strain), J. Path. Bact. *50*:17, 1940.

91. Greene, J. M.: Primary carcinoma of the liver. A ten year collective review, Int. Abstr. Surg. *69*:231, 1939.

92. Greene, L. S., and Schiff, L.: Primary carcinoma of the liver—a plea for earlier diagnosis with emphasis on the serum alkaline phosphatase values, Gastroenterology *40*:219, 1961.

93. Gregory, R.: Primary carcinoma of the liver. Tumor thrombus of the inferior vena cava and right auricle, Arch. Int. Med. *64*:566, 1939.

94. Griffith, J. F. C.: Primary carcinoma of the liver in infancy and childhood, Am. J. Med. Sci. *155*:79, 1918.

95. Grime, R. T., Moore, T., Nicholson, A., and Whitehead, R.: Cystic hamartomas and polycystic disease of the liver, Brit. J. Surg. *47*:307, 1959-60.

96. Gustafson, E. G.: An analysis of 62 cases of primary carcinoma of the liver based on 24,400 necropsies at Bellevue Hospital, Ann. Int. Med. *11*:889, 1937.

97. Gutman, A. B., Olson, K. B., Gutman, E. B., and Flood, C. A.: Effect of disease of the liver and biliary tract upon the phosphatase activity of the serum, J. Clin. Invest. *19*:129, 1940.

98. Hanot, V., and Gilbert, A.: Études sur les maladies du foie, Paris, Aseelin & Hauzeau, 1888.

99. Hansen, A. E., Ziegler, M. R., and Mc-Quarrie, I.: Disturbance of osseous and lipid metabolism in a child with primary carcinoma of the liver, J. Pediat. *17*:9, 1940.

100. Hartz, P. H.: Role of schistosomiasis in the etiology of cancer of the liver in the Chinese, Arch. Path. *39*:1, 1945.

101. Hartz, P. H., and Van der Sar, A.: Teratoma of the liver in an infant, Am. J. Clin. Path. *15*:159, 1945.

102. Hepatic carcinogenesis, a clinicopathologic conference; Case Report No. 24, Penn. Med. J. *62*:1344, 1959. Mercy Hosp., Pittsburgh; A. Cantarow, Guest Participant.

103. Herxheimer, G.: Leber Gewächse *in* Henke, F., and Lubarsch, O. (eds.): Handb. spez. path. Anat. Hist., vol. 10, pp. 797-987, Berlin, Springer, 1930.

104. Higginson, J.: Primary carcinoma of the liver in Africa, Brit. J. Cancer *10*:609, 1956.

105. Higginson, J., and Steiner, P. E.: Definition and classification of malignant epithelial neoplasm of the liver, Acta Un. int. Cancr. *17*:593, 1961.

106. Hoffman, H. S.: Benign hepatoma; review of the literature and report of a case, Ann. Int. Med. *17*:130, 1942.

107. Horta, J. de S.: Late lesions in man caused by colloidal thorium dioxide (Thorotrast): a new case of sarcoma of the liver 22 years after the injection, A.M.A. Arch. Path. *62*:403, 1956.

108. Hou, P. C.: A relationship between primary carcinoma of the liver and infestation with *Clonorchis sinensis*, J. Path. Bact. *72*:239, 1956.

109. Hou, P. C., and McFadzean, A. J. S.: Glycogen in primary carcinoma of the liver, J. Path. Bact. *72*:411, 1956.

110. Hoyne, R. M., and Kernohan, J. W.: Primary carcinoma of the liver. A study of 31 cases, Arch. Int. Med. *79*:532, 1947.

111. Hyams, V. J., Thomas, D. F., and Sarkisian, S. S.: Adrenal rest tumor of the liver, Am. J. Surg. *99*:960, 1960.

112. Ishak, K. G.: and Glunz, P. R.: Hepatoblastoma and hepatocarcinoma in infancy and childhood; report of 47 cases, Cancer *20*:396, 1967.

113. Jaffe, R. H.: Sarcoma and carcinoma of the liver following cirrhosis, Arch. Int. Med. *33*:330, 1924.

114. Jones, E.: Primary carcinoma of the liver with associated cirrhosis in infants and children; report of a case, Arch. Path. *70*:5, 1960.

115. Josephs, B. N., Robbins, G., and Levine, A.: Polycythemia secondary to hamartoma of the liver, J.A.M.A. *179*:867, 1962.

116. Kan, Y. W., McFadzean, A. J. S., Todd, D., and Tso, S. C.: Further observations on polycythemia in hepatocellular carcinoma, Blood *18*:592, 1961.

117. Kaplan, L., and Cole, S. L.: Fraternal primary hepatocellular carcinoma in three male, adult siblings, Am. J. Med. *39*:305, 1965.

118. Kay, S., and Talbert, P. C.: Adenoma of the liver, mixed type (hamartoma). Report of two cases, Cancer *3*:307, 1950.

119. Keen, W. W.: Removal of an angioma of the liver by elastic constriction external to the abdominal cavity with table of 59 cases of operation for hepatic tumors, Penn. Med. J. *1*:193, 1897.

120. Keith, W. D., and McNair, A. Y.: Haemochromatosis, diabetes mellitus and primary carcinoma of the liver, Canad. Med. Ass. J. *22*:528, 1930.

121. Kelsch, A., and Kiener, P. L.: Contribution à l'histoire de l'adenome du foie, Arch. physiol. norm. et path. *3*:622, 1876.

122. Kendrey, G.: Die Rolle der Virushepatitis bei der Entstehung des primären Leberkrebses, Beitr. Z. Path. Anat. *120*:1, 1958.

123. Kilfoy, E. J., and Terry, M. C.: Primary carcinoma of the liver in childhood, Surg., Gynec. Obstet. *48*:751, 1928.

124. Klatskin, G.: Adenocarcinoma of the hepatic duct at its bifurcation within the porta hepatis; an unusual tumor with distinctive clinical and pathological features, Am. J. Med. *38*:241, 1965.

125. Klein, H., and Klein, S. P.: Spontaneous hypoglycemia associated with massive hepatoma; a review of current concepts and report of a case, A.M.A. Arch. Int. Med. *103*:273, 1959.

126. Klotz, S. D.: An analysis of liver function by a simplified combination of laboratory tests, Bull. N. Y. Med. Coll. *6*:1, 1943.

127. Kunstadter, R. H.: Hemangio-endothelioma of the liver in infancy (case report

and review of the literature), Am. J. Dis. Child. 46:803, 1933.

128. Ladd, W. E., and Gross, R. E.: Abdominal Surgery of Infancy and Childhood, pp. 289-290, Philadelphia, Saunders, 1941.

129. Lanthier, P. L.: L'adenome solitaire du foie: son diagnostic, son traitement, son prognostic, vol. 48, 138 pp., Thèse de Paris, 1938.

130. Lembeck, F.: Über den Nachweis von 5-Oxytryptamin (Enteramin, Serotonin) in Carcinoidmetastasen, Arch. Exp. Path. Pharmak. 221:50, 1954.

131. Lemmer, K. E.: Primary carcinoma of the liver, Arch. Surg. 61:599, 1950.

132. Lennard-Jones, J. E., and Snow, P. J. D.: Metastasising carcinoid tumours, Gastroenterologia 85:169, 1956.

133. L'Esperance, E. S.: Atypical hemorrhagic malignant hepatoma, J. Med. Res. 27:225, 1915.

134. Lichtman, S. S.: New growth of the liver in Diseases of Liver, Gall Bladder and Bile Ducts, pp. 572-599, Philadelphia, Lea & Febiger, 1942.

135. Lindgren, A. G. H., Hansson, G., and Nilsson, L. A.: Primary carcinoma arising in congenital liver in conjunction with miliary cholangiomatosis; report of a case, Acta. path. microbiol. scand. 52:343, 1961.

136. Loesch, J.: Primary carcinoma of the liver, Arch. Path. 28:223, 1939.

137. Long, E. L., Nelson, A. A., Fitzhugh, O. G., and Hansen, W. H.: Liver tumors produced in rats by feeding safrole, Arch. Path. 75:595, 1963.

138. Longmire, W. P., and Marable, S. A.: Clinical experiences with major hepatic resections, Ann. Surg. 154:460, 1961.

139. Lubarsch, D.: Über die Bedeutung der pathologischen Glykogen Ablagerungen, Arch. path. Anat. 183:188, 1906.

140. Lucké, B.: The pathology of fatal epidemic hepatitis, Am. J. Path. 20:471, 1944.

141. MacDonald, R. A.: Cirrhosis and primary carcinoma of the liver; changes in their occurrence at the Boston City Hospital, 1874-1954, New Engl. J. Med. 255:1179, 1956.

142. ———: Primary carcinoma of the liver: a clinicopathologic study of 108 cases, A.M.A. Arch. Int. Med. 99:266, 1957.

143. MacDonald, R. A., and Mallory, G. K.: The natural history of postnecrotic cirrhosis; a study of 221 autopsy cases, Am. J. Med. 24:334, 1958.

144. MacMahon, H. E., Murphy, A. S., and Bates, M. I.: Endothelial cell sarcoma of liver following Thorotrast injections, Am. J. Path. 23:585, 1947.

145. Maier, W.: Das gestielte Hamartom der Leber. Ein Beitrag zur Diagnostik, Morphologie und Behandlung von Lebertumoren im Kindesalter, Z. Kinderheilk. 77:422, 1955.

146. Major, R. H., and Black, D. R.: A huge hemangioma of the liver associated with hemangiomata of the skull and bilateral cystic adrenals, Am. J. Med. Sci. 156:469, 1918.

147. Mason, H. H., and Andersen, D. H.: Glycogen disease of the liver (von Gierke's disease) with hepatomata; case report with metabolic studies, Pediatrics 16:785, 1955.

148. Matthews, W. F., and Abell, M. R.: Primary carcinoma of liver, Univ. Mich. Med. Bull. 25:313, 1959.

149. McFadzean, A. J. S., and Yeung Tse-Tse: Hypoglycemia in primary carcinoma of the liver, A.M.A. Arch. Int. Med. 98:720, 1956.

150. Mendelsohn, M. L., and Bodansky, O.: The value of liver function tests in the diagnosis of intrahepatic metastasis in the non-icteric cancer patient, Cancer 5:1, 1952.

151. Meranze, D. R., Meranze, T., and Rothman, M. M.: Serum phosphatase as an aid in the diagnosis of metastatic cancer to the liver, Penn. Med. J. 14:1160, 1938.

152. Miele, A. J., and Edmonds, H. W.: Calcified liver metastasis: a specific roentgen diagnostic sign, Radiology 80:779, 1963.

153. Miller, J. K.: Primary sarcoma of the liver: endothelioblastoma. Case report, Am. J. Surg. 44:458, 1939.

154. Milman, D. H., and Grayzel, D. M.: Mixed tumors of the liver. Report of a case with a review of the literature, A.M.A. Am. J. Dis. Child. 81:408, 1951.

155. Monaco, A. P., Hallgrimsson, J., and McDermott, W. V., Jr.: Multiple adenoma (hamartoma) of the liver treated by subtotal (90%) resection: morphological and functional studies of regeneration, Ann. Surg. 159:513, 1964.

156. Monier-Vinard, H. R.: Sur un nouveau

Type de Tumeur Primitive du Foie: l'Hépatome, 82 pp., Paris, Jouve, 1910.

157. Mori, W.: Cirrhosis and primary cancer of the liver; comparative study in Tokyo and Cincinnati, Cancer 20:627, 1967.

158. Mulligan, R. M.: Neoplasms of the Dog, Baltimore, Williams & Wilkins, 1949.

159. Nakamura, T., Nakamura, S., and Abe, S.: Hepatic angiography: hepatic venography and splenoportography, Vasc. Dis. 2:14, 1965.

160. Nettleship, A., and Fink, W. J.: Neoplasms of the liver following injection of Thorotrast, Am. J. Clin. Path. 35:422, 1961.

161. Nieburgs, H. E., Parets, A. D., Perez, V., and Boudreau, C.: Cellular changes in liver tissue adjacent and distant to malignant tumors, Arch. Path. 80:262, 1965.

162. Nissel, W.: Die Mischgeschwülste der Leber, Virchows Arch. path. Anat. 269:446, 1928.

163. Noeggerath, E.: Geburtshindernis in Folge eines Lebercarcinoms beim Neugeboren, Dtsch. Klin. 6:496, 1854.

164. Oettlé, A. G.: The incidence of primary carcinoma of the liver in the southern Bantu. I. Critical review of the literature, J. Nat. Cancer Inst. 17:249, 1956.

165. Oettlé, A. G., and Higginson, J.: The incidence of primary carcinoma of the liver in the southern Bantu. II. Preliminary report on incidence in Johannesburg, J. Nat. Cancer Inst. 17:281, 1956.

166. Orr, J. W.: The histology of the rat's liver during the course of carcinogenesis by butter yellow (p-dimethylamino-azobenzene), J. Path. Bact. 50:393, 1940.

167. Overton, R. C., Kaden, V. G., and Livesay, W. R.: The surgical significance of primary carcinoma of the liver: an analysis of 66 cases and a report of an unusual case of primary hepatic carcinoma, Surgery 377:519, 1955.

168. Pack, G. T., and LeFevre, R. G.: Age and sex distribution and incidence of neoplastic diseases at Memorial Hospital, J. Cancer Res. 14:167, 1930.

169. Pack, G. T., and Miller, T. R.: The treatment of hepatic tumors, New York J. Med. 53:2205, 1953.

170. Pack, G. T., and Molander, D. W.: Metabolism before and after hepatic lobectomy for cancer; studies in 23 patients, A.M.A. Arch. Surg. 80:685, 1960.

171. Packard, G. B., and Palmer, H D.: Primary neoplasms of the liver in infants and children, Ann. Surg. 142:214, 1955.

172. Paulson, M., and Wyler, C. I.: Multiple tests of hepatic function in gastroenteric malignancy. The value of the Bromsulphthalein, hippuric acid and the van den Bergh reaction in detecting hepatic metastasis, with an evaluation of the hippuric acid test, Ann. Int. Med. 16:872, 1942.

173. Phillipp, P. W.: Über Krebsbildungen in Kindesalter, Z. Krebsforsch. 5:361, 1907.

174. Phillips, R., and Murikami, K.: Primary neoplasms of the liver; results of radiation therapy, Cancer 13:714, 1960.

175. Pirie, J. H. H.: Carcinoma of the liver in natives and its frequent association with schistosomiasis, Med. J. S. Afr. 17:87, 1921.

176. Pizzolato, P., and Kistler, J. J.: Primary carcinoma of the liver with a report of a Kupffer cell sarcoma, Southern Med. J. 52:1423, 1959.

177. Potter, E. L.: Pathology of the Fetus and Newborn, Chicago, Year Book Pub., 1952.

178. Powell, L. D., Kaump, M. D., and Jenks, A. L.: Primary carcinoma of the liver with spontaneous rupture, J. Iowa M. Soc. 29:193, 1939.

179. Quattlebaum, J. K.: Hepatic lobectomy for benign and malignant lesions, Surg. Clin. N. A. 42:507, 1962.

180. Ramsey, T. L.: Primary hypernephroma of the liver, Ann. Surg. 90:41, 1929.

181. Ranke, E. J.: Eosinophilia and hepatocellular carcinoma; report of a case, Am. J. Dig. Dis. 10:548, 1965.

182. Ranström, S.: Miliary hepatocellular adenomatosis, Acta path. microbiol. scand. 33:225, 1953.

183. Ray, B. S.: Large cavernous hemangioma of the liver. Report of an inoperable case treated with roentgen therapy, Ann. Surg. 109:373, 1939.

184. Reeves, R. L., Tesluk, H., and Harrison, C. E.: Precocious puberty associated with hepatoma, J. Clin. Endocr. 19:1651, 1959.

185. Rewell, R. E.: Benign hamartoma of the liver, Arch. Dis. Child. 32:159, 1957.

186. Ribbert, H.: Über Bau, Wachstum, und Genese der Angiome, nebst Bemerkungen über Cystenbildung, Virchows Arch. path. Anat. 151:381, 1898.

187. ———: Das maligne Adenom der

Leber, Dtsch. med. Wsch. 35:1607, 1909.

188. Ricketts, W. E., and Green, J. W.: Atypical hepatic cirrhosis with angiomatous change. Report of a case, Gastroenterology 17:33, 1951.

189. Roberts, J. B. M.: Primary hepatic malignancy with particular reference to the embryoma of infancy, Brit. J. Surg. 49: 3, 1961.

190. Roberts, M. H., and Sullivan, C.: Influence of the liver on bone metabolism; report of two cases, J.A.M.A. 159:1002, 1955.

191. Rowen, H. S., and Mallory, F. B.: A multinucleated liver cell carcinoma, Am. J. Path. 1:677, 1925.

192. Ruebner, B. H., Green, R., Miyai, K., Caranasos, G., and Abbey, H.: The rarity of intrahepatic metastasis in cirrhosis of the liver; a statistical explanation with some comments on the interpretation of necropsy data, Am. J. Path. 39:739, 1961.

193. Ruprecht, A. L., and Kinney, T. D.: Esophageal varices caused by metastasis of carcinoma to the liver, Am. J. Dig. Dis. 1:145, 1956.

194. Ruzicka, F. F., Jr., Gould, H. R., Bradley, E. G., and Rousselot, L. M.: Value of splenic portography in the diagnosis of intrahepatic and extrahepatic neoplasm, Am. J. Med. 29:434, 1960.

195. Safdi, S. A., Gall, E. A., Kumpe, C. W., and Schiff, L.: Needle biopsy of the liver. II. Experiences with malignant neoplasm, Gastroenterology 11:93, 1948.

196. Samuelsson, S. M. and Werner, I.: Hepatic carcinoma simulating hyperparathyroidism, Acta med. scand. 173:539, 1963.

197. Sanes, S., and MacCallum, J. D.: Primary carcinoma of the liver. Cholangioma in hepatolithiasis, Am. J. Path. 18: 675, 1942.

198. Schatzki, R.: Roentgenological diagnosis of primary carcinoma of the liver, Am. J. Roentgenol. 46:476, 1941.

199. Schiff, L.: The clinical value of needle biopsy of the liver, Ann. Int. Med. 34: 948, 1951.

200. Schmorl, G.: Zur Kenntniss der accessorischen Nebennieren, Ziegler's Beitr. path. Anat. 9:523, 1891.

201. Schragen, V. L.: Surgical aspects of adenoma of the liver, Ann. Surg. 105:33, 1937.

202. Schumacher, H. B., Jr.: Hemangioma of the liver. Discussion of symptomatology and report of a patient treated by operation, Surgery 11:209, 1942.

203. Shallow, T. A., and Wagner, F. B.: Primary fibrosarcoma of the liver, Ann. Surg. 125:439, 1947.

204. Shanmugaratnam, K.: Primary carcinomas of the liver and biliary tract, Brit. J. Cancer 10:232, 1956.

205. Sheehan, H. L.: An embryonic tumour of the liver containing striated muscle, J. Path. Bact. 33:251, 1930.

206. Sheldon, J. H.: Hemochromatosis, London, Oxford, 1935.

207. Sherrick, J. C., Elias, H., and Krishna Murthy, A. S.: Reaction of the liver to metastatic carcinoma, Arch. Path. 77: 188, 1964.

208. Shorter, G., Baggenstoss, A. H., Logan, G. B., and Hallenbeck, G. A.: Primary carcinoma of the liver in infancy and childhood; report of 11 cases and review of the literature, Pediatrics 25:191, 1960.

209. Simmonds, M.: Die knotige Hyperplasie und das Adenom der Leber, Dtsch. Arch. klin. Med. 34:388, 1884.

210. Simpson, H. M., Jr., Baggenstoss, A. H., and Stauffer, M. H.: Primary sarcoma of the liver: a report of three cases, Southern Med. J. 48:1177, 1955.

211. Smith, J. C.: Diffuse intrasinusoidal metastatic cancer of the liver, Ann. Int. Med. 54:104, 1961.

212. Smith, L. W.: Four unusual malignant tumors of the liver, Arch. Path. 1:365, 1926.

213. Snow, P. J. D., Lennard-Jones, J. E., Curzon, G., and Stacey, R. S.: Humoral effect of metastasising carcinoid tumors, Lancet 2:1004, 1955.

214. Sobin, L. H.: Multiple congenital neoplasms, Arch. Path. 76:602, 1963.

215. Spiegel, H. A.: Pedunculated angioendothelioma of the liver. Report of an unusual case, Arch. Pediat. 46:188, 1929.

216. Stein, Y.: Detection of space occupying lesions of the liver by directional counting of Co^{60}-labeled B_{12}, J. Lab. Clin. Med. 56:290, 1960.

217. Steiner, M. M.: Primary carcinoma of the liver in childhood. Report of two cases, with a critical review of the literature, Am. J. Dis. Child. 55:807, 1938.

218. Steiner, P. E.: The etiology of human liver cancer in Africa and the United

States of America, Tr. Stud. Coll. Physicians, Phila. 28:61, 1960.

219. Steiner, P. E., and Higginson, J.: Cholangiocellular carcinoma of the liver, Cancer 12:753, 1959.

220. Stewart, H. L., Cantarow, A., and Morgan, D. R.: Changes in the liver of the cat following ligation of single hepatic ducts, Arch. Path. 23:641, 1937.

221. Storey, P. B., and Goldstein, W.: Pulmonary embolization from primary hepatic carcinoma, Arch. Int. Med. 110:262, 1962.

222. Stumpf, H. H., and Liber, A. F.: Hepatocellular adenomatosis, report of a case with liver function studies, Am. J. Med. 17:887, 1954.

223. Suckow, E. E., Henegar, G. C., and Baserga, R.: Tumors of the liver following administration of Thorotrast, Am. J. Path. 38:663, 1961.

224. Sutton, P. M.: Parenchymal cell damage and bile duct activity in the precancerous liver, Brit. J. Cancer, 16:619, 1962.

225. Swalm, W. A., Gault, E. S., and Morrison, L.: A rare case of primary liver cell carcinoma in liver fluke disease (Clonorchis sinensis), Am. J. Dig. Dis. 4:789, 1937-8.

226. Sweed, A., and Weinberg, T.: Hemangioendothelioma of the liver in infancy, Am. J. Dis. Child. 80:436, 1950.

227. Symmers, W. St. C., and Ward-McQuaid, J. N.: Successful resection of a large cavernous lymphangiomatoid lesion in the liver of a child aged 19 months, Brit. J. Surg. 38:12, 1950.

228. Teng, C. T., Daeschner, C. W., Jr., Singleton, E. B., and Rosenberg, H. S.: Liver diseases and osteoporosis in children. II. Etiological considerations, J. Pediat. 59:703, 1961.

229. Teng, C. T., Daeschner, C. W., Jr., Singleton, E. B., Rosenberg, H. S., Cole, V. W., Hill, L. L., and Brennan, J. C.: Liver diseases and osteoporosis in children. I. Clinical observation, J. Pediat. 59:684, 1961.

230. Tesluk, H., and Nordin, W. A.: Hemangioendothelioma of liver following thorium dioxide administration, A.M.A. Arch. Path. 60:493, 1955.

231. Thompson, C. M., and Hilferty, D. J.: Primary carcinoma of the liver (cholangi-

232. Thorson, A., Biörck, G., Björkman, G., and Waldenström, J.: Malignant carcinoid of the small intestine with metastases to the liver, valvular disease of the right side of the heart (pulmonary stenosis and tricuspid regurgitation without septal defects), peripheral vasomotor symptoms, bronchoconstriction, and an unusual type of cyanosis: a clinical and pathologic syndrome, Am. Heart J. 47:795, 1954.

233. Tio (Tiong Hoo), Leijnse, B., Jarrett, A., and Rimington, C.: Acquired porphyria from a liver tumour, Clin. Sci. 16:517, 1957.

234. Trites, A. E. W.: Peliosis hepatis: report of a case, A.M.A. Arch. Path. 63:183, 1957.

235. Tull, J. C.: Primary carcinoma of the liver. A study of 134 cases, J. Path. Bact. 35:557, 1932.

236. Viallet, A., Benhamou, J. P., Berthelot, P., Hartmann, L., and Fauvert, R.: Primary carcinoma of the liver and dysproteinemia, Gastroenterology 43:88, 1962.

237. Warvi, W. N.: Primary neoplasm of the liver, Arch. Path. 37:367, 1944.

238. Watson, A. J.: Diffuse intra-sinusoidal metastatic carcinoma of the liver, J. Path. Bact. 69:207, 1955.

239. Wells, J.: Calcified liver metastases, New Engl. J. Med. 255:639, 1956.

240. White, J., Dalton, A. J., and Edwards, J. E.: Pathology of rat hepatoma, J. Nat. Cancer Inst. 2:539, 1941-2.

241. Wilbur, D. L., Wood, D. A., and Willett, F. M.: Primary carcinoma of the liver, Ann. Int. Med. 20:453, 1944.

242. Willeford, G., and Stembridge, V. A.: Primary sarcoma of the liver; report of a case, Am. J. Dis. Child. 80:404, 1950.

243. Willis, R. A.: Carcinoma of the liver in Pathology of Tumours, pp. 430-437, St. Louis, Mosby, 1948.

244. Winters, R. W., Robinson, S. J., and Bates, G.: Hemangioma of the liver with heart failure: a case report, Pediatrics 14:117, 1954.

245. Wolbach, S. B.: The latent period in experimental carcinogenesis (Abstr.), Arch. Path. 22:279, 1936.

246. Yamagiwa, K.: Zur Kenntnis des pre-

mären parenchymatösen Leberkarzinoms ("Hepatoma"), Virchows Arch. path. Anat. *206*:437, 1911.

247. Yarbrough, S. M., and Evashwick, G.: Case of teratoma of the liver, with 14-year postoperative survival, Cancer *9*: 848, 1956.

248. Yoshida, T.: Über die experimentelle Erzeugung von Hepatom durch die Fetterung mit *o*-Amidoazotoluol, Proc. Imp. Acad. Japan *8*:464, 1932.

249. Yuhl, E. T., and Stirrett, L. A.: Clinical evaluation of the hepatic radioactivity survey, Ann. Surg. *138*:857, 953.

250. Zak, F. G.: Peliosis hepatis, Am. J. Path. *26*:1, 1950.

25

Surgery of the Liver

MICHAEL E. DE BAKEY, M.D., AND *GEORGE L. JORDAN, JR.*, M.D.

TRAUMA TO THE LIVER

The liver lies in a relatively protected area, for although it is an intra-abdominal organ it is enclosed within the costal cage unless enlarged. It is the largest intra-abdominal organ, however, and its consistency is such that it ruptures more readily than most other organs. The relative frequency of injury to intra-abdominal structures has been tabulated by a number of authors. Griswold and Collier tabulated several series of abdominal trauma and noted that the liver was the fourth in order of frequency among intra-abdominal organs injured, being preceded by spleen, kidney and intestine in that order.[71] The spleen leads the list in most series in which blunt trauma is the usual type of injury.[58, 131] The experience at the Baylor Affiliated Hospitals in Houston, Texas, has been tabulated by Beall, Crosthwait and De Bakey.[5] In this series, the liver was the organ most often injured, probably representing the high percentage of penetrating injuries.

Pathology. Penetrating injuries are the most common throughout the United States.[124] The hepatic wound varies with the type of wounding agent. Knife wounds, for example, usually make a sharp, relatively superficial incision while pistol or rifle wounds produce through-and-through perforations with associated contusion and at times stellate fracture. The degree of damage of gunshot wounds is proportional to the velocity of the missile. Shotgun wounds at close range may be immediately fatal due to the severe destruction of the organ.

Wounds resulting from blunt trauma range from small, subcapsular hematomas to large, stellate fractures which shatter an entire lobe.

The liver is a highly vascular organ and significant hemorrhage may occur from small wounds, while profuse hemorrhage should be anticipated from any large wound. Bile leakage occurs uniformly and if not controlled or drained properly results in bile peritonitis or intra-abdominal abscess. Hepatic reserve is such that rarely does a patient arrive at a hospital alive if his liver has been damaged to such an extent that it cannot support life when hemorrhage is controlled. Devitalized segments, however, may give rise to late complications. The most frequent is hemorrhage, which occurs as tissue sloughs. Rarely an intrahepatic abscess forms and rare traumatic cysts have been reported.

Hemobilia probably occurs to some degree in most hepatic wounds of any severity. Rarely, it is serious.[122, 207] In such instances it may represent dissolution of an intrahepatic hematoma with hemorrhage into the biliary tract occurring as a late complication.

Diagnosis. Initial examination of the wounded patient should include a careful history and physical examination. The patient should be totally disrobed and moved sufficiently to examine all areas of the body. This is extremely important because associated wounds are common. Also lateral and posterior entrance or exit wounds or identification of a subcutaneous missile may be missed if examination is not complete.

Penetrating wounds of the right upper

quadrant require no special diagnostic procedures. Patients with injuries of this type should undergo abdominal exploration immediately.

Diagnosis of a hepatic wound following blunt trauma may be extremely difficult in the absence of definite signs of hemorrhage or peritonitis. Pain is the most common symptom. Pain may be accentuated with respiration and referred to the shoulder as the result of diaphragmatic irritation. The usual signs of peritonitis are present if the peritoneal cavity has been contaminated, consisting of abdominal tenderness, rebound tenderness, muscle spasm and decreased or absent peristalsis. A fluid wave may be present due to free peritoneal fluid. If physical findings are not sufficiently definite to warrant exploration at the time of admission, examination should be repeated at frequent intervals.

Shock is present in most patients with severe wounds and this finding should suggest hepatic injury in patients with right upper quadrant pain following blunt trauma.

When clinical observations raise suspicion of injury but the signs are not sufficiently definite to warrant exploration, peritoneal tap should be performed. In the past a "four quadrant tap" was usually performed in which a needle was inserted into all four quadrants independently in search for free intraperitoneal fluid. Recently other technics have been described, including the placement of a relatively large rubber catheter and irrigation of the peritoneal cavity with large volumes of sterile saline.[188] We prefer the placement of a small plastic catheter which can be left in place for several hours. As the patient changes position and examinations are repeated, drainage may become evident which was not found at the time of the initial paracentesis.

Laboratory studies should include a hemoglobin concentration and hematocrit, white blood cell count and differential count. These are performed repeatedly if necessary. The presence of a high white blood cell count should make one suspicious of visceral injury, and a falling hematocrit should suggest intra-abdominal hemorrhage.

Roentgenograms taken in the supine and upright positions are indicated. Displacement of the stomach or hepatic flexure of the colon or elevation of the right leaf of the diaphragm may be seen with a perihepatic hematoma. Fracture of one of the lower ribs on the right should always raise suspicion. Diagnosis by angiography has been of recent interest.[3, 97] Freeark has suggested total abdominal angiography in patients with suspected abdominal wounds.[59]

Treatment. Initial therapy should be the same for all patients with severe intra-abdominal trauma regardless of the organ involved. Blood should be drawn immediately for typing and cross-matching as well as for laboratory studies, and intravenous therapy is instituted immediately. An arm or neck vein should be used, or a subclavian catheter inserted, because an associated vena caval wound may preclude proper fluid administration from the lower extremity. Large plastic catheters should be used, for they are less easily dislodged and allow administration of large volumes rapidly. If the patient is in shock, one of the catheters should be passed into the superior vena cava for central venous monitoring during fluid replacement. An airway must be assured, particularly in patients with associated chest trauma, and a thoracostomy tube should be placed before induction of anesthesia if associated chest trauma exists. A urinary catheter is inserted and fractures are splinted. If the patient is in shock, dextran administration should be instituted until whole blood is available. When hemorrhage is severe, uncrossmatched type specific blood or low titer O negative blood may be used until properly crossmatched blood is available. Excessive time should not be lost trying to "prepare the patient for surgery." In the presence of severe hemorrhage, operative control is perhaps the most important resuscitative measure. Unresponsive shock, therefore, is an urgent indication for surgery and in critical situations the abdomen should be opened in the emergency room without waiting for transport to the operating room.

Adequate exposure is mandatory. A midline incision allows rapid entrance into the abdomen and good exposure for most lesions. When injuries involve the dome, how-

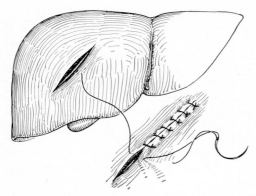

FIG. 25–1. Simple laceration of the right lobe of the liver and repair by suture.

ever, the incision should be extended into the right chest and the diaphragm divided as needed for adequate exposure of the entire organ. Control of hemorrhage takes first priority in treatment. Superficial lacerations are treated by simple suture using large, relatively blunt needles and a suture sufficiently large so that it will not cut through the liver substance (Fig. 25–1). When hemorrhage from deep lacerations is difficult to control, temporary occlusion of the hepatic artery and portal vein may be necessary. At normothermic conditions, 15 minutes should be the maximum time for a single period of occlusion. Occlusion time may be safely increased by local hypothermia, cooling the

liver with sterile iced saline. Obvious necrotic tissue should be debrided and the raw surface repaired with suture (Fig. 25–2). In some patients hemorrhage may be difficult to control even with adequate sutures. The use of hemostatic agents such as Gelfoam or Oxycel gauze should be minimized, for hemostasis is less secure, and these agents may be a focus for infection. Their use, however, is occasionally necessary to obtain good hemostatic control. Recent interest has developed in the use of plastic adhesives such as methyl 2-cyanoacrylate and other homologues of the cyanoacrylate compounds for hemostasis. These substances are still in an investigative phase but some success has been reported on the basis of use in the human as well as the experimental animal.[130, 231]

In the rare patient, a formal total lobectomy is necessary to remove a destroyed lobe, and McClelland and associates have advocated increased use of this technic (Fig. 25–3).[116, 132, 138, 179] Most surgeons, however, prefer simple debridement in most instances and limit formal resections to rare patients with unusually severe wounds.[5, 119, 123, 124, 225]

In some patients, even those with through-and-through bullet wounds, hemorrhage will have stopped before the abdo-

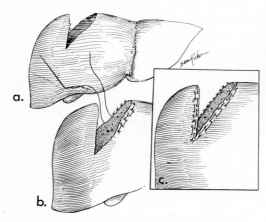

FIG. 25–2. a. Damaged area of right lobe has been débrided. b. and c. Repair with mattress sutures.

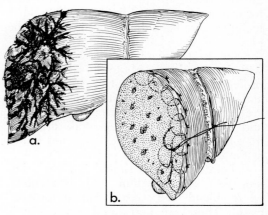

FIG. 25–3. a. Severe contusion and fracture of entire right lobe. b. Treatment by right lobectomy. (Redrawn from Shires, T.: Care of the Trauma Patient, New York. McGraw-Hill, 1966.)

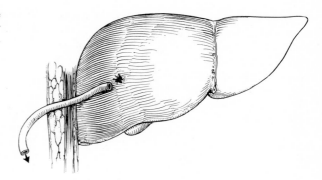

Fig. 25–4. Perforating wound of the liver resulting from passage of a low velocity bullet. After control of hemorrhage drainage is instituted.

men is opened, and treatment is limited to drainage (Fig. 25–4). Adequate drainage should be employed in all patients regardless of the severity of injury. Leakage of tissue fluid and bile will occur in all patients to some extent. Furthermore, some oozing occurs not infrequently despite apparently good hemostasis at the time of operation, and late bleeding may be diagnosed quickly if drains are in place.

To decrease bile drainage and the possibility of a biliary fistula, Merendino and associates have advocated placement of a T-tube in the common bile duct to prevent any increase in pressure in the ductal system.[137] This procedure, however, is rarely necessary.

Mortality. The mortality rate for hepatic wounds was extremely high prior to World War II, being more than 60 per cent in most series.[5, 9] Madding and Kennedy, however, reported a series of 829 patients treated during World War II with a mortality rate of only 27 per cent,[124] and since that time a definite decrease has occurred with rates of 8.9 to 17.3 per cent being reported by several authors.[5, 131, 208, 225] However, these figures represent the result of treatment of those patients who are alive when first seen by a physician. Fitzgerald and associates, in a study of patients with blunt trauma, found that 74 of 105 patients with hepatic injury had died before reaching the hospital.[58]

Several factors are particularly important in relation to the mortality rate. One is the severity of the injury, for the mortality rate is low in patients who have superficial lacerations. McClelland and associates state that

TABLE 25–1.

	MORTALITY RATE	
NUMBER OF ASSOCIATED ORGANS INJURED	Madding and Kennedy[124]	Beall and Associates[5]
0	9.7	4.6
1	26.5	10.9
2	39.7	23.0
3	54.8	29.6
4 (or more— Madding)	84.6	38.1
5 (or more)		87.5

the mortality rate should be 1 per cent or less in patients with small penetrating injuries which involve only the liver.[131] The mortality rate is high for those patients who require resection of large amounts of hepatic tissue. As a corollary, the mortality rate is higher for those patients who are in shock at the time of hospital admission. Of equal importance is the number of associated injuries, for there is a steady increase in mortality rate with each additional organ or vessel injured (Table 25–1).[5, 83, 124]

Mortality rate is related to the type of wounding agent, which has a direct bearing upon the severity of hepatic injury and the number of associated injuries. Thus, in the experience of Beall and associates, stab wounds resulted in a mortality rate of only 3.3 per cent, gunshot wounds, 25.5 per cent, and blunt trauma (mainly automobile accidents), 44.9 per cent.

Cause of Death. Hemorrhage with shock is the most common cause of death. In the series of Beall and associates, 71 per cent of deaths were due to this cause, but hemorrhage was more often from another organ or vessel than from the liver itself.[5] A variety of factors are responsible for other deaths. Extra-abdominal injury, such as cerebral trauma, renal insufficiency, pulmonary complications, and infections, are those that occur with greatest frequency. Bile peritonitis is a rare cause of death today and should not exist if proper peritoneal toilet is performed at surgery and adequate drainage instituted.

Complications. A high incidence of nonfatal complications can be anticipated. Mc-Clelland and associates reported a 20 per cent incidence.[131] The two most common are infection and pulmonary complications. Infections most often are seen in the abdominal wound. Subphrenic abscess, however, is second in frequency while other intra-abdominal abscesses and intrahepatic infections are uncommon. The pulmonary complications may be the result of the associated thoracic wounds while others are postoperative atelectasis and pneumonia.

Persistent biliary fistula is unusual, being recorded in only 3 per cent of the Houston series.[5]

CYSTS OF THE LIVER

POLYCYSTIC DISEASE

Polycystic disease of the liver is an embryologic maldevelopment similar to polycystic disease of the kidney.[30] In fact, when polycystic disease of the liver is found, the possibility of associated cysts of the kidney is high. In collected series the incidence has been approximately 50 per cent, and other cystic lesions may be found, including cysts of the pancreas, the lung, or the spleen (Fig. 25–5). Furthermore, other congenital abnormalities have been noted.[135] It is of particular significance that cerebrovascular aneurysms have been found in a number of these patients.[19, 195] Polycystic liver is diagnosed infrequently during life, but Brown reported 8 cases among 11,245 autopsies[19] while Feldman found 7 in only 1,319 autopsies.[53] The cysts vary in number from 2

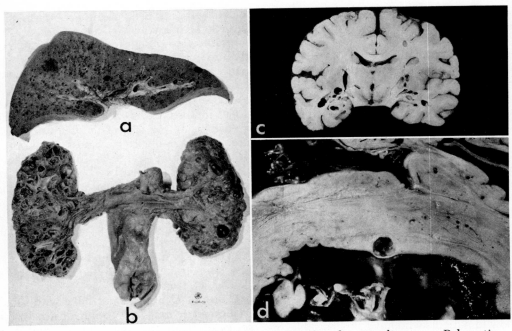

FIG. 25–5. Necropsy specimens from a patient with polycystic disease. a. Polycystic disease of the liver with multiple small cysts throughout both lobes. b. Bilateral polycystic disease of the kidney. c. Cysts of the brain. d. Cyst of the myocardium.

or 3 to multiple cysts which replace a large portion of hepatic tissue in both lobes (Fig. 25–6). They vary in size from those which are almost microscopic to cysts containing 1,000 cc. or more of fluid which usually is brownish in color. The hepatic tissue between the cystic lesions is normal in gross appearance and normal on histologic examination. Rupture, intracystic hemorrhage and infection represent the pathologic complications, but each of these complications is rare.[135, 142]

Clinical Features. In most reported cases there have been no symptoms and the cysts were an unsuspected finding at operation or necropsy. In an occasional patient the large size of the cyst produces abdominal pain due to its weight or due to pressure on surrounding structures. Jaundice due to the pressure of this cyst on bile ducts has been reported but this complication is rare. When the cysts are large, the liver becomes palpable; characteristically it is nontender. Although some nodularity may be appreciated, multiple cysts cannot be diagnosed with any degree of certainty on the basis of clinical grounds alone. Temperature is elevated only when infection has occurred or when there has been rupture, and in the latter circumstance there are signs of peritoneal irritation.

Diagnosis. Few patients have symptoms that warrant investigation, and rarely is the diagnosis made preoperatively. Hepatic function tests are usually normal. Roentgenographic studies of biliary tree and gastrointestinal tract may disclose pressure defects due to an adjacent mass, but there is no characteristic appearance to denote polycystic disease of the liver. Hepatic scan using radioactive materials may show multiple filling defects in the hepatic parenchyma, but no characteristic features differentiate such cysts from other space-occupying lesions. It has been stated that arteriography may suggest cysts by demonstrating filling defects in the liver in the absence of the "tumor stain," but the experience with this test is not sufficient to allow an absolute statement of its reliability.

Treatment. No treatment is necessary in most instances. When asymptomatic cysts are found incidentally at operation for other

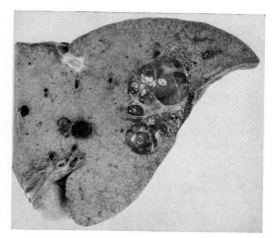

FIG. 25–6. Necropsy specimen of polycystic disease of the liver with several cysts in the left lobe only.

lesions, treatment is not indicated. When symptoms do exist, however, treatment may be directed toward the large cysts which are the cause of symptoms. Occasionally such cysts are present on the surface of the liver and may even be pedunculated so that they can be completely excised. If the cysts cannot be totally excised safely, they may be aspirated, and the cyst cavity managed by suture closure, external drainage or internal drainage through anastomosis to a Roux-en-Y loop of jejunum. Even in symptomatic patients, treatment is limited to the large symptomatic cysts and no effort should be made to eradicate all lesions deeper within the organ.

Other methods of therapy, including the injection of formalin to cause scarring of the cystic cavity, have been suggested, but these can be mentioned only to be condemned. Major hepatic resections have been performed when cysts are limited to one lobe of the liver, but operations of this magnitude are justified only when necessary to relieve life-endangering complications.

Prognosis. Hepatic cysts rarely progress to a point at which hepatic function is compromised. Prognosis is excellent, in contradistinction to that with cysts of the kidney, which often produce renal insufficiency and death. In fact, the most common cause of death in these patients is renal failure due to polycystic disease of the kidney. Surgi-

TABLE 25–2. CLASSIFICATION OF
HEPATIC CYSTS

I. Congenital
   A. Polycystic Disease
   B. Solitary Cysts
II. Acquired
   A. Traumatic
   B. Inflammatory
      1. Retention cysts due to inflamma-
        tory obstruction of bile ducts
      2. Hydatid
   C. Neoplastic
      1. Dermoid
      2. Degeneration of malignant neo-
        plasms

cal treatment of the large cysts will relieve symptoms and the need for a second operation because of enlargement of the remaining cysts is uncommon.

SOLITARY CYSTS OF THE LIVER

Solitary cysts of the liver may be true cysts with an epithelial lining or false cysts lined by fibrous tissue (Table 25–2). Most true cysts are congenital. Their formation was discussed in detail by Moschcowitz in 1906 and there has been little additional contribution to these concepts in the ensuing 62 years.[146] He presented evidence that cysts arose from aberrant bile ducts or from congenital obstruction caused by inflammatory hyperplasia. This would appear to be adequate explanation for the majority of the cysts. Other cysts may form, however, because of hemorrhage or trauma, inflammatory lesions with obstruction of the bile ducts, as dermoid cysts, or by degeneration of malignant neoplasms.[63, 85, 175]

The right lobe is reported to be involved approximately twice as often as the left, though such recordings in most cases are based upon the classic description, using the falciform ligament as the line of division of the right and left lobes, rather than the intrahepatic segmental distribution of bile ducts and vessels (Fig. 25–7). The solitary cyst of congenital origin is unilocular in most instances, for in a collection of 189 solitary cysts by Davis in 1937, only 20 were multilocular.[39] The cysts are often large, containing 500 ml. or more and occasionally they become extremely large. One patient with a cyst containing 17,000 cc. was reported by Burch and Jones.[21]

The contents of the cyst may be thin or thick and vary in color from a clear serous fluid to a bile-colored fluid with a specific gravity of 1.010 to 1.022. Grossly, these cysts are rounded or ovoid, usually well encapsulated and circumscribed. The cyst wall is usually comprised of an epithelial lining, containing in many instances all of the cellular types found normally within the liver. Schaack has best described the microscopic picture, noting that the cyst is usually lined with cuboidal epithelium. He also described three layers of connective tissue making up the wall of the cyst, but these may contain

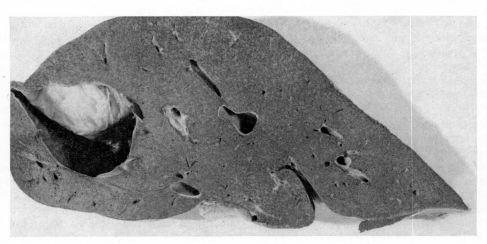

FIG. 25–7. Large single cyst of right lobe of liver found at necropsy.

numerous elements normally found in the liver.[192] Large blood vessels may extend into the cyst wall. The acquired cysts may represent retention cysts behind areas of obstruction, in which case the lining epithelium is the same as that of the biliary ductal system. Cysts that result from neoplasia are lined with neoplastic tissue, whereas those that result from intrahepatic hemorrhage or trauma are false cysts with a fibrous tissue lining. Complications that may occur include intracystic hemorrhage, infection, or rupture either into the biliary ductal system or into the free peritoneal cavity. Such complications are rare.

Clinical Features. Solitary cysts are found more frequently in females than in males in a ratio of 4 to 1. Most occur in the age range of 20 to 50 years, though occasionally, cysts are found in the very young or very old.[175] Glanzman and associates, for example, reported a cyst containing 2,500 cc. of fluid in a 2-year-old child.[65] According to Geist, the oldest patient found in a review of the literature was 82 years old.[63]

Solitary cysts, similar to polycystic lesions, are often asymptomatic and found incidentally at operation or necropsy. A review of the experience at the Mayo Clinic revealed only 38 patients in 47 years and only 11 of these were operated upon because of symptoms.[85] The rest of the lesions were found incidentally at operation for other conditions. When symptoms do exist the most common complaint is discomfort due to a large, heavy mass in the right upper quadrant. Thus vague abdominal discomfort, nausea and vomiting, and symptoms related to pressure on adjacent viscera are the most common symptoms. The presence of an abdominal mass may also be noted by the patients. Some cysts have presented so low in the abdomen that the diagnosis of ovarian cyst was entertained preoperatively.[21] The only physical abnormality is a palpable mass in the upper abdomen which moves with respiration. Although the cystic nature of the mass is apparent in some patients, in others it appears to be a hard, solid lesion. In most instances, the mass is located in the right upper quadrant, though extension to the left upper quadrant may be observed. Torsion with acute pain,

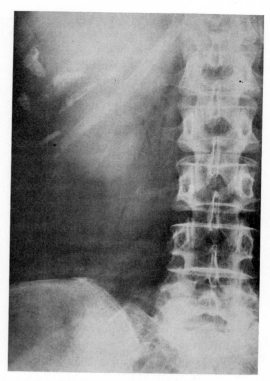

Fig. 25–8. Roentgenogram of a large single cyst arising from the inferior surface of the right lobe of the liver. The overlying renal shadow allows estimation of the large size of this cyst, which measured 5 inches in diameter. On the original film, calcification was visible in the wall, and the possibility of echinococcus cyst was considered.

strangulation, hemorrhage and rupture have been reported as complications.

Laboratory Studies. There are no diagnostic laboratory tests. Mild jaundice may occur when pressure on the common bile duct or hepatic ducts occurs, but this is uncommon.

Roentgenographic Findings. Roentgenographic abnormalities depend upon the location of the cyst. The leaf of the diaphragm may be elevated or adjacent organs displaced. Occasionally these cysts develop calcification of the wall, and this may cause confusion in differentiation from echinococcus cyst (Fig. 25–8).

Treatment. For cysts that are symptomatic, excision is the treatment of choice.

In some patients the cyst is so large and extends so deeply into hepatic tissue with proximity to large vessels and bile ducts that excision is hazardous. Therefore, some cysts have been aspirated and the cavity obliterated by suture. Few series are large enough to warrant a statement of risk of operative intervention. Beattie and Robertson in 1932 reported a mortality rate of 20 per cent in 62 cases, but Geist, in a review of 122 patients treated from 1924 to 1955, found a mortality rate of only 2.4 per cent.[6, 63] In a series reported from the Mayo Clinic there were no deaths.[85] Thus surgical mortality rates have fallen; and such cysts should be treated safely.

Prognosis. Following removal of the cyst the prognosis is excellent. Recurrence is rare.

HYDATID CYSTS

Based upon the world experience the most frequent cyst of the liver is the echinococcus cyst. In fact, in some countries, this probably represents the most common hepatic disease. Even in the United States, hydatid cysts are probably as common as other cysts of the liver though the majority of cases occur in immigrants from countries where the disease is endemic. Katz and Pan were able to find only 24 cases in which it appeared that infestation had occurred within the United States.[102] In some other countries of the world however, particularly where raising of sheep is common and dogs are used as shepherds, the disease is extremely common. In Greece, for example, 716 patients were operated upon for hydatid disease during a recent 1 year period, and a series as large as 6,000 consecutive cases has been reported from this country.[216] Other countries with a high incidence include Uruguay, Argentina, Australia, New Zealand and South Africa. As recently as 1965, Nicks estimated that 20 to 40 per cent of all dogs in Australia were infected.[150]

Epidemiology. The dog is the definitive host for this parasitic small tapeworm. The worm is approximately 0.5 cm. in length with the characteristic features being a head, commonly termed a scolex, on which are footlets and suckers, a short neck, and three proglottids. The tapeworm grows in the intestine of the dog as the primary host without apparent detriment to the animal. Ova develop in the terminal proglottid which ruptures and discharges the ova. The ova pass in the feces, thus infecting the intermediate host, the most common of which is the sheep. Pigs, cattle and man also serve as intermediate hosts. The intermediate host becomes infected by ingesting material in which ova have passed, and infestation in man often occurs in childhood because of handling of dogs as pets.

After the intermediate host has ingested the ovum, its outer shell is digested by gastric juice and the parasite passes through the portal circulation into the liver where it may either die or grow into an echinococcus cyst. Infestation may occur in the liver alone or there may be passage through the liver to involve other organs. At times, other organs are involved in the absence of hepatic disease. Cysts have been reported in virtually all organs of the body; the lungs and brain are two of the most common extrahepatic sites. This cycle is completed when the dogs eat the viscera of infected animals. Thus, this disease can be eliminated if all slaughtered meat is inspected properly and the dog is prevented from ingesting the viscera.[192]

Pathology. The liver is the most common site of echinococcus infestation, approximately 70 per cent of all cysts being found in this organ. The right lobe is most frequently involved, possibly because most of the portal blood from the upper gastrointestinal tract reaches this area. Usually the cysts are single, though multiple cysts may occur. Each cyst consists of an outer layer of adventitia representing a host reaction to the parasite and an inner membrane which contains the growing organism. Typically the cyst fluid is under high pressure and is colorless, though after the passage of time, bile contamination may occur. The cyst grows very slowly and, thus, even with infestation in childhood, symptoms may not occur until adulthood has been reached.

The most common complication is rupture of the cyst because of the high intracystic pressure (Table 25–3). Harris believes that rupture into the biliary tract is the most common complication.[80] He states that Deve recorded a 24 per cent incidence

TABLE 25–3. COMPLICATIONS OF
HYDATID CYSTS

I. Rupture
    A. Intrabiliary
    B. Intraperitoneal
    C. Through the diaphragm
        1. Into the pleural space
        2. Into the lung or bronchus
    D. Into other organs
II. Infection
III. Allergic Manifestations
    A. Urticaria
    B. Anaphylactic shock

of spontaneous cure following such rupture; there was a 30 per cent mortality rate within 6 weeks. In addition to spread of the disease, rupture into the biliary tract may produce obstructive jaundice. The most common site of rupture is into the intrahepatic ducts, though rupture into the common bile duct, cystic duct and gallbladder have all been reported. Rupture into the peritoneal cavity may occur as cysts are commonly subserosal in location. Following rupture into the peritoneum, the cyst may die and no further difficulty ensues. Hankins believes that the presence of bile decreases chances of peritoneal implantation.[77] The cysts may implant in the peritoneal cavity, however, and generalized infestation of the peritoneum occurs with slowly progressing size of the abdomen. Death may ultimately ensue. The rupture does not usually evacuate the cyst completely; therefore, it may seal with recurrence of the intrahepatic portion of the cyst. It is often stated that rupture of the cyst results in implantation in most instances. Schiller, however, in a long term follow-up study of 30 patients with documented ruptures of hydatid cysts, found positive evidence of dissemination in only 4.[193] Ten of the 30 patients were followed for more than 5 years. All were alive for periods up to 26 years and 9 were asymptomatic. It thus appears that statistically the chance of dissemination is less than often quoted, but it may constitute a severe problem when it occurs.

Cysts located at the dome of the diaphragm may rupture through the diaphragm into the pleural cavity or into the bronchus. Nicks, in a review of 91 patients with hydatid disease treated in a 5 year period, recorded 7 patients with intrapleural rupture from hepatic cysts.[150] This complication may result in a chronic hepatobronchial fistula or the development of an empyema containing both bile and the viable contents of the hepatic cyst. Rupture into other organs may occur because of adherence to the stomach or duodenum. Even rupture into the vena cava has been reported.

Infection. The contents of hydatid cysts are usually bacteriologically sterile. Secondary infection, however, can occur either from extension to the biliary tract or from septicemia. Active infection of the cyst may result in death of the parasite.

Allergic Manifestations. Allergic manifestations to the cyst fluid are common. Urticaria is probably the most common allergic manifestation, but true anaphylactic shock may be observed, particularly in association with rupture of the cyst. Schiller reported a 7 per cent mortality rate from anaphylactic shock following rupture into the peritoneal cavity.[193]

Clinical Features. Many patients with hydatid cysts have no symptoms and remain in good health even though the cyst becomes sufficiently large to be found by palpation on physical examination. In the absence of complications, the only symptoms are vague abdominal distress due to pressure on adjacent organs. With the development of complications, however, significant symptoms develop. Harris described a triad of symptoms typical of rupture into the biliary tract which included: (1) biliary colic in an adolescent or young adult, (2) jaundice, and (3) findings of the laminated membrane in the feces.[80] The symptoms are similar to those of cholelithiasis and cholecystitis and the diagnosis is suspected only if there is other evidence of hydatid disease or if the patient lives in an endemic area. Intraperitoneal rupture, on the other hand, is associated with severe symptoms usually consisting of abdominal pain. Shock may occur as may other signs of sensitivity, and the patient develops the physical findings of an acute abdominal catastrophe. Intrathoracic rupture may be acute or chronic and is also characterized by severe pain as well as dyspnea and coughing when rupture has occurred into the bronchus. When bronchial rupture has occurred the material expectorated may be bile stained.

Secondary infection should be suspected if the cyst becomes tender. Chills and fever may follow.

Diagnosis. Several laboratory tests aid in diagnosis. An increase in circulating *eosinophils* (over 7 per cent) is present in one quarter of patients and is less than 2 per cent in half of patients with echinococcosis.[181] Eosinophil counts are elevated in a higher percentage of patients with rupture than in those with simple intrahepatic cysts. The standardized *Casoni* test has the widest use and is considered the most reliable immunologic procedure by most investigators. This is performed by injection of 0.2 ml. of sterile hydatid fluid intradermally. The positive test is characterized by development of a wheal in 15 minutes, and should be compared with a control saline injection. A positive reaction may occur many years after treatment of this disease. In contradistinction, the *complement fixation test,* which also has a high incidence of positive reaction during the active stage of infection, usually becomes negative within a few months after removal of the cyst. Serologic tests including the indirect hemagglutination, bentonite flocculation and latex agglutination tests have been reported positive in 82 per cent of patients infected with *E. granulosa.*[98] After rupture into the biliary tract, elements of the parasite may be found in the stool or if there has been rupture into the tracheobronchial tree, the material produced by coughing will contain contents of this cyst.[195]

In endemic areas the roentgenographic findings of a calcific cystic lesion is suggestive of an echinococcus cyst. Uncalcified cysts may also be observed on plain roentgenograms of the abdominal cavity and may displace organs or diaphragm. When gas enters the cyst the inner membrane falls away from the adventitia and floats on the remaining cyst fluid, producing a picture virtually pathognomonic of the disease. Other roentgenographic technics include hepatic angiography, tomography and hepatic scan following the injection of radioactive materials. These tests demonstrate filling defects within the liver, but do not allow differentiation from other types of cysts or solid tumors of the same shape.[206] When operation is performed, aspiration of the contents of the cyst will allow identification of the parasite.

Treatment. Treatment of a hydatid cyst is surgical, for there is no known drug that can be administered orally or systemically to which the disease responds. Treatment is indicated whenever the diagnosis is made because of the high incidence of complications, many of which terminate fatally. Operation is performed under general anesthesia with an incision made as directly over the cyst as possible. The cyst must be sterilized and removed without contamination of the peritoneal cavity, for spillage of viable parasites may result in development of new cysts in the abdominal cavity. After the liver is well walled off with protective pads and towels, a needle is introduced into the cavity and material aspirated both to relieve pressure within the cyst and to obtain material for microscopic examination. A solution is then injected to kill the parasite before attempts at removal. In the past the most common solution was 2 per cent formalin, which kills the parasite rapidly. Unfortunately, this agent has resulted in the death of some patients and therefore is used much less frequently today. A variety of other substances may also kill the parasite. Absolute alcohol (96% alcohol) is as effective as formalin without the same degree of toxicity.[77] Harris advocates the use of 30 per cent saline.[80] After death of the parasite, the lining membrane and all cyst contents are removed. This can be accomplished by surgical resection or aspiration through a large trocar under high negative pressure. After the cyst cavity has been evacuated it may be filled with sterile saline and closed with suture unless it is infected or there is a significant communication with the biliary tree. Most authors advocate external drainage under these circumstances. Harris, however, advocates water-tight closure after filling the cyst with saline even when rupture into the biliary tree has occurred.[80] Other technics for obliteration of this cyst include filling the cyst with omentum, or obliteration around a catheter, producing a method of external drainage.[72]

When complications have occurred, the surgical procedure must be modified to control the problems that result from the complication as well as treatment of the primary cyst. When intrabiliary rupture has occurred, it is important to cleanse the biliary tree and to establish drainage. Following peritoneal rupture, careful cleansing of the peritoneal cavity is important in an attempt to prevent growth of the cyst, though such treatment may not be uniformly successful. Rupture into the pleural cavity may require open drainage and possible decortication, while rupture into the bronchus occasionally requires resection of pulmonary tissue for ultimate control.

HEPATIC ABSCESS

PYOGENIC ABSCESS OF THE LIVER

Pyogenic abscess was formerly of great importance because of its association with appendicitis. With improved treatment, however, appendicitis has become an infrequent cause of this lesion, and for a period the incidence of hepatic abscess seemed to be decreasing. Liver abscess resulting from bacterial infection is seen in many hospitals, however, with a frequency equal to that of the pre-antibiotic era, though the relative frequency of etiologic factors has changed. Many are cryptogenic and present difficult problems in diagnosis and management.

Incidence. The exact incidence of pyogenic hepatic abscess is not known because necropsy examination is not performed routinely and the diagnosis cannot be established with certainty on clinical grounds alone in many patients. Prior to 1938 (the beginning of the chemotherapeutic era) the reported postmortem incidence varied from 0.45 to 1.47 per cent,[108, 163] whereas the incidence based on total hospital admissions varied from 0.04 to 0.007 per cent.[108, 154] Of 186 cases of hepatic abscess reported by Ochsner and associates in 1938,[163, 164] pyogenic abscess constituted only 25 per cent, whereas amebic abscess comprised 75 per

cent. However, this incidence of amebic abscess was greater than that reported by others,[154] since the cases occurred in the South where the incidence of amebiasis was about 3 times greater than in the North. When all areas of the world are considered, amebic abscess is still more common than pyogenic abscess. In the United States, however, the incidence of amebiasis is decreasing. Pyogenic abscesses, though seen infrequently, constitute the majority of the hepatic abscesses. Among 146 patients with hepatic abscesses in two recent reports from hospitals in the North, almost 89 per cent were pyogenic, there being only 17 amebic abscesses.[13, 185] A similar change has occurred in our own locality. During the past 5 years 13 liver abscesses were diagnosed at the Ben Taub General Hospital, an incidence of 0.01 per cent of hospital admissions. Ten, 76 per cent of these, were pyogenic. Formerly, pyogenic hepatic abscess was encountered predominantly in male patients in the ratio of 6 to 4,[163] but in recent years the incidence of many of the predisposing conditions has declined so that today this sex difference probably does not exist. For the same reason, the distribution according to age has changed significantly. A reduction in the severity of appendicitis has lowered the incidence of complications associated with that disease, and the previous predominant occurrence of pyogenic abscess of the liver in the third and the fourth decades[163, 170] is now less striking. No racial susceptibility to pyogenic hepatic abscess has been demonstrated.

Etiology. Pyogenic abscess of the liver results from invasion of the liver by pus-producing micro-organisms. This may occur by any of several routes (Table 25–4).

Extension of Infection from Contiguous Structures. Suppurative cholangitis appears to have supplanted appendicitis as the commonest antecedent focal infection of pyogenic hepatic abscess. In 1948 Kinney and Ferrebee analyzed 222 pyogenic abscesses of the liver and found 22 per cent secondary to obstruction of the common bile duct. Of 133 abscesses involving both right and left lobes, 37 per cent were secondary to obstruction of the common duct.[107] More recent reports reveal a steadily increasing fre-

TABLE 25–4. ETIOLOGY OF PYOGENIC
HEPATIC ABSCESS

I. Extension of Infection from Contiguous
Structures
   A. Cholangitis
      1. Benign obstruction of the com-
         mon bile duct
      2. Malignant obstruction of the com-
         mon bile duct
   B. Cholecystitis
   C. Penetrating gastroduodenal ulcers
   D. Perihepatic abscess
II. Hematogenous
   A. Infection by way of the portal vein
      1. Appendicitis
      2. Inflammatory disease of stomach,
         intestine and rectum
      3. Inflammatory disease of pancreas
         and spleen
      4. Intra-abdominal abscesses
      5. Postoperative thrombophlebitis of
         portal system
      6. Omphalitis
   B. Infection by way of the hepatic artery
      1. Septicemia or bacteremia from any
         cause
III. Primary Hepatic Lesions
   A. Trauma
   B. Malignancy
   C. Miscellaneous
IV. Idiopathic or Cryptogenic

quency. Pyrtek and Bartus, for example,
found that 61 per cent of their patients had
obstruction of the biliary tree.[176] This increase may be due in part to the fact that
the complications of appendicitis and other
intra-abdominal inflammatory processes respond more readily to antibiotic therapy
than does obstructive cholangitis. It also
represents an actual increase in the number
of patients with both benign and malignant
biliary tract obstructions in our aging population.

Hepatic abscess may result also from
cholecystitis, the infection reaching the liver
by way of the lymphatic system, by penetration of gallstones, or by direct rupture of
the gallbladder itself into the adjacent liver
substance. Kinney and Ferrebee also reported 12 instances of hepatic abscess associated with inflammation of the gallbladder.[107] In 7 the abscess was due to metas-

tases, and in 5 it was the result of direct
extension. In addition, suppurative processes in the region of the pancreas may
extend directly into the liver substance.
Gastric or duodenal ulcers may penetrate
through the wall of the stomach into the
adjacent liver surfaces to produce localized
suppurative processes. However, these abscesses are almost always single, generally
small and of no clinical significance. Gastroduodenal ulcers may perforate and result in purulent collections about the liver.
These abscesses may extend directly to the
liver or indirectly by involvement of lymphatic or venous channels.

Hematogenous. INFECTION BY WAY OF
THE PORTAL VENOUS SYSTEM. Suppurative
appendicitis, complicated by portal thrombophlebitis or portal pyemia, was a common antecedent lesion in pyogenic abscess
of the liver prior to the advent of the antimicrobial agents. In fact, Ochsner and associates found that hepatic abscess secondary to suppurative appendicitis and pylephlebitis comprised 10 to 30 per cent of
their series of pyogenic hepatic abscesses.[163]
Petrén stated that hepatic abscess or suppurative pylephlebitis of the portal vein occurred in 0.3 to 0.4 per cent of all cases and
in at least 5 per cent of all fatal cases of
appendicitis.[170] Others have reported incidences of 0.09 to 0.36 per cent.[163] Pyogenic
hepatic abscess may result also from infec
tious processes in other areas drained by
the portal venous system. Less commonly
the source of infection is gastric or duodenal ulceration, enteritis, diverticulitis,
proctitis, infected hemorrhoids, as well as
infections of other intra-abdominal organs
such as the pancreas and spleen. Infectious
processes in the subhepatic region, particularly those in the lesser omental bursa, may
result in pyogenic hepatic abscess unless
surgical drainage is carried out early, for
in this region secondary involvement of
splenic and the superior mesenteric veins is
possible. Shallow has reported a pyogenic
liver abscess secondary to hemorrhagic pancreatitis and pancreatic abscess which ruptured into the splenic vein, thus infecting
the portal system.[197] Rarely, hepatic abscess occurs in infants as the result of exten-

sion of infection from the umbilicus through the umbilical veins. Of special note are the rare abscesses which follow surgery of intra-abdominal organs. Thrombophlebitis of the gastric veins, following gastrectomy, for example, has been incriminated as a cause of hepatic abscess.[129] The decreasing frequency of intra-abdominal disease as a cause for this lesion is emphasized by the fact that in the past 5 years we have encountered no patient with hepatic abscess secondary to appendicitis at the Ben Taub General Hospital despite treatment of over 150 patients with perforated appendicitis during this period.

INFECTION BY WAY OF THE HEPATIC ARTERY. A limited number of pyogenic abscesses of the liver are a result of extension, by way of the hepatic artery, of infection from processes elsewhere. These hematogenous infections may arise from osteomyelitis, subacute bacterial endocarditis, infection of the upper respiratory tract, or any other condition from which septicemia may result. Although a decrease in infection by this route would be anticipated as a result of increased availability of potent antimicrobial agents, such has not been the case, for this mode of infection is reported in 10 to 15 per cent of cases occurring in the past 25 years.

Primary Hepatic Lesions. TRAUMA. Although trauma is a rare cause of hepatic abscess, a number of cases have been reported in which injury was a predisposing factor. In the series collected from the Charity Hospital in New Orleans where a large number of injuries are seen, 10.6 per cent of the cases of hepatic abscess were secondary to trauma.[163] A review of 550 patients who survived hepatic trauma in Baylor affiliated hospitals disclosed 3 hepatic abscesses.[5] Hepatic abscess usually results from penetrating injuries that either were not treated surgically or were drained improperly. Following injury, blood and bile accumulate within the area of hepatic injury, and infection results either from micro-organisms introduced with the injuring agent or from micro-organisms already present in the hepatic parenchyma. Nonpenetrating crush injuries also may result

in pyogenic hepatic abscess. The mechanism is one of contusion of the liver substance, permitting growth of micro-organisms within the hepatic parenchyma.

MALIGNANCY. Intrahepatic malignancy, either primary or secondary, may undergo necrosis with superimposed secondary infection. In a series reported by Robertson and associates such lesions accounted for 16 per cent of all hepatic abscesses observed during a 25 year period.[185]

MISCELLANEOUS. Rare hepatic abscesses are secondary to schistosomiasis, ascaris infestation and tuberculous infections of the liver with superimposed growth of pyogenic organisms.[107, 109]

Idiopathic or Cryptogenic Hepatic Abscess. Approximately one half of all hepatic abscesses have no known predisposing cause. Although these are labeled "primary," since no distant infectious focal processes can be found, they probably are secondary abscesses which arise from infection through one of the aforementioned routes. Rothenberg and Linder are of the opinion that such abscesses are the result of hematogenous infections due to distant foci that may be so inconspicuous as to be overlooked completely.[189] Beaver, on the other hand, has expressed the belief that the idiopathic hepatic abscess is the result of unrecognized infections in the areas drained by the portal venous system.[7]

Bacteriology. Micro-organisms commonly found in pyogenic hepatic abscess are colon bacilli, streptococci and staphylococci. A number of cases due to Friedländer's bacillus have also been reported.[14, 44, 108, 153, 199] Unfortunately, detailed bacteriological studies have not been reported in all series. St. John in 1940 was of the opinion that anaerobic organisms would be found with greater frequency if proper culture technics were used.[191] A recent report by Block and associates supports this concept for in 5 of 12 patients with positive cultures, anaerobic organisms were found.[13] In several instances abscesses due to *Bacteroides funduliformis* have been encountered.[8, 68, 190] In many instances hepatic abscess that occurs without an obvious primary cause is due to *Staphylococcus aureus*.[55, 89] Frequently,

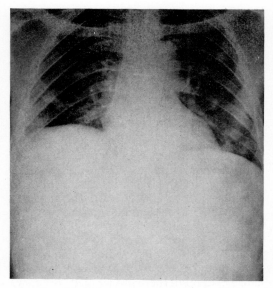

Fig. 25–9. Roentgenogram of the chest of a patient with carcinoma of the common bile duct. The right leaf of the diaphragm is elevated and the cardiophrenic sulcus is blunted slightly.

there is a long latent interval between the original infection, which is often insignificant, and the development of the hepatic abscess. Abscesses due to *Escherichia coli* may contain gas.[234] This organism is normally aerobic but is also a facultative anaerobe and gas producer, and the high glycogen count of the liver appears to be an ideal culture medium for *E. coli*. Pyogenic abscess associated with schistosomiasis and ascariasis[91, 109, 161] also has been reported. Other micro-organisms that rarely cause hepatic abscess are *Bacillus aerogenes capsulatus*, *B. pyocyaneus*, Leptothrix, Streptothrix, Salmonella, spirochetes and gonococci.

The purulent material obtained from pyogenic hepatic abscess frequently proves to be sterile when cultured. The pus was sterile in about 50 per cent of the cases reported by Elsberg[48] and Rothenberg and Linder[189] and in 40 per cent of the cases reported by Ochsner and associates.[164]

Pathogenesis and Pathology. The infrequency with which hepatic abscess occurs is somewhat surprising in view of the liver's direct vascular communications with the portal and the systemic circulations, its inti-

mate biliary system, and its communicating lymphatic channels. That infection is not encountered more commonly is due undoubtedly to the liver's rich blood supply, its characteristic sinusoidal vascular structure with freely moving blood, and the phagocytic reticuloendothelial cells that make up the parenchyma. These factors combine to provide a high degree of immunity against localization of infection and the subsequent development of abscess. As pointed out previously, infection by way of the portal and the systemic circulations was the commonest mode of development of pyogenic hepatic abscess prior to the advent of the antibiotic agents. However, the biliary system has come to play an increasingly important role in the pathogenesis of hepatic abscess, largely as a result of the relative increase in incidence of hepatic abscess secondary to biliary obstruction and ascending cholangitis. Common duct obstruction may be due to a variety of causes, such as gallstones, inflammatory strictures about the ampulla of Vater or inflammatory or neoplastic diseases of the pancreas. Infection of the biliary system commonly is superimposed upon biliary stasis secondary to common duct obstruction, and the spread of the inflammatory process through the biliary tract and into the substance of the liver follows rapidly (Figs. 25–9 and 25–10). When the bile ducts are the route of infection, the distribution of the infectious process corresponds to the architecture of the bile duct system, thus frequently resulting in multiple suppurative foci. Periphlebitis may be superimposed on suppurative cholangitis by extension of infection along the portal spaces through the lymphatics or the small veins of the bile ducts. Such a process may result in involvement of almost the entire liver and closely resembles the abscesses resulting from appendicitis and portal pyemia. In cholecystitis associated with cholelithiasis, occasionally the gallstones penetrate the gallbladder bed and directly involve the liver substance, or the gallbladder ruptures directly into the hepatic parenchyma with development of a localized hepatic abscess.

Although in the older literature acute suppurative appendicitis was considered as

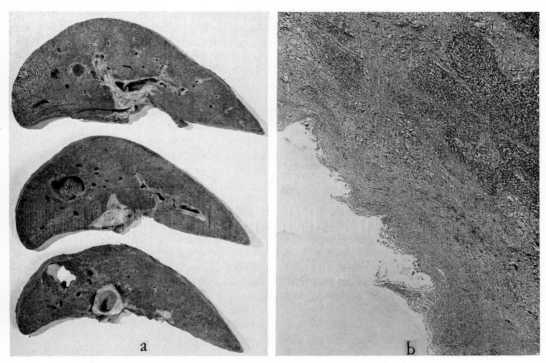

Fig. 25–10. (a) Postmortem examination of the patient represented in Fig. 25–9 disclosed a large pyogenic abscess occupying the right lobe of the liver and extending toward the diaphragmatic surface. (b) Photomicrograph of section taken from the wall of the abscess. The inner margin of the abscess is composed of cellular debris and infiltration of leukocytes. More peripherally, fibrous connective tissue and inflammatory cells are interspersed among islands of hepatic cells.

the most common antecedent lesion in pyogenic hepatic abscess, its frequency probably was overestimated. Today, with the decline of complications of acute appendicitis, its role in the production of pyogenic hepatic abscess has become even less important. Waller in 1846 reported probably the first instance of appendicitis complicated by multiple hepatic abscesses.[163] Later, Reginald Fitz, in his classic description of appendicitis, mentioned its occurrence.[57] The French clinicians, particularly, recognized the importance of appendicitis as an antecedent lesion.[43] The proper genesis of this infection is easy to follow. In the course of inflammation of the appendix, thrombophlebitis of the appendiceal intramural vessels occurs. The phlebitis can involve progressively the appendiceal veins and the mesoappendix, the ileocecal, the superior mesenteric and the portal veins, or

a small septic embolus can become detached from the thrombus in the immediate neighborhood of the inflamed appendix and be transported through the contributing venous channels and the portal vein to the liver. The abscesses are usually multiple and for the most part occupy the right lobe. The explanation for this latter fact lies in the experimental work of Sérégé,[196] Glenard,[66] Bartlett,[4] Copher and Dick,[35] and, more recently, Kinney and Ferrebee.[107] These investigators have demonstrated two currents of blood in the portal vein: one from the superior mesenteric vein, which flows to the right lobe, and one from the inferior mesenteric and splenic veins, which flows to the left lobe.

Other lesions in the portal area may cause pyogenic hepatic abscess by extension of infection via the portal route. Infected hemorrhoids, proctitis, diverticulitis, bacillary dysentery, carcinoma of the colon, and ulcerations of the intestinal tract are all potential causes of hepatic abscess. In addition, hepatic abscess may result from direct extension from contiguous suppurative processes. Gastric or duodenal ulceration with localized abscess formation may extend through the hepatic capsule and produce an abscess of the liver. Infection of the pleural cavity has been reported to penetrate the diaphragm and invade the substance of the liver.

Direct trauma to the liver, such as penetrating wounds, may give rise to hepatic suppuration. Injuries that produce the greatest destruction of hepatic tissue are more likely to be followed by infection and abscess formation. Blunt trauma to the body wall may also produce injury to the hepatic tissue, either by contusion with parenchymal hemorrhage and extravasation of bile, or by tear of the hepatic capsule and fracture of parenchyma. Then the traumatized portion of the liver may become invaded by pathogenic organisms that are always present in the liver substance. The abscesses resulting from trauma are usually single and well localized.

Pyogenic hepatic abscess may result also from penetration of foreign bodies. Bullet and stab wounds account for most, but unusual penetrating foreign bodies, such as a fishbone, a piece of glass, a fragment of straw and a toothpick have been reported.[145, 163]

Hepatic abscesses may be single or multiple. Multiple pyogenic abscesses of the liver usually result from involvement of the portal vein, the hepatic artery, or the biliary system. Ochsner and associates found multiple hepatic abscesses in 45.5 per cent of their cases, with involvement of the right lobe in 68.1 per cent, the left lobe in 2.2 per cent, and both lobes in 27.2 per cent,[163] whereas Kinney and Ferrebee reported an incidence of 32, 8 and 59 per cent for these respective lobes.[107] It has been suggested that many of the large solitary abscesses begin as multiple small lesions and increase in size and coalesce to form one large abscess cavity. Rothenberg and Linder found that the single abscess occurs 5 times more frequently in the right than in the left lobe

and is usually near the dome of the liver.[189] Chronic solitary hepatic abscess with fibrous tissue formation of the wall has been well described by Beaver.[7] In 8 cases reported by him the abscesses were extremely chronic in nature, varying in duration from 10 months to over 2 years. The granulomatous appearance of these lesions was striking.

In suppurative pylephlebitis the portal vein and its branches contain pus and disintegrated blood clots. Dilatation of the veins, which is due to weakening of the walls of the vessels resulting from the inflammatory process, with subsequent bulging is characteristic. Further involvement of the vessel may lead to perforation, which facilitates escape of pus into the surrounding hepatic parenchyma. The extent to which the portal vessels are involved may vary considerably. The liver containing a hepatic abscess is almost invariably enlarged (Figs. 25–10a and 25–11a). In some instances its weight is doubled. Because of involvement of Glisson's capsule, perihepatitis is common and occasionally may produce adherence to the diaphragm. Coagulation necrosis precedes suppuration and may give the erroneous impression of multiple metastatic nodules from a distant neoplasm. The organ may present a mottled appearance, the areas of abscess formation being pale yellow in contrast with the deep maroon color of the uninvolved hepatic tissue. On section, the abscesses, when multiple, may be seen scattered throughout the liver substance (Fig. 25–12a), although in some cases they are more or less confined to particular areas, the left lobe escaping involvement more often than the right. The necrotic areas may vary in size from a fraction of 1 mm. to 1 cm. or more. Coalescent small abscesses form larger cavities, or, in some cases, adjacent necrotic areas lend a honeycombed appearance to the diseased organ. The hepatic parenchyma may be destroyed so extensively as to leave only a shell of the organ.

Microscopically, pylephlebitis is characterized by round-cell infiltration of the venous wall, with leukocytes and cellular debris present in the lumen. Adjacent hepatic cells exhibit reaction to the inflammatory process, with various stages of degen-

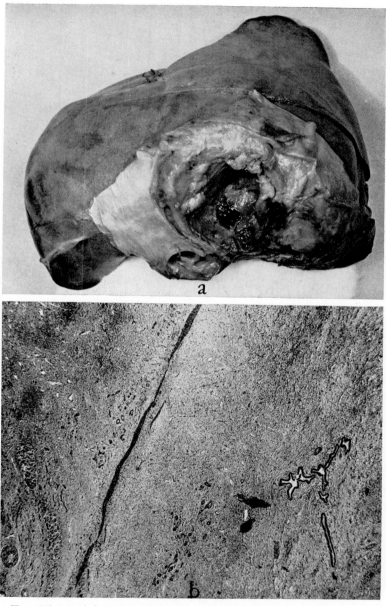

FIG. 25–11. (a) Postmortem examination of patient represented in Fig. 25–15 disclosed a large abscess in the right lobe of the liver that had extended through the diaphragm and into the right pleural space, producing thoracic empyema. (b) Photomicrograph of section taken from the wall of the abscess. There is extensive infiltration of hepatic parenchyma with fibrous connective tissue, and aggregations of lymphocytes, plasma cells and large mononuclear cells. Islands of hepatic cells and newly formed bile ducts are evident.

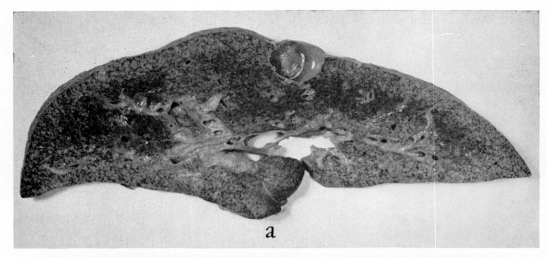

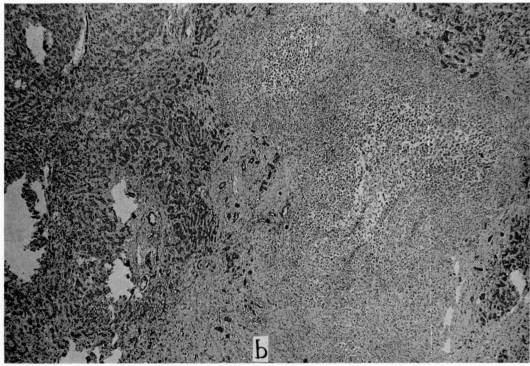

FIG. 25–12. (a) Postmortem examination of patient represented in Fig. 25–14 disclosed multiple, small cholangitic abscesses throughout the hepatic parenchyma. (b) Photomicrograph of section of hepatic parenchyma containing an abscess. A central area of necrosis is surrounded by leukocytic infiltration. On the periphery, fibrous connective tissue and infiltration of inflammatory cells are interspersed among hepatic cells.

eration usually demonstrable. Cellular necrosis characterizes the area of abscess formation (Fig. 25–10b). The central portions of the larger lesions contain practically nothing but cellular debris, whereas a fibrous capsule limits the periphery (Fig. 25–11b). The multiple abscess cavities occurring in suppurative cholangitis usually

LABORATORY FINDINGS

Leukocyte count - 20,100   BSP (retention 30') - 26%
Thymol Turbidity - 8 units   Serum Bilirubin - 1.9 mgm
Cephalin Flocculation - 2 +

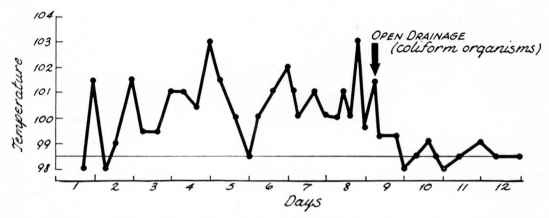

FIG. 25–13. Clinical chart of the patient with a large solitary abscess of the liver represented in Fig. 25–16. Following open drainage of the abscess, the symptoms subsided rapidly. Culture of purulent material removed during drainage disclosed coliform organisms.

are filled with bile-stained purulent material (Fig. 25–12b).

Clinical Manifestations. Symptoms. The symptoms of pyogenic hepatic abscess may be due primarily to involvement of the liver itself, the systemic response to hepatic sepsis, or the inflammatory process from which the hepatic abscess originated.

Fever is almost always the initial symptom. The temperature may be 100° to 105° F. Fever is remittent, intermittent or continuous, depending upon the type of abscess and the pathogenic organisms involved. Characteristically, multiple hepatic abscesses associated with cholangitis, pylephlebitis and suppurative appendicitis give rise to a fever of the "picket fence" type, which is accompanied by daily chills. The solitary pyogenic abscess generally produces a less severe febrile response, and chills occur less frequently (Fig. 25–13). The occurrence of chills followed by rapid rise of temperature during the course of appendicitis is strongly suggestive of pylephlebitis and hepatic abscess.

Malaise, anorexia, weakness, loss of weight and abdominal distention are common. Nausea and vomiting occur in about 20 per cent of patients.

Pain, usually dull and constant, is almost always present but is rarely the initial symptom. Pain occurs most commonly over the hepatic area, either anteriorly in the right hypochondrium or epigastrium, or laterally in the axillary line. It may extend to the right shoulder, probably as a result of phrenic irritation. About 40 per cent of Rothenberg and Linder's patients complained of pain on inspiration in the region of the lower right portion of the chest, probably as a result of involvement of the diaphragmatic pleura. Intercostal pain and development of pleural effusion have been noted also.

The average duration of symptoms depends upon the type of onset. About 6 per cent of Rothenberg and Linder's[189] patients had symptoms 3 weeks or less prior to hospitalization, whereas this group constituted approximately 40 per cent of the cases collected by Ochsner and associates,[163] the average duration being 11 days.

Physical Findings. Enlargement of the liver and tenderness in the hepatic area are the most constant physical signs. The liver is enlarged, in either an upward or a downward direction, in 60 to 90 per cent of patients with pyogenic hepatic abscess. This is one of the few conditions that produce upward enlargement of the liver. Tenderness over the hepatic area can be elicited in almost all patients with hepatic abscess. Occasionally, the abscess produces a localized, downward enlargement of the liver that can be palpated below the costal margin. Infrequently, the skin overlying the abscess is red and swollen; this indicates involvement of the abdominal parietes. Jaundice is a common sign of hepatic abscess associated with ascending cholangitis and of multiple abscesses of pylephlebitic origin but is rare in other types of hepatic abscess; when it occurs it is of grave prognostic import.

In the absence of pre-existing hepatic disease, ascites is rare except as a terminal event. When it does develop, it is more likely to be in cases of hepatic abscess originating in appendicitis and suppurative pylephlebitis.

If the abscess projects below the costal margin, spasm of the muscles in the upper right quadrant (epigastrium) may be present, and then the liver border is felt with difficulty. Tenderness in the intercostal spaces is common and is usually associated with limitation of expansion of the right lower portion of the chest. Generally, the patient prefers to lie on the right side because of the splinting effect which this position affords. In upward enlargement of the liver, dullness is increased over the right lower portion of the chest, and if the inflammatory process involves the diaphragm, rales at the base of the right lung or signs of pleural effusion may be elicited.

Laboratory Observations. Pyogenic hepatic abscess is associated characteristically with leukocytosis, which generally varies in degree with the acuteness of the suppurative process (Fig. 25–13). An average leukocyte count of 26,924 cells/cu.mm., with 89 per cent polymorphonuclear leukocytes in the most acute cases, has been reported.[163] In the more chronic cases the leukocyte count is slightly elevated, and the number of polymorphonuclear leukocytes

is also proportionately less. In a group of patients with solitary hepatic abscess, an average leukocyte count of 16,000 cells/cu.mm., with 86 per cent polymorphonuclear leukocytes, was found.[189] In the chronic hepatic abscesses the leukocyte count may be normal. Acute hepatic abscess may be associated with slight anemia, whereas in chronic abscesses almost invariably the erythrocyte count and hemoglobin are reduced.

Urinalysis generally reveals nothing abnormal. In patients with a severe septic course albuminuria may be present, and jaundice usually is associated with bile in the urine. Hirschowitz is of the opinion that excessive amounts of urobilin should be present in the urine, and that normal amounts practically exclude pyogenic hepatic abscess.[87]

If hepatic abscess results from septicemia, blood cultures are positive. In the usual patient hepatic function tests provide little information of diagnostic value with one exception. The serum alkaline phosphatase concentration may be elevated when all other tests of hepatic function are normal.[73] This test was abnormal in 3 of 4 cases reported by Matheson and associates.[129] The cause for this elevation, which may be observed also in intrahepatic malignancy, is not understood. Elevation of the serum bilirubin concentration and other abnormalities of hepatic function tests occur in those patients who develop jaundice. Rapidly occurring hepatic enlargement in a patient with normal liver function should suggest the presence of hepatic abscess. On the other hand, hepatic abscess occasionally may masquerade as portal cirrhosis.

Roentgenographic Observations. Roentgenographic examination is one of the most effective aids in the diagnosis of hepatic abscess. Characteristically, elevation and limitation or absence of motion of the diaphragm, particularly on the right, can be demonstrated fluoroscopically or roentgenographically. These changes have been emphasized by a number of observers.[42, 168] The characteristic changes in contour of the diaphragm in hepatic abscess were first noted by Granger[70] and subsequently emphasized by others.[156, 157, 159, 160, 162] Obliter-

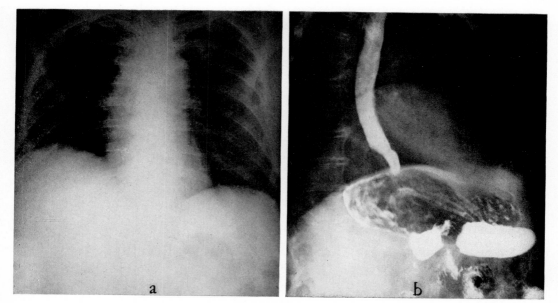

Fig. 25–14. (a) Posteroanterior roentgenogram of the chest of a patient with carcinoma of the pancreas and cholangitis. The right leaf of the diaphragm is elevated, and the cardiophrenic sulcus is partially obliterated. (b) Lateral roentgenogram taken during an upper gastrointestinal series 1 week later shows marked elevation of the right leaf of the diaphragm, particularly in its anterior portion, with obliteration of the anterior costophrenic sulcus.

ation of the cardiophrenic angle in the posteroanterior roentgenogram (Figs. 25–9 and 25–14a) and obliteration of the anterior costophrenic angle in the lateral view (Figs. 25–14b and 25–15c) are character-istic of hepatic abscess associated with subphrenic infection. On the other hand, in subphrenic abscess due to other causes, the posteroanterior view shows obliteration of the costophrenic angle; the lateral view shows

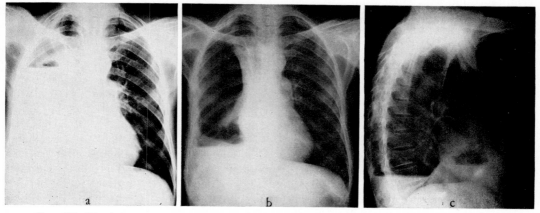

Fig. 25–15. (a) Posteroanterior roentgenogram of the chest reveals a loculated, right hydrothorax. (b) Following thoracentesis, almost complete collapse of the lung is noted. (c) Right lateral roentgenogram reveals elevation of the anterior portion of the right leaf of the diaphragm with obliteration of the anterior costophrenic sulcus. A cavity beneath the diaphragm appears to extend upward into the chest.

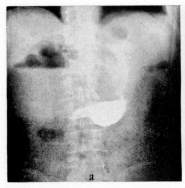
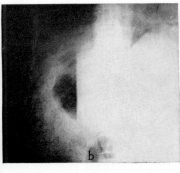
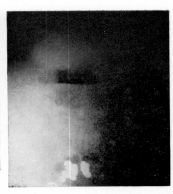

Fig. 25–16. Roentgenograms of the diaphragmatic region of a 54-year-old patient with vague, upper abdominal symptoms and impaired liver function. (a) Anteroposterior roentgenogram made during upper gastrointestinal series reveals a gas pocket with fluid level in the region of the right lobe of the liver. (b) With the patient in the lateral decubitus position, the roentgenogram shows the abscess occupies almost the entire thickness of the right lobe of the liver. (c) Right lateral roentgenogram indicates the anteroposterior extent of the abscess.

obliteration of the posterior costophrenic angle.[155, 159] Abscesses involving the left lobe of the liver may be more difficult to demonstrate roentgenographically, but, as pointed out by Miles,[139] abscesses of the left lobe may produce pressure deformities on the barium-filled stomach in which the lesser curvature assumes a crescentic shape and the cardia and the duodenal cap are displaced. When hepatic abscess is associated with subphrenic infection, pleural effusion is common. Indeed, pulmonary symptoms and roentgenographic signs may be so prominent as to obscure the symptoms and signs pointing to hepatic abscess.

In 40 per cent of the cases of single pyogenic hepatic abscess reported by Rothenberg and Linder,[189] elevation and fixation of the diaphragm were noted, and roentgenographic signs were positive in 82.1 per cent of the cases studied by Ochsner and associates.[163] When the hepatic infection is due to gas-producing organisms, fluid levels within the liver substance may be demonstrated roentgenographically (Fig. 25–16).

Roentgenographic examination following aspiration of a hepatic abscess and injection of radiopaque material or air has been suggested by a number of investigators. Wilmoth employed Lipiodol.[227] Reeves,[183] Huard,[91] and Carnot[25] advocated injection of thorium dioxide into the cavity. These methods determine the size, shape and position of the abscess. However, it is questionable whether such procedures have practical value in view of the potential hazard of thorium dioxide, and the possibility of contamination of pleural or peritoneal cavity by the aspirating needle. Hepatosplenography in cases of suspected hepatic abscess was suggested by Reeves and Stuck, as early as 1938[182] and during the next few years several investigators reported enthusiastically on the use of this procedure.[54, 110, 136, 183] This technic did not become popular because of the hazard from radioactivity and the granuloma formation which followed use of Thorotrast. Today, however, hepatic scan has become a very useful diagnostic tool. Two agents, radioactive rose bengal I[131] and radioactive colloidal gold, can be used safely and allow a high degree of accuracy in diagnosis (Fig. 25–17). Both anteroposterior and lateral scans should be made for localization. Block and associates have noted that this technic allows early diagnosis and results in prompt treatment with a decrease in mortality and morbidity.[13] Newer radioactive agents are under study which may prove to be superior to those now available. In our experience hepatography with radioactive materials has not given the high degree of diagnostic accuracy reported by some; nevertheless, it is a valuable procedure and, as noted, is safe.

Diagnosis. Although the diagnosis of pyogenic hepatic abscess should not be difficult if the condition is kept in mind and if adequate clinical and laboratory procedures are carried out, unfortunately many are not diagnosed prior to operation or autopsy and others are recognized only after prolonged observation of the patient, being a diagnosis of exclusion. In a patient with pain and tenderness localized in the hepatic area and with hepatomegaly, associated with chills and fever, the possibility of pyogenic hepatic abscess always should be considered. Pain and tenderness, although usually well localized to the right lower portion of the chest or the right upper abdominal quadrant, may be present in the epigastrium or may extend to the right shoulder. Occasionally, pain is confined to the lower portion of the chest and, in the presence of tenderness in the intercostal spaces and aggravation of pain by deep breathing and coughing, suggests some primary involvement of the respiratory system. In acute cases the leukocyte count should be fairly high with predominance of polymorphonuclear forms. Fluoroscopy and roentgenograms of the chest and the abdomen will reveal the characteristic changes already described. It is important that roentgenograms of the chest include the diaphragm and that the patient be in the erect position when the films are made. Both postero-anterior and right lateral exposures should be made. Nausea and vomiting are not common in hepatic abscess, except when they result from an associated intra-abdominal process. In fact, absence of nausea and vomiting in the presence of clinical manifestations of intra-abdominal sepsis points to a diagnosis of hepatic abscess.

It is of prognostic and therapeutic importance to determine the origin of the hepatic suppuration and the number of abscesses. In a patient with a history of suppurative appendicitis, the diagnosis of multiple hepatic abscesses associated with pylephlebitis should not be difficult. The preceding suppurative appendicitis, the sudden onset of chills and fever, pain and tenderness extending from the right iliac region up to the hepatic area, the high white blood count and the obvious sepsis constitute a classic clinical picture. Chills and fever and pronounced leukocytosis in a patient with biliary obstruction should suggest the development of multiple hepatic abscesses, particularly if there is pain and tenderness over the hepatic area. Lesions in the portal area other than acute appendicitis likewise may give rise to multiple hepatic abscesses, and the occurrence of this complication should be kept in mind when treating any intra-abdominal abscess. Hepatography should be performed whenever the diagnosis is considered but not proved by other means.

The single pyogenic hepatic abscess generally is associated with an insidious onset, and frequently it is impossible to determine the origin of the infection. Fever and chills are less prominent, and the leukocyte response is less striking. Jaundice is not common in the single pyogenic hepatic abscess unless it reaches a large size. Thus, in general, the solitary hepatic abscess is more difficult to diagnose than the multiple acute abscesses.

It is important to differentiate pyogenic hepatic abscess from amebic abscess. This may be difficult when the pyogenic hepatic abscess is of the solitary type and is somewhat chronic. The onset of the amebic hepatic abscess is usually insidious. The temperature may be elevated slightly or only moderately, chills rarely occur, and the patient does not appear to be ill. The presence of previous diarrhea and the finding of *Entamoeba histolytica* in the stools confirm the diagnosis. Amebic abscesses may become infected secondarily, in which case they should be treated as pyogenic abscesses. Aspiration of the liver as a diagnostic procedure probably is unwarranted in pyogenic hepatic abscess. Although with the use of antimicrobial agents this procedure carries less risk than formerly, in the majority of instances the diagnosis can be made by other means, and it is preferable to employ needle aspiration only when operative exposure of the liver has been carried out. Unfortunately, despite the clinical and laboratory procedures described above, many hepatic abscesses are not even suspected during life. Of 37 patients re-

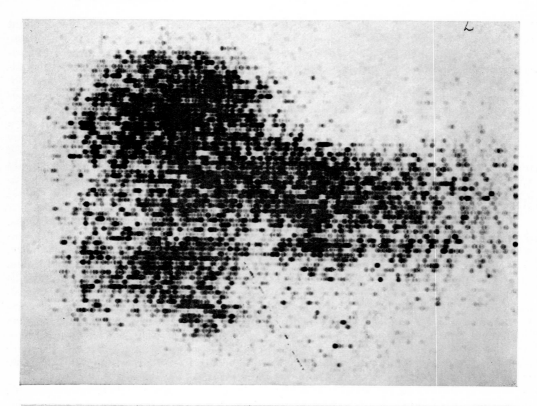

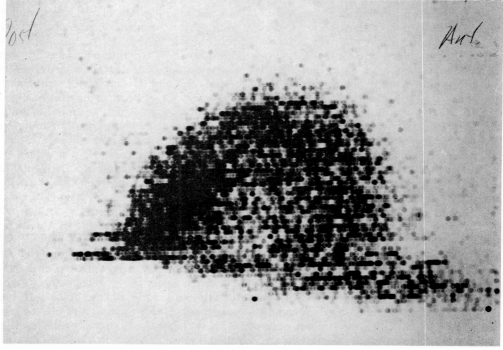

FIGURE 25–17. (*Caption on facing page.*)

ported by Robertson and associates in 1966, 24 were found at necropsy and only 9 were accurately diagnosed and treated.[185] The experience of Pyrtek and Bartus was similar, for 26 of 42 abscesses resulting from benign disease were diagnosed at autopsy—only 16 being treated.[176] Block and associates, however, using hepatic scans as a diagnostic tool, have improved their results and during 1962-1963 diagnosed and successfully treated eight consecutive patients.[13]

Complications. Complications of pyogenic hepatic abscess may result from rupture or extension into adjacent structures and, when present, add to the gravity of the condition. In a collected series of 258 cases and in 47 cases of their own, Ochsner and associates found the fatality rate to be, respectively, 60.8 and 36 per cent without complications and 90.7 and 90.9 per cent with complications.[163] The incidence of complications depends largely upon the extent of the hepatic involvement as well as the location of the abscess. Formerly, the incidence of complications was about 25 to 30 per cent.[163] The exact incidence since the introduction of the antibiotic agents is not known, but it probably has been lowered significantly.

Pleuropulmonary involvement, the most frequent complication of pyogenic hepatic abscess, occurs in 15 to 20 per cent of cases. It develops either by direct extension through the diaphragm or by embolism. The former route is usually responsible for extension of the infectious process. Pleuropulmonary complications are commonly associated with single pyogenic abscess of the liver, except in cases of septicemia, in which involvement of other organs is likely to occur. The solitary abscess most frequently occurs in the right lobe of the liver and usually near the dome. As the abscess cavity enlarges, it extends toward the diaphragm, and soon this structure is incorporated into the wall of the abscess. If the abscess enlarges rapidly before adherent

pleuritis develops, it may rupture directly into the pleural cavity with resulting empyema (Fig. 25–15). On the other hand, if it enlarges slowly, pleurisy with adhesions develops simultaneously, and the pleural cavity is obliterated. Thus, in the absence of a free pleural space, the abscess ruptures directly into the lung.

Peritonitis may complicate pyogenic hepatic abscess as a result either of rupture of the abscess into the peritoneal cavity or of contamination by transperitoneal drainage of the abscess. Because of the extremely high incidence of peritonitis following transpleural or transperitoneal drainage of hepatic abscesses, methods of avoiding contamination of pleural or peritoneal surfaces were devised with striking reduction in the incidence of pleural or peritoneal complications following drainage.[149, 155, 163]

Pyogenic hepatic abscesses are complicated by the development of a subphrenic abscess in 2 to 5 per cent of cases. If septicemia is the antecedent infection, lesions will be observed in other organs also, such as the lungs, the spleen, the kidneys and the brain. Formerly, this type of complication was reported to occur in about 4 per cent of cases, and the results were invariably fatal. Within recent years, however, with the striking improvement in the results of treatment of septicemia it is likely that some patients with multiple visceral abscesses are now recovering from this formerly fatal condition.

Rarely, pyogenic hepatic abscess ruptures into the pericardium,[235] vena cava,[163] hepatic vein,[95, 220] thoracic duct[151] or abdominal wall.[163]

Treatment. The treatment of pyogenic hepatic abscess may be considered conveniently under prophylactic and active measures.

Prophylactic Measures. Therapeutic measures directed toward control and eradication of the common antecedent infection are of great prophylactic value. Formerly,

FIG. 25–17. Hepatic scan using radioactive colloidal gold in a patient with pyogenic abscess of the right lobe. (*Top*) Scan in anteroposterior position revealing filling defect in right lobe. (*Bottom*) Scan in lateral position which localizes the abscess to the inferior aspect of the midportion of the lobe. (From John A. Burdine, M.D., Chief, Isotope Service, Ben Taub General Hospital, Houston, Texas)

it was considered essential in patients with appendicitis and preoperative history of chills to examine the appendiceal, ileocolic, inferior mesenteric vessels and portal vein during operation. This would permit detection of thrombosis in these vessels and its degree of extension, so that appropriate surgical therapy could be instituted and thus prevent the possible development of pylephlebitis and multiple hepatic abscesses. In the older medical literature there are a number of reports of operations for pylephlebitis occurring either in the pre- or postoperative period. Evacuation of the infected, thrombosed vein was advocated by Gerster[64] as early as 1903. Somewhat later, Wilms successfully treated a case by ligation of the veins at the ileocecal angle.[228] In 1913 Braun proposed ligation of the ileocolic vein and reported two cases successfully treated in this way.[17] Others unsuccessfully attempted ligation of the portal vein in pylephlebitis.[10, 29]

The necessity of these prophylactic operations is obviated by the routine employment of antimicrobial drugs in the treatment of infectious processes that give rise to pyogenic hepatic abscess. Thus, although at the time of appendectomy there may be evidence of involvement of the appendiceal or ileocolic veins, prompt institution of antibiotic therapy generally not only prevents dissemination of the infectious process but eradicates it entirely in most instances.

When suppurative cholangitis is a result of obstruction of the extrahepatic biliary ducts, it is imperative to provide biliary drainage to control the infection. Symptoms rapidly subside in most patients following surgical drainage combined with appropriate antibiotic therapy.

Active Measures. The active treatment of pyogenic hepatic abscess consists in drainage of the abscess, when feasible, and administration of appropriate antibiotic agents (Fig. 25–13). Surgical drainage is effective primarily in solitary abscesses. In most instances the abscess can be localized by appropriate studies. Formerly, drainage through an extraserous approach was emphasized in contrast with the transperitoneal or transpleural approaches, which were associated with an extremely high fatality rate. Today, however, there appears to be no increase in morbidity or mortality associated with transperitoneal drainage, which should be employed for abscesses localized in the anterior or antero-inferior surface of the liver. The abdominal cavity is entered through a cutaneous incision made just beneath and parallel with the costal margin. The involved area of the liver is located, and with the adjacent viscera protected by gauze packs, the abscess is opened and evacuated. Similarly, if a pyogenic abscess of the liver is discovered during laparotomy, it should be drained at that time. On the other hand, if there is no evidence of localization of the abscess in the anterior abdominal region, the best method of drainage is by the retroperitoneal approach.[149] The cutaneous incision is made over the twelfth rib, which is resected subperiosteally, and a transverse incision is made through its bed at the level of the spinous process of the first lumbar vertebra. The retroperitoneal space is entered through this incision between the upper pole of the kidney and the inferior surface of the liver. Then the parietal peritoneum is mobilized from beneath the diaphragm, and the abscess can be completely drained extraserously.

In most instances the cavity created by the abscess will rapidly fill in with granulation tissue following adequate drainage. However, in some cases drainage persists indefinitely, necessitating closure of the cavity with a flap constructed from the thoracic or the abdominal wall.

Broad-spectrum antibiotic therapy should be instituted when the diagnosis is made. At the time of drainage of the abscess the purulent material should be cultured to identify the specific organisms and to test them for sensitivity to antibiotics. Specific antimicrobial therapy should be instituted as soon as possible. Rarely a hepatic abscess located near the lower border of the liver can be completely excised.

Multiple hepatic abscesses usually cannot be drained surgically. For this reason, therapy must consist in intensive administration of antibiotics and supportive measures. In many instances the infecting organism can be identified by culture of material from the site of the antecedent infection. In other instances the multiple abscesses may be discovered at laparotomy, and aspiration of one of the abscesses will yield material for culture. Multiple liver abscesses that develop as a result of suppurative cholangitis are treated best by drainage of the extrahepatic biliary ducts combined with intensive antimicrobial therapy.

Schramel reports a case of suppurative cholangitis with multiple hepatic abscesses secondary to common duct obstruction. The infection was due to *Proteus vulgaris,* and over a period of 9 years had failed to respond to antibiotic therapy, although common duct obstruction was relieved. Finally, a catheter was placed in a tributary of the portal vein, and one of the nitrofurans was administered directly into the portal vein. The fever subsided promptly, and the patient has remained well during the 10 months since treatment.[194]

Complications. The complications resulting from pyogenic hepatic abscess usually are treated at the same time as the abscess, since hepatic abscess is diagnosed in many instances only after complications have developed. Thoracic empyema resulting from rupture of a pyogenic hepatic abscess through the diaphragm should be drained. Usually, the point of perforation through the diaphragm can be located at the time of thoracotomy, and the location of the abscess within the liver can be ascertained. Following evacuation of the pleural space and decortication of the pulmonary surfaces, the opening in the diaphragm is repaired if necessary. The thoracotomy wound is closed, and the chest is drained by an intercostal catheter connected to a water-seal suction bottle. Then the hepatic abscess is drained, usually through a separate incision, depending upon its location.

If thoracic empyema is due to lymphatic extension of the infectious process across the diaphragm from the liver, it is necessary only to drain the empyema and to re-expand the lung. The hepatic abscess is treated separately by drainage anteriorly or posteriorly.

Bronchohepatic fistula usually requires no therapy other than administration of appropriate antibiotic drugs, for the abscess cavity may be evacuated completely through the bronchial fistula. Persistence of symptoms following development of a bronchohepatic fistula is indicative of inadequate drainage. Under these circumstances the hepatic abscess should be drained surgically.

Pyogenic pulmonary abscess secondary to pyogenic hepatic abscess is managed conservatively. Abscesses not responding favorably to this type of therapy may require resection. Subphrenic abscesses can be drained simultaneously with a hepatic abscess. This is accomplished best by the extraserous route, either anteriorly or posteriorly.

Peritonitis resulting from rupture of a pyogenic hepatic abscess is treated by drainage of the hepatic abscess and evacuation of the purulent material from the peritoneal cavity at laparotomy followed by intensive antibiotic therapy.

Prognosis. The prognosis of pyogenic hepatic abscess depends on (1) the number of abscesses, (2) the type of infecting micro-organism, (3) adequacy of drainage, (4) resistance of the host, (5) presence or absence of complications and (6) nature of the antecedent infectious process. Multiple hepatic abscesses carry a graver prognosis than the solitary abscess. Prior to the advent of antibiotic drugs, multiple abscesses, especially those associated with suppurative appendicitis and pylephlebitis, were considered to be almost uniformly fatal, in striking contrast with the prognosis for the solitary abscess, largely because the single abscess usually could be drained adequately. Eliason[47] reported a case fatality rate of 50 per cent in a series of hepatic abscesses following appendicitis, but 58 per cent of these abscesses were solitary. Ochsner and associates reported a fatality rate of 95 per cent for multiple abscess and 37.5 per cent for solitary abscess.[163]

In 1939 Howard[90] collected from the literature 42 cases of hepatic abscess with recovery, of which 11 were multiple. Since then the increasing number of reports of recovery from hepatic abscess suggests that the use of antimicrobial agents has greatly altered the prognosis. This is particularly true of multiple abscesses that cannot be drained properly. For therapy to be most effective, the infecting micro-organisms must be identified bacteriologically, and antibiotic sensitivity studies must be made to determine the proper agent for therapy.

Even today the mortality rate remains extremely high because so many lesions are not diagnosed. There were only 6 survivors among 37 patients reported by Robertson and associates[185] and mortality rates as high as 69 per cent of the treated cases have been reported in recent years.[13] With accurate diagnosis and energetic therapy, however, favorable results are now being obtained. Block and associates[13] reported no deaths among the last 8 patients treated and we have had no fatalities among patients accurately diagnosed and treated during the past 5 years.

Adequate surgical drainage is one of the most effective measures in the treatment of hepatic abscess. When the abscess is solitary and can be localized properly in the liver, drainage usually brings about striking improvement in the condition of the patient and, when combined with appropriate antibiotic therapy, effects a cure in the majority of instances. When multiple abscesses are present, however, adequate surgical drainage is generally not feasible and the prognosis is not as good.

Advances in the use of adjuvant therapeutic measures have also played a significant role in the reduction of fatalities from infections. Careful maintenance of proper fluid and electrolyte balances, more liberal use of blood transfusions, and other supportive measures all tend to improve the resistance of the host to infection.

The presence or the absence of complications resulting from hepatic abscess also may affect the prognosis vitally. A fatality rate of 90.9 per cent in cases with complications as contrasted with 36 per cent in cases without complications has been reported.[163]

Finally, the nature of the antecedent infectious process influences the prognosis of hepatic abscess. If the primary infection can be controlled by antibiotic therapy, surgical drainage, or both, the prognosis is generally good. On the other hand, if the primary infection does not respond to these measures, it is unlikely that the hepatic abscess can be treated successfully, particularly if the abscesses are multiple. Infrequently, multiple hepatic abscesses develop because of septicemia which does not respond to antimicrobial therapy. Under these circumstances the hepatic involvement is simply a part of a generalized infectious process, and the prognosis is that of the septicemia. Thus, in those instances in which the infecting micro-organisms are resistant to available antibiotics, and in which drainage is not possible, the prognosis still remains grave.

HEPATIC AMEBIASIS

Kartulis is often given credit for the first description of amebic liver abscess in 1887.[50, 99] Only 4 years later Councilman and Lafleur[36] described the pathology and pathogenesis and in 1902 Rogers demonstrated ameba in the abscess wall.[186]

Formerly, amebiasis was believed to occur principally in tropical or subtropical localities. For this reason, amebic abscess of the liver commonly was called tropical abscess, and the nonamebic variety, due to pyogenic organisms, was called nontropical abscess.

It is now well recognized that amebiasis is endemic in the United States and other nontropical countries. Although more frequent in the South, amebic abscess is encountered in all areas of the United States. In fact, only 23 years ago Craig reported that 11.6 per cent of 49,336 persons examined in all parts of the United States were infected with *Entamoeba histolytica*, and 12.7 per cent of 189 American physicians were infected.[38] There is reason to believe that the incidence is much less today. Although comparable studies are not available, fewer patients are seen with clinical manifestations of the disease. Even today, however, amebiasis occurs with significant frequency in all parts of the United States, and it is a disease of major concern in many areas of the world where American troops are now stationed.

The most common site of extra-intestinal amebiasis is the liver. Amebic involvement of the liver may occur as a presuppurative stage, referred to as amebic hepatitis, and also as frank suppuration, which is designated as amebic hepatic abscess.

Incidence. The incidence of hepatic involvement varies considerably, depending upon the incidence and the relative control of the primary intestinal infection and the nature of the population from which the statistical material is derived. Studies based upon autopsy material show a much higher incidence of hepatic involvement than analyses based on clinical material alone, largely because cases in which autopsy is performed represent a more advanced stage of the disease. The incidence based on autopsy cases is 7.6 to 84.4 per cent, with an average of 36.6 per cent.[41] In clinical cases of intestinal amebiasis the incidence varies from less than 1 per cent to more than 25 per cent, with an average incidence of 8.1 per cent. In recent years the incidence of hepatic involvement in intestinal amebiasis has shown a decrease, which suggests that intestinal amebiasis is being recognized earlier and treated more effectively.

Amebic hepatic infection occurs predominantly in the male sex in a ratio of about 8 to 2. It is observed more frequently during adult life, the highest incidence occurring in the third, fourth and fifth decades of life. Rarely is the disease encountered in patients at the 2 extremes of life, although Wray and associates recently reported a case in a 2-month-old child.[232] All races are susceptible to infection with *Entamoeba histolytica* and no predisposition to the white or Negro races has been demonstrated in the United States. Some observers in the tropics, however, are of the opinion that clinical manifestations of the disease appear less often in natives than in individuals of the white race in these same areas. Craig believes that these natives acquire partial immunity from constant reinfections since childhood, accounting for the comparative mildness of symptoms of amebiasis and the relative infrequency of hepatic complications.[38]

Pathogenesis. It is generally agreed that amebas usually enter the liver by way of the portal system. In support of this hypothesis is the frequent observation of amebas in the capillaries and the venules of the intestinal submucosa and muscularis and in the portal tributaries of sections taken from patients with amebiasis.

Attempts to produce amebic involvement of the liver as a sequel to intestinal involvement in the experimental animal have been unsuccessful. Maegraith and Harinasuta, however, injected cultures of ameba into the mesenteric veins and directly into the portal vein of guinea pigs and produced amebic hepatic lesions in a large percentage of animals. These lesions appeared within the first 3 to 4 days following inoculation but disappeared rapidly after this time. These experiments tend to confirm the assumption that amebas gain entrance into the liver by way of the portal system.[125]

Two other possible routes of invasion of the liver are (1) direct extension through the intestinal wall, peritoneum and capsule of the liver and (2) the lymphatic system. However, it is unlikely that amebas enter the liver to any significant degree by other than the portal route.

Amebas probably are carried to the liver more frequently than is indicated by the incidence of amebic hepatic infection, for as Faust[51, 52] has shown, the hepatic parenchyma appears to possess an amebostatic factor. Actual invasion and growth of amebas in the liver are more likely if an overwhelming number of parasites with relatively increased virulence gain entrance to the liver, or if the resistance of the liver is lowered. The two most significant factors in actual development of amebic hepatitis and amebic hepatic abscess are (1) production by the amebas of intrahepatic portal thrombosis and infarction, and (2) cytolytic activity of the amebas. Amebas carried to the liver from the intestine via the portal circulation are filtered into the portal capillaries, and if they lodge in these smaller portal radicles in sufficient number, thrombosis with infarction and consequent focal necrosis may ensue. Thus, the way is paved for the cytolytic activity of the ameba, permitting lysis and destruction of the involved hepatic parenchyma at the earliest stage of abscess formation. Histologic studies of sections of the liver in various stages provide further evidence of this mode of development of amebic infection of the liver. In the early stage of the process Craig[38] described

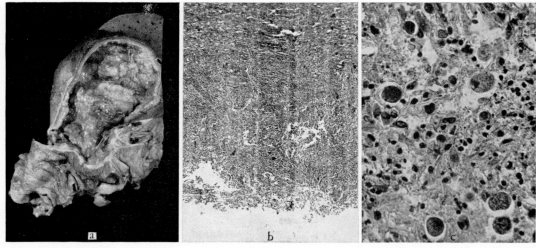

Fɪɢ. 25–18. (a) Photograph of the right lobe of a liver removed at necropsy. An abscess cavity measuring 15 by 10 cm. fills almost the entire lobe. The wall of the abscess is about 1 cm. thick. (b) Low-power photomicrograph of section taken from the wall of the abscess reveals a central zone of necrosis, a middle zone of destroyed hepatic cells in which only a fibrous connective-tissue stroma remains, and an outer zone of hepatic parenchyma which is infiltrated with inflammatory cells. (c) High-power photomicrograph of the section shown in (b) reveals *Entamoeba histolytica* in the middle and the outer zones of the abscess wall.

a peripheral zone of hyperemia surrounding an "area composed of cytolyzed tissue cells in which may be seen red blood corpuscles, degenerated liver cells, a few leukocytes, connective tissue cells, and granular debris, with now and then a trophozoite of Entamoeba histolytica lying in a zone of completely cytolyzed material." This early stage, without progressing any further, may heal by connective-tissue replacement, leaving focal areas of scar tissue representing healed small amebic abscesses. Thus, in the early phase a balance exists between progression of the process toward suppuration and true abscess formation or regression toward healing. The direction in which the infectious process proceeds is determined by a number of factors, including the virulence and the number of the organisms, the resistance of the host, the presence of pathogenic bacteria, and possibly detrimental factors, such as alcohol and trauma.

Pathology. The gross and microscopic appearances of the liver infected with amebas depend upon the extent and the stage of involvement. Characteristically, abscesses are single and occur in the right lobe near

the dome of the liver or on the inferior surface near the hepatic flexure of the colon (Fig. 25–18a). Multiple abscesses are encountered occasionally. It appears that involvement of the left lobe and the presence of multiple abscesses are more common when the disease is far advanced. This is borne out by the highest incidence of left-lobe involvement and multiple lesions in series based on autopsy cases.[41, 160] Obviously, extensive hepatic involvement is more likely in fatal cases in which necropsy is performed. Moreover, in clinical cases, small abscesses may resolve with appropriate therapy and remain unrecognized, whereas thorough postmortem examination will reveal these small lesions.

During the earlier stages of amebic hepatitis amebas are found most frequently in the focal areas of necrosis. As the process develops into true abscesses, the amebas become less evident and are more likely to be found in the zone of necrotic tissue surrounding the peripheral margins of the abscess. Microscopically, there are 3 zones in the active abscess: (1) an outer zone of relatively normal tissue that is being invaded by the amebas; (2) a middle zone in which the parenchymal cells have been destroyed and only the stroma remains; and (3) the necrotic center (Fig. 25–18b). The fact that amebas appear in the peripheral margins of the abscess accounts for the difficulty in demonstrating them in the "pus" more frequently than in one third of the cases (Fig. 25–18c).

Amebic hepatic abscess is also typically sterile, as shown by the fact that pathogenic organisms can be demonstrated in the purulent material in only a small number of cases, in which instances the organisms are probably secondary invaders. However, when an amebic hepatic abscess becomes infected secondarily the process assumes a pyogenic nature. Also the contents of the abscess change in appearance. The typical sterile amebic hepatic abscess contains a viscid, glary, yellowish-red to chocolate-brown material that resembles anchovy sauce or chocolate sauce. Its appearance is so characteristic that it may be considered as pathognomonic. However, once the lesion becomes infected secondarily, the contents become more purulent and have a grayish or grayish-yellow creamy appearance.

Clinical Manifestations. The clinical manifestations of amebic hepatic disease are extremely variable. Symptoms may occur suddenly or develop insidiously. They may appear during the acute phase of intestinal amebiasis or months or even years later. They may develop also in patients who never have had dysenteric symptoms, a fact which is not sufficiently understood. The erroneous impression exists that diarrhea is a common or accompanying manifestation af amebic hepatitis and hepatic abscess. However, experience has demonstrated that a relatively large proportion of patients give no history of diarrhea. In fact, diarrhea or dysentery is a symptom at the time of admission in only half of the patients with amebic hepatic disease, this symptom occurring with about equal frequency among patients with hepatitis and hepatic abscess.[41, 157, 160, 162, 164]

Although the nature of onset and the duration of symptoms in amebic hepatic disease may vary considerably, acute and chronic forms are usually distinguishable. It is particularly important to recognize the early stage of amebic hepatitis, since institution of appropriate therapy during this presuppurative period may prevent progression to abscess formation. In the acute form of the disease the clinical picture is usually more characteristic, with distinctive manifestations that develop more rapidly than in the chronic form. In about one third of the cases the onset of symptoms is acute (3 weeks or less).

The clinical manifestations of hepatic amebiasis may be classified into systemic and local. Systemic symptoms, in order of frequency, are fever, loss of weight, weakness, profuse chills and sweating, nausea, malaise and anorexia. Although fever is usually of a low grade, intermittent or remittent in nature, it may vary considerably, depending upon the onset and the occurrence of secondary infection or other complications. It is present almost invariably in the presuppurative form of the disease, whereas in the later stage of abscess formation it may be absent or of low grade. Chills and sweating also are encountered more frequently in the acute and the subacute forms and in abscesses associated with secondary infection. Weakness and loss of weight may appear early but are more prominent in advanced cases, whereas anorexia, nausea and vomiting are more likely to occur in the early stages of the disease. Although pallor is not uncommon, especially in the chronic form of the disease, jaundice occurs in a relatively small proportion of patients. When present, jaundice is more likely to be associated with abscess formation than with amebic hepatitis.

The earliest and most common local manifestations of hepatic amebiasis are pain and tenderness in the right upper abdominal quadrant in the region cf the liver. Pain is variable, ranging from a dull, aching discomfort to a sharp, stabbing pain. Although usually located directly over the liver, it may be more severe anteriorly below the right costal margin, in the epigastrium, in the axillary line, or posteriorly over the twelfth rib. At times the pain is pleuritic, more prominent in the right lower pulmonary area and accentuated by deep breathing. At other times, it is referred to the right shoulder. Pain in the chest and the shoulder is more likely to be encountered in amebic hepatic abscess than in amebic hepatitis.

Enlargement of the liver is another characteristic local sign which is present in over three fourths of the patients. Usually the liver margin can be felt readily below the right costal arch anteriorly, and on percussion liver dullness is found to extend higher than normal. Palpation of the liver margin may be difficult in some instances because of the acute tenderness and the rigidity of the abdominal muscles in the right upper quadrant. Manifestations of low pleuropulmonary involvement on the right side are not uncommon and result from compression of the lower portion of the right lung as well as from contiguous inflammatory changes. Thus, dullness, diminished breath sounds, crepitant rales, friction rub and signs of fluid in the pleural cavity may be elicited in the patient with amebic hepatic abscess.

When the abscess is in the left lobe, physical findings are those of tenderness in the epigastrium or left hypochondrium with enlargement of the left lobe. Pleuropulmonary involvement may be observed on the left. Alkan and associates found jaundice in 3 of 7 patients, a higher inidence than is reported with involvement of the right lobe.[1]

In the chronic form of the disease, symptoms may develop so insidiously as to be almost unrecognizable. Most patients complain only of slight malaise and anorexia, with no symptoms referable to the hepatic area. Only by careful examination can one elicit tenderness in the right upper abdominal quadrant or the lower portion of the right chest, and detect hepatic enlargement.

The clinical manifestations of hepatic amebiasis may occur in the absence of a demonstrable abscess. Under these circumstances the diagnosis of amebic hepatitis is usually made. Tandon and associates found a diffuse decrease in the uptake of radioactive rose bengal in patients with this diagnosis, and some had small filling defects suggesting small multiple abscesses.[211] The specificity of the clinical syndrome of amebic hepatitis has been questioned by Kean

and by Lamont and Pooler, however. Necropsy examination and hepatic biopsies in cases of amebiasis failed to reveal any anatomic changes in the liver which would confirm the specific diagnosis of amebic hepatitis.[103, 112] It is possible that this syndrome is nonspecific, and that the clinical diagnosis of amebic hepatitis may on occasion be made when there is no actual hepatic infection. On the other hand, there is a stage of amebic infestation before an actual abscess develops, and experience has indicated that patients with this diagnosis respond best to drugs effective against extraintestinal amebiasis.

Laboratory Findings. Hematologic studies and fecal examination may yield information of diagnostic significance. Characteristically, there is moderate leukocytosis in amebic hepatic abscess in contrast with the pronounced leukocytosis occurring in the pyogenic form of hepatic disease. Furthermore, in amebic hepatic abscess there is, as a rule, no concomitant increase in the polymorphonuclear leukocytes. In the acute form of the disease the leukocyte count averages 16,000/cu. mm., whereas in the chronic form it is about 13,000, with average polymorphonuclear percentages in these two forms of about 80 and 75, respectively.[41] In general, pronounced leukocytosis is suggestive of secondary infection. Furthermore, the total leukocyte count is greater in hepatic abscess than in amebic hepatitis, and anemia is more pronounced in the former.

As emphasized previously, only about half of patients with amebic hepatic disease have associated dysentery, and even with the most careful laboratory examination only about 45 per cent of patients show evidence of amebas or cysts in the stools. Frequent examinations yield positive results in a higher percentage of patients with amebic hepatitis than with amebic hepatic abscess.[203] Thus, De Bakey and Ochsner reported demonstration of amebas in the stools of 66 per cent of patients with amebic hepatitis and in only 47 per cent of those with amebic hepatic abscess.[41]

The specific complement-fixation test, first described by Craig[37] in 1927, is another diagnostic laboratory procedure. The test is similar to the standard complement-fixation test for syphilis. Terry and Bozicevich[212] are of the opinion that the complement-fixation test is far more reliable than a history of diarrhea, amebas in the stools, proctoscopic examination, or even a combination of these, in the presence of a clinical picture consistent with hepatic amebiasis. They also believe that it has prognostic value in determining response to therapy, as previously indicated by Craig. On the basis of investigations on 54 patients with amebiasis, 10 of whom had hepatic involvement, Montero and Uribe reached similar conclusions.[144] Kasliwal and associates found this test positive in only 15.5 per cent of patients with intestinal amebiasis; however, it was positive in all 5 cases of proven amebic abscess and in 83 per cent of 12 patients with a diagnosis of amebic hepatitis.[101]

Despite these favorable reports, difficulties with preparation of a potent antigen and proper performance of the test have limited its usefulness, so that it has been abandoned at the Communicable Disease Center in Atlanta.[140] Milgram and associates report that results have been more reliable with the hemagglutination test first described by Kessel and co-workers in 1961.[105, 140] Tests revealed that 96 per cent of 121 patients with amebic liver abscess had positive serology.[140]

In recent years other tests have been described which may be of diagnostic value. Powell and associates have evaluated a gel-diffusion precipitin test. A positive reaction was recorded in 96 per cent of 360 patients with proven liver abscess. They believe that the test is of great value in excluding hepatic abscess in patients with hepatomegaly.[172] Jeanes has used immunofluorescent technics for diagnosis of amebiasis.[96]

Healy has noted that amebae can be demonstrated in the material aspirated from a hepatic abscess in many instances if proper technic is used.[82] Only the last 10 to 15 cc. of material aspirated should be examined. Ten units of streptodornase per ml. of pus is added and the material is incubated for 30 minutes at 37° C. before examination.

Complete liver function studies should be performed on all patients suspected of having amebic hepatic disease. Rarely are these functions altered significantly. They are of value chiefly in differentiation of other types of hepatic disorders. Characteristically, significant enlargement of the liver with normal liver function is suggestive of amebic hepatic disease. However, in some instances, particularly in the presence of liver abscess involving a large part of the hepatic parenchyma, changes in hepatic functions may be observed. Chakravarti, who studied the plasma proteins in patients with amebic hepatitis and amebic hepatic abscess, noted that in all the albumin level was decreased and the globulin fraction increased, while the total protein level remained within normal limits.[26] The changes were greatest in patients with abscess, and in every instance the plasma protein returned to normal levels following recovery. Hare and Ritchey reported an instance of amebic hepatic abscess which, on the basis of clinical manifestations and laboratory observations, appeared to be portal cirrhosis.[78] In this instance all liver function values were depressed, and only at necropsy was the diagnosis of amebic hepatic abscess established.

Roentgenographic Findings. Roentgenography is a particularly useful diagnostic procedure in amebic hepatic infections.[41, 160] Fluoroscopic examination usually reveals elevation and immobility or restriction of motion of the right leaf of the diaphragm. Varying degrees of pulmonary and pleural reaction may be observed in the right basal area, since the portion of the liver most frequently involved is the area near the dome, which is in close contact with the diaphragm. In addition, in the presence of amebic hepatic abscess, distinct bulging of the diaphragm upward into the lower pulmonary field may be observed.

Roentgenographic examination is particularly useful in differentiating amebic infections of the liver and the subphrenic space from those due to other causes.[159] The most common site of pyogenic infections of the subphrenic space is the right postero-superior space, whereas amebic infections are located generally in the right lobe of the liver and near the dome, somewhat more anteriorly than posteriorly. Therefore, in the latter the roentgenogram characteristically shows, in the anteroposterior view,

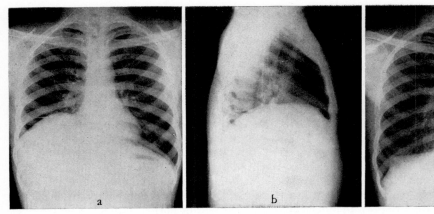

a   b   c

FIG. 25–19. (a) Posteroanterior roentgenogram of patient with an amebic hepatic abscess, showing elevation of the right leaf of the diaphragm and obliteration of the right cardiophrenic sulcus. (b) Lateral roentgenogram showing elevation of the right diaphragm in its central and anterior portions with blunting of the anterior costophrenic sulcus. (c) Posteroanterior roentgenogram made after aspiration of amebic hepatic abscess. The diaphragm has assumed its normal position, and only a stringlike adhesion remains as a residual of the hepatic abscess.

that the medial portion of the right leaf of the diaphragm is elevated and the cardiophrenic angle is obliterated (Fig. 25–19a and 25–20a). In the lateral roentgenogram, elevation is primarily anterior with a tendency toward obliteration of the anterior costophrenic angle (Fig. 25–19b and 25–20b). On the other hand, in pyogenic subphrenic infections, there is elevation particularly of the lateral portion of the diaphragm in the posteroanterior roentgenogram and obliteration of the costophrenic angle in the lateral roentgenogram. In amebic abscess of the left lobe of the liver these observations usually are not apparent, and the presence of this type of amebic hepatic infection is difficult to demonstrate in ordinary roentgenograms. However, it has been shown that abscesses in the left lobe produce characteristic pressure deformities on the stomach, which may be demonstrated following ingestion of barium.[139] The cardia, the lesser curvature and the duodenal cap are displaced downward, and the lesser curvature assumes a typical crescentic shape. The great value of roentgenography in establishing the diagnosis of hepatic amebiasis has been demonstrated repeatedly by many observers. The findings of De Bakey and Ochsner are particularly

striking in this regard, for of 225 cases of amebic hepatic disease 181 (80.5 per cent) had positive roentgenographic observations. For obvious reasons, the incidence of positive roentgenologic signs is much higher in hepatic abscess than in hepatitis.

Various modifications in technic have been proposed as an aid in the roentgenographic diagnosis of hepatic abscess. These include injection of air (Figs. 25–20c and d) or iodized oil into the abscess cavity following aspiration[23, 34, 93, 214, 236] and hepatography after pneumoperitoneum.[111] Hepatic scan after injection of radioactive rose bengal I[131] or colloidal gold has proved to be an excellent diagnostic aid in recent years (Fig. 25–21). As noted in the section in pyogenic abscess, these substances can be used safely, in contradistinction to Thorotrast which was associated with undesirable sequelae in many patients. Tandon and associates have reported a high incidence of correct diagnosis in proven hepatic abscesses. Furthermore, their findings suggest that many patients with the diagnosis of amebic hepatitis have small abscesses.[211]

Percutaneous splenic portography may be of value in amebic liver abscess. By this method the altered intrahepatic portal venous pattern can be demonstrated, abscesses can be located precisely when they cannot be reached by an aspirating needle, and the technic may be useful for follow-up examination after specific therapy.[20] Special procedures are necessary in occasional cases only, as the usual roentgenographic studies are adequate in most instances. Furthermore, some of these technics constitute an added risk to the patient and should not be used routinely.

Diagnosis. The diagnosis of amebic hepatic infection is usually made with relative ease once the condition is suspected.

However, a high index of suspicion must be maintained in all patients with symptoms localized to the hepatic area which have no other obvious explanation. Moreover, it must be kept in mind that amebic hepatitis and hepatic abscess frequently develop in patients who never have had dysenteric symptoms. In addition, the onset may vary considerably. Characteristically, symptoms consisting of low-grade fever, slight to moderate loss of weight, malaise, anorexia, and pain and tenderness in the right upper quadrant of the abdomen are suggestive of amebic hepatic disease. If the

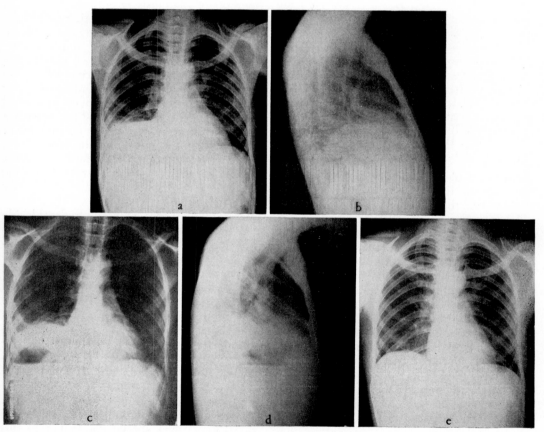

FIG. 25–20. Roentgenogram of the chest of a patient with an amebic hepatic abscess treated successfully by aspiration. (a) Posteroanterior view shows elevation of the right leaf of the diaphragm with blunting of both costophrenic and cardiophrenic sulci. There is evidence of a basal pneumonitis and pleural effusion. (b) Lateral view discloses elevation of the central portion of the diaphragm with slight blunting of the anterior costophrenic sulcus. (c and d) Following aspiration of the hepatic abscess, air was injected to outline the extent of the cavity. (e) Posteroanterior roentgenogram taken about 1 month after aspiration of the amebic hepatic abscess. The diaphragmatic contour now appears normal.

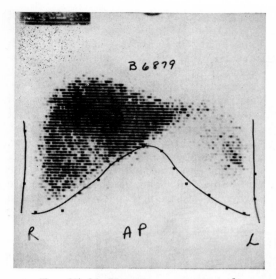

B 6879

R   A P   L

FIG. 25–21. Hepatic scan using radio-active colloidal gold which discloses a filling defect in the right lobe of the liver. This proved to be an amebic abscess. (From Philip C. Johnson, M. D., Director, Radioisotope Laboratory, The Methodist Hospital, Houston, Texas)

pain has a pleuritic or diaphragmatic component, the diagnosis is even more likely. Because of the frequency with which pain occurs in the lower pulmonary area, many cases of amebic hepatic disease are diagnosed originally as pneumonia (Fig. 25–22). Landsman reported 3 such cases.[113] The liver is almost always enlarged, and without this the diagnosis should be made with caution. Slight to moderate leukocytosis and normal results of liver function tests are of value in establishing the diagnosis. Since fecal examination may not disclose the presence of amebas, it cannot be relied upon to establish the diagnosis.

The complement-fixation, hemagglutination or gel diffusion tests should be employed when needed to help in differential diagnosis.

The diagnosis may be established firmly by roentgenographic and fluoroscopic observations. In early cases these changes may be mild, and only by careful examination are they detected. As the amebic hepatic infection progresses, however, the roent-

genographic changes become obvious (Fig. 25–22).

Demonstration of "chocolate-sauce" pus from material aspirated from the abscess usually establishes the diagnosis of amebic hepatic abscess even though amebae are not found on examination of the aspirated material. The method of examination described by Healy, however, may improve the incidence of positive identification of organisms. Aspiration should be performed whenever it is believed that the amebic process has reached the abscess stage. When the proper precautions are observed and the procedure properly performed, this method of diagnosis is entirely innocuous.

Treatment. Conservative therapy is effective in most instances of amebic hepatic infection. During the stage of simple amebic hepatitis treatment consists of administration of one or more of the drugs which are specific for extra-intestinal amebiasis. The amebacides commonly employed to control amebic infection of the intestinal tract are of little or no value in the treatment of amebic hepatic infection; therefore, it is extremely important that amebic hepatitis be recognized early in order that specific therapy in this presuppurative stage may be instituted.

For many years emetine hydrochloride has been the drug of choice in the therapy of extra-intestinal amebiasis. It is administered subcutaneously or intramuscularly in doses of 0.065 Gm (1 grain) daily until 0.39 to 0.65 Gm. (6 to 10 grains) have been given. Emetine is essentially a protoplasmic poison with an apparent selective action on muscles. Thus, if the drug must be administered in excessive amounts or over a prolonged period of time, there is danger of toxicity, particularly from its effect on the cardiac musculature. For this reason, care should be exercised in its use. If a second course is indicated, an interval of 20 to 30 days should elapse before this is administered, to avoid cumulative toxic effects.[202] If the drug is administered in the dosage already outlined, clinical manifestations of toxicity are rarely encountered, but electrocardiography should be performed during periods of administration.

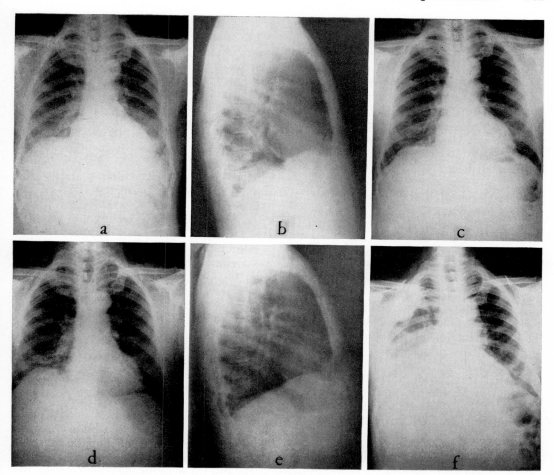

FIG. 25–22. Serial chest roentgenograms taken during a 7-month period and showing the gradual development of an amebic hepatic abscess.

(a) Posteroanterior view taken in January, 1952, because patient complained of pain in the right lower chest. There is slight elevation of the diaphragm and blunting of the cardiophrenic angle. The roentgenogram was reported to show "pneumonitis."

(b) The lateral projection, taken at the same time as (a), discloses elevation of the anterior portion of the diaphragm and obliteration of the anterior costophrenic sulcus.

(c) Posteroanterior roentgenogram taken in March, 1952, because of persistence of symptoms. There is irregularity of the right diaphragm and blunting of the cardiophrenic angle.

(d and e) In July, 1952, anteroposterior and lateral roentgenograms disclose progression of the diaphragmatic changes. There is now evidence of pulmonary parenchymal changes at the right base.

(f) Posteroanterior projection taken about 2 weeks after roentgenograms shown in (d) and (e). The right lung field is now obscured by a pleural effusion. The patient developed a bronchohepatic fistula, and after treatment with emetine and chloroquine, and thoracentesis, he recovered.

Chloroquine (7-chloro-4-[4-diethylamino-1-methylbutylamino]quinoline) is one of the nontoxic, highly active compounds of the 4-aminoquinoline series disclosed by the wartime antimalarial drug-research program. In the belief that its antiplasmodial activity might extend to other pathogenic protozoa and because it is highly concentrated in the liver (about 500 times its plasma concentration) and is almost completely absorbed from the gastrointestinal tract, its therapeutic effectiveness was investigated.[31-33] The striking results, particularly in hepatic amebiasis, led others to use this agent in amebic hepatic abscess.[49, 79, 148, 204] Chloroquine is administered orally (chloroquine diphosphate) in a dosage of 1 Gm. daily for 2 to 3 days followed by 0.5 Gm. daily for 2 to 3 weeks. No serious toxic manifestations have been observed even after repeated courses of therapy, although minor reactions such as headaches, pruritus, disturbances of visual accommodation, and gastrointestinal complaints are noted occasionally. Like emetine, chloroquine is not always effective in the treatment of amebic hepatic disease, and failure to respond to chloroquine does not rule out this condition.[52] If either emetine or chloroquine alone fails to eradicate the amebic hepatic infection, dual therapy with these drugs may be effective.[201]

In 1965 Powell and associates reported a comparative study of dehydroemetine, emetine hydrochloride and chloroquine in treatment of amebic liver abscess. They concluded that the treatment of choice is a combination of dehydroemetine plus chloroquine.[173] These investigators have also studied a new nitro-thiazole derivative, Ciba 32,644-BA. There were 3 relapses among 30 treated patients with amebic enteritis, but 100 per cent success among 15 patients with hepatic abscess.[174] Thus, at this time several drugs may be of value.

Upon completion of therapy for the liver abscess, a full course of treatment with one of the intestinal amebacides should be administered.

The iodochlorohydroxyquinolines, chiniofon and Diodoquin, have been employed extensively in the treatment of amebic colitis. Chiniofon is administered orally in dosage of 1 Gm. 3 times daily before meals for 7 to 8 days. Treatment with Diodoquin consists of administration of 2.5 Gm. daily in 3 or 4 divided doses for about 20 days. Milibis (bismuth glycolylarsanilate) is also a valuable antiamebic drug which is relatively insoluble and is absorbed rather slowly by the intestinal wall.[88, 203] Hence,

it is useful primarily in treatment of early acute amebic infections or in asymptomatic cases. Although it is reported to have a low toxicity, it should be prescribed with caution for patients who have an idiosyncrasy to arsenic.[201]

As mentioned previously, both emetine and chloroquine may be employed to advantage in the treatment of amebic hepatic abscess. Thus, emetine may be administered initially for 7 to 10 days followed by a course of therapy with chloroquine. During administration of chloroquine, one of the intestinal amebacides (chiniofon, Diodoquin or Milibis) may be given (Fig. 25-23).

Although many antibiotic agents have been employed in the treatment of amebiasis, the only 3 that appear to have any benefit are chlortetracycline (Aureomycin), oxytetracycline (Terramycin) and fumagillin.[106, 134] They have been employed primarily for the treatment of intestinal amebiasis. These agents however are best used in combination with another amebacide for the incidence of relapse when used alone is higher than with some of the other preparations.

If clinical manifestations persist after emetine or chloroquine is administered, or if there is evidence of hepatic abscess, aspiration is indicated. Although amebic hepatic abscess may be diagnosed at the onset, it is important to administer emetine or chloroquine for several days prior to aspiration.[40, 41] Aspiration always should be performed in the operating room under strict aseptic conditions to avoid contamination. Furthermore, open drainage may be done without delay in cases of secondary infection. Physical findings and roentgenographic studies will indicate the site of puncture. Local infiltration with a 1 per cent solution of procaine hydrochloride is preferable to general anesthesia. In the presence of localizing signs and pointing of the abscess, the aspirating needle may be inserted directly over the mass. It is important to avoid traversing the peritoneal or the pleural cavity. Thus, in the absence of localizing signs, the needle should be introduced through the tenth intercostal space in the anterior axillary line and di-

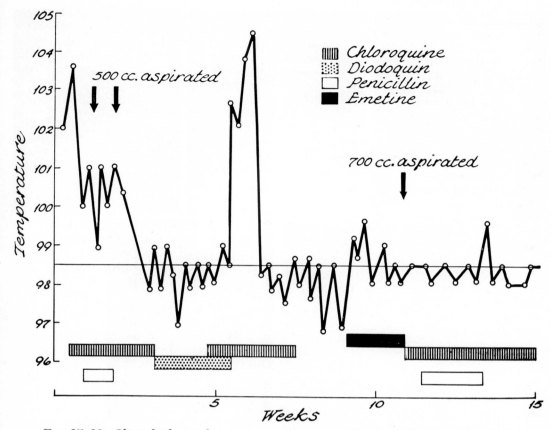

Fig 25–23. Clinical chart of a patient with an amebic liver abscess. Chloroquine, Diodoquin, emetine and penicillin were administered, and aspiration was performed on 3 occasions, resulting in resolution of the abscess.

rected upward, medially and backward. Should multiple aspirations become necessary, or if it is desirable to change the direction of the needle after it has been inserted, it should be removed entirely before it is reintroduced in order to avoid injury to the hepatic parenchyma. As much of the liquefied necrotic material is removed as possible, and smear and culture should be made immediately. If the smear contains numerous pyogenic organisms, the abscess should be drained openly and promptly, care being taken to avoid contamination of the uninvolved serous cavity. It is not necessary to inject an amebacide into the cavity following aspiration. Repeated aspirations, when necessary, can be accomplished through the site used for the initial aspiration.

Prior to aspiration, antibiotic therapy should be initiated. If the abscess is infected secondarily, the organism should be identified promptly by culture, and antibiotic sensitivity studies should be performed in order to determine the most suitable agent.

Rarely, an amebic hepatic abscess will not resolve completely following administration of emetine and chloroquine, and multiple aspirations are performed because of the large size of the abscess cavity and the extensive fibrosis in its wall, which prevent closure of the cavity following drainage. Under these circumstances it may become necessary to open the abscess widely and close it by the use of a muscular flap from the abdominal or the thoracic wall.

Complications. Secondary infection with

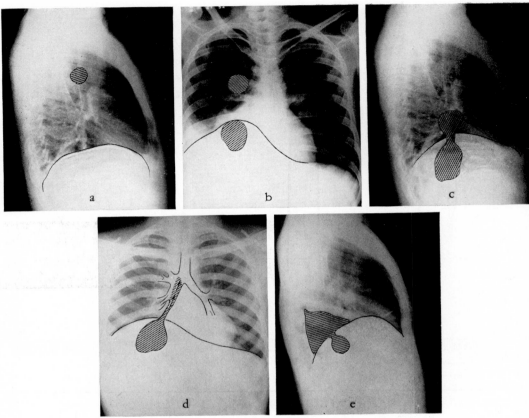

FIG. 25–24. Retouched roentgenograms demonstrating the types of pleuropulmonary complications of amebiasis. (a) Pulmonary abscess without hepatic involvement. (b) Independent pulmonary and hepatic abscesses. (c) Pulmonary abscess extending from hepatic abscess. (d) Bronchohepatic fistula. (e) Empyema extending from a hepatic abscess.

pyogenic organisms, direct extension, or rupture of the abscess into a serous cavity or an adjacent viscus are the most important complications of amebic hepatic infection. These almost invariably occur in association with abscess formation and consequently are seen in the later stages of amebic hepatic disease. Thus if an amebic hepatic infection is recognized early, in the presuppurative stage, it can be controlled with appropriate therapy and these serious complications can be prevented.

Secondary Infection with Pyogenic Organisms. True amebic hepatic abscesses are bacteriologically sterile and when pyogenic organisms are demonstrable, they are probably secondary invaders. Under these cir-

cumstances, a change occurs both in the nature of the abscess contents and in the clinical manifestations. The typical "chocolate-sauce" pus becomes purulent, may appear greenish-yellow or grayish-yellow and frequently is malodorous. The clinical manifestations become more severe with a higher, usually spiking, fever and leukocytosis. Most commonly, streptococci and staphylococci are found in the purulent material removed from the abscess, although pneumococci, enterococci and colon bacilli may be observed also. The incidence of secondary infection is 10 to 20 per cent.[41, 126] Secondary infection may affect the prognosis significantly, resulting in a great increase in mortality rate.

Although antimicrobial therapy should be vigorous in the treatment of a secondarily infected amebic hepatic abscess, in most instances this will not obviate the necessity for adequate prompt open drainage.

Pleuropulmonary Involvement. The next most frequent complication is pleuropulmonary involvement. Usually, this represents rupture or direct extension of the hepatic abscess through the diaphragm, although rarely it is due to systemic invasion.[158] Pleuropulmonary amebic infections may be divided into 5 types, according to their gross pathologic characteristics (Fig. 25–24): hematogenous pulmonary abscess without hepatic involvement; hematogenous pulmonary abscess and independent hepatic abscess; pulmonary abscess extending from hepatic abscess; bronchohepatic fistula; and empyema extending from a hepatic abscess. The last three are by far the most common.

Although there is convincing evidence that pleuropulmonary amebiasis results from systemic invasion by the ameba, most commonly it is the result of direct extension from an amebic hepatic abscess and usually follows perforation through the diaphragm or occasionally transphrenic migration by way of the lymphatics. Occurrence of this complication is dependent particularly upon virulence of the infection, resistance of the host and location of the process in the liver. Most amebic hepatic abscesses are located near the convex surface and in the posterior portion of the right lobe of the liver, and the adjacent diaphragm is invaded readily and incorporated by the abscess as it enlarges, thus permitting extension into the thoracic cavity (Fig. 25–25). The abscess may rupture into the base of the right lung or into the free pleural cavity, depending upon the severity of the process. A more rapidly progressing abscess largely associated with a pleural reaction of sufficient degree produces obliterative adhesions so that the abscess usually ruptures into the pleural cavity. Following rupture into the pulmonary parenchyma a bronchial fistula may result which permits evacuation of the contents of the abscess through the tracheobronchial tree (Fig. 25–26). This latter event usu-

ally occurs in abscesses that develop slowly and in which the pleural cavity has been obliterated by adhesions.

Pleuropulmonary complications occur only in patients with true amebic hepatic abscess, the incidence being about 15 to 20 per cent.[41] About 40 per cent of these complications are primarily pleural with empyema, the remainder being primarily pulmonary. The latter are divided about equally between bronchohepatic fistulas and pulmonary abscesses communicating with the hepatic abscess.

When the abscess involves the left lobe of the liver, pleuropulmonary complications may develop in the left hemithorax. Characteristically, pleuropulmonary complications are associated with pain in the right lower region of the chest, frequently extending to the right shoulder, unproductive cough, and slight or moderate dyspnea, in addition to the usual manifestations of amebic hepatic abscess, which become more pronounced as the abscess encroaches upon the chest. In some instances these symptoms suddenly become more prominent, and the patient begins to cough up large quantities of purulent "chocolate-sauce" material. This establishes the presence of a bronchohepatic fistula.

Physical examination discloses characteristic signs of consolidation or cavitation, particularly in the right lower pulmonary area. The diagnosis is confirmed by roentgenographic examination. Fluoroscopy may demonstrate that the diaphragm is elevated and immobilized. Roentgenograms usually reveal increased density in the lower right pulmonary field, and in both the anteroposterior and the lateral views a triangular shadow may be seen extending upward from the liver toward the hilum of the lung. If the abscess ruptures into the pleural cavity, the roentgenographic picture is one of pleural effusion or empyema. If iodized oil is introduced into the trachea a bronchohepatic fistula can be visualized accurately.

Treatment of pleuropulmonary complications is determined by the type of involvement and the presence or the absence of secondary infection. Emetine or chloroquine should be given to all patients. In the presence of a bronchohepatic fistula,

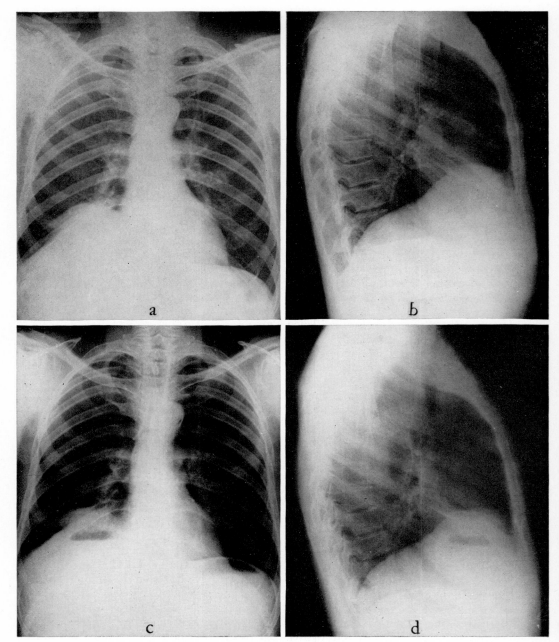

FIG. 25–25. Roentgenograms of patient with a pulmonary abscess extending from an amebic hepatic abscess. (a) Posteroanterior projection, showing elevation of the right leaf of the diaphragm and blunting of the cardiophrenic angle. A small abscess cavity is visible within the density at the right lung base. (b) Lateral projection reveals an abscess cavity above and immediately below the diaphragm. (c and d) Posteroanterior and lateral roentgenograms taken after aspiration of the hepatic abscess and institution of emetine and chloroquine therapy.

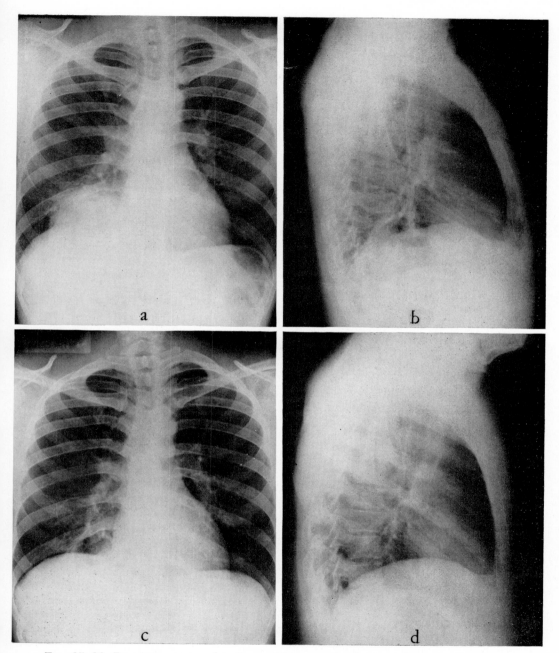

FIG. 25–26. Roentgenograms of patient with an amebic hepatic abscess complicated by a bronchohepatic fistula. (a) Posteroanterior projection, showing elevation of the right leaf of the diaphragm and obliteration of the right cardiophrenic angle. (b) Lateral view shows the elevation to involve primarily the anterior portion of the diaphragm. The anterior costophrenic sulcus is obliterated. (c and d) Posteroanterior and lateral roentgenograms taken after development of a bronchohepatic fistula. The hepatic abscess cavity is outlined by the air-fluid level. A triangular shadow extends from the diaphragm toward the pulmonary hilum and represents the course of the bronchohepatic fistula.

conservative therapy, consisting of administration of emetine or chloroquine and
postural drainage, is usually adequate. In
some instances bronchoscopy may help to
evacuate the abscess. If, after bronchohepatic fistula develops, the hepatic abscess
is still prominent, aspiration should be performed. In the absence of secondary infection conservative therapy, consisting of
aspiration of hepatic abscess and the pleural
effusion, also should be employed. The
value of more definitive surgical therapy in
certain forms of pleuropulmonary complications of amebic hepatic abscess has been
emphasized by Shaw.[198] He believed that
in the presence of empyema that does not
respond to repeated aspiration, in persistent bronchohepatic fistula or in chronic
pulmonary abscess, the most effective therapy is thoracotomy with removal of the
products of infection, including decortication of the lung and the diaphragm and
resection of the involved portion of the
lung.

Rupture of Amebic Hepatic Abscess. INTO
PERITONEAL CAVITY. Rupture of an amebic
hepatic abscess into the peritoneal cavity
is the next most frequent complication, occurring in 6 to 9 per cent of patients with
true abscess.[41] The seriousness of this complication is indicated by the mortality rate
of about 75 per cent. However, the prognosis in general depends upon whether
there is localized or generalized peritonitis
with extension of the abscess into the peritoneal cavity. If the abscess progresses
gradually, the peritoneal adhesions along
the inferior surface of the liver are stimulated so that the process becomes walled
off with the formation of localized peritonitis. If, on the other hand, the extension is
rapid, and particularly if the abscess is infected secondarily, perforation and rupture
into the virgin peritoneal cavity produce
generalized peritonitis. This type of complication is much more severe than the former type. In the treatment of the patients
emetine or chloroquine always should be
administered, and in the majority of cases
open drainage is necessary because of the
presence of secondary infection.

INTO PERICARDIAL CAVITY. Rupture of an
amebic hepatic abscess into the pericardial
cavity has been reported by several observers.[41] It usually occurs with an abscess
of the left lobe of the liver and is characterized clinically by sudden manifestations of pyopericardium and collapse. In
some instances associated pericarditis rather
than pericardial abscess has been reported.
Most reported cases of true perforation have
terminated fatally.

OTHER AREAS. Other unusual complications of amebic hepatic abscess include rupture of the abscess into the gastrointestinal
tract, into the biliary tract, into the portal
vein and the inferior vena cava, through the
abdominal wall, and extension to the spleen
and the kidneys. Cerebral abscess has been
reported,[128] but often it is preceded by hepatic and pleuropulmonary involvement.
Halpert and Ashley, who reviewed the literature on this subject in 1944, found that
only 5 cases, including their own, of the
61 reported up to that time were not associated with either hepatic or pulmonary involvement.[76] Since then, at least 6 cases
have been reported, of which all but 2 were
associated with hepatic or pleuropulmonary
involvement. All reported cases have terminated fatally, with the possible exception of
a case of Collard and Kendall in which the
diagnosis of cerebral amebiasis was based
essentially on the "dramatic response to
emetine."[28] These complications represent
far advanced and often neglected stages of
the disease, and the small number of such
instances reported in the recent literature
is perhaps indicative of the awareness of
amebic hepatic infection and the institution
of prompt therapy in the early stages.

Prognosis. The prognosis of hepatic
amebiasis is dependent upon (1) the relative virulence of the organism and resistance
of the host, (2) the stage of the infection,
(3) the multiplicity of lesions in the liver,
in the case of abscess, (4) the presence or
absence of secondary infection, and (5)
the type of therapy employed.

The prognostic importance of the extent
or the stage of infection is emphasized by
the fact that in the series of De Bakey and
Ochsner[41] the mortality rate was about 22
per cent for hepatic abscess, whereas for

amebic hepatitis there were no fatalities. This striking difference emphasizes the importance of recognizing the earlier phases of amebic hepatic disease, a fact pointed out more than 45 years ago by Rogers,[187] who described it as the "presuppurative" stage.

In the presence of abscess formation, multiple abscesses may affect the prognosis seriously. This is particularly true when multiple abscesses are clinically demonstrable.

The presence of complications also has a grave influence on the prognosis of amebic hepatic infections. The development of pleuropulmonary involvement and of secondary infection of the hepatic abscesses radically changes the characteristics of amebic hepatic infection and increases the difficulty of treatment. Many differences exist between the relatively benign and limiting features of the purely amebic abscess and the rapidly invasive and septic type of pyogenic lesion of the liver.

In 1951 De Bakey and Ochsner reported a mortality rate of 5 per cent for sterile abscesses, whereas that for abscesses secondarily infected was 40 per cent.[41] More recent experience indicates a decrease in the incidence of complications as well as improvements in treatment of uncomplicated abscesses. Several recent reports have tabulated small groups of patients treated with no mortality.[173, 174, 232]

The type of therapy employed is also of prognostic import. It has been suggested that the use of antimicrobial agents, along with emetine or chloroquine, allows closed drainage of amebic infections, and may be employed despite the presence of secondary infection. However, our experience does not confirm these observations. Although antibiotic agents are of value in preventing systemic invasion and limiting extension of the process in the presence of secondary infection, adequate drainage is necessary in most instances.

The superiority of conservative management with emetine and chloroquine, with or without aspiration, has been demonstrated clearly, and its prognostic importance is well documented.

When open drainage is necessary for complicated amebic hepatic abscesses, the prognosis is significantly better when drainage is accomplished without contamination of the pleural or the peritoneal cavity.

HEPATIC RESECTION

The century of the surgeon began with the discovery of general anesthesia. When operations could be performed painlessly, attempts to control disease by surgical intervention were soon encompassing almost all areas of the body. Thus, according to Brittain, in 1870 Bruns successfully resected a portion of the liver damaged by a gunshot wound, and only 18 years later Langenbuch excised a portion of the liver as treatment for tumor.[18, 114] Before 1900, less than 60 years after the first use of ether anesthesia, Keen had collected 76 cases of hepatic resection and reported a left hepatic lobectomy.[104] In 1911, Wendell performed a right lobectomy.[224] Despite these early operations, hepatic resection, with the exception of small excisions or biopsies, is not a common operation even today. This is partly due to the fact that lesions involving the liver which can be cured by resection do not occur as frequently as lesions in other intra-abdominal organs. Technics of hepatic resection, however, are now well established and an experienced surgeon does not hesitate to remove as much of the liver as is necessary to excise localized disease.

Anatomy. Current technics of hepatic resection awaited detailed anatomic studies. Although as early as 1897 Cantlie stated that the right and left lobes were divided in the region of the gallbladder fossa, many textbooks of anatomy continue to use the external appearance of the liver, particularly the location of the falciform ligament, as the basis for the descriptions of the lobular boundaries.[24] The earlier description by Cantlie and others, however, has been confirmed in recent years and expanded by the studies of Healey, Braasch and others. [15, 81, 180] These observations, which document the intrahepatic distribution of arteries, veins and bile ducts, have revealed a segmental division of the liver which can

TABLE 25–5.

I. Benign Lesions
    a. Trauma
    b. Inflammatory diseases
       1. Hepatic stones and abscess
       2. Benign obstruction of the hepatic ducts
       3. Tuberculosis
       4. Syphilis
       5. Plasma cell granuloma
    c. Cysts
    d. Tumors
       1. Adenoma
       2. Hemangioma
II. Malignant Lesions
    a. Primary
       1. Hepatoma
       2. Cholangiocarcinoma
       3. Cancer of major intrahepatic ducts
       4. Sarcoma
    b. Hepatic involvement by contiguous spread
       1. Gallbladder
       2. Stomach
       3. Colon
    c. Metastatic
       1. Colon
       2. Melanoma
       3. Carcinoid

be compared to segmental divisions of lobes of the lungs. They allow a rational, planned approach to resection of various segments of the liver based upon an understanding of the distribution of the vessels and bile ducts. On this basis, the liver can be divided into two major lobes, right and left, by a line extending through the gallbladder fossa to the vena cava. The right lobe can be further subdivided into anterior and posterior segments, while the left lobe is divided into medial and lateral segments. The falciform ligament is at the junction of medial and lateral segments of the left lobe rather than at the division of the right and left lobes. Further subdivisions are also possible, but at this time, attempts at the resection of smaller, specific segments are rarely made.

INDICATIONS FOR RESECTION

Benign lesions. A number of benign lesions may require major hepatic resection (Table 25–5). Total removal of a lobe may be the best technical maneuver for control of hemorrhage and debridement of devitalized tissue in severe trauma involving an entire lobe, for example.[132] This problem is discussed in more detail in the section under trauma. A number of inflammatory lesions have been treated by hepatic resection. All of these represent rare indications for this operation. Nevertheless, hepatic stones with abscess and benign obstruction of the hepatic ducts with hepatic atrophy may, on occasion, be best treated by removal of the involved hepatic tissue. Tuberculomas, syphilis and plasma cell granuloma also are rare lesions which require major hepatic resection infrequently.[62, 86, 133, 141, 171, 178] Major hepatic resections have been performed for polycystic disease of the liver as well as for multiple hydatid cysts localized to one lobe. Few such cases have been reported and it is an exceptional circumstance under which these lesions justify this operation.[27] Benign tumors may require resection. McDermott and Ottinger reported removal of 90 per cent of the liver for multiple adenomata.[133] A number of authors have reported resection of hemangiomas. In fact, only a few years ago, some authors believed that hemangioma was the lesion most commonly treated by hepatic resection. Hemangioma is of particular significance in the newborn, for rupture with fatal hemorrhage is a common complication. Thus, presence of this tumor represents a particularly important indication for hepatectomy in childhood when the lesion is limited to one lobe.[200]

Malignant lesions. Malignant lesions confined to one lobe have been the disease processes most often treated by hepatic lobectomy. Unfortunately, experience in the United States indicates that most primary malignant hepatic tumors including hepatoma (hepatic cell carcinoma) and cholangiocarcinomas are rapidly fatal and most have involved both lobes of the liver prior to the time that the diagnosis is made. Consequently, in the majority of cases, the only possible treatment would be total resection of the liver and transplantation. This operation is being performed today, but this represents an experimental procedure, and at present is not recommended for routine treatment. Fortunately, some of the lesions are localized to one lobe.[2, 218]

Overton and associates in a review of 66 patients with this diagnosis found that approximately 10 per cent of patients could have been considered candidates for lobectomy on the basis of distribution of the disease in the liver found at necropsy; however, in only 2 was lobectomy performed.[165] None of their patients survived for 5 years and 5-year survivals have been infrequent. In a review of the world literature, up to 1957, Reifferschied found 103 reports of resection for primary carcinoma of the liver. Three patients survived for 1 year and 16 for over 2 years.[184] Yvergneaux and colleagues found reports on 20 patients with hepatic cell carcinoma with survival for longer than 3 years by 1962.[233] This included a 7-year survival in a 56-year-old woman who had left hepatectomy for carcinoma. This patient subsequently underwent resection for what was presumed to be a new tumor, 7 years later. Our own experience indicates a poor prognosis for this lesion, for in a review of 100 patients with carcinoma of the liver, there has yet been no 5-year survival. One patient underwent resection in Houston, Texas, however, in which a left lobectomy was performed as an emergency procedure because of spontaneous rupture of a malignant hepatoma with hemorrhage. The patient has been alive and well for three and one half years.[84]

The most encouraging report is that of Lin and associates who reported a resectability rate of 46.1 per cent among 121 patients treated in Formosa.[115] Eight of the 42 patients who underwent lobectomy were alive at the time of the report, 3 having survived 5 or more years. Thus, all patients suspected of having primary malignant disease of the liver deserve exploration with resection of the tumor when technically possible, for there is no other known effective treatment.

Primary cancer of the major intrahepatic ducts can be differentiated from cholangiocarcinoma. This is at times a slowly growing lesion and relatively prolonged survival is occasionally recorded even when there has not been resection. Although there is little experience with major hepatic resections for this lesion, its natural course would suggest that hepatic resection should be associated with a better survival rate than with the usual primary hepatic tumor.

Primary sarcomas of the liver are so rare that there is little experience on which to base statements concerning treatment. Resection has been successfully performed for this tumor, however, and there is no other method of treatment that can be attended by success. Thus, the operation is indicated when the lesion is localized.[178]

The liver is occasionally involved by spread from contiguous carcinomas, and in selected patients with carcinoma of the colon or stomach, resection of a large segment of liver is justified to encompass all of the tumor. Extension of the tumor by contiguous spread appears to represent an entirely different process from extension by distant metastatic spread. The chances of successful treatment are much greater. Of particular significance is direct spread from the gallbladder into the liver adjacent to the gallbladder bed. This highly malignant tumor is only occasionally amenable to resection, but when localized to this area, hepatic lobectomy would appear to be the treatment of choice, for there are reports of successful operations with 5-year survival.[16]

The management of metastatic disease involving the liver is a subject of some debate in the literature at present. There are those who advocate major hepatic resections for metastases from lesions that are growing slowly, particularly those in the colon, as well as lesions that have a less predictable course, such as single metastatic lesions from melanoma in the absence of other known metastatic disease.[60, 62, 221] Major hepatic resections have also been performed for metastatic lesions from more malignant tumors such as the stomach, and some have even advocated second-look operations in asymptomatic patients to determine the presence or absence of metastatic involvement of the liver with resection of these lesions when found.[60] Most surgeons do not believe that such operations are indicated in the treatment of

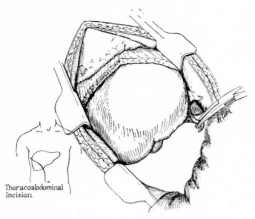

Thoracoabdominal
Incision

FIG. 25–27. Resection of the right lobe of the liver: after exposure through a thoraco-abdominal incision, ligaments are divided.

metastatic hepatic disease, and limit resection of the liver to the unusual circumstance where a single metastasis is found from a slowly growing tumor several years after apparent successful treatment of the primary growth. Thus, it would appear that resection of the liver for a single mestastasis might be accomplished in a similar way as treatment of a single metastatic lesion in the lung. When multiple metastases are present, even though apparently localized to one lobe of the liver, the likelihood of success would appear to be extremely small. One tumor, however, represents a special indication for resection even when multiple metastases are present if the tumor is limited to one lobe. Carcinoid tumor usually grows slowly and after hepatic metastases occur, the carcinoid syndrome frequently develops, which may be quite disabling. Resection of the involved portion of liver may not only result in prolongation of life, but may relieve disabling symptoms as well.[229]

HEPATIC RESECTION IN CHILDREN

Resections in children represent a special problem. Technically, resection is much easier than in the adult. In addition, resection of tumors that occur in children apparently produces better results than can be anticipated in adults. A variety of names has been attached to tumors in childhood

and the terminology is somewhat confusing. However, the terms *malignant teratoma, embryonal hepatoma* and *hepatoblastoma* all refer to tumors that may grow relatively slowly and for which hepatic resections have been successful.

Peterson, Varco and Good, for example, reported a five and a half year survival of an infant following excision of embryonal hepatoma.[169] Successful reports have been recorded by a number of other authors.[56, 75, 94, 100, 117] Fish and McCary reported an experience with 6 personal cases and a review of 130 patients collected from the literature between 1953 and 1965. The tumor was localized to one lobe in more than half of these patients (70 patients), and there was coexistent cirrhosis in only 5 in contradistinction to the frequency of cirrhosis associated with hepatic tumors in adults. Surgical resection had been performed in 47 of these patients, and at the time of review, 22 patients were alive, 7 with metastases and 15 without evidence of recurrence.[56]

Thus an aggressive approach to the management of childhood tumors of the liver is warranted.

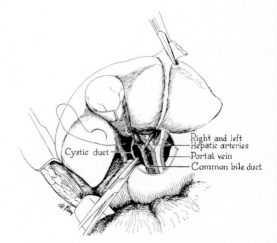

Cystic duct

Right and left Hepatic arteries
Portal vein
Common bile duct

FIG. 25–28. Structures in the porta hepatis are exposed. The right hepatic duct has been divided and the end closed with suture. Lines indicate planned division of the branches of the hepatic artery and portal vein to the right lobe. The cystic duct has been divided to remove the gallbladder with the specimen.

TECHNIC

Simple wedge excision of small amounts of hepatic tissue requires control of hemorrhage and bile drainage by placing mattress sutures along the cut edge of the liver or by suture approximation if the defect is small.

Formal lobectomy, however, is an operation of considerable magnitude.[147, 180, 230] Exposure is best obtained through a thoraco-abdominal incision, dividing the diaphragm to expose the superior surface of the liver. The hepatic ligaments are divided. (Fig. 25–27). The porta hepatis is dissected to identify the hepatic artery and its two major branches, the portal vein and its right and left branches, and the right and left hepatic ducts joining to form the common hepatic duct. The branches of the artery and vein and bile duct to the diseased lobe are divided (Fig. 25–28). The ends of these structures are best closed with suture, rather than with ties. Attention then is directed to the under side of the liver, where the hepatic veins are identified, ligated and divided. Ligature with suture, rather than a simple tie is recommended (Fig. 25–29). The liver is transected bluntly, using a knife handle rather than a

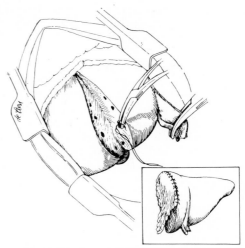

FIG. 25–30. The lobe is removed by blunt division of the liver substance, placing suture ligations around vessels and bile ducts as they are encountered. Insert shows completion of procedure with omentum covering the liver surface. In some patients the falciform ligament can be used.

blade. Areas of resistance representing vessels or ducts can be identified in this manner, allowing individual ligature before division, thereby decreasing blood loss (Fig. 25–30). Transection is made along the line extending through the gallbladder fossa to the vena cava, including removal of the gallbladder as a part of the procedure. In some patients the liver must be transected before the hepatic veins are ligated because of difficulty in exposure, and the need to insure protection of the venous drainage from the opposite lobe. Weeping from the raw surface may be decreased by placing multiple interlocking sutures. Approximation of a piece of omentum against the raw surface may also decrease drainage from this area. Currently there is increasing interest in the use of plastic adhesives to help control hemorrhage from the liver. These agents may be used to aid in approximation of the omentum to the transected liver surface. Adequate drainage should be insured.

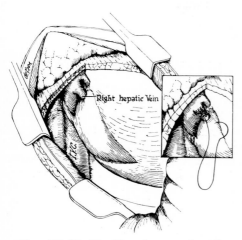

FIG. 25–29. The liver is rotated to the left and the posterior parietal peritoneum incised. The hepatic veins are identified and ligated. This illustration demonstrates the main right hepatic vein near the superior border of the liver. The insert demonstrates division and control with sutures. I.V.C., inferior vena cava.

MORTALITY AND COMPLICATIONS

The mortality rates reported in the literature vary from 11.9 to 20 per cent.[115,133]

Complications common to all operations may be encountered following hepatic surgery, but several complications constitute a special hazard.

Hemorrhage is the most common serious complication and is one of the most common causes of death. Therefore, hemostasis must be meticulous and it is for this reason that most surgeons recommend adequate control of both the inflow and outflow vascular structures prior to actual transection of the liver. On the other hand, Lin and associates have developed a technic of direct transection of the liver, controlling hemorrhage as it is encountered; their mortality rate is one of the best reported.[115] A second problem is that of *air embolism,* for many venous structures are opened during this procedure. This is best avoided by ligation of the hepatic veins before the liver is transected, but as stated above, this may not always be possible, depending upon the anatomy and difficulty of identifying the major hepatic branches to the left lobe. Some *bile drainage* is to be anticipated during the first few days. Occasionally, if large bile ducts are not ligated adequately, a *persistent biliary fistula* occurs. If adequately drained and no infection ensues, spontaneous closure is the rule. If inadequately drained, *bile peritonitis* or *subphrenic abscess* may further complicate the postoperative course.

Impairment of hepatic function as measured by the usual tests may occur in the early postoperative period, depending upon the status of the remaining hepatic tissue. In the normal liver, the entire lobe may be resected without significantly altering measurable hepatic function, though jaundice is not uncommon. On the basis of animal experiments, it has been estimated that approximately 75 per cent of functioning hepatic tissue must be removed before there is significant alteration in hepatic function which can be measured by usual technics. In the cirrhotic liver, however, removal of an entire lobe may reduce significantly the amount of functioning tissue available, and postoperative care of the patient may be extremely difficult. In patients with known impaired hepatic function, therefore, a major hepatic resection may be contraindicated. When remaining hepatic function is normal, even more than a lobe may be removed with survival. Monaco and co-workers, for example, removed an estimated 90 per cent of the liver in a human with survival.[143] When this amount of tissue is removed, abnormalities of hepatic function tests and jaundice are to be expected in the postoperative period, but if a patient survives through the immediate postoperative period, the long-term prognosis is excellent insofar as return of hepatic function is concerned. The liver is the only organ in the abdomen for which there is unequivocal evidence of significant regeneration with an increase in cell mass. In the cases reported by McDermott and Ottinger, reexploration or hepatic scan taken 1 year following resection revealed that the hepatic mass had returned virtually to normal by regeneration of the liver, similar to that observed in the dog.[133] Pack and colleagues have reported a similar experience.[166, 167]

These data indicate that hepatic resection can be performed with sufficient safety to make it a standard surgical procedure, and the results of resection are sufficiently good to warrant use for treatment of trauma as well as for certain benign and malignant lesions.[118, 147, 230]

HEPATIC TRANSPLANTATION

There is current interest in transplantation of many organs, for increasing success has been reported in the use of renal transplants in the human. Transplantation of the liver is a much more complex problem than transplantation of the kidney because the liver is a large, single organ located immediately beneath the diaphragm, with a dual blood supply. The venous drainage is into the vena cava above the level of the renal veins. For these reasons, the liver posed a number of technical problems which were solved successfully only a few years ago, in contradistinction to the solution of technical problems of renal transplantation in the early part of this century.[222]

Two different approaches have been used in liver transplantation. In one, the recipient's own liver is removed and an entire donor liver is implanted into the same site. In the other all or part of a donor liver is transplanted in an ectopic site, to supplement the residual function of the host's own liver.

It has been demonstrated that transplantation in the animal is feasible and that acute rejection can be prevented with immunosuppressive regimens similar to those used for protection of renal transplants. The most commonly used drugs have been Imuran and corticosteriods. Currently, there is increasing interest in the use of antilymphocyte globulin, though the exact place of this agent is yet to be delineated.[22, 210]

Human experience to date is limited and hepatic transplantation is experimental. Less than 10 persons underwent orthotopic hepatic transplantation prior to 1967 and all died in less than 1 month postoperatively. During 1967, however, 7 transplants were performed by Starzl and associates and all survived longer than 1 month. Three are still alive, one being 9 months postoperatively.[209] Halgrimson and associates are of the opinion that orthotopic transplantation is superior to ectopic auxiliary transplantation because the transplanted liver atrophies unless portal blood is supplied.[74] If portal blood is diverted into the homograft, away from the host liver, the recipient's own liver atrophies. These authors suggest, therefore, the possibility of a hepatotrophic substance in splanchnic blood which is essential for maintenance of morphologic and functional integrity of hepatic tissue.

A liver may be rejected as any other homograft. A special problem is the development of intrahepatic abscesses. This complication may well represent a problem of rejection with sufficient damage of hepatic tissue to allow bacterial sepsis. It is also possible, however, that the hepatic abscesses are the result of technical problems at the time of transplantation with some death of hepatic tissue due to impaired blood supply.

Progress in this field is very encouraging, but much refinement in technic and immunosuppressive regimens are necessary before widespread clinical application is possible.

HEPATIC PERFUSION

The multiple complicated functions of the liver have precluded serious attempts to construct an artificial liver which could function in a manner comparable to an artificial kidney. Consequently, attempts have been made in other directions to find methods by which the liver can be supported during periods of acute disease when improvement of function could be anticipated if life were preserved over a relatively short term. These attempts have centered primarily around the use of extracorporeal perfusion of a homologous or heterologous liver to serve this function. In addition to human cadavers, a number of experimental animals have been investigated as possible donors. Studies in the dog indicate that in this animal hepatic outflow block develops relatively early in the course of perfusion and dog livers have not proved to be particularly satisfactory. Recently, studies have involved livers from the pig and from the calf. Both of these animals have relatively large organs, more nearly the size of the human, and these livers can be subjected to perfusion with a high likelihood of success and a lower incidence of technical difficulties than were experienced in canine perfusion experiments.[12, 46, 153, 217] It has been demonstrated that the perfused liver can function as an extracorporeal organ: it forms bile, clears metabolic waste products from the perfused blood, as well as synthesizes some new compounds.

Following experiments in animals, extracorporeal perfusion has been accomplished in a number of humans with hepatic disease. In most of the recent experiences, the pig liver has been used. Norman and associates[152] reported the use of the porcine liver in studies on several patients entering end stage hepatic failure with severe preterminal hepatic disease. These authors found that the bile produced by the perfused porcine liver contained human proteins and no demonstrable porcine protein. No long-term survivals were obtained but one patient lived as long as 18 days after 5 serial perfusions. None of these patients showed a demonstrable antibody response to circulating porcine antigens, though other studies have indicated that porcine protein may be found in the blood of patients who were subjected to perfusion for as long as 20 days following this procedure.[152, 219]

Eiseman and associates have reported an experience with 27 perfusions in 16 patients and demonstrated that marked improvement may be observed after perfusion for 4 to 5 hours, and that such improvement may last for as long as 4 days. Re-perfusion has been advocated at intervals of 5 to 7 days as indicated on the basis of the clinical response.[46] Watts and associates have used this technique in 3 patients. Little improvement was observed in 2 patients but in the third patient with acute hepatic insufficiency associated with pregnancy, perfusion appears to have contributed to the survival. Two perfusions were performed in 9 and 8 hours respectively resulting in a marked reduction in serum bilirubin and serum ammonia concentrations as well as striking clinical improvement. At the time of discharge hepatic functions were essentially normal.[219]

As technics are improved, this treatment modality holds promise for increasing applicability.

REFERENCES

1. Alkan, W. J., Kalmi, B., and Kalderon, M.: The clinical syndrome of amebic abscess of the left lobe of the liver, Ann. Int. Med. 55:800, 1961.
2. Anbe, D. T., Smith, R. F., Patton, R. B., and Monto, R. W.: Primary hepatoma with apparent successful surgical resection, Arch. Int. Med. 111:10, 1963.
3. Baker, R. J., Taxman, P., and Freeark, R. J.: An assessment of the management of nonpenetrating liver injuries, Arch. Surg. 93:84, 1966.
4. Bartlett, F. K., Corper, H. J., and Long, E. R.: The independence of the lobes of the liver, Am J. Physiol. 35:36, 1914.
5. Beall, A. C., Jr., Crosthwait, R. W., and De Bakey, M. E.: Traumatic injuries to the liver in Moseley, H. F. (ed.): Accident Surgery, Vol. III, Chap. 9, pp. 101-112, New York, Appleton-Century-Crofts, 1965.
6. Beattie, D. A., and Robertson, H. D.: A case of simple cyst of the liver; with an analysis of 62 other cases, Lancet 2: 674, 1932.
7. Beaver, D. C.: Granulomatous abscess of the liver of pyogenic origin, Am. J. Path. 7:259, 1931.
8. Beaver, D. C., Henthorne, J. C., and Macy, J. W.: Abscesses of liver caused by Bacteroides funduliformis; report of two cases, Arch. Path. 17:493, 1934.
9. Beebe, G. W., and De Bakey, M. E.: Battle Casualties, Springfield, Ill., Charles C Thomas, 1952.
10. Beer, E.: Ligation of the portal vein in suppurative phlebitis, Am. J. Med. Sci. 150:548, 1915.
11. Berberian, D. A., Dennis, E. W., and Korns, R. F.: Drug prophylaxis of amebiasis, J.A.M.A. 148:700, 1952.
12. Bibler, D. D., Condon, R. E., and Nyhus, L. M.: Temporary use of the ex-vivo heterologous liver for hepatic insufficiency: metabolic effects and sensitivity to perfused protein in dogs. Ann. Surg. 164:61, 1966.
13. Block, M. A., Schuman, B. M., Eyler, W. R., Truant, J. P., and DuSault, L. A.: Surgery of liver abscesses, Arch. Surg. 88:602, 1964.
14. Boettiger, C., Weinstein, M., and Werne, J.: Primary suppuration of liver due to Friedländer's bacillus, J.A.M.A. 114: 1050, 1940.
15. Braasch, J. W.: The surgical anatomy of the liver and pancreas, Surg. Clin. N. Amer. 38:747, 1958.
16. Brasfield, R. D.: Right hepatic lobectomy for carcinoma of the gallbladder; a five year cure, Ann. Surg. 153:563, 1961.
17. Braun, H.: Die Unterbindung der Vena ileocolica bei mesenterialer Pyamie nach Appendicitis, Beitr. klin. Chir. 86:314, 1913.
18. Brittain, R. S.: Liver trauma, Surg. Clin. N. Amer. 43:433, 1963.
19. Brown, R. A. P.: Polycystic disease of the kidneys and intracranial aneurysms, Glasgow, M. J. 32:333, 1951.
20. Bunnag, T. S., Kaoparisuthi, V., Arthachinta, S., Chienpradit, K., and Binbakaya, L.: Percutaneous splenic portography in amebic liver abscess, Am. J. Roentgenol. 80:324, 1958.

21. Burch, J. C., and Jones, H. E.: Large nonparasitic cyst of the liver simulating an ovarian cyst, Am. J. Obstet. Gynec. 63:441, 1952.

22. Calne, R. Y., White, H. J. O., Yoffa, D. E., Binns, R. M., Maginn, R. R., Herbertson, R. M., Millard, P. R., Molina, V. P., and Davis, D. R.: Prolonged survival of liver transplants in the pig, Brit. Med. J. 4:645, 1967.

23. Cameron, J. D. S., and Lawler, N. A.: Aspiration, air replacement and radiology in the diagnosis and prognosis of hepatic abscess, J. Roy. Army Med. Corps, 80:1, 1943.

24. Cantlie, J.: On a new arrangement of the right and left lobe of the liver, J. Anat. Physiol. 32:4, 1897.

25. Carnot, P., and Cachéra, R.: Le diagnostic et la surveillance radiologiques des grands abcès du foie par ponctions et injections aérolipiodolées, Arch. mal. appar. dig. 24:988, 1934.

26. Chakravarti, H.: Studies on plasma protein. II. Amoebic dysentery and liver disease, Indian Med. Gaz. 85:394, 1950.

27. Clay, R. C., and Finney, G. G.: Lobectomy of the liver for benign conditions, Ann. Surg. 147:827, 1958.

28. Collard, P. J., and Kendall, D.: Cerebral amebiasis treated with emetine, Lancet 2:17, 1947.

29. Colp, R.: The treatment of pylephlebitis of appendicular origin; with a report of three cases of ligation of the portal vein, Surg. Gynec. Obstet. 43:627, 1926.

30. Comfort, M. W., Gray, H. K., Dahlin, D. C, and Whitesell, F. B., Jr.: Polycystic disease of the liver: study of 24 cases, Gastroenterology 20:60, 1952.

31. Conan, N. J.: Chloroquine in amebiasis, Am. J. Trop. Med. 28:107, 1948.

32. ———: The treatment of amebic hepatitis with chloroquine, Bull. N. Y. Acad. Med. 24:545, 1948.

33. ———: The treatment of hepatic amebiasis with chloroquine, Am. J. Med. 6: 309, 1949.

34. Convers, F.: El examen radiológico en los abscesos amibianos del hígado, Rev. Fac. Med. (Bogotá) 15:727, 1947.

35. Copher, G. H., and Dick, B. M.: "Stream line" phenomena in the portal vein and the selective distribution of portal blood in the liver, Arch. Surg. 17:408, 1928.

36. Councilman, W. T., and Lafleur, H. A.: Amoebic dysentery, Johns Hopkins Hosp. Rep. 2:395, 1891.

37. Craig, C. F.: Observation upon the hemolytic, cytolytic, and complement-binding properties of extracts of Endamoeba histolytica, Am. J. Trop. Med. 7:225, 1927.

38. ———: The Etiology, Diagnosis, and Treatment of Amebiasis, Baltimore, Williams & Wilkins, 1944.

39. Davis, C. R.: Non-parasitic cysts of the liver, Am. J. Surg. 35:590, 1937.

40. De Bakey, M. E., and Ochsner, A.: Surgical treatment of amebiasis, Wisconsin Med. J. 48:243, 1949.

41. ———: Hepatic amebiasis; a 20 year experience and analysis of 263 cases, Surg. Gynec. Obstet. (Int. Abstr. Surg.) 92:209, 1951.

42. Dickinson, J. C.: Radiographic findings in hepatic abscess, amebic in type, Radiology, 4:273, 1925.

43. Dieulafoy, A.: Le foie appendiculaire; abcès du foie consecutifs à l'appendicite, Sem. méd. prof. 18:449, 1898.

44. DiFiglia, S. E., and Cramer, C.: Friedländer's bacillus meningitis in case with liver abscess and recurrent bacteremia and analysis of cases receiving specific therapy, New York J. Med. 51:761, 1951.

45. Doshi, J. C.: Amebic abscess of the left lobe of the liver, Indian J. Med. Sci. 19: 670, 1965.

46. Eiseman, B., Van Wyck, J., and Griffen, W. O., Jr.: Methods for extracorporeal hepatic assist, Surg. Gynec. Obstet. 123: 522, 1966.

47. Eliason, E. L.: Pylephlebitis and liver abscess, Surg. Gynec. Obstet. 42:510, 1926.

48. Elsberg, C. A.: Solitary abscess of the liver, Ann. Surg. 44:209, 1906.

49. Emmett, J.: Refractory amebic abscess of the liver treated with chloroquine, J.A.M.A. 141:22, 1949.

50. Fariss, B. L.: Amebic liver abscess, Am. J. Gastroenterol. 44:559, 1965.

51. Faust, E. C.: Some modern conceptions of amebiasis, Science 99:45, 1944.

52. ———: Amebiasis (Am. Lect. Series), Springfield, Ill., Charles C Thomas, 1954.

53. Feldman, M.: Polycystic disease of the liver, Am. J. Gastroenterol. 29:83, 1958.

54. Ficklen, E. A.: Undescribed fluoroscopic finding in solitary abscess of liver; case report, New Orleans med. surg. J. 94: 587, 1942.

55. Fink, A. A.: Staphylococcic actinophyto-

tic (botryomycotic) abscess of the liver with pulmonary involvement, Arch. Path. *31*:103, 1941.

56. Fish, J. C., and McCary, R. G.: Primary cancer of the liver in childhood, Arch. Surg. 93:355, 1966.

57. Fitz, H. R.: Perforating inflammation of the vermiform appendix, Am. J. Med. Sci. 92:321, 1886.

58. Fitzgerald, J. B., Crawford, E. S., and De Bakey, M. E.: Surgical considerations of non-penetrating abdominal injuries, Am J. Surg. *100*:22, 1960.

59. Freeark, R. J., Love, L., and Baker, R. J.: The role of aortography in the management of blunt abdominal trauma, J. Trauma 8:557, 1968.

60. Friesen, S. R., Hardin, C. A., and Kittle, C. F.: Prolonged survivals after partial hepatectomies and second-look procedures for primary and secondary carcinoma of the liver, Surgery 61:203, 1967.

61. Fuss, E. M., and Fuhrman, M.: Multiple gaseous liver abscesses due to anaerobic *Streptococcus viridans* with recovery, New York J. Med. 50:1142, 1950.

62. Gans, H., Koh, S.-K., and Aust, J. B.: Hepatic resection: results in 39 patients operated on during the 11-year period from 1952 to 1963, Arch. Surg. 93:523, 1966.

63. Geist, D. C.: Solitary non-parasitic cyst of the liver, Arch. Surg. 71:867, 1955.

64. Gerster, A. G.: On septic thrombosis of the roots of the portal vein in appendicitis and on pylephlebitis, together with some remarks on "peritoneal sepsis," Med. Rec. 63:1005, 1903.

65. Glanzman, S., Cally, J. R., and Hammett, J. E.: Treatment of solitary nonparasitic cyst of the liver, New York J. Med. *60*:3684, 1960.

66. Glenard, F.: Note sur les localisations lobaires hépatiques, Bull. Soc. méd. Paris 3:186, 1901.

67. Gondring, W. H.: Solitary cyst of the falciform ligament of the liver, Am. J. Surg. *109*:526, 1965.

68. Goodnough, C. F.: Liver abscess caused by *Bacteroides funduliformis*, Am. J. Surg. 53:506, 1941.

69. Gracey, L.: Tuberculous abscess of the liver, Brit. J. Surg. 52:442, 1965.

70. Granger, A.: Radiological signs of subdiaphragmatic abscess, New Orleans Med. Surg. J. 82:748, 1930.

71. Griswold, R. A., and Collier, H. S.: Blunt abdominal trauma, Surg. Gynec. Obstet. *112*:309, 1961.

72. Guedj, P., Gairoard, J., Morvan, F., and Bogaert, J.: Le traitement chirurgical actuel du kyste hydatique du foie et de ses principales complications; à propos d'une statistique de 600 kystes opérés, J. Chir. (Paris) 93:191, 1967.

73. Gutman, A. B., Olson, K. B., Gutman, E. B., and Flood, C. A.: Effect of disease of liver and biliary tract upon phosphatase activity of serum, J. Clin. Invest. *19*:129, 1940.

74. Halgrimson, C. G., Marchioro, T. L., Faris, T. D., Porter, K. A., Peters, G. N., and Starzl, T. E.: Auxiliary liver transplantation: effect of host portacaval shunt; experimental and clinical observations, Arch. Surg. 93:107, 1966.

75. Haller, J. A., Jr., and Stowens, D.: Right hepatic lobectomy in infancy, Surgery 53:368, 1963.

76. Halpert, B., and Ashley, J. D., Jr.: Amebic colitis complicated with abscess of the brain, Arch. Path. 38:112, 1944.

77. Hankins, J. R.: Management of complicated hepatic hydatid cysts, Ann. Surg. *158*:1020, 1963.

78. Hare, L., and Ritchey, J. O.: Amebiasis masquerading as portal cirrhosis, J. Indiana Med. Ass. *39*:347, 1946.

79. Harris, J. B., and Wise, R. A.: Chloroquine treatment of amebic liver abscess, Am. Practit. 3:128, 1952.

80. Harris, J. D.: Rupture of hydatid cysts of the liver into the biliary tracts, Brit. J. Surg. 52:210, 1965.

81. Healey, J. E., Jr.: Clinical-anatomical aspects of radical hepatic surgery, J. Internat. Coll. Surg. 22:542, 1954.

82. Healy, G. F.: The laboratory diagnosis of amebiasis, Am. J. Gastroenterol. *42*:191, 1964.

83. Hellstrom, G.: Lesions associated with closed liver injury; clinical study of 192 fatal cases, Acta Chir. Scand. *131*:460, 1966.

84. Henley, W. S.: Personal communication.

85. Henson, S. W., Jr., Gray, H. K., and Dockerty, M. B.: Benign tumors of the liver. III. Solitary cysts, Surg. Gynec. Obstet. *103*:607, 1956.

86. Hicken, N. F., McAllister, A. J., and Nilsson, J.: Resection of entire left lobe of liver. Intrahepatic abscesses, stones and foreign bodies, Am. J. Surg. *105*:278, 1963.

87. Hirschowitz, B. I.: Pyogenic liver abscess: a review with a case report of a solitary abscess caused by *Salmonella enteritidis*, Gastroenterology 21:291, 1952.

88. Hoekenga, M.: The prophylaxis of malaria and amebiasis with Milibis-Aralen, J. Lab. Clin. Med. 39:267, 1952.

89. Holmes, A. H.: Non-tropical solitary abscess of liver, Brit. Med. J. 2:991, 1934.

90. Howard, R. N.: Portal pyemia following acute appendicitis: case of multiple liver abscesses with recovery, Aust. New Zeal. J. Surg. 10:31, 1940.

91. Huard, P., Renucci, N., and Huynh-tan-Doi: Les abcès du foie non amibiens, Bull. Soc. méd.-chir. Indochine 13:849, 1935.

92. Hudson, E. K.: Obstructive jaundice from solitary hepatic cyst, Am. J. Gastroent. 39:161, 1963.

93. Hunt, R. S.: Secondarily infected liver abscess treated with penicillin, Lancet 2:138, 1945.

94. Ishak, K. G., and Glunz, P.: Hepatoblastoma and hepatocarcinoma in infancy and childhood; report of 47 cases, Cancer 20:396, 1967.

95. Jacobs, C. A., St. Onge, J. A., Starry, A. C., and Summers, M. P.: Rupture of liver abscess into hepatic vein causing sudden death; report of a case, J. Iowa Med. Soc. 38:447, 1948.

96. Jeanes, A. L.: Immunofluorescent diagnosis of amoebiasis, Brit. Med. J. 2:1531, 1964.

97. Judkins, M. P., and Dotter, C. T.: Angiographic diagnosis of intrahepatic rupture secondary to blunt trauma, Northwest Med. 64:577, 1965.

98. Kagan, I. G., Osimani, J. J., Varela, J. C., and Allain, D. S.: Evaluation of intradermal and serologic tests for the diagnosis of hydatid disease, Am. J. Trop. Med. 15:172, 1966.

99. Kartulis, S.: Zur aetiologie der leberabscesse. Labende dystentevie-amöben im eiter der dysenterischen Leberabscesse, Zbl. Bakt. Parasit. 2:745, 1887.

100. Kasai, M., Kimura, S., Sasaki, M., and Ouchi, H.: Successful total right hepatic lobectomy for primary hepatoma in an infant, Surgery 54:351, 1963.

101. Kasliwal, R. M., Kenney, M., Gupta, M. L., Sethi, J. P., Tatz, J. S., and Illes, C. H.: Significance of the complement-fixation test in diagnosis of amoebiasis in an endemic area, Brit. Med. J. 1:837, 1966.

102. Katz, A. M., and Pan, C.-T.: Echinococcus disease in the United States, Am. J. Med. 25:759, 1958.

103. Kean, B. H.: Amebic hepatitis; absence of diffuse lesions at autopsy and in biopsies, A.M.A. Arch. Int. Med. 96:667, 1955.

104. Keen, W. W.: Report of a case of resection of the liver for removal of a neoplasm, with a table of 76 cases of resection of the liver for hepatic tumors, Ann. Surg. 30:267, 1899.

105. Kessel, J. F., Lewis, W. P., Ma, S., and Kim, H.: Preliminary report on a hemagglutination test for entamoebae, Proc. Soc. Exp. Biol. Med. 106:409, 1961.

106. Killough, J. H., and Magill, G. B.: Terramycin in epidemic typhus, amebic dysentery, and typhoid, J.A.M.A. 147:1737, 1951.

107. Kinney, T. D., and Ferrebee, J. W.: Hepatic abscess—factors determining its localization, Arch. Path. 45:41, 1948.

108. Kinney, T. D., and Ginsberg, H. S.: Pyogenic liver abscesses due to *Klebsiella pneumoniae* (Friedländer's bacillus), New Engl. J. Med. 228:145, 1943.

109. Konar, N. R., and Saha, A. K.: Ascaris liver abscess, J. Indian Med. Ass. 45:450, 1965.

110. Koster, H.: Thorium dioxide as aid in differential diagnosis of pylephlebitis, Radiology 35:728, 1940.

111. Lal, H. B.: Pneumoperitoneum in the study of hepatic abscess, Indian Med. Gaz. 85:90, 1950.

112. Lamont, N. McE., and Pooler, N. R.: Hepatic amoebiasis, Quart. J. Med. 27:389, 1958.

113. Landsman, J. B.: Liver abscess; report of three cases, Glasgow Med. J. 28:320, 1947.

114. Langenbuch, C.: Ein Fall von Resection eines linksseitigen Schnürlappens der Leber; Heilung, Berl. klin. Wschr. 25:37, 1888.

115. Lin, T.-Y.: The results of hepatic lobectomy for primary carcinoma of the liver, Surg. Gynec. Obstet. 123:289, 1966.

116. Lin, T.-Y., and Chen, C.-C.: Metabolic function and regeneration of cirrhotic and non-cirrhotic livers after hepatic lobectomy in man, Ann. Surg. 162:959, 1965.

117. Lin, T.-Y., Chen, C.-C., and Lin, W.-P.: Primary carcinoma of the liver in infancy

and childhood; report of 21 cases with resection in 6 cases, Surgery 60:1275, 1966.

118. Longmire, W. P., Jr.: Hepatic surgery: trauma, tumors, and cysts, Ann. Surg. 161:1, 1965.

119. Longmire, W. P., Jr., and Marable, S. A.: Clinical experiences with major hepatic resections, Ann. Surg. 154:460, 1961.

120. MacKenzie, W. C., and Gray, H. K.: Single pyogenic abscess of liver; report of case, Proc. Mayo Clin. 12:596, 1937.

121. Macris, G. J., and Galanis, N. N.: Rupture of echinococcus cysts of the liver into the biliary ducts, Am. Surg. 32:36, 1966.

122. MacVaugh, H., III, Haupt, G. J., Myers, R. N., and Daly, J. W.: Traumatic hemobilia, Surgery 60:547, 1966.

123. Madding, G. F.: Wounds of the liver, Surg. Clin. N. Amer. 38:1619, 1958.

124. Madding, G. F., and Kennedy, P. A.: Trauma to the Liver, Philadelphia, Saunders, 1965.

125. Maegraith, B. G., and Harinasuta, C.: Experimental amoebic infection of the liver in guinea pigs; infection via mesenteric vein and via portal vein, Ann. Trop. Med. 48:421, 1954.

126. Manson-Bahr, P.: Secondary bacterial infections of amebic abscess of the liver, Trop. Dis. Bull. 45:519, 1948.

127. ————: The treatment of amebic liver abscess with chloroquine, J. Trop. Med. 52:91, 1949.

128. Marray, A. M., and Philipzs, G. L. C.: Report of a case of amoebic abscess of liver, lung, and brain, Glasgow Med. J. 144:116, 1945.

129. Matheson, N. A., Gardner, D. L., and Dudley, H. A. F: Liver sepsis, Brit. J. Surg. 51:363, 1964.

130. Matsumoto, T., Hardaway, R. M., Heisterkamp, C. A., Pani, K. C., and Leonard, F.: Higher homologous cyanoacrylate tissue adhesives in surgery of internal organs, Arch. Surg. 94:861, 1967.

131. McClelland, R. N., Jones, R. C., Shires, G. T., and Perry, M. O.: Liver trauma in Shires, G. T.: Care of the Trauma Patient, Chap. 18, pp. 374-383, New York, McGraw-Hill, 1966.

132. McClelland, R. N., Shires, G. T., and Poulos, E.: Hepatic resection for massive trauma, J. Trauma 4:282, 1964.

133. McDermott, W. V., Jr., and Ottinger, L. W.: Elective hepatic resection, Am. J. Surg. 112:376, 1966.

134. McHardy, G., and Frye, W. W.: Anti

135. Melnick, P. J.: Polycystic liver, A.M.A. Arch. Path. 59:162, 1955.

136. Meredith, R. H., Cooper, L. F., and Yater, W. M.: Thorotrast hepatosplenography as diagnostic aid in solitary liver abscess: report of 4 cases, Med. Ann. D.C. 11:382, 1942.

137. Merendino, K. A., Dillard, D. H., and Cammock, E. E.: The concept of surgical biliary decompression in the management of liver trauma, Surg., Gynec. Obstet. 117:285, 1963.

138. Michels, N. A.: Newer anatomy of the liver and its variant blood supply and collateral circulation, Am. J. Surg. 112: 337, 1966.

139. Miles, J. M.: The roentgenological diagnosis of abscess of the concave surface of the liver, Am. J. Roentgenol. 34:65, 1936.

140. Milgram, E. A., Healy, G. R., and Kagan, I. G.: Studies on the use of the indirect hemagglutination test in the diagnosis of amebiasis, Gastroenterology 50:645, 1966.

141. Mistilis, S., and Schiff, L.: A case of jaundice due to unilateral hepatic duct obstruction with relief after hepatic lobectomy, Gut 4: 13, 1963.

142. Mody, A. E., Desai, H. G., and Bhanusali, H. S.: Polycystic disease of the liver; a case report, Indian J. Med. Sci. 19:130, 1965.

143. Monaco, A. P., Hallgrimsson, J., and McDermott, W. V., Jr.: Multiple adenoma (hamartoma) of the liver treated by subtotal (90%) resection, Ann. Surg. 159:513, 1964.

144. Montero, E., and Uribe, V.: Correlación endoscópia, parasitológica y serológica en el diagnóstico de la amebiasis, Rev. méd. Chile 77:143, 1949.

145. Morris, R. W.: Liver abscess, J.A.M.A. 114:2369, 1940.

146. Moschcowitz, E.: Non-parasitic cysts (congenital) of the liver with a study of aberrant bile ducts, Am. J. Med. Sci. 131:674, 1906.

147. Moseley, R. V.: Primary malignant tumors of the liver; a review of the clinical and pathologic characteristics of 47 cases and a discussion of current diagnostic techniques and surgical management, Surgery 61:674, 1967.

148. Murgatroyd, F., and Kent, R. P.: Refractory amebic liver abscess treated by chlo

biotics in management of amebiasis, J.A.M.A. 154:646, 1954.

roquine, Tr. Roy. Soc. Trop. Med. *42*:15, 1948.

149. Nather, K., and Ochsner, A.: Retroperitoneal operation for subphrenic abscess, Surg., Gynec. Obstet. *37*:665, 1923.

150. Nicks, R.: Intrapleural rupture of hydatid cysts, Med. J. Aust. *1*:352, 1965.

151. Nieweg, G. A.: Abscess of the liver and right psoas muscle secondary to gangrenous appendix, U.S. Vet. Bur. M. Bull. *5*:58, 1929.

152. Norman, J. C., Saravis, C. A., Brown, M. E., and McDermott, W. V., Jr.: Immunochemical observations and clinical heterologous (xenogeneic) liver perfusions, Surgery *60*:179, 1966.

153. Norman, J. K., and Binford, C. H.: Liver abscess due to Friedländer's bacillus (*K. pneumoniae*) complicating adenocarcinoma of ampulla of Vater, Am. J. Clin. Path. *15*:534, 1945.

154. Norris, G. W., and Farley, D. L.: Abscess of the liver, Med. Clin. N. Amer. *10*:17, 1926.

155. Ochsner, A.: Subphrenic abscess, New Orleans med. surg. J. *81*:102, 1928.

156. Ochsner, A., and De Bakey, M. E.: Diagnosis and treatment of amebic abscess of the liver, Am. J. Dig. Dis. *2*:47, 1935.

157. ———: Liver abscess; amebic abscess: analysis of 73 cases, Am. J. Surg. *29*:173, 1935.

158. ———: Pleuropulmonary complications of amebiasis, J. Thoracic Surg. *5*:225, 1936.

159. ———: Subphrenic abscess: collected review and an analysis of 3,608 collected and personal cases, Surg. Gynec. Obstet. (Int. Abstr. Surg.) *66*:426, 1938.

160. ———: Amebic hepatitis and hepatic abscess, Surgery *13*:460, 612, 1943.

161. Ochsner, A., De Bakey, E. G., and Dixon, J. L.: Complications of ascariasis requiring surgical treatment; report of a case with abdominothoracic complications, Am. J. Dis. Child. *77*:389, 1949.

162. Ochsner, A., De Bakey, M. E., Kleinsasser, L., and De Bakey, E. G.: Amebic hepatitis and hepatic abscess, Rev. Gastroent. *9*:438, 1942.

163. Ochsner, A., De Bakey, M. E., and Murray, S.: Pyogenic abscess of the liver; an analysis of 47 cases with review of the literature, Am. J. Surg. *40*:292, 1938.

164. ———: Amebic hepatic abscess; analysis of 139 cases with review of literature, J. internat. Chir. *4*:1, 1939.

165. Overton, R. C., Kaden, V. G., and Livesay, W. R.: The surgical significance of primary carcinoma of the liver, Surgery *37*:519, 1955.

166. Pack, G. T., Islami, A. H., Hubbard, J. C., and Brasfield, R. D.: Regeneration of human liver after major hepatectomy, Surgery *52*:617, 1962.

167. Pack, G. T., and Molander, D. W.: Metabolism before and after hepatic lobectomy for cancer, Arch. Surg. *80*:685, 1960.

168. Pancoast, H. K.: The roentgenological diagnosis of liver abscess with or without subdiaphragmatic abscess, Am. J. Roentgenol. *16*:303, 1926.

169. Peterson, R. D., Varco, R. L., and Good, R. A.: Five-year survival of an infant after surgical excision of an embryonal hepatoma, Pediatrics *27*:474, 1961.

170. Petrén, G.: Ueber Leberabscesse als Komplikation zu akuter Appendicitis, Beitr. Klin. Chir. *94*:225, 1914.

171. Pickrell, K. L., and Clay, R. C.: Lobectomy of the liver: report of three cases, Arch. Surg. *48*:267, 1944.

172. Powell, S. J., Maddison, S. E., Wilmot, A. J., and Elsdon-Dew, R.: Amoebic gel-diffusion precipitin test, Lancet *2*:602, 1965.

173. Powell, S. J., Wilmot, A. J., Macleod, I. N., and Elsdon-Dew, R.: A comparative trial of dehydroemetine, emetine hydrochloride and chloroquine in the treatment of amoebic liver abscess, Ann. Trop. Med. Parasit. *59*:496, 1965.

174. ———: The effect of a nitro-thiazole derivative, Ciba 32,644-Ba in amebic dysentery and amebic liver abscess, Am. J. Trop. Med. *15*:300, 1966.

175. Prussin, G., and Schiffmann, A.: Solitary nonparasitic cyst of the liver, Am. J. Gastroent. *42*:425, 1964.

176. Pyrtek, L. J., and Bartus, S. A.: Hepatic pyemia, New Engl. J. Med. *272*:551, 1965.

177. Quattlebaum, J. K.: Massive resection of the liver, Ann. Surg. *137*:787, 1953.

178. ———: Hepatic lobectomy for benign and malignant lesions, Surg. Clin. N. Amer. *42*:507, 1962.

179. Quattlebaum, J. K., and Quattlebaum, J. K., Jr.: Technic of hepatic lobectomy, Ann. Surg. *149*:648, 1959.

180. ———: Technique of hepatic resection, Surgery *58*:1075, 1965.

181. Rakower, J.: Echinococcosis; a survey of

100 cases, Harefuah (Jerusalem) 59:261, 1960; Abstract: Trop. Dis. Bull. 58:344, 1961.

182. Reeves, D. L., and Stuck, R. M.: Clinical and experimental results with Thorotrast, Medicine 17:37, 1938.

183. Reeves, R. J., and Youngstrom, K. A.: Diagnosis of liver abscess by means of Thorotrast hepatosplenography, Texas J. Med. 42:310, 1946.

184. Reifferscheid, M.: Chirurgie der Leber, p. 150, Stuttgart, Georg Thieme, 1957. (Quoted by Moseley.[147])

185. Robertson, R. D., Foster, J. H., and Peterson, C. G.: Pyogenic liver abscess studied by cholangiography, Am. Surgeon 32:521, 1966.

186. Rogers, L.: Tropical or amoebic abscess of the liver and its relationship to amoebic dysentery, Brit. Med. J. 2:844, 1902.

187. ———: Lettsonian Lectures on amebic liver abscess, Lancet 1:463, 569, 677, 1922.

188. Root, H. D., Hauser, C. W., McKinley, C. R., LaFave, J. W., and Mendiola, R. P., Jr.: Diagnostic peritoneal lavage, Surgery 57:633, 1965.

189. Rothenberg, R. E., and Linder, W.: Single pyogenic liver abscesses; a study of 24 cases, Surg. Gynec. Obstet. 59:31, 1934.

190. Rubin, S. H., Bornstein, P. K., Perrine, C., Rubin, A. D., and Schwimmer, D.: Aureomycin treatment of recurrent cholangitis with liver abscesses due to *Bacteroides funduliformis*, Ann. Int. Med. 35:468, 1951.

191. St. John, F. B., Pulaski, E. J., and Ferrer, J. M.: Primary abscess of liver due to anaerobic nonhemolytic streptococcus, Ann. Surg. 166:217, 1942.

192. Schaak, W.: Zurfrage der nicht parasitären Lebercysten, Arch. Klin. Chir. 125:183, 1923.

193. Schiller, C. F.: Complications of *echinococcus* cyst rupture, J.A.M.A. 195:220, 1966.

194. Schramel, R. J.: Personal communication.

195. Schwartz, S. I.: Surgical Diseases of the Liver, New York, McGraw Hill, 1964.

196. Sérégé, H.: Contribution à l'étude de la circulation du sang fort dans le foie et des localisations lobaires hépatiques, J. méd. Bordeaux 31:271, 291, 312; 1901. Etude sur l'indépendance anatomique et physiologique des lobes du foie, J. méd. Bordeaux 32:327, 341, 357; 1902.

197. Shallow, T. A., Eger, S. A., and Wagner, F. B., Jr: Suppurative pancreatitis with associated liver abscess, Ann. Surg. 121:853, 1945.

198. Shaw, R. R.: Thoracic complications of amebiasis, Surg. Gynec. Obstet. 88:753, 1949.

199. Sheridan, E. P.: Liver abscess, pneumonia and empyema due to Friedländer's bacillus in diabetes mellitus, New Engl. J. Med. 223:528, 1945.

200. Siderys, H., Moore, T. C., and Schumacker, H. B., Jr.: Left hepatic lobectomy for hemangioma of the liver in the newborn, Surgery 52:502, 1962.

201. Sodeman, W. A.: Some recent advances in the diagnosis and treatment of amebiasis, Med. Ann. D.C. 20:409, 1951.

202. ———: Amebiasis *in* Conn, H. F. (ed.): Current Therapy, Philadelphia, Saunders, 1952.

203. Sodeman, W. A., and Beaver, P. C.: A study of the therapeutic effects of some amebacidal drugs, Am. J. Med. 12:440, 1952.

204. Sodeman, W. A., Doerner, A. A., Gordon, E. M., and Gillikin, C. M.: Chloroquine in hepatic amebiasis, Ann. Int. Med. 35:331, 1951.

205. Sodeman, W. A., and Lewis, B. O.: Amebic hepatitis, Am. J. Trop. Med. 25:35, 1945.

206. Sodeman, W. A., Jr., and Haynie, T. P.: Hepatic photoscanning in hydatid liver cysts, J.A.M.A. 188:318, 1964.

207. Sparkman, R. S.: Massive hemobilia following traumatic rupture of the liver, Ann. Surg. 138:899, 1953.

208. Sparkman, R. S., and Fogelman, M. J.: Wounds of the liver; review of 100 cases, Ann. Surg. 139:690, 1954.

209. Starzl, T. E., Groth, C. G., Brettschneider, L., Penn, I., Fulginiti, V. A., Moon, J. B., Blanchard, H., Martin, A. J., Jr., and Porter, K. A.: Orthotopic homotransplantation of the human liver, Ann. Surg. 168:392, 1968.

210. Stuart, F. P., Torres, E., Hester, W. J., Dammin, G. J., and Moore, F. D.: Orthotopic autotransplantation and allotransplantation of the liver; functional and structural patterns in the dog, Ann. Surg. 165:325, 1967.

211. Tandon, B. N., Choudhury, A. K. R., Tikare, S. K., and Wig, K. L.: A study of hepatic amebiasis by radioactive rose

bengal scanning of the liver, Am. J. Trop. Med. 15:16, 1966.

212. Terry, L. L., and Bozicevich, J.: The importance of the complement fixation test in amebic hepatitis and liver abscess, Southern Med. J. 41:691, 1948.

213. Thakur, C. P.: Successful conservative management of spontaneous intraperitoneal rupture of amebic liver abscess; a case report, Indian J. Med. Sci. 19:766, 1965.

214. Theron, P.: Surgical aspects of amebiasis, Brit. Med. J. 2:123, 1947.

215. Tinker, M. B., and Tinker, M. B., Jr.: Resection of the liver, J.A.M.A. 112:2006, 1939.

216. Toole, H., Propatoridis, J., and Pangalos, N.: Intrapulmonary rupture of hydatid cysts of the liver, Thorax 8:274, 1953.

217. Van Wyk, J., Liem, D. S., and Eiseman, B.: Function of cadaver liver, Surgery 58:120, 1965.

218. Wallace, R. H.: Resection of the liver for hepatoma, Arch. Surg. 43:14, 1941.

219. Watts, J. McK., Douglas, M. C., Dudley, H. A. F., Gurr, F. W., and Owen, J. A.: Heterologous liver perfusion in acute hepatic failure, Brit Med. J. 2:341, 1967.

220. Webber, R. J., and Coe, J. I.: Rupture of pyogenic hepatic abscess into hepatic vein, Surgery 27:907, 1950.

221. Welch, C. E., and Burke, J. F.: Carcinoma of the colon and rectum, New Engl. J. Med. 266:211, 1962.

222. Welch, C. S.: A note on transplantation of the whole liver in dogs, Transplantation Bull. 2:54, 1955.

223. Wellman, G. O.: Solitary pyogenic abscess of liver; report of case due to anaerobic streptococci cured by penicillin, Illinois Med. J. 93:327, 1948.

224. Wendell, W.: Beitrage zur Chirurgie der Leber, Arch. Klin. Chir. 95:887, 1911.

225. Williams, L. F., Jr., and Byrne, J. J.: Trauma to the liver at Boston City Hospital from 1955–1965, Am. J. Surg. 112:368, 1966.

226. Wilmoth, C. L.: The use of the exploring needle and shadow casting media in the diagnosis of hepatic and perihepatic abscesses, Ann. Surg. 93:722, 1931.

227. ———: Diagnosis and treatment of abscess in and about the liver, Penn. Med. J. 45:123, 1941.

228. Wilms, M.: Venenunterbindung bei eitriger Pfortaderthrombose nach Appendicitis, Zbl. Chir. 36:1041, 1909.

229. Wilson, H., Storer, E. H., and Star, F. J.: Carcinoid tumors, Am. J. Surg. 105:35, 1963.

230. Wilson, H., and Wolf, R. Y.: Hepatic lobectomy; indications, technique and results, Surgery 59:472, 1966.

231. Wojnar, V. S., German, A. I., Moghul, T. H., and Scarano, D.: Liver, spleen and kidney wounds: experimental repair with topical adhesive, Arch. Surg. 89:237, 1964.

232. Wray, C. H., Stark, C. E., Jr., Brackney, E. L., and Moretz, W. H.: Surgical problems in amebiasis, Am. Surg. 30:780, 1964.

233. Yvergneaux, E., Van de Vijver, W., Yvergneaux, J. P., and Boddaert, J.: Hepatocarcinoma traité par résection atypique du segment III, Acta Gastro-ent. Belg. 26:372, 1963.

234. Zingaro, A. A.: Pyopneumohepatitis, Am. J. Roentgenol. 64:785, 1950.

235. Zodikoff, R.: Multiple liver abscesses with rupture into the pericardium, Am. Heart J. 33:375, 1947.

236. Zuckerbrod, M., Litwins, J., Rogliano, F. T., and Jellinger, D.: Amebic liver abscess, Ann. Int. Med. 32:798, 1948.

26

Liver Disease in Infancy and Childhood

WOLF W. ZUELZER, M.D., AND *A. JOSEPH BROUGH*, M.D.

INTRODUCTION

In early life the liver differs significantly from the adult organ in structure, function and response to local and systemic influences. Though designed ultimately to assume a central role in metabolism, it is still predominantly an organ of hemopoiesis as late as in mid-gestation. Its erythropoietic activity does not cease entirely until birth and may be substantial in premature infants at that time. Under pathologic conditions the infantile liver may continue or resume its hemopoietic function. At birth the circulatory conditions in the liver are modified to some extent by the closure of the ductus venosus. What is more important, the hitherto largely untried organ is now subjected to newly arising metabolic demands of extra-uterine life.

A lag in the ability of the neonatal liver to meet at least one such demand is manifested by the phenomenon of physiologic jaundice. The unique situation reflected by the temporary accumulation of bilirubin in the body fluids and tissues of the newborn infant has largely been elucidated in the last few years and is one of the principal reasons for giving separate consideration to the liver and its diseases in the pediatric age group. The genesis of physiologic jaundice must be understood because the same mechanisms may be operative in a variety of pathologic conditions associated with icterus in the first few weeks of life and because in the newborn period any form of jaundice and any disturbance in hepatic function is always superimposed on a situation physiologically conducive to icterus.

Many of the disturbances likely to affect the liver in earliest extra-uterine life are thus characteristic of the age group and rarely, if ever, occur in later life; or, if they do occur, they produce different manifestations. Moreover, the distant effects of severe jaundice and hyperbilirubinemia, especially those known as kernicterus or bilirubin encephalopathy, are restricted almost entirely to the newborn period.

The common diseases of the adult liver are rare in infancy and childhood. On the other hand, conditions that arise from the interrelationship between mother and child during and after gestation—immunologic differences, infections transplacentally or postnatally acquired and directly or indirectly affecting the liver, congenital malformations, neoplasms of congenital or developmental origin and genetically determined abnormalities of metabolism—these are the disturbances likely to manifest themselves first or exclusively in early life. Therefore, familiarity with these problems is essential for the successful management of hepatic disorders of early life in the clinic and in the laboratory.

DEVELOPMENT AND STRUCTURE OF THE LIVER

The liver develops as an outgrowth of the entodermal tube in the region of the future duodenum. The primary branching of the hepatic diverticulum furnishes the liver anlage proper, the gallbladder and the cystic duct. Disturbances of development in this region are not uncommon and produce the varied patterns of atresia of the extrahepatic bile ducts. The liver anlage proper is formed by branching cell cords which invade the splanchnic mesoderm and differentiate proximally into the hepatic ducts and distally into secretory hepatic tubules. The intertubular spaces are filled by sinusoidal vessels that arise from the breakup of the omphalomesenteric veins as they pass through this region. The radial growth of secretory tubules from the branches of the hepatic ducts produces the secretory lobules, the center of which is formed by the bile ducts accompanied by branches of the portal vein and the hepatic artery. The overlapping radial system of growth of the hepatic veins simultaneously produces the vascular lobules of the liver which are visualized more readily and are more familiar to the student of histology. These structures are centered around the hepatic veins from which a radiating pattern of polygonal cells extends toward the portal tracts.[111] Since according to this classic theory the hepatic cell cords develop from the hepatic ducts in the centers of the secretory lobules, it is difficult to accept the occasional reports of isolated atresias of the intrahepatic bile ducts in the presence of normal lobular patterns in the liver.[2, 121] Failure of development of these ducts should lead to agenesis of the secretory lobules normally arising from them. Moreover, such a process would require that one accept the assumption of identical defects arising simultaneously in millions of separate units of the hepatic anlage.

At birth, in the full-term infant, the central veins and the portal triads are well defined, but the radial pattern of the cell cords is less distinct, and the lobular boundaries are less well-defined than in the adult liver. In the premature infant and under pathologic circumstances in the full-term baby as well, the presence of more or less extensive hemopoietic foci further tends to obscure the architecture. These foci are composed of erythrocyte precursors developing within the cell cords and also found scattered in the lumens of the sinusoids. Their presence correlates well with nucleated red cells circulating in the peripheral blood. Hepatic hemopoiesis is frequently marked in erythroblastosis fetalis, in which condition it appears to represent a compensatory phenomenon in the presence of hemolysis. For less well known reasons it also occurs in infants born to diabetic mothers[104] and in many infections, notably congenital syphilis. Granulocyte precursors also may be found under these conditions but are limited to the connective tissue about the portal triads.

The gross shape of the liver at birth is essentially that of the adult organ, but the two lobes are more nearly equal in size than those of the adult liver. Occasionally, right and left lobes differ strikingly in appearance due to greater or lesser congestion, fat content or even hemorrhage or necrosis in one or the other lobe. These differences have been attributed to the entry of arterial blood from the umbilical vein into the left but not the right lobe of the liver.[60]

The capsule is thin and easily lifted or even ruptured by hematomas collecting underneath as the result of mechanical trauma sustained during birth. The weight of the liver is greater in proportion to total body weight than that of the adult liver but is highly variable, as is, of course, the birth weight itself. The figure given by Coppoletta and Wolbach[32] for the weight of the organ at birth (78 Gm.) is probably too low; that given by Potter and Adair (150 Gm.) is on the high side.[114] Only very large deviations are significant, and it must be kept in mind that the enormous dilatation of the sinusoids of the liver seen especially in asphyxiated infants may rapidly increase the weight of the organ. More meaningful figures have been developed by Potter by relating the weight of the organ to total body weight.[113] Even in healthy infants the liver is normally palpable at birth and remains so to a greater or lesser degree for about 2 years, a fact which tends to make the clinical appraisal of hepatomegaly hazardous at times.

NEONATAL JAUNDICE

MECHANISMS

The central fact in any consideration of the neonatal liver is the occurrence of icterus as a physiologic phenomenon. Although in the light of the newer knowledge concerning the nature and the metabolism of the bile pigments, a sharp line can no longer be drawn between physiologic icterus and many other conditions associated with hyperbilirubinemia in the newborn period, the term is firmly embedded in medical usage and is not easily replaced. It can be defined roughly by the time of its onset and disappearance, by the degree of the bilirubinemia and by the assumption that it can be explained solely in terms of the limited capacity of the neonatal organism to metabolize bilirubin. These terms can now be given the specific meaning of the activity of enzymatic processes in which the fetal and neonatal liver compares unfavorably with the mature organ.

For many years one of the most puzzling aspects of physiologic icterus was the fact that the *elevation of serum bilirubin* is due almost entirely to an increase in the "indirect-reacting" fraction as determined by the diazo reaction. Generally the prevalence of this fraction in later life is associated with hemolytic states, yet an acceleration of the breakdown of fetal and neonatal erythrocytes sufficient to explain the retention of bilirubin in the normal newborn infant could never be demonstrated.[106] It was necessary, therefore, to postulate a special functional inadequacy of the neonatal liver with regard to the excretion of bilirubin, but the nature of the functional defect could not be defined until the chemical differences between the "indirect-reacting" and the "direct-reacting" fractions were recognized and the enzymatic steps by which the liver converts one form into the other were uncovered. Then it could be shown that the fetal and to a lesser extent the neonatal liver are lagging in the capacity to perform the enzymatic reactions now known to be prerequisite to bilirubin excretion. This lag is now generally accepted as the limiting factor in the bilirubin metabolism of the newborn infant and as the basis of physiologic icterus.

Bilirubin in the plasma is in two forms: the so-called free, i.e., unconjugated pigment and the conjugated pigment, i.e., bilirubin diglucuronide. The former is highly insoluble and gives an indirect van den Bergh reaction, i.e., it must be solubilized by alcohol. The diglucuronide is highly soluble and conjugation must precede the excretion of the pigment. For a time it was believed that bilirubin existed in the plasma in the third form, bilirubin monoglucuronide,[14] and that it contributed a variable but often substantial fraction of the pigment in neonatal jaundice. It is now clear that the third fraction ("fraction I") extracted by column chromotography or solvent partition[48] is in fact the product of variable complexing of free and fully conjugated pigment[15, 59, 96, 108, 146] and plays no part in the physiologic processes. Conjugation involves the transfer of glucuronide molecules from uridine diphosphoglucuronic acid (UDPGA) and is catalyzed by a hepatic microsomal enzyme, glucuronyl transferase.[128] This enzyme is virtually inactive in the fetal liver until about mid-gestation and is of low activity at birth compared with that in the mature organ.[20, 46, 93] Following birth it increases rapidly, and in the experimental animal reaches adult levels in approximately 3 weeks. However, not only does the activity of the glucuronyl transferase lag in the liver of the newborn infant and animal, but the key substance UDPGA itself, formation of which is in turn dependent on a series of enzymatic steps, is present in decreased amounts in the neonatal liver as compared with that of the adult, and the penultimate step by which the precursor substance UDP-glucose is oxidized to UDPGA is likewise performed inadequately, apparently because of the limited activity of the enzyme UDPG dehydrogenase which catalyzes this reaction.[23] This enzyme, too, rapidly becomes more active after birth.

On the basis of these facts, failure of the hepatic conjugating mechanisms for bilirubin has been generally accepted as the basis of physiologic icterus, and there can be little doubt that this view is substantially correct, though other mechanisms may also be involved as will be shown shortly. The factors that influence the presence, the state of activity and the development of the enzymes and the substrates required by the neonatal liver for the conjugation of bilirubin are unknown. Stated in a general way, the *maturity* of the neonate determines to a large extent the ability to metabolize and excrete bilirubin, for in general premature infants tend to exhibit a more profound and longer-lasting hyperbilirubinemia and this tendency is inversely related to birth weight. It is a fair assumption that this relationship reflects the state of activity of the hepatic enzyme systems involved, but it is not known whether the enzymes themselves undergo a process of increase and adaptive maturation or whether their activity increases because of changing metabolic conditions such as the withdrawal of inhibitory influences, possibly of maternal origin, at the end of gestation, or other endocrine or general metabolic stimuli. In any event the transition from an intra- to an extra-uterine environment affects the activity of the systems involved, since even in small premature infants jaundice ceases after a week or two, long before the conceptual age of a mature newborn infant is reached.

Two other factors appear likely to influence the metabolism of bilirubin in the newborn infant. One is the state of *carbohydrate metabolism* or perhaps more specifically the availability of glucose for the synthesis of the key substance UDPGA. This assumption is rendered likely by a number of clinical observations that relate to the development of hyperbilirubinemia in diverse conditions, in infants born to diabetic mothers, in infants with pyloric stenosis and intestinal obstruction, in galactosemia and in cretinism. One is tempted to speculate that the common denominator in all these situations might well be lack of available carbohydrate reserves.[156]

The second factor, likewise suggested by clinical observations, is *hypoxia*, since both full-term and premature infants with otherwise unexplained hyperbilirubinemia frequently have a history of respiratory difficulties and the like.[22] Since oxygen is required for most enzymatic reactions involved in the conjugation of bilirubin, this, too, is a reasonable assumption. However, possibly the hyperbilirubinemia of such infants is related not so much directly to lack of oxygen as to depletion of carbohydrate stores due to excessive muscular activity in respiratory distress.

Finally, the assumption that the excretion

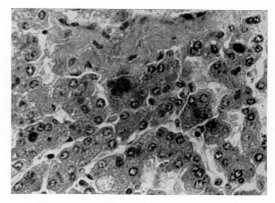

Fig. 26–1. Plugs of inspissated bile. From 8-day-old infant dying after unsuccessful operation for congenital atresia of jejunum. No icterus. Liver otherwise normal.

of fully conjugated bilirubin presents no problem for the neonatal liver needs to be re-examined in the light of the data obtained with the solvent partition method. In premature infants at least, it is not uncommon to find significant amounts of bilirubin diglucuronide in the serum often amounting to absolute concentrations of 1.0 to 3.0 mg. in 100 ml.[159] Under pathologic conditions, e.g., in severe hemolytic disease, in which a greatly increased load of pigment must be excreted by an organ likely to be damaged by the effects of severe anemia, direct-reacting bilirubin is often even more markedly increased in full-term infants.[75] In both situations, in the apparently normal premature infant and in the patient with severe hemolytic disease, so-called bile thrombi are commonly found in histologic sections of the liver (Fig. 26–1). All these observations suggest that at times the excretory capacity of the neonatal liver is exceeded in the absence of organic liver disease. The significance of this interpretation for the evaluation of "obliterative" jaundice in newborns is discussed subsequently.

Further evidence that the neonatal liver is handicapped with respect to its excretory functions was established by Mollison and Cutbush[107] and Yudkin and co-workers[151] who showed that *Bromsulphalein excretion* is impaired in the majority of newborn infants. Brown and Brauer have carried these observations a step further by showing that conjugated as well as unconjugated dye appears in the plasma of the newborn infant after 5 mg./kg. of Bromsulphalein is administered.[21]

That extrahepatic factors influence the distribution of bilirubin in the body needs to be stressed. Bilirubin is solely bound to *albumin* and when the binding capacity of the plasma is exceeded it enters into the tissues. In the neonate and the premature infant whose serum albumin concentrations are apt to be relatively low, the binding capacity thus has potential clinical significance because it determines the proportion of pigment that may be relieved into the tissues, since it must be remembered that bilirubin competes with other formed substances (e.g., certain drugs) for binding sites. The fate of the pigment in the tissues necessarily depends on the cellular composition, i.e., on the availability of certain substances in which it may be soluble, e.g., fat. The size of the potential reservoir of *adipose tissue* sites may serve to hold extravascular bilirubin, so that it does not accumulate at critically susceptible sites such as the brain; thus it is another particularly significant factor in premature infants whose fat stores are as yet poorly developed.

CLASSIFICATION

As the foregoing discussion indicates, physiologic icterus cannot be sharply distinguished from abnormal conditions in which the same handicap is exaggerated; the same mechanisms may be involved. The physiologic state in theory is defined as jaundice of a type, time of onset, duration and degree that can be explained solely in terms of the limited capacity of the neonatal liver to metabolize bilirubin.[156] In practice this type is determined—in the absence of hemolysis or other evidence of disease—chiefly by the demonstration that the pigment in the serum is wholly or almost wholly indirect-reacting bilirubin. The other parameters must be based on statistical evaluation, and here one must allow for variation related to maturity; i.e., different standards apply to the premature and to the full-term infant.

When this is done and when abnormal hemolytic processes have been excluded, a large category remains in which bilirubin is of the indirect-reacting variety but the somewhat arbitrary limits of physiologic icterus are clearly exceeded, a category in which various etiologic factors not always clearly definable play a role but are perhaps less important than the common mechanism; i.e., a further depression of the same functions that are lagging even in entirely normal newborn infants. For lack of a better term one might call this category "exaggerated physiologic jaundice."

This category is distinguished on clinical and hematologic evidence from that in which an excessive load of bilirubin is imposed on the neonatal liver by an abnormal breakdown of hemoglobin, as in hemolytic disease of the newborn, other hemolytic anemias and occasionally the resorption of extravasated blood. Except for severe hemolytic disease in which, as mentioned, the excretory capacity of the liver may also be affected, with a consequent rise of the direct-reacting bilirubin in the serum, in this category as in those preceding, indirect-reacting bilirubin predominates in the serum, but its concentration usually rises at a more rapid rate, and the peak levels are often higher.

By contrast, elevation of the direct-reacting bilirubin in the serum and the concomitant appearance of bile in the urine generally denote organic hepatocellular damage, frank liver disease or anatomic obstruction. It is well to keep in mind that invariably under these circumstances the indirect-reacting bilirubin is also substantially elevated in the newborn infant and, for reasons already discussed, may even far exceed the direct-reacting fraction. Table 26–1 slightly modified from that presented by Zuelzer and Brown,[156] attempts to relate clinical and etiologic factors to underlying mechanisms as they can be visualized—or hypothesized at present.

PHYSIOLOGIC ICTERUS

The classic studies of Davidson, Merritt and Weech[40] established that the bilirubin level is elevated in the cord blood of most newborn infants. After birth the curve of

TABLE 26–1. CLASSIFICATION OF NEONATAL HYPERBILIRUBINEMIA

| Principal Mechanism | SERUM BILIRUBIN PRINCIPALLY INDIRECT-REACTING | | SERUM BILIRUBIN DIRECT AND INDIRECT-REACTING INADEQUATE EXCRETION AND INADEQUATE CONJUGATION | |
	Inadequate Conjugation	Increased Hemoglobin Degradation	Primarily Hepatocellular	Primarily Biliary
Etiology:				
Immaturity	"Physiologic" jaundice Prematurity			
Anatomic				Extrahepatic atresia
Perinatal hazards	Hypoxia Difficult delivery ?Breast feeding	Extravasations (cephalhema- toma, etc.)		
?Metabolic	Maternal diabetes Delayed CHO feeding Dehydration Pyloric stenosis Cretinism Mongolism	Pyknocytosis		
Genetic	Crigler-Najjar syndrome ?Familial transient hyperbili- rubinemia	Congenital spherocytosis Nonspherocytic anemia, etc.	Galactosemia ?Dubin-John- son[43, 45, 132] ?Rotor- Schiff[123, 44]	
Toxic	?Antihyper- tensives	Hemolytic ane- mia with vitamin K, naphthalene, G6PD defi- ciency, etc.	Chlorpromazine	
Infectious	?Depressing effect of bacterial infections	Bacterial hemolysis	Viral hepatitides "Toxic hepatitis" secondary to bacterial sepsis and diarrheal disease	"?Intrahepatic biliary atresia" (cholangiolitis)
Immunologic		Hemolytic disease (Rh, ABO, etc.)	Excretory failure after hemolytic disease	

the serum bilirubin rises rapidly, reaching a peak about the 3rd or 4th day and de-clining fairly rapidly thereafter. The degree of bilirubinemia observed in seemingly nor-mal infants varies considerably, and it is somewhat arbitrary to set an upper limit. The values obtained at any given moment must be interpreted in terms of the time elapsed since birth, and a bilirubin level which might well be physiologic for an infant 3 or 4 days old might be grossly abnormal in an infant less than 24 hours old. In the widely quoted study by Hsia et al. the range is 1.4 to 3.2 mg./100 ml. for cord bloods and levels of 0.6 to 13.2 mg. for specimens obtained on the 3rd and 4th days.[73] Since, as discussed above, it is difficult to decide whether the metabolic situation of a given infant with respect to bilirubin is in fact entirely normal, the peak values of 10 to 12 mg. which are apparently accepted by most students are probably too high for truly physiologic icterus.[156] From a practical point of view it seems wise to accept this range, but such levels should always be viewed with some degree of suspicion.

For premature infants, peak levels up to 15 mg. are regarded as physiologic in the authors' laboratory,[22] but it would be dangerous to be dogmatic on this point; other investigators have reported widely scattered values, which is not surprising in view of the inherent variation in any group of such babies and the variables in their management that are likely to influence the metabolism of bilirubin.

Although hyperbilirubinemia is a universal phenomenon in the newborn period, clinical jaundice is not. Depending somewhat on conditions of observation, icterus is observed in one to two thirds of newborn infants. When the concentration of bilirubin in the serum exceeds 4 to 5 mg./100 ml., the vast majority of infants show frank icterus. Below this level the presence of clinical jaundice is highly variable and seems to depend largely on capillary permeability and other factors connected with the circulatory system and the state of the skin and other tissues. The time of onset is somewhat variable. In most cases icterus becomes apparent on the 3rd or 4th day, sometimes on the 2nd. It is universally recognized that jaundice in the first 24 hours of extra-uterine life can never be regarded as physiologic but always as an indicator of an abnormal condition, however mild, and usually as a sign of hemolytic disease.

In the full-term infant physiologic icterus is clinically mild and unaccompanied by clinical symptoms. It usually disappears within 1 to 3 days, and correspondingly, the bilirubin level of the plasma decreases rapidly once the peak has been passed, so that by the end of the first week of life values of less than 2 mg./100 ml. are to be expected. A duration of jaundice and hyperbilirubinemia beyond the first week should be regarded as abnormal, even though it may not be possible to demonstrate the cause of such prolonged icterus in the individual case. In the premature infant, jaundice and hyperbilirubinemia are apt to persist longer, often well into the 2nd week of life, but accurate information on the end point seems to be lacking.

HYPERBILIRUBINEMIA

This heading refers to severe and usually prolonged jaundice and a corresponding hyperbilirubinemia exceeding the arbitrarily defined limits of physiologic icterus and characterized by an elevation of the indirect-reacting fraction of the plasma bilirubin in infants in whom neither organic liver disease nor accelerated hemolysis can be demonstrated. In the section on Classification of Neonatal Jaundice this type was referred to as "exaggerated physiologic jaundice." From what has been said, it is clear that the pertinent cases do not form a homogeneous group but represent instances of various conditions than can affect unfavorably the normally marginal conjugating capacity of the neonate for bilirubin. In many instances the causative factor or factors remain obscure, but an effort should always be made to analyze the situation, because the subsequent course cannot always be predicted; and if the jaundice persists, at a later stage when the differential diagnosis is even more difficult it may be crucial to have information pertaining to the early phase. Usually the hyperbilirubinemia subsides spontaneously by the 2nd or 3rd week, although in many clinics, levels in excess of 20 mg./100 ml. are not permitted to develop, and exchange transfusions are performed on the indication of averting the potential danger of kernicterus.

As mentioned above, apart from prematurity, respiratory distress and perhaps other conditions conducive to hypoxia in the perinatal period, including fetal distress from various causes such as prolonged and difficult labor, have most often been found to be associated with otherwise unexplained hyperbilirubinemia. In such infants, whether premature or full-term, the study of the serum bilirubin usually discloses predominantly unconjugated pigment, the most insoluble and therefore theoretically the most dangerous fraction.[158]

Next in frequency among the associated conditions are, in the authors' experience, *maternal diabetes* (which should be suspected especially if the infant is unusually large), and *intestinal obstruction*, which in turn is often associated with prematurity. Several observers have been impressed with the possible effect on the intensity of neonatal icterus of certain drugs given to the mother prior to delivery, such as antihypertensives, tranquilizers and perhaps others.[41, 98, 156] Documentation on this point is inadequate, but it seems plausible that pharmacologic and toxic factors can depress the marginally functioning conjugating mechanisms of the newborn infant more readily than those of the adult, whether by competing for glucuronides[147] or in other ways.

Breast-fed infants appear to be generally more susceptible to hyperbilirubinemia than bottle-fed infants, and the presence in breast milk of *progestins* that inhibit glucuronide conjugation has been incriminated for this phenomenon.[3] Reportedly, withdrawal of breast feeding is followed by a prompt decrease of jaundice in affected infants, but this has been rare in the authors' experience, and it may be that at least some of these cases remain inadequately understood.

General genetic factors may also be involved, for under circumstances presumably excluding environmental factors and hemolytic disorders, different racial groups vary considerably in the incidence of hyperbilirubinemia.[24]

A genetically determined condition, though rare, should always be considered in the presence of unexplained hyperbilirubinemia of this type. This is the familial syndrome described by Crigler and Najjar[38] under the name of *familial nonhemolytic jaundice* and now known to be due to a genetic defect in the activity of the key enzyme, glucuronyl transferase.[126] It is not clear how this condition is related to the type of familial nonhemolytic jaundice of adults known as Gilbert's disease.[56, 57, 115] If, as reported, the same enzyme defect is involved in both, the question remains as to why the Crigler-Najjar syndrome is so much more severe in early life, leading apparently without exception to the development of kernicterus, whereas Gilbert's disease does not seem to be associated with strikingly severe neonatal icterus and does not affect the central nervous system. It appears likely from pedigree data that the two disorders involve different genetic factors.[115]

Treatment. The treatment of hyperbilirubinemia not associated with hemolytic anemia disease has not been standardized. While the same basic considerations apply as in the control of jaundice in hemolytic disease, i.e., the prevention of kernicterus, the criteria for evaluating the threat cannot be the same, because the rate at which the pigment accumulates is slower and equivalent serum levels may not be indicative of equivalent total body concentrations. Kernicterus does at times occur in premature infants and, of course, in patients with the Crigler-Najjar syndrome and must be guarded against, but no fixed levels of serum bilirubin can be seen. Some clinics do not treat premature infants in the absence of a hemolytic process. On the other hand, the authors and others[109] have seen kernicterus develop in premature infants whose maximal observed bilirubin concentrations were less than 15 mg.%, and in our clinic exchange transfusion is frequently performed in jaundiced premature infants. No numerical values can be proposed at this time, but the size of the infant, the presence of unfavorable factors (e.g., respiratory distress or infection), the clinical condition of the infant and the duration of the hyperbilirubinemia as well as the pigment levels influence the decision. Generally, but not invariably, a single exchange transfusion suffices in simple hyperbilirubinemia. In full-term infants the criteria are far less stringent.

HEMOLYTIC DISEASE

After what has been said about the limited capacity of the neonatal liver to conjugate and excrete bilirubin, it is not surprising that in this age group jaundice is more often the expression of systemic conditions that affect the balance between capacity and load than of primary disease of the liver or the biliary tract. Apart from physiologic icterus, the commonest and most important disorder to be considered is hemolytic disease of the newborn, because it represents a combination of factors uniquely conducive to the development of severe jaundice and rapidly increasing and potentially dangerous levels of bilirubin in the body fluids and tissues. The more-or-less rapid and often greatly increased catabolism of hemoglobin resulting from the destruction of erythrocytes sensitized by maternal antibodies creates a markedly increased load of bilirubin to be handled by a system which normally operates with marginal efficiency at best. This system may be depressed further by concomitant direct effects on the liver such as hypoxia, vascular congestion and stasis, and perhaps antigen-antibody reactions.

Characteristically, the onset of jaundice is earlier than in physiologic icterus of hyperbilirubinemia not associated with accelerated hemolysis, usually on the first day of life; the rate of rise is apt to be more rapid, and the peak levels of bilirubin in the serum, in the absence of therapeutic intervention, are likely to be higher. When hemolysis is not a factor (and organic liver disease is not present), the concentration of the serum bilirubin rarely rises by more than 5 mg./100 ml. in any 24-hour period.[156] The diazo reaction does not usually help to differentiate qualitatively between hemolytic disease and simple or exaggerated physiologic jaundice. In both instances, it is usually the indirect-reacting bilirubin which alone is elevated, although for reasons to be discussed, in severe hemolytic

disease, usually of the type due to Rh antibodies, the direct-reacting pigment may also be increased.

ABO. The commonest form of hemolytic disease and of early and severe neonatal jaundice is ABO hemolytic disease, usually a rather mild disturbance as indicated by the name chosen by Halbrecht,[63] the first author to describe the condition, icterus praecox. The chief and often the sole clinical feature is icterus, usually apparent within 24 hours after birth. The serum bilirubin level may rise rapidly in the ensuing 3 to 4 days and exceed 20 or even 30 mg./100 ml. In untreated cases kernicterus develops with an appreciable frequency[158] which is the chief reason why the condition is of any concern at all.

The hematologic manifestations are usually rather mild, severe anemia is distinctly rare and even normoblastemia is uncommon and seldom marked. However, in cases severe enough to deserve the appellation of hemolytic disease, there is some degree of reticulocytosis in excess of that found in normal neonatal blood, and not infrequently this feature becomes striking. More characteristic is the presence of spherocytosis.[61]

Physical examination may show slight hepatic but only rarely splenic enlargement. In the presence of the clinical and hematologic features described, the serologic confirmation of the diagnosis offers a few problems. A detailed discussion of these problems is beyond the scope of this chapter. Suffice it to say that in the overwhelming majority of cases of clinically significant disease the mother is of blood group O and the infant of group A or B.[120] In heterospecific pregnancies which result in ABO hemolytic disease of the offspring, the maternal serum usually contains an increased concentration of "immune" (7 S) iso-antibodies as opposed to the "natural" (19 S) agglutinins. The former, which can cross the placenta, are responsible for varying degrees of hemolysis. From a practical point of view, the demonstration of maternal immune iso-antibodies in ABO hemolytic disease is laborious and less important than the few simple tests on the infant's blood needed to confirm the diagnosis.[157]

The direct Coombs' test is weakly positive or negative, but the serum of the infant can usually be shown to contain free homologous antibody, i.e., antibody that reacts more or less strongly with adult erythrocytes of the infant's own blood group when tested with the indirect antiglobulin test. It is essential when anti-A hemolytic disease is to be diagnosed to use test cells of subgroup A_1, since the maternal anti-A antibody usually has anti-A_1 specificity. In doubtful cases it may be necessary to elute the antibody from the infant's erythrocytes.[62] Such eluates must give a positive indirect Coombs' test with homologous adult erythrocytes if the diagnosis is to be substantiated.

Rh. Rh hemolytic disease is ordinarily not difficult to diagnose. In most cases the mother is Rh negative, and in modern obstetric practice a tentative prenatal diagnosis is usually made on serologic grounds and often on the basis of a history of the disease in siblings. It has become possible by means of amniocentesis to obtain prenatal information concerning the severity of the disease in the fetus[97, 100]; this procedure is used only if the history and/or the maternal status provides valid indications.[154]

At birth, all that is required for a definitive diagnosis is a positive direct antiglobulin test on the cord blood. This test is the cornerstone of the diagnosis and is almost invariably strongly positive in contrast with the weak reaction obtained in ABO hemolytic disease. This is also true when the sensitization of the fetal erythrocytes is due to antibodies less common than anti-D (anti-Rh$_o$), such as anti-c (anti-hr'), anti-E (anti-rh''), and those not related to the Rh system of antigens. In all such cases the mother may be Rh positive and therefore may have escaped the prenatal screening process. In this situation the antiglobulin test becomes even more important, much more so for initial diagnostic and therapeutic purposes than the antigenic analysis of mother and child.

The *clinical picture* of Rh hemolytic disease is more variable than was realized before the advent of reliable serologic procedures for diagnosis, ranging from the occasional completely asymptomatic state followed perhaps belatedly by anemia, through a picture characterized by manifest anemia with icterus and hepatosplenomegaly to severe anemia with edema and evidence of circulatory failure and, of course, stillbirth of a hydropic fetus. The commonest symptom is *jaundice*, which usually develops within a few hours after birth and progresses rapidly. At least a moderate degree of anemia is present in most cases, although it does not necessarily parallel the degree of jaundice and in fact may not be apparent even in babies with marked icterus until several days later. However, the blood picture in the average case does clearly reflect the hemolytic process by reticulocytosis, polychromasia and often normoblastemia.

The bilirubin level of the cord blood is usually elevated beyond the physiologic range. In a few hours and days after birth it is apt to rise rapidly and to levels sometimes almost unparalleled. In most cases the pigment is almost entirely of the indirect-reacting variety. However, there are cases in which from the beginning the direct-reacting fraction is also substantially increased, albeit to a lesser degree than the indirect and rarely accounting for more than a quarter of the total concentration. As a rule these are instances of severe hemolytic disease as judged by the degree of anemia and the clinical condition of the infant at birth or shortly thereafter.

Prior to the widespread use of exchange transfusion, a sustained and even progressive elevation of both the total and the direct-reacting serum bilirubin was not uncommon, and sometimes such infants developed the clinical and laboratory picture of obstructive jaundice; bile appeared in the urine, the stools were acholic, and the skin assumed a greenish tinge instead of the earlier orange-yellow. Not uncommonly jaundice persisted for 4 to 6 weeks in such cases. This syndrome used to be referred to as the "inspissated bile syndrome,"[75] a term relating to the presence of bile casts in histologic sections of the liver and reflecting the concept that these casts represented abnormally viscid secretion of bile into the intercellular bile canaliculi with consequent mechanical obstruction. It was

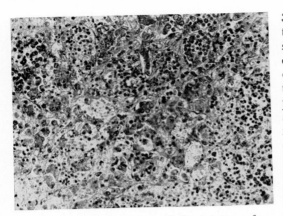

Fig. 26–2. Necrosis and dissociation of polygonal cells, congestion, extensive hemopoiesis. Liver of 15-hour-old infant dead of hydropic-anemic form of erythroblastosis fetalis. This is an example of unusually severe liver damage in this disease.

realized that the same clinical syndrome could occur in conditions not associated with hemolytic disease. The term "inspissated bile syndrome" should be abandoned (and has been by most authors), partly because it is apt to confuse and conceal etiologic conditions, but more importantly because it is not in keeping with current views on cholestasis, which has come to be regarded as the result rather than the mechanical cause of hepatic excretory failure. Considering the hepatocellular damage (Fig. 26–2), congestion, disruption of architecture and infiltration, changes that may equal or surpass in morphologic equivalents those of acute hepatitis, it is not difficult to conceive of excretory failure in severe hemolytic disease as the expression of organic liver damage superimposed on the hemolytic process. While evidence of excretory failure in the early acute stage of severe hemolytic disease is still seen, the late and prolonged phase of jaundice with obstructive features has become rare since exchange transfusion has been introduced.

In connection with the problem of excretory failure on the part of the liver in hemolytic disease, two kinds of observations should be mentioned. One is the frequent appearance of direct-reacting bilirubin in moderately severe cases about the 3rd or 4th day after birth, which under these circumstances presages a rapid subsequent decline of the total bilirubin level of the plasma and disappearance of jaundice. Such a sequence of events suggests that with improved liver function for conjugating the pigment presented as the result of hemolysis—to the extent to which it equals or even exceeds the load—the capacity to excrete conjugated bilirubin is temporarily surpassed.[156] In the absence of significant liver damage this functional disability is overcome rapidly, and the transient appearance of small amounts of direct-reacting bilirubin in such infants is thus a favorable prognostic sign.

More problematical are the rare instances in which hemolytic disease of moderate severity, as judged by the hematologic findings, is accompanied from the start by severe hyperbilirubinemia which persists and recurs despite multiple exchange transfusions and is characterized by excessively high levels of direct-reacting pigment in the plasma, often amounting to 50 per cent or more of the total bilirubin measured.[153] This feature and the marked discrepancy between the amount of pigment that can be accounted for by the apparent rate of hemolysis on the one hand, and the very high plasma levels actually observed on the other, suggest that such cases do not represent uncomplicated instances of hemolytic disease but most likely a combination of the latter with organic primary disease of the liver such as hepatitis. This is how we have interpreted examples of this type that we have observed, and it would seem to be wise not to accept such cases as mysterious deviations from the usual course of hemolytic disease but to search for evidence of primary liver disease. Unfortunately, no laboratory test clearly distinguishes hepatitis from hepatic damage secondary to hemolytic disease. In both situations the SGO transaminase may be markedly increased and liver function tests may yield abnormal results. Liver biopsy is helpful but is rarely resorted to under these circumstances.

The *histologic changes* in the liver in hemolytic disease vary greatly, depending on the severity as well as the stage of the disease. Some degree of hemosiderosis is usually found. Erythrophagocytosis within the Kupffer cells is an inconstant but sometimes striking feature.[156] Hematopoietic foci, though by no means pathognomonic for hemolytic disease, are present if hemolysis is at all marked and may be so abundant as to create the impression of having largely replaced the parenchymal cells. Combined with greater or lesser degrees of congestion, they contribute to the sometimes enormous gross enlargement of the organ seen clinically or at autopsy. The parenchymal cells may show swelling, granularity of the cytoplasm, droplets of bile pigment which presumably represent conjugated bilirubin, an amorphous iron-negative pigment which is believed to be unconjugated bilirubin, and outright necrosis. Canalicular bile stasis is often seen. Whether the hepatic changes that may result from uncomplicated hemolytic disease alone ever lead to permanent residues such as cirrhosis is unknown. Such a sequence is described in the older literature,[68] but the diagnosis of hemolytic disease rested on uncertain grounds at that time, and more recently few such reports have appeared.[35] The writer leans toward the view that cirrhosis in the wake of proved hemolytic disease represents the sequel of a coexisting hepatitis such as was discussed above.

A complication of jaundice that is peculiar to newborn infants and formerly was most common in, though not specific for, hemolytic disease, is the encephalopathy known as *kernicterus*. The clinical picture varies from mild spasticity and lethargy to loss of the Moro reflex, respiratory irregularities, opisthotonus and frequently death. In survivors, athetosis, spastic paralysis, 8th nerve deafness and mental retardation may be observed. The brain of infants who have died in the acute stage shows more or less extensive bright-yellow pigmentation of certain typical areas, notably the thalamus, the hypothalamic nuclei, the cornu Ammonis of the hippocampus, the flocculi of the cerebellum, the dentate nuclei and the floor of the 4th ventricle. Histologically, the involved areas exhibit pigmentation of nerve cells and fibers and necrobiosis, nu-

clear pyknosis and sometimes outright necrosis.

The pathogenesis of kernicterus has been largely clarified by clinical, biochemical and experimental studies. The pigment has been definitely identified as bilirubin, and the condition has been universally accepted as a bilirubin encephalopathy,[144] for it occurs in conditions unassociated with antigen-antibody reactions or even with accelerated hemolysis—for example, in the Crigler-Najjar[38] syndrome and the comparable lesions found in the so-called Gunn strain of rats which have a similar genetic defect in glucuronyl transferase.[83] A rough quantitative correlation between the intensity of the hyperbilirubinemia and the risk of kernicterus has been demonstrated. Moreover, kernicterus can be almost completely prevented by exchange transfusion, which prevents bilirubin from accumulating in excessive concentration in the tissues and body fluids. Unresolved questions that are of critical importance in regard to the development of kernicterus have been partially clarified;[26] for example, the blood brain barrier appears to be more permeable in the newborn and especially in the premature infant. It is, however, safe to say that this encephalopathy represents the main hazard of the inadequate conjugating capacity of the liver in the neonatal period.

Treatment. A full discussion of the treatment of hemolytic disease is beyond the scope of this chapter. It may suffice to restate that the aim is the prevention of bilirubin encephalopathy and the substitution of the residually vulnerable erythrocyte population (and to a lesser extent of bilirubin), and the indications for exchange transfusion rest on the evaluation of serum bilirubin levels, however limited the information that can be gained from this parameter.

OTHER ANEMIAS

Hemolytic anemias other than hemolytic disease proper can lead to profound jaundice in the newborn period and cause diagnostic difficulties. A detailed description is beyond the scope of this chapter. Such anemias must be considered in the differential diagnosis of severe and rapidly developing neonatal jaundice whenever the antiglobulin test is negative. Morphologic study of the erythrocytes often yields the correct answer as in congenital spherocytosis, in the toxic hemolytic anemias caused in susceptible individuals with a genetic deficiency of erythrocyte glucose-6-phosphate dehydrogenase and glutathione instability,[152] and in the remarkable, unexplained acute hemolytic anemia with bizarre distortion of the red corpuscles recently described under the name of infantile pyknocytosis.[140] Pyruvate-kinase deficiency of the red cells in its severe form may simulate the clinical and hematologic features of hemolytic disease.

INFECTIOUS PROCESSES

In any discussion of neonatal jaundice, sepsis and congenital syphilis formerly figured prominently. Today, at least under standard conditions prevailing in this country, neither condition is a major problem. Still, they must be considered in the differential diagnosis.

In current pediatric practice, *sepsis* denotes a variable symptom complex rather than either a demonstrable bacteremia or any etiologic or pathologic entity. It implies the spread of microorganisms from a portal of entry or primary focus by way of the blood stream and the likelihood of metastatic suppuration. It is not always possible to demonstrate anatomic lesions, nor can bacteremia be shown to exist in every case. Moreover, organisms not ordinarily considered as pathogenic, particularly members of the *E. coli* group, may be obtained in blood cultures; and unless such bacteria prove to be present on several occasions it may be impossible to decide whether they are contaminants or play a significant role in the illness.

The portal of entry may be the umbilicus, but there are many other possible sites, such as skin abrasions, mucous membranes, respiratory tract and genitalia. Often it is impossible to demonstrate the portal of entry by the time the clinical manifestations of a systemic illness have appeared.

The clinical picture is variable, depending on, among other things, the localization of single or multiple metastatic lesions which may involve many organs or systems. Fever is not always present; in fact, the temperature is often subnormal or merely unstable. Leukocytosis is not a constant finding. Anemia is likely to develop rapidly. The infant with sepsis appears toxic and lethargic, nurses poorly, often vomits and may have a hemorrhagic tendency. Jaundice often is among the first symptoms, and both the liver and spleen may be enlarged. Icterus attributable to sepsis rarely appears before the 3rd or 4th day of life. Sepsis is particularly likely if jaundice develops toward the end of the first week or becomes marked in an infant whose initial physiologic icterus has begun to subside.

The mechanism or mechanisms responsible for the development of jaundice in association with sepsis may not always be the same and are not clearly understood. If the onset falls into the period of physiologic icterus, the jaundice may in fact represent nothing more than that condition itself, at least at first, and subsequently may be prolonged for a variety of reasons: increased hemolysis as the direct or indirect result of bacterial infection, the effects of vomiting and starvation on the hepatic conjugating mechanism, the direct influence of dehydration on the concentration of bilirubin in the plasma and conceivably specific or nonspecific inhibition of the hepatocellular enzyme systems by bacteria or bacterial products. If any or all of these factors were operating, one would expect that the jaundice is of the retention type and the bilirubin in the plasma is essentially of the indirect-reacting variety. Since an evaluation in terms of the newer concepts of bilirubin metabolism has become feasible, the writers have seen a few instances in which this was true, but there have been too few cases to permit any conclusions.

On the other hand, a recent study by Bernstein and Brown[11] of sepsis due to *E. coli infections*, verified by autopsy in infants who became jaundiced after the period in which physiologic icterus may occur, disclosed that in such cases characteristically the jaundice was regurgitative in type, that is, not only the indirect-reacting but the direct-reacting bilirubin was elevated in the plasma, often markedly so. Several of the patients had frank choluria. Histologically, the livers of such infants showed cholestasis, both intra- and extracellular, toxic hepatocellular changes amounting in some instances to necrosis, and occasionally slight pericholangitis. Thus in *E. coli* sepsis which, in the material studied, was the commonest infection of young infants to be associated with jaundice, depression of the hepatic conjugating mechanism, though always evident, was not an adequate explanation for the icterus. Rather, a relatively gross and presumably toxic hepatocellular injury with morphologic changes and obvious impairment of hepatic excretory function was demonstrated. Conversely, in the presence of such a pattern of jaundice in young infants, *E. coli* sepsis must be considered high on the list of diagnostic possibilities.

Diarrheal Disease. With the advent of modern diagnostic and therapeutic as well as preventive methods, severe, prolonged diarrheal disease is rare, and few fatalities occur. When it was prevalent, it was associated with jaundice not uncommonly. At

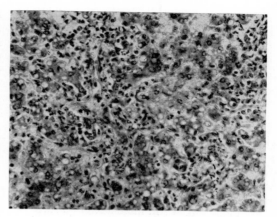

Fig. 26–4. More severe changes of the type illustrated in Fig. 26–3. Note the rather severe infiltration with leukocytes. From a 6-week-old infant dying from renal insufficiency due to congenital hydronephrosis and complicated by severe diarrhea.

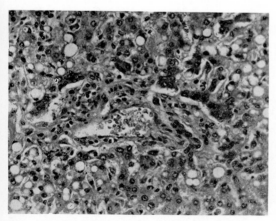

Fig. 26–3. Changes at the periphery of the hepatic lobules consisting of fatty metamorphosis, early proliferation of ducts and minimal infiltration with inflammatory cells. This is a common picture in severe or prolonged infantile diarrhea. Grossly, the liver was icteric in this 3-month-old infant dying of bronchopneumonia complicated by severe diarrhea.

that time little was known regarding mechanisms of infantile jaundice, and no attention was paid to the pattern of the serum bilirubin in such patients. From the clinical descriptions and from the similarity of the lesions found in the liver at autopsy with those seen in *E. coli* sepsis, it appears likely that the jaundice was likewise regurgitative in character and that changes in the liver were toxic in origin, as was believed by Wainwright, who in 1950 described the condition as hepatitis associated with infantile diarrhea.[143] Cholestasis is a prominent feature in sections of the liver; cellular changes range from fatty metamorphosis to necrosis and at the periphery of the lobules where these changes tend to be maximal, inflammatory cell infiltration, periportal edema, proliferation of bile ducts and even fibrosis may be found (Figs. 26–3 to 26–5). The development of such a toxic hepatitis and clinically the appearance of jaundice in infants with diarrheal disease is a grave prognostic sign. The therapy is primarily that of the basic disease process.

Congenital Syphilis. This disease has become almost a medical curiosity. Its effect on the liver is variable and depends largely on the extent and the duration of the transplacental sphirochetal invasion, which in

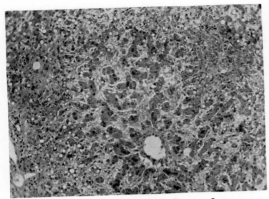

FIG. 26–5. A still more advanced stage of the lesions shown in Figs. 26–3 and 26–4. The lobules are surrounded by wide bands of fibrosis; the newly formed fibrous tissue is infiltrated by leukocytes; the polygonal cells at the periphery have undergone fatty changes and necrosis; the central portions show atrophy and marked inspissation of bile. From a 2-month-old infant with vomiting due to a congenital peritoneal band. The infant acquired severe diarrhea and became distended, dehydrated and icteric.

turn is determined by the stage and the control of the maternal infection. In severe cases the liver of the newborn infant is literally riddled with spirochetes and shows a picture of so-called miliary gummata, actually acute foci of necrosis, and inflammation, usually in association with a diffuse intralobular fibrosis and cirrhosis (Fig. 26–6).

At the other extreme are cases in which the liver does not change structurally and at most contains small numbers of spirochetes. Severe involvement of the liver in congenital syphilis usually is accompanied by icterus, hepatosplenomegaly, anemia and often spontaneous hemorrhages. The diagnosis is made on the basis of clinical evidence such as coryza, cutaneous and mucous lesions, osteochondritis and periostitis with their characteristic radiologic appearance and, of course, positive serologic tests. In every unexplained case of icterus in the newborn period, syphilis should be excluded by a suitable serologic method.

Viral Infections. The occurrence of infectious (epidemic) hepatitis and serum hepatitis in the neonatal period and early infancy is poorly documented, but this age is susceptible to several other more or less well-defined types of hepatitis. The observation of Stokes et al.[135] who reported the transmission of hepatitis from the mother of an infant with the disease and from the infant itself has not been repeated. Follow-up studies of infants born to mothers with infectious hepatitis have in no instance uncovered the development of overt disease. It would appear, therefore, that in the age group under discussion the viral agents responsible for adult hepatitis play a minimal role and that transmission of maternal epidemic and transfusion hepatitis is virtually nonexistent.

On the other hand, several viral agents that ordinarily do not affect the liver in older subjects may do so in the fetus, neonate and young infant, which indicates a special susceptibility of this age group. The agents in question—cytomegalovirus, herpes simplex, coxsackie and rubella—may involve other organs or systems and cause symptoms not specifically related to the liver. Frequently, however, hepatic involvement may be the principal manifestation of such infections and the main source of symptoms.

Cytomegalovirus. This virus has been identified as the cause of the striking cellu-

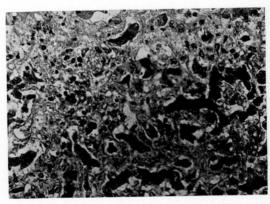

FIG. 26–6. Congenital syphilis, diffuse hepatic fibrosis and focal inflammatory changes. A 1-month-old infant, admitted with coryza, bleeding, desquamation of skin, hepatosplenomegaly and anemia. Kahn test positive. Innumerable spirochetes were found in liver and other tissues.

lar alterations (gigantism, nuclear and cyto-plasmic inclusions, etc.) that were first dis-covered with some frequency in the sali-vary glands of newborn infants and that gave rise to the name of the agent. It is as a rule widespread in the body, affecting such unrelated organ systems as kidney, liver, pancreas, brain and respiratory tract, and is transmittable in utero from asymp-tomatic mothers. The association of the general infection with clinical disease has been recognized only in comparatively re-cent times. The susceptibility of the fetus and neonate to an agent that behaves ordi-narily as an occult virus in early life be-speaks the special immunologic vulnerabil-ity of these subjects.

The classic picture is variable, depending on the organs involved, the degree of in-volvement and evidently the time and in-tensity of the infection. In its classic form the disease resembles severe hemolytic dis-ease of the newborn in that hemolytic ane-mia and jaundice are outstanding features. There is, however, thrombocytopenia, usu-ally a characteristic rash,[19] and encephalop-athy of varying degree, often associated with calcification. The virus may be iso-lated from urine, blood[138] and tissues, and characteristic inclusion-bearing renal epi-thelium may be at times demonstrated in

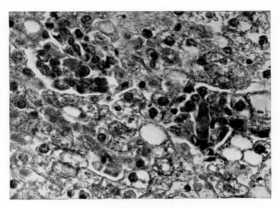

FIG. 26–8. Focal necrosis of inclusion-bearing cells surrounded by granuloma-like inflammatory reaction. Liver of 7-month-old infant with hepatomegaly, diarrhea and acidosis.

the urinary sediment.[54] Liver function tests are grossly abnormal and the serum bili-rubin shows marked increases in both the free and conjugated fractions.

On histologic examination, the liver is variable, depending on the stage of severity of the infection, but the characteristic in-clusion-bearing giant cells are rarely found in the parenchyma although they may be seen in the biliary epithelium (Fig. 26–7). On the other hand, the parenchyma shows the severe alterations generally described under the heading of giant cell hepatitis (Fig. 26–15). In its classic form this pic-ture was first decribed by Craig and Land-ing.[37] The most striking feature is a giant cell transformation of virtually the entire parenchyma associated with loss of the in-tralobular radial pattern, cellular swelling, cholestasis, glycogen and iron accumula-tion, pseudo-acinar formation and variable degrees of individual cellular necrosis (Fig. 26–8). The syncytium-like structures are multinucleated and the enlarged nuclei al-most invariably show prominent bodies which we have interpreted as inclusions rather than nucleoli.[161] Canalicular bile stasis and extramedullary hemopoiesis are prominent features which are apt to persist well beyond the neonatal period. The portal areas show relatively little involvement.

The later stages are variable. In infants who survive severe, generalized neonatal

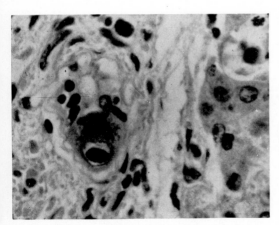

FIG. 26–7. Typical intranuclear and cytoplasmic inclusions in epithelial cell of small intrahepatic bile duct of 1-month-old icteric infant who had shown pur-pura, anemia, hepatosplenomegaly, ter-minal bleeding and cyanosis.

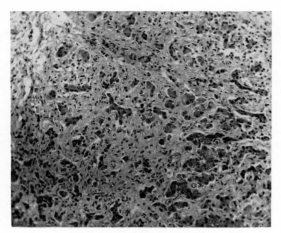

FIG. 26–9. Advanced stage of cytomeg-alic inclusion disease. Diffuse fibrosis of liver. Note similarity to picture in con-genital syphilis (see Fig. 26–6). From 2-month-old infant with icterus, micro-cephalus, hepatosplenomegaly, diarrhea and dehydration. Innumerable cytome-galic inclusions in kidneys, pancreas, in-testine, but rare in liver. Serologic tests and stains for spirochetes were negative.

disease, intralobular fibrosis may progress to extensive cirrhosis of postnecrotic type, yielding an end-stage that is reminiscent of the hepatic lesions of severe congenital syphilis (Fig. 26–9). Less severe postne-crotic cirrhosis may be seen in other sur-vivors and in infants who appear to acquire the disease later in prenatal or in postnatal life. Complete resolution and restitution of normal hepatic structure and function may take place.

The question as to the specificity of neo-natal (giant cell) hepatitis is not com-pletely resolved. The almost invariable as-sociation of generalized cytomegalovirus in-fection with this form of hepatic histology on the one hand and the isolation of the virus from a high percentage of cases of giant cell hepatitis as such in infants by Hanshaw and Weller[64] would seem to fa-vor the view that the lesions are the char-acteristic transformations of this particular agent in the liver, comparable to the gi-gantism of the affected cells in other or-gans. On the other hand, giant cells as such are found in variable numbers in other con-ditions, e.g., biliary atresia, adjacent to neo-

plasms and whenever hepatic injury is followed by regeneration, e.g., in toxic and other viral disorders. The distinguishing features in our view reside in the extent of the transformation and the severe architec-tectural change. The fact that gross giant cell transformation has been seen in asso-ciation with biliary atresia may be explained by the co-existence of viral infection and the anatomic condition, and does not in it-self militate against the viral etiology of the transformation.

In older infants, giant cell hepatitis oc-curs more commonly as an isolated hepatic disorder, at least in the clinical sense, and is characterized by gradual onset of hepa-tocellular type of jaundice, acholic stools, often diarrhea, failure to thrive, hepatosple-nomegaly and almost invariably an anemia of hemolytic type.[161] The prognosis is highly variable. A significant percentage of pa-tients die, often unexpectedly, and the pro-portion of cases with residual cirrhosis is undetermined. The differential diagnosis is discussed in conjunction with biliary atresia.

Herpes Simplex. For many years the virus of herpes simplex was thought to cause only relatively trivial infections of the epi-thelial surfaces of skin and mucous mem-branes. In 1935 Hass described inclusions in the liver and the adrenals of a premature infant that were indistinguishable from those caused by the herpes virus.[66] In 1952 Quilligan and Wilson,[117] and independently

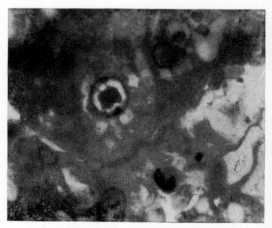

FIG. 26–10. Typical herpetic inclusion body and ballooning of cytoplasm of polygonal cell in liver.

Zuelzer and Stulberg,[160] isolated herpes simplex virus from the livers of newborn infants. The latter authors described 5 cases, and since then we have observed additional cases of herpes simplex hepatitis in newborn infants in which the virus was isolated. The nature of the condition was recognized by the typical intranuclear inclusions (Fig. 26–10). Though the disease is generalized with evidence of the presence of virus in many organs and tissues, the involvement of the liver is particularly marked and largely seems to determine the clinical picture.

The disease has been observed chiefly in premature infants. The virus may enter through the skin, the umbilicus or the mucous membranes when infective material, usually from the mother or a nurse, is present. The lesion at the portal of entry may be hidden or inconspicuous, and the disease does not become apparent until the virus has propagated extensively in the liver and other organs. The liver enlarges rapidly, the infant becomes lethargic, and there is rapidly deepening icterus, cyanosis, dyspnea, bleeding from various sites and severe hypoprothrombinemia. At autopsy the liver appears to be studded with white or yellow nodules (Fig. 26–11) which prove on histologic examination to be areas of coagulation necrosis (Fig. 26–12). However, the intervening parenchyma is not normal but shows degenerative changes, disruption of cell cords, beginning necrosis and hemorrhage. In several of the cases described, more than 75 per cent of the hepatic

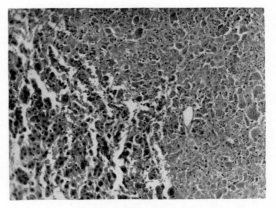

FIG. 26–12. Border zone between completely necrotic and partially preserved parenchyma in herpetic hepatitis.

parenchyma was completely destroyed.

On occasion the diagnosis is made on clinical grounds. The development of a sepsis-like picture in an infant after the first 5 to 6 days of life should arouse the suspicion of herpetic hepatitis and of viremia, especially if exposure to an adult with active herpes can be established. If vesicles are found on skin or mucous membranes, their contents should be studied. If no bacteria are found, the probability of viral lesions, i.e., herpes simplex, is great. As yet therapy is experimental. Gamma globulin or a hyperimmune anti-herpes serum may be employed along with supportive measures such as transfusions.

In older infants with herpetic stomatitis, a focal hepatitis with herpes inclusions has been found in several patients who died.[160] In one instance the clinical picture 2 weeks after the onset of stomatitis became one of lethargy, coma, vomiting of bile and blood-stained material, hematemesis and uncontrollable epistaxis and icterus. The histologic appearance of the liver indicated patchy necrosis of the parenchymal cells, many herpetic inclusions in the nuclei of the survivors and innumerable mitotic figures. While only a few cases of herpetic hepatitis have been recorded until recently, the true incidence of liver involvement in primary herpes simplex infections may be assumed to be much larger, although unrecognized, since few patients die, and few have been studied with respect to liver

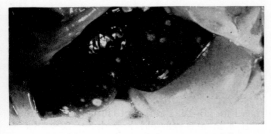

FIG. 26–11. Gross appearance of herpetic hepatitis. Multiple umbilicated whitish nodules in hemorrhagic liver. A 12-day-old premature infant with clinical picture of "sepsis." Icterus, bleeding, hemorrhages.

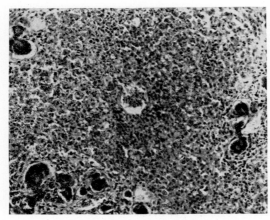

FIG. 26–13. Fulminating hepatitis in 3½-month-old infant transfused at 1 month of age. The symptoms were massive bleeding, hypoprothrombinemia, icterus, edema, ascites, death in respiratory failure. Cephalin flocculation 3+, serum bilirubin 3.5 mg./100 ml. The histologic picture is that of acute atrophy. Only the bile ducts have survived.

function. The recent finding of disseminated herpes simplex infections with prominent hepatic involvement in 32 infants of 6 to 36 months of age in a malnourished African population[5] bears this out and points up the importance of depressed immunologic function in the genesis of clinical disease caused by this occult virus.

Coxsackie Virus. Coxsackie virus may be transmitted transplacentally or acquired postnatally by young infants, and may cause widespread organic lesions among which myocarditis is the most constant and characteristic, but hepatitis or severe hepatic necrosis may be the most striking.[7] Clinically, the illness usually takes the course of a severe systemic infection with fever, cardiac and respiratory symptoms, often with manifestations of central nervous system involvement and a high fatality rate.[71, 86] Hepatomegaly has been reported, and we have knowledge of a case in which icterus was a prominent feature, but ordinarily the liver plays an inconspicuous role in the clinical symptomatology. However, the massive necrosis found at autopsy may present a diagnostic problem for the pathologist.

Older children may present with a symptom complex consisting of fever, anorexia, nausea and vomiting, lymphadenopathy, pharyngitis, conjunctivitis and hepatomegaly occasionally associated with splenomegaly and infrequently by a morbilliform eruption. Despite varying degrees of hepatic tenderness, liver function tests are usually normal.[130] Presumably, many of these children have a transient anicteric hepatitis and only occasionally is there clinical and biochemical evidence of hepatic injury.

Rubella Virus. Intrauterine rubella infection can result in pansystemic tissue alterations accompanied either by protean or specifically related clinical symptoms.[91] More than 70 per cent of those infants with the congenital syndrome may have varying degrees of hepatomegaly, almost consistently associated with splenomegaly which may persist for as long as 6 months.[31] Jaundice is present in at least 25 per cent of cases and has been attributed to hepatocellular disease. Approximately one-third of the patients have purpura which is attributed to thrombocytopenia,[31] but in other cases it appears to be related to hepatocellular disease. Recent evidence suggests that in some cases the purpuric rash is due to intradermal erythropoiesis.[19]

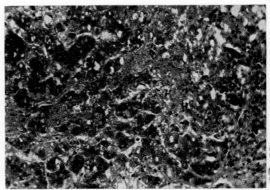

FIG. 26–14. Fatal acute infectious hepatitis in a 6-year-old boy dying 3 weeks after the onset of fever followed by vomiting, melena, icterus, lethargy, extreme hepatomegaly, anemia, hypoprothrombinemia and other marked abnormalities in liver function. Ascites, edema and coma supervened.

Biopsy and postmortem liver specimens have shown a variety of hepatic lesions, the morphologic character of which appears to be related to both the time of observation and the character of the disease process as it affects individual patients. The changes described include swelling with vacuolization of liver cells,[89] cellular bile stasis without cellular change,[131] typical giant cell hepatitis,[51, 134, 137] cholangiolitic hepatitis[137] and posthepatitic cirrhosis with lobular disarray and lobular bile stasis.[131] Progression to clinically manifest cirrhosis may occur after a period of years.[145]

Positive isolations of rubella virus from liver tissue are variable, appearing to be related in part to the activity of the hepatitis despite its recovery from other sites such as stool and nasopharyngeal secretions.[131, 134] In addition to hepatocellular damage, rubella virus may damage the bile duct system sufficiently to produce histopathologic and anatomic changes indistinguishable from those of classic biliary atresia.[137]

Infectious Hepatitis. In later infancy, perhaps from the age of 4 to 6 months on through childhood, both infectious hepatitis and homologous serum jaundice may occur; the clinical features and pathology are generally the same as for these conditions in later life. Therefore, it is unnecessary in a book devoted to diseases of the liver to dwell at length on hepatitis in childhood.

The recognition of infectious hepatitis in early childhood has increased with the awareness among physicians of its occurrence in this age group. It has been said that there are few adequate descriptions of the clinical and laboratory findings of infectious hepatitis in young children. The impression of most experienced clinicians that the disease is generally mild in children seems to be supported by the paucity of published records of fatalities. This is not to say that infectious hepatitis in children is invariably benign. Fulminating and fatal forms do occur. In this laboratory, a number of cases of fatal hepatitis have been seen (Figs. 26–13 and 26–14). On the other hand, the studies of Bennett and associates have established that the endemic form of infectious hepatitis may be predominantly

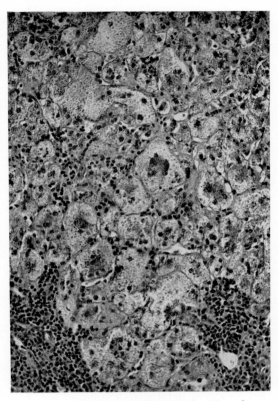

FIG. 26–15. Liver biopsy of a 5-week-old Negro male, jaundiced since 2 days of age. No other physical abnormalities. Admitted because of respiratory tract infection. Stools normal. Urine contained bile. Serum bilirubin 11 mg./100 ml. total; direct fraction 7.5. Cephalin flocculation 1 +, thymol turbidity 3.2 units. Alkaline phosphatase 29 Bodansky units. Serum protein, calcium and phosphorus in normal limits. SGO transaminase 750 units. Hemoglobin 8.8 Gm.%. Direct and indirect Coombs test negative. Operative cholangiogram normal. Liver biopsy shows above picture of giant cell hepatitis. Subsequent uneventful recovery.

nonicteric in early life.[8] In a study of a chronic epidemic in an orphanage, only 1 of 26 infants with sufficient evidence to establish the diagnosis had bilirubinemia. The disease was recognized only because of an outbreak of clinically manifest hepatitis among the adult personnel. Similar, but more extensive, studies of importance primarily for the epidemiology of the disease have been conducted by Krugman et al.[92]

BILIARY ATRESIA

Extrahepatic. Several anatomic variants of atresia occur. The entire extrahepatic biliary tree may be absent, including the gallbladder, or the hepatic duct or the common duct alone may be occluded. These conditions can be ascertained only by surgical exploration[125] and even then only with difficulties which even the use of operative and postoperative cholangiography cannot always overcome. Unfortunately, the majority of the cases can not be corrected surgically, and death results ultimately from biliary cirrhosis and its complications. Cases in which correction is possible must be promptly diagnosed and treated. In this section the details of surgical management are not considered but only the clinical and diagnostic features.

Interest in this condition, aroused largely because it was frequently confused with other forms of "obstructive" jaundice, has led to many detailed studies and made it necessary to revise earlier ideas, often based on preconception rather than observation, concerning the clinical and especially the laboratory findings. There is considerable variability in the rate at which the changes progress in biliary atresia and consequently in the picture obtained at any given age. This variability is of theoretical interest in itself and is an unsolved puzzle. It may reflect the variable onset of an inflammatory process at different stages of intrauterine and perhaps early postnatal development and thus provides a possible clue to the nature of the condition as possibly of viral origin, as opposed to "true," e.g., genetic, malformations.

Generally, jaundice is not a striking feature in the neonatal period, and most cases do not come to the attention of the physician until several, sometimes many, weeks after birth. Once icterus is established, it is persistent, and the skin has a greenish tinge; but, earlier ideas notwithstanding, the intensity of the jaundice may fluctuate noticeably and the plasma bilirubin levels may show rises and falls.[27] The stools eventually become clay-colored; but in many instances, too numerous to be disregarded, a history of normally colored stools is obtained, a confusing fact which can often be verified even in later stages by demonstration of at least small amounts of bile in the laboratory. Presumably, this is due to the diffusion of bile pigment into such secretions as tears and intestinal juices when the concentration of bilirubin in the plasma and the tissues is elevated over a long period of time.

The urine contains bile at all times. Urobilinogen which one would not expect to be present has been demonstrated in both stools and urine. The liver gradually increases in size and eventually becomes nodular. The spleen may not become palpable until several months after birth. The general state of health of the patients is often surprisingly good for many months and occasionally even for years, though ultimately malnutrition, rickets due to inadequate absorption of vitamin D, hypoprothrombinemia and portal hypertension develop, and the child succumbs to hepatic failure or intercurrent infection—unless, of course, it is corrected at an early age. Just how early this must be in order to prevent irreversible cirrhotic changes is a moot point, evidently because of the variable rate of progression of secondary hepatocellular damage, but clearly the earlier the better. When the differentiation from hepatitis is not possible on the basis of clinical and laboratory findings, liver biopsy is indicated after a reasonable period of observation, ideally not later than at 6 weeks of age.

Although there has been much controversy concerning the value of biopsy for histologic diagnosis, the objection to this procedure stems largely from three sources: failure to recognize the specific changes associated with anatomic biliary obstruction; performance of the biopsy at a stage when extensive secondary changes may obscure the original picture; and confusion between the regenerative changes encountered with hepatic injury in atresia as opposed to the more characteristic picture of giant cell hepatitis. Moreover, hepatitis superimposed on atresia must be recognized. The salient feature is proliferation of bile ducts at the periphery of the lobules with fibrosis and variable inflammatory response about the portal triads (Fig. 26–16). The larger bile ducts in the portal areas often show distention and bile stasis, but later they may be difficult to demonstrate. Stowens[136] regards enlargement of the branches of the hepatic artery as characteristic of atresia; however, the same change is encountered in a small number of hepatitis cases.[18] Cholestasis within the parenchyma is widespread, and the cells may undergo toxic alterations and irregular focal necrosis.

The laboratory findings of the earliest phase have been studied inadequately. In our experience the usual liver profile is normal in the first few weeks, except that the serum bilirubin is moderately elevated and, surprisingly, the indirect-reacting fraction is predominant but the direct-reacting bilirubin is always elevated, to the extent of several milligrams. Usually the SGO transaminase is only slightly elevated and at first rises only slowly,[90] though there are exceptions when high levels occur as early as 3 to 4 weeks. Later, very high concentrations are observed, and by that time abnormal results may be obtained with nearly all the tests employed.

From what has been said, the value of early and serial observations should be apparent. At present one cannot be dogmatic about the diagnostic features of the condition in the first few weeks of life. If reasonable doubt exists, most authors favor a simple exploratory laparotomy for the purpose of obtaining a biopsy, but in our experience needle biopsy often obviates this requirement. If the pathologic diagnosis eliminates hepatitis and establishes biliary atresia, cholangiograms are taken and eventually the extrahepatic biliary system is explored surgically in detail.

Intrahepatic Biliary Atresia. A condition in infancy and early childhood described

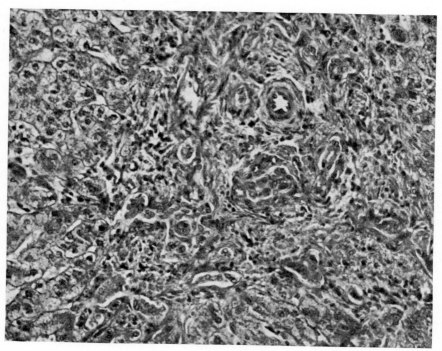

Fig. 26–16. Liver biopsy of 8-week-old female with persistent neonatal jaundice of obstructive type, showing characteristic portal changes. Liver moderately enlarged. Spleen not palpable. Exploratory laparotomy and cholangiogram revealed absence of hepatic ducts. The patient died at age 6 months with advanced biliary cirrhosis.

under this and similar names and characterized by prolonged jaundice with onset in the neonatal period, "obstructive" features and a high incidence of hypercholesterolemia and xanthomatosis seems to be well established.[121] However, considerable doubt must be expressed concerning the nature of this disease which those who originally described it regard as a congenital agenesis of the intrahepatic bile ducts.[2] This doubt is based in part on embryologic considerations, as mentioned earlier. Perhaps more important is the fact that the few cases reported thus far have been studied histologically at a relatively late stage, in late infancy or even in childhood. Consequently, possible early acquired lesions such as inflammatory changes that might lead to the obliteration of originally normally formed bile ducts cannot be excluded. Harris and Anderson[65] have described cases in which they attributed the disappearance of the bile ducts to disuse, atrophy or direct damage to their epithelium in the wake of a prolonged disturbance in the elimination of bilirubin through the hepatic ducts into the biliary canaliculi.

Personal observation of a case clinically resembling hepatitis in the first few weeks has led us to an even simpler explanation: direct damage to the epithelium of the bile ducts by a variant of hepatitis or cholangiolitis with subsequent fibrosis and occlusion. In the case in question the hepatic parenchyma appeared to be normal, but there was an inflammatory reaction in and about the biliary ducts associated with partial necrosis and atrophy of the epithelium and periductal fibrosis. The case was that of a young infant who died, and the appearance of the lesions suggested that, had the infant survived, precisely those residual changes would have developed which have been interpreted as agenesis of the intrahepatic bile ducts.

The prognosis is poor, although survival is longer than in extrahepatic biliary atresia, perhaps because the obstruction is usually not complete, but surgical correction is manifestly impossible (other perhaps than hepatic transplantation). Therapy is only supportive. The development of hypercholesteremia and of xanthomatosis is highly suggestive of the diagnosis which otherwise can be made only by histologic examination.

DIFFERENTIAL DIAGNOSIS OF OBSTRUCTIVE JAUNDICE IN INFANCY

The term and concept of the "inspissated bile syndrome" is today of historic interest only. Jaundice of "obstructive" or regurgitative type is common in early infancy and frequently presents diagnostic problems. There is no evidence, however, that mechanical obstruction by viscid intrahepatic bile thrombi plays any part in the genesis of the icterus, as was implied by the older term. Rather, current knowledge suggests that the accumulation of bile pigment visible in the liver of infants with various types of nonanatomic obstructive jaundice represents the result of excretory failure rather than its cause. With the exception of anatomic obstruction, the primary mechanism underlying the various etiologic subgroups of this type of jaundice is hepatocellular damage. Apart from genetic defects with the accumulation of hepatotoxic metabolites, e.g., galactosemia, which is referred to below, the majority of cases represent hepatitis, either infectious (viral) or toxic (e.g., associated with *E. coli* infections, etc.), or circulatory and anoxic damage, as in severe hemolytic disease. Though rare nowadays, congenital syphilis must not be forgotten in the differential diagnosis. From a practical point of view, the most important single criterion for distinguishing between any of these forms of jaundice on the one hand and the types of neonatal icterus due to failure of conjugation of bilirubin is the presence of direct-reacting pigment in the serum, usually accompanied by choluria and often by acholic stools.

In differentiating further between the various forms of regurgitation jaundice, hemolytic disease is usually evident on hematologic-serologic grounds. The recognition of galactosemia, though rare, is of prime importance because its results, e.g., cataracts, hepatic cirrhosis and mental deficiency are largely preventable, and the single symptom of jaundice may be the first sign of this condition which is readily diagnosed by the appropriate test for reducing substances in the urine. Any viral form of hepatitis is more difficult to diagnose, and must be differentiated from anatomic obstruction. Cases in which systemic viral disease is manifest, e.g., cytomegalovirus, rubella, etc., rarely present a diagnostic problem, but isolated cases of hepatitis do, especially when the onset is gradual. In our hands liver biopsy offers a highly reliable method of diagnosis; usually a Vim-Silverman needle can be used, provided the patient does not have a bleeding tendency. The reliability, based on follow-up studies, approaches 98 per cent.[18] Histologically, extrahepatic obstruction caused by choledochal cysts or, in one exceptional instance by a bile duct "plug" in the common duct (neonatal choledocholithiasis), cannot be distinguished from extrahepatic atresia, but since in either case the biopsy will lead to open exploration, this is not of practical concern. Needle biopsy appears to be a safe procedure[18] and offers the advantage of avoiding any theoretical risks of prolonged surgery and anesthesia, as well as the opportunity for serial studies. The rose-bengal test is always positive in atresia, in the sense that no dye is excreted, but in a few cases of severe giant cell hepatitis we have also observed it to be positive. It is therefore apt to fail as a differential test where it is most needed.

INFANTILE AND JUVENILE CIRRHOSIS

Cirrhosis of the liver in the pediatric age group is not as rare as was formerly believed and may be on the increase. If so, this may be due in part to an increase in the viral forms of hepatitis, which are now universally recognized as one of the leading causes of cirrhosis in the pediatric age group, and in part to the prolonged survival of patients with fibrocystic disease of the pancreas, a condition in which cirrhosis is prone to develop. On the other hand, it appears likely that increasing interest in hepatic disease in children and improved diagnostic methods have led to better recognition of the condition and to more frequent publications of the subject. Still, in comparison

with cirrhosis in the adult, the disease is rare in children.

There are other important differences between the cirrhosis of children and that of adults. In the pediatric age group Laennec's cirrhosis appears to be exceedingly rare, and most cases can be classified as either postnecrotic or obstructive biliary in type. Which type prevails seems to depend on the age group and the case material studied. Thus Craig and associates,[36] in a series of 98 cases, reported 61 as secondary to biliary obstruction and attributed 30 to hepatitis, whereas in the series of 27 cases reviewed by Ruggieri et al.,[124] 26 were classified as posthepatitic. In any event, these two categories represent the two largest groups of juvenile cirrhosis, at least in countries where parasitic and nutritional disease of the liver are uncommon.

Other etiologic factors in juvenile cirrhosis are largely genetic in origin and account at least in part for the occasional familial occurrence of the disease. In this category, galactosemia, which was briefly discussed above, occupies a prominent position. The so-called storage diseases, Gaucher's disease, Niemann-Pick disease and the hepatic form of glycogen storage disease can give rise to cirrhosis of the liver. Hepatolenticular degeneration is well known and presents few diagnostic problems when neurologic abnormalities are present. It has been suggested that some instances of familial juvenile cirrhosis without evidence of neurologic involvement represent abortive cases of this condition[99]; this seems plausible, though it cannot account for all cases of juvenile cirrhosis. A different, though likewise genetically determined, type of cirrhosis occurs, as mentioned, in some cases of fibrocystic disease of the pancreas. The condition, first described by Farber[53] in support of his mucoviscidosis theory of that disease, seems to vary in incidence. In our experience, as in that of Craig et al.[36] and of Hsia and Gellis,[74] cirrhosis is an uncommon complication, though focal intrahepatic biliary obstruction with fibrosis and proliferation is common (Fig. 26–17). By contrast di Sant'-Agnese and Blanc reported an incidence of 20 per cent in their case material.[42] Whether this reflects a different selection or difference

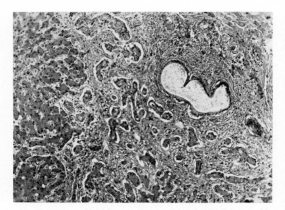

FIG. 26–17. Obstruction of intrahepatic bile duct with inspissated secretion in a 3-year-old child dying of pancreatic fibrosis (mucoviscidosis). Note dilatation of a larger duct with mucous-like secretion and proliferation and fibrosis about smaller ducts, some of which are also filled with inspissated secretions.

in management of the basic condition is unknown.

The literature contains references to so-called *congenital "idiopathic" cirrhosis*,[139] the explanation being that this group is etiologically unrelated to prior hepatitis. This inference seems to be based largely on the lack of giant cell transformation in histologic sections of the liver at the time the diagnosis of "idiopathic cirrhosis" is made. We doubt the validity of such criteria in that, firstly, subsidence of the initial infectious process, if any, should be associated with the disappearance of giant cells while scarring and cirrhosis are progressing, and, secondly, the development of cirrhosis requires time so that the initial inflammatory response is likely to have subsided at the time of the diagnosis. However, the persistence of such viral agents as cytomegalovirus may well continue to be associated with continuing active hepatitis (and giant cell structures) even while cirrhosis is developing. To assume that these cases are essentially different from those in which acute changes are no longer seen is to go beyond the available evidence.

The *clinical course* of cirrhosis in children is variable and obviously depends largely

on the etiology. The obstructive form, which is almost invariably due to congenital atresia of the bile ducts, develops at a variable rate in direct continuation of the prolonged obstructive jaundice characteristic of that condition. The patients remain icteric, and sooner or later the liver function tests become grossly abnormal, the spleen enlarges and ascites and esophageal varices are common in the later stages. The liver becomes increasingly nodular. The nutritional state sometimes remains surprisingly good for long periods of time, though rickets due to poor absorption of vitamin D is apt to develop ("hepatic rickets"). Death supervenes from hemorrhage, intercurrent infection or hepatic coma.

In contrast with the cirrhosis following biliary atresia, posthepatitic cirrhosis is most often separated in its clinical manifestations from the original disease by an interval ranging from a few months to many years and its onset is gradual. In some cases the accidental discovery of an enlarged spleen is the first clue. Other patients present with thrombopenic purpura or other hematologic manifestations of "hypersplenism" or with anemia. Portal hypertension may be advanced when the condition is first discovered, and massive bleeding from esophageal varices may be the first symptom (Fig. 26–18). Jaundice occurs in a high

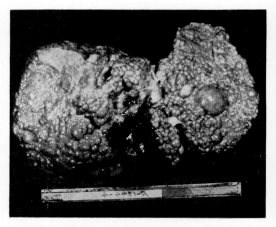

FIG. 26–18. Coarse nodular cirrhosis in a 6-year-old boy with de Toni-Fanconi syndrome.

Fig. 26–19. Splenoportogram of 5-year-old male with portal venous obstruction. Note collateral circulation through paravertebral plexus and azygous system.

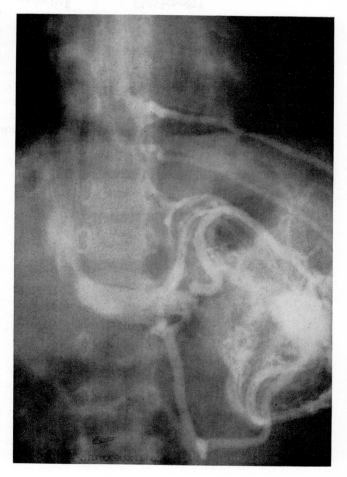

proportion of the cases at some stage of the disease but is relatively uncommon as a presenting symptom.

Cirrhosis that develops in patients with untreated galactosemia sometimes progresses extremely rapidly, with jaundice continuing after the neonatal period and ascites and failure to thrive occurring in months or even weeks.

The *diagnosis* of cirrhosis of the liver in the pediatric age group offers peculiar difficulties and challenges. The first requirement is a high index of suspicion, particularly in cases with a history of prolonged jaundice in early infancy, in cases of otherwise unexplained splenomegaly or hepatomegaly or both and in children who generally fail to grow and thrive without other apparent reason. The second requirement is awareness of the various etiologic conditions that are likely to produce cirrhosis in children. Thus it is never sufficient to establish the diagnosis of cirrhosis, but appropriate tests must be carried out to establish or exclude the diagnosis of galactosemia, Wilson's disease, fibrocystic disease and the various storage diseases. Therefore, not only are the customary tests of liver function required but also the proper chemical determinations of blood, urine and sweat, and studies of the bone marrow. A history of neonatal or infantile jaundice is likely to be significant. Rarely, one sees cirrhosis in infants who had hemolytic disease of the newborn and received exchange transfusions. Whether the development of cirrhosis in such patients

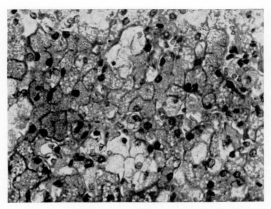

Fig. 26–20. Liver in Niemann-Pick disease. Note large foam cells in sinusoids, but also enlargement and plant cell-like contours of polygonal cells.

reflects (a) direct, irreversible damage caused by severe hemolytic disease or (b) transfusion hepatitis, cannot as a rule be determined.

The long-range *prognosis* of most of the etiologic types of juvenile cirrhosis is poor, particularly if portal hypertension develops. In our experience, however, many children reach puberty without serious impairment of health.

In the differential diagnosis of *portal hypertension* in childhood, the possibility of isolated occlusion ("cavernous transformation" or thrombosis) of the splenic and/or portal vein must be considered, since in our experience this cause is of the same order or frequency as posthepatitic cirrhosis. The simplest means of excluding cirrhosis is a needle biopsy; however, since a splenoportogram is an essential part of the diagnostic work-up, a radiologic diagnosis usually suffices.

The management of portal hypertension cannot be dealt with in detail in this chapter. The general approach should be conservative, for (1) fatal hemorrhage from bleeding esophageal or gastric varices is rare, (2) in the growth phase the establishment of surgical shunts is often unsatisfactory and (3) the spontaneous development of collateral venous circulation often surpasses the capacity of the anastomoses which the surgeon can hope to create (Fig. 26–19).

HEPATOMEGALY

The conditions that cause enlargement of the liver in infants and children are legion. For the most part they do not represent primary or localized disease of the liver itself but involve the liver as the result of a distant or generalized process. Usually, the reason for the hepatomegaly is clear or at least can be suspected from the history, general clinical picture, blood picture or other laboratory findings. Hepatomegaly secondary to cardiac failure, to blood disorders such as erythroblastosis fetalis, other hemolytic anemias, leukemias, Letterer-Siwe disease and the like rarely presents a diagnostic problem. This is true also of infectious processes that involve the liver or affect its size, such as generalized histoplasmosis, malaria, acute septicemias and certain viral infections, including infectious mononucleosis.

It is more difficult to diagnose cases in which systemic manifestations are lacking, and hepatomegaly is an isolated finding or is associated with splenomegaly in a child who otherwise appears to be normal. Such cases must be diagnosed properly, even if one must resort to laparotomy or liver biopsy. When hepatomegaly is accompanied by splenomegaly and the usual diagnostic procedures have been exhausted, one should suspect one of the lipoid storage diseases, Gaucher's disease or Niemann-Pick disease (Fig. 26–20). The presence of the characteristic cells in preparations of aspirated bone marrow usually established the diagnosis. In Hurler's syndrome (gargoylism) the diagnosis is usually suggested by skeletal anomalies, and characteristic cells may be found in the bone marrow or elsewhere, while urinary chromatograms show elevations of chondroitin sulfate. If the spleen is not enlarged, marked enlargement of the liver that cannot be accounted for by cardiac, hematologic or infectious disorders is likely to indicate fatty liver, glycogen storage disease, neoplasm or parasitism.

Fatty Liver

In autopsy material from infants and children the presence of visible fat in the polygonal cells of the liver is an extremely common finding. The extent of the fatty changes and the size of the fat droplets are highly variable. It is likely that these variations have a quantitative rather than a qualitative meaning. The distinction between fatty degeneration and fatty infiltration has been largely abandoned as unreliable. What should be called fatty liver is somewhat a question of definition. In many infants dying with a variety of diseases, notably infections and conditions associated with malnutrition and hypoxia, mild to moderately severe, usually zonal or spotty fat deposits are found. As a rule, these changes do not contribute significantly to enlargement of the liver and are probably without functional or clinical significance. If one designates as fatty liver only the markedly enlarged, grossly yellow, greasy liver in which virtually every cell is distended with fat globules, the condition is relatively rare.

Among the chief causes of such fatty metamorphosis in early life (fatty hepatomegaly would be a better term) are severe malnutrition; severe prolonged infection such as generalized tuberculosis, poorly controlled diabetes with lipemia and other conditions associated with long-standing hyperlipemia; and certain poisonings, notably aspirin and carbon tetrachloride poisoning. Under the heading of malnutrition one should include not only deficiencies in dietary intake but conditions that interfere with the absorption of foodstuff, such as untreated fibrocystic disease of the pancreas.

Little is known about liver function in such severe states of fatty metamorphosis in children. As a rule, there is surprisingly little clinical evidence of impairment in hepatic function, and the condition is recognized more often at autopsy than suspected during life. It is likely from observations in adults with comparable fatty liver that such infants are subject to the hazard of sudden hepatic failure (Fig. 26–21). Such a mechanism has been invoked as the cause of death in a syndrome of infants in which fatty liver is the chief pathologic finding and is designated variously as kwashiorkor,[72, 129] infantile pellagra,[58] malignant malnutrition and fat disease of the liver. The disease is rare in the continental United States but has been reported from nearly all tropical countries, including

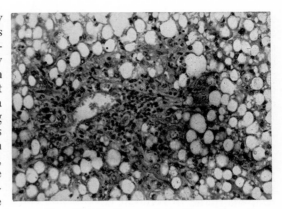

Fig. 26–21. Severe fatty liver. From a 5-month-old infant dying 10 days after onset of extensive bronchiolitis and bronchopneumonia. The terminal picture was suggestive of hepatic failure because of marked hepatomegaly, melena, coma, convulsions, edema and an acidotic type of breathing. The renal tubules likewise showed severe fatty changes.

Puerto Rico. Kwashiorkor is caused by prolonged inadequacy of protein intake, but probably the pure form of the disease is rare and many cases are complicated by associated dietary deficiencies. The characteristic clinical symptoms are diarrhea, edema, irritability and focal depigmentation of the skin. Depigmentation of the hair in Negroes produces a reddish color. The liver is greatly enlarged. Cheilosis, stomatitis, anemia and signs that indicate involvement of the central nervous system are probably manifestations of accompanying vitamin deficiencies. Prophylaxis and therapy are directed toward establishing an adequate protein intake by feeding milk. The prognosis is generally good unless complications supervene, but sudden death may occur.

Recently, interest has been revived in a clinicopathologic syndrome of encephalopathy with fatty degeneration and metamorphosis of the viscera, notably the liver and kidneys (see Chap. 17, Fatty Liver).[118] Described originally by Brain et al.,[17] the features of the disorder have been well summarized by Bradford and Latham.[16] Respiratory tract infections with fever are common. Occasionally there is a nonspecific erythematous cutaneous eruption. Nonspecific and nonlocalizing signs of central nervous system deterioration consisting of emesis, decerebrate-like rigidity and convulsions follow in a few days. In 40 to 65 per cent of cases, laboratory examinations show hypoglycemia, hypoglycorrhachia, ketonuria, metabolic acidosis, azotemia and minor selective alterations in liver functions.[16, 47, 84]

The pathologic alterations of the brain are nonspecific, consisting of swelling with vascular congestion, petechial hemorrhages, pericellular and perivascular pallor and swelling of astrocytes and neurons.[117] Fat droplets found in cerebral vessel walls and endothelial cells are considered as nonspecific changes.[117] The effects of superimposed hypoxia obscure a precise interpretation of these findings.

Hepatomegaly is usually marked and consists of a uniform, diffuse, microvacuolar, hepatocellular accumulation of lipid (Fig. 26–22). Focal necrosis and inflammatory infiltration have been noted.[47] The slightly enlarged kidneys show accumulation of finely divided lipid, primarily in swollen proximal convoluted tubules and to a lesser extent in other segments of the nephron.

The etiology and pathogenesis are unknown. Toxicologic studies have been unrewarding.[16] Antemortem and postmortem bacteriologic surveys have yielded no common pathogens. Viral agents have been implicated in 47 of 83 cases. In a summary of the attempted cultures, there were only 12 successful isolates, consisting primarily of adenovirus, reovirus and Coxsackie virus.[16] Eighty per cent of the cases terminated fatally. Only 2 of 46 patients under age 2 years survived. Whether the surviving cases had similar pathologic changes is problematical. The consensus is that the pathologic alterations are the result of several diverse agents including viral, toxic and nutritional factors.

GLYCOGEN STORAGE DISEASE

Diffuse hepatomegaly is one of the salient clinical features of the glycogen storage diseases. Currently nine types have been reported, six of which (I-VI) are generally recognized and thoroughly described. Each is biochemically characterized by a deficiency (invariably total and rarely partial) or a decrease in activity of a specific enzyme

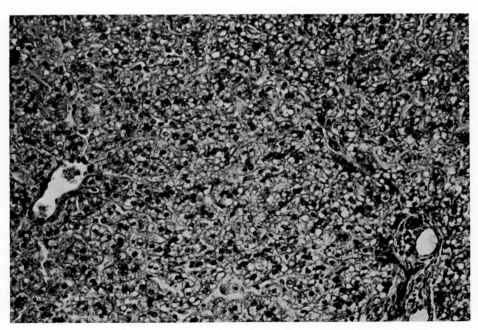

Fig. 26–22. Liver of 3-year-old male dying with encephalitis-like picture (convulsions and coma) and moderate hepatomegaly. Note the fine, diffuse, hepatic fatty metamorphosis.

involved in either the degradation or synthesis of glycogen. One or more organ or cellular systems is affected in each type and, excepting type V, all involve liver with the resultant accumulation of a normally (I, II, VI, VII, VIII, IX) or abnormally (III, IV) structured glycogen.

Type I, hepatorenal, von Gierke's disease or glucose-6-phosphatase deficiency, is characterized generally by moderate to marked hepatonephromegaly, growth retardation, episodic postprandial hypoglycemia with seizures, acidosis and hyperlipemia. Although death in early childhood is common, usually due to infection, some patients have few or no symptoms and survive to adulthood usually with regression in liver size.[34, 142]

Type II, generalized glycogen storage disease, Pompe's disease, acid maltase or lysosomal alpha-1, 4-glucosidase deficiency, involves all organ systems; it usually terminates fatally prior to age 2 years.[70] Hepatomegaly is moderate and the predominating signs are related primarily to involvement of the central nervous system, heart and peripheral skeletal muscle, all of which show characteristic and/or pathognomonic alterations.[25, 102] The disease is more complex than that of a simple carbohydrate metabolic dysfunction, since an acid mucopolysaccharide moiety is found in the skeletal musculature.[12]

Type III, debrancher deficiency, limit dextrinosis, Cori's disease or amylo-1, 6-glucosidase deficiency, is characterized by marked hepatomegaly with the accumulation of an abnormal glycogen, primarily in the liver and leukocytes, erythrocytes and occasionally in heart and skeletal muscle. Hypoglycemia, acidosis and hyperlipemia are mild or absent and there is a tendency toward pulmonary infection and liver failure.[33, 77, 141]

Type IV, debrancher deficiency, Anderson's disease or amylo-1,4-1,6 transglucosidase deficiency, is a rare type characterized by the generalized deposition of an abnormal glycogen (amylopectin?) notably in the liver, but also heart, skeletal muscle, spleen, lymph node and erythrocytes. Cirrhosis, presumably due to histotoxic effect of the abnormal carbohydrate, with hepatic failure results in early death.[76, 80]

Type VI, Her's disease or hepatic phosphorylase insufficiency, is characterized by marked hepatomegaly, frequently with severe hypoglycemia, moderate acidosis and slight growth retardation.[127]

Type VII, or phosphoglucomutase deficiency, has to date been reported in only two patients and is not yet well described as a clinical entity. Liver and muscle are reported to be affected.[81]

Recently described are solitary examples of types VIII and IX which are characterized by a reduction in hepatic phosphorylase activity. In type VIII there is moderate hepatomegaly without hypoglycemia, acidosis or hyperlipemia. Phosphorylase activity is increased to normal by the administration of glucagon or epinephrine. The reported patient also displayed progressive cerebral disease with increased urinary excretion of catecholamines. In contrast, phosphorylase activity in type IX did not increase with the administration of glucagon or epinephrine, but activity could be restored *in vitro*. Hepatomegaly was marked and there was an inconstant asymptomatic hypoglycemia during glucose tolerance testing.[76]

The diagnosis is based on the constellation of hepatomegaly, a tendency to acidosis and hypoglycemia, the biopsy findings and characterization of the stored carbohydrate and the enzymatic defect. For therapy, consult the pertinent articles.

TUMORS

Hepatic tumors are relatively uncommon in childhood and are represented by both malignant, primary and metastatic lesions and benign neoplastic and non-neoplastic hamartomatous or developmental masses.

Malignant Tumors. *Primary malignant epithelial neoplasms* are almost exclusively of hepatocellular origin and rank as the seventh most common form of pediatric neoplasia. The majority of cases are encountered prior to age 2 years. There is a male predominance varying from 2.5 to 11:1.[82] Most of the reported cases indicate a predilection for Caucasian children in spite of the high incidence of carcinoma in adults in non-Caucasian countries where hepatic carcinoma is seen infrequently in children. One type occurs commonly in premature[55, 82] and newborn[82] infants, indicating a dysontogenetic origin.[149] Antecedent hepatic disease such as hepatitis,[52, 122] extrahepatic biliary duct atresia[1, 110] and cirrhosis[82] is infrequently observed in juvenile hepatic carcinoma in contrast to adults, in whom cirrhosis is frequent. Coincidental metabolic dysfunctional states, including galactosemia,[49] glycogen storage disease[101] and the de Toni-Fanconi syndrome[29, 95] have also been reported.

Clinically, the most common presenting features are abdominal enlargement and a palpable mass, the latter being frequently indistinguishable from that encountered in neuroblastoma or nephroblastoma. Hepatic enlargement is generally asymmetrical or lobar in distribution. Rarely are discrete nodules palpable. Nonspecific manifestations include digestive disturbances such as anorexia, emesis and constipation as well as weight loss, cachexia and abdominal discomfort or pain. Splenomegaly is rare. Rare systemic and localized related manifestations and coincidental alterations include virilization[6, 78] or delayed sexual maturation in males,[13] macroglossia[94] and hemihypertrophy.[82] General laboratory examinations including liver function tests are generally of no diagnostic aid, but may show minor variations from normal values. X-ray studies with gastrointestinal examinations aid in defining the site of the mass and occasionally intrahepatic calcification is seen. Chest x-rays may demonstrate metastatic pulmonary lesions.

Grossly, the majority of tumors are solitary masses measuring up to 20 cm. in diameter and are found in the right lobe. Less frequently, multiple nodules are scattered throughout the entire liver rendering it impossible to determine whether or not a multicentric neoplasm or intrahepatic metastasis is present. Lobulation, trabeculation, focal necrosis and satellite nodularity are frequent. Calcification is present occasionally.

Primary malignant hepatocellular neoplasms have been separated on a morphologic basis into two major subtypes, hepatoblastoma and hepatocarcinoma,[82, 148, 150]

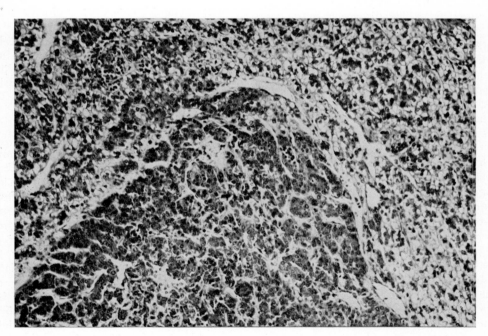

Fig. 26–23. Mixed, nonglycogenated and glycogenated cellular proliferation in hepatoblastoma.

(Fig. 26–23), a division that for the time being appears to be warranted also on clinical grounds.[82] The hepatoblastic type is further subdivided into a pure epithelial and a mixed epithelial and mesenchymal form. Both forms are constituted primarily by a dimorphic cellular population consisting of light and dark polyhedral glycogen-containing "fetal type cells" which form canalicular and sinusoidal complexes and small dark staining elongated, nonglycogenated "embryonal type cells" arranged in sheets. The mixed epithelial/mesenchymal type in addition contains foci of primitive mesenchyme, osteoid and squamous epithelium.[82] Juvenile hepatocarcinoma is morphologically indistinguishable from adult hepatocarcinoma.

Clinicopathologic correlations indicate that hepatoblastoma is invariably encountered prior to age 2 years and largely in males. Pallor and anemia are frequent. Occasionally the liver is calcified. Endocrine abnormalities as described may be present. Similarly, from an analysis of the reported 2 year survivals, the biologic activity appears to differ substantially from hepatocarcinoma, for approximately two-thirds of the salvaged cases are of hepatoblastic type.[82]

Early surgical resection offers the greatest chance of cure at present. Radiotherapy[9, 103, 112] and chemotherapy[28, 82] have been disappointing. The clinical course following discovery is rapid. Frequently the neoplasm extends into the portal vein or inferior vena cava.[133] Metastasis to regional portal and mediastinal lymph nodes, lungs, pleura and pericardium is common.

Other malignant neoplasms are extremely rare and present difficulties in precise classification and interpretation. Undifferentiated spindle cells and differentiated rhabdomyoblastic sarcomas occur. The latter presumably represents a neoplasm of intrahepatic bile duct origin analogous to that of the extrahepatic ducts.[87]

Teratomas of benign or malignant character may represent a unique neoplasm[105]; however, a relationship to hepatocellular neoplasms has been suggested.[82]

Metastatic Lesions. These lesions of the liver are far more frequent than primary malignant neoplasms and are discussed in Chapter 24. Leukemias, lymphomas, neuroblastoma, gonadal tumors and nephroblastoma are the most common types encountered in childhood. Physical examination, laboratory studies including peripheral blood and bone marrow examination, determination of urinary vandemandelic acid levels, x-ray studies, including intravenous pyelography and liver biopsy when necessary, may readily serve to disclose the nature of the lesion. With respect to neuroblastoma, we have encountered six examples of massive neonatal hepatomegaly accompanied by abdominal distention with variable degrees of fever, anemia and jaundice in whom needle and open liver biopsy yielded tissue almost completely replaced by cellular forms and configurations morphologically consistent with neuroblastoma. X-ray therapy, supplemented in some cases with systemic chemotherapy (Cytoxan and Vincristine), resulted in a complete and remarkable regression of these neoplasms, leaving variable degrees of hepatic fibrosis. One case was not treated. Two patients expired from intercurrent infections. Postmortem analysis showed in one no obvious primary site, whereas in the other, a microscopic focus of scarring was found in an otherwise normal left adrenal gland. The possibility that these clinically unique lesions represent true primary neuroblastoma cannot be entirely discounted in view of the speculative tridermal potentiality of hepatic tumors[82] and the frequently observed unidermal expression of teratoid tumors in other sites.

Benign Tumors. Benign tumors of clinical importance, in our experience, are encountered less frequently than primary malignant forms and include in decreasing frequency, hemangiomas, nonparasitic or biliary duct retention cysts, mesenchymal hamartoma/lymphangioma, benign epithelial lesions and adenomas. The neoplastic character of the majority of these is strongly disputed.

Cavernous hemangiomas, while fairly common in adults, usually as an incidental postmortem finding, are relatively rare in children, thus suggesting an etiology of an acquired nature. True cavernous hemangiomas do rarely occur and present as a mass lesion or diffuse hepatomegaly and are indistinguishable clinically from other hepatic tumors. Rupture with fatal exsanguinating intraperitoneal hemorrhage occurs[67, 69, 88] frequently unless surgical resection is undertaken.[10, 116]

Hemangioendothelioma occurs more commonly than cavernous hemangioma. They generally present with hepatomegaly and occasionally are associated with cutaneous angiomas and cardiomegaly with congestive heart failure.[119] Hepatic pulsation and bruit may present.[30] The cardiovascular alterations are attributed to multiple arteriovenous shunts. Grossly, solitary and/or multiple confluent nodules frequently replacing much of the normal parenchyma are present and may resemble carcinoma. The microscopic appearance is variable, ranging from delicate, thin-walled endothelialized channels similar to that of hemangiomatous hamartomatosis to highly cellular lesions which may be erroneously interpreted as an endothelial sarcoma (Fig. 26–24). The clinical course is variable and some patients expire from cardiac failure. Spontaneous regression with complete cure occurs rarely.[39, 50] Deep x-ray therapy may promote or hasten involution of the process. Malignant variants with lymph node and pulmonary metastasis have been reported.[85]

Mesenchymal hamartoma[50] is a rare lesion consisting of multiple endothelial lined and unlined spaces filled with proteinaceous fluid, chemically similar to liver lymph. The spaces are supported by both mature collagen and primitive mesenchyme. These characteristics suggest a lymphangiomatous lesion; however, others indicate a mesothelial lining and suggest a coelomic origin. Small collections of liver cells and bile ducts are present in all cases, particularly at the periphery (Fig. 26–25). Most cases occur in males prior to age 2 years. Our own experience and that of others indicates a lesion readily amenable to surgical excision.

Nonparasitic cysts or bile duct retention cysts are non-neoplastic cystic mass lesions most frequently encountered on the anterior-inferior surface of the right lobe of

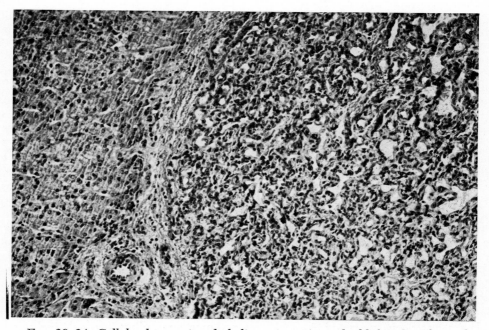

Fig. 26–24. Cellular hemangioendothelioma in a 5-month-old female infant who presented with marked hepatomegaly. Tumor nodules replaced 50 per cent of the liver. X-ray therapy was associated with complete regression.

the liver. They may be attached by a pedicle, but more frequently lie partially within the substance of the liver. The majority are surgically resectable and grossly consist of solitary or multiple communicating cystic spaces filled with clear mucinous fluid. Histologically, these spaces are generally lined by columnar epithelium of bile duct type which is supported by fibrous tissue in which there are occasional collections of atrophic liver cells and bile ducts (Fig. 26–26).

Focal nodular hyperplasia[50] is a rare lesion and most frequently consists of a solitary, circumscribed, multinodular gray to tan mass with a central depressed area of fibrosis and peripheral radiating fibrous trabeculations. Microscopically the lesion consists of masses of glycogen-ladened hepatic cells having no lobular orientation surrounded by fibrous tissue strands containing small bile ducts and lymphocytes. The pathogenesis is unknown.

Adenomas[50] are extremely rare lesions consisting of an encapsulated gray to brown mass of well-differentiated liver cells. They differ from focal nodular hyperplasia in that portal tracts and bile ducts are absent. Prognosis should be guarded, for even after meticulous study it may be impossible to exclude a well-differentiated hepatoblastoma.

PARASITISM

Hepatomegaly resulting from parasitic involvement of the liver is relatively rare in this country with the exception of *Toxocara canis* infection. A well-recognized syndrome involving multiple organ systems, originally described by Zuelzer and Apt,[155] defined by Beaver et al.[4] and designated as visceral larval migrans is established. The condition affects predominantly young children, approximately 2 to 3 years of age. Ninety per cent have a history of pica.[79] The chief manifestations consist of cough, wheezing respiration, fever, hepatomegaly, malnutrition and papulopustular skin lesions. The condition may be asymptomatic, but frequently various manifestations suggest allergy such as urticaria or evanescent arthralgia. Some cases have a history of convulsive seizures.[79] Hepatomegaly, while relatively common, is not

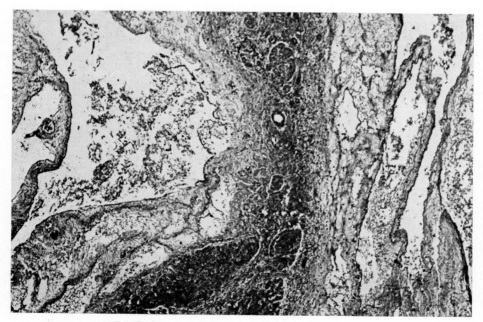

FIG. 26–25. Segment of large multicystic mass from the left lobe of the liver in a 1-year-old male. Chemical analysis of cyst fluid with the addition of small amounts of bilirubin, approximated that of lymph.

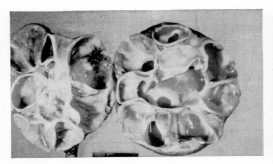

FIG. 26–26. Multilocular cystic mass (bile duct retention cyst) from the right lobe of an 8-year-old male. The lumen contained clear mucinous fluid and the lining consisted of simple columnar epithelium of bile duct type.

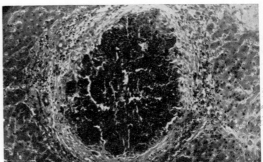

FIG. 26–28. Healed stage of lesions shown in Figures 26–27 and 26–29, walled off and calcified. Numerous active lesions were present at the same time.

invariably present. Varying degrees of anemia, usually microcytic, hypochromic type, may be present; the anemia is related more to age and nutritional factors than to the etiologic agent. Leukocyte counts may be as high as 150,000/mm.[3] and extreme degrees of eosinophilia as high as 80 per cent may be seen. Formerly such findings were often thought to indicate eosinophilic leukemia.

Impaired hepatic function is not usually demonstrable despite the presence, in some cases, of rather widespread granulomatous abscesses of the parenchyma (Figs. 26–27 and 26–28). Larvae can, on occasion, be demonstrated within these lesions[79] (Fig. 26–29), but more frequently parasitic elements cannot be found even after an exhaustive search.[155] Other laboratory tests show hypoalbuminemia and hyperglobulinemia. There is a significant increase in total gamma globulin, primarily due to an elevation in the gamma M fraction. Precipitating antibodies to A and B blood group substances and helminthic antigen are present in half the patients. Iso-agglutinin A and B titers are elevated (greater than 1:256) in 66 and 56 per cent of patients, respectively. Sheep cell agglutination titers are slightly elevated and 50 per cent of patients have heat stable antiglobulins.[79] As might be expected from the pathogenesis of the disorder, cross reactions with other helminthic antigens are encountered.[79] Precipitin and intradermal skin tests

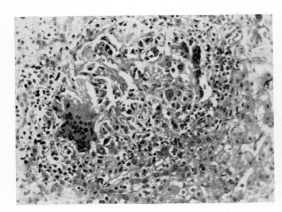

FIG. 26–27. Granuloma-like lesion in liver from a 3-year-old child with marked eosinophilia and hepatomegaly.

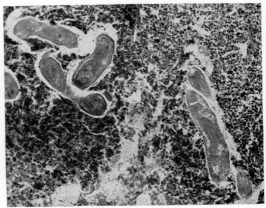

FIG. 26–29. Larvae, presumably *Toxocara canis*, in eosinophilic abscess of liver.

may also be employed in establishing the diagnosis. There is no specific therapy for this condition. It is essential to prevent further ingestion of infective material by appropriate means. Although the prognosis is generally good, hepatosplenomegaly and eosinophilia may persist for months or years.[155] Rarely is the disease fatal.

REFERENCES

1. Absolon, K. B., Rikkers, H., and Aust, J. B.: Thoracic duct lymph drainage in congenital biliary atresia, Surg. Gynec. Obstet. *120*:123, 1965.
2. Ahrens, E. H., Jr., Harris, R. C., and MacMahon, H. E.: Atresia of intrahepatic bile ducts, Pediatrics *8*:628, 1951.
3. Arias, I. M., and Gartner, L. M.: Production of unconjugated hyperbilirubinemia in full-term new-born infants following administration of pregnane-3(alpha),20(beta)-diol, Nature *203*:1292, 1964.
4. Beaver. P. C., Snyder, C. H., Carrera, G. M., Dent, J. H., and Lafferty, J. W.: Chronic eosinophilia due to visceral larva migrans, Pediatrics *9*:7, 1952.
5. Becker, W. B., Kipps, A., and McKenzie, D.: Disseminated herpes simplex virus infection, Am. J. Dis. Child. *115*:1, 1968.
6. Behrle, F. C., Mantz, F. A., Jr., Olson, R. L., and Trombold, J. C.: Virilization accompanying hepatoblastoma, Pediatrics *32*:265, 1963.
7. Benirschke, K., Kibrick, S., and Craig, J. M.: The pathology of fatal Coxsackie infection in the newborn (Abst.), Am. J. Path. *34*:587, 1958.
8. Bennett, A. M., Capps, R. B., Drake, M. E., Ettinger, R. H., Mills, E. H., and Stokes, J., Jr.: Endemic infectious hepatitis in an infants' orphanage; Part II, A.M.A. Arch. Int. Med. *90*:37, 1952.
9. Benson, C. D., Mustard, W. T., Ravitch, M. M., Snyder, W. H., and Welch, K. J.: Pediatric Surgery, vol. 1, part IV, p. 628, Chicago, Year Book Pub., 1962.
10. Berman, J. K., Kirkhoff, P., and Levene, N.: Hepatic lobectomy for hemangioma of the liver in a five-day-old infant, Arch. Surg. *71*:249, 1955.
11. Bernstein, J., and Brown, A. K.: Sepsis and jaundice in early infancy, Pediatrics *29*:873, 1962.
12. Bernstein, J., Gomez, M. R., and Brough,

A. J.: Storage of acid mucopolysaccharides in skeletal muscles of patients with generalized glycogenosis, Proc. Soc. Pediatric Res., Seattle, Wash., February, 1964 (unpublished).
13. Beynon, A. E.: Primary carcinoma of the liver in a boy aged 15, Lancet *2*:528, 1948.
14. Billing, B. H.: The 3 serum bile pigments in obstructive jaundice and hepatitis, J. Clin. Path. *8*:130, 1955.
15. Billing, B. H., Cole, P. G., and Lathe, G. H.: Excretion of bilirubin as diglucuronide giving direct van den Bergh reaction, Biochem. J. *65*:774, 1957.
16. Bradford, W. D., and Latham, W. C.: Acute encephalopathy and fatty hepatomegaly, Am. J. Dis. Child. *114*:152, 1967.
17. Brain, W. R., Hunter, D., and Turnbull, H. M.: Lancet *1*:221, 1929, quoted by Reye, R. D. K., and Morgan, G.: Letters to the editor, Lancet *2*:1061, 1963.
18. Brough, A. J., and Bernstein, J.: Liver biopsy in the diagnosis of infantile obstructive jaundice. (Pediatrics, In Press.)
19. Brough, A. J., Jones, D., Page, R. H., and Mizukami, I.: Dermal erythropoiesis in neonatal infants. A manifestation of intrauterine viral disease, Pediatrics *40*:627, 1967.
20. Brown, A. K.: Studies on the neonatal development of the glucuronide conjugating system (Abst.), A.M.A. J. Dis. Child. *94*:510, 1957.
21. Brown, A. K., and Brauer, R.: Unpublished observations.
22. Brown, A. K., and Zuelzer, W. W.: Studies in hyperbilirubinemia. I. Hyperbilirubinemia of the newborn unrelated to isoimmunization, A.M.A. J. Dis. Child. *93*:263, 1957.
23. ———: Studies on the neonatal development of the glucuronide conjugating system, J. Clin. Invest. *37*:332, 1958.
24. Brown, W. R., and Boon, W. H.: Ethnic group differences in plasma bilirubin levels of full-term healthy Singapore newborns, Pediatrics *36*:745, 1965.
25. Cardiff, R. D.: A histochemical and electron microscopic study of skeletal muscle in the case of Pompe's disease (glycogenosis II), Pediatrics *37*:249, 1966.
26. Chen, H., Lin, C., and Lien, I.: Vascular permeability in experimental kernicterus. An electron-microscopic study of the blood brain barrier, Am. J. Path. *51*:69, 1967.

27. Christy, R. A., and Boley, J. O.: The relation of hepatic fibrosis to concentration of bilirubin in the serum in congenital atresia of the biliary tract, Pediatrics 21:226, 1958.

28. Clatworthy, H. W., Jr., Boles, E. T., Jr., and Newton, W. A.: Primary tumours of the liver in infants and children, Arch. Dis. Child. 35:22, 1960.

29. Cleland, R. S.: Benign and malignant tumors of the liver, Pediat. Clin. N. Amer. 6:427, 1959.

30. Cooper, A. G., and Bolande, R. P.: Multiple hemangiomas in an infant with cardiac hypertrophy; postmortem angiographic demonstration of the arteriovenous fistulae, Pediatrics 35:27, 1965.

31. Cooper, L. Z., Green, R. H., Krugman, S., Giles, J. P., and Mirick, G. S.: Neonatal thrombocytopenic purpura and other manifestations of rubella contracted in utero, Am. J. Dis. Child. 110:416, 1965.

32. Coppoletta, J. M., and Wolbach, S. B.: Body length and organ weights of infants and children, Am. J. Path. 9:55, 1933.

33. Cori, G. T.: Biochemical aspects of glycogen deposition disease, Mod. Probl. in Paediat. 3:344, 1957.

34. Cori, G. T., and Cori, C. F.: Glucose-6-phosphatase of the liver in glycogen storage disease, J. Biol. Chem. 199:661, 1952.

35. Craig, J. M.: Sequences in the development of cirrhosis of the liver in cases of erythroblastosis fetalis, Arch. Path. 49:665, 1950.

36. Craig, J. M., Gellis, S. S., and Hsia, D. Y. Y.: Cirrhosis of liver in infants and children, A.M.A. Am. J. Dis. Child. 90:299, 1955.

37. Craig, J. M., and Landing, B. H.: A form of hepatitis in the neonatal period simulating biliary atresia, A.M.A. Arch. Path. 54:321, 1952.

38. Crigler, J. F., Jr., and Najjar, V. A.: Congenital familial non-hemolytic jaundice with kernicterus, Pediatrics 10:169, 1952.

39. Crocker, D. W., and Cleland, R. S.: Infantile hemangioendothelioma of the liver; report of 3 cases, Pediatrics 19:596, 1957.

40. Davidson, L. T., Merritt, K. K., and Weech, A. A.: Hyperbilirubinemia in the newborn, Am. J. Dis. Child. 61:958, 1941.

41. Diamond, L. K.: Maternal medication vs. neonatal jaundice, New Engl. J. Med. 260:393, 1959.

42. di Sant'Agnese, P. A., and Blanc, W. A.: A distinctive type of biliary cirrhosis of liver associated with cystic fibrosis of the pancreas: recognition through signs of portal hypertension, Pediatrics 18:387, 1956.

43. Dubin, I. N.: Chronic idiopathic jaundice. A review of 50 cases, Am. J. Med. 24:268, 1958.

44. ———: Rotor syndrome and chronic idiopathic jaundice, Arch. Int. Med. 110:823, 1962.

45. Dubin, I. N., and Johnson, F. B.: Chronic idiopathic jaundice with unidentified pigment in liver cells; a new clinico-pathologic entity with report of 12 cases, Medicine 33:155, 1954.

46. Dutton, G. J.: Foetal and gastro-intestinal glucuronide synthesis (Abst.), Biochem. J. 69:39P, 1958.

47. Dvorackova, I., Vortel, V., and Hroch, M.: Encephalitic syndrome with fatty degeneration of viscera, Arch. Path. 81:240, 1966.

48. Eberlein, W. R.: A simple solvent-partition method for measurement of free and conjugated bilirubin in serum, Pediatrics 25:878, 1960.

49. Edmonds, A. M., Hennigar, G. R., and Crooks, R.: Galactosemia—report of case with autopsy, Pediatrics 10:40, 1952.

50. Edmondson, H. A.: Differential diagnosis of tumors and tumor-like lesions of liver in infancy and childhood, A.M.A. J. Dis. Child. 91:168, 1956.

51. Esterly, J. R., Slusser, R. J., and Ruebner, B. H.: Hepatic lesions in the congenital rubella syndrome, J. Pediatrics 71:676, 1967.

52. Fajers, C. M., Falkmer, S., Frissell, E., and Pehrson, M.: Primary carcinoma of the liver and giant cell hepatitis in infancy, Acta Paediat. 49:96, 1960.

53. Farber, S.: Pancreatic function and disease in early life. V. Pathologic changes associated with pancreatic insufficiency in early life, Arch. Path. 37:238, 1944.

54. Fetterman, G. H.: A new laboratory aid in the clinical diagnosis of inclusion disease of infancy, Am. J. Clin. Path. 22:424, 1952.

55. Florentin, P., Rauber, G., and Macinot, C.: Hépatoblastome chez un nouveau-né, Ann. Anat. path. (Paris), 1:507, 1956.

56. Gilbert, N. A., and Lereboullet, P.: La

cholémie simple familiale, Sem. méd. (Paris) *11*:241, 1901.

57. Gilbert, N. A., Lereboullet, P., and Herscher, M.: Les trois cholémies congénitales, Bull. Soc. méd Hôp. Paris *24*: 1203, 1907.

58. Gillman, T., and Gillman, J.: Methionine and fatty liver in infant pellagrins, Nature *155*:634, 1945.

59. Gregory, C. H.: Studies of conjugated bilirubin. III. Pigment I, complex of conjugated and free bilirubin, J. Lab. Clin. Med. *61*:917, 1963.

60. Gruenwald, P.: Degenerative change in right half of liver resulting from intrauterine anoxia, Am. J. Clin. Path. *19*: 801, 1949.

61. Grumbach, A., and Gasser, C.: ABO Inkompatibilitaten und Morbus haemolyticus neonatorum, Helv. paediat. Acta *3*:447, 1948.

62. Haberman, S., Hill, J. M., and Soules, D. E.: The use of the elution test for demonstration of A and B produced hemolytic disease of the newborn, Rev. hemat. *9*:510, 1954.

63. Halbrecht, I.: Role of hemagglutinins anti-A and anti-B in the pathogenesis of jaundice of the newborn (icterus neonatorum praecox), Am. J. Dis. Child. *68*:248, 1944.

64. Hanshaw, J. B., Betts, R. F., Simon, G., and Boynton, R. C.: Acquired cytomegalovirus infection: association with hepatomegaly and abnormal liver-function tests, New Engl. J. Med. *272*:602, 1965.

65. Harris, R. C., and Anderson, D. H.: Intrahepatic bile duct atresia (Abst.), Am. J. Dis. Child. *100*:783, 1960.

66. Hass, G. M.: Hepato-adrenal necrosis with intranuclear inclusion bodies, Am. J. Path. *11*:127, 1935.

67. Hatten, D. F., and Werthammer, S.: Hemangioma of the liver causing death in a newborn infant, W. Virginia Med. J. *59*:8, 1963.

68. Hawksley, J. C., and Lightwood, R.: A contribution to the study of erythroblastosis: icterus gravis neonatorum, Quart. J. Med. *3*:155, 1934.

69. Hendrick, J. G.: Hemangioma of the liver causing death in a newborn infant, J. Pediat. *32*:309, 1948.

70. Hers, J. C. *in* Whelan, W. J., and Cameron, M. P. (eds.): Ciba Foundation on the Control of Glycogen Metabolism, Boston, Little, Brown, 1964, pp. 354-363.

71. Hosier, D. M., and Newton, W. A., Jr.: Serious Coxsackie infection in infants and children: myocarditis, meningoencephalitis and hepatitis, A.M.A. J. Dis. Child. *96*:251, 1958.

72. Howard, F. H., and Meriwether, W. A.: Fat disease of the liver in infants on the Isthmus of Panama, Pediatrics *10*:150, 1952.

73. Hsia, D. Y. Y., Allen, F. H., Jr., Diamond, L. K., and Gellis, S. S.: Serum bilirubin levels in the newborn infant, J. Pediat. *42*:277, 1953.

74. Hsia, D. Y. Y., and Gellis, S. S.: Portal hypertension in infants and children, A.M.A. Am. J. Dis. Child. *90*:290, 1955.

75. Hsia, D. Y. Y., Patterson, P., Allen, F. H., Diamond, L. K., and Gellis, S. S.: Prolonged obstructive jaundice in infancy. I. General survey of 156 cases, Pediatrics *10*:243, 1952.

76. Hug, G., Garancis, J. C., Schubert, W. K., and Kaplan, S.: Glycogen storage disease, Types II, III, VIII and IX, Am. J. Dis. Child. *111*:457, 1966.

77. Hug, G., Krill, C. E., Jr., Perrin, E. V., and Guest, G. M.: Cori's disease (amylo-1,6-glucosidase deficiency): report of a case in a Negro child, New Engl. J. Med. *268*:113, 1963.

78. Hung, W., Blizzard, R. M., Migeon, C. J., Camacho, A. M., and Nyhan, W. L.: Precocious puberty in a boy with hepatoma and circulating gonadotropin, J. Pediat. *63*:895, 1963.

79. Huntley, C. C., Costas, M. C., and Lyerly, A.: Visceral larva migrans syndrome: Clinical characteristics and immunologic studies in 51 patients, Pediatrics *36*:523, 1965.

80. Illingworth, B.: Glycogen storage disease, Am. J. Clin. Nutr. *9*:683, 1961.

81. Illingworth, B., and Brown, D. H. *in* Whelan, W. J., and Cameron, M. P. (eds.): Ciba Foundation on the control of glycogen metabolism, Boston, Little, Brown, 1964, pp. 336-349.

82. Ishak, K. G., and Glunz, P. R.: Hepatoblastoma and hepatocarcinoma in infancy and childhood, Cancer *20*:396, 1967.

83. Johnson, L., Sarmiento, F., Blanc, W. A., and Day, R.: Kernicterus in rats with inherited deficiency of glucuronyl transferase, A.M.A. J. Dis. Child. *97*:591, 1959.

84. Joske, R. A., Keall, D. D., Leak, P. J., Stanley, N. F., and Walters, M. N. I.: Hepatitis—encephalitis in humans with

reovirus infection, Arch. Int. Med. *113*: 811, 1964.

85. Kauffman, S. L., and Stout, A. P.: Malignant hemangioendothelioma in infants and children, Cancer *14*:1186, 1961.

86. Kibrick, S., and Benirschke, K.: Severe generalized disease (encephalohepato-myocarditis) occurring in the newborn period and due to infection with Coxsackie virus, group B: evidence of intrauterine infection with this agent, Pediatrics *22*:857, 1958.

87. Kissane, J. M., and Smith, M. G.: Pathology of Infancy and Childhood, p. 284, St. Louis, Mosby, 1967.

88. Kissinger, C. C., Sternfeld, E., and Zuker, S. D.: Rupture of a cavernous hemangioma as a cause of death in a newborn infant, Ohio St. M. J. *36*:383, 1940.

89. Korones, S. B., Ainger, L. E., Monif, G. R. G., Roane, J., Sever, J. L., and Fuste, F.: Congenital rubella syndrome: study of 22 infants; myocardial damage and other new clinical aspects, Am. J. Dis. Child. *110*:434, 1965.

90. Kove, S., Perry, R., and Wroblewski, F.: Diagnosis of neonatal jaundice by patterns of serum transaminase, Am. J. Dis. Child. *100*:47, 1960.

91. Krugman, S. (ed.): Rubella symposium, Am. J. Dis. Child., *110*:345, 1965.

92. Krugman, S., Ward, R., and Giles, J. B.: The natural history of infectious hepatitis, Am. J. Med. *32*:717, 1962.

93. Lathe, G. H., and Walker, M.: An enzyme defect in human neonatal jaundice and in Gunn's strain of jaundiced rats, Biochem. J. *67*:9P, 1957.

94. Leffers, I.: Uber eine seltene, maligne Mischgeschwulst der Leber bei einem 16 Monate alten Knaben, Beitr. Path. Anat. *105*:203, 1941.

95. Lelong, M., Alagille, D., Vinh, L. T., Colin, J., Roux, M., Gentil, C., and Gabilan, J. C.: Cirrhose congénitale et familiale rachitsme vitamino-resistant avec diabète gluco-phospho-amine, hépatome terminal, Pediatrie *16*:221, 1961.

96. Lester, R., and Schmid, R.: Bilirubin metabolism, New Engl. J. Med. *270*:779, 1964.

97. Liley, A. W.: The use of amniocentesis and fetal transfusion in erythroblastosis fetalis, Pediatrics *35*:836, 1965.

98. Lucey, J. F.: Hyperbilirubinemia of prematurity, Pediatrics *25*:690, 1960.

99. Lygren, T.: Hepatolenticular degeneration (Wilson's disease) and juvenile cirrhosis in the same family, Lancet *1*:275, 1959.

100. Mandelbaum, B., LaCroix, G. C., and Robinson, A. R.: Determination of fetal maturity by spectrophotometric analysis of amniotic fluid, Obstet. and Gynec. *29*:471, 1967.

101. Mason, H. H., and Andersen, D. H.: Glycogen disease of the liver (von Gierke's disease) with hepatomata; case report with metabolic studies, Pediatrics *16*:785, 1955.

102. McAdams, A. J., and Wilson, H. E.: The liver in generalized glycogen storage disease; light microscopic observations, Am. J. Path. *49*:99, 1966.

103. McDougal, R. A., and Gatzimos, C. D.: Primary carcinoma of the liver in infants and children, Cancer *10*:678, 1957.

104. Miller, H. C.: Effect of diabetic and prediabetic pregnancies on the fetus and newborn infant, J. Pediat. *29*:455, 1946.

105. Misugi, K., and Reiner, C. B.: A malignant true teratoma of liver in childhood, Arch. Path. *80*:409, 1965.

106. Mollison, P. L.: Physiologic jaundice of the newborn, Lancet *1*:513, 1948.

107. Mollison, P. L., and Cutbush, M.: Bromsulphalein excretion in the newborn, Arch. Dis. Child. *24*:7, 1949.

108. Nosslin, B.: Direct diazo reaction of bile pigments in serum: Experimental and clinical studies, Scand. J. Clin. Lab. Invest. *12*(Supp. 49):1-176, 1960.

109. Odell, G. B.: Personal communication.

110. Okuyama, K.: Primary liver cell carcinoma associated with biliary cirrhosis due to congenital bile duct atresia, J. Pediat. *67*:89, 1965.

111. Patten, B. M.: Human Embryology, Philadelphia, Blakiston, 1946.

112. Phillips, R., and Murikami, K.: Primary neoplasms of the liver—results of radiation therapy, Cancer *13*:714, 1960.

113. Potter, E. L.: Pathology of the Fetus and Infant, ed. 2, Chicago, Year Book Pub., 1961.

114. Potter, E. L., and Adair, F. L.: Fetal and Neonatal Death, Chicago, Univ. Chicago Press, 1940.

115. Powell, L. W., Hemingway, E., Billing, B. H., and Sherlock, S.: Idiopathic unconjugated hyperbilirubinemia (Gilbert's syndrome). A study of 42 families, New Engl. J. Med. *277*:1108, 1967.

116. Pryles, C. V., and Heggestad, G. E.: Large cavernous hemangioma of the liver: Successful resection in an 18-

month-old infant, A.M.A. Am. J. Dis. Child. 88:759, 1954.

117. Quilligan, J. J., Jr., and Wilson, J. L.: Fetal herpes simplex infection in a newborn infant, J. Lab. Clin. Med. 38:742, 1951.

118. Reye, R. D. K., Morgan, G., and Baral, J.: Encephalopathy and fatty degeneration of the viscera—a disease entity in childhood, Lancet 2:749, 1963.

119. Robbins, B. H., and Castle, R. F.: Letter to the editor, Pediatrics 35:868, 1965.

120. Rosenfield, R. E.: A-B hemolytic disease of the newborn, Proc. Ann. Meeting, Am. Assoc. Blood Banks, 1953.

121. Rosenthal, I. M., Spellberg, M. A., McGrew, E. A., and Rozenfield, I. H.: Absence of interlobular bile ducts, Am. J. Dis. Child. 101:228, 1961.

122. Roth, D., and Duncan, P. A.: Primary carcinoma of the liver after giant-cell hepatitis of infancy—report of a case, Cancer 8:986, 1955.

123. Rotor, A. B., Manahan, L., and Florentin, A.: Familial nonhemolytic jaundice with direct van den Bergh reaction, Acta Med. Philipinna 5:37, 1948.

124. Ruggieri, B. A., Baggenstoss, A. H., and Logan, G. B.: Juvenile cirrhosis: a clinico-pathologic study of 27 cases, A.M.A. J. Dis. Child. 94:64, 1957.

125. Santulli, T. V., Harris, R. C., and Reemtsma, K.: Surgical exploration in obstructive jaundice of infancy, Pediatries 26:27, 1960.

126. Schmid, R.: in Stanbury, J. B., Wyngaarden, J. B., and Fredrickson, D. S. (eds.): The Metabolic Basis of Inherited Disease, New York, McGraw-Hill, 1960.

127. ———: in Whelan, W. J., and Cameron, M. P. (eds.): Ciba Foundation on the Control of Glycogen Metabolism, Boston: Little, Brown, 1964, pp. 305-318.

128. Schmid, R., Hammaker, L., and Axelrod, J.: The enzymatic formation of bilirubin glucuronide, Arch. Biochem. 70:285, 1957.

129. Scrimshaw, N. W., Behar, M., Arroyave, G., Viteri, F., and Tejada, C.: Characteristics of kwashiorkor (sindrome pluricarencial de la infancia), Fed. Proc. 15:977, 1956.

130. Siegel, W., Spencer, F. J., Smith, D. J., Toman, J. M., Skinner, W. F., and Marx, M. B.: Two new variants of infection with Coxsackie virus group B, type 5, in young children: a syndrome of lymphadenopathy, pharyngitis and hepatomegaly or splenomegaly or both, and one of pneumonia, New Engl. J. Med. 268:1210, 1963.

131. Singer, D. B., Rudolph, A. J., Rosenberg, H. S., Rawls, W. E., and Boniuk, M.: Pathology of the congenital rubella syndrome, J. Pediatrics 71:665, 1967.

132. Sprinz, H., and Nelson, R. S.: Persistent nonhemolytic hyperbilirubinemia associated with lipochrome-like pigment in liver cells; report of 4 cases, Ann. Int. Med. 41:952, 1954.

133. Steiner, M. M.: Primary carcinoma of the liver in childhood, Am. J. Dis. Child. 55:807, 1938.

134. Stern, H., and Williams, B. M.: Isolation of rubella virus in a case of neonatal hepatitis, Lancet 1:293, 1966.

135. Stokes, J., Wolman, I. J., Blanchard, M. C., and Farquhar, J. D.: Viral hepatitis in the newborn: clinical features, epidemiology and pathology, A.M.A. Am. J. Dis. Child. 82:213, 1951.

136. Stowens, D.: Diseases of the extrahepatic biliary system in Pediatric Pathology, Baltimore, Williams & Wilkins, 1959.

137. Strauss, L., and Bernstein, J.: Neonatal hepatitis in congenital rubella, a histopathologic study, Arch. Path. 86:317, 1968.

138. Stulberg, C. S., Zuelzer, W. W., Page, R. H., Taylor, P. E., and Brough, A. J.: Cytomegalovirus infections with reference to isolations from lymph nodes and blood (31651), Proc. Soc. Exp. Biol. Med. 123:976, 1966.

139. Thaler, M. M.: Fatal neonatal cirrhosis: entity or end result, Pediatrics 33:721, 1964.

140. Tuffy, P., Brown, A. K., and Zuelzer, W. W.: Infantile pyknocytosis: a common erythrocyte abnormality of the first trimester, A.M.A. J. Dis. Child. 98:227, 1959.

141. Van Hoof, F., and Hers, H. G.: The subgroups of type III glycogenosis, European J. Biochem. 2:265, 1967.

142. van Creveld, S., and Huijing, F.: Glycogen storage disease. Biochemical and clinical data on 16 cases, Am. J. Med. 38:554, 1965.

143. Wainwright, J.: Hepatitis associated with infantile diarrhea, Arch. Dis. Child. 25:286, 1950.

144. Waters, W. J., and Bowen, W. R.: Bilirubin encephalopathy: studies related to

cellular respiration (Abst.), A.M.A. J. Dis. Child. 90:603, 1955.

145. Watson, J. R. H.: Hepatosplenomegaly as complication of maternal rubella: a report of 2 cases, Med. J. Australia 1: 516, 1952.

146. Weber, A. Ph., Schalm, L., and Witmans, J.: Bilirubin monoglucuronide (pigment I) complex, Acta med. Scand. 173:19, 1963.

147. Williams, R. T.: Detoxification Mechanisms: The Metabolism of Drugs and Allied Organic Compounds, New York, Wiley, 1947.

148. Willis, R. A.: Pathology of Tumours, 2nd ed., St. Louis, C. V. Mosby, 1953.

149. ———: The Borderland of Embryology and Pathology, London, Butterworth, 1958.

150. ———: The Pathology of the Tumours of Children, Springfield, Ill., Thomas, 1962.

151. Yudkin, S., Gellis, S. S., and Lappen, F.: Liver function in newborn infants, Arch. Dis. Child. 24:12, 1949.

152. Zinkham, W. H., and Childs, B.: Effect of naphthalene derivatives on glutathione metabolism of erythrocytes from patients with naphthalene hemolytic anemia (Abst.), J. Clin. Invest. 36:938, 1957.

153. Zuelzer, W. W.: Unpublished observations.

154. Zuelzer, W. W., Al-Rashid, R., and Teruya, J.: Relevance of parameters for pre- and postnatal therapy in hemolytic

disease, Am. J. Obstet. Gynec. 92:925, 1965.

155. Zuelzer, W. W., and Apt, L.: Disseminated visceral lesions associated with extreme eosinophilia, Am. J. Dis. Child. 78:153, 1949.

156. Zuelzer, W. W., and Brown, A. K.: Neonatal jaundice: a review, Am. J. Dis. Child. 101:87, 1961.

157. Zuelzer, W. W., and Cohen, F.: ABO hemolytic disease and heterospecific pregnancy, Pediat. Clin. N. Amer., pp. 405-428, 1957.

158. Zuelzer, W. W., Kaplan, E., and Evans, M.: ABO heterospecific pregnancy and hemolytic disease: A study of normal and pathologic variants. IV. Pathologic variants, A.M.A. Am. J. Dis. Child. 88:319, 1954.

159. Zuelzer, W. W., Reisman, L. E., and Brown, A. K.: Studies in hyperbilirubinemia. III. Separate metabolic defects in premature infants reflected in the partition of serum bilirubin, Am. J. Dis. Child. 102:815, 1961.

160. Zuelzer, W. W., and Stulberg, C. S.: Herpes simplex virus as cause of fulminating visceral disease and hepatitis in infancy, A.M.A. Am. J. Dis. Child. 83:421, 1952.

161. Zuelzer, W. W., Stulberg, C. S., Page, R. H., Teruya, J., and Brough, A. J.: Etiology and pathogenesis of acquired hemolytic anemia, Transfusion 6:438, 1966.

27

Amyloidosis of the Liver

MAURICE H. STAUFFER, M.D., AND *DAVID C. DAHLIN*, M.D.

The term "amyloid" was first used in 1853 by Virchow for a substance, present in many organs of a patient with an unusual disease, that gave a starchlike staining reaction. At first, generalized amyloidosis was recognized only when associated with various infectious, malignant and mesenchymal diseases. Hepatic involvement was common, being recognized in 60 per cent of cases,[13] but more recently in as high as 80 per cent of certain forms.[38] The fact that the disease was rare and often not noted prior to necropsy seems to emphasize the difficulty of clinical diagnosis. In recent years, improved diagnostic methods and more awareness of the disease among clinicians and pathologists have increased the percentage of correct diagnoses prior to death.[44]

In spite of much study, the etiology and many aspects of the disease remain obscure. Experimentally, amyloidosis has been produced in various animals by the injection of bacteria,[3] casein and other protein substances.[17] In some of the animals there has been an associated hyperglobulinemia to which has been attributed an etiologic role.[16] Some studies indicate that amyloid may be related to an antigen-antibody complex. The frequent observation of amyloidosis in association with plasmacytic disease, such as multiple myeloma, in which there may be hyperglobulinemia, lends some evidence to the suggested idea of an obscure derangement of protein metabolism. However, in many cases the absence of recognizable systemic disease and of measurable changes in serum or urinary protein emphasizes the unknown aspects.

The chemical nature is not completely known, but usually the amyloid material has been considered to be a complex protein combined with chondroitin sulfuric acid. Amyloid is a homogenous, amorphous, eosinophilic material that stains metachromatically with dyes such as methyl violet and methyl green.[22] It usually has an affinity for Congo red and stains yellow or faintly pink by the van Gieson connective-tissue technic. The appearance of amyloid when stained with hematoxylin and eosin is ordinarily quite characteristic. A stain to show metachromasia may be desired for confirmation. The van Gieson technic differentiates amyloid from brilliantly red-staining hyalin or collagen in the occasional troublesome case.

Cohen, in 1967, stated the belief that sections stained with Congo red and viewed in the polarizing microscope were the most satisfactory for diagnosing amyloid; a unique, green birefringence characterizes the substance.[11] The fluorescence of the amyloid in sections stained with thioflavine T[48] is considered by some to be an aid in the recognition of amyloid.

CLASSIFICATION

Since the clinical and pathologic manifestations of amyloidosis are variable, classification of the different forms has been suggested by several authors such as Lubarsch,[33] Reimann and co-workers[37] and Dahlin.[14] Dahlin suggested the following main groups:

1. Primary amyloidosis
2. Amyloidosis complicating myeloma
3. Secondary amyloidosis

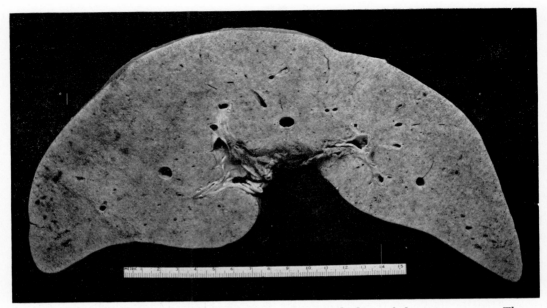

Fig. 27–1. A 4,000-Gm. liver with severe diffuse amyloidosis of the primary type. The predominant clinical signs had been related to hepatic involvement.

The first two categories in addition to being systemic may have focal or tumefactive lesions.[14] In recent years, a fourth type has been recognized in elderly patients at necropsy in which the amyloid is localized in the heart. The familial type,[26] often having vitreous opacities[29] and peripheral neuritis[1] with an apparent specific serum electrophoretic pattern described by Block and associates,[6, 7, 38] may constitute a fifth category. No less than 6 variants of heredofamilial amyloidosis were included in Cohen's classification in 1967.[11]

PRIMARY AMYLOIDOSIS

By definition, primary amyloidosis ("paraamyloidosis" or "atypical amyloidosis") occurs in the absence of any predisposing disease. Formerly, it was the rarest form of the disease—only 70 cases were reported up to 1950.[12] However, about 1956 Rukavina and co-workers[38] collected 154 cases from the literature; this number emphasizes its increased recognition. In a recent 11-year period, the amyloidosis in 27 of 63 patients with systemic amyloidosis seen at the Mayo Clinic was primary.[44]

Widespread deposition, leading to a bizarre clinical picture,[14] is the rule. There is a predilection for mesenchymal structures, such as muscle, blood vessels and the heart.

The heart is involved in most cases and is the basis for the death of 50 per cent of patients in congestive heart failure, the commonest form of death. Unexplained cardiac failure, especially if associated with marked albuminuria, should make one think of amyloidosis as a possible cause. In some instances, the clinical picture resembles that of constrictive pericarditis[18]: high venous pressure, hepatomegaly and atypical cardiac findings. In cases with involvement of other organs, such as the lungs, liver and kidneys, cardiac failure may appear to be more marked than it is. Abnormal electrocardiographic findings are noted in almost all cases of primary amyloidosis.[44]

The spleen, kidneys, adrenal glands and liver are infiltrated less commonly than the heart in primary amyloidosis. Although hepatic involvement was noted in only one third of cases by Dahlin in 1949,[13] Rukavina and co-workers found evidence of such involvement in 80 per cent of cases from the literature which they reviewed.[38] Recent observations indicate that hepatic signs and symptoms may dominate the clinical picture.[52] Jaundice, hepatomegaly, ascites and edema are the reported findings indicating hepatic involvement,[53] and most cases simulate cirrhosis of the liver.[20] The liver is usually hard, smooth and large, extending into the left upper quadrant; there may be a hepatoma-like enlargement on the surface of the liver near the costal margin.[44] Hepatic enlargement with ascites and debilitation of the patient may suggest metastatic carcinoma, but the association of marked albuminuria should lead one to suspect amyloidosis, since albuminuria is uncommon in cirrhosis or metastatic carcinoma. Although the liver is frequently involved in systemic amyloidosis, relatively few deaths are directly attributable to the hepatic disease.

The liver containing amyloid is firmer than normal; it may be somewhat translucent and brittle, owing to the waxy deposits of amyloid (Fig. 27–1). Histologic study reveals this substance on the reticular framework that separates the cords of hepatic cells from the sinusoids (27–2 to 27–4). When this intralobular deposition is

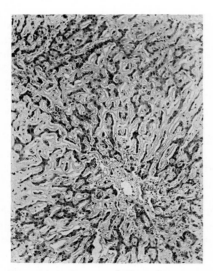

FIG. 27–2. Severe, diffuse, hepatic parenchymal amyloidosis of the primary type, histologically quite like the secondary variety. (Hematoxylin and eosin. × 85.)

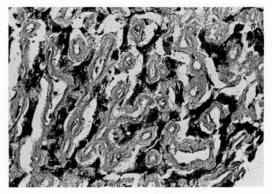

FIG. 27–3. Needle biopsy specimen with pale-staining amyloid between the sinusoids and the dark-staining hepatic cords. Detail of the hepatic cells has been altered by the special stain (Mallory's phosphotungstic acid hematoxylin. × 325.)

marked, the hepatic cells atrophy. The arteries and the veins of the portal triads usually have thickened walls and narrowed lumens, owing to amyloid deposition in the media. Heavy infiltration in these vessels is more common in primary than in secondary amyloidosis and may be a helpful differential feature.

Since amyloid interferes with function of the liver only by pressure and consequent secondary atrophy of the hepatic cells, patients with hepatic signs usually have pronounced hepatomegaly with severe infiltration. Jaundice has been reported in only 2 cases of secondary amyloidosis, but Stauffer found reports of jaundice in 6 patients with primary amyloidosis.[42] Of the 8, those with primary amyloidosis seemed to have more severe involvement of the liver. Portal hypertension is a rare complication; Kapp reviewed 4 cases from the literature in 1965 and reported 1 case associated with esophageal varices.[28] Petechiae and purpuric areas are noted frequently; and because of them, some cases of primary amyloidosis have been diagnosed erroneously as thrombocytopenic purpura. Periorbital subcutaneous blue-black discolorations are often seen.

Patients with hepatic involvement ordinarily have coexisting renal deposits of amy-

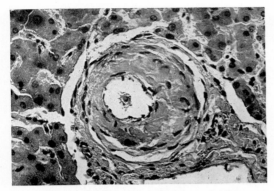

FIG. 27–4. Vessel of portal triad, showing prominent amyloid infiltration in a case of primary systemic amyloidosis. (Hematoxylin and eosin. × 400.)

loid which result in albuminuria. When this is severe, the complete nephrotic syndrome may result. Renal biopsy has shown infiltration of the kidneys to be more common than was previously suspected.[8]

Macroglossia is a prominent feature in one third of the cases of primary amyloidosis[12]; however, in the experience of one of us (MHS), it is noted more commonly in amyloidosis complicating myeloma. In combination with other findings, such as albuminuria, skin lesions, congestive heart failure and hepatomegaly, macroglossia certainly suggests primary amyloidosis.

The mucosa or the muscle of the gastrointestinal tract is found involved in more than 50 per cent of the cases of primary amyloidosis.[12] This may cause hemorrhage and, in advanced cases, can simulate gastric carcinoma. Chronic diarrhea may be noted, sometimes mimicking the nontropical sprue syndrome. Infiltration of the skin has led to a picture called "pseudoscleroderma" in some cases.

Neurologic features of primary amyloidosis were described by Kernohan and Woltman in 1941.[30] Chambers and associates reported 6 cases and reviewed the neurologic aspects.[10] The familial form of the disease, as described by Andrade[1] and Rukavina and co-workers,[38] has been especially noted to be associated with atypical neuritides and a much more benign course than other forms. Stauffer and associates have observed patients in whom postural hypotension was

a prominent symptom.[44] It apparently resulted from involvement of blood vessels, visceral nerves, or both.

AMYLOIDOSIS COMPLICATING MYELOMA

Although this form of amyloidosis might logically be considered secondary, ordinarily it is afforded a special place in the classification for two reasons: (1) it is a remarkably common complication of myeloma; (2) when there is a systemic distribution of amyloid in patients with myeloma, the deposition is greatest usually in the organs most involved in primary systemic amyloidosis. Apitz first strongly contended that a plasma cell dyscrasia was the etiologic basis of both diseases,[2] and Osserman emphasized this relationship.[34] More recently, Kyle and Bayrd stated that plasmacytic disease of some form may be present in many or most cases of so-called primary amyloidosis.[31] This theory is gaining favor. Every patient with a diagnosis of primary amyloidosis should have an aspiration of sternal marrow, since in several instances the authors have found myeloma, clinically unsuspected,[43, 44] to be present by this method of study. Many cases reported in the literature as primary amyloidosis undoubtedly would have been designated myeloma or plasmacytic disease if additional studies had been made. Careful scrutiny for myeloma should be made in patients with amyloid disease, in spite of some difference of opinion which may result, depending on the criteria for the diagnosis of myeloma.[31]

It has been estimated that 5 to 10 per cent of patients with disseminated myeloma harbor deposits of amyloid.[4] With or without a systemic distribution, these deposits may assume the local or tumefactive form. Such tumorous deposits of amyloid may appear in various organs, including bone, or within the myelomatous masses themselves. Severe involvement of the liver with production of signs and symptoms of hepatic disease is rare. We observed a case in which marked hepatomegaly due to amyloid was present for 1 year prior to signs establishing the diagnosis of multiple myeloma.[43]

Any significant degree of hepatomegaly associated with myeloma usually proves to be due to amyloid infiltration. Macroglossia is most commonly noted in amyloidosis complicating myeloma.

SECONDARY AMYLOIDOSIS

Formerly, this was the commonest form of the disease and occurred as a complication of chronic diseases, such as tuberculosis, bronchiectasis, osteomyelitis, syphilis, malignant tumors, lymphosarcoma and rheumatoid arthritis. In some series as high as 88 per cent of the cases of secondary amyloidosis have been associated with tuberculosis.[36] In recent years antibiotics, surgical treatment and control of infectious diseases have lowered the incidence of this type of amyloidosis. At the Mayo Clinic, in a recent 10-year period, secondary amyloidosis was the least common form.[44] Only 14 of the 63 cases of systemic amyloidosis were secondary; and among these, rheumatoid arthritis was the commonest primary disease.[43]

The liver is one of the organs most frequently involved. Hepatic infiltration, noted in 60 to 87 per cent of cases in various reported series,[12, 42] usually is seen in combination with involvement of the spleen, the kidneys and the adrenal glands—the organs most often attacked in secondary amyloidosis. Although involvement of the liver is frequent and may be severe, hepatic failure is most unusual, since the underlying disease is the cause of death in a majority of the cases, with a small percentage of patients dying in uremia. Hepatomegaly occurs in 60 to 75 per cent of cases of secondary amyloidosis, but jaundice and ascites of hepatic origin are rare.[42]

Pathologically, the liver in secondary amyloidosis is grossly indistinguishable from the liver in primary amyloidosis. It tends to be firm and large—Pearlman reported weights of more than 4,000 Gm. in 9 cases.[36] Microscopically, primary and secondary amyloidosis of the liver cannot be differentiated from each other with certainty. Parenchymal deposition in Disse's spaces is identical in both forms. The small vessels in the portal triads are affected in most cases of secondary amyloidosis and at times may be the only location of hepatic amyloid, but the involvement tends to be minimal compared with that of the primary form. Renal infiltration is the most consistent feature of secondary amyloidosis.

Clinical manifestations of secondary amyloidosis are not so variable as in the primary form and most commonly are related to renal dysfunction with marked albuminuria. In advanced cases hepatomegaly, splenomegaly and edema or the full nephrotic syndrome are present. Because of a combination of hepatic and renal diseases, it is usually not possible to determine the cause of the reduced serum albumin leading to edema. Addison's disease resulting from destruction of the adrenal glands is rare.

The reversibility of secondary amyloidosis,[47, 50] in some instances after treatment of the primary disease, is its most unique feature. Involvement of mesodermal structures, such as blood vessels and the heart, is absent or minimal so that cardiac insufficiency does not constitute a threat in secondary amyloidosis.

LABORATORY FEATURES

In primary and secondary amyloidosis and in the amyloidosis complicating myeloma, laboratory findings are similar but nonspecific. Hepatic dysfunction is shown best by use of the Bromsulphalein excretion test, but the degree of dye retention varies. In 4 cases reported by Stauffer and associates the Bromsulphalein test was normal despite amyloid infiltration of the liver proved by needle biopsy.[44] Jaundice is rare, but small amounts of direct-reacting serum bilirubin may be found.[44] Although reduced serum albumin[45] has been called the most common laboratory abnormality, it is not a constant feature, and the values for serum proteins may be extremely variable. Ordinarily, serum globulin is not increased and, even in amyloidosis associated with myeloma, hyperglobulinemia is not a common feature.

Block and associates, in 1955, reported an unusual peak in the alpha-2-globulin area on electrophoresis of serum of patients con-

sidered to have familial primary amyloidosis.[6] Subsequently, this was also found in
unaffected members of a family of a patient with the disease.[7] In patients with
familial amyloidosis, no abnormalities have
been elicited by the starch gel technic of
Smithies,[41] by immuno-electrophoresis, or
by paper electrophoretic analysis for lipoproteins and glycoproteins.[25] In 1959
Calkins and Cohen found the serum hexosamine levels elevated in nonhereditary primary amyloidosis but not in the familial
variety.[9] This would substantiate the views
of Kaufman and Thomas (1959), suggesting
that the hereditary disease differs from the
cases of sporadic primary amyloidosis.[29]

Results of the thymol turbidity and
cephalin-cholesterol flocculation tests usually are normal. An increase in the serum
alkaline phosphatase is frequently noted.
Stauffer and associates observed an elevated
cholesterol in 3 patients.[44] In 1 of these the
serum was grossly fatty, and the total serum
lipid value was 3,360 mg./100 ml.[44] In amyloidosis associated with myeloma, the latter
diagnosis is established in the usual manner, on the basis of such findings as Bence
Jones proteinuria and characteristic sternal
marrow.

DIAGNOSIS

Congo Red Test

Other than the staining of sections of tissue, the Congo red test is the only method
of diagnosis based on the affinity that certain types of amyloid have for a dye. In the
Congo red test, as originated by Bennhold,[5]
the amount of Congo red in the blood 1
hour after its intravenous injection is compared with a standard based on the amount
present 4 minutes after injection. The dose
used is 3 mg./kg. of body weight. Although
originally removal of 60 per cent of the
dye in 1 hour was considered to be diagnostic of amyloidosis, later reports showed that
90 to 100 per cent removal offered a much
more accurate basis for diagnosis. Paunz
suggested a simpler method which avoided
use of the standard: After injecting a
smaller dose (1.2 mg./kg. body weight),

he read the result as positive if 100 per
cent was removed at the end of 1 hour, or
negative if any dye was found in the
blood.[35] In our experience with the Paunz
technic, no false positives have been noted.
A positive result with the Paunz test or 90
per cent removal of the dye with the
quantitative Congo red test is nearly always
indicative of amyloidosis.

One of the most important observations
is that the test often gives a negative result
in primary systemic amyloidosis because in
this form of the disease the amyloid has
little affinity for Congo red.[15] For instance,
a negative Paunz test was found in 5 cases,
although tissue obtained from the liver by
needle biopsy revealed amyloid.[44] In patients with skin lesions, this test should not
be used, because it can result in a permanent red discoloration of the cutaneous
areas. Dermatologists have used a local injection to prove the affinity for Congo red
in these cases.[15] The radioactive iodine uptake tests has been used since amyloid has
some affinity for iodine, but results have
proved to be too erratic for the test to be
of value.

Biopsy

Since amyloid infiltrates many of the organs and tissues of the body, tissue biopsy
has long been used to verify the diagnosis.
Josefson in 1916 employed needle biopsy
of the spleen,[27] and Waldenström in 1928
first used needle biopsy of the liver to diagnose amyloidosis.[50] Since secondary amyloidosis involves the liver diffusely and is
present in two thirds of cases, needle biopsy
of the liver is currently used. Sherlock,[40]
Volwiler and Jones,[49] Topp and co-workers,[46] Iversen and Roholm,[24] Stauffer and
associates[44] and Wold[51] are among those
reporting positive diagnoses from needle
biopsy of this organ. The diagnosis also can
be made by this method in some cases of
primary systemic amyloidosis and of amyloidosis associated with myeloma when the
Congo red test is negative.[43, 44]

One death has been reported from hemorrhage subsequent to needle biopsy of the
liver in amyloidosis.[49] However, Stauffer
and associates[44] have reported 18 cases in

which the diagnosis was made by needle biopsy of the liver, with only one minor hemorrhage.

We believe that needle biopsy of the liver has proved to be one of the important methods for diagnosis of primary amyloidosis.[44] In cases in which cardiac involvement is associated with an elevated venous pressure, attempts should be made to lower the pressure by the use of digitalis and diuretics prior to hepatic biopsy. Frequently, the diagnosis has been made by biopsy of the liver at laparotomy. The pathologist may miss extensive deposits in sections of an aspirated specimen unless he is alerted to the possibility of its presence.[10, 15] The material is closely adherent to the cords of hepatic cells and may be difficult to recognize unless special stains are used. The most helpful are methyl violet and methyl green, in our experience. As indicated previously, some workers believe that viewing in the polarizing microscope of sections properly stained with Congo red or observing the fluorescence produced by thioflavine T provides useful diagnostic adjuncts.

Selikoff and Robitzek have found that gingival biopsy gives positive results in proved cases of secondary amyloidosis.[39] When macroglossia is present, biopsy of the tongue is useful. Skin, striated muscle, mucous membranes and lymph nodes are all reported as sites of positive biopsy specimens in primary amyloidosis.

Needle biopsy of the kidneys has been used to establish the diagnosis of amyloidosis.[8] Renal biopsy may be positive when other methods of diagnosis have failed. Frequently, a positive diagnosis is obtained from the kidney in amyloidosis with myeloma.

A new and safe method of obtaining tissue is biopsy of the small intestine with the Crosby capsule. Six cases of primary amyloidosis diagnosed in this manner were reported by Green and associates.[21] Gafni and Sohar reported cases of amyloidosis diagnosed by biopsy of the rectal mucosa.[19] Many of their patients were considered to have secondary amyloidosis associated with familial Mediterranean fever.[23] Tissue removed for biopsy provided diagnostic deposits of amyloid in the rectal submucosa or mucosa in 17 of 20 patients with primary systemic amyloidosis studied at our institution.[32]

PROGNOSIS AND TREATMENT

Numerous substances, including cortisone, have been used to treat primary amyloidosis and that associated with myeloma, but thus far all have been fruitless. In our experience systemic amyloidosis is fatal within a year, although some patients reportedly have lived longer. Patients with the more recently described familial type of amyloidosis with vitreous opacities[29] and peripheral neuritis[1, 7] may live as long as 10 years. In amyloidosis associated with myeloma the underlying disease ordinarily governs the patient's progress, but occasionally patients die of the complicating amyloidosis even before the myeloma becomes clinically evident.

In secondary amyloidosis the outlook is variable. In several cases, amyloidosis has reportedly regressed or disappeared after successful treatment of the associated disease. In 1928 Waldenström showed by aspiration biopsy that amyloid had disappeared completely from the liver in 3 patients after surgical treatment of tuberculous lesions.[50] A few spontaneous "cures" have been reported. Stauffer and associates mentioned that 1 patient was still living 10 years after amyloid was found in the liver by needle biopsy.[44] Amyloidosis should not be considered a contraindication to treatment of the primary disease, whether by surgical or other means.

REFERENCES

1. Andrade, C.: A peculiar form of peripheral neuropathy: familial atypical generalized amyloidosis with special involvement of peripheral nerves, Brain 75:408, 1952.
2. Apitz, K.: Die paraproteinosen (über die Störung des Eiweisstoffwechsels bei Plasmocytom), Virchows Arch. path. Anat. 306:631, 1940.
3. Bailey, C. H.: The production of amyloid disease and chronic nephritis in rabbits

by repeated intravenous injections of living colon bacilli, J. Exp. Med. 23:773, 1916.

4. Bayrd, E. D., and Bennett, W. A.: Amyloidosis complicating myeloma, Med. Clin. N. Amer. 34:1151, 1950.

5. Bennhold, H.: Über die Ausscheidung intravenös einverleibten Kongorotes bei den verschiedensten Erkrankungen insbesondere bei Amyloidosis, Dtsch. Arch. klin. Med. 142:32, 1923.

6. Block, W. D., Rukavina, J. G., and Curtis, A. C.: An atypical electrophoretic peak in serum of patients with familial primary systemic amyloidosis (21748), Proc. Soc. Exp. Biol. Med. 89:175, 1955.

7. ———: Serum electrophoretic studies on patients with familial primary systemic amyloidosis, J. Lab. Clin. Med. 47:357, 1956.

8. Broadbent, J. G., and Daugherty, G. W.: Personal communication.

9. Calkins, E., and Cohen, A. S.: Similarity of serum protein changes in primary and secondary amyloidosis, J. Clin. Invest. 38:993, 1959.

10. Chambers, R. A., Medd, W. E., and Spencer, H.: Primary amyloidosis: with special reference to involvement of the nervous system, Quart. J. Med. 27:207, 1958.

11. Cohen, A. S.: Amyloidosis, New Engl. J. Med. 277:522; 574; 628, 1967.

12. Dahlin, D. C.: Primary amyloidosis: with report of six cases, Am. J. Path. 25:105, 1949.

13. ———: Secondary amyloidosis, Ann. Int. Med. 31:105, 1949.

14. ———: Amyloidosis, Proc. Mayo Clin. 24:637, 1949.

15. Dahlin, D. C., Stauffer, M. H., and Mann, F. D.: Laboratory and biopsy diagnosis of amyloidosis, Med. Clin. N. Amer. 34:1171, 1950.

16. Dick, G. F., and Leiter, L.: Experimental amyloidosis and hyperglobulinemia, Trans. Ass. Am. Phycns. 52:246, 1937.

17. Eklund, C. M., and Reimann, H. A.: The etiology of amyloid disease: with a note on experimental renal amyloidosis, Arch. Path. 21:1 (Jan.) 1936.

18. Findley, J. W., Jr., and Adams, W.: Primary systemic amyloidosis simulating constrictive pericarditis: with steatorrhea and hyperesthesia, Arch. Int. Med. 81:342, 1948.

19. Gafni, J., and Sohar, E.: Rectal biopsy for the diagnosis of amyloidosis, Am. J. Med. Sci. 240:332, 1960.

20. Graham, W.: Primary amyloidosis simulating cirrhosis of liver, Canad. med. Ass. J. 66:58, 1952.

21. Green, P. A., Higgins, J. A., Brown, A. L., Jr., Hoffman, H. N., II, and Sommerville, R. L.: Amyloidosis: appraisal of intubation biopsy of the small intestine in diagnosis, Gastroenterology 41:452, 1961.

22. Hass, G. M., Huntington, R., and Krumdieck, N.: Amyloid. III. The properties of amyloid deposits occurring in several species under diverse conditions, Arch. Path. 35:226, 1943.

23. Heller, H., Sohar, E., and Scherf, L.: Familial Mediterranean fever, A.M.A. Arch. Int. Med. 102:50, 1958.

24 Iversen, P., and Roholm, K.: On aspiration biopsy of the liver, with remarks on its diagnostic significance, Acta med. scand. 102:1, 1939.

25. Jackson, C. E., Block, W. D., and Ratliff, W. C.: Serum hexosamine content and urinary acid mucopolysaccharide excretion in hereditary primary amyloidosis, J. Lab. Clin. Med. 56:544, 1960.

26. Jackson, C. E., Falls, H. F., Block, W. D., Rukavina, J. K., and Carey, J. H.: Inheritance of primary systemic amyloidosis, Am. J. Hum. Genet. 12:434, 1960.

27. Josefson, A.: Quoted by Waldenström.[50]

28. Kapp, J. P.: Hepatic amyloidosis with portal hypertension, J.A.M.A. 191:497, 1965.

29. Kaufman, H. E., and Thomas, L. B.: Vitreous opacities diagnostic of familial primary amyloidosis, New Engl. J. Med. 261:1267, 1959.

30. Kernohan, J. W., and Woltman, H. W.: Amyloid neuritis, Trans Am. Neurol. Ass. 67:236, 1941.

31. Kyle, R. A., and Bayrd, E. D.: "Primary" systemic amyloidosis and myeloma: discussion of relationship and review of 81 cases, Arch. Int. Med. 107:344, 1961.

32. Kyle, R. A., Spencer, R. J., and Dahlin, D. C.: Value of rectal biopsy in the diagnosis of primary systemic amyloidosis, Am. J. Med. Sci. 251:501, 1966.

33. Lubarsch, O.: Zur Kenntnis ungewöhnlicher Amyloidablagerungen, Virchows Arch. path. Anat. 271:867, 1929.

34. Osserman, E. F.: Plasma-cell myeloma. II. Clinical aspects (concluded), New Engl. J. Med. 261:1006, 1959.

35. Paunz: Quoted by Németh, L.: Über den klinischen Wert des Nachweises der Amy-

loidose durch die Kongorotprobe, Klin. Wschr. 5:1040, 1926.

36. Pearlman, A. W.: Amyloidosis: a clinical and pathological study of 135 cases, Quart. Bull. Sea View Hosp. 6:295, 1941.

37. Reimann, H. A., Koucky, R. F., and Eklund, C. M.: Primary amyloidosis limited to tissue of mesodermal origin, Am. J. Path. 11:977, 1935.

38. Rukavina, J. G., Block, W. D., Jackson, C. E., Falls, H. F., Carey, J. H., and Curtis, A. C.: Primary systemic amyloidosis: a review and an experimental, genetic and clinical study of 29 cases with particular emphasis on the familial form, Medicine 35:239,1956.

39. Selikoff, I. J., and Robitzek, E. H.: Gingival biopsy for the diagnosis of generalized amyloidosis, Am. J. Path. 23:1099, 1947.

40. Sherlock, S.: Aspiration liver biopsy: technique and diagnostic application, Lancet 2:397, 1945.

41. Smithies, O.: Zone electrophoresis in starch gels: group variations in the serum proteins of normal human adults, Biochem. J. 61:629, 1955.

42. Stauffer, M. H.: Hepatic manifestations in secondary amyloidosis, Med. Clin. N. Amer. 34:1165, 1950.

43. Stauffer, M. H., and Dahlin, D. C.: Unpublished data.

44. Stauffer, M. H., Gross, J. B., Foulk, W. T., and Dahlin, D. C.: Amyloidosis: diagnosis with needle biopsy of the liver in eighteen patients, Gastroenterology 41:92, 1961.

45. Tiber, A. M., Pearlman, A. W., and Cohen, S. E.: Hepatic function in patients with amyloidosis, Arch. Int. Med. 68:309, 1941.

46. Topp, J. H., Lindert, M. C. F., and Murphy, F. D.: Needle biopsy of the liver, Arch. Int. Med. 81:832, 1948.

47. Trasoff, A., Schneeberg, N., and Scarf, M.: Recovery from multiple rheumatoid arthritis complicated by amyloidosis in a child: report of a case and review of the literature, Arch. Int. Med. 74:4, 1944.

48. Vassar, P. S., and Culling, C. F. A.: Fluorescent stains, with special reference to amyloid and connective tissues, Arch. Path. 68:487, 1959.

49. Volwiler, W., and Jones, C. M.: The diagnostic and therapeutic value of liver biopsies: with particular reference to trocar biopsy, New Engl. J. Med. 237:651, 1947.

50. Waldenström, H.: On the formation and disappearance of amyloid in man, Acta chir. scand. 63:479, 1928.

51. Wold, L. E.: Amyloid disease with two case reports, J. Lancet 72:8, 1952.

52. Wollaeger, E. E.: Primary systemic amyloidosis with symptoms and signs of liver disease; diagnosis by liver biopsy: report of a case, Med. Clin. N. Amer. 34:1113, 1950.

53. Zetzel, L.: Hepatomegaly with jaundice due to primary amyloidosis, Gastroenterology 8:783, 1947.

28

Roentgen Aspects of
Liver and Biliary Tract Diseases

DAVID G. BRAGG, M.D., AND *JOHN A. EVANS*, M.D.

Few other organ systems within the body provide the radiologist with as great a scope in evaluation of function as does the liver and biliary tree. Much of the progress in this regard has been forthcoming within the past 15 years. The advent of oral and intravenous cholangiography has provided an excellent means of evaluating the integrity of the biliary tree in the nonjaundiced patient. More recently, the addition of hepatic angiography and radioisotopes has afforded other avenues through which to assess the hepatic region. Future advances will almost certainly match the progress within recent years, particularly with regard to the liver's neighbor, the pancreas.

The methods for evaluating the biliary tree which are covered in this chapter include plain film examination, barium studies, physiologic cholangiography, instrumentive cholangiography and radionuclide hepatography. The angiographic approach is covered in Chapter 10. Little emphasis is placed on technics of examination, since these can be gained from references cited in the bibliography.

PLAIN FILM EVALUATION OF THE LIVER AND BILIARY TREE

Reports began to appear in the medical literature soon after the roentgen beam was applied to medical uses. The first preoperative demonstration of an opaque biliary calculus was recorded prior to the turn of the century. Technical improvements in radiographic equipment provided additional in-

formation, for exposure times could be shortened and kilovoltage increased. Subsequently, contributions were rapidly added describing the significant role of x-ray evaluation of the liver.

The *normal liver silhouette* has been the subject of numerous investigations with varied conclusions.[40] It is generally agreed that plain film evaluation of hepatic size is often inaccurate and therefore of limited clinical usefulness. Splenic size is usually accurately assessed. Its lower margin is almost always visible and its enlargement causes downward displacement of the adjacent splenic flexure of the colon with medial displacement of the air-filled gastric fundus.

The many variations in the shape of the liver preclude much significance being attached to abnormalities in contour of the hepatic silhouette. With more recent radiopharmaceutical evaluation, both hepatic size and shape are more accurately estimated.[52]

Diffuse increase in the overall density of the hepatic silhouette is produced by Thorotrast and hemochromatosis. The increase in density associated with Thorotrast is more striking radiographically, presenting a granular appearance rather than a uniform homogeneous increase in density. The liver in hemochromatosis more often presents a diffuse increase in density, occasionally recognized as it contrasts against the diaphragmatic border on the chest x-ray (Sosman's line).

Hepatic calcifications. These may be classified as to their inflammatory, neoplastic

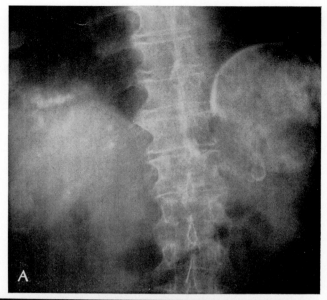

FIG. 28–1. Hydatid cysts of the liver and spleen antemortem (A) and in the postmortem specimen (B).

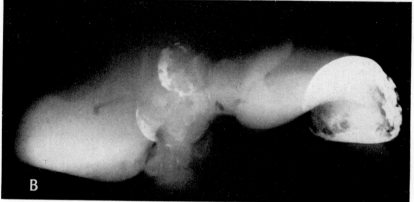

or non-neoplastic origin. Non-neoplastic varieties are related to abnormalities of the biliary tree and are discussed subsequently.

Inflammatory lesions within the liver seldom calcify. These include: (1) Hydatid cyst. These striking, densely calcified, oval masses are usually plainly visible with heavily calcified rims and amorphous calcareous interiors. (2) Granulomatous lesions. Abdominal tuberculosis and histoplasmosis are occasionally manifest by oval calcific densities, more commonly recognized in the splenic area. (3) Syphilis. A few scattered case reports disclose a nonspecific appearance of calcific densities related to proved syphilitic gummas.[19] (4)

Hepatic abscesses. Rare sequelae of intrahepatic abscesses present themselves as calcific densities, reportedly nonspecific in character (Fig. 28–1 A and B).

Vascular calcifications are uncommonly observed in the liver. Occasional calcification within an hepatic artery aneurysm can be recognized. A more characteristic appearance is described in association with portal vein thrombosis and subsequent calcification. Since this condition is usually associated with significant portal hypertension, the splenic contour is inevitably enlarged in combination with these portal vein calcifications.[19]

Neoplastic hepatic calcifications provide

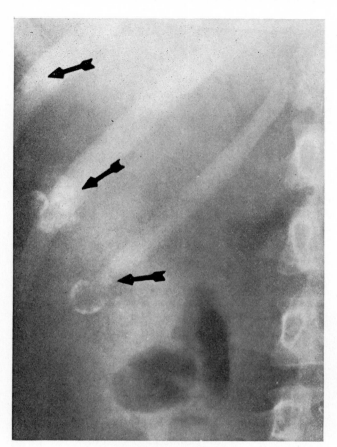

FIG. 28–2. Calcified ovarian metastases. These are somewhat more dense than the usual ovarian lesions which tend to be "cloud-like" and indistinct.

a unique opportunity in roentgen differential diagnosis. Both primary and metastatic lesions calcify and thus can be detected. Of the primary hepatic tumors that may calcify, the cavernous hemangioma represents one of the benign counterparts. These tumors show spicules of calcification which tend to radiate out from a central core.[41] Hamartomas of the liver occur in young females and present with curvilinear calcific densities surrounding the margins of these cystic lesions. Primary malignant hepatic tumors calcify infrequently, which suggests this diagnosis on occasion in a patient with known underlying cirrhosis.

Metastatic hepatic lesions that calcify include the mucin-producing adenocarcinomas and neuroblastoma. The more commonly observed calcified carcinomas with spread to the liver originate from the ovary and the left colon. The ovarian metastases provide a characteristic "cloud-like" density

which is often overlooked. The calcified gastrointestinal metastases appear denser and are more easily visualized, for no shadows obscure them in this area.[33] Metastatic hepatic implants of a neuroblastoma occasionally show stippled calcific densities as well as calcification of the primary tumor which is superimposed on the hepatic silhouette when arising in the right suprarenal area.[42] It is variously quoted that nearly half of the abdominal neuroblastomas reveal calcifications (Figs. 28–2 and 28–3).

Air as Contrast Medium. Air is an excellent contrast medium with which to detect many abnormalities within the liver and its adjacent bed. Air within the biliary tree can easily be appreciated radiographically, conforming to the distribution of this branching duct system. The gas is usually apparent centrally near the region of the porta hepatis and fades gradually as the finer ramifications of the biliary tree are

FIG. 28–3. Calcified mucin-producing carcinoma from the sigmoid colon. The visible lesion (*arrow*) resembles closely in appearance the calcified ovarian lesions (FIG. 28–2).

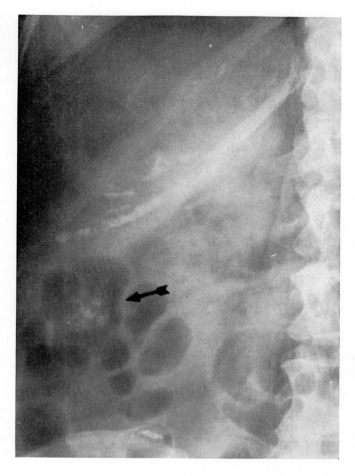

reached. Air within the portal venous system, on the other hand, can be confused with this appearance. This latter situation presents in an entirely different fashion, with the gas outlining tubular structures along the periphery of the liver, disappearing at the midportion of the liver. Differentiation of these two entities is of obvious importance as their prognostic implications differ so widely. Air within the biliary tree is seen following recent passage of a stone, in fistula formation subsequent to perforation of a peptic ulcer or passage of a stone, and postoperatively. Air in the biliary tree is seen inconstantly subsequent to diverting surgical procedures and its absence is not evidence of obstruction (Figs. 28–4 and 28–5). Portal vein gas is a grave prognostic sign seen subsequent to bowel infarction and necrosis or a childhood enterocolitis.

Emphysematous cholecystitis is an unusual radiographic entity. Gas outlines the walls and lumen of the gallbladder, occasionally extending well into the cystic duct, providing its characteristic roentgen appearance[4] (Fig. 28–6). This is caused by gas forming organisms.

Both subphrenic and intrahepatic abscess collections may have associated pockets of gas which provide air fluid levels visible with a horizontal x-ray beam. Subphrenic collections are obviously much more common. In the radiographic evaluation of a suspected subphrenic abscess, fluoroscopy for diaphragmatic motion is occasionally helpful. Diaphragmatic motion may, however, be normal with a well-documented subphrenic abscess. X-ray films should be obtained in the erect or decubitus projections to evaluate both the adjacent lung volume for small pleural effusions and dis-

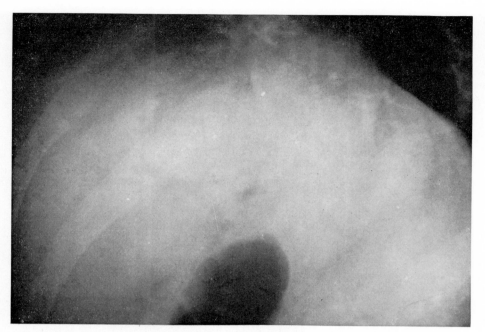

Fig. 28–4. Air in the biliary tree. Note the central collection in the common duct and proximal radicles as opposed to the peripheral location with portal vein gas (Fig. 28–5).

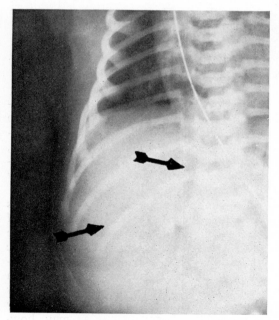

Fig. 28–5. Air in the portal and hepatic venous system. In this child the peripheral location (*arrow*) is not as striking, whereas the gas in the larger veins are (*arrow*).

coid zones of atelectasis, as well as fluid levels beneath the diaphragm. Probably the most helpful single study, however, is combined lung and liver scanning, with a subphrenic collection widening the interval between them. Pneumoperitoneography is effective in the evaluation of subphrenic lesions. Unfortunately, the patient with a suspected abscess is often too ill to tolerate this study. It usually is relatively simple to differentiate intrahepatic from subphrenic collections with CO_2 in the abdomen (approximately 500 cc. injected in the mid-abdomen below the umbilicus, utilizing erect films in at least two planes). With a subdiaphragmatic abscess, adhesions and inflammatory by-products prevent the gas from dissecting between the liver and diaphragm. Intrahepatic abscess cavities, even those in close proximity to the surface, tend not to evoke significant extrahepatic changes which might obliterate the subphrenic space. The need to differentiate these two entities is not infrequent due to the predilection of amebic abscess cavities for the right hepatic lobe, often in a peripheral location.[10]

FIG. 28–6. Emphysematous cholecystitis. Note the air within both
the lumen and the wall of the
gallbladder.

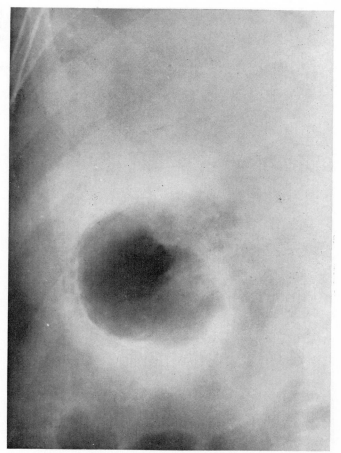

The abdomen that is filled with *ascitic fluid* has a "ground glass" radiographic appearance; the air-filled small intestinal loops float centrally. The air-filled colonic loops often appear "squared off" as they frame the abdomen. Fluid collecting in the lateral gutters widens the distance between the lateral colonic walls and the properitoneal fat. With large collections of ascitic fluid the retroperitoneal landmarks are usually camouflaged. The ability to detect small amounts of fluid is often helpful. In a supine film of the abdomen, the true pelvis collects the available dependent fluid. This can be recognized as it dissects between the air-filled intestinal loops.[15] With larger ascitic collections, the right abdominal gutter directs the fluid to the inferior and lateral

hepatic angle, silhouetting this usually clearly visible landmark.[25]

Biliary calculi may be detected radiographically by either their calcium or gas content. Approximately 15 per cent of these stones contain sufficient calcium to be seen on plain films. Calcific densities often confused in differential diagnosis include: renal calculi, costal cartilage calcification, mesenteric lymph node calcification, enteroliths and cutaneous and intrahepatic calcifications (previously described). The simple expedient of a right posterior oblique film eliminates most of these differential considerations. The more anterior location of biliary densities and their propensity to move with the hepatic flexure of the colon indicate the true nature of these calcifica-

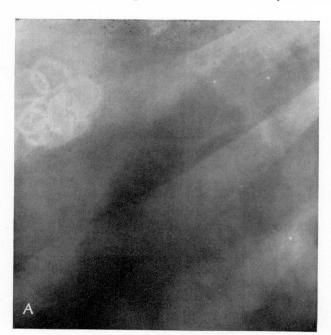

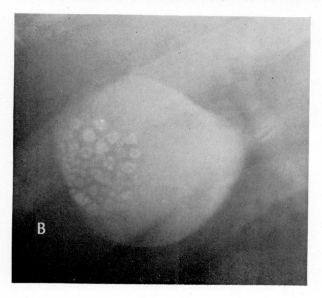

FIG. 28–7. A, B, C. Mixed stones. Examples of opaque mixed stones of varying numbers and shapes.

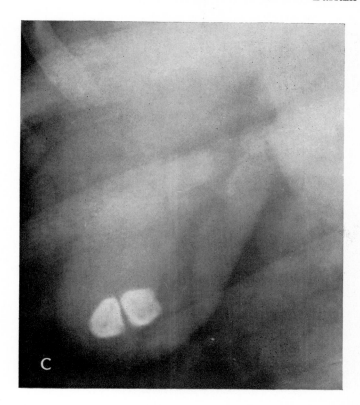

tions. Rare biliary stones are recognized by the stellate collection of gas in the center of a nonopaque stone leading to many descriptive titles such as the "star" or "Benz" signs.[32]

The four types of biliary calculi as seen radiographically are the pigment, cholesterol, calcium carbonate and mixed or composite stones. Of these, the most common is the mixed stone, which contains all three ingredients. These calculi present with the characteristic appearances of biliary stones: polyhedral, multifaceted and laminated. Pigment stones are small, multiple and radiolucent, whereas the pure cholesterol stone usually appears solo, is large and cannot be visualized on the plain film. The calcium carbonate stone is least common; it is radiopaque and said to accompany low grade obstructive biliary disease[47] (Figs. 28–7 and 28–8).

Milk of calcium, or "limewater" bile, is an unusual radiologic hallmark of cystic duct obstruction. Pathologically the material is semi-fluid with a sandy texture and is composed almost entirely of calcium carbonate.[36] Films must utilize a horizontal beam to recognize the radiopaque fluid level in the right upper abdomen with this entity.

Calcification of the gallbladder wall, the so-called "porcelain gallbladder," infrequently occurs as a response to long-standing cholecystitis with obstruction of the cystic duct as a constantly associated feature. The calcification may occur within the muscular coat or within the mucosa in the glandular spaces and Rokitansky-Aschoff sinuses.[38] The rim-like calcific margins and amorphous calcareous interior of the porcelain gallbladder may be mistaken for a large calculus (which should show evidence of lamination or faceting) as well as for other previously mentioned hepatic calcific masses such as hydatid cysts (Fig. 28–9).

BARIUM STUDIES

The esophagram has unquestionable value in the search for varices. The accuracy of this method varies with the technics uti-

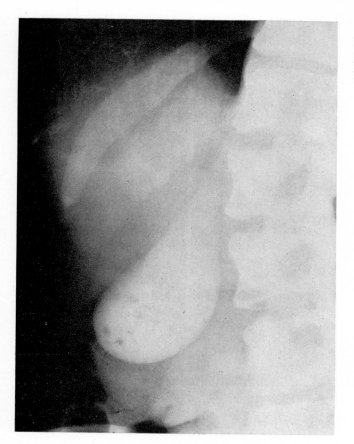

FIG. 28–8. Bile pigment stones on an oral cholecystogram, with a laminated stone near the neck of the gallbladder found at surgery to be in the pancreas.

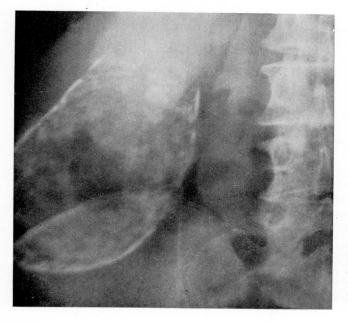

FIG. 28–9. Porcelain gallbladder. Note the densely calcified margins and amorphous calcareous interiors. The calcific pattern resembles that seen with hydatid cysts (see Fig. 28–1A, B) but the contour and position reveals its true origin.

FIG. 28–10. Esophageal and gastric fundal varices in a young male with a hepatoma and multiple pulmonary metastases. Splenomegaly is an almost constant companion with radiographically demonstrable varices as in this patient.

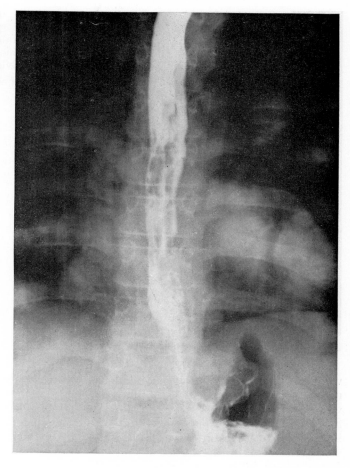

lized. Success depends on obtaining multiple spot films of the collapsed and resting esophagus during quiet breathing. Fluoroscopically, large varices not uncommonly completely disappear during esophageal contraction and distension. The frequent association of gastric varices is often overlooked, for they usually resemble large gastric rugae (Fig. 28–10).

The impression of an enlarged common bile duct is occasionally recognized as it causes an indentation against the junction of the first and second duodenum. The gallbladder also is adjacent to this area and may deform the duodenum in a similar location.

The impressions of periampullary masses upon the medial portion of the descending duodenum are well known. The "Frostberg" or inverted 3 sign indicates that a mass has encroached into the duodenal lumen, whether it be inflammatory or neoplastic in character.[16] The double contour of the medial wall of the second portion of the duodenum together with the smoothing out of mucosal folds locally are more frequently encountered radiographic signs of pancreatic mass lesions. Widening of the duodenal loop is a late manifestation of enlargement of the pancreatic head, as is the impression upon the greater curvature of the gastric antrum ("pad sign").

PHYSIOLOGIC CHOLANGIOGRAPHY

With the report in 1924 of an injectable radiopaque media excreted by the biliary system, Graham and Cole brought a new perspective to hepatic radiography.[18] The phthalein compounds which they utilized

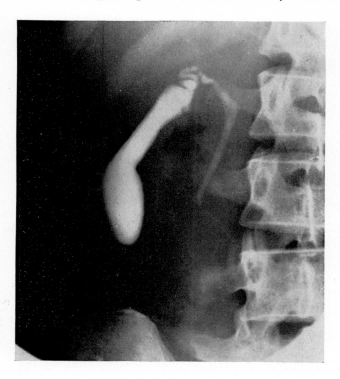

FIG. 28–11. Normal oral cholecystogram 10 minutes following the fatty meal. Note the excellent opacification of the cystic and common bile ducts.

were poorly tolerated, however, and not until 1940, when Priodax was introduced, was nonoperative cholecystography made feasible. Priodax provided excellent visualization of the gallbladder but little information concerning the duct system. Some 10 years later, iopanoic acid was added and is still the most widely used cholecystographic agent. Several reports recently have commented upon the nephrotoxic effects of these agents.[5, 48] As a result, bunamiodyl sodium was withdrawn from the market and dose schedules of iopanoic acid were realistically lowered. We no longer recommend a "double dose study." With newer oral cholecystographic compounds, the gallbladder and biliary tree can be opacified more rapidly.

Successful *intravenous cholangiography* was made feasible through the introduction of sodium iodipamide in 1953. Reports the following year endorsed the application of this agent.[17] The presently used contrast material, iodipamide methylglucamine, replaced the sodium salt as it was found to be better tolerated.

These agents are all substituted triiodo-

benzoic acid derivatives. It is felt that such compounds with incompletely substituted rings bind to serum albumin, are filtered by the liver and excreted into the bile. The unbound fraction is then rapidly removed by glomerular filtration.[29] Normally, approximately 90 per cent of iodipamide methylglucamine is excreted into the bile and 10 per cent is found in the urine. Virtually none is reabsorbed from the intestinal tract once excreted in the bile. Once within the liver, iopanoic acid combines to form a glucuronide ester, whereas iodipamide methylglucamine is extracted intact and excreted.[28] The relative toxicity of these agents therefore depends to a degree on the integrity of the hepatobiliary system. In severe liver disease or biliary obstruction, the risk of nephrotoxicity greatly increases.[14]

Success of *oral cholangiography* is directly related to the care by which the examination is executed. Carefully coned-down views with both horizontal and vertical x-ray beams of low kilovoltage and high milliamperage are essential. Not infrequently, special views are necessary to avoid competing shadows usually origi-

FIG. 28–12. Effect of the "repeat dose" oral cholecystogram. The faintly visualized gallbladder (A) is converted to a diagnostic study (B) in this case, following a second dose.

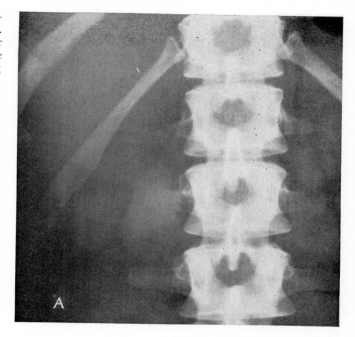

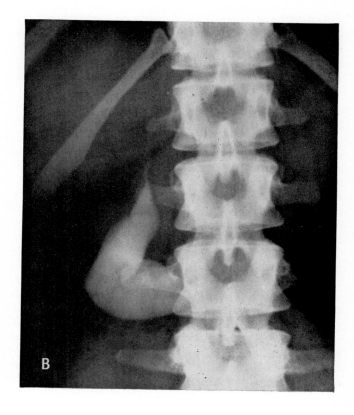

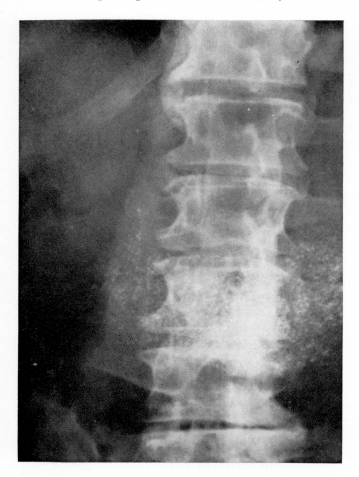

FIG. 28–13. Gastric outlet obstruction (pre-pyloric ulcer) shown following an oral cholecystogram. The retention of the fragmented but unabsorbed iopanoic acid should suggest gastric obstruction. The gallbladder of course cannot be visualized in these situations because the contrast cannot be absorbed from the stomach.

nating from the bowel. The challenge of a fatty stimulus is essential both to shrink the target organ and to better enable one to see certain abnormalities such as adenomyomas and Rokitansky-Aschoff sinuses. By this maneuver the distal duct system can also be visualized in a significant percentage of cases. Examinations of this quality have a diagnostic accuracy of 98 percent[1] (Fig. 28–11).

In our hands, a repeat dose study has been useful when faint visualization resulted from a single dose. In these instances, the patient should be instructed to remain on a fat-free diet while awaiting the repeat dose study. If nonvisualization results from the initial dose, it is unusual to obtain a diagnostic study from an additional dose. Nonvisualization resulting from a single dose is said to be associated with a 95 per cent incidence of gallbladder disease which will not be better opacified with a repeat dose[50] (Fig. 28–12).

The causes of nonvisualization are varied and can be grouped into hepatic and extrahepatic categories. Assuming good patient cooperation, various functional and anatomic explanations become obvious. Gastric outlet obstruction is one of the most significant abnormalities which can be suspected during the course of an oral cholecystogram. The opaque but unabsorbed particles of the contrast agent are clearly confined in the gastric antrum where they cannot be absorbed. Subsequent gastrointestinal evaluation almost invariably reveals a significant gastric outlet obstruction in these instances (Fig. 28–13).

The intrahepatic causes of nonvisualization in the nonjaundiced patient almost exclusively relate to gallbladder disease and cystic duct obstruction. Recently the concept that a diseased or obstructed gallbladder cannot concentrate the contrast material and thus become radiopaque has been challenged. Berk and Lasser have demonstrated in an experimental model that the gallbladder reabsorbs conjugated iopanoic acid if it is inflamed but not if it is normal.[3] This provides an interesting theory to explain radiographic nonvisualization in cholecystitis.

The various *filling defects* apparent in the gallbladder during cholecystography can be subdivided into fixed and movable lesions. The previously described calculi form the movable group. The necessity to demonstrate this feature is one reason why both horizontal and vertical x-ray beam studies are essential. Evaluation of these films will show that the filling defect is mobile, and that, not infrequently, the stones of similar density "layer out" within the contrast-bile mixture (Fig. 28–14).

The fixed filling defects form a complex and confused radiographic differential list. Discrepancies in classification began with the original description of a "papilloma" of the gallbladder in 1931.[26] A complete radiologic-pathologic description of these lesions was published by Ochsner in 1966.[37] The radiologic diagnosis of a polypoid filling defect of course depends upon its unchanging location and appearance on multiple films in varying positions. Solitary lesions are far more common and usually represent cholesterol polyps.

Jutras recently clarified the radiographic appearance of *adenomyomatosis*.[23, 24] He has shown that this interesting entity presents 3 patterns: (1) localized (a single indentation usually at the gallbladder fundus often with a central fleck of contrast and surrounded by small outpouchings or diverticuli filled with contrast) (Fig. 28–15), (2) segmental (narrowing usually near the neck of the gallbladder with small surrounding outpouchings of contrast)

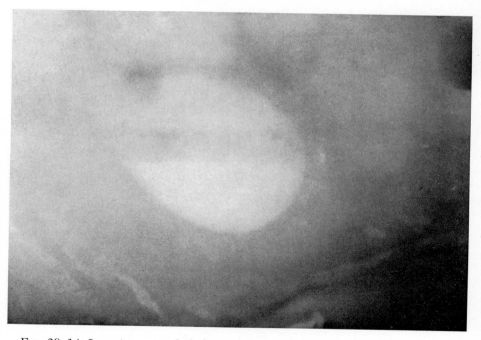

Fig. 28–14. Layering on oral cholecystogram. Note the band of decreased density which represents small calculi. This case was selected because the morphology of the individual stones is not apparent but the diagnosis becomes obvious with knowledge of the layering phenomenon. On intravenous studies, layering is physiologic and of no significance.

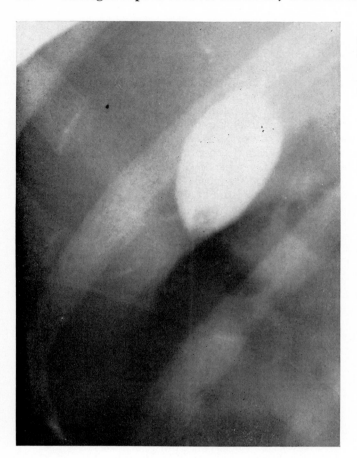

FIG. 28–15. Localized adeno-myoma. Note the radiolucent defect in the gallbladder fundus. The associated findings of contrast-filled diverticuli are not evident.

(Fig. 28–16), or (3) generalized (resembling the segmental form but scattered over the entire surface of the gallbladder). If these lesions are present, the gallbladder is densely opacified with contrast. The response to the fatty meal is also occasionally exaggerated when the small outpouchings of contrast with their associated filling defects are made more apparent.

The many other pathologic types of fixed filling defects in the gallbladder wall usually cannot be differentiated radiographically. Virtually all of these lesions are benign, for cholangiography has little to add in the case of carcinoma of the gallbladder.[51]

Cholecystitis may present during cholangiography with nonvisualization by either failure to concentrate or through reabsorption of the contrast. Indirect evidence of cholecystitis may be gained even though visualization is faint. Rokitansky-Aschoff sinuses are seen as diverticulum-like outpouchings from the wall of the opacified organ. Occasionally the margins of the gallbladder appear dull or finely spiculated. On close inspection the explanation for this is chronic cholecystitis, often manifested by some thickening of the wall and filling of Rokitansky-Aschoff sinuses. Poor or nonvisualization alone is insufficient evidence of cholecystitis. In Baker and Hodgson's series, 3 per cent of "nonfunctioning" gallbladders and 9 per cent of "poorly functioning" organs were found by pathologic exam to be normal[1] (Fig. 28–17 A and B).

Finally, *alterations in appearance and position* may be significant. Congenital anomalies of position and number are rare. A large film should thus be obtained of the entire abdomen before the conclusion of "nonvisualization" is reached. True dupli-

Fig. 28–16. Segmental adenomyomatosis. Note the constricted zone near the gallbladder neck with faintly visualized diverticular recesses filled with contrast (*arrow*).

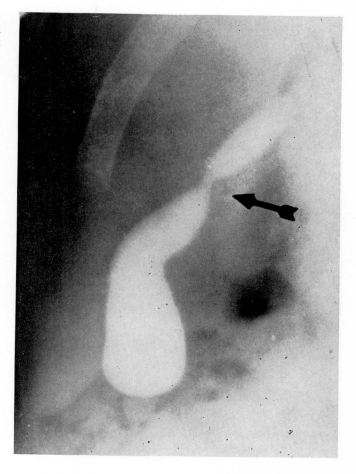

cation of the gallbladder is rare and is over-diagnosed on cholecystography, being mistaken for examples of bilobed organs. Septation of the gallbladder is caused by duplication of a mucosal fold producing a compartmentalized appearance. The best-known example of this is the phrygian cap. These segments must be visualized clearly because they may harbor calculi or possibly predispose to adenomyomatous lesions.

Bile duct calculi are rarely radiopaque and therefore are a challenge to diagnosis. Most opaque stones are thought to be formed in the gallbladder with less than 5 per cent of biliary duct calculi visible on plain films.[44] To render these calculi opaque, Salzman and Warden recommend the "4 day study." A 3 Gm. dose of iopanoic acid is repeated daily for 4 days; the contrast agent is allowed to react with the biliverdin coating of the calculus, making it radiopaque.[45] This procedure is occasionally successful in spite of the previously mentioned precautions concerning high dose cholangiograms.

Iodipamide methylglucamine is generally well tolerated by the nonjaundiced patient. The liver function studies best correlating with the odds of visualization are serum bilirubin and BSP values. If the total bilirubin is greater than 3.0 mg., the percentage of visualization will be 9.3 per cent. If BSP retention is greater than 20 per cent, the odds of visualization are 26.2 per cent.[55, 56] Theoretically, the direct bilirubin level should provide the most accurate prediction of duct visualization. The trend of the laboratory values and clinical picture is also more important than any single absolute figure.

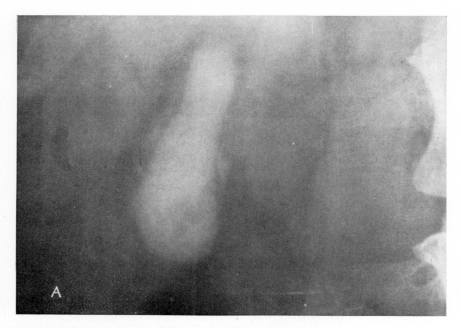

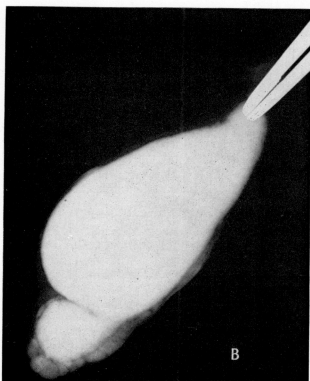

Fig. 28–17. Rokitansky-Aschoff sinuses seen in a gallbladder opacified with a "repeat dose" technic (A) and in a surgical specimen of another patient (B). A mucosal duplication is also present near the gallbladder fundus (B).

The contrast should be injected over a 10-minute period following a 1 cc. intravenous test dose, thereby avoiding many uncomfortable side effects such as nausea and vomiting. The only contraindications to intravenous cholangiography are severe hepatic and renal disease or iodide sensitivity.

Radiographic technic plays an equally important role with *intravenous cholangiography*. Careful collimation of the x-ray beam which again is of a low kilovoltage is imperative. The filming sequence which has proven successful in our hands calls for films at 20-minute intervals. If the gallbladder is visualized and a nondilated common duct is seen, a fatty meal is given and the examination treated as an oral study. Following cholecystectomy or in the presence of a dilated common bile duct, laminography of the duct is recommended.[2] The body section films in patients with intact gallbladders are best obtained 40 to 60 minutes following the injection. Following cholecystectomy, the unobstructed duct drains more rapidly and laminograms should be obtained earlier.

Since the level of contrast density is often less than ideal, particularly if the common duct is dilated, the morphology of the distal segment of the duct may be impossible to evaluate. Incompletely obstructing stones, tumors, and fibrotic changes near the sphincter of Oddi can thus be concealed. Secondary evidence of incomplete obstruction is therefore necessary if one is to detect these abnormalities.

Common duct size has been the subject of many papers. Suffice it to say that duct size alone is not sufficient evidence of a current obstructing process. The normal common duct caliber (measured at the cystic duct level) is 5.0 to 7.0 mm.[31, 49] Contrary to earlier reports, the common duct is not dilated in the absence of obstruction following cholecystectomy. If the ducts increase in size postoperatively, an obstruction should be suspected.

Wise has proposed a "time-density-retention" concept to aid in predicting *obstructing common duct lesions*. Assuming identical film qualities (a situation often difficult to achieve), one compares the radiographic density of the opacified ducts on the 60- and 120-minute films. The unobstructed ducts should show a progressive decrease in contrast density, with the 120-minute film showing a less opaque common duct than the 60-minute film.

With significant common duct obstruction, Wise summarizes the following findings, alone or in combination, which might be expected:[56]

1. Decrease in the contrast density or volume noted in the intestinal tract. This observation is of limited value.

2. Increase in common duct size. As mentioned, this alone does not often help except in extreme dilatation. If the gallbladder is intact, however, we have found that common duct diameters in excess of 9 mm. are almost invariably associated with significant obstructive lesions.

3. The common duct is more opacified on the 120-minute film than on the 60-minute study (time-density-retention concept).

4. The time in which the ducts opacify is noted. With obstruction, the ducts tend to visualize later in the course of the study.

5. Morphologic changes. Normal ducts taper as the ampullary region is approached; almost none of the intrahepatic segment of the ducts is opacified. In the obstructed biliary tree, the common duct loses its tapered contour as it dilates, and progressively more of the intrahepatic system becomes visible. The left hepatic duct dilates earlier and more markedly than the right.

Using these criteria, Wise has been about 90 per cent accurate in predicting obstruction. He identified the obstructing stone when present in only 59.2 per cent of cases.[56] Thus these indirect signs must play a significant role in the identification of significant obstructing lesions of the common duct.

Intravenous cholangiography often plays an important part in evaluation of the acute surgical abdomen. If the gallbladder cannot be visualized on delayed films (4 and 24 hours) associated with opacification of the duct system, one may presume that the cystic duct is obstructed. In rare examples, the cystic duct is found to be patent. In these instances, viscid bile combined with

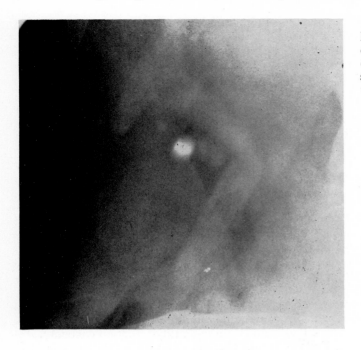

FIG. 28–18. Intravenous cholangiogram showing a dilated common bile duct and an opaque cystic duct stone which is obstructing the gallbladder and preventing it from filling.

stasis probably explains the nonvisualization. The study remains as an effective adjunct to the clinical evaluation of the acute surgical abdomen with signs pointing toward a possible biliary origin (Fig. 28–18).

Recently, infusion cholangiographic studies have been recommended to enhance the visualization of the biliary tree. This is performed with 40 cc. of iodipamide methylglucamine diluted in 50 cc. of normal saline infused intravenously over a 30-minute period.[13] We find that this helps in a similar manner as does the repeat-dose oral cholecystogram: if visualization is poor, the ducts are more densely opacified but contrast density is usually not enhanced with previous nonvisualization.

Common pitfalls in the interpretation of intravenous cholangiograms include superimposition of contrast-filled bowel loops and the "layering phenomenon." The duodenal bulb and gastric antrum frequently collect excreted contrast material and exactly mimic an opacified gallbladder. If this occurs, a few sips of cold water will flush the material away and prove this to be the case. As opposed to the similar observation with oral cholecystography, layering of contrast against the nonopaque bile is physio-

logic and normal. The admixture of bile and contrast is less complete here and readily separates.

INSTRUMENTIVE CHOLANGIOGRAPHY

The biliary tree was opacified directly long before the previously described oral and intravenous methods were conceived. In 1918 Reich was first to demonstrate the biliary tree antemortem by instilling bismuth and petrolatum into a fistulous communication.[46] The first successful percutaneous study was reported 3 years later by Burckhardt and Muller, who injected the biliary tree through the gallbladder.[6] Mirizzi reported the first operative cholangiogram in 1931.[34] The operative studies were popularized in the United States by Hicken, Best and Hunt some 5 years subsequently.[20]

In spite of its early success, percutaneous cholangiography was not generally accepted until the early 1950's. Some of this delay undoubtedly was due to the advent of physiologic cholangiography as earlier described. The problem remained, however, of the jaundiced patient who could not be evaluated by intravenous methods. Percutaneous studies are therefore designed to evaluate the status of the biliary tree in patients whose elevated bilirubin values preclude successful oral or intravenous studies. This procedure is extremely useful in differentiating obstructive from non-obstructive jaundice as well as in defining the nature of the obstructing lesion when present. Occasionally, the duct system can also be decompressed when necessary by leaving a small polyethylene catheter in place.[35]

The study is generally performed in the radiology department under image-amplified fluoroscopic control. A 7 inch, 20-21 gauge needle is inserted subcostally in the midclavicular line under local anesthesia. When the needle enters the duct system, bile is withdrawn and contrast instilled with appropriate films obtained. It is vital to be able to see the distal common bile duct in cases of obstructive jaundice to determine the nature of the obstruction and allow the surgeon to better plan the surgical approach. The patient ordinarily is explored following the procedure at which time any complications such as bleeding or bile leakage can be corrected. Technically, the greater the dilatation or more complete the obstruction, the easier it becomes to enter a bile duct. In experienced hands, the procedure was successful in 92 per cent of patients with dilated systems but in only 43 per cent of individuals with a normal biliary tree.[35]

On percutaneous studies common duct stones appear either as a meniscus defect if impacted near the ampulla or they float more proximally within the dilated ducts (Figs. 28–19 and 28–20). The degree of

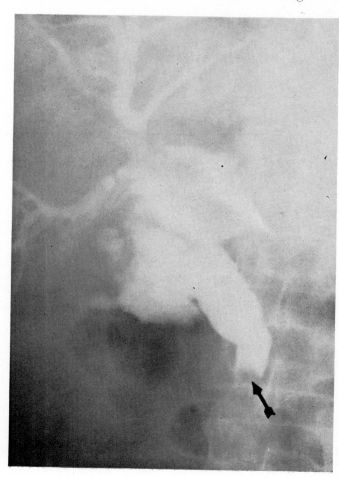

FIG. 28–19. Impacted common duct stone. Percutaneous cholangiogram showing the typical meniscus defect caused by the calculus.

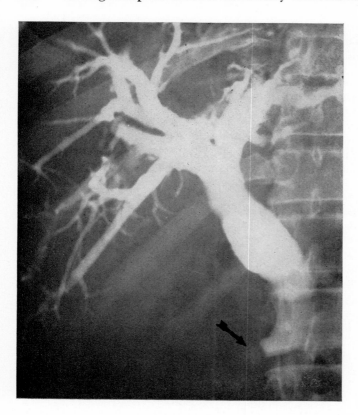

FIG. 28–20. Impacted opaque common duct stone on percutaneous cholangiogram.

obstruction seen with ampullary neoplasms often is less marked than with pancreatic head tumors. With the former, the distal opacified segment of the common duct may be seen to have a shallow meniscus (resembling an impacted stone) or appear with a ragged, uneven stump. Carcinoma of the pancreatic head is associated with the largest duct calibers. An irregular narrowing or tapering to the duct is seen, occasionally with an uneven, amputated margin. Differentiation from an ampullary carcinoma is often impossible.[11] The diagnostic accuracy of the transhepatic cholangiogram in the New York Hospital series of pancreatic carcinoma was 98 per cent (34 cases). A perfect record has been recorded with the ampullary lesions although the group was small (7 cases)[35] (Figs. 28–21 and 28–22).

Carcinoma of the bile ducts is often overlooked both by the surgeon and radiologist. The lesion is usually best seen on instrumentive cholangiograms as a short segment stenosing lesion with abrupt, rigid margins[9]

(Fig. 28–23). This appearance should not be confused with the changes of ascending cholangitis which show uneven narrowing and dilatations of the intrahepatic ducts, often with lack of filling of the tributary ducts ("leafless tree") (Fig. 28–24).

This study is extremely helpful in planning the management of the jaundiced patient. It is not intended to be a substitute for routine oral or intravenous methods of evaluation, for obvious reasons. The complication rates have been acceptably low, with only 4 deaths attributable to the procedure in more than 800 cases.[35]

Operative cholangiography is not discussed in detail here. Refer to the excellent and complete review of these procedures by Schein, Stern and Jacobson.[46] Suffice it to say that the operative studies when properly performed, through cooperative efforts of radiologist, surgeon and anesthesiologist, provide invaluable assistance in the subsequent management of these patients. With present-day equipment, advantages of more sophisticated operating room

FIG. 28–21. Carcinoma of the pancreas. Note the severe obstruction as evidenced by the more dilated intrahepatic ducts.

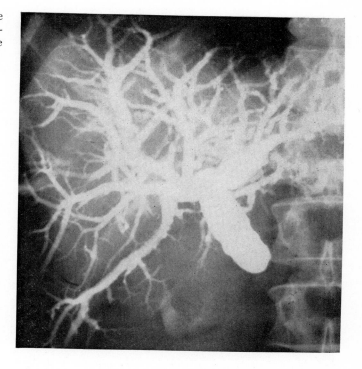

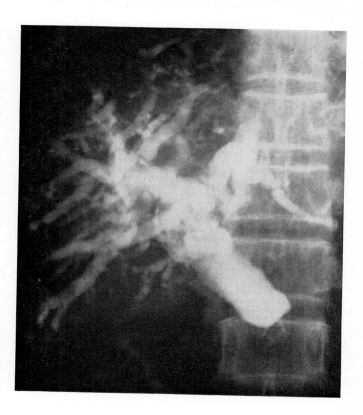

FIG. 28–22. Carcinoma of the pancreas. Percutaneous cholangiogram showing the obstructed biliary tree with amputation of the common duct.

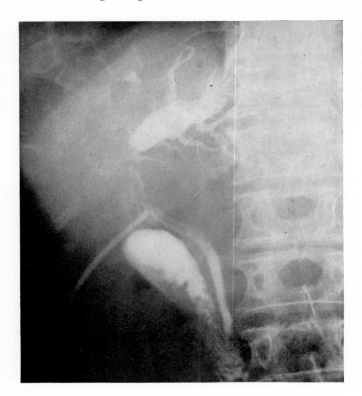

FIG. 28–23. Carcinoma of the left hepatic duct. The stenotic lesion can be seen incompletely near the bifurcation of the ducts, extending distally. Note the greatly dilated left hepatic duct and normal common bile duct.

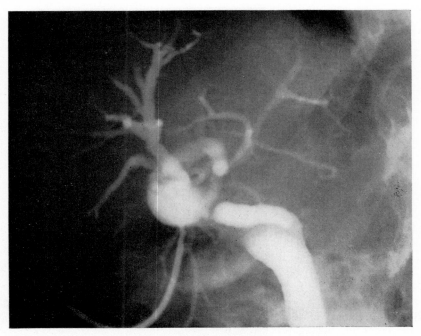

FIG. 28–24. Ascending cholangitis. "T" tube cholangiogram showing the appearance of the biliary tree with a cholangitis. Note the irregular dilatation and lack of branching tributaries (leafless tree" appearance).

radiographic units and rapid (90 second) processing, the surgical procedure should not be significantly delayed.

Intrahepatic and common duct stones are reportedly overlooked at surgery in 16 to 25 per cent of cases.[43] With this in mind, the simple expedient of operative and post-operative cholangiography seems justified when feasible. The examinations are often hasty and incomplete, and in these cases may serve to provide a false sense of security.

Postoperative cholangiograms are performed in the radiology department under careful fluoroscopic control. A water-soluble contrast agent is used and low kilovoltage spot films in multiple positions are vital. Overhead, uncontrolled films are of limited usefulness, for the degree of filling (or emptying) is not under observation and therefore random. The two most important projections include lateral and right posterior oblique views emphasizing the distal common duct. The lateral view allows one to fill the then dependent and anterior left hepatic radicles as well as visualize the cystic duct remnant to best advantage. It is well to remember that the posterior and medial insertion of the cystic duct often shares its lateral wall with the common bile duct. A cystic duct "stump" is therefore inevitable or the surgeon will enter the common duct during his dissection (Fig. 28–25). Multiple views of the distal common duct in the right posterior oblique projection are necessary so that one can visualize the ampullary and transduodenal segments of the common duct. These are seen to actively fill and empty fluoroscopically and are often difficult to evaluate.

The primary purpose of the postoperative studies is to search for residual calculi as well as to follow the status of chronic biliary tract changes of stenosis or infection. Air bubbles frequently interfere with the search for stones; every effort should be made to clear the tubes of contained air prior to the examination. We subject the ducts to dependent drainage 12 hours preceding the study and document suspected calculi by a repeat examination (Fig. 28–26).

A satisfactory cholangiogram requires that the bile ducts be adequately visualized. Undue pressure must be avoided during filling of the duct system. Gravity pressure alone may be sufficient and should be tried before positive hand pressure is used. Post-procedure fever and discomfort can certainly be minimized if this course is fol-

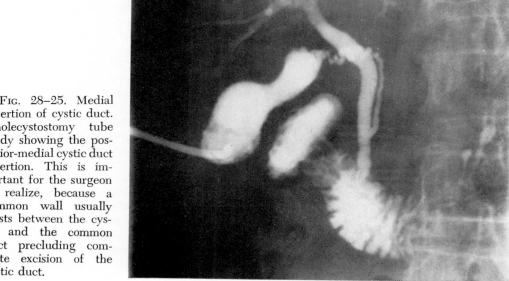

FIG. 28–25. Medial insertion of cystic duct. Cholecystostomy tube study showing the posterior-medial cystic duct insertion. This is important for the surgeon to realize, because a common wall usually exists between the cystic and the common duct precluding complete excision of the cystic duct.

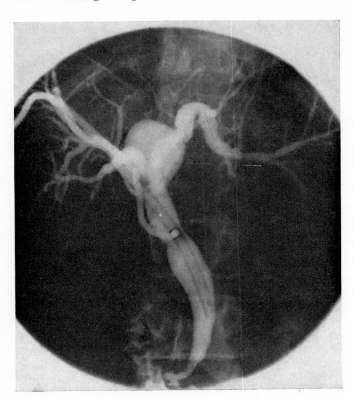

FIG. 28–26. Choledochal cyst. "T" tube cholangiogram showing a choledochal cyst appearing as a sac-like dilation arising from the common hepatic duct.

lowed. Extravasation and reflux into the duct of Wirsung are probably related to the intraductal injection pressures. These complications undoubtedly affect post-cholangiogram morbidity.

RADIONUCLIDE HEPATOGRAPHY

The impetus for the use of radioisotopes in organ scanning was provided by Cassen et al. in 1951.[7] They introduced a prototype scintillation scanner to detect the activity of nuclides selectively tagged to substances whose metabolic fate could be predicted. Subsequent improvements in detection equipment and production of organ specific short lived radiopharmaceutical agents have been responsible for the present position of liver scanning in clinical medicine.

Most scanning equipment provides only a rectilinear potential. The more recent application of units such as the gamma ray scintillation camera has added more versatility to organ scanning. With this expedient, short lived isotopes can be rapidly followed with multiple scans in varied projections over short time periods.

Attempts to improve the resolution of the recorded information have centered upon both mechanical and computer aids as well as improved isotopes. Kuhl and Edwards have applied principles analogous to tomography to organ scanning, allowing better resolution and providing information concerning lesion depth.[27] More recently, the group at Memorial Sloan-Kettering have added digital and computerized readouts to translate the data into more useable forms. This format changes the visual data into raw numbers (reflecting actual count rates) and allows one to more accurately judge the significance of counting variations.[53]

Radioisotopes. The radioisotopes most commonly used in liver scanning may be grouped into those that seek the reticulo-endothelial system and those that are handled through the polygonal cells, similar to bile. The most commonly used agent of the former group is *colloidal gold* (^{198}Au).

It is prepared from purified gold foil and has a physical half-life of 2.7 days. The principal energy used in scanning is its gamma emission (0.4 Mev). The gold is retained by the reticuloendothelial cells indefinitely. Its selective affinity for the liver is dependent upon the hepatic blood flow, with more being shunted to the extrahepatic reticuloendothelial tissues of the spleen and marrow with portal hypertension. The average dose utilized is 2 microcuries/kg. body weight, with larger increments advised in cirrhotic individuals. The longer half-life of [198]Au allows multiple scans as well as delayed evaluation as long as 1 to 3 days later. In these dose ranges, the hepatic radiation amounts to approximately 4 rads[52] (Fig. 28–27).

Colloidal aggregates of *human serum albumin* [131]I also have an affinity for the Kupffer cells of the liver and are used in hepatic scanning. This material tends to aggregate and thus is distributed without uniformity in the liver. The hepatic dose is significantly less with this agent than with [198]Au.

In the continuing search for a radionuclide with an acceptable energy level and short half-life, *technetium* has been found to fulfill these criteria (technetium-99m sulfur colloid). It is also withdrawn by the reticuloendothelial system. Since its half-life is short, large doses can be given, effecting higher hepatic activity. The statistical advantages of a higher count rate provide increased accuracy in recognition of lesions.

Radiopharmaceuticals removed by the polygonal cells provide an advantage in the differential diagnosis of obstructive and parenchymal jaundice. Since the metabolic pathways of these agents resemble that of bile, counting over the liver and lower abdomen provides information concerning the integrity of the biliary tree.[12] *Rose bengal* [131]I is the principal agent used in this group of isotopes. The hepatic dose is less than with [198]Au (0.25 rad).[52] In the absence of obstructive jaundice, however, its presence in the gastrointestinal tract places it in proximity to the gonads, increasing the dose to these organs to a greater level than agents with an affinity to reticuloendothelial tissue. The other available radiopharmaceutical in this group is iodipamide ^{131}I which is little used today. Practical disadvantages of this group of compounds relate to their presence in the bowel and gallbladder with subsequent interference in

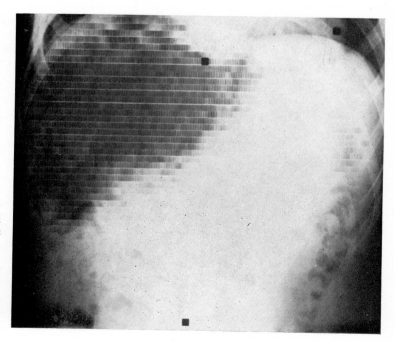

FIG. 28–27. Normal [198]Au liver scan. This is shown superimposed on a "demagnified" film of the abdomen obtained at 100 inches. Note the small amount of splenic uptake with no visible vertebral marrow activity.

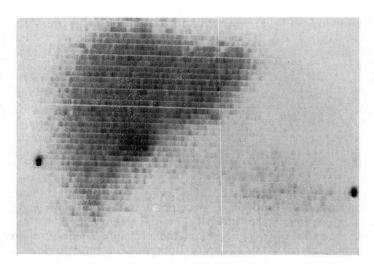

Fig. 28–28. Normal rose bengal ^{131}I liver scan. Note the increased activity within the gallbladder and ill-defined uptake below the hepatic silhouette which represents activity in the large intestine.

scanning resolution. Also, its shorter biologic half-life (duration in the liver) precludes delayed scans as possible with [198]Au (Fig. 28–28).

Application of Hepatic Scanning. Hepatic scanning is used to recognize and localize space-occupying lesions, to determine liver size, shape and integrity and to assess and follow-up the effects of treatment (Fig. 28–29).

It is used principally to recognize and localize lesions. The accuracy of this effort relates to many variables. The threshold size of a detectable lesion depends on counting statistics, on the depth and location of the mass as well as on the integrity of the surrounding hepatic parenchyma. The various etiologies of these solitary filling defects can usually not be discriminated on the scan alone. Reportedly, however, primary liver tumors may be suspected by the appearance of a filling defect superimposed on a cirrhotic background.[21] Multiplicity of filling defects of course favor a metastatic etiology with good reliability.[30, 39] False-positive results become possible with the decreased counting statistics associated with cirrhosis.[22]

The procedure is often extremely helpful in the differential diagnosis of intra- and extrahepatic mass lesions. As mentioned, with suspected right subphrenic ab-

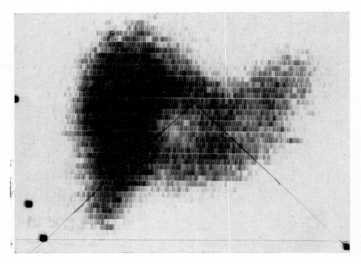

Fig. 28–29. [198]Au liver scan with a metastatic deposit. A single large central defect is easily seen with decreased uptake over the area of the left lobe of the liver. The curvilinear impression on the upper margin of the liver is produced by the heart.

Fig. 28–30. ^{198}Au liver scan in a patient with cirrhosis. Note the intense splenic activity as well as the vertebral marrow uptake.

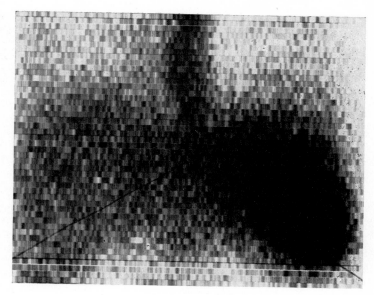

scess collections the liver scan alone, superimposed on film of the abdomen or combined with lung scans, provides invaluable assistance.

The hepatic scan equivalent of cirrhosis has received a great deal of attention in the recent past. The inhomogeneous or "mottled" appearance is not specific, whereas the extrahepatic distribution of the nuclide as well as its perihilar concentration is said to be characteristic.[8] The increased extrahepatic uptake of agents directed to the reticuloendothelial tissues is presumably the effect of portal hypertension with resultant increased blood flow to such areas as the spleen and marrow (Fig. 28–30).

Common pitfalls in the interpretation of liver scans relate to variations in normal liver size and shape. There is a well visualized notch near the porta hepatis in 15 per cent of cases.[30] The left hepatic lobe varies in its presentation both in size and appearance. The hepatic periphery is difficult to evaluate. Respiratory motion often produces serrations, particularly along the superior and lateral liver margins. Low counting statistics, as mentioned, whatever the cause, make interpretation difficult. The greater the count rate, the less is the chance of false-negative results with regard to the

prediction of hepatic parenchymal disease and filling defects.

REFERENCES

1. Baker, H. L., Jr., and Hodgson, J. R.: Oral cholecystography: an evaluation of its accuracy, Gastroenterology 34:1137, 1958.
2. Bell, A. L. L., Immerman, L. L., and Arcomano, J.: Body-section cholangiography with new intravenous medium (Cholografin^R), Radiology 66:84, 1956.
3. Berk, R. N., and Lasser, E. C.: Altered concepts of the mechanism of nonvisualization of the gallbladder, Radiology 82:296, 1964.
4. Blum, L., and Stagg, A.: Emphysematous cholecystitis, A. J. Roentgenol. 89:840, 1963.
5. Blythe, W. B., and Woods, J. W.: Acute renal insufficiency after ingestion of a gallbladder dye: report of a case, New Engl. J. Med. 264:1045, 1961.
6. Burckhardt, H., and Muller, W.: Versuche über die Punktion der Gallenblase und ihre Röntgendarstellung, Dtsch. Z. Chir. 162:168, 1921.
7. Cassen, B., Curtis, L., Reed, C., and Libby, R.: Instrumentation for I^{131} use in medical studies, Nucleonics 9:46, 1951.
8. Christie, J. H., MacIntyre, W. J., Crespo, G. G. and Koch-Weser, D.: Radioisotope

scanning in hepatic cirrhosis, Radiology 81:455, 1963.

9. Clemett, A. R.: Carcinoma of the major bile ducts, Radiology 84:894, 1965.

10. Ellman, B., McLeod, I. N., and Powell, S. J.: Diagnostic pneumoperitoneum in amoebic liver abscess, Brit. Med. J. 2: 1406, 1965.

11. Evans, J. A.: Specialized roentgen diagnostic technics in the investigation of abdominal disease, Radiology 82:579, 1964.

12. Eyler, W. R., Du Sault, L. A., Poznanski, A. K., and Schuman, B. M.: Isotope scanning in the evaluation of the jaundiced patient, Radiol. Clin. N. Amer. 4:589, 1966.

13. Feldman, M. I., and Keohane, M.: Slow infusion intravenous cholangiography, Radiology 87:355, 1966.

14. Fischer, H. W.: Physiologic and pharmacologic aspects of cholangiography, Radiol. Clin. N. Amer. 4:625, 1966.

15. Frimann-Dahl, J.: Roentgen Examinations in Acute Abdominal Diseases, Springfield, Ill., Thomas, 1960.

16. Frostberg, N.: A characteristic duodenal deformity in cases of different kinds of peri-vaterial enlargement of the pancreas, Acta Radiol. 19:164, 1938.

17. Glenn, F., Evans, J., Hill, M., and McClenahan, J.: Intravenous cholangiography, Ann. Surg. 140:600, 1954.

18. Graham, E. A., and Cole, W. H.: Roentgenologic examination of the gallbladder: preliminary report of a new method utilizing intravenous injection of tetrabromophenolphthalein, J.A.M.A. 82:613, 1924.

19. Haddow, R. A., and Kemp-Harper, R. A.: Calcification in the liver and portal system, Clin. Radiol. 18:225, 1967.

20. Hicken, N. F., Best, R. R., and Hunt, H. B.: Cholangiography: visualization of the gallbladder and bile ducts during and after operation, Ann. Surg. 103:210, 1936.

21. Johnson, P. M., and Grossman, F. M.: Radioisotope scanning in primary carcinoma of the liver, Radiology 84:868, 1965.

22. Johnson, P. M., and Sweeney, W. A.: The false positive liver scan, J. Nuclear Med. 7:375, 1966.

23. Jutras, J. A., and Lévesque, H.-P.: Adenomyoma and adenomyomatosis of the gallbladder; radiologic and pathologic correlations, Radiol. Clin. N. Amer. 4:483, 1966.

24. Jutras, J. A., Longtin, J. M., and Lévesque, H.-P.: Hyperplastic cholecystoses, Am. J. Roentgenol. 83:795, 1960.

25. Keeffe, E. J., Gagliardi, R. A., and Pfister, R. C.: The roentgenographic evaluation of ascites, Am. J. Roentgenol. 101:388, 1967.

26. Kirklin, B. R.: Cholecystographic diagnosis of papillomas of the gallbladder, Am. J. Roentgenol. 25:46, 1931.

27. Kuhl, D. E., and Edwards, R. Q.: Cylindrical and section radioisotope scanning of the liver and brain, Radiology 83:926, 1964.

28. Lasser, E. C.: Pharmacodynamics of biliary contrast media, Radiol. Clin. N. Amer. 4:511, 1966.

29. Lasser, E. C., Farr, R. S., Fujimagari, T., and Tripp, W. N.: The significance of protein binding of contrast media in roentgen diagnosis, Am. J. Roentgenol. 87:338, 1962.

30. McAfee, J. G., Ause, R. G., and Wagner, H. N.: Diagnostic value of scintillation scanning of the liver, Arch. Int. Med. 116: 95, 1965.

31. McClenahan, J. L., Evans, J. A., and Braunstein, P. W.: Intravenous cholangiography in the postcholecystectomy syndrome, J.A.M.A. 159:1353, 1955.

32. Margulis, A., and Joachim, H. (eds.): Alimentary Tract Roentgenology, St. Louis, Mosby, 1967.

33. Miele, A. J., and Edmonds, H. W.: Calcified liver metastases: a specific roentgen diagnostic sign, Radiology 80:779, 1963.

34. Mirizzi, P. L.: La cholangiografia durante las operaciones de las vias biliares, Bol. Soc. Cirug. B. Aires 16:1133, 1932.

35. Mujahed, Z., and Evans, J. A.: Percutaneous transhepatic cholangiography, Radiol. Clin. N. Amer. 4:535, 1966.

36. Nolan, B., Ross, J. A., and Samuel, E.: Lime-water bile, Brit. J. Surg. 48:201, 1960.

37. Ochsner, S. F.: Solitary polypoid lesions of the gallbladder, Radiol. Clin. N. Amer. 4:501, 1966.

38. Ochsner, S. F., and Carrera, G. M.: Calcification of the gallbladder ("porcelain gallbladder"), Am. J. Roentgenol. 89:847, 1963.

39. Ozarda, A., and Pickren, J.: Topographic distribution of liver metastases: its relation to surgical and isotope diagnosis, J. Nuclear Med. 3:149, 1962.

40. Pfahler, G. E.: Measurement of the liver

by means of roentgen rays, based upon a study of 502 subjects, Am. J. Roentgenol. 16:558, 1926.

41. Plachta, A.: Calcified cavernous hemangioma of the liver, Radiology 79:783, 1962.

42. Ross, P.: Calcifications in liver metastases from neuroblastoma, Radiology 85:1074, 1965.

43. Sachs, M. D.: Routine cholangiography, operative and postoperative, Radiol. Clin. N. Amer. 4:547, 1966.

44. Salzman, E.: Opacification of bile duct calculi, Radiol. Clin. N. Amer. 4:525, 1966.

45. Salzman, E., and Warden, M. R.: Telepaque opacification of radiolucent biliary calculi: the "rim sign," Radiology 71:85, 1958.

46. Schein, C. J., Stern, W. Z., and Jacobson, H. G.: The Common Bile Duct, Operative Cholangiography, Biliary Endoscopy, and Choledocholithotomy, Springfield, Ill., Thomas, 1966.

47. Schiff, L. (ed.): Diseases of the Liver, Chap. 28, Philadelphia, Lippincott, 1956.

48. Seaman, W. B., Cosgriff, S., and Wells, J.: Renal insufficiency following cholecystography, Am. J. Roentgenol. 90:859, 1963.

49. Shehadi, W. H.: Intravenous cholecystocholangiography, J.A.M.A. 159:1350, 1669, 1955.

50. ———: Radiologic examination of the biliary tract: plain film of the abdomen; oral cholecystography, Radiol. Clin. N. Amer. 4:463, 1966.

51. Thorbjarnarson, B., and Glenn, F.: Carcinoma of the gallbladder, Cancer 12:1009, 1959.

52. Wagner, H. N., Jr, McAfee, J .G., and Mozley, J. M.: Diagnosis of liver disease by radioisotope scanning, Arch. Int. Med. 107:324, 1961.

53. Weber, D. A., Kenny, P., Pochaczevsky, R., Corey, K. R., and Laughlin, J. S.: Liver scans with digital readout, J. Nuclear Med. 6:528, 1965.

54. Wiot, J. F., and Felson, B.: Gas in the portal venous system, Am. J. Roentgenol. 86:920, 1961.

55. Wise, R. E.: Current concepts of intravenous cholangiography, Radiol. Clin. N. Amer. 4:521, 1966.

56. ———: Intravenous Cholangiography, Springfield, Ill., Thomas, 1962.

29

Diseases of the Gallbladder and the Extrahepatic Bile Ducts

ROGER D. WILLIAMS, M.D., AND *JAY C. FISH*, M.D.

The problems associated with the gallbladder and extrahepatic bile ducts are some of the most frequently encountered by the clinician. Biliary tract surgery now exceeds that for hernia and other common procedures in most hospitals.[5] Fortunately, improvements in diagnosis, anesthesia and pre- and postoperative care, and better graduate education of surgeons have significantly decreased the morbidity and mortality of biliary tract surgery.[20, 21] Asymptomatic gallstones soon produce complications in the majority of patients[52] and there is little reason, excepting specific contraindications, to delay elective surgery. There is some room for improvement in the management of jaundiced patients, in selection of the optimum time for surgery, in preventing complications and in decreasing the number of patients who are dissatisfied with surgery because of continued abdominal symptoms. Improved results may be anticipated if patients are carefully selected for surgery which is meticulously performed with a thorough knowledge of anatomic, physiologic and pathologic variations in the diseased biliary tract.

SURGICAL ANATOMY

Although the anatomy of the liver and biliary tract are discussed in Chapter 1, a brief review is indicated in order to delineate normal from diseased states. Few congenital abnormalities occur in either the gallbladder or bile ducts; however, there are more anatomic variations in the area of the cystic and hepatic duct communication than any area of similar size in the body. Surgeons must know these variations and relate them to the pathologic findings at the time of surgery.

Gallbladder. The normal gallbladder is a thin-walled, elongated sac containing 30 to 60 cc. of bile. It lies in a fossa in the medial inferior surface of the right lobe of the liver. Attachments vary from almost complete embedding within the liver substance to a thin pedicle suspending the gallbladder from the under surface of the liver. The tip of the gallbladder may be deformed or partially segmented to form the phrygian cap, a radiologic and anatomic finding of no pathologic significance. The gallbladder tapers to the cystic duct, usually curving in a sigmoid fashion to form an ampulla (Hartman's pouch). This pouch often folds over the cystic duct, less often the common duct; and it is attached by avascular adhesions to the duodenum and/or colon. This relationship provides shortening and thickening of these attachments with inflammation and explains the occasional spontaneous fistulization between gallbladder and duodenum or colon preceding gallstone ileus.[3]

Major variations of the gallbladder seldom occur. As attachments to the liver range from imbedding to pedicle formation, the division of the arterial supply also varies. Most often there are two branches, the division occurring at the ampulla or upper part of the cystic duct. The location of the cystic artery in relation to the cystic duct and hepatic artery is more variable. Congenital absence of the gallbladder without atresia of the bile ducts, as well as duplication, are rare.

Bile Ducts. There are numerous variations in length and relationship among cystic, hepatic and common bile ducts. The usual *cystic duct* is about 3 cm. long with a lumen compromised by spiral folds (Heister's valves) which impede stones and attempted instrumentation. The cystic duct joins the hepatic duct about 2.5 cm. from the junction of the right and left branches. It may, however, enter the left hepatic duct or at any place below it including the duodenum. Several of the variations are shown in Figure 29–1. The difficulties in exploring the common duct, dangers of peritonitis or bile fistula from leaving untied an accessory duct, and the possibility of injury to hepatic or common bile ducts are increased by the combination of anatomic variation and severe biliary tract disease.

The normal *common bile duct* is thin-walled and 4 to 12 mm. in diameter (average, 7.4 mm.).[34] Along its anterior border courses a small artery and vein while the hepatic artery lies medial and the portal vein posterior. Its length, usually 9 to 11 cm., varies according to the cystic duct junction. The middle third of this duct lies behind the first portion of the duodenum approximately 2 cm. from the pylorus. The lower third passes through the head of the pancreas curving anteriorly to terminate in the posteromedial aspect of the second portion of the duodenum. The duct passes obliquely through the duodenal wall and is joined by the pancreatic duct. The short common reservoir, the ampulla of Vater, narrows considerably before opening into the duodenum. Two longitudinal and two annular, muscular sheaths shorten and erect the papilla and apparently control bile pressure, relaxing to permit emptying and contracting to encourage filling of the gallbladder.

Variations of anatomy of the common duct are uncommon, excepting atresia, relationship to the cystic duct and variation of the length of the hepatic ducts. Biliary atresia usually involves both the intra- and

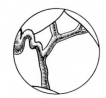

A. NORMAL 3 to 5 cm.   B. SHORT CYSTIC DUCT

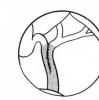

C. EXCESSIVE MOBILITY   D. CYSTIC PARALLEL WITH
   OF COMMON DUCT   COMMON DUCT

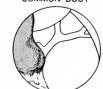

E. ACCESSORY CYSTIC   F. LARGE PENDULOUS
   OR HEPATIC DUCT   AMPULLA

FIG. 29–1. Variations of gallbladder and extrahepatic bile ducts.

(A.) The length and the insertion of the cystic duct vary considerably, but on the average it is 3 cm. long and descends to join the lateral aspect of the common hepatic duct approximately 1 inch below the junction of the right and the left hepatic ducts. Possible anomalies include variations shown in B to F.

(B.) A short but wide cystic duct which predisposes to trauma.

(C.) If the common duct is excessively mobile, traction on the gallbladder may tent the ductal system and may result in accidental injury.

(D.) The cystic duct descends for varying distances parallel with the common hepatic duct in nearly 1 out of every 4 patients.

(E.) Accessory cystic ducts may join the hepatic, common hepatic, main cystic or common bile ducts.

(F.) When the ampulla is large and pendulous or the site of an impacted stone, it may obscure the bile ducts and hepatic arteries.

extrahepatic bile ducts. The gallbladder is frequently present and connects with the duodenum through a small common duct.[45]

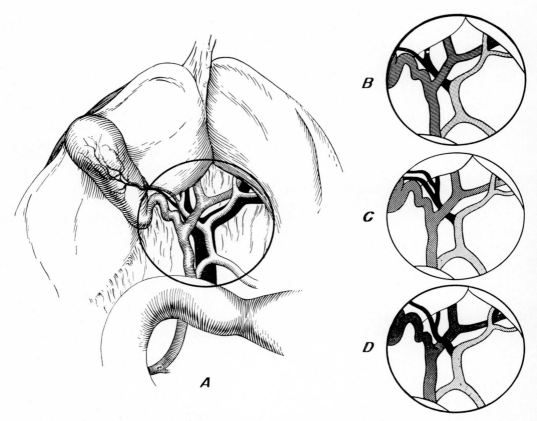

FIG. 29–2. (A) Normal anatomic relations of the gallbladder and the extrahepatic bile ducts. (B) The right hepatic branch lies parallel with and in close proximity to the cystic duct itself in nearly 1 out of every 5 patients. (C) Vessels corresponding to the anterior and the posterior branches of the cystic artery originate as separate vessels from the right hepatic artery in 15 per cent of patients. (D) The right hepatic artery passes in front of the common hepatic duct in some 12 per cent of cases.

In only about 10 per cent of infants are ducts found at the liver hilum for anastomosis, and most of these infants already have biliary cirrhosis. Choledochal cysts occur as a result of either reduplication from retention cysts or as an enlargement due to partial obstruction of the duct during the development of its lumen.[1] Considerable difference of opinion exists as to the frequency of a common channel for entrance of pancreatic and bile ducts at the ampulla, probably due to the methods of study. A common channel, important in the development of both pancreatitis and cholecystitis,[11, 47] has been found in 60 to 90 per cent of patients.[7, 10, 37, 43]

Arteries of the Extrahepatic Bile Ducts.

The hepatic artery proper ascends in the hepatoduodenal ligament and, at varying distances from the liver, divides into right and left branches. It lies medial to the common duct and anterior to the portal vein and can be readily compressed by a finger inserted through the foramen of Winslow against the thumb. The hepatic artery and several of its variations are shown in Figure 29–2. There are numerous other minor variations of the blood supply to the gallbladder and major variations of supply to the liver, including a right hepatic branch, and less often the entire blood supply from the superior mesenteric artery. These variations are nicely demonstrated by Michels.[36]

Lymphatics. The lymphatic drainage

from the gallbladder and bile ducts is to three rather constant lymph nodes, at the neck of the gallbladder, at the junction of the cystic and hepatic ducts and near the termination of the common duct. These nodes may be confused with the common duct stones and are important in infection and tumor spread. In addition, small lymphatic channels connect with liver lymphatics[4] and are important in the spread of gallbladder cancer.

PATHOPHYSIOLOGY OF BILIARY TRACT

It is important to appreciate the changes that occur in the gallbladder and bile ducts as a result of the two most frequent pathologic states: obstruction and inflammation. These changes should be noted at the time of surgery and correlated with factors in the history as well as laboratory data. Generally, obstruction without inflammation results in distention, the gallbladder and extrahepatic ducts remaining rather thin-walled. Infection preceding obstruction usually produces sufficient reaction and fibrosis in the duct and gallbladder walls to prevent dilatation.

The gallbladder serves primarily as a concentrating reservoir and the ducts as conduits. Although the gallbladder contracts, there is no evidence that spasm or contraction of the common duct can occur in man.[33] Contrary to opinions otherwise, there is no evidence that the ductal system in man[26] dilates after cholecystectomy as it does in dogs.[28] On the other hand, there is increasing evidence that the capacity of the gallbladder and ductal system nearly doubles after vagotomy and this is associated with an increased incidence of gallstones.[29]

Pathophysiologic changes in the biliary tract can be related to the degree of extrahepatic ductal obstruction and to biliary pressure as well as infection.[53] Serum levels of alkaline phosphatase and bilirubin are greater and more rapidly reach peak levels with high bile pressure. The alkaline phosphatase may be elevated at pressures slightly above normal (100 mm. water), whereas serum bilirubin remains normal. In the absence of infection, the extrahepatic ductal

system and gallbladder dilate greatly; the higher the pressures, the greater the dilatation. Infection within the ductal system after it dilates only thickens the ductal walls. If infection and inflammation precede obstruction, dilatation may not occur but the duct walls thicken. Once the ducts dilate, they do not return to normal even when pressure becomes normal and jaundice clears. Liver damage associated with extrahepatic obstruction is slow to develop unless there is superimposed infection.

CHOLELITHIASIS

Cholelithiasis is one of the most common abnormalities of man today. As the older age group increases, the incidence of gallstones and the problems they present are multiplied. It is estimated that over 10 per cent of the adult population has stones, and this increases to over 30 per cent of persons over 65 years. The sex incidence greatly favors women in the first four decades of life, after which there is little difference in incidence between men and women. The incidence is increased to 20 to 40 per cent in hemolytic anemias.

Causes, Types and Location of Gallstones. Although one of the most common metabolic and pathologic abnormalities of man, the specific mechanisms of gallstone formation are not defined.[19] Reviews of the causes of gallstone formations suggest that infection, general metabolic disorders and stasis are primarily the etiologic factors.[30, 41] There has been considerable interest in the factors causing stratification of bile[46] and the relationship of bile constituents to stone formation. It seems well established that bacteria play a significant role in stone formation experimentally[18] and, with or without parasites, clinically.[35]

Stasis appears to be the primary factor in gallstone formation. Experimental production of stones has always been associated with bile stasis. Bacteria grow better during bile stasis. Vagotomy has been associated with an increased incidence of gallstones[29]; after this procedure the biliary tract becomes atonic, a state supposedly conducive to stasis. It remains to be determined what effect pressure, a variable with changing bile flow and other biliary dynamics, will have on cell proliferation or shedding, which are altered by distention,[27] and the secretion or excretion of various constituents of the bile by the liver.

Although the incidence of various kinds of gallstones varies geographically, the so-called mixed stone accounts for approximately three-fourths of those noted in the United States. These stones are a combination of all three stone-forming constituents of bile; cholesterol, bilirubin and calcium. They vary in size and shape but more often are polyhedral, multifaceted and yellow-brown to black. Crystalline cholesterol and calcium bilirubinate stones each account for about 10 per cent of surgically removed gallstones, whereas calcium carbonate stones are rare. The radio-opacity of stones depends upon the calcium content; less than 10 per cent are seen in routine recumbent or upright roentgenograms.

Gallstones may be found anywhere in the biliary tract. They are usually formed in the gallbladder and pass into the common bile duct. Approximately 20 per cent of patients with cholelithiasis have choledocholithiasis. Rarely stones are found in the common duct when none were noted in the gallbladder. Of importance to the surgeon, stones are found in the hepatic ducts in 7 per cent of patients with cholelithiasis.[61]

CHOLECYSTOGRAPHY

Since only a small percentage of gallstones are radiopaque, cholecystography is usually required to visualize stones. If the examination is carefully performed and evaluated, one may also evaluate gallbladder disease accurately. Visualization of the gallbladder by Graham and Cole in 1924[22] after the intravenous injection of an iodine-containing compound was nearly as satisfactory as today; the safety of new compounds has permitted use in nearly all patients suspected of gallbladder disease. The problem today, as in the early use of cholecystography, lies in interpretation.

Several precautions are required in recommending and interpreting cholecystography. Sensitivity to iodides prohibits this test, particularly intravenous cholangiog-raphy which is also dangerous in the presence of renal disease. Although renal failure has been ascribed to this test, previous renal disease, shock from a reaction to the injection of the iodide and dehydration are contributing factors. The failure of the gallbladder to fill by oral cholecystography may be due to failure to take the iodides, poor absorption, liver disease, partial biliary tract obstruction with or without jaundice, obstruction of the cystic duct or gallbladder disease affecting concentration. Since pancreatitis, as well as other disorders that produce partial biliary obstruction, may prevent concentration in the gallbladder for several weeks, a single failure to visualize the gallbladder is of little value unless the typical symptoms of biliary colic alone are an indication for surgery.

Stones may be overlooked unless special technics are used. The right lateral decubitus position employing horizontal x-ray beams is useful in detecting the layering of stones in the top, bottom or between the layers of bile or contrast media. Occasionally oral cholecystography repeated for several days leads to "opacification" of stones in the common duct.[50] Intravenous cholangiography, popular during the last decade,[23] is of most value in patients whose gallbladder has been removed and who have evidence of partial bile duct obstruction, usually due to stones. This examination, like the oral cholecystogram, is not feasible in the presence of clinical jaundice unless the bilirubin is rapidly falling.

CHOLECYSTITIS

Acute, recurrent and chronic cholecystitis, is extremely common and may be confused clinically with appendicitis, duodenal ulcer, acute and chronic pancreatitis and other abdominal disorders as well as pneumonia and coronary heart disease. At least 90 per cent of cases are associated with gallstones; however, inflammation of the gallbladder can occur without stones.

Pathogenesis. Although the exact cause of gallbladder inflammation is not always obvious, bile outflow is usually obstructed. This obstruction may occur from causes other than stones.[25] It was formerly thought that bacterial invasion of the gallbladder wall was responsible for cholecystitis; however, except in its late stages, even in acute cholecystitis, the gallbladder contents and wall may be free of bacteria.[6] It has also been suggested that acute cholecystitis results primarily from chemical irritation following obstruction of the cystic duct. After an initial concentration of bile, this concentrated bile mixture becomes irritating; osmotic pressure is increased within the gallbladder associated with enlargement, edema and, finally, occlusion of small blood vessels leading to necrosis. Pressure within the gallbladder is greatly increased (Fig. 29–3).

More recent studies suggest that acute cholecystitis is due to enzymatic changes combined with cystic duct obstruction.[47] Experimentally, simple obstruction of the gallbladder results in hydrops. When pancreatic juice, trypsin or chymotrypsin is added to the bile, obstruction leads to acute inflammation, often progressing to gangrenous cholecystitis. A high enzyme content of gallbladder bile at the time of surgery was earlier demonstrated by Popper.[39] The frequent association of cholecystitis and pancreatitis suggests that the mechanism of their production through a mixture of bile and pancreatic juice is similar.[11]

Symptomatology. The symptoms of cholecystitis are so variable as to confuse this disorder with hiatus hernia, pancreatitis, appendicitis, duodenal ulcer, angina pectoris, regional enteritis and right-sided colon lesions. In other words, the symptoms vary with the severity of inflammation and the pain resulting from obstruction or local peritonitis.

In acute cholecystitis the pain may begin gradually or suddenly as biliary colic. It is generally assumed that pain referral to the epigastrium is via the splanchnic nerves originating in T_{7-10} and that subscapular pain may result from somatic referral by summation over the dorsal nerve roots beneath the scapula. Pain and tenderness in the right upper abdomen is secondary to parietal peritoneal involvement by an inflamed gallbladder (Fig. 29–4). During early stages, acute cholecystitis may simulate lesions which involve any portion of the foregut. Colic usually results from acute

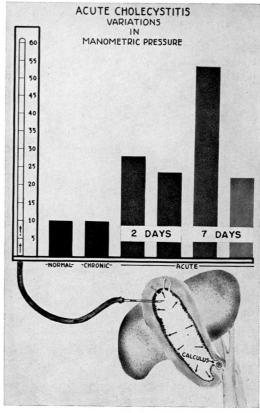

Fig. 29–3. Pressure measurements within the gallbladder at operation are increased greatly and are directly proportional to the duration of obstruction.

obstruction of the cystic or common bile ducts.

Experimental observations after mechanical distention of the gallbladder and common duct by means of a balloon introduced at the time of surgery have helped to explain biliary pain.[58] Overdistention of the gallbladder produced the feeling of indigestion or deep epigastric discomfort (Fig. 29–4). Pain was felt in the epigastrium rather than the right upper quadrant. Nausea, vomiting and referred pain to the back did not occur. Distention of the cystic and common ducts produced epigastric pain characteristic of biliary colic and accompanied by nausea and vomiting. More recent observations confirmed these findings but failed to explain the irregularity of occurrence of subscapular pain or why some

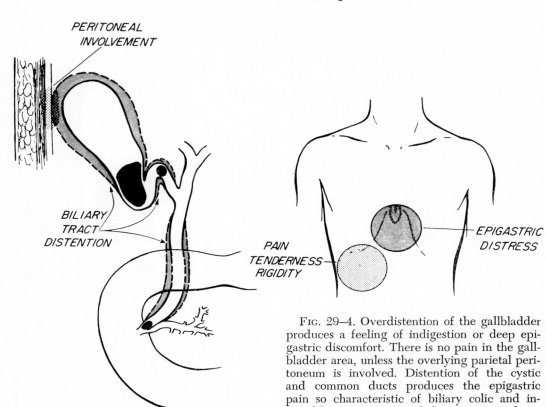

PERITONEAL
INVOLVEMENT

BILIARY
TRACT
DISTENTION

PAIN
TENDERNESS
RIGIDITY

EPIGASTRIC
DISTRESS

FIG. 29–4. Overdistention of the gallbladder produces a feeling of indigestion or deep epigastric discomfort. There is no pain in the gallbladder area, unless the overlying parietal peritoneum is involved. Distention of the cystic and common ducts produces the epigastric pain so characteristic of biliary colic and invariably is accompanied by nausea and involuntary vomiting.

patients fail to have any pain with acute distention of the bile ducts.

In chronic cholecystitis the symptoms may be vague. Abdominal distention and eructation may be due to air swallowing occasioned by mild discomfort due to temporary or partial occlusion of the cystic duct without acute inflammation. These symptoms more often follow ingestion of fat or a large meal. Since similar discomfort occurs with chronic pancreatitis, duodenal ulcer, hiatus hernia, carcinoma of the right colon and, rarely, diverticulitis of the colon, the history of onset, relation to meals, exact pain distribution and method of achieving relief is best for establishing a diagnosis. If an acute attack of colic pain is associated with jaundice the diagnosis is simple. Multiple acute attacks of pain may be due to the passage of small stones or an accompanying angina pectoris; the differential diagnosis may be difficult. The pain of angina occurs reflexly

from stimulation of the common bile duct[42]; electrocardiographic changes may also be noted.

Physical Examination. The physical findings are helpful only in the presence of common duct stone, hydrops or acute cholecystitis. Rarely is tenderness present with asymptomatic gallstones or uncomplicated cholecystitis. In acute cholecystitis the gallbladder occasionally is palpable and tender on deep inspiration. More often there may be either enough guarding and increased muscle tone to prevent delineation of a mass or the omentum surrounds the gallbladder and a poorly defined tender mass is noted in the right upper abdomen. Due to splinting of the right diaphragm, basalar atelectasis occurs and the presence of rales may lead to confusing the diagnosis of cholecystitis with pneumonia unless the examination is carefully performed.

Laboratory Data. Laboratory determinations are used to follow the course of acute cholecystitis, in the diagnosis of both acute and chronic cholecystitis, and as aids in differential diagnosis. The white blood count is almost invariably elevated with acute cholecystitis and a further increase after hydration of the patient suggests progression of the disease process and possible gangrene. The serum amylase may be slightly elevated; however, if the level exceeds 400 Somogyi units, pancreatitis is present. Pancreatitis accompanies approximately 15 per cent of cases of acute cholecystitis. Other laboratory tests should include the prothrombin time, determination of the blood urea nitrogen and blood sugar. In diabetics, cholecystitis may more rapidly progress to gangrene.

Roentgenographic examinations are of importance in both acute and chronic cholecystitis. Recumbent and supine abdominal as well as chest films help to differentiate other lesions such as pneumonia or perforated ulcer. When appendicitis or acute duodenal ulcer are considered in the differential diagnosis the intravenous cholangiogram has been used to eliminate cholecystitis.[23] This examination is of help only if the gallbladder shows clearly and, even so, can be misleading since an inflamed gallbladder is rarely visualized. In chronic cholecystitis, oral cholecystography must be accompanied by a thorough evaluation of the entire gastrointestinal and urinary tracts and occasionally the spine for other causes of pain. Unless such studies are performed, removal of the gallbladder will leave many patients with residual postcholecystectomy symptoms that were actually due to lesions outside the gallbladder.

Management. Patients with acute cholecystitis should be hospitalized for careful management. Although opinions vary between early and late surgical intervention, a selective approach has been found safer.[60, 62] After admission, patients are given intravenous fluids, antibiotics, atropine and nasogastric suction. The temperature, pulse, respirations, white blood count as well as changes in vital capacity and physical signs are recorded every 4 hours. Failure to subside or worsening after hydration demonstrated by increased pain and tenderness,

a white blood count above 20,000 or temperature over 101° F. are indications for surgical intervention. Care must be taken to differentiate increasing signs and white blood count due to pneumonia. Since four of five patients progressively improve on this management, their surgery can be deferred, thus permitting better evaluation before elective cholecystectomy.

Patients with chronic cholecystitis and cholelithiasis should have elective cholecystectomy unless there are specific contraindications. Even if gallstones are asymptomatic, more than one-third of these patients will develop complications within a decade of diagnosis.[52] Every effort should be made to improve operative risks and eliminate other disorders whose symptoms may mimic cholecystitis. Obesity should be corrected if possible, diabetes brought under control, and the tracheal-bronchial tree cleared. Angina pectoris is not a contraindication to elective surgery and may be greatly improved after cholecystectomy.

JAUNDICE

Jaundice is a major complication of disorders of the gallbladder and extrahepatic bile ducts. It may be difficult to determine its cause and to differentiate it from hepatocellular disease or intrahepatic obstruction. Since differential diagnosis including laboratory tests are discussed elsewhere, only a few comments are necessary here.

The relative frequency of various causes of jaundice noted in approximately 500 patients are shown in Figure 29–5. The pain pattern of stones is similar when they block the cystic or common ducts but nausea and vomiting are more common with common duct colic. Jaundice caused by stones is more often intermittent, whereas that due to tumor is usually progressive or constant. Common duct stones occur rarely without stones in the gallbladder. They are found in the common duct in approximately 20 per cent of patients with gallbladder stones. Of patients with choledocholithiasis, roughly 40 per cent are jaundiced at the time of surgery, 20 per cent have previously been jaundiced, but another 40 per cent have never been jaundiced before surgery.

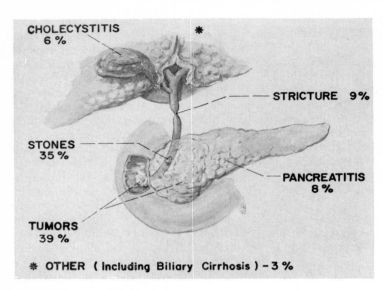

CHOLECYSTITIS
6 %

*

STRICTURE 9%

STONES
35%

PANCREATITIS
8%

TUMORS
39 %

* OTHER (Including Biliary Cirrhosis) – 3 %

FIG. 29–5. Frequency of causes of extrahepatic biliary tract obstruction is shown from nearly 500 surgical cases. Most cases of cholecystitis with jaundice have evidence of extrahepatic obstruction. (Fish, J. C., Williams D. D. and Williams, R. D.: Arch. Surg. 96:875, 1968.)

Percutaneous transhepatic cholangiography has been frequently used in recent years to determine the site and cause of obstruction or to differentiate intra- from extrahepatic causes of jaundice.[8] This technic, in which a long Teflon needle is inserted into either the left or right lobe of the liver, provides excellent cholangiograms. The examination is of most help in determining an inoperable malignant obstruction (Fig. 29–6); however, even in these patients a tissue diagnosis is often sought. Unfortunately, complications of this examination are fairly frequent.[8, 16, 17] Since leakage of bile is frequent, the examination must be performed just prior to surgery. The pressure should be lowered and not raised in the bile ducts if septicemia is to be avoided.

Jaundice associated with cholecystitis is common. It has been estimated that jaundice occurs in over 30 per cent of patients with acute cholecystitis but common duct stone is found in only 10 to 15 per cent of them.[20] Other causes of jaundice include pancreatitis, tumors, hepatitis and drug sensitivity producing intrahepatic obstruction. In many cases the cause remains unknown because of inadequate exploration or failure

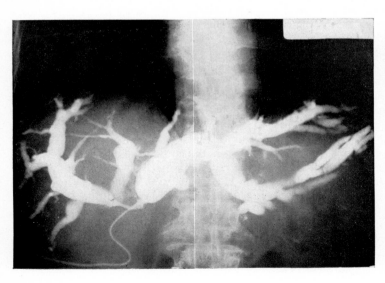

FIG. 29–6. Percutaneous transhepatic cholangiogram shows a carcinoma of the hepatic ducts found to be inoperable at surgery.

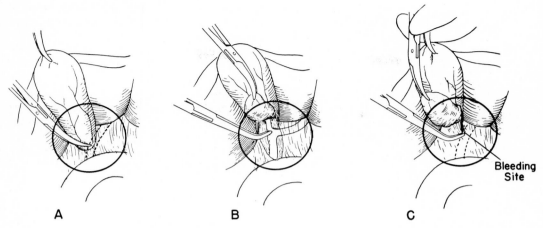

A   B   C

FIG. 29–7. Accidental injury to the common duct may result from: (A) failure to mobilize the ampulla, (B) angulation of the common duct, (C) blind application of clamp to bleeding point.

to biopsy the liver. Although it has been suggested that pancreatic enzymes cause cholangitis and jaundice,[17a] cholangitis as a cause of jaundice in the absence of bile duct obstruction must be rare. A review of the basis of icterus in patients requiring surgery for cholecystitis[15] suggests that it is usually obstruction of the common bile duct. A careful exploration of the pancreas, common duct and duodenum is necessary before assuming that the stone has passed or that cholangitis caused the jaundice.

PRINCIPLES OF SURGERY OF THE GALLBLADDER AND BILE DUCTS

Although the technic of cholecystectomy and choledochotomy may be found described elsewhere,[59] a few principles involved in surgery of the gallbladder and extrahepatic bile ducts will be mentioned. The mortality in biliary tract surgery varies from less than 0.5 per cent for elective cholecystectomy to over 10 per cent in jaundiced patients. Preoperative preparation may be as important as the surgery. Correction of obesity or a smoker's cough with chronic bronchitis significantly decreases complications. Vitamin K is needed in most jaundiced patients. If the patient is icteric and has lost weight or has even a mild anemia, preoperative transfusions are imperative.[12] Hypotension in jaundiced pa-

tients has been shown to more readily produce renal damage, and the resulting azotemia is poorly tolerated.[54] During the period of diagnostic evaluation a high protein and high caloric diet should be supplemented with bile salts or pancreatic extracts as needed to increase intestinal absorption.

The principles of surgical technic are shown in Figures 29–7, 29–8 and 29–9. Care must be exercised with full knowledge of the variations in anatomy to prevent accidental injury to the common or hepatic ducts. The common bile duct should be explored if enlarged or thickened or if jaundice is present. The use of operative cholangiography[40] either via the cystic duct or needle puncture of the common duct decreases the necessity of choledochotomy if the technic is carefully employed. Correct positioning with preliminary films to assure exposure and prevent the common duct from overlying the spine, cleansing of barium from the colon, and the use of a small amount of dilute (25 to 35 per cent) iodide solution are but a few of the important factors in obtaining good roentgenograms of the ductal system. Sloppy preparation and execution of this adjunct to biliary surgery will make cholangiography valueless. The same principles apply to postoperative cholangiograms (Fig. 29–10).

The usual procedure for cholelithiasis and

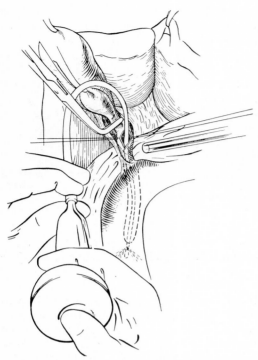

Fig. 29–8. It is advisable to irrigate the passages in an effort to dislodge and wash downward any overlooked stones in the hepatic ducts. Patency of the ampulla of Vater must be proved before closure.

cholecystitis is cholecystectomy. Cholecystostomy is rarely preferred in elderly, poorrisk patients and can be accomplished under local anesthesia. After removing the stones and inserting a catheter into the gallbladder it is preferable to suture the gallbladder to the anterior peritoneum. Exploration of the common duct will be indicated in the presence of jaundice, a history of recurrent jaundice, chills or fever, pancreatitis, or findings at surgery suggesting partial obstruction.

The common duct must be explored gently but thoroughly. Small, malleable pituitary scoops are preferable to remove stones. French woven catheters with gentle tapered olive tips of various sizes permit irrigation while sounding the bile ducts (Fig. 29–9). Forceful irrigation with cold or hot saline or forceful dilatation of the ampulla assures no better chance of remov-

ing the elusive stone, but does increase the chances of postoperative pancreatitis. Although the pancreatic head must be adequately examined in many cases by mobilization of the duodenum, duodenotomy for stone removal is rarely necessary if common duct exploration is gentle and thorough. The common duct should be drained with a simple catheter or a T tube whose limbs are short and do not pass through the ampulla to block the pancreatic duct. Although primary closure of the common duct has been advocated under special conditions,[44] this technic is not popular.

After surgery, close observation for potential complications is necessary. Atelectasis, bleeding, pancreatitis and bile leaks are the most significant complications. Pancreatitis is usually the most serious and may be overlooked if serum amylase determinations are not made. A drain placed along the gallbladder bed may be removed in 48 hours if there is no bile drainage. Should bile leak along this drain, it may come from an accessory duct, the cystic duct stump or around the T tube in the common duct; leakage should stop unless obstruction was overlooked. If a tube was left in the common duct it should never be clamped unless it is to remain a long time as a stint. It can safely be determined when to remove this tube; clamping is dangerous and only pain, bile leakage or fever can result if there is obstruction. If bile flows through the duct with the tube elevated 10 to 12 cm. above duct level (i.e., on the abdomen) or if sterile saline perfuses through the duct readily at pressures less than 12 cm. of water, the tube can be safely removed. If not, cholangiography and a thorough evaluation of the cause of obstruction must be carried out.

SUPPURATIVE CHOLANGITIS

Acute suppurative cholangitis is a severe complication of biliary tract obstruction. Bacterial growth in bile is inhibited until partial or complete obstruction alters the bile and permits E. coli, Pseudomonas, Klebsiella or even clostridia to proliferate. The basis for diagnosis of acute suppurative cholangitis includes an acute illness, evidence of obstruction and frank pus in the common duct.[24] Charcot's triad (jaundice, chills and fever and pain in the right upper abdomen) is still considered by some as necessary for the diagnosis; however, all patients may not fulfill the criteria.

Since suppurative cholangitis carries a high mortality, attention to factors causing infection and septicemia is important in its management. In most cases the obstruction is due to a common duct stone and gram-negative organisms are present. Septicemia and bacteremia occur rather suddenly, apparently due to an increase in the degree of obstruction of the bile ducts. If intrahepatic abscesses have not formed, decom-

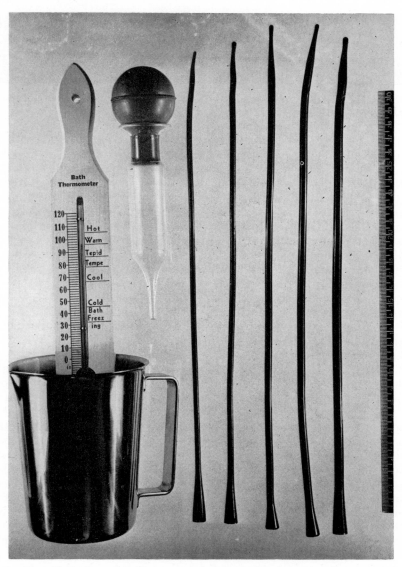

FIG. 29–9. French, silk-woven, olive-tipped catheters and an Asepto syringe are used to inject warm saline into the ductal system. Under no circumstances should saline be injected without first determining its exact temperature by a thermometer reading. The temperature should not exceed 110°F.

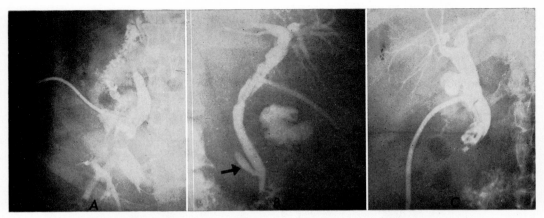

FIG. 29–10. Postoperative cholangiograms. (A) Blood clot in dilated duct simulating overlooked stone. (B) Common channel. (C) Overlooked stones with long-armed T tube which prevents washing out by irrigation.

pression of the common duct gives dramatic results. Recent observations in our laboratory show that bacteremia is related to the pressure in the bile ducts.[57] Bacteria enter the bloodstream via the hepatic veins or lymph when intraductal pressures rise above 200 mm. water and this bacteremia may be rapidly fatal. Emergency decompression of the common duct appears to be mandatory if mortality in cholangitis is to be lowered. On the other hand, since mortality is higher in patients with increasing rather than stable or decreasing jaundice who do not have infection, cholangitis is the only indication for emergency surgery in jaundiced patients.

CHOLESTEROLOSIS AND HYDROPS

Cholesterolosis, or a "strawberry gallbladder," is a metabolic disease characterized by polypoid enlargement of the villi which contain yellowish deposits of cholesterol which are visible grossly. Seedlike projections from the mucosa may break off, float free in the gallbladder and act as a central nidus for crystallization of bile pigments, cholesterol or calcium. The lesion is of little clinical importance, and cholecystectomy is not indicated unless stones are present.

Hydrops of the gallbladder is produced by chronic obstruction of the cystic duct in the absence of acute inflammation. The pig-

ment is absorbed from the contained bile, and the gallbladder distends because of continued mucous secretion from its lining, and may be palpable as a smooth, tender mass. The contents of the obstructed viscus are sterile and are known as "white bile." However, if the contents become infected, empyema results, and operative intervention becomes urgent.

CHOLECYSTOENTERIC FISTULA

Acute recurrent bouts of cholecystitis usually lead to adhesions between the gallbladder, duodenum and colon. Occasionally there is adherence to the anterior gastric wall. After many years or following gangrenous cholecystitis large stones repeatedly obstructing the gallbladder outlet may erode from the gallbladder into the intestine. The fistula more often occurs between gallbladder and duodenum. The large stones usually obstruct the intestine[49]; this can be diagnosed more readily if suspected (Fig. 29–11). Most patients with gallstone intestinal obstruction are over age 65, have vague upper abdominal symptoms for many years, develop intermittent obstruction which in a period of a few days becomes complete as the stone tumbles down the gut, and may have the typical diagnostic radiographic finding of air in the biliary tree. The obstruction is readily removed by enterotomy. Due to the patient's age, complicating dis-

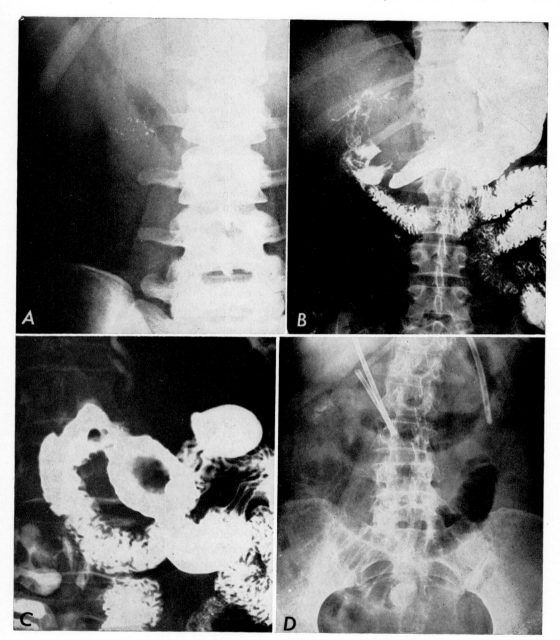

F IG. 29–11. Internal biliary fistulae. X-ray examination of the abdomen may demonstrate (A) air or (B) barium in the biliary tree. (C) Large solitary gallstone outlined in duodenum by barium swallow. (D) Gallstone ileus. Note radiopaque gallstones in the right upper quadrant and near the midline anterior to the sacrum. The latter stone is impacted in the terminal ileum.

eases and delays in diagnosis, the mortality remains above 10 per cent. Repair of the fistula at the time of enterotomy is rarely indicated and may increase mortality. Late symptoms of biliary fistula may require subsequent repair.

SCLEROSING CHOLANGITIS (SECONDARY)

Occasionally during surgery for cholelithiasis or suspected chronic cholecystitis the bile ducts are found markedly thickened, yet of normal diameter while the gallbladder is relatively uninvolved. More often these patients present with chronic mild jaundice. A cholangiogram may show narrowed intrahepatic bile ducts and irregularity of the extrahepatic ducts. The cause of this disorder is unknown, and treatment, including prolonged drainage of the common bile duct and administration of steroids, has been disappointing. Biopsy of the ducts will show chronic inflammation involving the ductal glands, mucosa and the entire duct wall with bile pigmentation in areas of inflammation. The inflammation may spread into the small intrahepatic ducts which show periductal sclerosis. Cholestatic jaundice may persist in spite of the patent main bile duct.[32] Biopsy of the bile ducts may prove particularly helpful in excluding sclerosing carcinoma.[2]

INJURY AND STRICTURE OF THE BILE DUCTS

Except those that occur during surgery, traumatic injuries to the extrahepatic bile ducts and gallbladder are infrequent.[9] The majority of violent traumatic injuries are penetrating and occur more often in men. If the gallbladder is injured, it is preferable to remove it. Since bile duct injuries are so uncommon and variable, no outline for treatment, other than to avoid simple closure, can be readily presented.

Injuries to the bile ducts occurring during surgery are most unfortunate. They usually are the result of hasty surgery, lack of exposure and unfamiliarity with the variable anatomy in the area of the junction of the cystic and common ducts. Jaundice usually occurs shortly after surgery and is progressive. Occasionally jaundice develops late and, since the degree of stenosis varies, it may be mild or intermittent.

Since over half of these injuries involve the hepatic ducts, the theory that they are due to "tenting" of the common duct and clamping it during dissection of the cystic duct may not be plausible.[48] Stricture probably results from direct damage to the ducts rather than subsequent bile leaks or infection. The surgical procedures used in the management of bile duct strictures are too varied to discuss adequately here. Although bile duct injury should be recognized and repaired immediately, even then the repair may be unsuccessful.[31] Despite numerous attempts to find substitutes for damaged, strictured or absent extrahepatic bile ducts, biliary dynamics[51] are not conducive to success with these prosthetics.

TUMORS OF THE GALLBLADDER

Benign tumors of the gallbladder are uncommon, but papillomas, adenomas, fibromas, lipomas and cystadenomas have been described. The papilloma and adenoma are the most frequent. The former consists of hyperplastic mucosal villi filled with cholesterol and having the strawberry appearance of cholesterolosis. Adenomas occur primarily in the fundus where they may be seen on a cholecystogram or palpated during surgery. Most benign tumors are incidental findings of surgery and are cured by cholecystectomy.

Carcinoma of the gallbladder is a serious lesion considered by some surgeons to be a complication of gallstones. This cancer occurs in 0.2 to 0.4 per cent of the population and approximately 2.5 per cent of patients requiring surgery of the gallbladder and bile ducts. Its incidence increases with age. Cholelithiasis occurs in 70 to 90 per cent of patients with this carcinoma. Although tumors have been produced experimentally in animals with foreign bodies in the gallbladder, the relationship between gallstones and cancer in man remains primarily statistical.

Since carcinoma of the gallbladder is such an insidious disease, the diagnosis is seldom made before surgery. Symptoms vary from those of acute cholecystitis to weight loss progressing to painless jaundice. Unless the lesion is far advanced, no clinical or laboratory data differentiate carcinoma from cholecystitis. Despite late diagnosis and considerable pessimism in the past, gallbladder cancer can often be successfully treated surgically if liver and node resection are adequate.[13]

TUMORS OF THE EXTRAHEPATIC BILE DUCTS

Although primary cancer of the biliary tract can occur anywhere, the most common sight outside of the gallbladder is at the ampulla. This lesion occurs in patients somewhat older than those with gallbladder cancer. A correct diagnosis is rare before surgery since it may be confused with pancreatic carcinoma or common duct stone. The papillomatous type of carcinoma which obstructs early has a better prognosis than nodular infiltrating lesions.

The most common presenting complaints are pain and jaundice. Formerly considered uncommon in malignant obstruction of the bile ducts, pain is present in more than three-fourths of these patients. The pain may be in the epigastrium, referred to the subscapular region or penetrating into the high lumbar back region. The majority of patients lose considerable weight because of pain and poor utilization of food before hospitalization.

Jaundice is acute in onset and progressive. By the time of hospitalization the physical and laboratory signs of complete biliary obstruction may be present. Since the gallbladder is enlarged in 80 per cent or more of cases, the so-called positive Courvoisier's law (Fig. 29–12) is of help in differentiating tumor obstruction from common duct stone. (See also Chapter 8, Jaundice.)

Surgical intervention must be carefully planned. Blood volume deficits are usual and require preoperative replacement to prevent operative or postoperative hypotension followed by azotemia. If there is evidence of malabsorption due to combined bile and pancreatic duct obstruction, preoperative high caloric feedings will require pancreatic and bile supplements. Water-soluble vitamin K will be necessary to raise and maintain prothrombin levels. The intestinal and urinary tracts must be evaluated carefully to exclude a primary carcinoma which has metastasized and caused bile duct obstruction. Just before surgery, percutaneous cholangiography helps to define

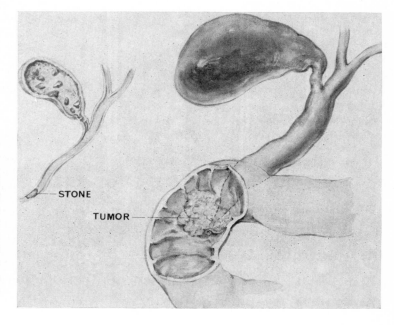

FIG. 29–12. Courvoisier's law. The thick-walled, indurated gallbladder, usually associated with cholelithiasis, cannot distend with extrahepatic duct obstruction. Tumor obstruction results in marked dilatation of the gallbladder which is often palpable. (Williams, R. D., and Fish, J. C.: Arch. Surg. 95:374.)

STONE

TUMOR

the site and cause of obstruction and perhaps shorten the operation.

Surgical exploration may permit either resection[14] or only biopsy and relief of jaundice.[55] A tissue diagnosis should be made if at all possible. It may be impossible to differentiate bile duct and pancreatic carcinoma; resection gives better results with the former. Rarely resection of carcinoma outside the ampulla is successful.[38] Since the majority of procedures are palliative only and many do not even relieve jaundice, an expeditious approach should be made to establish a diagnosis and to provide, if possible, internal bile drainage.

REFERENCES

1. Alonzo-Lej, F., Rever, W. B., Jr., and Pessagno, D. J.: Congenital choledochal cyst: collective review, Int. Abstr. Surg. *108*:1, 1959.
2. Altemeier, W. A., Gall, E. A., Culbertson, W. R., and Inge, W. W.: Sclerosing carcinoma of the intrahepatic (hilar) bile ducts, Surgery *60*:191, 1966.
3. Amoury, R. A., and Barker, H. G.: Multiple biliary enteric fistulas, Am. J. Surg. *111*:180, 1966.
4. Bartlett, R. W., Crile, G., Jr., and Graham, E. N.: A lymphatic connection between the gallbladder and the liver, Surg. Gynec. Obstet. *61*:363, 1953.
5. Beal, J. M.: Present status of biliary tract surgery, Surg. Clin. N. Amer. *46*:69, 1966.
6. Branch, C. D., and Zollinger, R. M.: Acute cholecystitis, New Engl. J. Med. *214*:1173, 1936.
7. Cameron, A. L., and Noble, J. L.: Reflux of bile up the duct of Wirsung caused by an impacted biliary calculus, J.A.M.A. *82*:1410, 1924.
8. Castiglioni, G. C., and Petronio, R.: Percutaneous intrahepatic cholangiography as a diagnostic aid in posthepatic jaundice, Surgery *56*:635, 1964.
9. Diethrich, E. B., Beall, A. C., Jr., Jordan, G. L., Jr., and DeBakey, M. E.: Traumatic injuries to the extrahepatic biliary tract, Am. J. Surg. *112*:756, 1966.
10. Doubilet, H., and Mulholland, J. H.: Eight year study of pancreatitis and sphincterotomy, J.A.M.A. *160*:521, 1956.
11. Elliott, D. W., Williams, R. D., and Zollinger, R. M.: Alterations in the pancreatic resistance to bile in the pathogenesis of acute pancreatitis, Ann. Surg. *146*:669, 1957.
12. Ellison, E. H., Zollinger, R. M., Cedars, N., and Britt, C. I.: Value of blood volume determinations in gastrointestinal disease, A.M.A. Arch. Surg. *66*:869, 1953.
13. Fahim, R. B., Ferris, D. O., and McDonald, J. R.: Carcinoma of the gallbladder: appraisal of its surgical treatment, Arch. Surg. *86*:334, 1963.
14. Fish, J. C., and Cleveland, B. R.: Pancreaticoduodenectomy for periampullary carcinoma: an analysis of 38 cases, Ann. Surg. *159*:469, 1964.
15. Fish, J. C., Williams, D. D., and Williams, R. D.: Jaundice with cholecystitis, Arch. Surg. *96*:875, 1968.
16. Flemma, R. J., Capp, M. P., and Shingleton, W. W.: Percutaneous transhepatic cholangiography, Arch. Surg. *90*:5, 1965.
17. Flemma, R. J., Flint, L. M., Osterhout, S., and Shingleton, W. W.: Bacteriologic studies of biliary tract infection, Ann. Surg. *166*:563, 1967.
17a. Foley, J. J., and Ellison, E. H.: Infusion of pancreatic enzymes into the biliary radicals of the liver, Arch. Surg. *88*:589, 1964.
18. Frey, C., Thorpe, C., and Abrams, G.: Gallstone formation in germ-free mouse, Am. J. Surg. *115*:75, 1968.
19. Friedman, G. D., Kannel, W. B., and Dawber, T. R.: Epidemiology of gallbladder disease: observations in the Framingham study, J. Chronic Dis. *19*:273, 1966.
20. Glenn, F.: Chronic and acute cholecystitis and common duct stone, Am. J. Gastroent. *44*:232, 1965.
21. Glenn, F., and Hays, D. M.: The causes of death following biliary tract surgery for non-malignant disease, Surg. Gynec. Obstet. *94*:283, 1952.
22. Graham, E. A., and Cole, W. H.: Roentgenologic examination of the gallbladder. Preliminary report of a new method utilizing intravenous injection of tetrabromophenolphthalein, J.A.M.A. *82*:613, 1924.
23. Harrington, O. B., Beall, A. C., Jr., Noon, G., and De Bakey, M. E.: Intravenous cholangiography in acute chole-

cystitis: use in differential diagnosis, Arch. Surg. 88:585, 1964.

24. Haupert, A. P., Carey, L. C., Evans, W. E., and Ellison, E. H.: Acute suppurative cholangitis, Arch. Surg. 94:460, 1967.

25. Hoerr, S. O., and Hazard, J. B.: Acute cholecystitis without gallbladder stones, Am. J. Surg. 111:47, 1966.

26. Hughes, J., LoCurcio, S. B., Edmunds, R., and Finby, N.: The common duct after cholecystectomy; initial report of a 10 year study, J.A.M.A. 197:247, 1966.

27. Jacoby, F.: Mitotic activity in the gallbladder epithelium in the guinea pig after ligation of the common bile duct, J. Physiol. (London) 119:21P, 1953.

28. Judd, E. S., and Mann, F. C.: The effect of removal of the gallbladder: an experimental study, Surg. Gynec. Obstet. 24:437, 1917.

29. Lagache, G., Leplat, F., Combemale, B., and Proye, C.: Retentissement biliaire de la vagotomie pour ulcère, Ann. Chir. 20:607, 1966.

30. Large, A. M.: On the formation of gallstones, Surgery 54:928, 1963.

31. Longmire, W. P., Jr.: Early management of injury to the extrahepatic biliary tract, J.A.M.A. 195:623, 1966.

32. Longmire, W. P., Jr., Joseph, W. L., Levin, P. M., and Mellinkoff, S. M.: Diagnosis and treatment of cholangiolitic hepatitis (primary biliary cirrhosis), Ann. Surg. 162:356, 1965.

33. Ludwick, J. R., and Bass, P.: Contractile and electric activity of the extrahepatic biliary tract and duodenum, Surg. Gynec. Obstet. 124:536, 1967.

34. Mahour, G. H., Wakim, K. G., and Ferris, D. O.: The common bile duct in man: its diameter and circumference, Ann. Surg. 165:415, 1967.

35. Maki, T., Pathogenesis of calcium bilirubinate gallstone, Ann. Surg. 164:90, 1966.

36. Michels, N. A.: The hepatic cystic and retroduodenal arteries and their relation to the biliary ducts, Ann. Surg. 133:503, 1951.

37. Millbourn, E.: On acute pancreatic affections following gastric resection for ulcer or cancer and possibilities of avoiding them, Acta chir. scand. 98:1, 1949.

38. Monge, J. J., and Rudie, P. S.: Segmental resection of the common hepatic duct for carcinoma, Arch. Surg. 93:1015, 1966.

39. Popper, H. L.: Pankreassaft in den Gallenwegen. Seine pathogenetische Bedeutung für die Entstehung der akuten Pankreaserkrankungen, Arch. klin. Chir. 175:660, 1933.

40. Pyrtek, L. J., and Bartus, S. H.: Critical evaluation of routine and selective operating room cholangiography, Am. J. Surg. 103:761, 1962.

41. Rains, A. J. H.: Researches concerning the formation of gallstones, Brit. Med. J. 2:685, 1962.

42. Ravdin, I. S., Royster, H. P., and Sanders, G. P.: Reflexes originating in the common duct giving rise to pain simulating angina pectoris, Ann. Surg. 115:1055, 1942.

43. Rienhoff, W. F., Jr., and Pickrell, K. L.: Pancreatitis: an anatomic study of the pancreatic and extrahepatic biliary systems, Arch. Surg. 51:205, 1945.

44. Sawyers, J. L., Herrington, L. J., Jr., and Edwards, W. H.: Primary closure of the common bile duct, Am. J. Surg. 109:107, 1965.

45. Sterling, J. A.: Biliary tract morphology and prognosis of biliary atresia, Am. J. Gastroent. 45:261, 1966.

46. Thureborn, E.: The stratification of bile and its importance for the solubility of cholesterol, Gastroenterology 50:775, 1966.

47. Wagner, D. E., Elliott, D. W., Endahl, G. L., and MacPherson, C. T.: Specific pancreatic enzymes in the etiology of acute cholecystitis, Surgery 50:259, 1962.

48. Warren, K. W., and McDonald, W. M.: Facts and fiction regarding strictures of the extrahepatic bile ducts, Ann. Surg. 159:996, 1964.

49. Warshaw, A. L., and Bartlett, M. K.: Choice of operation for gallstone intestinal obstruction, Ann. Surg. 164:1051, 1966.

50. Watkins, D. H., and Salzman, E.: Opacifying gallstones: utility of a new examination for the demonstration of duct stones useful in the presence of jaundice, A.M.A. Arch. Surg. 80:986, 1960.

51. Watts, J. McK., and Dunphy, J. E.: The role of the common bile duct in biliary dynamics, Surg., Gynec. Obstet. 122:1207, 1966.

52. Wenckert, A., and Robertson, B.: Natural course of gallstone disease, Gastroenterology 50:376, 1966.

53. Williams, R. D.: Partial and intermittent biliary tract obstruction, Am. Surgeon 32:479, 1966.

54. Williams, R. D., Elliott, D. W., and Zollinger, R. M.: The effect of hypotension in obstructive jaundice, A.M.A. Arch. Surg. 81:334, 1960.

55. ———: Surgery for malignant jaundice, A.M.A. Arch. Surg. 80:992, 1960.

56. Williams, R. D., and Fish, J. C.: The significance of biliary pressure, Arch. Surg. 95:374, 1967.

57. Williams, R. D., and Huang, T. T.: Effect of bile duct pressure on bacteremia and septicemia in experimental cholangitis. (Surgery, 1969. In press.)

58. Zollinger, R. M.: Observations following distention of the gallbladder and common bile duct in man, Proc. Soc. Exp. Biol. Med. 30:1260, 1932-33.

59. Zollinger, R. M., and Cutler, E. C. (eds.): Atlas of Surgical Operations, 3rd ed., New York, Macmillan, 1961.

60. Zollinger, R. M., and Gross, H. T.: The acute gallbladder, Ohio St. Med. J. 44: 473, 1948.

61. Zollinger, R. M., and Sirak, H. D.: Gallbladder surgery in patients in the older age group, J. Am. Geriat. Soc. 2:46, 1954.

62. Zollinger, R. M., and Williams, R. D.: Cholecystectomy, J.A.M.A. 190:145, 1964.

30

Miscellaneous Disorders

Jaundice During Pregnancy

URS PETER HAEMMERLI, M.D.

THE LIVER IN NORMAL PREGNANCY

The liver functions well during pregnancy. However, most "liver function tests" show some deviations from the accepted normal for nonpregnant subjects. These disturbances are usually of minor degree, are more common in the later weeks of pregnancy and are rapidly rectified after delivery.

Table 30–1 summarizes these changes in relation to the stage of gestation. During pregnancy it is best to accept for all laboratory tests an intermediary range between certainly normal and certainly abnormal results. In this intermediary range a laboratory result may or may not have pathologic significance because physiologic deviations from the accepted normal occur only in some pregnant women. For this reason the most valuable tests to assess liver function are those that remain normal in all cases of uncomplicated pregnancies, i.e., the serum transaminases and 5-nucleotidase and the prothrombin time. For the same reason liver biopsy may be used more often than outside pregnancy in order to clarify some puzzling biochemical findings. Main diagnostic difficulties will be encountered with raised serum alkaline phosphatase levels and pathologic turbidity and flocculation tests, as well as in most cases with mild jaundice.

The liver is difficult to palpate toward term, for the enlarging uterus displaces the liver upward, backward and to the right. A readily palpable liver in the third trimester nearly always has pathologic significance. It is equally difficult to palpate the spleen. Spider angiomatas occur in up to two thirds of normal pregnancies, and may appear as early as the second month of gestation, increasing sharply between the second and fifth month and more slowly thereafter. They are usually inconspicuous and are missed by most obstetricians. After delivery most of these angiomata disappear. Palmar erythema is also found in about two thirds of normal gestations, and about half of the cases have both spider angiomata and palmar erythema.

Liver histology in uncomplicated pregnancy reveals only minor nonspecific changes. There is some variation in size and shape of liver cells and nuclei, a slight increase in binucleated cells, rarely an incipient ballooning of centroacinar liver cells, a mild increase in glycogen content, and occasionally slight lymphocytic infiltration and minor ductular proliferation in the normal-sized portal spaces. The Kupffer cells may be slightly proliferated and mobilized and contain more PAS positive granules than normal. In PAS stains treated with diastase the framework is somewhat thicker than in the absence of pregnancy.

Pregnancy leads to an increase in total body water of approximately 20 per cent, an increase in total blood volume and plasma volume of 50 to 65 per cent and a relatively minor increase in total red cell mass. Cardiac output is increased 30 to 50

1. *No changes*
   Serum transaminases
   Serum 5-nucleotidase
   Prothrombin time
   Oral galactose tolerance test
   Liver blood flow
2. *Minor nonspecific changes*
   Liver displacement by enlarging uterus
   Liver histology
3. *Progressive decrease toward term*
   Hemoglobin
   Hematocrit
   Total erythrocyte count
   Total serum proteins
   Serum albumin
   Serum gamma globulin
   Serum cholinesterase
   Intravenous bilirubin tolerance test
   Maximal Bromsulphalein excretory
      capacity (T_m)
4. *Progressive increase toward term*
   Spider nevi and palmar erythema
   Total white cell count
   Segmented and nonsegmented granulo-
      cytes
   Myelocytes and metamyelocytes
   Erythrocyte sedimentation rate
   Serum alkaline phosphatase
   Serum leucine aminopeptidase
   Serum cholesterol
   Total serum lipids
   Alpha- and beta-lipoproteins
   Phospholipids
   Serum alpha- and beta-globulins
   Serum fibrinogen
   Coagulation factors VII, VIII, IX, X
   Bromsulphalein retention
   Hepatic Bromsulphalein storage capacity
      (S)
   Total body water
   Cardiac output
   Total blood volume
   Plasma volume
   Erythrocyte volume
5. *Occasional increase not dependent on stage
   of gestation*
   Urinary bile pigments
   Serum bilirubin
   Serum turbidity and flocculation tests
6. *Erratic behavior, both abnormally low and
   high levels*
   Serum iron

per cent. Liver blood flow remains quantitatively unchanged but decreases in relation to cardiac output. The excess blood volume is shunted through the placenta. These changes reach their maximum in the 7th month.

Among the laboratory examinations, the most marked deviations from the accepted normal are found in the peripheral blood counts. In only about half of all normal pregnancies are the white cell and differential counts normal. Total white cell counts increase in about 20 per cent of gestations, and levels of 10,000 to 15,000 white cells/ cu.mm. are considered normal in the last trimester. Both segmented and nonsegmented granulocytes may increase, and myelocytes and metamyelocytes can be found, sometimes independent of any "shift to the left." Hemoglobin levels and hematocrit fall progressively to about 85 to 90 per cent of levels considered normal in nonpregnant women. During the last trimester, anemia is defined as a hemoglobin value below 10 Gm./100 ml. Serum iron concentrations remain on the whole constant, but may fluctuate widely between 50 and 300 mcg./100 ml. in individual cases. There is no correlation between serum iron and hemoglobin levels. Iron-binding capacity increases and iron saturation falls correspondingly.

Changes in serum proteins are reflected in an increasing erythrocyte sedimentation rate. Total serum proteins fall progressively toward term and levels below 6 Gm./100 ml. are found in about half of pregnant women. On serum electrophoresis, there is a distinct fall in serum albumin, a slight increase in alpha and beta globulins and a minor decrease in gamma globulins. The albumin/globulin ratio falls correspondingly, on the average from 1.3 to 0.7. The reports on serum turbidity and flocculation reactions are more conflicting. Thymol turbidity, cephalin flocculation, Takata reaction and cadmium reaction are normal in some series, in others they give pathologic results in 5 to 40 per cent of cases. It is possible that the results of the tests are greatly affected by differences in technic and reagents used. The positive reactions usually occur independent of the stage of gestation.

The prothrombin time remains normal, but fibrinogen and coagulation factors VII, VIII, IX and X are often increased toward term.

Serum cholesterol starts to rise in the 4th month and reaches a maximum in the 8th month. More than half of all uncomplicated pregnancies are characterized by a level of more than 250 mg./100 ml. and values of up to 500 mg./100 ml. are still considered normal at term. There is a corresponding rise in total serum lipids, phospholipids and alpha- and beta-lipoproteins.

Among the serum enzymes, the changes in alkaline phosphatase are most often noted. Mean values for all uncomplicated pregnancies rise slowly during the first half of pregnancy, then sharply during the 7th month and reach a peak at term. The observed rise depends on the method used. Mean values at term reach the upper limit of normal with the King-Armstrong method, slightly surpass the upper limit of normal with the Bodansky, Buch and Buch, Bessey-Lowry and Shinowara-Jones-Reinhart technics and reach twice the upper limit of normal with the Roberts and the Vermehren methods. Many individuals of course surpass these mean values, whereas others remain normal. The same holds true for serum leucine aminopeptidase. During gestation the observed rise of both these enzymes apparently originates from the placenta and not from the hepatobiliary tract. Serum 5-nucleotidase, an enzyme paralleling the liver-specific component of alkaline phosphatase, remains normal throughout pregnancy and has therefore a special diagnostic value. Serum lactic dehydrogenase and serum ornithyl carbamyl transferase may become elevated in some cases toward term. Serum tributyrinase and serum cholinesterase decrease toward term and the latter may be abnormally low in about two fifths of all cases in the 3rd trimester. SGOT and SGPT remain normal throughout pregnancy and are therefore the most useful serum enzymes to detect parenchymal liver disease during gestation.

An impairment of hepatic excretory capacity is reflected by an increased Bromsulphalein retention during the last month of gestation. Mean retention after 45 minutes at term is about 10 per cent, and values up to 15 per cent must be considered normal. With the Bromsulphalein infusion technic of Wheeler, the maximal Bromsulphalein excretory capacity (T_m) decreases after the 5th month of pregnancy, whereas hepatic storage capacity (S) increases. Similarly, bilirubin is retained in the second half of pregnancy on intravenous bilirubin tolerance tests. In 2 to 6 per cent of uncomplicated pregnancies the serum bilirubin may be elevated to between 1 and 2 mg./100 ml., and in about 20 per cent of women with normal total serum bilirubin the direct-reacting fraction is increased. In these cases the serum bilirubin does not rise further toward term; in fact the subclinical icterus occurs independent of the stage of gestation. Data on urinary bile components are scanty. In a small percentage of cases urinary bilirubin, urobilinogen and/or urobilin may be present or increased. In contrast to the impaired Bromsulphalein excretion the oral galactose tolerance test remains normal.

During labor, there is a further increase in alkaline phosphatase, serum transaminases, lactic dehydrogenase and Bromsulphalein retention. After delivery, most deviations from the pre-pregnancy norm are rectified within 2 weeks. Elevated alkaline phosphatase levels may become normal in 4 to 6 weeks, and serum protein, 6 to 12 weeks.

INCIDENCE AND CLASSIFICATION OF JAUNDICE DURING PREGNANCY

Jaundice during pregnancy is rare. In a collective series from the world literature the incidence of jaundice was 0.067 per cent among 822,842 pregnancies, or 1 case per 1,500 gestations. In single series, the incidence varies between 1 per 300 to 1 per 5,000 cases. At least 40 per cent of all cases of jaundice during pregnancy are due to infectious hepatitis and at least 20 per cent to intrahepatic cholestasis of pregnancy. In about 10 per cent, jaundice is a consequence of another complication of pregnancy. Rare causes of jaundice during gestation are obstructive gallstone disease and hemolysis. Many patients with mild jaundice and few

TABLE 30–2. JAUNDICE DURING PREGNANCY
(ICTERUS GRAVIDARUM)

A. Jaundice in pregnancy (Synonyms: icterus in graviditate, concomitant jaundice, coincidental jaundice, ictère intercurrent)
  I. Usual forms of jaundice that occur also in nonpregnant persons
    1. Hepatic parenchymal disease (especially viral hepatitis)
    2. Intrahepatic cholestasis (i.e., drug jaundice)
    3. Extrahepatic cholestasis (i.e., common duct stones)
    4. Congenital "idiopathic" hyperbilirubinemias
    5. Hemolytic disorders
  II. Jaundice in typical medical complications of pregnancy
    1. Jaundice in severe pyelonephritis
    2. Jaundice in pyelonephritis and tetracycline toxicity
    3. Delayed chloroform poisoning
    4. Jaundice after (criminal) abortions (Clostridium perfringens septicemia, quinine toxicity, etc.)
B. Jaundice of pregnancy (Synonyms: icterus e graviditate, icterus graviditatis, icterus peculiar to pregnancy, ictère lié à la grossesse)
  I. Idiopathic jaundice of pregnancy
    1. Intrahepatic cholestasis of pregnancy ("jaundice of late pregnancy," "recurrent jaundice of pregnancy")
    2. Acute fatty metamorphosis of pregnancy ("obstetric acute yellow atrophy")
  II. Jaundice as a complication of another disease linked to pregnancy
    1. Jaundice in hyperemesis gravidarum
    2. Jaundice in severe toxemia of pregnancy
    3. Jaundice with hydatiform mole
    4. Jaundice in megaloblastic anemia of pregnancy
    5. Jaundice in hemolytic anemia of pregnancy
C. Nonclassified cases

symptoms are difficult to classify without liver biopsy; most of these are mild forms of viral hepatitis.

A classification of jaundice during pregnancy is given in Table 30–2. The following definitions are used: Jaundice *during* pregnancy designates all forms of jaundice, jaundice *in* pregnancy all forms of icterus that may also occur in nonpregnant persons, and jaundice *of* pregnancy those forms of jaundice that are observed only in pregnant women. The two main categories are both subdivided into primary forms of jaundice and those that occur as a complication of another disease.

JAUNDICE IN PREGNANCY

Any disease that causes jaundice may by chance occur during pregnancy. Theoretically, the course of this disease could be altered by gestation, and, vice versa, the disease might affect the course of pregnancy and the health of the unborn child. Such mutual influences are, however, surprisingly few. The effect is clearly deleterious only in the combination of gestation and certain hemoglobinopathies. An impression not supported by facts is that in an icteric disease itching is more frequent in pregnant than in nonpregnant persons. Any form of jaundice during pregnancy predisposes to premature delivery. Survival of the newborn in these cases depends on the degree of maturity and not on the cause of the mother's disease.

Infectious viral hepatitis is the most frequent cause of jaundice during pregnancy. Pregnant women are, however, no more susceptible to infection than the same age class in the general population; in fact they may be less often afflicted. Viral hepatitis occurs in all trimesters of gestation. The course of the disease is not necessarily more severe than in the nonpregnant female and symptoms and jaundice are often surprisingly mild. Mortality from hepatitis during pregnancy was 1.8 per cent in a collective European series, which is somewhat less than in the general population. An exception to this rule is found among the indigent population of the North African Mediterranean area with a mortality of 24 per cent and in Asia with a mortality of 50 per cent. In these countries, the course of hepatitis during pregnancy is extremely severe and most patients are admitted to hospital already in hepatic coma. The general debility and undernutrition of this population makes the combination of pregnancy and hepatitis hazardous. The high mortality figures may be

FIG. 30–1. Clinical course in cases of recurrent intrahepatic cholestasis of pregnancy documented by liver biopsy and serial laboratory determinations. (Haemmerli[1])

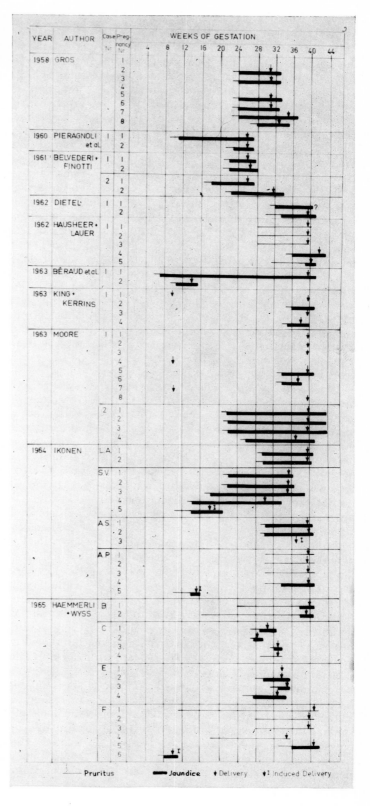

darker. Urine color may fluctuate during the disease. Stools are occasionally light colored, but in many cases feces are normal. The liver is not palpable and is normal in size and consistency. The spleen is not enlarged. Itching and jaundice never regress before delivery. After delivery, pruritus usually disappears within 2 days in many, within 1 week in most and within 2 weeks in all cases. Jaundice disappears as a rule within 1 to 2 weeks, but may last up to 4 weeks postpartum in exceptional cases.

The biochemical features of cholestasis are present. Serum bilirubin never surpasses 8 mg./100 ml. and remains below 5 mg./100 ml. in the majority of cases. Direct-reacting bilirubin constitutes the major fraction. Urobilinogen is never absent from the urine; bilirubinuria is probably always present, but may be transient or intermittent and can be missed. Serum alkaline phosphatase is, with few exceptions, elevated to a moderate extent, with a highest recorded level of 28 Bodansky units per cent. This is paralleled by an increase in serum 5-nucleotidase. Serum cholesterol is rarely normal and is usually elevated to up to 590 mg./100 ml., but levels up to 500 mg./100 ml. are also seen in uncomplicated pregnancies. Esterification of cholesterol is normal. Serum bile acids are increased. Serum electrophoresis shows an exaggeration of the changes seen in uncomplicated pregnancy. Serum albumin is decreased, alpha-2-globulins are mildly and beta-globulins markedly increased. Beta-globulins are always higher than gamma-globulins. Turbidity and flocculation tests are usually normal.

Prothrombin time may be prolonged, especially in cases with long duration of jaundice. The lowest observed level was 27 per cent of normal, but signs of hemorrhagic diathesis are never present. Prolongation of prothrombin time is due to a decrease in the vitamin K-dependent coagulation factors II, VII, IX and X, whereas factor V and fibrinogen remain normal. Bromsulphalein retention after 45 minutes is increased to between 10 and 30 per cent, while oral galactose tolerance remains normal. The serum transaminases are increased up to 300 Wroblewski units. In about half the cases SGPT is slightly higher than SGOT. In 3 unverified cases in the literature, transaminases rose to 900 Wroblewski units. Serum 1-phosphofructaldolase and serum sorbit dehydrogenase rise parallel to the transaminases. There is no correlation between serum bilirubin, alkaline phosphatase, cholesterol and transaminases. Serum iron may be low, normal or high and often fluctuates. Hemoglobin and white cell counts are within the normal range for uncomplicated pregnancies. There is no hemolysis and no impairment of renal function.

After delivery, serum bilirubin and transaminases start to decrease immediately while alkaline phosphatase may rise further for the next 2 weeks. When close serial laboratory determinations are performed, a transient dip of serum bilirubin and transaminases to completely normal values may be observed within the first 24 hours after delivery (Fig. 30–2). The levels then rapidly rise again to decline more slowly over succeeding days. Permanent normalization occurs first for bilirubin and transaminases, next for cholesterol, while BSP retention and especially alkaline phosphatase normalization may take 1 to 3 months after delivery.

At laparatomy (done under mistaken diagnosis) the liver is of normal shape, size, consistency and color, as is the spleen. The extrahepatic biliary system is unobstructed and bile flow and secretory pressures are normal. On liver biopsy, the liver architecture, liver cells and portal tracts are intact, without signs of necrosis or inflammation. Apart from the minor nonspecific changes seen also in uncomplicated pregnancies there is only a mild, focal and irregular intrahepatic cholestasis. It is so inconspicuous, that it can easily be missed and the slides are often read as normal. Cholestasis in this disease is best looked for on unstained slides. In the pericentral area of the liver lobules some bile canaliculi contain bile plugs, but few canaliculi are dilated. The surrounding liver cells contain some bile pigments and an accumulation of fine basophilic granules. Not all lobules

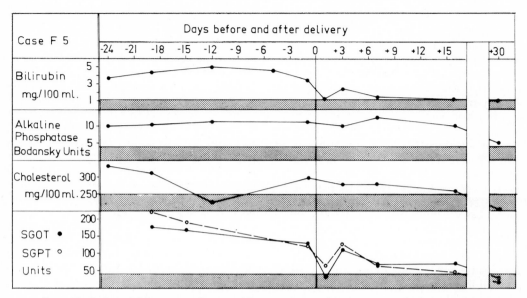

Fɪɢ. 30–2. Serial laboratory data in 5th pregnancy of a woman with recurrent intrahepatic cholestasis of pregnancy. Note transient dip to normal of serum bilirubin and serum transaminases on first postpartum day, and slight further rise of serum alkaline phosphatase after delivery. (Haemmerli and Wyss.[2])

are involved. Electron microscopy reveals only the same findings that are seen in other forms of intrahepatic cholestasis.

In this disease, cholestasis is clinically marked (pruritus), biochemically moderate (obstructive pattern) and histologically minimal.

There are no obstetric complications during labor and delivery. Uterine bleeding is not excessive, not even when the maternal prothrombin time is prolonged. Premature delivery occurs in about a third of the affected mothers. Child survival depends solely on the degree of maturity. The babies are not jaundiced or otherwise affected by the mothers' disorder. Some have extremely prolonged prothrombin times, but so do babies born of normal mothers.

Intrahepatic cholestasis of pregnancy needs little treatment. Diet and bed rest are not indicated, nor any other forms of "liver therapy." Vitamin K should be given when prothrombin time is prolonged or prophylactically in cases with jaundice of long duration. The main therapy is directed toward relief of itching. Cholestyramine is

the drug of choice. About 10 Gm./day must be given initially. After 1 to 2 weeks the dose can usually be reduced to 6 Gm./day. Pruritus is relieved, but does not completely disappear. Nilevar and Dianabol may also be successfully employed, but both drugs can intensify jaundice and are therefore not recommended. Antihistaminics are of no avail. Therapeutic abortion will "cure" the patient, but should never be resorted to because the disorder is benign and resolves after spontaneous delivery.

Pruritus gravidarum (defined as diffuse itching and excluding localized abdominal, vulvar or anal pruritus) appears to be a "forme fruste" of intrahepatic cholestasis of pregnancy. Total serum bilirubin remains normal per definition, but the direct-reacting fraction may be somewhat elevated. Prothrombin time is also normal. All other laboratory tests which are abnormal in intrahepatic cholestasis of pregnancy may be elevated to a minor degree, including serum transaminases. Treatment consists of cholestyramine.

Pruritus gravidarum and intrahepatic

cholestasis of pregnancy tend to recur with successive pregnancies. In the individual woman the disorder tends to run a similar course regarding time of onset of pruritus, time of onset of jaundice and time of delivery in relation to stage of pregnancy, but intensity of both pruritus and jaundice may vary. In some women the course is identical, in others jaundice becomes more intense with each successive gestation, whereas in a third group jaundice becomes milder and only pruritus is present in the last pregnancy. In rare cases an anicteric pruritic or even a completely asymptomatic pregnancy is interspaced between two icteric ones. Completely asymptomatic gestations may also follow several gestations with icterus. In cases with many recurrent episodes of intrahepatic cholestasis of pregnancy, it is remarkable that premature delivery is a feature of the individual woman and not the disease. Many women with recurrent jaundice always deliver at term, whereas others with premature delivery during jaundice deliver prematurely during the same week of pregnancy in gestations unaccompanied by pruritus and jaundice.

The pathogenesis of intrahepatic cholestasis of pregnancy is unknown. In some instances the same disorder occurs in the patient's mother or sister, but this is far from the rule. Most likely an influence of gestational hormones on an especially sensitive liver has to be postulated. This theory has received new impetus by the observation that probably all women with previous intrahepatic cholestasis of pregnancy will develop jaundice when exposed to contraceptive drugs. In fact this exposure has been proposed as a diagnostic test in cases where the nature of jaundice during pregnancy has remained unclear. Otherwise contraceptive drugs should not be employed in these patients.

This unusual cholestatic reaction to a natural or unknown steroid produced during pregnancy probably represents just an exaggeration of a process that occurs naturally in the liver during gestation as evidenced by the impaired Bromsulphalein excretory capacity and the impaired excretion of an intravenous bilirubin load during the second half of normal pregnancies.

No permanent liver impairment occurs even after many recurrent episodes of intrahepatic cholestasis of pregnancy. There is, however, a tendency for increased gallstone formation in these patients.

Acute fatty metamorphosis of pregnancy is extremely rare; and mortality is high. It occurs at any age in the childbearing period, but mostly in primiparas. Occasionally it is observed as late as in the 12th gestation. Clinically the disease is virtually indistinguishable from fulminant viral hepatitis. The onset of symptoms is usually between the 36th and 40th and always after the 30th week of gestation. Severe, persistent vomiting occurs suddenly, occasionally accompanied by severe headaches and/or abdominal pains, followed in a few days by jaundice and tachycardia but no fever. The jaundice becomes rapidly intense, the patient somnolent, the vomiting assumes a coffee-ground aspect and may progress to frank hematemesis. About half of the patients develop oliguria, anuria, uremia and acidosis. In most cases premature labor sets in, the patient delivers a stillborn child, then develops high fever and coma and dies within 3 days to 4 weeks after the onset of symptoms and 2 to 4 days after delivery. In exceptional cases, the patient dies rapidly before becoming jaundiced or before having delivered; whereas in others the whole clinical picture starts only after delivery. Few patients and infants survive.

Laboratory features are consistent with obstructive jaundice except that urine bilirubin may be absent except terminally. In most cases serum bilirubin remains below 10 mg./100 ml., but may reach 26 mg./100 ml. The serum alkaline phosphatase is mildly or markedly elevated and the turbidity and flocculation tests are usually negative. Serum transaminases remain mostly below 300 Wroblewski units. Prothrombin time is extremely impaired. The white cell count is 20,000 to 30,000 cells/cu. mm. Hypoglycemia may occur. In patients with oliguria, azotemia with a disproportionate rise of creatinine and uric acid is seen.

The liver histology shows a characteristic picture. The liver architecture is intact and there is a striking absence of postmortem

FIG. 30–3. Acute fatty metamorphosis of pregnancy, postmortem examination. (*Top*) pericentral fatty metamorphosis with periportal rim of intact liver cells (dark bands). (*Bottom*) Liver cells in pericentral zone contain fine lipid-laden vacuoles around centrally placed nucleus. Irregularity and duplication of nuclei. Sinusoids are compressed. (Courtesy of Kühn, H. A., Wegener, F., and Hahn, J.: Acta hepatosplenol. *14*:65.)

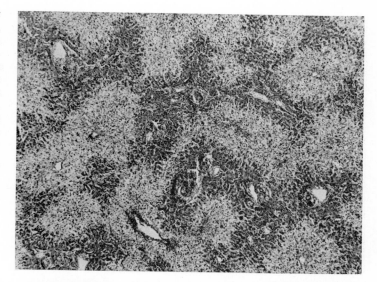

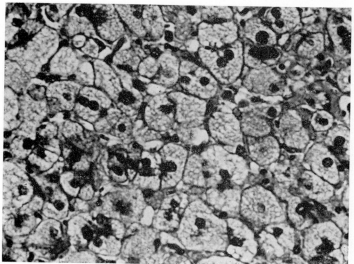

autolysis. There is no necrosis and no inflammation. The portal tracts are intact. The liver cells show a diffuse fatty change, usually with a small ring of peripheral liver cells remaining intact (Fig. 30–3). Bile thrombi may be seen in the centroacinar area. In survivors followed by serial biopsies, regeneration of liver tissue starts from the periphery toward the center of the lobule. The fatty metamorphosis consists of fine intracytoplasmic lipid-laden vacuoles arranged around the centrally placed normal nucleus. Electron microscopy shows a striking honeycomb appearance of the smooth endoplasmic reticulum, which suggests nutritional or toxic liver injury. The cause of the disease is, however, unknown. The histologic similarity to tetracycline toxicity has been mentioned. Tetracycline causes depression of protein formation and generally inhibits cell metabolism. At autopsy fatty degeneration of the kidney tubules is seen and a clinically unsuspected acute hemorrhagic pancreatitis is often found.

Treatment is symptomatic for hepatic and renal failure. The use of a Sengstaken tube has been tried in cases with frank hema-

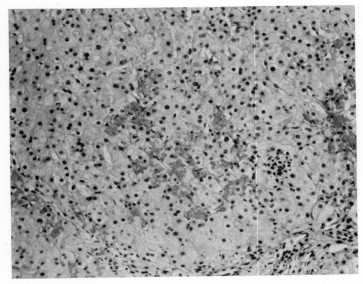

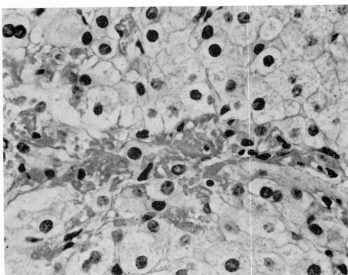

FIG. 30–4. Jaundice in toxemia of pregnancy with spontaneous improvement on bed rest and diet. Liver biopsy; author's observation with Prof. Held and Prof. Uehlinger, Zürich. (*Top*) Dark patches are fibrin thrombi in intermediary zone of liver lobules. (*Bottom*) The fibrin thrombi are located within Disse's spaces and compress the sinusoids. Occasionally single liver cell necrosis and mild portal infiltration.

temesis. Corticosteroids are of no value. A few mothers and babies have survived spontaneously, a few others after cesarean section: this procedure may be tried when the diagnosis is confirmed early in the course. Unfortunately this can only be achieved with certainty by liver biopsy which is often contraindicated because of the markedly disturbed blood coagulation. The clinical picture of fulminant hepatitis near term should, however, always arouse the suspicion of acute fatty metamorphosis of pregnancy.

The disease is potentially reversible. In the few survivors, liver function has been restored to normal.

Hyperemesis gravidarum is rarely accompanied by mild jaundice. Serum bilirubin may reach a maximum of 8 mg./100 ml., but usually stays below 4 mg./100 ml. Urine urobilinogen is increased and bilirubinuria may be present. Same patients have elevated serum alkaline phosphatase and serum transaminases. Thymol turbidity remains normal. Liver biopsies have not been performed. Jaundice in hyperemesis gravidarum has no prognostic significance and needs no special therapy. Diagnostically, viral hepatitis has to be considered, as well as chlorpromazine-induced jaundice whenever this drug is used for the treatment of hyperemesis.

Toxemia of pregnancy is often accompanied by an increased abnormality of liver function tests. Thymol turbidity and cephalin flocculation tests are positive in about half the cases. Elevation of serum alkaline phosphatase and serum transaminases parallel the severity of the clinical course and are most abnormal in cases with convulsions. Jaundice is rare, occurs late in the course and has often a grave prognostic significance. Liver biopsy is normal in many cases with icterus. Fibrin thrombi can sometimes be found in the sinusoids of the periportal zone and perhaps a cluster of necrotic hepatic cells (Fig. 30–4). Inflammation is absent. This is in contrast to the striking findings at autopsy, where fibrin thrombi obstruct many sinusoids and lead to hemorrhagic necrosis which then becomes confluent and involves large liver areas.

Treatment is directed at the toxemia.

Hydatiform mole on a rare occasion is associated with jaundice, which occurs in most cases after hospitalization for the primary disease. Liver function tests are little disturbed and liver biopsy in a single case showed no specific abnormality. The cause of this jaundice is not clear; it resolves spontaneously after passage of the mole.

Megaloblastic anemia of pregnancy, usually due to folic acid deficiency, and **hemolytic anemia of pregnancy** are extremely rare. Subicterus may be a feature of the more severe cases.

Recurrent Jaundice During Pregnancy

Recurrent jaundice during pregnancy is nearly always due to recurrent intrahepatic cholestasis of pregnancy. However, recurrence of jaundice in successive pregnancies is not a proof of this diagnosis, especially

Table 30–3. Recurrent Jaundice During Pregnancy

A. Recurrent jaundice in pregnancy
   I. Recurrent jaundice recurring also in nonpregnant persons
      1. Recurrent viral hepatitis or exacerbation of anicteric chronic hepatitis
      2. Recurrent jaundice in primary biliary cirrhosis
      3. Recurrent posthepatitic hyperbilirubinemia
      4. Recurrent common bile duct obstruction due to gallstones
      5. Recurrent exacerbations of familial nonhemolytic jaundice
      6. Recurrent hemolytic jaundice
   II. Recurrent jaundice due to medical complications of pregnancy
      1. Recurrent jaundice in severe pyelonephritis
B. Recurrent jaundice of pregnancy
   I. Recurrent idiopathic jaundice of pregnancy
      1. Recurrent intrahepatic cholestasis of pregnancy
   II. Recurrent jaundice as complication of disease linked to pregnancy
      1. Recurrent jaundice in hyperemesis gravidarum
C. Recurrent jaundice during pregnancy due to different diseases causing jaundice during pregnancy.
   Example: Hepatitis in one, hemolytic jaundice in the other gestation
D. Nonclassified cases of recurrent jaundice during pregnancy

when some features of the icterus do not fit into the typical and uniform picture. Table 30–3 lists all verified causes for recurrent jaundice during pregnancy reported in the literature.

Indications for Interruption of Pregnancy Because of Jaundice

Interruption of pregnancy is clearly indicated in S-C, S-S and C-C hemoglobinopathies, in rare cases of toxemia of pregnancy and perhaps hyperemesis gravidarum. The indication for interruption in these cases is never based on the usually mild jaundice but on the severity of the underlying disease.

The only possibly valuable indication for interruption of pregnancy because of jaundice is in acute fatty metamorphosis of pregnancy. This is a personal opinion based on the few reported survivors after cesarean section in this usually fatal disease. Experience on a larger scale is, however, lacking, and some patients have survived after spontaneous delivery.

Interruption of pregnancy "cures" intrahepatic cholestasis of pregnancy, but is definitely contraindicated, because the disease is benign, resolves always after spontaneous delivery, carries no risk for the child and causes no impairment of health and general activity during the jaundiced stage for the mother, whereas any operation entails a potential hazard.

Interruption of pregnancy for jaundice is probably most often performed in severe cases of viral hepatitis. It does not ameliorate the course of the disease; furthermore, anesthesia and operation of any type are poorly tolerated in patients with viral hepatitis.

The same reasoning holds true for the rare patients with cirrhosis of the liver. The only indication for a cesarean section is massive uncontrollable hematemesis near term when a portacaval shunt can technically not be performed because of the large uterus.

Termination of pregnancy is not indicated in pyelonephritis, tetracycline toxicity, drug-induced cholestasis or chronic idiopathic hyperbilirubinemias. In common duct obstruction due to gallstones, surgery on the biliary tract can be performed before the 36th week, after which it should be deferred until after delivery.

Interruption of pregnancy because of jaundice is practiced far too often. Better knowledge of the different forms of jaundice during pregnancy should improve this situation.

REFERENCES

1. Haemmerli, U. P.: Jaundice during pregnancy, with special emphasis on recurrent jaundice during pregnancy and its differential diagnosis, Acta med. scand. Suppl. *444*: 1-111, 1966. (Reprinted 1967 by Springer Verlag, New York, Inc.)
2. Haemmerli, U. P., and Wyss, H. I.: Recurrent intrahepatic cholestasis of pregnancy; report of six cases, and review of the literature, Medicine *46*:299, 1967.
3. Ikonen, E.: Jaundice in late pregnancy, Acta obstet. gynec. scand. Suppl. *5*:1-130, 1964.
4. Thorling, L.: Jaundice in pregnancy; a clinical study, Acta med. scand. Suppl. *302*:1-123, 1955.

Postoperative Jaundice

LEON MORGENSTERN, M.D.

Jaundice in the postoperative period is probably more frequent than is generally realized and its incidence seems to be rising.[16, 58] It may be mild and transient, and thus overlooked by the casual clinical observer; or its onset may be abrupt and dramatic, denoting a serious complication. Most frequently, significant postoperative jaundice appears gradually and poses complex questions in diagnosis and management. The patterns of postoperative jaundice, as characterized by clinical course and biochemical profile, frequently permit an accurate etiologic diagnosis. The watchword in management of jaundice occurring during this period is conservatism.

POSTOPERATIVE LIVER FUNCTION

Much has been written concerning the effect of anesthesia and surgery on liver function.[18, 30, 36, 37, 48, 86, 109, 140, 148] The great majority of studies show that the general effects of a surgical procedure on liver structure and function are minimal, in the absence of pre-existent liver disease or operative shock. Conventional light microscopy of sections of liver taken during the operative period showed only a mild degree of polymorphonuclear leukocytic infiltration in the hepatic sinusoids.[87, 138] Ultrastructural changes involving all elements have been described[91] following operative procedures, but their significance is difficult to assess.

Liver function, as measured by the usual biochemical tests in the postoperative period, also shows little or no derangement, again providing that pre-operative liver function is normal and surgery is uneventful. Serum bilirubin and alkaline phosphatase are not significantly affected by the uncomplicated operative procedure.[18, 37] SGOT is elevated transiently, however, after major abdominal or thoracic operations.[2, 10, 27, 64, 72] Such elevations rarely exceed 2 to 3 times the normal range (8 to 40 U) and are short-lived, rarely persisting beyond 48 to 72 hours.

Following severe injury or operative trauma, however, particularly when complicated by shock[132, 133, 135, 149] and the administration of multiple transfusions, moderate to marked rises in the serum bilirubin may occur.[48, 60, 128] Each transfusion imposes an additional bilirubin load of 250 mg. or more due to the "storage deficit" of bank-blood[79, 93, 112, 122] and the postoperative hyperbilirubinemia merely reflects the inability of the liver to handle a greatly increased bilirubin load. Changes in alkaline phosphatase are neither constant nor significant. Several studies have shown abnormal Bromsulphalein retention following severe injury or operative trauma[48, 87, 109] but this is not a useful test in the study of postoperative jaundice.

The three most valuable tests in following a patient with postoperative jaundice are serum bilirubin, alkaline phosphatase[53, 67, 71, 104] and SGOT.[64] Coupled with the clinical history and the physical examination, they best delineate the pattern and extent of liver dysfunction. Also useful are the urinary and fecal urobilinogen, prothrombin time and protein electrophoresis. Liver biopsy frequently fails to differentiate between jaundice of obstructive and nonobstructive etiology and may be followed by a serious bile leak in the obstructed patient. For this reason it should be reserved for cases that do not resolve in several weeks and in which the etiology of the jaundice is more likely to be hepatocellular in origin.

PATTERNS OF POSTOPERATIVE JAUNDICE

JAUNDICE OF BILIARY TRACT ORIGIN

Following Operations for Severe Acute Cholecystitis. An acute and significant rise in the serum bilirubin, with or without a concomitant rise in the alkaline phosphatase, may follow operations for severe acute cholecystitis, with or without choledocholithiasis (Figs. 30–5 and 30–6). Occasionally, the SGOT may rise to moderate levels, but the rise is usually mild and transient. Hyperbilirubinemia and hyperphosphatasemia are moderate and short-lived, rarely lasting more than 1 week in the absence of true obstruction. The mechanism is probably hepatocellular, but not readily evident on light-microscopy studies of liver biopsies. Triaditis and even liver cell necrosis occur in the region of the gallbladder bed with severe, acute cholecystitis.[31] This may explain transient elevations of the SGOT but not the hyperbilirubinemia and hyperphosphatasemia. It is sometimes assumed that the latter are manifestations of common duct stones which pass spontaneously, but frequently these cannot be demonstrated by exploration or subsequent x-ray.[108] Some other mechanism for the jaundice, as yet unexplained, must exist. In any event, judicious temporization is in order in these cases, rather than ill-advised re-exploration.

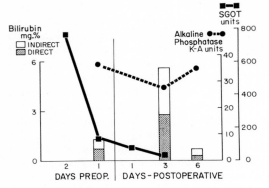

FIG. 30–5. Jaundice following acute cholecystectomy. Male, age 60. Cholecystectomy for suppurative cholecystitis. Common duct negative for calculi. No halothane or transfusions. Note high initial SGOT.

Due to Retained Common Duct Stone or Duct Stricture. With postoperative jaundice due to stone or accidental surgical narrowing of the common duct, the hyperbilirubinemia is mild to moderate and characteristically waxes and wanes.[51, 52, 89, 98] Urobilinogen appears intermittently in the urine and stools; the alkaline phosphatase, however, continues to rise and remains elevated.

Most patients with retained common duct stone are relatively asymptomatic in the early postoperative period. As time passes, recurrent hyperbilirubinemia, fixed or rising hyperphosphatasemia and episodes of recurrent cholangitis substantiate the diagnosis. Obstruction of one main hepatic duct, either left or right, will result in the same syndrome.[92, 121, 142] This course is in marked contrast to the short-lived hyperbilirubinemia which occurs following operation for acute severe cholecystitis of the necrotizing variety described immediately above.

Due to Complete Ductal Ligation. Fortunately, this complication is rare in good surgical practice. Jaundice secondary to complete ductal obstruction proceeds inexorably at the rate of 0.5 to 2.0 mg.%/day, reaching a peak and leveling off at 20 to 30 mg.%. The alkaline phosphatase rises steadily to high levels. With acute ductal obstruction a temporary, but high, elevation (up to 1,000 U) of SGOT can occur.[46] Fre-

quently this pattern is interrupted by the formation of an external or internal biliary fistula, or the supervention of bile peritonitis. Clinically, the patients manifest more deep-seated pain, discomfort, restlessness and tachycardia than patients with more benign forms of postoperative jaundice.

The management of patients with jaundice following biliary tract surgery should be conservative, and not based on laboratory findings alone. Jaundice *per se* is not a prime indication for re-exploration. Since radiologic demonstration of the biliary tract (in the absence of a T tube) is not possible in the jaundiced patient, the decision for re-exploration must be based on careful clinical observation as well as the laboratory findings. Abdominal discomfort, deep tenderness, recurrent attacks of chills and fever, waxing and waning hyperbilirubinemia, rising alkaline phosphatase and finally unrelenting jaundice over many weeks, are more proper indications for re-exploration than early postoperative jaundice alone.

JAUNDICE OF HEPATOCELLULAR ORIGIN

"Benign Postoperative Cholestasis." A form of moderately severe or severe postoperative jaundice that has been reported more frequently in the recent American and foreign literature has been given the name

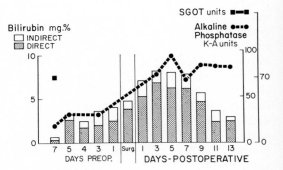

FIG. 30–6. Jaundice following cholecystectomy and choledochotomy. Female, age 37. Cholecystectomy and choledochotomy for ulcerative cholecystitis and impacted common duct calculus. Negative T-tube cholangiogram on 9th postoperative day. No halothane. No transfusions.

of "benign postoperative cholestasis." This term is perhaps unfortunate since morphologic evidence of cholestasis is not constant.[39] The condition was first described in fair detail by Caroli in 1956,[21] who reported 14 such cases, by Sevitt[129] in injured and burned subjects and, more recently by Schmid,[126] Kantrowitz[69] and others.[100, 125, 127] The syndrome may bear some relationship to other benign cholestatic syndromes which have received much recent attention.[9, 63, 120, 121, 131, 137]

The jaundice generally follows major operations on severely ill patients who receive a number of blood transfusions (Fig. 30–7). It occurs early in the postoperative period, persists for a week or more and may be accompanied by hyperphosphatasemia. Elevation of SGOT, if it occurs at all, is mild. Liver biopsies may show cholestasis of varying degree, erythrophagocytosis by Kupffer cells and some degenerative hepatocellular changes. Morphologic derangement is not proportionate to the severity of the clinical jaundice.

The process is benign and self-limited, in most cases being due to bilirubin overload imposed on a liver whose excretory capacity is impaired on the cellular level by shock, sepsis or unrecognized hepatotoxic agents. Since these patients are, or have

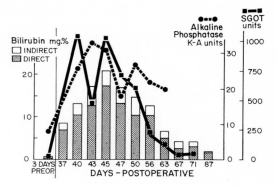

FIG. 30–8. Homologous serum hepatitis. Female, age 70. Radical mastectomy for carcinoma of breast. Onset of malaise, anorexia and jaundice 37 days postoperatively. Note elevation of alkaline phosphatase.

been, very ill and subject to many therapeutic measures, it is difficult to accurately dissect the multiplicate etiology of their jaundice. What is important is the realization that severe jaundice may occur under these conditions and its occurrence is neither reason for undue prognostic pessimism nor premature surgical activism.

Hepatitis or Cirrhosis. Homologous serum hepatitis may occur any time from several weeks to several months after surgery.[55, 57] A typical example is shown in Figure 30–8. It is not a cause of jaundice in the immediate postoperative period, unless it appears coincidentally due to the administration of blood, plasma, fibrinogen[85] or other virus-carrying inoculum several weeks to months prior to the surgical procedure. It can be differentiated from jaundice of obstructive etiology by history, clinical symptoms and the high transaminase values of the latter.

Similarly, infectious hepatitis may become coincidentally manifest in the postoperative period. The incidence of infectious hepatitis has risen in the past several decades, prompting several authors to explain the increasing incidence of massive postoperative hepatic necrosis in this way. Massive hepatic necrosis due to viral hepatitis is in no way distinguishable from a process due to certain hepatotoxic drugs. Again, the clinical course,[76] high trans-

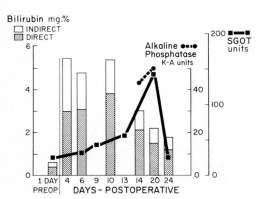

FIG. 30–7. "Benign postoperative cholestasis." Male, age 72. Massive upper gastrointestinal hemorrhage due to Rendu-Osler-Weber disease, requiring multiple transfusions. Near-total gastrectomy. Note rapid postoperative onset of jaundice, elevated alkaline phosphatase. Biliary tract negative.

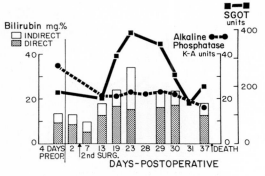

FIG. 30–9. Chronic active hepatitis. Female, age 19. Laparotomy and liver biopsy. No halothane. Tolerated first procedure well. On 4th postoperative day developed perforated steroid ulcer and generalized peritonitis. Course following second surgery poor. Death on 38th postoperative day.

aminase values and lack of other etiologic factors should permit this diagnosis to be made by exclusion in the postoperative period.

Mild cases of active, subacute or chronic active hepatitis which are subjected to minimal operative procedures rarely suffer serious consequences from the operative procedure *per se*, save for a transient rise in bilirubin and elevation in enzymes. Complicated operative procedures or postoperative complications, however, are not well tolerated.[56] An example of the latter instance is shown in Figure 30–9.

Similarly, mild or moderate cases of cirrhosis fare surprisingly well after uncomplicated surgical procedures, showing only a slight transient rise in bilirubinemia.[28, 83] Frequently jaundice is undetectable clinically.

Even the more severe hepatitides and cirrhoses may escape the consequences of ill-advised or mandatory operative procedures, but complicated procedures or untoward complications often eventuate in liver failure or death.[54, 75, 113] In the cirrhotic this train of events sometimes follows a successful portacaval shunting operation (Fig. 30–10). A steadily rising serum bilirubin or a persistently high serum bilirubin is a bad prognostic sign.

Hepatic Necrosis due to Hepatic Arterial

Ligation. A fair number of instances of hepatic arterial ligation or hepatic infarction have been reported in man,[13, 41, 70] although this too is fortunately a rare complication of upper abdominal surgery. The common hepatic artery is susceptible to injury during gastrectomy, portacaval shunt or operations on the common bile duct. The right hepatic artery is most frequently injured during cholecystectomy. Occlusion of the left hepatic artery is usually the result of thrombus or embolus[22]; I have observed one case of this.

If the hepatic artery is occluded, hepatic infarction in man does not invariably result. Collateral pathways and the dual hepatic circulation are probably responsible for the variable outcome after this accident. In dogs, hepatic de-arterialization almost invariably results in clostridial infection of the liver, but in man this is a rare consequence. I have seen two cases of clostridial hepatitis following ligation of the common hepatic artery and occlusion of the left hepatic artery.

As the pattern of response is variable, so has the pattern of the jaundice been variable. In complete infarction of a lobe, the elevations in serum bilirubin and SGOT are swift and high; when ligation of the artery does not result in infarction, the

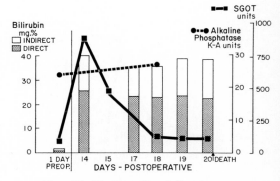

FIG. 30–10. Jaundice following portacaval shunt. Male, age 41. Emergency portacaval shunt for bleeding esophageal varices, requiring many transfusions. No halothane. Gradual rise and persistence of marked hyperbilirubinemia. Autopsy: Extensive cirrhosis; bile thrombi; occasional foci of polymorphonuclear cells.

bilirubin and SGOT are only transiently and moderately elevated.[13]

The consequences of elective hepatic de-arterialization in metastatic liver disease are well described by Almersjö.[2] The serum bilirubin rises only slightly or moderately; alkaline phosphatase is not significantly affected. SGOT and SGPT rise to moderate or high levels within the 1st week.

POSTOPERATIVE JAUNDICE DUE TO HEMOLYSIS

One pattern of early, severe postoperative jaundice following operations on the upper abdomen is especially noteworthy, namely that due to severe clostridial sepsis. I have observed several such cases in the past decade and sporadic reports have appeared in the surgical literature.[1, 19, 20, 61, 130, 144] This variety of postoperative jaundice, swift in onset and severe, occurs within 24 to 72 hours following surgery on the biliary tract, colon or stomach. The patient is restless, apprehensive, hypotensive and tachycardic, although characteristically alert. Fever and leukocytosis are not prominent. The etiology is most frequently seeding of the operative area with clostridial organisms from the biliary tract, colon or stomach, although rarely it may be due to hepatic arterial ligation as mentioned above.

The clue to diagnosis is the swift, acute rise in bilirubin associated with the clinical signs of clostridial sepsis. Although it might be expected that the chief component of such a rise would be unconjugated bilirubin, the rise may be predominantly in the direct fraction (Fig. 30–11). This should not obscure the true nature of the hyperbilirubinemia. If clostridial sepsis is suspected, one should search carefully for wound crepitus which can easily be missed on casual examination. If the wound is aspirated, one may obtain enough fluid to identify the gram-positive bacilli on direct smear. This complication, if promptly recognized and treated with appropriate antibiotics (massive doses of penicillin) and the use of hyperbaric oxygen, is remediable and not necessarily fatal.

Localized clostridial cellulitis or myositis, milder in nature than the fulminant variety just described, need not necessarily result

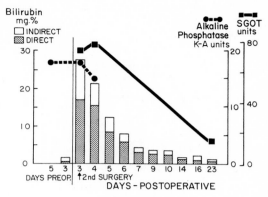

FIG. 30–11. Clostridial sepsis. Male, age 52. Cholecystectomy for cholelithiasis. Abrupt onset of severe jaundice 72 hours postoperatively. *Clostridium perfringens* isolated from bile, wound and blood. Recovered after wide incision and drainage of cellulitic areas, massive doses of penicillin and hyperbaric oxygen.

in generalized clostridial sepsis, hemolysis and hyperbilirubinemia.

Hemolytic transfusion reactions can be immediate or delayed following transfusion[93] and may be responsible for an immediate postoperative hyperbilirubinemia or one that occurs later, following transfusion during operation. Maximum bilirubin levels are not reached before 3 to 6 hours after the hemolytic episode. If the jaundice is suspected to be due to incompatible transfusion (major blood groups or rarer subgroups), residues of all units of blood transfused as well as pre- and post-transfusion venous blood samples of the patient should be secured. Hemoglobinemia, hemoglobinuria, estimation of serum hepatoglobin and the elevated indirect hyperbilirubinemia substantiate the diagnosis. A direct component higher than 15 per cent of the total bilirubin usually denotes associated hepatic dysfunction.[143]

Hemolytic syndromes may occur late after open heart surgery and artificial valve replacement on a mechanical and autoimmune basis.[84, 101] Anemia and jaundice made worse by transfusions within weeks following such surgery are diagnostic of this condition even before the more esoteric laboratory tests return. Fever and high indirect bilirubinemia follow each transfusion

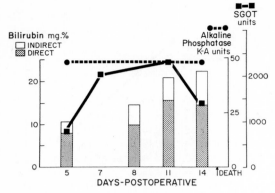

FIG. 30–12. Massive hepatic necrosis. Double halothane anesthesia. Female, age 41. Near total glossectomy for carcinoma of the tongue (halothane 1 hr., 45 min.). Radical neck dissection 38 days later (halothane 3 hrs.). Icterus noted on 5th postoperative day progressing to lethargy, coma and death on 16th postoperative day.

for the worsening anemia. Positive antiglobulin tests help substantiate the autoimmune nature of the disorder, and a favorable response to steroid therapy may be anticipated. Other causes of postoperative jaundice following open heart surgery have been described in recent reports,[73, 114, 117] since jaundice is not an infrequent early or late sequela of such surgery.

Pre-existent hemolytic syndromes may be aggravated by major surgical procedures. Sickle-cell disease is an example of a syndrome in which severe hemolytic crises may be precipitated by surgery,[116] with marked aggravation of the jaundice in the postoperative period. Biliary lithiasis, frequently coexistent in these syndromes, renders the postoperative jaundice pattern even more complex. Renal failure, occurring in consequence of such a crisis, may result in extraordinarily high levels of serum bilirubin (above 50 mg.%) due to retention of direct bilirubin which is ordinarily excreted in the urine.[43]

POSTOPERATIVE JAUNDICE DUE TO DRUGS

The use of potentially hepatotoxic drugs such as the phenothiazines, anabolic steroids, certain antibiotics and others which comprise a huge and ever-growing list is commonplace in surgical patients today.[24, 35, 40, 103, 118, 119] Thus they are potential causal factors in any case of jaundice of obscure etiology that occurs in the postoperative period. The hepatotoxic drugs and their actions are well described in Chapter 14. The great majority of postoperative jaundice cases that I have seen have not been thought to be primarily related to drug toxicity.

The anesthetic halothane has been the subject of rather heated controversy in the past few years. The first reports of massive hepatic necrosis associated with halothane appeared early in 1958, shortly after halothane was introduced.[146] Since then in a number of reports halothane has been associated with fatal postoperative massive hepatic necrosis or nonfatal hepatic dysfunction.[14, 15, 82, 134] Outnumbering the case reports implicating halothane as a hepatotoxin are numerous articles that refute such a relationship.[25, 29, 32, 38, 50, 58, 66, 111, 134, 139] The matter is still unsettled.

In 1965 I reported 5 cases of fatal hepatic necrosis and 4 cases of nonfatal hepatic dysfunction believed to be associated with halothane.[95] Since then, the number of cases has risen to 37, with 5 additional fatalities.

The pattern of the jaundice is variable. Usually its onset is before the 5th postoperative day, or at least this is when it

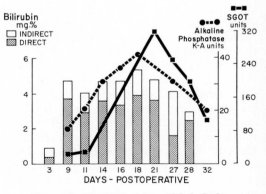

FIG. 30–13. Probable mild halothane jaundice. Male, age 64. Underwent vagotomy and hemigastrectomy under halothane anesthesia (4¼ hrs.). No transfusions or hepatotoxic drugs. Jaundice noted on 9th postoperative day.

becomes clinically apparent. Fever, often septic in character, is common. In the acute massive necrosis group the course is one of inexorable worsening with progressive jaundice, lethargy, coma and death (Fig. 30–12). At autopsy, the findings are in no way distinguishable from those of acute, fulminating viral hepatitis. In all these cases the transaminase values have been high.

In a second group of cases the onset is more insidious and the course less dramatic (Fig. 30–13 and 30–14). Fever, malaise and anorexia accompany the jaundice. The alkaline phosphatase may rise moderately. The transaminases may not be markedly elevated. The course relents within 7 to 28 days, and, should liver biopsy be done, again it is not distinguishable from other types of hepatitis.

A third group exhibits minimal hyperbilirubinemia, fever, anorexia, nausea or vomiting and high transaminase values. These cases may be missed if the appropriate laboratory tests are not done.

In 47 per cent of our cases, jaundice followed the administration of a second halothane anesthesia, a pattern frequently cited in other published reports.

The 1966 National Halothane Study concluded that it "had not entirely ruled out a rare relationship between halothane and massive hepatic necrosis."[17, 45] Regarding such a relationship, a persistent disquietude has arisen from a continuing number of published and unpublished reports. The First Progress Report of the Fulminant Hepatic Failure Surveillance Study from the Thorndike Memorial Laboratory in Boston, December, 1967, included 24 patients (out of 75) in whom hepatic failure followed operations under general anesthesia. Nineteen, only two of whom survived, received halothane. Four had received halothane only once, 8 twice, and 7 three or more times. Eleven had unexplained fever within 1 to 4 days after the next to the last exposure.

Perhaps 60 million or more halothane anesthesias have been administered. It has superior qualities as an anesthetic agent. The rare instances of hepatic damage that occur following its use should not preclude its wide, general usage. It is unwise, however, to completely disregard its possible association with hepatic damage. It should probably not be administered to people with known liver disease; repeated use should be restricted particularly in those patients who have had a fever of unknown cause after the first administration; finally,

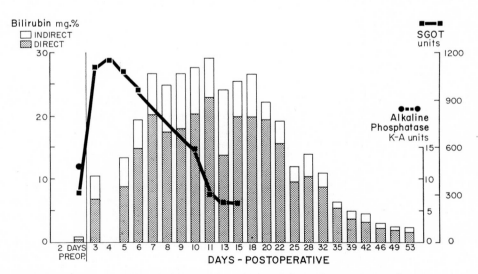

Fig. 30–14. Probable halothane jaundice, moderately severe. Male, age 61. Endarterectomy, halothane anesthesia (9¼ hours). One year and 4 days later, coloproctectomy for carcinoma of rectum under halothane anesthesia. Fever, jaundice and leukopenia noted on 3rd postoperative day.

until we have better means of predicting, preventing or identifying this entity, its association with postoperative hepatic dysfunction should be considered a possibility when other likely causes have been ruled out.

Miscellaneous Causes of Postoperative Jaundice

Severe sepsis is often a cause of unexplained jaundice, particularly when intraperitoneal.[96, 107] Mild hyperbilirubinemia occurs in these cases more often than is generally realized. Occasionally the jaundice is unaccountably more severe, and on biopsy or autopsy, liver sections show a moderate degree of centrilobular necrosis and cholestasis.

Wound infection may also delay a resolving jaundice, or cause a worsening of an existent jaundice.

Familial or congenital jaundice, such as Gilbert's disease or the Dubin-Johnson syndrome, may not be recognized preoperatively.[33, 78, 105, 123, 124] A transient postoperative hyperbilirubinemia is generally the rule in such cases, but of no particular consequence.

Inflammatory diseases of the small and large intestine, such as regional enteritis and ulcerative colitis, can be associated with postoperative liver dysfunction[7, 12, 88, 90, 136, 145] Jaundice is by no means the rule following operations on such patients, but mild degrees of icterus can be discerned frequently by chemical test. In others, unaccountably, the postoperative hepatic dysfunction is more severe, as manifested by hyperbilirubinemia and hyperphosphatasemia. Liver biopsy may show nonspecific triaditis, granulomata, cirrhosis, fatty change, cholestasis, hepatitis or amyloidosis.[34]

The resorption of massive hematomata, such as occurs in major soft part trauma, or following retroperitoneal hemorrhage, for example, may result in modest elevations of the serum bilirubin, without corresponding hyperphosphatasemia.

Acute postoperative pancreatitis[4, 42] may result in significant hyperbilirubinemia and hyperphosphatasemia.

Infantile pyloric stenosis has been reported to be associated with jaundice,[23, 47]

which may be present preoperatively as well as in the postoperative period. Mechanical factors alone seem insufficient to account for the hyperbilirubinemia, which is of the nonhemolytic, acholuric type. Some abnormality of bile pigment metabolism has been postulated in these patients.[5, 26]

Heart failure in the postoperative period may be associated with mild to moderate hyperbilirubinemia. Abnormal BSP retention is frequent but alkaline phosphatase is seldom elevated.[110]

Pulmonary embolism, particularly when associated with pre-existent liver dysfunction or congestive failure, has been known to produce mild degrees of hyperbilirubinemia.

Major hepatic resections are followed by varying degrees of hyperbilirubinemia, hyperphosphatasemia and elevated SGOT, depending on the extent of resection. Postoperative hepatic function in such patients has been summarized well by Pack and associates.[62, 99]

Pattern of Jaundice Following Operative Relief of Pre-existent Obstruction

Carcinoma of the Head of Pancreas. A brief postoperative *rise* in bilirubin frequently follows relief of the obstruction by either bypass or resection. Thereafter, the average case shows a progressive fall of 1 to 2 mg.%/day, providing hepatic function is not too deranged.

The decline is most rapid in the first week, after which a slow decline may persist for several weeks. Completely normal levels are usually reached within 1 month. Rundle reported a group of patients in whom the bilirubin reached half its preoperative value in 17.4 days.[115] In a comparable series, I reported the average time to reach half the pre-operative level as 7.5 days.[94] Such decline curves are subject to great variation due to the many complex variables involved.

The alkaline phosphatase generally falls more slowly than the bilirubin. Cases that cannot be relieved of complete obstruction level off at bilirubin levels between 20 and 30, but the alkaline phosphatase may rise to levels of 300 U (K.A.) and above. Obstructive jaundice in the previously healthy adult may be tolerated for surprisingly long periods of time providing proper supportive care is given and cholangitis does not supervene.

Common Duct Stone. The levels of hyperbilirubinemia reached with common duct stone are generally not as high as with carcinoma. Barring cholangitis, retained stone, pre-existent liver damage or wound infection, the serum bilirubin should fall rapidly to normal, followed closely by a declining alkaline phosphatase. Transient elevations in both these values, as well as the transaminases, are often seen acutely following the operative procedure. Subsequently, the fall in bilirubin is most rapid when the pre-operative elevation has been abrupt and of short duration. Decline curves are more rapid than is seen with relief of a malignant obstruction.

Following operations for obstructive jaundice, whether the obstruction is benign or malignant, there is not infrequently a post-decompression oligocholia followed by choleresis.[65] This may be responsible for the transient rise in serum bilirubin which is frequently seen following operative decompression.

CONCLUSIONS

Postoperative jaundice has no special characteristics except that it occurs in the postoperative period and may be causally related to factors related to the surgical procedure. Conditions that predispose to it should be known; conditions that cause it should be recognized and avoided if possible.

Once postoperative jaundice is present, the chief danger to the patient is that this sign alone will worry the surgeon into an ill-advised second operative procedure. Conservatism and watchful waiting should be the rule. Daily, elaborate biochemical profiles are not only unnecessary, but deplete the patient without cause. Laboratory values alone should not be sufficient reason for operation.

All icterogenic drugs should be stopped. A good urinary output should be maintained, using mannitol-induced diuresis if

necessary. Operation should be a measure of last resort and only if obstruction is reasonably certain. In doubtful cases transhepatic cholangiography may preclude unnecessary surgery.

Finally, if surgery is unavoidable, halothane should be avoided as an anesthetic especially if it has been used previously. And if on exploration the diagnosis appears to be hepatocellular rather than obstructive, operation should be gentle, conservative and not too prolonged.

REFERENCES

1. Aldrete, J. S., and Judd, E. S.: Gas gangrene: a complication of elective abdominal surgery, Arch. Surg. 90:745, 1965.
2. Almersjö, O., Bengmark, S., Engevik, L., Hafström, L. O., Loughridge, B. P., and Nilsson, L. A. V.: Serum enzyme changes after hepatic dearterialization in man, Ann. Surg. 167:9, 1968.
3. Alter, A. A., Prutting, D., and Selirio, E:. Hemolytic anemia caused by penicillin. Letters to the journal, J.A.M.A. 204:635, 1968.
4. Anderson, M. C.: Hepatic morphology and function: alterations associated with acute pancreatitis, Arch. Surg. 92:664, 1966.
5. Arias, I., Schorr, J. B., and Fraad, L. M.: Clinical conference—congenital hypertrophic pyloric stenosis with jaundice, Pediatrics 24:338, 1959.
6. Arias, I. M.: Studies of chronic familial non-hemolytic jaundice with conjugated bilirubin in the serum with and without an unidentified pigment in the liver cells, Am. J. Med. 31:510, 1961.
7. Atkinson, A. J., and Carroll, W. W.: Sclerosing cholangitis; association with regional enteritis, J.A.M.A. 188:183, 1964.
8. Babior, B. M., and Davidson, C. S.: Postoperative massive liver necrosis; a clinical and pathological study, New Engl. J. Med. 276:645, 1967.
9. Biempica, L., Gutstein, S., and Arias, I. M.: Morphological and biochemical studies of benign recurrent cholestasis, Gastroenterology 52:521, 1967.
10. Blodgett, R. C., Jr., Anderson, M. W., McGuckin, W. F., and Fleisher, G. A.: Glutamic oxaloacetic transaminase: activity in serum after transurethral pro-

static resection, Arch. Int. Med. *114*:344, 1964.

11. Braasch, J. W., and Preble, H. E.: Unilateral hepatic duct obstruction, Ann. Surg. *158*:17, 1963.

12. Braasch, J. W., and Ross, J. R.: The colon surgeon looks at jaundice, Dis. Colon Rectum *1*:405, 1958.

13. Brittain, R. S., Marchioro, T. L., Hermann, G., Waddell, W. R., and Starzl, T. E.: Accidental hepatic artery ligation in humans, Am. J. Surg. *107*:822, 1964.

14. Brody, G. L., and Sweet, R. B.: Halothane anesthesia as a possible cause of massive hepatic necrosis, Anesthesiology *24*:29, 1963.

15. Brunson, J. G., Eckman, P. L., and Campbell, J. B.: Increasing prevalence of unexplained liver necrosis, New Engl. J. Med. *257*:52, 1957.

16. Bunker, J. P., and Blumenfeld, C. M.: Liver necrosis after halothane anesthesia: cause or coincidence? New Engl. J. Med. *268*:531, 1963.

17. Bunker, J. P. et al.: Summary of the national halothane study: possible association between halothane anesthesia and postoperative hepatic necrosis (a cooperative study), J.A.M.A. *197*:775, 1966.

18. Burdette, W. J., Stevens, L. E., and Groschel, U.: Stability of hepatic metabolism during surgery, Am. J. Surg. *107*: 239, 1964.

19. Cabrera, A., Tsukada, Y., and Pickren, J. W.: Clostridial gas gangrene and septicemia in malignant disease, Cancer *18*: 800, 1965.

20. Canipe, T. L., and Hudspeth, A. S.: Gas gangrene septicemia, Arch. Surg. *89*:544, 1964.

21. Caroli, J. *et al.*: Les ictères de la gastrectomie, Arch. Mal. Appar. Dig. *39*:1057, 1950.

22. Case 5–1963. Case records of the Massachusetts General Hospital: Hepatic arterial thrombosis, New Engl. J. Med. *268*: 153, 1963.

23. Chaves-Carballo, E., Harris, L. E., and Lynn, H. B.: Jaundice associated with pyloric stenosis and neonatal small-bowel obstructions, Clin. Pediat. *7*:198, 1968.

24. Cook, G. C., and Sherlock, S.: Jaundice and its relation to therapeutic agents, Lancet *1*:175, 1965.

25. Council on Drugs: Liver necrosis after halothane anesthesia: post hoc, ergo propter hoc? J.A.M.A. *185*:204, 1963.

26. Cracco, J. B., Dower, J. C., and Harris, L. E.: Bilirubin metabolism in the newborn, Mayo Clin. Proc. *40*:868, 1965.

27. Craver, W. L., Johnson, G., Jr., and Beal, J. M.: Alterations in serum glutamic-oxalacetic transaminase activity following operations, Surg. Forum *8*:77, 1957.

28. Da Silva, L. C., De Godoy, A., Mendes, F. T., Leite, G. M., and Pontes J. F.: Indirect reacting hyperbilirubinemia after portosystemic shunt: its relation to other complications, Gastroenterology *39*:605, 1960.

29. Davidson, C. S., Babior, B., and Popper, H.: Concerning hepatotoxicity of halothane, New Engl. J. Med. *275*:1497, 1966.

30. Dawson, B., *et al.*: Hepatic function tests: post-operative changes with halothane or diethyl ether anesthesia, Mayo Clin. Proc. *41*:599, 1966.

31. Deaver, J. B., and Reimann, S. P.: Excursions into Surgical Subjects, pp. 95–96, Philadelphia, Saunders, 1923.

32. De Backer, L. J., and Longnecker, D. S.: Prospective and retrospective searches for liver necrosis following halothane anesthesia, J.A.M.A. *195*:157, 1966.

33. Dollinger, M. R., Brandborg, L. L., Sartor, V. E., and Bernstein, J. M.: Chronic familial hyperbilirubinemia: hepatic defect(s) associated with occult hemolysis, Gastroenterology *52*:875, 1967.

34. Dordal, E., Glagov, S., and Kirsner, J. B.: Hepatic lesions in chronic inflammatory bowel disease. I. Clinical correlations with liver biopsy diagnoses in 103 patients, Gastroenterology *52*:239, 1967.

35. Dujovne, C. A., Chan, C. H., and Zimmerman, H. J.: Sulfonamide hepatic injury: review of the literature and report of a case due to sulfamethoxazole, New Engl. J. Med. *277*:785, 1967.

36. Dunlap, R. W., Jr., Dockerty, M. B., and Waugh, J. M.: Hepatic changes occurring during upper abdominal operations: biopsy studies, Surg. Gynec. Obstet. *99*: 220, 1954.

37. Dykes, M. H. M., and Walzer, S. G.: Preoperative and postoperative hepatic dysfunction, Surg. Gynec. Obstet. *124*: 747, 1967.

38. Dykes, M. H. M., Walzer, S. G., Slater, E. M., Gibson, J. M., and Ellis, D. S.: Acute parenchymatous hepatic disease following general anesthesia; clinical appraisal of hepatotoxicity following ad-

ministration of halothane, J.A.M.A. *193*: 339, 1965.

39. Editorial: The spectrum of jaundice, New Engl. J. Med. *276*:635, 1967.

40. Fekety, F. R., Jr.: Gastrointestinal complications of antibiotic therapy, J.A.M.A. *203*:210, 1968.

41. Fitch, E. A., and Denman, F. P.: Infarction of the entire right lobe of the liver, Arch. Surg. *77*:235, 1958.

42. Frieden, J. H.: The significance of jaundice in acute pancreatitis, Arch. Surg. *90*:422, 1965.

43. Fulop, M.: Bilirubinemia and renal failure, New Engl. J. Med. *276*:1208, 1967.

44. Galambos, J. T.: Evaluation of the jaundiced patient in the postoperative period, Southern Med. J. *53*:1263, 1960.

45. Gall, E. A.: Report of the pathology panel—national halothane study, Anesthesiology *29*:233, 1968.

46. Gardner, B.: Marked elevation of serum transaminases in obstructive jaundice, Am. J. Surg. *111*:575, 1966.

47. Garrow, E., and Hertzler, J.: Hypertrophic pyloric stenosis with jaundice; a case report of one family, J. Pediat. Surg. *1*:284, 1966.

48. Geller, W., and Tagnon, H. J.: Liver dysfunction following abdominal operations; the significance of postoperative hyperbilirubinemia, Arch. Int. Med. *86*: 908, 1950.

49. Gilbert, F. I., Jr.: Cholestatic hepatitis caused by esters of erythromycin and oleandomycin, J.A.M.A. *182*:1048, 1962.

50. Gingrich, T. F., and Virtue, R. W.: Postoperative liver damage: is anesthesia involved? Surgery *57*:241, 1965.

51. Glenn, F.: Complications of biliary tract surgery, Surg. Gynec. Obstet. *110*:141, 1960.

52. ———: Postoperative strictures of the extrahepatic bile ducts, Surg. Gynec. Obstet. *120*:560, 1965.

53. Gutman, A. B.: Serum alkaline phosphatase activity in diseases of the skeletal and hepatobiliary systems: a consideration of current status, Am. J. Med. *27*: 875, 1959.

54. Hamilton, J. E.: The management of bleeding esophageal varices associated with cirrhosis of the liver, Ann. Surg. *141*:637, 1955.

55. Hampers, C. L., Prager, D., and Senior, J. R.: Post-transfusion anicteric hepatitis, New Engl. J. Med. *271*:747, 1964.

56. Harville, D. D., and Summerskill, W. H. J.: Surgery in acute hepatitis: causes and effects, J.A.M.A. *184*:257, 1963.

57. Havens, W. P., Jr.: Viral hepatitis: Clinical patterns and diagnosis, Am. J. Med. *32*:665, 1962.

58. Henderson, J. C., and Gordon, R. A.: The incidence of postoperative jaundice with special reference to halothane, Canad. Anaesth. Soc. J. *11*:453, 1964.

59. Herber, R., and Specht, N. W.: Liver necrosis following anesthesia, Arch. Int. Med. *115*:266, 1965.

60. Howard, J. M., and Hughes, C. W. (eds.): Battle casualties in Korea: Studies of the surgical research team, vol. 1, parts 1, 2, 3, 4. The systemic response to injury, Army Medical Service Graduate School, Walter Reed Army Medical Center, Washington, D.C., U.S. Govt. Printing Office, 1955.

61. Isenberg, A. N.: *Clostridium welchii* infection; a clinical evaluation, Arch. Surg. *92*:727, 1966.

62. Islami, A. H., Pack, G. T., Miller, T. R., Vanamee, P., Randall, H. T., and Roberts K. E.: Postoperative course following total right hepatic lobectomy, Surgery *39*:551, 1956.

63. Javitt, N. B., and Arias, I. M.: Intrahepatic cholestasis: a functional approach to pathogenesis, Gastroenterology *53*: 171, 1967.

64. Jensen, J. S.: Serum glutamic oxalacetic transaminase in surgical patients, Ugeskr. Laeg. *123*:838, 1961.

65. Jesseph, J. E.: Oligocholia and choleresis after operations for obstructive jaundice, Rev. Surg. *19*:312, 1962.

66. Johnstone, M.: Liver injury in the surgical patient: a critical review, Brit. J. Anaesthesiol. *36*:718, 1964.

67. Jonsson, G.: Relative diagnostic significance of bilirubin and phosphatase values in the postcholecystectomy syndrome, Acta chir. scand. *115*:299, 1958.

68. Jordan, G. L., Jr., and Skelton, E. L., Jr.: Significance of jaundice following pancreatoduodenal resection, J.A.M.A. *162*:196, 1956.

69. Kantrowitz, P. A., Jones, W. A., Greenberger, N. J., and Isselbacher, K. J.: Severe postoperative hyperbilirubinemia simulating obstructive jaundice, New Engl. J. Med. *276*:591, 1967.

70. Karasewich, E. G., and Bowden, L.: He-

patic artery injury, Surg. Gynec. Obstet. *124*:1057, 1967.

71. Karl, M. M.: The serum alkaline phosphatase, J.A.M.A. *203*:591, 1968.

72. Killen, D. A.: Serum enzyme elevations: a diagnostic test for acute myocardial infarction during the early postoperative period, Arch. Surg. *96*:200, 1968.

73. Kingsley, D. P. E.: Hepatic damage following profound hypothermia and extracorporeal circulation in man, Thorax *21*: 91, 1966.

74. Klein, N. C., and Jeffries, G. H.: Hepatotoxicity after methoxyflurane administration, J.A.M.A. *197*:1037, 1966.

75. Koenemann, L. C., and Ceballos, R.: Massive hepatic necrosis following portacaval shunt; report of 2 cases and considerations of liver hemodynamics after shunt, J.A.M.A. *198*:138, 1966.

76. Krugman, S., Ward, R., and Giles, J. P.: The natural history of infectious hepatitis, Am. J. Med. *32*:717, 1962.

77. Kunelis, C. T., Peters, J. L., and Edmondson, H. A.: Fatty liver of pregnancy and its relationship to tetracycline therapy, Am. J. Med. *38*:359, 1965.

78. Levine, R. A., and Klatskin, G.: Unconjugated hyperbilirubinemia in the absence of overt hemolysis, Am. J. Med. *36*:541, 1964.

79. Lewis, G. P., and Brown, M.: The output of bilirubin in bile: response to experimental hemoglobinaemia, Gastroenterology *54*:159, 1968.

80. Lewis, G. P., and Rogers, K. M.: Physiological concepts in relation to drug toxicity *in* Thomson, T J., and Gillespie, I. E. (eds.): Postgraduate Gastroenterology, Proc. of Conf., Glasgow, 1965; pp. 77–86, London, Bailliere, Tindall & Cassell, 1966.

81. Lindenauer, S. M., and Child, C. G., III: Disturbances of liver function in biliary tract disease, Surg. Gynec. Obstet. *123*: 1205, 1966.

82. Lindenbaum, J., and Leifer, E.: Hepatic necrosis associated with halothane anesthesia, New Engl. J. Med. *268*:525, 1963.

83. Lindenmuth, W. W., and Eisenberg, M. M.: The surgical risk in cirrhosis of the liver, Arch. Surg. *86*:235, 1963.

84. Lynch, E., Alfrey, C. P., Nevaril, C. G., and Hellums, J. D.: Hemolysis and artificial heart valve. Report to the Southern Soc. for Clin. Res. *16*:80, 1968.

85. Mainwaring, R. L., and Brueckner, G. G.: Fibrinogen-transmitted hepatitis, J.A.M.A. *195*:437, 1966.

86. Massarrat, S.: The influence of surgery on the biliary system, especially in diseases of the liver, on the serum level of the enzymes sorbitol dehydrogenase, glutamic-pyruvic transaminase, lactic dehydrogenase, and glutamic dehydrogenase, Acta Hepatosplen, (Stuttg.) *9*:86, 1962.

87. Mateer, J. G., Hartman, F. W., Baltz, J. I., Fallis, L. D., McGraw, A. B., and Steele, H. H.: Combined liver biopsy and liver function study in 132 cases of cholelithiasis and 31 cases of peptic ulcer (operated cases), Gastroenterology *11*: 284, 1948.

88. Maurer, L. H., Hughes, R. W., Jr., Folley, J. H., and Mosenthal, W. T.: Granulomatous hepatitis associated with regional enteritis, Gastroenterology *53*:301, 1967.

89. McKenzie, A. D.: Strictures of the common bile duct: a report of 12 cases, Canad. J. Surg. *2*:135, 1968.

90. McKenzie, C. G.: Pyogenic infection of liver secondary to infection in the portal drainage area, Brit. Med. J. *2*:1558, 1964.

91. Minio, F., and Gardiol, D.: Hépatopathie peropératoire, Ann. d'Anat. Path. *10*:301, 1965.

92. Mistilis, S., and Schiff, L.: A case of jaundice due to unilateral hepatic duct obstruction with relief after hepatic lobectomy, Gut *4*:13, 1963.

93. Mollison, P. L.: Blood Transfusion in Clinical Medicine, ed. 4, pp. 553-589, Philadelphia, Davis; Oxford, Blackwell, 1967.

94. Morgenstern, L.: Jaundice in the postoperative period, Am. Surg. *29*:111, 1963.

95. Morgenstern, L., Sacks, H. J., and Marmer, M. J.: Postoperative jaundice associated with halothane anesthesia, Surg. Gynec. Obstet. *121*:728, 1965.

96. Neale, G., Caughey, D. E., Mollin, D. L., and Booth, C. C.: Effects of intrahepatic and extrahepatic infection on liver function, Brit. Med. J. *1*:382, 1966.

97. Nesmith, L. W., and Davis, J. W.: Hemolytic anemia caused by penicillin, J.A.M.A. *203*:27, 1968.

98. Norcross, J. W., and Dadey, J. L.: Medical complications of operative bile-duct injuries, New Engl. J. Med. *257*:1216, 1957.

99. Pack, G. T., and Molander, D. W.: Pre-

operative and postoperative management of patients subjected to hepatic lobectomy, in Pack, G. T., and Ariel, I. M.: Treatment of Cancer and Allied Diseases, V, ed. 2, pp. 370-379, New York, Hoeber, 1962.

100. Pichlmayr, I., and Stich, W.: Der bilirubinostatische Ikterus, eine neue Ikterusform beim zusammentreffen von Operation, Narkose und Bluttransfusion, Klin. Wschr. 13:665, 1962.

101. Pirofsky, B., Sutherland, D. W., Starr, A., and Griswold, H. E.: Hemolytic anemia complicating aortic-valve surgery: an autoimmune syndrome, New Engl. J. Med. 272:235, 1965.

102. Popper, H.: Hepatic drug reactions simulating viral hepatitis, in McIntyre, N., and Sherlock, S.: Therapeutic Agents and the Liver, pp. 81-97, Oxford, Blackwell; Philadelphia, Davis, 1965.

103. Popper, H., Rubin, E., Gardiol, D., Schaffner, F., and Paronetto, F.: Drug-induced liver disease, Arch. Int. Med. 115:128, 1965.

104. Posen, S.: Alkaline phosphatase, Ann. Int. Med. 67:183, 1967.

105. Powell, L. W., Hemingway, E., Billing, B. H., and Sherlock, S.: Idiopathic unconjugated hyperbilirubinemia (Gilbert's syndrome); a study of 42 families, New Engl. J. Med. 277:1108, 1967.

106. Pruzanski, W.: The influence of steroids on serum bilirubin, leucine aminopeptidase and alkaline phosphatase in extrahepatic obstructive jaundice: the possible diagnostic importance, Am. J. Med. Sci. 251:685, 1966.

107. Pyrtek, L. J., and Bartus, S. A.: Hepatic pyemia, New Engl. J. Med. 272:551, 1965.

108. Reinus, F. Z., and Kesseler, H. J.: Jaundice complicating acute cholecystitis, Surgery 48:522, 1960.

109. Rhoads, J. E., and Howard, J. M.: The Chemistry of Trauma, pp. 151-165, Springfield, Thomas, 1963.

110. Richman, S. M., Delman, A. J., and Grob, D.: Alterations in indices of liver function in congestive heart failure with particular reference to serum enzymes, Am. J. Med. 30:211, 1961.

111. Rodgers, J. B., Mallory, G. K., and Davidson, C. S.: Massive liver cell necrosis, Arch. Int. Med. 114:637, 1964.

112. Ross, J. F., Finch, C. A., Peacock, W. C., and Sammons, M. E.: The in vitro preservation and post-transfusion survival of stored blood, J. Clin. Invest. 26:687, 1947.

113. Rubin, E.: Studies in hepatic injury induced by experimental portacaval shunts, Israel J. Med. Sci. 4:155, 1968.

114. Rubinson, R. M., Holland, P., Schmidt, P. J., and Morrow, A. G.: Hepatitis after open-heart surgery, J. Thorac. Cardiovasc. Surg. 50:575, 1965.

115. Rundle, F. F., Perry, D., Cass, M., and Oddie, T. H.: Rise in serum bilirubin with biliary obstruction and its decline curve after operative relief, Surgery 43:555, 1958.

116. Salisbury, P. F.: Recovery from acute renal failure and acidosis in sickle-cell disease, J.A.M.A. 174:356, 1960.

117. Sanderson, R. G., Ellison, J. H., Benson, J. A., Jr., and Starr, A.: Jaundice following open-heart surgery, Ann. Surg. 165:217, 1967.

118. Schaffner, F.: Iatrogenic jaundice, J.A.M.A. 174:1690, 1960.

119. ————: Diagnosis of drug-induced hepatic damage, J.A.M.A. 191:466, 1965.

120. Schaffner, F., and Popper, H.: Morphologic studies of cholestasis, Gastroenterology 37:565, 1959.

121. Schapiro, R. H., and Isselbacher, K. J.: Benign recurrent intrahepatic cholestasis, New Engl. J. Med. 268:708, 1963.

122. Schenk, W. G., Jr., and Bow, T. M.: Post-transfusion erythrocyte survival: an evaluation of the radio-chromate method, Arch. Surg. 82:391, 1961.

123. Schiff, L., and Billing, B. H.: Congenital defects in bilirubin metabolism as seen in the adult, Gastroenterology 37:595, 1959.

124. Schiff, L., Billing, B. H., and Oikawa, Y.: Familial nonhemolytic jaundice with conjugated bilirubin in the serum: a case study, New Engl. J. Med. 260:1315, 1959.

125. Schmid, M., and Hefti, M. L.: Benign postoperative jaundice, a form of intrahepatic cholestasis, Zschr. Gastroent. 4:89, 1966.

126. Schmid, M., Hefti, M. L., Gattiker, R., Kistler, H. J., and Senning, A.: Benign postoperative intrahepatic cholestasis, New Engl. J. Med. 272:545, 1965.

127. Schniefers, K. H., and Wenn, B.: Icterus following operative interventions, Dtsch. Med. Wschr. 92:540, 1967.

128. Scott, R., Howard, J. M., and Olney, J.

M., Jr.: Hepatic function of the battle casualty: the systemic response to injury, Internat. Abstr. Surg. *102*:209, 1956.

129. Sevitt, S.: Hepatic jaundice after blood transfusion in injured and burned subjects, Brit. J. Surg. *46*:68, 1958.

130. Shapiro, B., Rohman, M., and Cooper, P.: Clostridial infection following abdominal surgery, Ann. Surg. *158*:27, 1963.

131. Sherlock, S.: Biliary secretory failure in man: the problem of cholestasis, *in* Taylor, W. (ed.): The Biliary System, Symposium of NATO Advanced Study Inst. pp. 585-599, Oxford, Blackwell, 1965.

132. Shoemaker, W. C., and Fitch, L. B.: Hepatic lesion of hemorrhagic shock, Arch. Surg. *85*:492, 1962.

133. Shoemaker, W. C., Szanto, P. B., Fitch, L. B., and Brill, N. R.: Hepatic physiologic and morphologic alterations in hemorrhagic shock, Surg. Gynec. Obstet. *118*:828, 1964.

134. Slater, E. M., Gibson, J. M., Dykes, M. H. M., and Walzer, S. G.: Postoperative hepatic necrosis: its incidence and diagnostic value in association with the administration of halothane, New Engl. J. Med. *270*:983, 1964.

135. Smith, L. L., and Veragut, U. P.: the liver and shock, *in* Progress in Surgery, vol. 4, pp. 55-107, New York, Karger, 1964.

136. Stauffer, M. H., Sauer, W. G., Dearing, W. H., and Baggenstoss, A. H.: The spectrum of cholestatic hepatic disease, J.A.M.A. *191*:829, 1965.

137. Summerskill, W. H. J.: The syndrome of benign recurrent cholestasis, Am. J. Med. *38*:298, 1965.

138. Sunzel, H., and Zettergren, L.: Histological liver lesions developing during abdominal operations; a study of their aetiology and pathogenesis in 69 cases of partial gastrectomy, Gastroenterologia *105*:45, 1966.

139. Thompson, D. S., Eason, C. N., and Thompson, B. W.: An evaluation of the effect of halothane on liver function and disease, Am. J. Surg. *114*:658, 1967.

140. Thum, H. J.: Investigations on serum enzyme activities in surgery of bile ducts, Langenbeck Arch. klin. Chir. *297*:91, 1961.

141. Ticktin, H. E., and Zimmerman, H. J.: Hepatic dysfunction and jaundice in patients receiving triacetyloleandomycin. New Engl. J. Med. *267*:964, 1962.

142. Tiesenga, M. F., Neal, R. H., and Hemwall, G. A.: Jaundice due to right hepatic duct obstruction, J.A.M.A. *187*:367, 1964.

143. Tisdale, W. A., Klatskin, G., and Kinsella, E. D.: The significance of the direct-reacting fraction of serum bilirubin in hemolytic jaundice, Am. J. Med. *26*: 214, 1959.

144. Turner, F. P.: Fatal *Clostridium welchii* septicemia following cholecystectomy, Am. J. Surg. *108*:3, 1964.

145. Vinnik, I. E., and Kern, F., Jr.: Biliary cirrhosis in a patient with chronic ulcerative colitis, Gastroenterology *45*:529, 1963.

146. Virtue, R. W. and Payne, K. W.: Postoperative death after fluothane, Anesthesiology *19*:562, 1958.

147. Walker, C. O., and Combes, B.: Biliary cirrhosis induced by chlorpromazine, Gastroenterology *51*:631, 1966.

148. Wanke, M., and Ehlers, C. T.: Clinical and biochemical investigation of hepatic function after gastric resections, Langenbeck Arch. klin. Chir. *303*:215, 1963.

149. Williams, R. D., Elliott, D. W., and Zollinger, R. M.: The effect of hypotension in obstructive jaundice, Arch. Surg. *81*: 334, 1960.

150. Wruble, L. D., Ladman, A. J., Britt, L. G., and Cummins, A. J.: Hepatotoxicity produced by tetracycline overdosage, J.A.M.A. *192*:6, 1965.

Diseases of the Liver
Associated with Ulcerative Colitis

STEVEN P. MISTILIS, M.D.

Liver disease may occur in acute and chronic inflammatory disorders of the bowel such as ulcerative colitis, [1, 3, 4, 7-9, 11, 12, 14, 17, 20-22, 24-29, 31, 34, 36, 37, 43, 49-51] Crohn's disease,[11, 35] typhoid fever, tuberculous enteritis and diverticulitis. Hepatic lesions may also be found in numerous intra-abdominal conditions such as pancreatitis, appendiceal abscess, suppurative portal phlebitis[39] and obstruction to the biliary ducts from a stone, stricture or carcinoma.[6] The reported incidence of liver involvement in patients with chronic inflammatory lesions of the bowel has varied considerably. Based on autopsy material or biopsies in a selected group of patients, the incidence of liver involvement is high[21, 22, 29]; based on clinical evidence of liver disease it is low.[11, 12, 25-28]

Most studies have been concerned with liver changes in two common forms of chronic inflammatory bowel disease, namely, ulcerative and granulomatous colitis. The hepatic lesions reported in ulcerative colitis [25-28] include pericholangitis,[3, 11, 22, 24, 49, 51] fatty liver,[17, 21, 34, 25-28] active chronic hepatitis,[1, 14, 25-28, 42, 55] cirrhosis,[1, 17, 20-22, 25-28, 34, 36, 47, 50] nonspecific hepatitis, bile duct carcinoma,[25, 40] primary biliary cirrhosis,[3, 24, 34, 49] viral hepatitis[34] and primary sclerosing cholangitis.[52] The incidence of these hepatic changes in two large studies based on aspiration liver biopsies has been between 10 and 15 per cent.[11, 25-28] Similar changes have been reported in Crohn's disease.[11]

Fatty metamorphosis used to be considered the commonest hepatic lesion in ulcerative colitis.[17, 21, 34] This belief was based on material obtained from patients at operation or postmortem and fatty liver was probably related to nutritional deficiencies in a fulminant or long-standing debilitating disease. I found that pericholangitis was the commonest hepatic change in patients with ulcerative colitis[25-28]; this has been confirmed.[11] The other lesions seen in order of frequency are active chronic hepatitis, fatty liver and cirrhosis. There also appears to be a definite association between ulcerative colitis and sclerosing cholangitis[52] and cholangio-carcinoma.[25, 40]

PERICHOLANGITIS AND ULCERATIVE COLITIS

Pathology. The changes of pericholangitis are not specific for ulcerative colitis. Identical liver changes may be seen in pancreatitis,[39] Crohn's disease,[11, 35] extrahepatic bile duct obstruction, diverticulitis, typhoid fever, septicemia[39] and primary sclerosing cholangitis.[52] The changes may superficially resemble those encountered in primary biliary cirrhosis,[6, 23, 30, 38, 54] benign recurrent cholestasis[10, 45-48] and some forms of drug-induced hepatitis, tuberculosis, sarcoid, brucellosis and lymphomas.[39]

Although the term pericholangitis focuses attention on bile duct involvement, other structures in the portal tract may be affected and changes may also extend into the hepatic lobule. The most striking changes, however, are in the portal tracts and the severity varies considerably from one portal tract to another. All biliary radicles may be involved but the small and medium sized perilobular bile ducts are most affected. The changes may not be confined to the perilobular biliary system but may extend to include the extrahepatic bile ducts. The disease may be acute, subacute or chronic and a combination of these changes is often found in the one histologic section.

In the *acute stage* (Fig. 30–15) the portal tracts are swollen from inflammatory exudate, edema and infiltration with lymphocytes, histiocytes, polymorphonuclear leu-

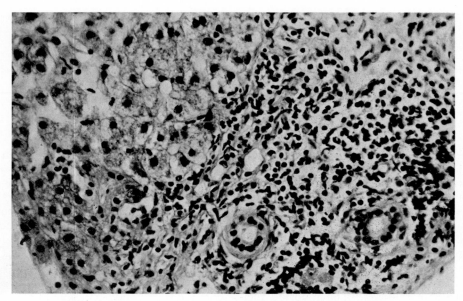

FIG. 30–15. Acute pericholangitis with marked swelling of the portal tract, intense inflammatory cell infiltration, perilymphangitis and ductular changes. × 100.

kocytes and plasma cells. Inflammation is concentrated about the perilobular bile ducts which occasionally show evidence of mucosal damage. Perilymphangitis and some endophlebitis may also be present. Intra-

lobular changes include pericentral bile stasis, Kupffer cell proliferation, small foci of inflammation and necrosis, and occasional parenchymal degenerative change in in the form of acidophilic bodies.

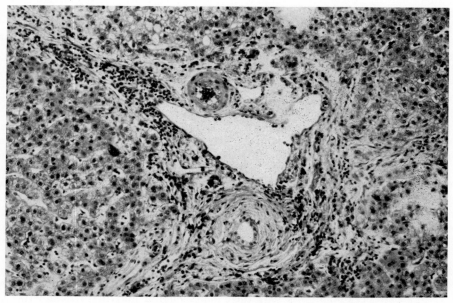

FIG. 30–16. Subacute pericholangitis. Inflammatory reaction has lessened. Considerable edema is still present and early fibrosis is evident. × 125.

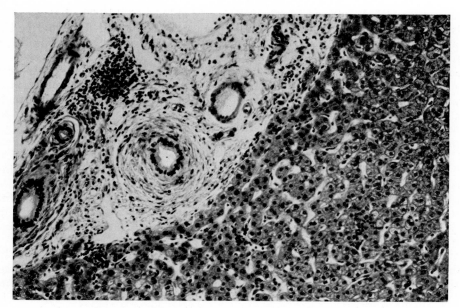

Fig. 30–17. Chronic pericholangitis; circumductal fibrosis can be seen to involve the small and medium sized perilobular bile ducts. The fibrosis is confined to the portal tract. The portal inflammatory reaction has subsided but some inflammatory cells are present within the lobule. × 75.

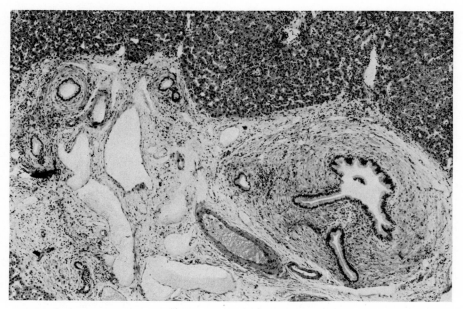

Fig. 30–18. Chronic pericholangitis. There is advanced circumductal fibrosis involving biliary radicles of all sizes. Lymphangiectasis is prominent and some phlebosclerosis can be seen. There is union of several portal tracts in the advanced fibrotic change. Parenchymal dissolution has occurred and there is an approximation of the fibrotic process to central veins. Inflammatory cells can be seen concentrated about several central veins. × 40.

In subacute pericholangitis (Fig. 30–16) there is less inflammation but mild peribiliary and periportal fibrosis. These changes represent a transition between acute and chronic stages.

The *chronic stage* (Figs. 30–17 to 30–19) is characterized by concentric circumductal fibrosis, dilated lymphatic vessels, mild phlebosclerosis, varying portal and septal fibrosis and a marked reduction of inflammation in the portal tracts. Some cases show a few areas of piecemeal necrosis in the perilobular region or at the junction of the hepatic lobules and fibrous bands. Fibrosis is usually confined to the portal tracts but may spread to the interlobular septa or traverse the hepatic lobules. Broad bands of fibrous tissue with a histologic pattern characteristic of postnecrotic cirrhosis appear to result from progressive destruction of the hepatic parenchymal tissue.

Changes seen early in the disease may resolve *spontaneously* or in response to therapy. Once pericholangitis with fibrosis is established, progression to the chronic stage is probably inevitable. The lesion eventually becomes inactive and the usual end result is periportal fibrosis of a varying degree. A few patients may develop cirrhosis.

Clinical Features. The disease may be classified clinically into three groups[25-28]; namely, asymptomatic, cholestatic and cholangitic. However, these appear to be merely clinical variants of the same pathologic process. The liver disease appears at a variable interval after the onset of ulcerative colitis and there is no correlation between its severity and that of colitis. When the liver disease becomes manifest the colitis is often in a chronic inactive phase (Fig. 30–20) and may persist after the colon has been resected.

The term pericholangitis might imply that episodes of clinical *cholangitis* form the predominant clinical pattern. This is not so, and although typical cholangitis episodes consisting of fever, abdominal pain, toxemia, a tender enlarged liver and leukocytosis may be seen, this is an unusual pattern. Recurrent cholangitis associated with

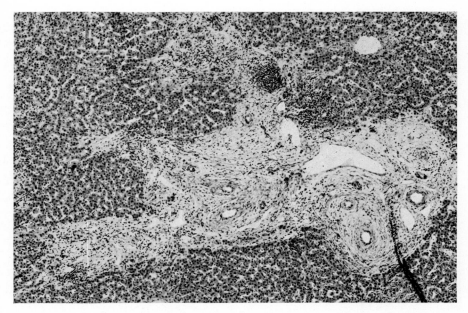

Fig. 30–19. Chronic pericholangitis with post-necrotic cirrhosis. The inflammatory reaction can be seen along a "broad front" concentrated at the junctional zone of portal tracts and hepatic lobules. Large accumulations of inflammatory cells of almost pseudogranulomatous proportions are present. There is piecemeal necrosis with dissolution of parenchymal cells in consecutive lobules. × 100.

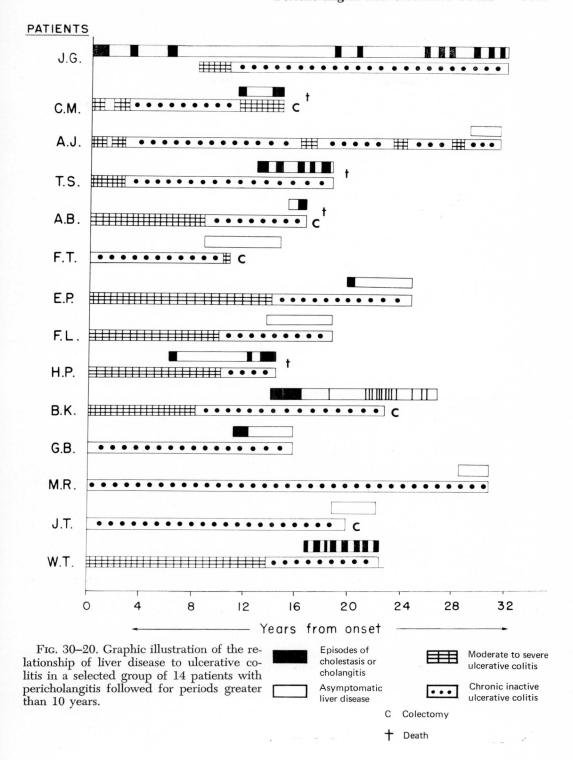

Fig. 30–20. Graphic illustration of the relationship of liver disease to ulcerative colitis in a selected group of 14 patients with pericholangitis followed for periods greater than 10 years.

Episodes of cholestasis or cholangitis

Asymptomatic liver disease

Moderate to severe ulcerative colitis

Chronic inactive ulcerative colitis

C   Colectomy

†   Death

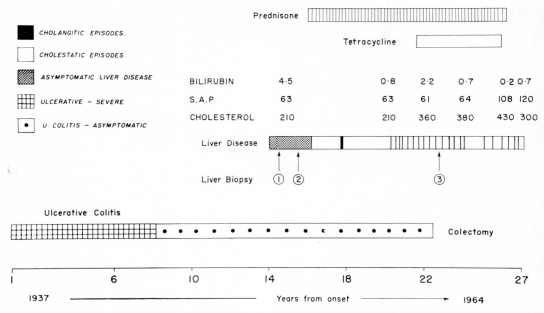

FIG. 30–21. Graphic illustration of the effect of prednisone, tetracycline and colectomy on the clinical course in a case of ulcerative colitis and pericholangitis.

ulcerative colitis is a relatively benign disease since, for example, as many as 25 attacks have been documented in one patient for a period of 33 years. The onset of the attack is entirely unpredictable and its duration variable. Patients may remain symptom-free for long periods.

Among *symptomatic patients*, episodes of cholestasis constitute the commonest clinical group. These episodes are often sudden in onset; many recur and are characterized by jaundice, intense pruritus, hepatomegaly and occasionally mild fever. Jaundice and pruritus may persist for as long as 2 years but eventually subside.

Asymptomatic pericholangitis is the commonest form of the disease and is characterized by hepatomegaly, a normal serum bilirubin, a persistent elevation of the serum alkaline phosphatase, hypercholesterolemia and abnormal BSP retention. The patients may develop splenomegaly and esophageal varices from obstruction to portal venous flow at a presinusoidal level.

The three clinical forms of the disease may be encountered in the one patient (Fig. 30–21). A patient who presents with cho-

lestasis may subsequently have an attack of cholangitis. During the intervening periods, the clinical picture and biochemical and histologic changes resemble those of patients in whom the disorder remains asymptomatic throughout.

The most significant biochemical change is a persistent elevation of the serum alkaline phosphatase. This is usually associated with abnormal BSP retention and hypercholesterolemia. The unimpressive transaminase levels may help to distinguish the cholestatic form of the disease from acute infectious hepatitis. Marked serum protein disturbances do not occur: this is important in the differentiation from active chronic hepatitis. Serum cholesterol, while usually persistently raised, is not as high as in primary biliary cirrhosis.

Etiology. Portal bacteremia had been documented in cases of ulcerative colitis,[5] and is probably significant, since portal blood is normally sterile.[32] Irritating material or bacteria reaching the liver via the portal vein are apparently drained from the interstitial spaces by the portal lymphatics.[39] This might explain the presence of polymorphonuclear leukocytes in the acute stage of the disease and perilymphangitis and lymphangiectasia in the subacute and chronic stages.[25] Assuming bacterial infection becomes established in the portal tracts, the pathologic changes appear to be self-perpetuating despite antibiotics and colectomy.[25-28] A similar situation has been noted in animals given alpha-naphthylisothiocyanate, an agent that induces ductular damage.[13] The subsequent inflammatory reaction, ductular proliferation and periductular fibrosis progress as a response to the initial ductular injury.

It is of interest to speculate on the similarity of the pathologic findings in patients with pericholangitis and the changes in animals given large amounts of lithocholic acid.[18, 33] This bile acid is highly insoluble and under normal circumstances is not reabsorbed from the gastrointestinal tract in man. It may be that significant amounts, however, are absorbed when the bowel mucosa is damaged as in ulcerative colitis. Alternatively lithocholic acid may be produced from its precursor chenodeoxycholic acid by bacterial action in the portal tracts.

Treatment. The various therapeutic measures available include long-term tetracycline therapy, corticosteroids, colectomy and biliary drainage. Since patients with pericholangitis may develop cirrhosis or extensive periportal fibrosis with presinusoidal portal hypertension,[25] every effort should be made to arrest this process early in its course. The effectiveness of therapy may depend on early detection of the lesion. In asymptomatic patients considerable reliance must be placed on an enlarged liver or a raised serum alkaline phosphatase. Liver biopsy establishes the diagnosis.

Results of these therapeutic measures so far reported have been disappointing, but treatment has usually been instituted well *after* the disease was established. In my series,[27] tetracycline therapy given for periods of up to 6 years, in a dose of 500 mg./day, did not appear to affect the clinical course but in a dosage of 2.0 Gm./day it does appear to shorten the cholangitis episodes. Neither biliary drianage nor steroids

appear to relieve the jaundice and episodes of jaundice recurring after colectomy.

CIRRHOSIS AND PORTAL HYPERTENSION

The reported incidence of cirrhosis in ulcerative colitis has varied from 1.5 to 19 per cent.[1, 17, 20-22, 25, 34, 36, 47, 50] Although portal and biliary cirrhosis have been reported, postnecrotic cirrhosis is commonest.[25] Cirrhosis is inevitable in active chronic hepatitis and occurs in a significant number of patients with pericholangitis. In some cases the cause of the cirrhosis is not known and has been possibly related to serum or infectious hepatitis.[25, 34]

In ulcerative colitis portal hypertension may develop.[4, 26, 28, 47] Apart from its occurrence with cirrhosis, presinusoidal portal hypertension can be shown to be secondary to an extensive periportal fibrosis.[28] If the portal venous blood flow is obstructed, esophageal varices may result, but in patients who have had a total colectomy, varices may appear on the abdomen at the ileostomy stoma (Fig. 30–22) or in the rectum at the site of an ileorectal anastomosis. In such patients the possibility of portal hypertension should be considered if there is bleeding from the ileostomy or rectum; inflammation in the remaining small bowel is uncommon. A portacaval shunt prevents further bleeding, for in most cases of pericholangitis portal hypertension is due to an obstruction of portal venous flow at the presinusoidal level and there is no significant parenchymal disease.

PRIMARY BILIARY CIRRHOSIS

Primary biliary cirrhosis[3, 24, 34, 49, 50] reportedly has occurred in ulcerative colitis, but recent studies show that most of these cases were probably examples of chronic pericholangitis. Since both disorders involve the biliary system at a similar level, it is not surprising to find many features common to both diseases. However, it is important to distinguish between these entities, for in primary biliary cirrhosis the long-term prognosis is poor.

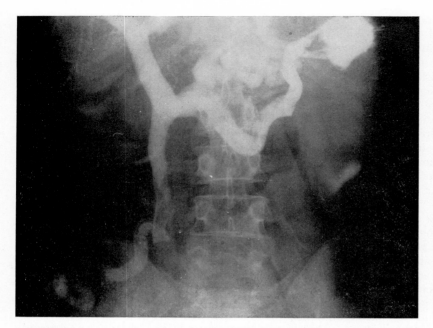

FIG.   30–22. (*Top*) Splenoportogram in a patient with pericholangitis and ulcerative colitis. The portal hypertension developed after colectomy. Note the varices at the ileosveins with distal dilated mesenteric tomy stoma. (*Bottom*) Subcutaneous varices can be seen on the abdomen at the ileostomy site. (Published by courtesy of Dr. Alan Cameron of Green Bay Hospital, Auckland, New Zealand.)

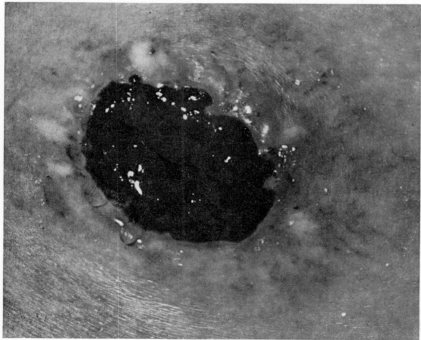

Pruritus, hepatosplenomegaly, jaundice,langitis, hepatic tenderness, leukocytosis hypercholesterolemia, abnormal BSP reten-and the absence of marked hypercholestion, marked elevation of the serum alkalineterolemia, xanthomata, tuberous skin lephosphatase and presinusoidal portal hyper-sions and severe pigmentation distinguishes tension occur in both disorders. However,pericholangitis from primary biliary cirrhothe presence of fever, abdominal pain, cho-sis. Although patients with **pericholangitis**

may have persistent cholestasis for up to 2 years, the jaundice eventually subsides. Antinuclear, smooth muscle and antimitochondrial antibodies are frequently detected in patients with primary biliary cirrhosis but are not found in ulcerative colitis with persistent cholestasis.

In primary biliary cirrhosis, ductular involvement is initially confined to medium sized intrahepatic biliary radicles (see Chapter 20), polymorphonuclear leukocytes are unusual in the inflammatory reaction, bile stasis more peripheral in distribution, ductular proliferation is absent early in the disease, normal bile ducts are reduced in number and granulomas with giant cells are frequently present. These changes are to be contrasted with pericholangitis or ulcerative colitis where bile ducts are prominent, inflammation surrounds ducts of all sizes, polymorphs are seen in the portal tracts, bile stasis, if present, is centrilobular, and there are lymphangiectasia and mild phlebitic changes without a granulomatous reaction. These two diseases cannot be distinguished histologically later in the course of the disease when cirrhosis has been established.

PRIMARY SCLEROSING CHOLANGITIS

Primary sclerosing cholangitis is a rare disease characterized by partial or total involvement of the extrahepatic biliary ducts by a progressive inflammatory sclerosing and obliterative process. The disease may involve the intrahepatic bile ducts and biliary radicles in the portal tract. Patients present with chronic biliary obstruction and later develop all the features of secondary biliary cirrhosis with portal hypertension and liver cell failure. Gastrointestinal bleeding from esophageal varices is a common terminal event.

In a large series of patients with sclerosing cholangitis,[52] approximately 30 per cent were found to have associated ulcerative colitis. No cause could be found for the remaining cases. Some of these patients had had previous biliary tract surgery and some were found to have cholelithiasis. Sclerosing cholangitis is occasionally seen in patients with a generalized vasculitis, retroperitoneal fibrosis[2, 15, 16, 41, 44] Reidel's thyroiditis,[2] mediastinal fibrosis and pseudo-tumor of the orbit.[53] It may often be seen, however, without intra-abdominal or a general systemic disease.[52]

Primary sclerosing cholangitis should not be confused with suppurative cholangitis, benign stricture or primary biliary cirrhosis. Every attempt should be made to exclude cholangiocarcinoma, for the disorders may have an identical clinical picture and similar findings at laparotomy.

Although patients with ulcerative colitis may have a sclerosing cholangitis of the extrahepatic biliary tree, this association is not common; it was found in only 0.8 per cent of 1,474 patients with ulcerative colitis.[52] In most cases the colitis is moderately severe and the sclerosing cholangitis usually appears after an interval of 3 to 25 years.

The clinical manifestations of sclerosing cholangitis are the same whether or not there is associated disease. Patients give a history of jaundice, intermittent epigastric and right upper quadrant pain, pruritus and occasionally nausea, vomiting and febrile episodes. Jaundice may initially be intermittent or fluctuate in intensity but later becomes chronic and progressive. The liver is enlarged and occasionally tender, and patients often show signs of secondary biliary cirrhosis with portal hypertension. The laboratory tests are those of obstructive jaundice with an increase in the serum bilirubin, alkaline phosphatase and serum cholesterol levels with essentially normal serum proteins.

Diagnosis can usually be made only by exploratory laparotomy. The extrahepatic ducts are thickened, indurated and in an advanced case the common bile duct appears as a cord-like structure with a pinpoint lumen. In most cases the entire biliary tree is involved, but in others the disease process is confined to one portion of the common bile duct or may involve the right or left hepatic duct. Operative cholangiography will outline the extent of duct involvement but this procedure may be technically difficult in cases where the duct lumen is virtually occluded. A preoperative

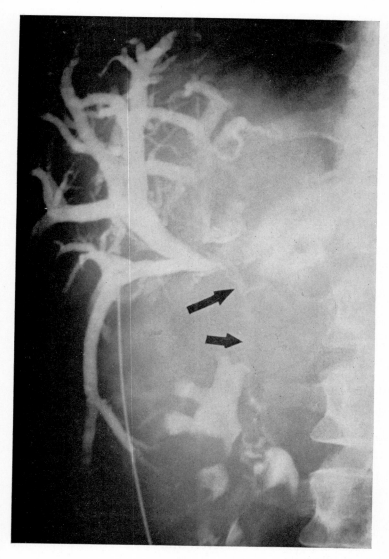

FIG. 30–23. Transhepatic cholangiogram in a case of idiopathic sclerosing cholangitis. The common duct lumen is narrowed and the proximal right and left hepatic ducts are dilated.

transhepatic cholangiogram sometimes provides a more adequate picture of the biliary tree and intrahepatic bile ducts (Fig. 30–23).

Multiple biopsies and sections of the enlarged glands and ducts must be taken at operation to exclude ductal carcinoma. The pathologic changes are identical regardless of the cause. Marked fibrosis is found in the submucosa and subserosa and this is accompanied by edema and infiltration with lymphocytes, plasma cells and histiocytes. The ductular epithelium is initially intact but

may later become involved in the inflammatory and fibrotic process.

Medical treatment with steroids and broad-spectrum antibiotics has been suggested and may induce temporary improvement. Treatment should however be directed toward decompressing the biliary system to prevent further liver damage. The duct should be dilated and drained where possible but this may not be feasible when the common bile duct is completely occluded. The proximal ducts are then dilated, and a hepatico-jejunostomy or cholecystojejunostomy with jejunojejunostomy over a T or Y tube may provide adequate internal drainage of bile.

ACTIVE CHRONIC HEPATITIS

Patients with active chronic hepatitis frequently give a history of chronic diarrhea, and a proportion of these can be shown to have ulcerative colitis. The association of these two diseases is well established.[1, 14, 25-28, 42, 55] Clinical, laboratory and histologic features of active chronic hepatitis are similar regardless of the presence or absence of colitis. However, associated ulcerative colitis worsens the overall prognosis.

Active chronic hepatitis must be distinguished from pericholangitis, for these two diseases demand different treatment. Spider nevi, acne, amenorrhea, Cushingoid facies, L.E. cells, hyperglobulinemia, mlutiple skin rashes, glomerulonephritis, arthralgia, markedly elevated zinc sulfate turbidity levels, perilobular piecemeal necrosis and inflammation in liver biopsy sections together with abnormal serologic reactions occur in active chronic hepatitis but rarely in pericholangitis. Occasionally the pathologic features of both diseases are encountered in the same section; here the clinical picture is usually that of active chronic hepatitis. Steroids or azathioprine are frequently effective in active chronic hepatitis but not in pericholangitis.

REFERENCES

1. Bargen, J. A.: Disease of the liver associated with ulcerative colitis, Ann. Int. Med. 39:285, 1953.
2. Bartholomew, L. G., Cain, J. C., Woolner, L. B., Utz, D. C., and Ferris, D. O.: Sclerosing cholangitis; its possible association with Reidel's struma and fibrous retroperitonitis; report of two cases, New Engl. J. Med. 269:8, 1963.
3. Boden, R. W., Rankin, J. G., Goulston, S. J. M., and Morrow, W.: The liver in ulcerative colitis: the significance of raised serum alkaline phosphatase levels, Lancet 2:245, 1959.
4. Brooke, B. N., Dykes, P. W., and Walker, F. C.: A study of liver disorder in ulcer-

ative colitis, Postgrad. Med. J. 37:245, 1961.
5. Brooke, B. N., and Slaney, G.: Portal bacteraemia in ulcerative colitis, Lancet 1: 1206, 1958.
6. Cameron, R., and Hou, P. C.: Biliary Cirrhosis, p. 87, London, Oliver; Springfield, Ill., Thomas, 1962.
7. Clinical Pathological Conference, Massachusetts General Hospital, New Engl. J. Med. 239:635, 1948.
8. ———: New Engl. J. Med. 240:388, 1949.
9. ———: New Engl. J. Med. 270: 206, 1964.
10. De Groote, J., Goubeau, P., and Vandenbroucke, J.: Ictère cholostatique recidevant, Acta gastroenterol. 23:747, 1960.
11. Dordal, E., Glagov, S., and Kirsner, J. B.: Hepatic lesions in chronic inflammatory bowel disease, Gastroenterology 52:239, 1967.
12. Edwards, F. C., and Truelove, S. C.: The course and prognosis of ulcerative colitis. III. Complications, Gut 5:1, 1964.
13. Goldfarb, S., Singer, E. J., and Popper, H.: Experimental cholangitis due to alpha-naphthyl-isothiocyanate (A.N.I.T.), Am. J. Path. 40:685, 1962.
14. Gray, N., Mackay, I. R., Taft, L. I., Weiden, S., and Wood, I. J.: Hepatitis, colitis and lupus manifestations, Am. J. Dig. Dis. 3:481, 1958.
15. Hardy, J. D.: Some lesions of the biliary tract; idiopathic retroperitoneal fibrosis and other problems, Am. J. Surg. 103:457, 1962.
16. Hellstrom, H. R., and Perez-Stable, E. C.: Retroperitoneal fibrosis with disseminated vasculitis and intrahepatic sclerosing cholangitis, Am. J. Med. 40:184, 1966.
17. Hoffbauer, F. N., Dennis, C., and Karlson, K.: The liver in ulcerative colitis, Univ. Minn. Med. Bull. 23:129, 1951.
18. Holsti, P.: Cirrhosis of the liver induced in rabbits by gastric instillation of 3-monohydroxycholanic acid, Nature 186:250, 1960.
19. Hunt, R. D.: Proliferation of bile ductules (the ductular cell reaction) induced by lithocholic acid, Fed. Proc. 24:431, 1965.
20. Jones, G. W., Baggenstoss, A. H., and Bargen, J. A.: Hepatic lesions and dysfunction associated with chronic ulcerative colitis, Am. J. Med. Sci. 221:279, 1951.
21. Kimmelstiel, P., Large, H. L., Jr., and

Verner, H. D.: Liver damage in ulcerative colitis, Am. J. Path. 28:259, 1952.

22. Kleckner, M. S., Stauffer, M. H., Bargen, J. A., and Dockerty, M. B.: Hepatic lesions in the living patient with chronic ulcerative colitis as demonstrated by needle biopsy, Gastroenterology 22:13, 1952.

23. MacMahon, H. E.: Biliary cirrhosis: differential features of the five types, Lab. Invest. 4:243, 1955.

24. McCarthy, C. F., and Read, A. E.: Bleeding esophageal varices in ulcerative colitis, Gastroenterology 42:325, 1962.

25. Mistilis, S. P.: Pericholangitis and ulcerative colitis. I. Pathology, etiology and pathogenesis, Ann. Int. Med. 63:1, 1965.

26. Mistilis, S. P., and Goulston, S. J. M.: Liver disease in ulcerative colitis in Badenoch, J., and Brooke, B. N. (eds.): Recent Advances in Gastroenterology, London, Churchill; Boston, Little, Brown, 1965.

27. Mistilis, S. P., Skyring, A. P., and Goulston, S. J. M.: Effect of longterm tetracycline therapy, steroid therapy, colectomy and biliary drainage in pericholangitis associated with ulcerative colitis, Aust. Ann. Med. 14:286, 1965.

28. ———: Pericholangitis and ulcerative colitis. II. Clinical aspects, Ann. Int. Med. 63:17, 1965.

29. Monto, A. S.: The liver in ulcerative disease of the small intestinal tract: functional and anatomical changes, Ann. Int. Med. 50:1385, 1959.

30. Moschcowitz, E.: Morphology and pathogenesis of biliary cirrhosis, Arch. Path. 54:259, 1952.

31. Olhagen, L.: Ulcerative colitis in cirrhosis of the liver, Acta med. Scand. 162:143, 1958.

32. Orloff, M. J., Peskin, G. W., and Ellis, H. L.: A bacteriologic study of human portal blood: implications regarding hepatic ischaemia in man, Ann. Surg. 148:738, 1958.

33. Palmer, R. H., and Hruban, Z.: Production of bile duct hyperplasia and gall stones by lithocholic acid, J. Clin. Invest. 45:1255, 1966.

34. Palmer, W. L., Kirsner, J. B., Goldgraber, M. B., and Fuentes, S. S.: Disease of the liver in chronic ulcerative colitis, Am. J. Med. 36:856, 1964.

35. ———: Disease of the liver in regional enteritis, Am. J. Med. Sci. 246:663, 1963.

36. Parker, R. G. F., and Kendall, E. J. C.: The liver in ulcerative colitis, Brit. Med. J. 2:1030, 1954.

37. Pollard, H. M., and Block, M.: Association of hepatic insufficiency with chronic ulcerative colitis, Arch. Int. Med. 82:159, 1948.

38. Popper, H., Rubin, E., and Schaffner, F.: The problem of primary biliary cirrhosis (Editorial), Am. J. Med. 33:807, 1962.

39. Popper, H., and Shaffner, F.: Liver: Structure and Function, pp. 240-248, New York, McGraw-Hill, 1957.

40. Rankin, J. G., Skyring, A. P., and Goulston, S. J. M.: Liver in ulcerative colitis; obstructive jaundice due to bile duct carcinoma, Gut 7:433, 1966.

41. Raper, F. P.: Idiopathic retroperitoneal fibrosis involving the ureters, Brit. J. Urol. 28:436, 1956.

42. Read. A. E., Sherlock, S., and Harrison, C. V.: Active "juvenile" cirrhosis considered as a part of systemic disease and the effect of corticosteroid therapy, Gut 4:378, 1963

43. Ross, J. R., and Swarts, J. M.: Hepatic dysfunction and cirrhosis in chronic ulcerative colitis, Gastroenterology 10:81, 1948.

44. Schneider, C. F.: Idiopathic retroperitoneal fiibrosis producing vena caval, biliary, ureteral and duodenal obstructions, Ann. Surg. 159:316, 1964.

45. Shapiro, R., and Isselbacher, K. J.: Benign recurrent intrahepatic cholestasis, New Engl. J. Med. 268:708, 1963.

46. Summerskill, W. H. J, and Walshe, J. M.: Benign recurrent intrahepatic "obstructive" jaundice, Lancet 2:686, 1959.

47. Tumen, H. J., Monaghan, J. F., and Jobb, E.: Hepatic cirrhosis as a complication of chronic ulcerative colitis, Ann. Int. Med. 26:542, 1947.

48. Tygstrup, N.: Intermittent possibly familial intrahepatic cholestatic jaundice, Lancet 1:1171, 1960.

49. Vinnik, I. E., and Kern, F., Jr.: Biliary cirrhosis in a patient with chronic ulcerative colitis, Gastroenterology 45:529, 1963.

50. ———: Liver diseases in ulcerative colitis, Arch. Int. Med. 112:41, 1963.

51. Vinnik, I. E., Kern, F., Jr., and Corley, W. D.: Serum 5-nucleotidase and pericholangitis in patients with chronic ulcera-

tive colitis, Gastroenterology *45*:492, 1963.

52. Warren, K. W., Athanassiades, S., and Monge, J. I.: Primary sclerosing cholangitis; a study of 42 cases, Am. J. Surg. *111*:23, 1966.

53. Wenger, J., Gingrich, G. W., and Mendeloff, J.: Sclerosing cholangitis—a manifestation of systemic disease, increased serum gamma globulin, follicular lymph node hyperplasia, and orbital pseudotumor, Arch. Int. Med. *116*:509, 1965.

54. Williams, G. E. G.: Pericholangiolitic biliary cirrhosis, J. Path. Bact. 89:23, 1965.

55. Willoxc, R. G., and Isselbacher, K. J.: Chronic liver disease in young people; clinical features and course in 33 patients, Am. J. Med. *30*:185, 1961.

Idiopathic Benign Recurrent Intrahepatic Cholestasis

LEON SCHIFF, M.D.

In 1958 Summerskill and Walshe described two patients who had multiple episodes of jaundice accompanied by chemical and histologic evidence of cholestasis, a syndrome they designated as benign recurrent intrahepatic obstructive jaundice.[13] By 1967, over 20 cases of this disease had been recorded.[1-4, 8, 9, 11-17]

The age of onset varies from 1 to 27 years. The disease has been reported in siblings.[3, 8, 16] The clinical features are characterized by recurrent attacks of pruritus, ano-

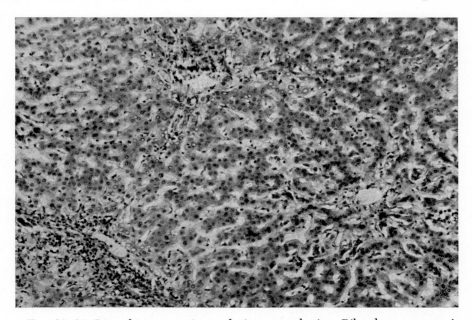

FIG. 30–24. Liver biopsy specimen, during exacerbation. Bile plugs are seen in mid-zone canaliculi and some pseudoacinar alteration is evident. Small collections of inflammatory cells are seen, usually in portal areas. Nuclear "glycogen" vacuolization, of unknown significance, is prominent. Hematoxylin and eosin. × 150,

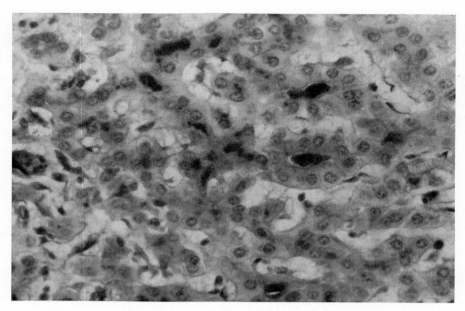

FIG. 30–25. Higher magnification of Figure 30–24. × 500.

rexia and weight loss followed within a period of 1 to 3 weeks by the development of obstructive jaundice with clay-colored stools and dark urine. Abdominal pain and chills and fever do not occur. Hepatomegaly is usually absent. Despite numerous episodes of jaundice dating from as early as 1 year of age and extending over a period

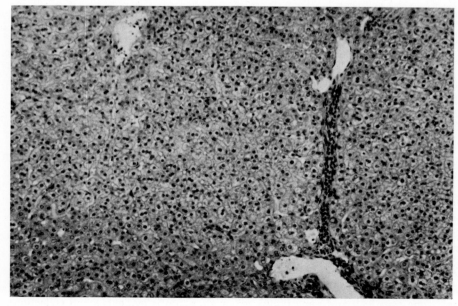

FIG. 30–26. Liver biopsy specimen, during remission, 90 days later than in Figures 30–24 and 30–25. The liver is essentially normal, save for granules of pigment, histochemically of lipofuscin type, in a few cells. Hematoxylin and eosin. × 150.

of 38 years in one case, there may be no persistent impairment of liver function or persistent pathologic changes.[9]

The average duration of an attack is 3 to 4 months, although some have reportedly lasted up to 2 years. An interval of 9 years between attacks has been recorded.[12] The exacerbations may be seasonal and seasonal pruritus may recur for years prior to the initial appearance of jaundice.[11]

The depth of icterus may vary from one attack to another. In most cases the serum bilirubin is 10 to 20 mg.% with a major increase in the conjugated fraction. There is decrease in Bromsulphalein storage and Tm,[1, 17] increase in serum alkaline phos-

phatase, serum bile acids, and alpha-2 and beta-globulins, with a slight rise in the serum transaminase. During remission, there is a return to normal in the results of these laboratory tests.

Contradictory results have been reported on the rate at which injected unconjugated bilirubin disappears from the plasma. Williams et al.[17] found a normal disappearance rate in two cases in contrast with Brodersen and Tygstrup,[2] who reported an abnormally rapid disappearance in two cases and postulated a hyperactive bilirubin conjugating mechanism. The mechanism of the icterus which occurs in recurrent intrahepatic cholestasis has been assumed to be

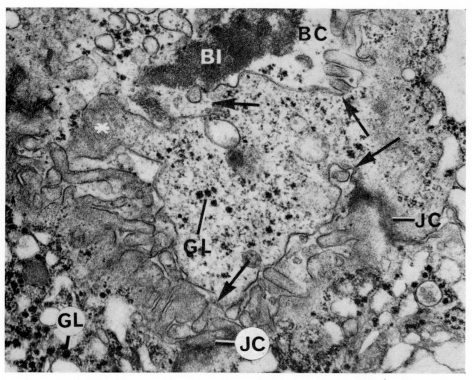

Fig. 30–27. Thin section stained with uranium and lead. A bile canaliculus (BC) lies within four continuous cells. A large, clear bleb protrudes into the canalicular lumen with its membrane continuous with the microvilli at the long arrows. The asterisk shows a mass of protruded cytoplasm that may be an enlarged microvillus. Inside the bleb, glycogen aggregates (GL) are evident. A dense granular material (BI) like the bile pigment described by others, is present in the lumen. Glycogen aggregates are seen inside the lumen, possibly a preparative artifact or a result of leakage from the bleb. The canalicular membrane is broken in areas of the bleb (short arrows), but junctional complexes (JC) are well preserved. × 23,000. (From Biempica, Gutstein and Arias, Gastroenterology 52:521, 1967.)

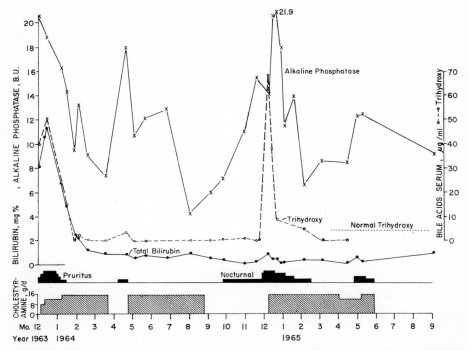

FIG. 30–28. Cholestyramine effect on levels of bile acids, bilirubin, alkaline phostase and pruritus. (This figure appeared, in part, *in* Spiegel *et al.*: Am. J. Med. 39:682, 1965.)

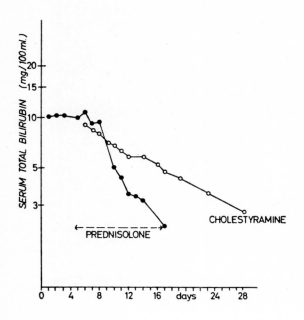

FIG. 30–29. The effect of prednisolone therapy in Case 4 (23rd attack) contrasted with the rate of fall in serum bilirubin level observed during a previous attack (22nd) when he was treated with cholestyramine. (Williams et al.: Quart. J. Med. 33:387, 1964)

due to a block in the excretion of bilirubin into the bile with consequent regurgitation of the pigment into the blood as is assumed to be true in other forms of cholestasis.

Biopsy specimens of liver obtained during symptomatic periods show marked centrilobular bile stasis and cellular infiltration of the portal areas as viewed under light microscopy (Figs. 30–24 and 30–25). These changes usually disappear during a remission (Fig. 30–26). Studies of the electron microscopic changes have been carried out by a number of authors.[1, 3, 10, 13] During periods of exacerbation, bile canalicular changes are similar to those seen in other forms of cholestasis with distortion and reduction of the microvilli. Other changes include mitochondrial alterations, almost complete cessation of nucleoside phosphatase activity, reduction in the number of acid phosphatase-rich lysosomes, abundance of lipid spheres and glycogen-rich nuclei and intracanalicular and intracellular bile pigment[1] (Fig. 30–27). Numerous vesicles, mainly intracellular and of variable size, have been described.[13] During clinical remission, the ultrastructural changes in general return to normal, although small amounts of intracellular and intracanalicular bile pigment, some glycogen-rich nuclei and crystalloid nucleoids with the microbodies may still be present.[1] The round bodies described by Summerskill as disappearing during remission may still be found in the anicteric phase of the disease.[3]

Extrahepatic biliary obstruction must be excluded by laparotomy and operative cholangiography. Klatskin has been impressed with the smallness of the bile ducts as revealed in the operative cholangiograms obtained from several of the reported cases.[7]

Contradictory results have been recorded on the effects of cholestyramine on the pruritus. This may be explained by inadequate doses in some cases, as exemplified in our own experience, in which it was necessary to increase the dose up to 16 Gm./day in order to obtain relief.[11] Of considerable interest was the simultaneous lowering of the serum bilirubin, serum bile acids, and serum alkaline phosphatase which followed the institution of cholestyramine therapy, in this patient suggesting the possibility of a cor-

rective effect on the basic disturbance present (Fig. 30–28). The role of bile salts in the experimental production of cholestasis,[5, 6] indistinguishable from that which occurs clinically, suggests that they play an etiologic role in the idiopathic recurrent form. Further study in this regard would appear unwarranted.

The serum bilirubin has been reported to drop with the use of steroids (Fig. 30–29) and maintenance of such therapy has been advocated with the hope of reducing the frequency of recurrence.[17]

REFERENCES

1. Biempica. L., Gutstein, S., and Arias, I. M.: Morphological and biochemical studies of benign recurrent cholestasis, Gastroenterology 52:521, 1967.
2. Brodersen, R., and Tygstrup, N.: Serum bilirubin studies in patients with intermittent intrahepatic cholestasis, Gut 8:46, 1967.
3. Da Silva, L. C., and De Brito, T.: Benign recurrent intrahepatic cholestasis in two brothers. A clinical, light, and electron microscopy study, Ann. Int. Med. 65:330, 1966.
4. De Groote, J., Goubeau, P., and Vandenbroucke, J.: Recurring cholestatic icterus, Acta Gastroenterol. Belg. 23:747, 1960.
5. Javitt, N. B.: Cholestasis in rats induced by taurolithocholate, Nature 210:1262, 1966.
6. Javitt, N. B. and Arias, I. M.: Intrahepatic cholestasis: a functional approach to pathogenesis, Gastroenterology 53:171, 1967.
7. Klatskin, G.: Personal communication.
8. Kühn, H. A.: Intrahepatic cholestasis in two brothers, German Med. Monthly 8:185, 1963.
9. Schapiro, R. H., and Isselbacher, K. J.: Benign recurrent intrahepatic cholestasis, New Engl. J. Med. 268:708, 1963.
10. Schubert, W. K., Garancis, J., and Perrin, E.: Idiopathic benign recurrent cholestasis: biochemical and histologic changes induced by cholestyramine therapy, Clin. Res. 13:409, 1965.
11. Spiegel, E. L., Shubert, W., Perrin, E., and Schiff, L.: Benign recurrent intrahepatic cholestasis, with response to cholestyramine, Am. J. Med. 39:682, 1965.

12. Stathers, G., Reed, C. S. H., and Hirst, E.: Idiopathic recurrent cholestasis, Gastroenterology 52:536, 1967.

13. Summerskill, W. H. J.: The syndrome of benign recurrent cholestasis, Am. J. Med. 38:298, 1965.

14. Summerskill, W. H. J., and Walshe, J. M.: Benign recurrent intrahepatic "obstructive" jaundice, Lancet 2:686, 1959.

15. Tygstrup, N.: Intermittent, possibly famil-ial, intrahepatic cholestatic jaundice, Lancet 1:1171, 1960.

16. Tygstrup, N.: Discussion in Taylor, W.: The Biliary System, p. 598, Philadelphia, Davis, 1965.

17. Williams, R., Cartter, M. A., Sherlock, S., Scheuer, P. J, and Hill, K. R.: Idiopathic recurrent cholestasis: a study of the functional and pathological lesions in four cases, Quart. J. Med. 33:387, 1964.

Index

Page numbers in **bold face** indicate illustrations. Page numbers followed by the letter "t" indicate tabular material.

Antibody(ies)
 in biliary cirrhosis, 756
 in drug-induced hepatitis, 509
 reactions in liver diseases, 654t
Anticoagulant therapy, hepatic changes due to, 831
 in hepatocellular disease, 152
Anticonvulsants, hepatitis due to, 538-540
Antiemetics, in viral hepatitis, 465
Antiglobulin test, in hemolytic anemias, 933, 936
Antihemophilic factor (AHF), in hepatic disease, 157
Anti-infection agents, hepatitis due to, 540-547
Antimetabolites, hepatitis due to, 547-548
Antimony, hepatitis due to, 540-541
Antinuclear factor (A.N.F.), in liver diseases, 654, 654t
Anti-ovulatory drugs, hepatic diseases and, 465
Antistreptolysin O levels, in hepatobiliary disease, 604
Antisyphilitic therapy, Laennec's cirrhosis due to, 695
Antithyroid drugs, hepatitis due to, 553
Apiol derivatives, hepatitis due to, 565
Apoferritin, 779
Apoproteins, 674
Appendicitis, pyogenic hepatic abscess and, 875, 876, 879, 883, 887
Arginine, in hepatic coma, 402
Arsanilic acid, hepatitis due to, 542
Arsenic(als)
 biliary cirrhosis due to, 756
 hepatitis due to, 541-542
 hypersensitivity to, 541
 jaundice due to, 412
 Laennec's cirrhosis due to, 695
Arteriography. See also Angiography.
 emergency selective, in intestinal hemorrhage, 346-347
 in hepatic polycystic disease, 869
Arteriovenous fistulae, splanchnic, portal hypertension and, 278-279
Artery(ies). See specific artery; for example, Cystic artery.
Arthralgia, in active chronic hepatitis, 649
 in drug-induced hepatitis, 512
Arthritis, in active chronic hepatitis, 649
 rheumatoid, amyloidosis secondary to, 969
 effect of icterus on, 412
Ascariasis, pyogenic hepatic abscess due to, 877, 878
Ascites, 355-377
 adrenal function in, 359
 after portal-systemic shunt, 295
 complications of, 365
 diet and nutrition in, 361
 differential diagnosis of, 356
 diuretic therapy in, 361-364
 due to constricted inferior vena cava, 35
 glomerular filtration rate in, 359
 hypoalbuminemia and, 357, 358
 hyponatremia in, 370
 in amyloidosis, 967
 in cirrhosis, biliary, 759, 765
  Laennec's, 702, 711, 713
  postnecrotic, 733
 in heart failure, 825
 in hemochromatosis, 777, 778
 in hepatitis, active chronic, 648
  subacute, 460
 in pericarditis, 830
 in pyogenic hepatic abscess, 884
 in sarcoidosis, hepatitis-associated, 633
 intra-abdominal factors in, 357-359

Ascites (Cont.)
 jaundice and, 249
 lymph in, 358
 pathogenesis of, 357-360
 peritonitis and, 356
 physical findings in, 355
 portal hypertension and, 282, 283, 357
 potassium metabolism in, 369
 prognosis of, 365
 renal function in, 359, 360
 Starling's equilibrium in, 357
 surgical management of, 364-365
 treatment of, 293, 360-365
 water and electrolyte metabolism in, 369
Ascitic fluid
 abdominal roentgenography of, 979
 hemorrhagic, 249
Aspergillosis, hepatic carcinoma and, 838
 hepatitis with, 549, 625
Aspirin poisoning, fatty liver due to, 951
Asterixis, in hepatic coma, 379
Atelectasis, in liver injury, 868
ATP. See Adenosine triphosphate.
ATP-ase activity, of littoral cells. 20
Auscultation, in liver diseases, 248
Autoimmune complement fixation test. 646
Autoimmune disorders, criteria for, 757
 primary biliary cirrhosis as, 756
Autumnal fever, 613
Azathioprine, hepatitis due to, 547
 in active chronic hepatitis, 659, 664-665
Azotemia
 ammonium metabolism and, 389
 diuretics in, 370
 hepatic coma and, 390
 hyponatremia in, 369
 in fatty liver of pregnancy, 681
 in hepatic failure. 366
  prognosis of, 370
 in hepatitis. carbon tetrachloride-induced, 518
  viral, 459
 in Laennec's cirrhosis, 715
 treatment of, 370

Bacillus, Friedländer's, pyogenic hepatic abscess due to, 877
Bacteremia
 due to suppurative cholangitis, 1015
 in Laennec's cirrhosis, 715
 portal, in ulcerative colitis with pericholangitis, 1056
Bacteria. intestinal, effect on bile salts, 110
  fecal bile pigments and, 233
Bacterial infections. hepatitis with. 603-608
Bacteroides funduliformis, pyogenic hepatic abscess due to, 877
BAL. See Dimercaprol.
Balloon cells, in viral hepatitis, 439, 440
Balloon tamponade, in hemorrhagic esophageal varices. 289, 290, 291
Banti's syndrome, 279
Barbiturates. in hepatic coma, 393
Barium studies. in hepatic and biliary roentgenography, 981-983. 983
Barium swallow, to demonstrate esophageal varices, 285
Benz sign, 981
Berylliosis
 hepatic poisoning in, 514-516
 occupations related to, 515
Bessey-Lowry test, 183
Biguanidines, hepatitis due to, 556

Hepatic coma (*Cont.*)
blood nonprotein nitrogen in, 390
calorie requirements in, 398-399
chlorothiazides in, 395
clinical manifestations of, 378-381, 397
collateral circulation in, 31
course of, 381
differential diagnosis of, 384-385
diseases ending in, 378
diuretics in, 395-396
electroencephalographic abnormalities in, 380, 381
electrolyte intake in, 397-398
exchange transfusions in, 402
fluid intake and output in, 397-398
general therapeutic measures in, 396-401
hemodialysis in, 402
high-protein diets and, 361
histologic liver changes in, 383
hypnotics in, 392-394
hypoglycemia in, 382, 388
impending, 378, 379-380
in alcoholism, 384
in cirrhosis, Laennec's, 715
treatment of, 711
secondary biliary, 759
in diuretic therapy, 364
in heart failure, 826
in hepatitis, active chronic, 648, 656
fulminant, 459
toxic, **505**
viral, impending, 451
in hyponatremia, 390
in pregnancy, 1027
in renal circulatory failure, 367
laboratory findings in, 382-383, 385, 388, 397
metabolic abnormalities and, 388
metabolic hypotheses of, 391
mortality in, 378
neuropsychiatric syndromes in, 380-381
nursing care in, 396
nutrient intake in, 397-398
oliguria in, 382, 390
onset and development of, 378-381
paracentesis in, 395
pathogenesis of, 385-392
pathology of, 383-384
potassium deficiency in, 389, 390, 396
precipitating factors in, 381t, 381-382
prevention of, 392-396
prodrome of, 378-379
prognosis of, 381
protein intake in, 386, 399-400
renal function and, 390
spontaneous, 390, 391
spontaneous abortion due to, 1027
treatment of, 392-403
tremor in, 379
water tolerance in, 398
Wilson's disease and, 387
Hepatic cords, 17
Hepatic cyst, 335, **335**, 872-875
calcification in, 975, **975**
clinical features of, 873-874
complications of, 872, 873t
diagnosis of, 874
epidemiology of, 872
pathology of, 872-873
resection in, 910
symptoms of, 873
treatment of, 874-875
splenic, 975, **975**

Hepatic disease(s). See also specific disease; for example, *Cirrhosis.*
antibody reactions in, 654t
antihemophilic factor in, 157
childhood. See under *Infant(s).*
chronic, infections and, 602
portal-systemic shunt in, 299-300
correction of, future, 258
course of, needle biopsy in, 218
electron microscopy in, 60-71
ending in hepatic coma, 378
erythrocyte survival in, 234, **234**
fibrinogen deficiency in, 153-155
galactosemia and, 946, 947
hemostasis in, 147-165
laboratory tests for, 198, 199-200
lithocholic acid in, 129
obstructive versus parenchymal, alkaline phosphatase versus 5'-nucleotidase in, 188
leucine aminopeptidase in, 189
oral contraceptives and, 465
parenchymal, portal hypertension in, 275-277
vitamin K-dependent factors and, 152
platelet abnormalities and, 157-159
proaccelerin deficiency in, 153
prognosis of, serum protein levels and, 193
prothrombin time in, 152, 197
renal failure in, 366-367, 367t
renal function in, 367-369
ulcerative colitis associated with. See under *Ulcerative colitis.*
urobilinogen in, 171
vitamin K-dependent clotting factor deficiency and, 150
Hepatic duct(s)
anomalies of, 39
benign obstruction of, resection in, 910
bifurcation of, carcinoma of, 257
cancer of, instrumentive cholangiography in, 1012, **1012**
resection in, 911
common, 36
histology of, 38
ligation of, postoperative jaundice due to, 1038
stricture of, biliary cirrhosis due to, 759
Hepatic injury
amino acids administered in, 507
bile peritonitis in, 868
bile salt ratio and, 128
drug-induced, electron microscopy of, 63
due to chloroform, dietary protein and, 502
fluid replacement in, 865
lithocholate blood levels in, 128
Hepatic necrosis. See also *Toxic hepatitis.*
cordotomy and, 501
healed, after toxic hepatitis, 504
in drug-sensitive hepatitis, 511
in heart failure, 816, 823-824, 823t
in viral hepatitis, 444-445, **444**, 459-460
ischemic, 22, **23**, 501
prothrombin time in, 197
subacute. See *Hepatitis, active chronic.*
submassive, 468
vitamin E deficiency and, 500
Hepatic perfusion, 915-916
Hepatic phosphorylase insufficiency, 953
Hepatic plates, 17
Hepatic resection, 909-914. See also *Lobectomy.*
air embolism in, 914
anatomic aspects of, 909-910
complications in, 913-914

Wilson's disease (*Cont.*)
  splenic manifestations of, 801
  surgery in, 807
  transaminase levels in, 802
  treatment of, 807-811

Xanthelasma, in biliary cirrhosis, 742, 758, 759
Xanthomatosis, in biliary atresia, 946
  in biliary cirrhosis, 739, 740, **741**, 742, 744, **747**, **748**, 756, 758
  in drug-induced hepatitis, 511, 512
X-ray examination. See *Roentgenography.*

X-ray therapy. See *Radiotherapy.*

Yellow atrophy. See *Postnecrotic cirrhosis.*
Yellow fever virus, in Kupffer cells, 436

Zenker's disease, Weil's disease versus, 617
Zieve's syndrome, 680
Zuckergussleber, 830
Zuckerkandel's plexus, 39
Zwischenstück, 17